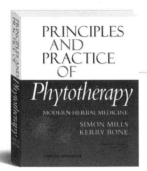
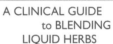
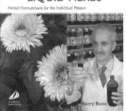

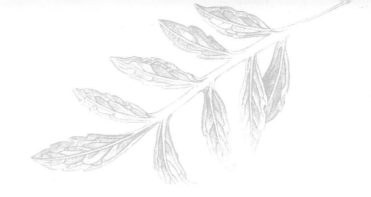

THE ESSENTIAL GUIDE
TO HERBAL SAFETY

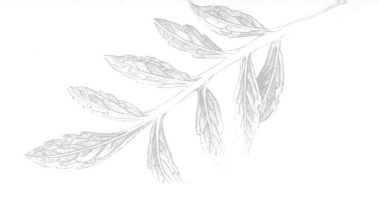

The Essential Guide to Herbal Safety

Simon Mills, MA, MCPP, FNIMH
Peninsula Medical School
Universities of Exeter and Plymouth
Exeter, United Kingdom

Kerry Bone, BSc (Hons), Dip Phyto, FNIMH, FNHAA, MCPP
Director, Research and Development, MediHerb
Adjunct Associate Professor, School of Health
University of New England
Armidale, Australia

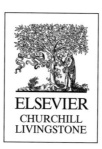

ELSEVIER
CHURCHILL
LIVINGSTONE

CHURCHILL LIVINGSTONE

An imprint of Elsevier Limited

The Essential Guide to Herbal Safety
© 2005, Elsevier Limited. All rights reserved.

First edition 2005
Reprinted 2005

ISBN 0 443 07171 3

British Library Cataloguing in Publication Data
A catalogue record for this book is available from the British Library

Library of Congress Cataloging in Publication Data
A catalog record for this book is available from the Library of Congress

Notice
Herbal Medicine is an ever-changing field. Standard safety precautions must be followed, but as new research and clinical experience broaden our knowledge, changes in treatment and drug therapy may become necessary or appropriate. Readers are advised to check the most current product information provided by the manufacturer of each drug to be administered to verify the recommended dose, the method and duration of administration, and contraindications. It is the responsibility of the licensed practitioner, relying on experience and knowledge of the patient, to determine dosages and the best treatment for each individual patient. Neither the Publisher nor the editors/contributor assumes any liability for any injury and/or damage to persons or property arising from this publication.

The Publisher

your source for books,
journals and multimedia
in the health sciences
www.elsevierhealth.com

Working together to grow
libraries in developing countries

www.elsevier.com | www.bookaid.org | www.sabre.org

ELSEVIER   BOOK AID International   Sabre Foundation

Publishing Director: Linda Duncan
Acquisitions Editor: Kellie White
Senior Development Editor: Kim Fons
Publishing Services Manager: Pat Joiner
Project Manager: David Stein
Senior Designer: Amy Buxton

Printed in the United States of America

Last digit is the print number: 9 8 7 6 5 4 3 2

The
Publisher's
policy is to use
**paper manufactured
from sustainable forests**

CONTRIBUTORS

SIMON MILLS, *MA, MCPP, FNIMH*

Simon Mills has practiced herbal medicine since 1977 and has been in the forefront of the movement for establishing high professional standards of practice in the United Kingdom for much of that time. He is now both Teaching Fellow in Integrated Healthcare at the Peninsula Medical School at the Universities of Exeter and Plymouth in the United Kingdom and Director of the Masters Program in Botanical Healing at the Tai Sophia Institute, Maryland, in the United States. He is President of the British Herbal Medicine Association and Secretary of the European Scientific Cooperative on Phytotherapy (ESCOP) and as such has been involved in setting scientific standards for herbal remedies in the United Kingdom and across Europe for many years. He is currently developing with Kerry Bone a major on-line evidence-based resource for professional use of herbal remedies (http://www.phytotherapy.info).

KERRY BONE, *BSc (Hons), Dip Phyto, FNIMH, FNHAA, MCPP*

Kerry Bone was an experienced research and industrial chemist before studying herbal medicine full-time in the United Kingdom where he graduated from the College of Phytotherapy and joined the National Institute of Medical Herbalists. He is a practising herbalist (20 years' experience), head of Research and Development at MediHerb, and Principal of the Australian College of Phytotherapy.

Working for the Australian College of Phytotherapy, and in conjunction with the University of New England (Australia), Kerry has developed a Masters degree program in clinical herbal medicine. In relation to this work he has been appointed adjunct Associate Professor by the university.

He is a regular contributor to various journals and has published several books including the best-selling text *Principles and Practice of Phytotherapy: Modern Herbal Medicine,* which he co-authored with Simon Mills.

JOANNE BARNES, *BPharm, PhD, MRPharmS, FLS*

Joanne Barnes is a Lecturer in Phytopharmacy at the Centre for Pharmacognosy and Phytotherapy, School of Pharmacy, University of London, in the United Kingdom.

BERRIS BURGOYNE, *BHScNat, MNHAA, MANTA*

Berris Burgoyne is one of Australia's most popular presenters on herbal medicine practice. She is known to many therapists for her articles and presentations at postgraduate courses. Berris runs a busy naturopathic practice in Brisbane, and lectured in herbal medicine at the Australian College of Natural Medicine for over 10 years. She also works as a technical consultant for MediHerb.

JANICE MCMILLAN, *BSc (Pharmacology), Adv Dip Health Sci (Naturopathy), Dip Health Sci (Herbal Med), MNHAA*

Janice McMillan has a Science degree majoring in Pharmacology and is a qualified Naturopath and Herbalist. She worked as a Naturopath for 2 years prior to her position as Assistant Technical Writer with MediHerb for over 2 years. She assisted in the research and writing of the herbal medicine text, *A Clinical Guide to Blending Liquid Herbs: Herbal Formulations for the Individual Patient,* published by Churchill Livingstone in 2003 and contributed to the EXTRACT database, an interactive clinical evidence database of medicinal plants. Janice currently supervises the production of herbal tablets and concentrated extracts at MediHerb.

MICHELLE MORGAN, BSc (Chemistry), Dip App Sci (Herbal Medicine), MATMS

Michelle Morgan has a Bachelor of Science degree majoring in Chemistry, and worked as a laboratory technician and Quality Assurance Chemist before joining MediHerb in 1995. As Technical Writer at MediHerb she is responsible for literature searching, technical and marketing writing, some regulatory functions, editing, and the organisation of technical publications including those on MediHerb's websites.

She assisted in the research and writing of several herbal medicine textbooks including *A Clinical Guide to Blending Liquid Herbs: Herbal Formulations for the Individual Patient*, published by Churchill Livingstone in 2003. Michelle is a qualified herbalist and practises part-time in Warwick, Queensland, in Australia.

STEPHEN MYERS, PhD, BMed, ND

Stephen Myers is the Director of the Australian Centre for Complementary Medicine Education and Research (ACCMER), a joint venture of the University of Queensland and Southern Cross University. Until 2001, he was the Foundation Head of the School of Natural and Complementary Medicine at Southern Cross University, where he still plays an active role. He initially qualified as a naturopathic practitioner and later in Western medicine. He has a PhD in basic and clinical pharmacology. His current passion is to play a role in building an active research culture in complementary medicine.

MATHIAS SCHMIDT, PhD

Mathias Schmidt earned his PhD in pharmaceutical chemistry and instrumental analysis at the University of Tübingen, Germany. He has 10 years of experience in medicinal plant research in the German pharmaceutical industry, where as the head of the scientific department in two pharmaceutical companies specialising in herbal medicine, he was responsible for pharmacological and clinical research as well as pharmacovigilance. As such, he was deeply involved in the recent German drug safety protocols against kava (*Piper methysticum*) and St. John's wort (*Hypericum perforatum*).

In February 2004, he began working on consultancy projects in the quality assessment of herbal medicines, with a special focus on pharmacovigilance and pharmacological, clinical, and toxicological research, as well as traceability and medicinal plant cultivation under Good Agricultural and Collection Practice conditions. Dr. Schmidt is author and co-author of more than 80 publications and abstracts including two books.

DEBBIE SHAW, BSc (Hons)

Debbie Shaw is a Research Scientist on the pharmacovigilance and safety of herbal medicines at the Medical Toxicology Unit, Guy's and St Thomas' Hospital Trust, London, in the United Kingdom.

TRINA WARD, BSc (Hons), MPhil

Trina Ward is a Chinese herbalist and acupuncturist and is a researcher at the Acupuncture Research Resource Centre at the Centre for Complementary Healthcare and Integrated Medicine, Thames Valley University, London, in the United Kingdom.

HANS WOHLMUTH, BSc, ND, MNHAA

Hans Wohlmuth is a lecturer in Pharmacognosy and Phytotherapy in the School of Natural and Complementary Medicine at Southern Cross University, Lismore, New South Wales, Australia. He holds qualifications in natural medicine and biology and is a former practitioner of herbal medicine. He has taught herbal medicine for more than a decade and is actively engaged in medicinal plant research.

FOREWORD

In Europe the use of "herbal medicinal products" is an integral part of the medical system and also of my work. I have been in orthodox medical practice for over 50 years. For many of these I have directed the medical toxicology department at the University of Münster and have worked intensively on safety issues on behalf of the European Commission. My whole professional life has therefore been devoted to improving the safe use of medicines and resolving consumer health problems. Moreover I am also Chairman of the Board of the European Scientific Cooperative on Phytotherapy (ESCOP), a scientific research network whose members are national associations of phytotherapy or herbal medicine across Europe.

Since 1989 ESCOP has taken the lead in setting standards for the safe and effective use of herbal medicinal products in Europe. ESCOP is best known for its harmonised European monographs. It has recently published 80 revised and updated monographs and formally submitted them to the European Medicines Evaluation Agency (EMEA) and its Committee on Herbal Medicinal Products as a basis for establishing core data on the leading herbal medicinal products in Europe. Moreover this vital work has been built on strong foundations. In 1994 ESCOP received a grant from the European Commission BIO-MED programme. As well as supporting the work of monograph production, this funding also enabled ESCOP to take the initiative on the safety of herbal medicines. We started to explore the risks involved in taking herbs, looked for those that might be hidden, interviewed physicians and users, and set up a new adverse reporting scheme. Some people asked,

"Why should the herbal sector look for risks associated with its own products?" Our answer has been clear: there are no two sides to safety. It is our duty to establish exactly the level of risk of our medicines. Indeed there is no one better able to do this than the experts in the field.

It is for this reason that I welcome this book with enthusiasm and also with the expectation that it will be widely used. It provides a realistic risk/benefit analysis of phytomedicine in the clinical context and thus truly demonstrates its potential for many indications.

The book is written by acknowledged experts. The editors actually use herbal medicines in their clinical practice and have done so for many years. Yet they are also prominent in developing a scientific rationale for this work, Simon Mills in part as Secretary of ESCOP. This inside knowledge and their academic expertise have allowed the authors to explore some of the most important general issues: idiosyncratic reactions and contact sensitivity, the xenobiotic debate, the negative placebo effect, and the adverse herb-drug interactions and the identification of potential adverse reactions including pharmacovigilance data. Technical expertise is shown also in the important sections on the impact of herb quality on safety.

They do us all a service in exposing some of the damaging media scares on the hazards of herbs and as an exemplar have thoroughly criticised the recent unfortunate prohibition of kava-kava. What emerges is a stimulating contribution to an area that we all need to understand better.

Most importantly this text is another sign of the maturity of phytomedicine, that it can provide real experts that are not afraid to ask difficult questions.

Fritz H. Kemper

Professor Dr. med. Dr. h.c. mult.

Chairman of the Board of ESCOP

May 2004

In the early to mid 1990's, with the rapid growth of the herbal medicine industry as consumers became more and more interested in complementary and alternative medicine (CAM), a number of different viewpoints were prevalent within various sectors of society. Consumers, who were moving in significant numbers to consultation of natural medicine practitioners and also to self-medication, were in general assuming that herbal medicines, being of natural origin, were therefore safe. The practitioners of orthodox medicine, having not been exposed to herbal medicine to any great extent in their medical course or training, and increasingly not being consulted by their patients about their use of herbal medicine, took a defensive approach. A common response was to declare that "there was nothing much in it" and that the consumer interest was largely based on belief and mythology. When various science-based groups started to look more closely at herbal medicines, some disturbing findings emerged, particularly related to the quality of the herbal medicines. These findings were widely reported in the popular media (usually in a highly sensationalised form), and it fuelled a growing consumer concern that quality and safety were perhaps not always of paramount concern to at least some portions of the prospering industry. Following a number of such reports in the late 1990's, the public concern led people to turn again to their trusted healthcare professionals for advice about the safety and efficacy of the products and practices that they had embraced or that were being recommended to them. Parts of the orthodox profession, seizing on this disquiet, saw the opportunity to respond, and articles appeared in mainstream medical journals with provocative titles implicating herbal medicines in particular with adverse findings on safety and lack of efficacy. This in turn heralded the acceptance that herbal medicines consisted of complex chemical mixtures with potentially profound pharmacology and toxicology.

The current book arises out of the ashes of this seeming chaos and a recognition of the need to examine rationally and carefully issues of safety of phytomedicines, or rational herbal medicines The book follows the tradition of the very successful collaboration between Simon Mills and Kerry Bone in the definitive text, *Principles and Practice of Phytotherapy: Modern Herbal Medicine,* which has had an important role in providing valuable background information and analysis on the chemistry and pharmacology of herbal medicines. The standards set by that book have been maintained in this text, which has added additional expert contributors and is written with an emphasis on analysis of issues of safety. These issues came to the forefront of consumer and healthcare practitioner awareness following new information appearing from clinical experience and clinical investigation of St. John's wort (*Hypericum perforatum*), which followed its rapid rise in use when clinical trials provided the evidence for its effectiveness in mild to moderate depression. Despite results demonstrating a lower incidence of side effects compared to other pharmaceutical agents used for this condition, case studies and some clinical evaluations uncovered interactions between St. John's wort and other medications being used concomitantly. The occurrence of these herb-drug interactions became widely known, and with their mechanisms easily rationalised, it was accepted that such interactions were possible with many other medicines. This realisation led to the need for more information and research, but also a rational analysis of the data on safety already existing in the literature. As practitioners and scholars in this field, Mills, Bone, and their colleagues have undertaken such an analysis. The stated goal of the current book is to undertake an objective appraisal of the safety and associated risks of phytomedicines, maintaining a balanced view and realistic appraisal. As such, it is aimed at providing pharmacists, herbalists, naturopaths, medical doctors, chiropractors, and other healthcare professionals with reliable information and analysis for counselling and treatment of patients.

The book has a variety of useful information for the reader, with emphasis on the balance that was sought. The early part of the book provides the backdrop in which the information needed is addressed. The style uses discussion rather than being encyclopaedic, although valuable and informative tables are also provided. I was particularly interested in the section on herb-drug interactions, specifically in how a balance between the established and potential interactions was reconciled with the need to counsel practitioners on how to advise their patients. I believe this balance has been achieved admirably in this section and throughout the book. Thus the criteria for establishing the significance of the herb-drug

interaction are clearly stated, and in the tables information is provided on the potential interaction: the basis for any concern about that interaction is stated and a recommended action is given. The categorisation of risk and recommendation has in my view shown an appropriate concern for both the quality of the information and the health and safety needs of the patient. Overall, this book provides rational views on the safety of phytotherapy agents and presents an invaluable source of knowledge, understanding, and information for the busy scientist and practitioner.

BASIL ROUFOGALIS
Professor of Pharmaceutical Chemistry
University of Sydney
NSW Australia

PREFACE

There are some good reasons to use herbal products in healthcare and it is clear that more professionals are being drawn to do so. As these ancient medicines come under closer modern scrutiny, there are many enticing prospects that indeed they genuinely could combine gentleness with efficacy. The rationales for their potential benefits are now often well-developed and the professional debates rich and promising. For the first time since they dropped out of mainstream medicine behind the rush of new pharmaceuticals in the early 20th century, herbal medicines are serious contenders in professional healthcare. Approximately 70% of medical doctors in Germany prescribe herbal products, while in France they make up over 10% of all prescriptions. When we wrote *Principles and Practice of Phytotherapy: Modern Herbal Medicine* we were able to reflect these developments and to describe a sophisticated professional strategy for healthcare with herbs. We are gratified to see that this work has been taken up in more and more educational programmes and professional workshops, reinforcing signs that the professional future of phytotherapy is ensured.

Modern scrutiny of herbal medicine cuts both ways. The modern world has also become risk-averse and safety concerns are generally much more acute than they were a generation ago. For many years, proponents of herbal practice were comforted by the idea that their remedies were generally safe and well-tried over centuries of use and that whole plants lacked the inherent potential toxicity of single chemical entities. Such comfortable assumptions have increasingly been challenged. There have been specific shocks, among them: the sudden emergence of St. John's wort as a pow-

erful cytochrome P450 inducer with significant potential for interaction with many modern drugs, the disturbing association of aristolochia with serious kidney disease, and the prohibition of kava around the world. More widely, with the lack of consistent external regulation around the world, there has been a growing media and medical focus on the safe manufacture of herbal products, with evidence that some may not be exactly what the label states. Perhaps most significantly in the long term, the increasing sophistication of drug-monitoring schemes around the world means that rare adverse effects associated with the use of herbal products are more likely to be noticed.

Some herbal practitioners may think that the world has become a little less comfortable. There are mutterings of a plot ("Why are the two most successful herbal remedies, St. John's wort and kava, with the most impact on conventional pharmaceutical consumption, the ones that have been withdrawn or impugned?"). However an enlightened view is that all this is part of the coming of age of phytotherapy. If herbs are really going to cut it in the real world, then their proponents also need to do so. There should be no two sides to safety.

In the early 1990's, as Professor Kemper outlines in his Foreword to this book, the main phytotherapy association in Europe agreed to be proactive in the search for evidence of adverse effects. The European Scientific Cooperative on Phytotherapy (ESCOP), representing national associations of herbal medicine, embarked on a number of initiatives to explore the extent of adverse reports for herbs and the difficulties in quantifying them. We set up a website to encourage herbal practitioners to report them, and we sought a panel of independent toxicologists to assess any information we found. This was all part of a genuine attempt to seek out any safety issues associated with the use of herbs. Since herbal products are already approved for use in most countries, this represented the most sensible approach to addressing uncertainties over safety. It is heartening to see that considerable progress is now being made in the field of herbal "pharmacovigilance".

This book represents an extensive discussion of the current major issues that relate to the safe use of herbs. It additionally contains comprehensive reviews of the published safety data for 125 common herbs. Many experts have contributed to arriving at a balanced perspective on the complex safety challenges relating to self-prescribed or professional herbal use. Most importantly the editors of this work have a practical working knowledge of the use of medicinal plants, and hence any theoretical distortions, which are common in the herbal safety literature and in the media, are avoided.

Simon Mills
Kerry Bone

ACKNOWLEDGEMENTS

The editors would like to acknowledge the input and support of secretarial staff, Jan Frousheger and Petra Moroney, who provided invaluable assistance throughout the preparation of this text.

But once again our greatest debt is to our wives Rachel and Patricia who have contributed directly to this work and most importantly provided moral support for this and so many other of our professional involvements. This book represents another example of the tangible results of their sacrifices.

CONTENTS

PART

I

SAFETY ISSUES

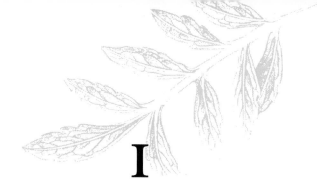

I

INTRODUCTION: WHAT IS HERB SAFETY?

Simon Mills

We live in a perilous world. Wheat, rye, barley, and oats contain a protein called gluten that is hydrolysed in the digestive system to yield a peptide α-gliadin, a well-established intestinal irritant,[1,2] leading to a condition known as coeliac disease that affects 1 person in every 250,[3] is particularly common in people with diabetes,[4] and has caused thousands of deaths around the world. Apple seeds, the kernels of apricots, plums, and other stone fruits, and bitter almonds contain significant quantities of glycosides that on hydrolysis yield cyanide,[5] a process that also occurs in the digestive system. Potatoes are members of the deadly nightshade family: when the tuber turns green under the influence of light it produces teratogenic alkaloids.[6,7] Many common household pulses, like red kidney bean[8] and haricot bean (used in "baked beans"), contain various toxins, notably types of lectins called phytohaemagglutinins,[9] and trypsin inhibitors,[10] which can only reliably be neutralised by boiling for at least 30 minutes. Cereals, nuts,[11] dried fruit, spices,[12] and beer[13] are particularly prone to aflatoxins and other mycotoxins produced by moulds on the food in storage; these

may also find their way into breast milk in women[14] and also cow's milk,[15,16] eggs, and poultry[17] via contaminated animal feeds.[18] There is a positive association between dietary exposure to mycotoxins and an increased incidence of hepatitis and primary hepatocellular carcinoma.[19,20] Dangerous type I hypersensitivity reactions are increasingly recorded to peanuts, shrimp and other crustaceans, and spices.[21]

One could speculate what would happen to the consumption levels of such foods if their dangers were widely publicised. Currently cigarettes sold in developed countries carry prominent labels on packs warning that they can kill or at least seriously damage the health of the smoker's own children. Evidence suggests that in the face of such appalling risks, reductions in smoking in some quarters are compensated by increases in others, notably women and adolescents. Conversely, growing anxieties in the same countries (but probably in different sections of the population) about the perceived but unproven risks of agricultural chemicals and genetically modified foods have led to a growing business for organically grown food sold at significantly higher prices. In developing countries these issues disappear entirely: cigarette smoking increases dramatically and modern agribusiness investments flourish.

It appears that the public perception of risk is not consistent with its calculated level. Real risks can be ignored; fears can exaggerate theoretical risks. The opinions of those who may guide society are of little effect: the experts are widely ignored or disbelieved, and the media are seen as entertainment rather than as educational (one herbal manufacturer in the United Kingdom routinely noted increases in sales of products after safety alarms were splashed across the newspapers, perhaps reflecting the adage that any news is good news). It is possible that publicity about the dangers of common foods would be seen as ridiculous scientism by the majority ("they will soon be telling us that nothing is safe") and would merely add to the anxieties of those susceptible to them.

In this book the authors examine the issues of herbal safety. Faced with such irrationalities in perceptions of risk the first question might be who needs this information? It probably is not the public. It is not clear whether the frequent media stories about herbal threats to health have directly affected their consumption: the use of Chinese and ayurvedic medicine, the herbal approaches most frequently questioned in the United Kingdom, continues to grow faster than other therapies. In the United States, where there has been a decrease in consumer confidence in herbs, it is likely because the exaggerated health claims there did not match the often paltry herbal substances behind the label in the absence of consistently applied quality or dosage standards. (One professional observer of the United States herb scene recently reported that 75% of herbal products in the United States were judged as being of poor quality.[22]) Negative media attention may simply have reinforced a consumer protest about oversold dodgy goods. In other parts of the world, the public again seems to swim in a current that is different from the professional or even media view.

Do the regulators need more information? Faced with the banning of kava in many coun-

tries, some may argue that there is a deficit of information at the highest level. However, kava has been much an exception to a wider rule, that proscriptions on herbs have been few. Experts in herbal safety have been remarkably sanguine about the risks to public health in herb use. Recorded cases of harm after herb use remain remarkably low, even allowing for obvious underreporting in this sector. Some herbalists may spot a conspiracy against them, but all the evidence suggests remarkable calmness in the corridors of health ministries about herbs.

The wider health care community certainly needs more facts about herbal safety, and there are many anecdotes of unreasonable conclusions being drawn about the risks of herb use by physicians and pharmacists in the absence of good data (see Chapter 6 for some examples). However, it may be that what is first required for this community is well-presented and convincing evidence of benefit. The herbal sector is familiar with the benefit-risk assessment of a herbal remedy being distorted based on zero (or nonproven) efficacy (as was certainly the case with kava).

A manual on herb safety should assume a readership that is inclined to take the remedies seriously. Therefore, this book is dedicated to the reader who already uses herbal remedies or at least would like to do so. The number of practitioners using herbs continues to grow, and wider professional interest increases perhaps even faster. What actual practitioners need is a realistic assessment of the risks in their work, practical guidance to reduce risks, and tools to articulate the issues to patients, fellow professionals, and regulators.

In this text the issues are examined carefully with clinical realities in mind. The authors are closely involved in their subject but are not misled by this proximity. Their main intention is to seek clarity and to sift through and organise the evidence fairly. The opening chapters address the relevant topics systematically. For example, the authors are well aware that the food scares that introduce this chapter are exaggerated. The real point of these examples is to show how difficult it is to predict the toxicity of a plant only from the presence of toxic constituents. As with other phytopharmacologic questions, the action of the whole plant and the way in which it is normally consumed count for more than any individual constituent list.

Nevertheless there clearly are safety issues in herbal medicine. Chapter 2, which introduces the *dossier of adverse reactions* to herbal remedies that the sector has to address, was written by Debbie Shaw, a senior researcher at a leading toxicology unit who advises the British medicine agency on herb safety. General herbal safety issues are reviewed, including the potential for harm to liver, kidney, heart, and other body systems, issues of quality and adulteration, risks of phototoxicity, allergic reaction, and harm to particular groups of patients. Major known adverse reactions to herbs are also introduced.

Chapter 3 is the first to offer a comprehensive response to these challenges. It introduces types of adverse reaction that may owe more to the constitution of the person at the time of the consumption than to the properties of the medicine itself: the adverse placebo (or *nocebo*) effect and the usually minor *transient adverse reactions in treatment*, including those sometimes referred to as "healing crises."

Many other cases of adverse reactions involving herbs are also less often caused by toxicity of the plant than by unpredictable, *idiosyncratic* reactions by the body. They may even account for the majority of serious reactions to herbs. The body's constitution is at least as relevant as the properties of the plant. Chapter 4 reviews the issues involved in medicine and patient and ways in which idiosyncratic reactions may better be understood and even reduced.

Chapter 5 explores the idea that natural plant constituents are often foreign to the body's primary metabolic pathways ("xenobiotics") and are thus treated by the same mechanisms as many pharmaceutical agents and synthetic substances. The main mechanism for xenobiotic metabolism, the *cytochrome P450 enzyme system*, is introduced as an element in the possible coevolution of mutual defences between plants and animals. Potential for interactions within the cytochrome P450 system between drugs and food and herb constituents are highlighted to put recent findings about St. John's wort and grapefruit into

context. An obvious conclusion is that many plants and foods have the potential to interact with the body's machinery for metabolising drugs: rather than be surprised by the next St. John's wort it may be more useful to understand the risks generally of taking powerful drugs with a narrow therapeutic window.

This leads to a comprehensive review of *adverse herb-drug interactions* (AHDIs). The first priority is a critique of the AHDI information found in the media and other texts and professional literature. This is an area in which there is an astonishing amount of alarmist misinformation, even from authors who specialise in the field. To counteract this a rational basis for appreciating the risk of interaction is proposed, and practical guidance is provided. A table lists the most credible interactions for remedies that are likely to be used by herbal practitioners.

A leading safety question is how safe herbal remedies are during *pregnancy and lactation*. In the absence of much reliable data there has been a confusion of advice. In Chapter 7 evidence on the effects of plants during pregnancy and lactation is reviewed, and a rational and flexible classification system is developed (and then applied in the herb monographs later in this book).

Poor herb *quality* has probably been the main safety problem. The many issues, including substitution, contamination, and adulteration, are comprehensively reviewed in Chapter 8. It is unfortunate that much of the supply of herbal remedies to practitioners has effectively escaped the discipline of good manufacturing practice (GMP). The herbal practitioner scanning the catalogues of tinctures should be aware that the cheapest option may not be worth giving to a patient and may even be unsafe. In the United States and Europe new laws will force manufacturers of practitioners' herbal supplies in coming years to meet these standards. In Australia this has been mandatory for many years, and a relatively prosperous herbal sector shows that it is not only practicable but also builds confidence among the public. Practitioners should be willing to pay premium prices for assured quality products and to put pressure on their suppliers not to wait for the law.

These concerns are even more pressing in another herbal sector. In a research project sponsored by the leading organisation of practitioners of *Chinese herbal medicines* in the United Kingdom, Trina Ward reviewed the safety profile of these remedies. This project coincided with repeated media reports of adulteration and substitutions and negative industry reports on quality standards of oriental products, and her review is not entirely reassuring. Practitioners who choose to use Chinese remedies must read this review and apply the appropriate cautions, particularly if they use finished formulations imported directly from Asia. The sooner that regulators in China and other exporters of traditional medicines raise standards of quality and apply transparent GMP standards (including traceable and reliable certificates of analysis), the sooner will they arrest the growing crisis of confidence in this important herbal resource.

Probably the most common type of adverse reactions reported to herbal products involves hypersensitivity or *allergic* reactions. In Chapter 10 by Professor Stephen Myers and Hans Wohlmuth from Australia, these adverse reactions are classified by clinical presentation, and conclusions are drawn about the risks of allergic responses.

Chapter 11, written by Dr. Joanne Barnes from the University of London, outlines the current initiatives in herbal *pharmacovigilance*. In the absence of much toxicologic data for herbs and because they are already well established in humans, it is important to improve the careful monitoring of human use. If, as the statisticians advise, one needs to see 30,000 cases to have a 95% chance of seeing an adverse case for which there is a 1 in 10,000 risk, then only concerted action by the health care community is possible. Many of the initiatives come from Europe, where herbal remedies are classified as medicinal products and are fitted into the conventional postmarketing surveillance schemes. These form the core of this review. The herbal sector should not be afraid to be proactive in searching for adverse reactions. Only an open and transparent acknowledgment of the real risks will assure the public that we have nothing to hide.

Chapter 12, which ends Part 1, focuses closely on the most dramatic case history in the story of herbal safety. The association of *kava* consumption with adverse hepatic reactions has led to widespread restrictions on its use around the world. Dr. Mathias Schmidt leads a thorough review of the case for the prosecution against kava, considering all the evidence that has been available. Serious gaps are apparent in the assessment of the benefit-risk balance for herbal remedies, even for one with an impressive traditional reputation and an accumulating dossier of conventional clinical trial data. It is clear that regulators need to be helped to weigh the arguments more pragmatically in the future.

The second and largest part of this book provides a review of the individual safety monographs for 125 herbal remedies most used by herbal practitioners in the English-speaking developed world and Europe. All the pertinent information in the literature for the plants or their major constituents is drawn together, and then taking advantage of the authors' many years in practice, it is summarised to provide an effective clinical guide for practitioners. The results are realistic rather than just theoretical assessments of risk and include practical steps to reduce any that may be apparent.

This book is a safety manual for the herbal practitioner. We need a level-headed understanding of the risks of our remedies to alert us to the problems we face and to put these into real-life clinical perspective. This text is our contribution.

REFERENCES

1. Clemente MG, De Virgiliis S, Kang JS, et al: Early effects of gliadin on enterocyte intracellular signalling involved in intestinal barrier function, *Gut* 52:218-223, 2003.
2. Giovannini C, Matarrese P, Scazzocchio B, et al: Wheat gliadin induces apoptosis of intestinal cells via an autocrine mechanism involving Fas-Fas ligand pathway, *FEBS Lett* 540:117-124, 2003.
3. Fasano A, Berti I, Gerarduzzi T, et al: Prevalence of celiac disease in at-risk and not-at-risk groups in the United States: a large multicenter study, *Arch Intern Med* 163:286-292, 2003.
4. Troncone R, Franzese A, Mazzarella G, et al: Gluten sensitivity in a subset of children with insulin dependent diabetes mellitus, *Am J Gastroenterol* 98:590-595, 2003.

5. Holzbecher MD, Moss MA, Ellenberger HA: The cyanide content of laetrile preparations, apricot, peach and apple seeds, *J Toxicol Clin Toxicol* 22:341-347, 1984.

6. Harvey MH, McMillan M, Morgan MR, et al: Solanidine is present in sera of healthy individuals and in amounts dependent on their dietary potato consumption, *Hum Toxicol* 4:187-194, 1985.

7. Friedman M, Henika PR, Mackey BE: Effect of feeding solanidine, solasodine and tomatidine to non-pregnant and pregnant mice, *Food Chem Toxicol* 41:61-71, 2003.

8. Venter FS, Thiel PG: Red kidney beans—to eat or not to eat? *S Afr Med J* 85:250-252, 1995.

9. Santidrian S, de Moya CC, Grant G, et al: Local (gut) and systemic metabolism of rats is altered by consumption of raw bean (Phaseolus vulgaris L var athropurpurea), *Br J Nutr* 89:311-319, 2003.

10. Brandon DL, Bates AH, Friedman M: ELISA analysis of soybean trypsin inhibitors in processed foods, *Adv Exp Med Biol* 289:321-337, 1991.

11. Jimenez M, Mateo R, Querol A, et al: Mycotoxins and mycotoxigenic moulds in nuts and sunflower seeds for human consumption, *Mycopathologia* 115:121-127, 1991.

12. Patel S, Hazel CM, Winterton AG, et al: Survey of ethnic foods for mycotoxins, *Food Addit Contam* 13:833-841, 1996.

13. Scott PM: Mycotoxins transmitted into beer from contaminated grains during brewing, *J AOAC Int* 79:875-882, 1996.

14. Wild CP, Pionneau FA, Montesano R, et al: Aflatoxin detected in human breast milk by immunoassay, *Int J Cancer* 40:328-333, 1987.

15. Rodriguez Velasco ML, Calonge Delso MM, Ordonez Escudero D: ELISA and HPLC determination of the occurrence of aflatoxin M(1) in raw cow's milk, *Food Addit Contam* 20:276-280, 2003.

16. Skrinjar M, Stubblefield RD, Vujicic IF, et al: Distribution of aflatoxin-producing moulds and aflatoxins in dairy cattle feed and raw milk, *Acta Microbiol Hung* 39:175-179, 1992.

17. Bintvihok A, Thiengnin S, Doi K, et al: Residues of aflatoxins in the liver, muscle and eggs of domestic fowls, *J Vet Med Sci* 64:1037-1039, 2002.

18. Wood GE: Aflatoxins in domestic and imported foods and feeds, *J Assoc Off Anal Chem* 72:543-548, 1989.

19. Groopman JD, Scholl P, Wang JS: Epidemiology of human aflatoxin exposures and their relationship to liver cancer, *Prog Clin Biol Res* 395:211-222, 1996.

20. Jackson PE, Groopman JD: Aflatoxin and liver cancer, *Baillieres Best Pract Res Clin Gastroenterol* 13:545-555, 1999.

21. De Maat-Bleeker F: (Etiology of hypersensitivity reactions following Chinese or Indonesian meals), *Ned-Tijdschr-Geneeskd* 136:229-232, 1992.

22. Mahady G: WHO Collaborating Center, University of Illinois, speaking to the British Toxicology Society Meeting, June 23, 2002.

2

Adverse Effects of Herbal Remedies: The Case to Answer

Debbie Shaw

For those charged by the public with monitoring drug safety and adverse reactions, the popular view that herbal remedies are generally safe needs qualification. In this chapter recent safety concerns involving herbal remedies are summarised. Many of these are elaborated and addressed elsewhere in this text, and some constructive measures are identified. Tighter regulatory controls on the supply of herbal remedies in Europe and the United States were largely framed as a result of safety concerns, and the prospects of herbal products as a useful health care option may be judged by the way that such problems are minimised in the future.

In the United States and many other countries herbal remedies are regulated as dietary supplements, and consumers may be unaware that many of these herbs may be registered as medicinal products in another country. In one country the same herb may be classified as a health food or dietary supplement and a licensed herbal medicine. The label of "dietary supplement" (i.e., supplementary to a normal

diet) leads to important misconceptions: first, as a food supplement these products will have no side effects and are safe and free from unwanted effects at any dose; therefore, second, these products are "tonics" devoid of pharmacologic activity and have no therapeutic benefits. This contributes to possible misuse and overdose of botanical products and resulting underestimation of the possible risks and benefits from herbal remedies.

Herbal remedies, even single herbs, contain complex mixtures of chemicals, many of which have active pharmacologic properties. These confer the beneficial medicinal properties on the herbs but can also cause side effects or adverse reactions. However, even skeptics, who doubt that herbal remedies have physiologic activity or any therapeutic benefit, need to be aware of issues affecting patient safety. Anecdotal reports of efficacy or adverse reactions may not provide conclusive evidence of either but do provide some guidance on potential benefits or necessary cautions. Whereas the procedures for adverse reaction monitoring of drugs has developed rapidly since the 1960s, the monitoring of unwanted effects of herbal remedies is a recent phenomenon resulting from their considerable increase in use and concerns on safety. Generally these remedies do not fit easily within existing adverse drug reaction (ADR) schemes; there are problems identifying adverse effects, for which neither patient nor physician may make the association between use of a herbal remedy and unexpected health effects or appreciate the need to investigate and report suspected adverse effects. Technical difficulties arise in adding these to existing electronic database systems because they are complex botanical mixtures, with a variety of Latin, common, or pharmaceutical names and synonyms, complex chemistry, and different formulations.

ADVERSE EFFECTS OF DRUGS AND HERBS: A COMPARISON

Adverse reactions are defined as a response to a drug that is noxious and unintended and which occurs at doses normally used in humans. They can be classified as type A (augmented) or predictable reactions; type B (bizarre), unpredictable or idiosyncratic reactions; type C (chronic), reactions that develop with long-term therapy; type D, delayed effects such as carcinogenicity or teratogenicity; type E (end of use), reactions occur after stopping use, such as withdrawal symptoms; and type F (failure) applies to unexpected failure of treatment.[1] Type A is dose dependent, and type A and C reactions can be predicted based on the known pharmacology of the drug. Type B reactions, which cannot be explained based on the known pharmacology of the drug, include immune reactions such as anaphylaxis but also include toxicity from reactive metabolites and may affect any organ (see Chapter 4). Type D reactions are difficult to identify because of the delayed onset of months or years.[1] The active constituents and mechanisms of action of orthodox drugs are scientifically investigated, and for these it may be relatively easy to make the distinction between types of adverse effects and side effects.

With herbal remedies, acute reactions may be recognised if the effects occur soon after use of the product, and the association of cause and effect can be relatively easy. For most herbs, however, neither the active principles nor mechanisms of action have been identified so correlation with pharmacologic plausibility is seldom possible. Details of metabolism with bioavailability and production of active or inactive metabolites have rarely been studied. Therefore, it is not generally possible to separate adverse reactions from side effects or to differentiate between type A and B reactions.

Adverse effects of herbal remedies may be caused by the pharmacologic activity of the constituents or by intrinsically toxic components, overdose (acute or chronic), interactions between herbal remedies, or herb-drug interactions. Patient susceptibility (genetic or medical) or misuse may also lead to unwanted effects. Supply of intrinsically toxic herbs may be restricted in countries with active regulatory systems, but this cannot prevent the cultivation or importation of these herbs by consumers for their own use. Restricted herbs are often supplied through the Internet. Other problems may result from use of poor quality products, incorrect processing, misidentification or substitution of herbal ingredients, variability of levels of active ingredients, or adulteration or contamination during manufacture.

THERAPEUTIC DOSE VERSUS OVERDOSE

Orthodox drugs are generally single chemical compounds with clearly identified dose regimens. The effects of an overdose are not considered as an ADR. For any herbal remedy, the many variables make this distinction difficult, namely, plants have a complex chemistry modified by many factors ranging from genotype to all the different conditions during growth, harvesting, storage, and processing. Herbal practitioners of different traditions may use different plant parts, types of extract, combinations, and therapeutic dose according to their training. However, when products are self-prescribed and obtained as over-the-counter (OTC) products these limitations may not apply. Consumers may not be aware of the different uses of the various plant parts or implications of the type of extract or quality of the product, and they may not be able to correlate these factors with the guidance given in herbal medicine textbooks. There is a belief among some users that because these products are safe, then "if one tablet is good, two are better." This can lead to chronic or acute overdose with the intention of increasing beneficial effects. Unless there is clear evidence of overdose from patient information, it is rarely possible for medical professionals to differentiate between an overdose and therapeutic dose; therefore, all tend to be reported as adverse effects in the literature.

Other Causes of Adverse Effects

Use of poor quality products, with problems of adulteration, substitution, or use of incorrect starting materials, is not normally a concern for adverse effects with orthodox drugs. The medicine licensing structure does not allow for errors, and when there are any problems in manufacture, batches of drugs are rapidly withdrawn from supply or distribution is stopped. A significant proportion of herbal side effects reported in the literature are related to the use of incorrect plants or products adulterated with pharmaceutical agents or heavy metals. The issues of quality control of herbal materials are covered in Chapter 8.

The majority of herbal remedies are obtained as OTC products, self-prescribed by consumers. Such self-prescription can also lead to inappropriate use of a remedy, including use of the incorrect herb for a condition or a misdiagnosed condition, misidentification of herb collected or cultivated by patients, use of many different herbal products with overdose or interactions, or deliberate use of doses greater than recommended because of the belief that these are safe and have greater efficacy. Chronic misuse or abuse of products can lead to adverse health effects, and health care professionals need to be aware of how these remedies are being used by their patients. Diagnosis of toxicity may be delayed if the patient does not disclose details of herbal remedy use to the health care professional, and active questioning may be needed.

Botanical Identity

Identity is not an issue in orthodox drug monitoring. However, for any herbal remedy, confirmation of botanical identity is essential for any serious evaluation of reports of efficacy or toxicity. Ideally plant material should be properly identified with the correct Latin binomial, plant part, any processing, and type of extract. When herbal remedies are misidentified there can be serious consequences, and clinical effects will be attributed to the wrong plant. Recent instances include plantain contaminated with digitalis in the United States[2]; *Aristolochia* species as substitutes for *Stephania*, *Akebia*, or *Clematis* species[3]; and kava substituted with 1,4 butanediol, an industrial solvent that is metabolised to γ-hydroxybutyrate.[4] The identity of some crude herbal material may be relatively easy to confirm with simple tests. Powders, extracts, or herbal products containing combinations of herbs are more difficult and require laboratory analysis. However, few physicians have funding or contacts with phytochemical laboratories or botanic gardens with the relevant experience to analyse the material and confirm identity if they need to investigate the herbs used by a patient. For more discussion of these issues, see Chapter 8.

Assessing Reports of Adverse Effects

Reports of adverse effects of herbal remedies in the literature often cause much controversy. These are usually single cases with incomplete data provided. In any review of a suspected adverse reaction it is not always possible to exclude all other causes, especially for illnesses with nonspecific symptoms. If there is reasonable temporal relationship, herbal remedies may be labelled as the causative agent in part because the association cannot be excluded either by knowledge of mechanism of action or biochemical analysis providing evidence of toxins in blood or urine. In other words, herbal remedies are identified as the causative agent because the association cannot be excluded rather than there being positive evidence of toxicity. Details of the pattern of recovery of the patient may be significant in excluding other causes but are rarely presented. There may be questions about the botanical identity of the herbal ingredient and doses used. The value of such reports is often questioned. However, when physicians are concerned about a serious adverse event thought to result from an herbal remedy whose use was not essential for the patient's well-being, they may feel obliged to publish warnings to alert colleagues.

MONITORING ADVERSE EFFECTS

The most extensive database of adverse effects from herbal therapies is held by the Uppsala Monitoring Centre (UMC), the coordinating centre for the World Health Organisation (WHO) International Drug Monitoring Programme. Their role is to identify drugs with problematic side effects and to maintain a single global database for drug safety data. The data come from national centres in 72 countries and include reports on traditional and herbal remedies.[5] These comprise a relatively small component of the database with 11,716 reports compiled over 20 years compared with >3 million records on orthodox medicines.[6]

In a review of these reports the most common critical term was anaphylaxis, followed by facial oedema, bronchospasm and oesophageal stricture, and angioedema. Of the noncritical terms, pruritus was followed by rash and urticaria, nausea and vomiting, and diarrhea and abdominal pain. There were 21 fatal outcomes (2487 reports with single ingredient products), 3 each associated with senna (intestinal perforation) and psyllium mucolloid or ispaghula husk (respiratory failure).[5] The remaining reports are associated with a wide range of herbs, and no "problem" herbs are identified. However, it must be noted that the quality of assessment of these reports varies. These reports are not evidence of association but generate a signal. To make any more valid assessment of causal effect requires detailed evaluation of individual reports.[5] For more information on the issues surrounding the collection of pharmacovigilance data and various adverse reaction reporting mechanisms for herbs, see Chapter 11.

It is important to identify and properly document any adverse effects from herbal remedies. Although most have been used extensively and some have been used for hundreds of years, it must be borne in mind that the methods and patterns of use are changing.

Traditionally many medicinal herbs were used as teas with seasonal availability; however, now most herbal products are concentrated capsules or tablets. These are often specialist extracts that either concentrate or remove certain chemical constituents to increase potency and/or reduce side effects. However, these types of products may have a different chemical profile from the herb and give rise to previously unreported side effects. One of the theories of the recently reported hepatotoxicity of kava, an herb previously considered safe, is that high concentrations of kavalactones in some types of extracts contributed to toxicity (see Chapter 12). Many herbs are traditionally only used short term; therefore, long-term use may lead to unexpected adverse reactions, especially herbal stimulants or herbs used for weight loss. Concentrated formulations (e.g., extracts, capsules, tablets) also make it easier for consumers to use high doses chronically.

Reported Adverse Effects

The following incidents of adverse effects associated with herbal remedies are notable. Some are covered in detail elsewhere in this text and are only listed briefly here (e.g., see the various safety monographs and Chapter 9 for an extensive review of the Chinese herb issue).

Hepatic Effects

There is a perception that herbal remedies are prone to causing liver toxicity; however, this is not surprising because the liver is the primary organ involved in metabolism of foreign compounds and is the first organ (after the digestive tract) that is exposed to these compounds. Because relatively high concentrations of the compounds may be present, the liver is a target for different types of toxicity. Early symptoms may be relatively nonspecific and remain unrecognized for some time, and there are no special diagnostic tests for herbal hepatotoxicity. General symptoms include abdominal pain, tiredness, weakness, nausea, vomiting, and jaundice. Rash, arthralgias, fever, leucocytosis, and eosinophilia can occur in hypersensitivity reactions. The picture on histologic examination is also nonspecific and similar to other liver diseases. Causes of toxic hepatitis are difficult to identify because symptoms may be similar to naturally occurring liver disease.

Investigation usually involves standard screens of liver function (alanine aminotransferase [ALT], aspartate aminotransferase [AST], alkaline phosphatase (AP), γ-glutamyl-transferase (GGT), bilirubin) and exclusion of chronic alcohol ingestion, viral hepatitis, autoimmune disease, Wilson's disease, and so on. Once all likely causes are excluded, liver damage caused by drug actions is usually diagnosed by identifying temporal relationship, onset of damage, and response to drug withdrawal; therefore, evidence may be circumstantial rather than confirmed.

Differentiating liver damage from drug hepatotoxicity, idiosyncratic reactions, and viral hepatitis is notoriously difficult. Hepatitis viruses are not all serologically defined and can be difficult to exclude with certainty. Acute hepatitis of whatever cause is often caused by the formation of reactive metabolites in the liver and may take the following forms.

Cholestatic

This response is produced by flucloxacillin, phenothiazines (notably chlorpromazine), antithyroid drugs, and oral hypoglycaemic drugs. The latent period is 1 to 4 weeks; the main symptom, jaundice, may sometimes resolve although the patient keeps taking the drug. Other symptoms include fever, chills, anorexia, nausea, and a rash; there may be itching and dark urine and pale stools; and liver biopsy shows bile stasis, perhaps eosinophil infiltration, but usually little hepatocellular necrosis.

Hepatocellular

This response is seen with monoamine oxidase inhibitors (MAOIs) and other hydrazine derivatives like phenylbutazone, isoniazid, sulphonamides, and the anaesthetic halothane, especially after repeated administration. Hepatic granulomas may be a prominent feature.

Mixed Hypersensitivity Reactions

Apart from eosinophil infiltration or granuloma formation, there are no specific histologic features on liver biopsy to suggest drug sensitivity.

Metabolite formation may lead to predictable toxic hepatitis after large overdoses (e.g., paracetamol) or to idiosyncratic toxic hepatitis after therapeutic doses (e.g., isoniazid).

Prolonged, drug-induced cellular necrosis may also lead to subacute hepatitis, chronic hepatitis, or even cirrhosis; again the causes of each of these are difficult to differentiate. In many cases the main clinical problem is to distinguish drug-induced hepatic disease from that caused by viral hepatitis; in others the lesion produced is a more chronic one and may resemble chronic aggressive hepatitis or cirrhosis.

These difficulties in diagnosis in modern times underline how difficult it would have been in former times to link exposure to herbal medicines with liver damage. Traditional reputations for herbal safety have to be qualified by this major uncertainty.

Known adverse hepatic effects of herbal products include the following.

Pyrrolizidine Alkaloids

Long-term use of plants such as *Symphytum officinale* (comfrey), *Tussilago farfara* (coltsfoot), or *Senecio* species that contain unsaturated pyrrolizidine alkaloids (PAs) has been associated with the development of specific liver damage, namely, veno-occlusive disease.[7] The toxicity is caused by conversion of the PAs to cytotoxic pyrroles, which damage the sinusoidal and endothelial cells. The vasculature is occluded, and this reduction in blood flow results in ischaemic damage and centrilobular necrosis. Symptoms include arterial hypertension, right ventricular hypertrophy, abdominal pain, ascites, hepatomegaly and increased serum transaminase levels, jaundice, liver cirrhosis, and liver failure. Some of the PAs have been shown to be carcinogenic and mutagenic, and renal toxicity may also occur.[8-10]

The concentration of PAs varies between species and different parts of the plants; for example, young leaves have higher concentrations, and the level in the roots can be between 10 and 100 times greater than in the leaves of *Symphytum* species.[11,12] Oral use of concentrated products and the root has been restricted in Europe and the United States. Comfrey is mainly recommended for topical application on unbroken skin. However, the leaves have continued to be used as a tea, and plants are readily available from garden centres and can be used as home remedies. Unexpected toxicity may occur because of misidentification of the leaves: *Symphytum* and *Digitalis* leaves look similar in young plants when not in flower. Mistaken use of the *Digitalis* leaves may cause cardiac effects.

It should be noted that the saturated PAs found in plants such as *Echinacea* are not converted to the toxic pyrroles and are therefore not associated with veno-occlusive disease.

Teucrium chamaedrys (germander)

This herb was used in weight-loss products in France until approximately 20 cases of hepatotoxicity, including cytolytic hepatitis and fulminant hepatitis, were reported. Toxicity is thought to be caused by the metabolic activation by cytochrome P450 of the furano neoclerodane diterpenoids into hepatotoxic epoxides.[13,14] These may be partly inactivated by glutathione and epoxide hydrolase. Although this herb is no longer in general use medicinally, there are concerns that different species are still supplied because of inaccurate botanical identification. A documented example is *Teucrium canadense*, which has been supplied as *Scutellaria lateriflora* (skullcap).[15] This substitution is thought to have led to erroneous reports of liver toxicity of *Scutellaria* and valerian (also see the relevant safety monographs in this text) because unfortunately the multi-ingredient products that were used were not analysed to confirm botanical identity. These reports have led to much confusion, and analysis of the product is recommended in any suspected cases of liver toxicity with *Scutellaria* or valerian to check the identity of the plant used (see also Chapter 8). More commonly, though, it has been found that other species of *Scutellaria* have been used in place of *S. lateriflora*. There are no obvious safety issues associated with this replacement.

Chelidonium majus (greater celandine)

This herb is used to manage gastric and biliary disorders. At least 10 cases of acute hepatitis with marked cholestasis have been reported. All patients recovered after discontinuation of the herb. There was one unintentional rechallenge, which led to recurrence of liver inflammation (see the monograph on this herb).[16]

Piper methysticum (kava)

Details of this issue are covered in Chapter 12.

Larrea tridentata (chaparral)

There have been reports of acute hepatitis associated with the ingestion of chaparral (see the monograph on this herb).

Ephedra Spp. (ma huang)

A case of acute hepatitis associated with the use of ma huang (*Ephedra* spp.) was reported in the United States.[17] The time course, worsening of symptoms after unsupervised rechallenge, recovery on stopping the product, and exclusion of other causes indicated a causal relationship with use of the product. Unfortunately the contents of the product were not analysed to confirm botanical identity. Given the lack of reports in the literature of hepatotoxicity with ma huang and ephedrine, it is possible that the product concerned contained some other ingredient or contaminant or was misidentified. A second report detailed exacerbation of autoimmune hepatitis.[18] In both cases the product was used for weight loss, not the traditional therapeutic use to manage respiratory conditions. The main concerns of long-term use of high doses of ma huang are myocardial infarction, seizures, and stroke.

Chinese Herbal Medicine and Liver Toxicity

In traditional Chinese medicine, approximately 2000 different natural substances—plant, animal, or mineral—are commonly used medicinally. Prescriptions use complex formulations of up to 25 different ingredients to manage a range of medical conditions. In view of this range and combination of ingredients, it can be seen that any "global" labels of the toxicity of Chinese medicine are inaccurate. This also complicates any investigation of suspected adverse effects because of the complexity of the formulas used. Details of Chinese herbal medicine are covered in Chapter 9.

Case Reports

There have been a number of reports of liver toxicity of Chinese herbal medicine in the medical literature, and other cases have been reported to the Medical Toxicology Unit, Guy's & St. Thomas' NHS Trust in London.[19-23] Details of at least 20 cases of hepatotoxicity after the use of Chinese herbal medicine for skin conditions, lipomas, and arthralgia have been reviewed. These do not appear to be related to age, sex, or ethnic origin. The cases ranged from asymptomatic elevated liver enzymes to symptoms of jaundice, hepatitis, and acute liver failure. Two patients died after unsuccessful liver transplantation[21,22]; the remainder recovered after stopping use of the herbs. In two patients unsupervised rechallenge resulted in more rapid and severe recurrence of symptoms.[20,21] Using the WHO definitions, the causal relationship was assessed as "possible" in the remaining cases based on time course, recovery on stopping use of Chinese herbs, and exclusion of other causes.[1] In the majority of cases ALT or AST was >10 times normal. A thorough review of the prescriptions used by these patients showed 107 different ingredients, but no common herb was used in all cases. At present, because no dose or time dependency has been identified, it is thought to be an idiosyncratic reaction.

Concerns of liver toxicity have led to at least two detailed studies of liver effects. In a review of 1507 patients using Chinese herbal medicine for chronic pain at a hospital in Kotzing, Germany, only 14 showed minor elevations of ALT >2 times normal, and all returned to normal after 8 weeks, even with continued treatment with Chinese herbs. There was no evidence of interaction with the prescribed pharmaceutical drugs that were taken at the same time.[24]

In another study of 1265 patients attending a single herbal practitioner, 1 developed hepatitis, and 106 developed slightly increased ALT levels (<3 times normal). In 95% of the patients this returned to normal within 2 weeks and remained elevated (at 2 to 3 times normal) in only three patients.[25]

Because this appears to be an idiosyncratic reaction with no predictive factors and because changes in liver function are easily detected, many practitioners of Chinese herbal medicine in the United Kingdom have introduced regular liver function monitoring of patients before and during treatment. They also provide guidelines for patients on liver toxicity.

Until more is known about the active constituents and their metabolism, any association of specific herbs with liver toxicity will be difficult to prove or disprove.

Other Herbal Treatments

A report from Denver, Colorado described the cases of three children and three adults in whom severe toxic effects developed after ingestion of a Chinese herbal medication, jin bu huan, sold as a safe natural anodyne. Jin bu huan produced distinct clinical syndromes: a single, acute ingestion in children rapidly produced life-threatening central nervous system and respiratory depression, whereas long-term use in adults was associated with hepatitis. Jin bu huan contains only levo-tetrahydropalmatine (L-thp), a potent neuroactive substance. L-thp has been registered as a pharmaceutical agent in mainland China; therefore, it is questionable whether jin bu huan should be considered a herbal product or pharmaceutical agent.[26] In the reports of toxicity, investigation was further complicated because the plant ingredients were misidentified on the package, resulting in significant delay in identifying the constituent responsible for its toxicity. The highly concentrated formulation and the lack of childproof packaging contributed to the development of toxic reactions.[27]

Renal Effects

The kidneys have spare capacity, and symptoms may only occur when renal function becomes severely impaired. For example, in patients with chronic renal failure symptoms may only occur when the glomerular filtration rate is reduced to as low as 10%.[28] This implies that there may be a considerable time delay between use of the causative agent and development of symptoms. Any such time delay can lead to difficulties in identifying the cause.

The role of the kidney in excretion makes it a target for toxicity. Active transport of compounds and reabsorption of water and sodium, especially in the tubules, leads to concentration of compounds in the tubular cells and interstitial fluid, leaving the kidney exposed to higher concentration of metabolites than any other organ. The cytochrome P450 content of the kidney is much less than the liver, but this is still sufficient for some metabolic activation causing local toxicity. The proximal tubule is the most common site of damage. Specific drugs such as the aminoglycosides can damage the glomeruli.[28]

Aristolochic Acid Nephropathy

Various species of *Aristolochia* have been used in many traditions of herbal medicine around the world. Although there was some traditional knowledge of possible renal toxicity of these herbs, this has only been extensively investigated since 1993. In what is the most serious incident of herbal injury in recent times, a slimming clinic in Belgium erroneously used *Aristolochia fangchi* in a combination therapy with other herbs and drugs including acetazolamide, diethylpropion, and fenfluramine.[29] This resulted in approximately 105 patients with acute renal failure requiring dialysis and at least half of whom required kidney transplantation.[30] Subsequently reports worldwide have provided details on approximately 65 additional cases associated with different species, reported when no comparable additional drug treatment was used.[31-35]

This has led to a syndrome called "Chinese herb nephropathy" (CHN) being described in the medical literature, although it is more correctly termed "aristolochic acid nephropathy" (AAN) because it is associated with ingestion of aristolochic acids and not Chinese herbs in general.[36] Its features are rapidly progressive renal fibrosis with the development of renal cell carcinoma.

Patients may present with acute renal failure. Symptoms include mild to moderate hypertension, anaemia, mild tubular proteinuria, glycosuria, and elevations in plasma creatinine. Renal biopsy shows interstitial fibrosis with atrophy and loss of tubules, relative sparing of the glomeruli with mild collapse of the capillaries, and wrinkling of the basement membranes. Progression to end-stage renal disease is faster than in other interstitial nephropathies.[37] Onset of symptoms of renal damage may be delayed for up to 3 years after stopping use of the preparation; therefore, it is important to obtain a complete medical history from the patient. Steroid therapy has been reported to slow the deterioration of renal function.[38] The presence of the aristolochic acids (the nephrotoxic component) can be confirmed by laboratory analysis of the herbal products, and when this is suspected samples of the product should be kept for analysis. DNA-aristolochic acid adducts may be detected in the removed kidney and can provide a lifelong biological marker of exposure.[36]

Because there were concerns about the increased risk of cancer from ingestion of aristolochic acid, some of the Belgian AAN patients were advised to have their native kidneys and ureters removed. Of the 39 patients who agreed to prophylactic surgery there were 18 cases of urothelial carcinoma and 19 cases with mild to moderate dysplasia. In only two patients were no lesions found.[30] In one of the three AAN cases reported in the United Kingdom, transitional cell carcinoma was found in the renal pelvis and ureter 3 years after transplantation.[39] There is now a suggestion that urothelial carcinoma may develop even without associated renal failure after a single case report from Belgium.[40] All tissue samples analysed contained aristolochic acid-related DNA adducts. The presence of DNA adducts[41] provides a disturbing mechanism for carcinogenesis: some AAN cases were marked by the overexpression of p53, a tumour-suppressor gene, which suggests a possible p53 gene mutation.[42] Nortier and Lord recommend removal of both native kidneys and ureter in transplantation patients with AAN. Continued screening for urothelial cancer is advised for any patient diagnosed with AAN.[30]

The use of the combination treatment by the slimming clinic (herbs with anorectic, diuretic, tranquilizer, laxative, and atropinergic drugs) is likely to have contributed to the severity of the AAN cases reported in Belgium. However, the subsequent reports show that combination therapy is not an essential factor for the development of renal damage associated with AAN. Individual patient susceptibility, genetic polymorphism, and cumulative dose of aristolochic acid appear to be significant factors in toxicity.[36,43] The contribution of these factors is supported by evidence from Japan and China where AAN is characterized by development of Fanconi syndrome, whereas this has only a single report in Europe.[44-46] In China the effects of dose on the clinical manifestations of AAN have been further defined according to long-term, short-term, or intermittent ingestion of aristolochic acids.[47]

Oxalates

Oxalates are found in plants such as *Rheum palmatum* (rhubarb species) and *Rumex* spp. Ingestion of the needlelike crystals cause immediate pain and local irritation; however, the soluble form has no such effect, and these plants may be used in herbal remedies. Oxalic acid may combine with calcium after absorption and form insoluble calcium oxalate crystals. These can cause mechanical injuries in the kidneys. Acute renal failure may occur if the calcium is precipitated in the renal tubules. Development of symptoms may take 24 to 48 hours. The urinary concentrations of calcium and oxalate are important for the crystallization of calcium oxalate.

Poisoning by ingestion of oxalate-containing plants, such as raw rhubarb, is infrequent, and such deaths are rare.[48] There is one report of a fatal poisoning in a 53-year-old man who ingested a large quantity of *Rumex crispus* leaf as a salad vegetable.[49]

There are other data showing a link with herb consumption and renal cell carcinoma: a Uruguayan epidemiologic study showed that heavy consumption of maté tea (*Ilex paraguayensis*) was associated with a threefold increase in risk (marginally less than a high red meat intake!).[50]

Cardiac Toxicity

The therapeutic benefits of the cardiac glycosides derived from *Digitalis* spp., such as digoxin, are well known. Other steroid glycosides are found in *Apocynum*, *Asclepias*, and *Convallaria* spp. that have medicinal uses. These glycosides have a narrow margin of safety with a low therapeutic index. To further complicate use, patient sensitivities vary, requiring careful

dose monitoring. For these reasons these plants are not generally available in OTC products for self-use by consumers. However, there are occasional case reports of toxicity, usually related to the misidentification of the plant material. In the United States the accidental contamination of *Platago major* (plantain) with *Digitalis lanata* in a cleansing-weight-loss product resulted in cases of cardiac arrhythmias.[2] When not in flower, many plants can look similar to the untrained eye, and other examples include comfrey (*Symphytum* spp.) and foxglove (*Digitalis* spp.). Adverse effects of the cardiac glycosides include vomiting, diarrhoea, visual disturbances, hypotension, and ventricular arrhythmias and ventricular tachycardia with fibrillation and sinoarterial block.

Aconitum Spp. (Aconite)

Various species of aconite have been used in many traditions of herbal medicine for conditions such as rheumatism and joint pain, and also to dilate the coronary, cerebral, and peripheral arteries and improve capillary circulation. It is used topically as a liniment for muscular pains.[51,52] These plants contain potent cardioactive constituents, the aconitine alkaloids, which can be toxic at low doses. Onset of symptoms is within 30 minutes of ingestion, and symptoms include numbness, paraesthesia, muscle weakness, metabolic and/or respiratory acidosis, hypotension, palpitations, tachyarrhythmia, and reduced consciousness.[53,54] There is no antidote, and treatment is symptomatic and supportive. Although deaths have been reported in Hong Kong, early supportive treatment, in patients without underlying cardiac conditions, has resulted in positive outcomes.[54,55] In traditional Chinese medicine the root is boiled repeatedly to hydrolyse the alkaloids and significantly reduce toxicity by up to 1000-fold.[56] In a controlled trial, heated aconite preparation demonstrated positive inotropic, positive chronotropic, and vasodilator effects in patients with left ventricular failure.[57] Aconite is restricted for use in OTC products but may still be found in imported products. Toxicity has been reported when liniments have been ingested in error because of poor labelling or instructions.

Allergic Reactions

Anaphylaxis and allergic reactions are the most common reports to the UMC.[5] Herbs suspected to be associated with these types of reports include asparagus root, silymarin, bromelain, echinacea, fennel oil, fenugreek seed, garlic, ginkgo biloba, psyllium mucilage, and ispaghula. The validity of such reports depends on correct identification of the herbs and correct assessment of the case details.

Ginkgo biloba fruits have caused allergic reactions with erythema, oedema, blisters, and itching. The fresh seeds are potentially toxic, but roasted seeds are eaten like peanuts in parts of China, although in limited quantities of up to 10 per day because greater amounts can cause skin disorders, irritation of mucous membranes, and other toxicity. Gingko seed is used in Chinese medicine after processing by steaming, stir-frying, or roasting.[58-60]

Echinacea (e.g., *Echinacea angustifolia, Echinacea pallida,* and *Echinacea purpurea*) is commonly used to support and boost the immune system. Combinations of plants and plant parts are used in the wide range of products. It is thought that the acute hypersensitivity reactions most likely occur with use of the above ground parts of the plant. However, it may be difficult to confirm this because it is not possible to identify either the part of the plant or the species used in many products. For a detailed discussion of allergic reactions, see Chapter 10.

Haematologic Disturbances

Herbs such as *Salvia miltiorrhiza* (dan shen) and *Angelica sinensis* (dang gui) have been reported to interact with warfarin treatment and increase prothrombin time, although neither herb shows this activity if used alone.[61] Dang gui should only be used with professional supervision by patients with bleeding or clotting disorders. It is contraindicated before surgery. Because it has uterine effects, it should be avoided during pregnancy, unless under medical supervision.[62] A recent study from Denmark has shown that *Ginkgo biloba* used in combination with warfarin does not increase international normalised ratio (INR).[63] However, there have been some anecdotal reports of haematologic effects of ginkgo,

including two case reports of subdural haematoma,[64,65] one of subarachnoid haemorrhage,[66] one of bleeding iris,[67] and one report of interaction with warfarin.[68] The evidence from these reports is not always complete or conclusive, but physicians need to be aware of reported risks. Because ginkgo is one of the top selling herbs, many more similar reports would have been expected, and this may be an idiosyncratic effect only affecting a subset of predisposed patients. Additional observation or monitoring may be appropriate when there are concerns or before surgery.

Gastrointestinal Disorders and Diarrhoea

Diarrhoea can occur with many herbs (other than laxatives), and reports include silymarin, evening primrose oil, peppermint oil, feverfew, Chinese medicines, ginkgo, and caffeine-containing plants. With these and many other herbs, the effect is transient and only occurs during the first few days of use. Herbal remedies can be taken with meals to prevent or reduce gastrointestinal effects. However, prolonged diarrhoea is a health risk with dehydration, muscle cramps, and electrolyte imbalance with potential heart disorders caused by potassium loss. These effects can be particularly serious for children.

Herbal laxatives, such as senna or cascara, are popular remedies for constipation. As well as having laxative properties, these may cause abdominal pains. It is interesting to note that some consumers become concerned about these effects of these products, even at therapeutic doses, and will seek medical attention.

Phototoxicity

Phototoxicity can be caused by topical application of herbal extracts but is also considered a risk if large amounts of certain foods or herbs are eaten. The furanocoumarins (psoralens) are the photosensitising constituents present in plants such as celery, parsnip, parsley, rue, citrus species (bergamot), and *Psoralea corylifolia*. This latter herb is used topically to manage vitiligo or other skin conditions. The psoralens sensitise the skin to subsequent exposure to ultraviolet (UV) light, with increased pigmentation on the treated area.[69] This is similar to psoralen and UVA (PUVA) therapy used in orthodox medicine to manage dermatologic conditions: an oral dose of methoxalen is followed by exposure to a period of UVA light. Serious burns or blisters may be caused if the dose of psoralens is too high and the light exposure is not carefully regulated. In herbal therapy the dose applied will depend on the type of extract and the herb used. UV exposure is often not a controlled period under a UV lamp but depends on sunlight. In countries with fluctuating light levels this increases the difficulties in regulating exposure. In the United Kingdom there have been two reports of severe burns when high-strength psoralen extracts were used, followed by exposure to UV lamps.[70]

Even ingestion of large amounts of soup made from vegetables including parsley, celery, or parsnip have resulted in reports of phototoxic burns after exposure to UV light.[71] *Hypericum perforatum* and *Angelica archangelica* have been reported to cause photosensitivity at much higher doses than normally used therapeutically (see also the monograph on St. John's wort).[72] The phototoxic reaction requires exposure to UV light; therefore, when there are concerns about the use of a topical lotion or dose of herb ingested, risks can be reduced by washing the treated area and avoiding UV light (e.g., long-sleeved clothes and staying indoors) for at least 24 hours after ingestion.

Herbs with Toxic Volatile Oil Constituents

The essential oils in some medicinal plants contain potentially toxic constituents. Often these are aromatic or flavourings also used for culinary purposes, and limiting the level of a constituent allowed in a food product ensures safe use. These oils are highly concentrated extracts produced by distillation or other solvent extraction. Toxicity of the oil is likely to be different to that of the original plant material or water decoctions. This clearly illustrates the need to differentiate between types of extracts that are used because these will have different safety implications. Several plants contain potentially toxic volatile oils, but only a few are described here.

Sassafras albidum (safrole)

Sassafras albidum is used as a carminative and for gout, rheumatic pain, and dermatologic conditions.[73] Sassafras has been used in foods and beverages. Studies in mice with high doses of the aqueous or ethanolic extracts have resulted in ataxia, central nervous system depression, and hypothermia.[74] It also causes dose-related induction and inhibition of liver enzymes.[75,76] The main concerns about toxicity relate to use of the volatile oil and its principal constituent, safrole. As with other essential oils, even very small amounts are highly toxic, and even one teaspoon has proved fatal in an adult. Symptoms include vomiting, stupor, and collapse. Large amounts are reported to be psychoactive and hallucinogenic.[77] Safrole, an allylbenzene, is a procarcinogen that is converted into toxic substances by the liver. Potential toxicity is reduced because some of these active metabolites are subsequently detoxified by further metabolism.[78] Evidence of carcinogenicity of safrole comes from in vitro studies showing covalent binding to DNA.[79] In the United States, only safrole-free extracts can be used in foods. Sassafras is contraindicated during pregnancy and lactation. The herbal extract should not be used for extended periods.

Other culinary herbs that contain safrole include cinnamon, nutmeg, and basil, although toxicity issues are related to therapeutic use and not amounts in culinary use.

Acorus calamus and *Asarum* spp. (β-asarone)

Acorus root has been used medicinally to stimulate digestion, for anorexia and gastric ulcers, and as an antispasmodic agent.[73,80] Even short-term use of high doses of *Asarum* or *Acorus* spp. has caused nausea and vomiting.[81] As with sassafras, toxicity is related to a single constituent, the β-asarone in the volatile oil. It is also an allylbenzene and a procarcinogen. However, there is considerable variation in the β-asarone content of the different genetic species. *Acorus americanus* and *Acorus calamus* contain only trace amounts, but the Indian species, *Acorus angustatus*, contains between 80% and 96% of β-asarone.[80,82] It is recommended that only roots with trace amounts of β-asarone should be used therapeutically.

Ingestion of the volatile oil is not recommended. Topical use of the oil in bath preparations has been reported to cause erythema and dermatitis.[83]

Herbs containing β-asarone should not be used long term and should be avoided during pregnancy and lactation.

Estragole is another allylbenzene and is a constituent of culinary herbs such as tarragon, fennel, basil, and chervil. The level of estragole is limited in foods, and toxicity is not related to normal culinary use.

Juniperus communis (Juniper)

The essential oil of juniper is sometimes labelled as a renal irritant and abortifacient. Reports on overdose include pain near the kidney, strong diuresis, albuminuria, haematuria, purplish urine, tachycardia, hypertension, and rarely convulsions, menorrhagia, and abortion.[77] However, the evidence is conflicting. From some early publications dating back to 1920s it appears that there has been confusion between *Juniper communis* and *Juniper sabina* (Savin) and possible adulteration of juniper oil with other species. Savin is known to be dangerous during pregnancy and in patients with renal disease.[84,85] A more recent study by Hiel and Schilcher[86] suggests that the essential oil of the ripe berries is safe. Owing to the contradictory nature of the published studies, caution is still required, and juniper should be avoided during pregnancy or be used with professional supervision by patients with renal disease.

Juniper oil is not phototoxic but may be an irritant after topical application.

Miscellaneous Herbal Cautions

Phytolacca americana (pokeroot)

Pokeroot has been used for inflammatory conditions such as rheumatism or laryngitis and as a purgative or externally on abscesses.[73] It should be used with professional supervision because safe doses can be easily exceeded especially with ingestion of tinctures. The irritant phytolaccatoxins (triterpenoid saponins) are responsible for severe gastrointestinal irritation and intense abdominal cramping.[87] The toxins are also absorbed through broken skin

or conjunctival membranes.[88] Systemic exposure to the lectins found in all parts of the plant can cause haematologic aberrations.[89,90] Symptoms of ingestion include nausea, vomiting, abdominal pain and cramping, watery diarrhoea, haematemesis and bloody diarrhoea, hypotension, and tachycardia.[91] Because of risks of toxicity, extreme caution is required; therefore, this herb may not be suitable for self-prescription.

Viscum album (mistletoe)

Mistletoe preparations have been used for hypertension, arteriosclerosis, tachycardia, and hysteria.[73] The cytotoxic and immunostimulant properties have been shown in in vitro and animal studies.[92] In Europe, it has been used as a cancer treatment alongside conventional treatment, and some limited benefits have been shown with a fermented plant juice product. There were no reports of serious toxicity in 1000 patients using this product.[93]

The viscotoxins are low molecular weight proteins with cytotoxic and cardiotoxic properties.[94] The lectins are the other toxic constituent, and these inhibit protein synthesis and are associated with the agglutinating activity. Symptoms include hypotension, coma, seizures, myosis, mydriasis, and death.[95] The lectins and viscotoxins are not known to be hepatotoxic. Additional monitoring may be required for patients undergoing cardiac and blood pressure–regulating treatment and/or immune suppression and coagulation therapy. The berries are highly poisonous.[96] Owing to concerns about toxicity mistletoe may not be suitable for self-prescription. It should also be avoided during pregnancy and lactation.

Trichosanthes kirilowii (tian hua fen)

Root, fruit, and seeds are used in Chinese medicine for conditions, including jaundice, diabetes, mastitis, and haemorrhoids. There have been concerns about safety because the fresh root contains a polypeptide, trichosanthin (approximately 0.05%), which has been used to induce abortion.[58,97] It is unlikely that oral use of either the dried plant material or decoctions would have this effect. Because it is a peptide, trichosanthin is unstable and is likely to be inactivated on drying or cooking or broken down in the digestive tract. However, deaths have been reported in China after vaginal administration of the plant material. Infection is likely to be a major contributory factor to the severity of these cases.

Salicylates

Plants including *Salix* spp. (willow), *Filipendula ulmaria* (meadowsweet), and *Populus tremuloides* (poplar) contain salicylates. They are used for rheumatism and other inflammatory conditions, fevers, and headaches.[98] However, they are not thought to be effective inhibitors of platelet aggregation. The anticlotting property of aspirin is reportedly caused by the acetyl group (acetylsalicylic acid), which is absent in the plant extracts. Therefore, these herbs are unlikely to be effective alternatives to aspirin for patients with cardiac disorders. This also means that standard warnings in books on herbal medicine against the use of salicylate-containing herbs with anticoagulants may be unduly cautious.[98] Although interactions are theoretically unlikely, physicians may wish to carry out additional therapeutic drug monitoring or check clotting parameters if there are concerns about patients either maintained on anticoagulant therapy or before surgery. Adverse effects for willow bark in a small proportion of patients have included abdominal pain, nausea, dizziness, sweating, and rash.[99]

Cyanogenic Glycosides

Cyanogenic glycosides are widely distributed through many plant species. An example is amygdalin found in bitter almond and the seeds of apples, apricots, and peaches among others. Hydrogen cyanide is released by chewing or crushing the plant tissue or during digestion. Laetrile, derived from amygdalin in apricot kernels, was promoted for management of cancer in the 1970s. However, subsequent trials have found no demonstrable antitumour activity.[100,101] Even moderate consumption of the seeds of apricot, peach, or bitter almond can cause severe toxic reactions. Symptoms of nonlethal doses include nausea, vomiting, headache, and dizziness. With ingestion of approximately 150 mg (e.g., 60 apricot kernels), the lethal dose, symptoms progress to hyperventilation, collapse, convulsions,

coma, and respiratory failure. Chronic poisoning with sublethal doses (either in the diet or cyanogenetic drugs) causes agranulocytosis, increased blood thiocyanate, goiter, thyroid cancer, optic nerve lesions, ataxia, hypertonia, cretinism, and mental retardation.[100] The antidote for cyanide poisoning has to be administered immediately after ingestion for it to be effective. Use should be avoided during pregnancy because even low levels are considered teratogenic. Herbs containing cyanogenic glycosides should not be used long term.

Weight-Loss Products

These are not always strictly herbal remedies, but herbs are often used as OTC weight-loss products because consumers consider them to be natural and safe. Psychological stresses may lead consumers to overuse these products or to use them long term regardless of instructions or warnings on the bottles. There are a number of herbs that are used in this way, and these can be subdivided into three groups: laxatives, diuretics, and stimulants. Short-term use of these may not lead to any adverse reactions. However, it is long-term use, especially of high doses, that is of most concern.

Laxative herbs include senna, aloes, and cascara. Long-term use of any laxative drug can lead to electrolyte imbalance, dehydration and muscle cramps, albuminuria, and haematuria. The loss of potassium can lead to heart disorders and may increase the effects of cardiac glycosides.[102] Prescribed diuretic drugs have similar effects, and if used with laxatives they will potentiate these effects. Chronic overstimulation of the bowel by use of laxatives can also lead to dependence or "lazy bowel," which may require larger doses of laxative to maintain bowel function. Such misuse can lead to adverse effects from herbs normally considered safe. (For more discussion of these issues, see the monograph on senna.)

Herbal diuretic agents do not have a strong effect and are not comparable in potency with prescribed thiazide or loop diuretic agents. Therefore, they are unlikely to cause electrolyte imbalance, but long-term use of high doses should be avoided.

Products containing stimulants such as ephedrine (e.g., *Ephedra* spp. or ma huang) or caffeine (e.g., guarana, maté tea, and kola nut) are used for weight loss and as energy sources for athletes or euphoriants in herbal highs. The main concern comes from abuse of these products because doses tend to be higher than for medicinal use. The active constituent of the most widely used products is often ephedrine, which is available in some cold remedies. Reported adverse effects of *Ephedra* include palpitations, myocardial infarction, psychiatric symptoms such as anxiety and aggression, autonomic hyperactivity, insomnia, hepatitis, and even death in the United States.[17,103] These cases have caused much debate on dose and duration of use, use of synthetic ephedrine in "herbal" products, and also the variable quality of the reports. Concerns about the adverse effects resulting from use of excessive doses of *Ephedra* for weight loss or to improve athletic performance have contributed to the restrictions on sale and use of products containing this herb. This has limited even the therapeutic uses by herbal practitioners for its beneficial effects in patients with lung problems, febrile disease, and allergic conditions.

Health care providers should be aware of the potential for misuse or abuse of these types of products by their patients. Some patients using these products will disregard warnings and continue to use high doses long term despite minor side effects as long as they believe that they are losing weight. (For more information on *Ephedra*, see the safety monograph in this text.)

SPECIAL PATIENT GROUPS

It is generally recognized that changes in metabolic functions in the very young and very old populations and in pregnant and lactating women require more cautious prescription because of the greater risk of adverse effects from medicines. Herbal remedies are generally considered to be milder than pharmaceutical drugs and less likely to cause adverse effects. Unfortunately there is a general lack of objective information on the safety of herbs in special patient groups, including children, the elderly population, pregnant or lactating women, and those with renal or hepatic diseases. Caution is required for use of any herbal

remedies in these groups, especially those herbs with known toxicity because the differences in metabolism may change a safe dose into a toxic dose. During pregnancy, when there are changes in metabolic rate and volume of distribution, this can also affect the level of dose required for therapeutic effects of some drugs. A number of herbs are traditionally used as emmenagogues to stimulate and promote menstruation. These should be avoided during pregnancy because the uterine stimulant properties may induce miscarriage. The full safety profile of any herb to be used during pregnancy or lactation needs to be carefully considered and should only be used when benefits exceed risk. Drug interactions are a concern among the elderly population and those with chronic diseases because they may be taking a range of prescribed medicines.

Some herbs have traditional uses as abortifacients. These are often potentially toxic herbs used at high doses. For example, use of high doses of pennyroyal oil has resulted in death from fulminant liver failure with massive necrosis.[104] Other serious complications include renal or multiorgan failure.[105] Because some are cytotoxic and teratogenic these may cause severe developmental abnormalities.

CONCLUSIONS AND RECOMMENDATIONS

Any review of the adverse effects of herbal medicine will focus on the negative aspects of these therapies. However, it is important for physicians and consumers to maintain a balanced perspective on the value of herbal remedies: they may have health benefits and risks. Many hundreds of herbs are used medicinally with different chemical constituents and different pharmacologic activity; they are at least as varied as the range of drugs used in orthodox medicine. Therefore, as with orthodox drugs, broad sweeping statements on the efficacy or toxicity of herbs are an oversimplification.

In the interests of patient well-being, health care professionals need to establish an open dialogue with their patients about their use of herbal remedies. In any discussion the appropriate use of any herb is an important consideration; as with any OTC drugs, due attention should be paid to the choice of the correct medicinal herb (i.e., drug), dose, duration of use, and reasons for use. If recommended doses are exceeded or the remedy is used inappropriately, the occurrence of side effects should not be surprising.

Some patients may be reluctant to disclose such information to their orthodox health care provider if they anticipate a negative response or if they perceive a lack of understanding of herbal therapy. Such fears need to be allayed, possibly by routinely including direct questions on the use of any herbs or supplements when taking a medical history. This information may be needed in case unexplained symptoms occur, to reduce the risk of interactions with prescribed drugs, or if the patient becomes pregnant. Herbs may be misused for recreational purposes, in sports or athletics, or for slimming; therefore, knowledge of dose and reasons for use can identify cases in which additional vigilance is advisable. If patients are under the impression that their health care providers disapprove of the use of herbal remedies, they may be too afraid to seek medical assistance if they suffer an adverse effect. This may delay medical treatment, complicate diagnosis, or lead to incorrect drug therapy if the patient has given misleading or inadequate information.

Generally there is a lack of authoritative information on the safety of most medicinal herbs. Relatively few medicinal herbs have been investigated in clinical trials or postmarketing surveillance; therefore, information on adverse effects largely depends on spontaneous or anecdotal reports. Unfortunately, many of these anecdotal reports lack adequate data for proper evaluation. To rectify this situation, when any suspected adverse effect does occur it needs to be fully investigated and reported to the appropriate local or national ADR monitoring system.

In addition to the standard questions on an ADR reporting form, additional details are needed to ensure that an herbal report is valid. The correct identification of all the herbs used is essential, including Latin binomial, part of plant used, type of extract, and formulation. Brand name and manufacturer are also needed

for any herbal product because of variability in products. Well-documented case reports are often not differentiated from those lacking adequate medical or botanical validation. Better standards of reporting will improve the available safety information.

To improve patient safety, health care professionals need to be more aware of the full spectrum of possible unwanted health effects from the use of herbal remedies. Correspondingly, most texts on herbal safety in the medical reference literature err on the side of caution to ensure that details of theoretical risks and documented reports are provided. However, it should be appreciated that the difference between these types of evidence may not be clear. In some instances the theoretical concerns are based only on the overall chemistry of the plant and presence of a potentially toxic constituent without verifying the pharmacokinetic or pharmacodynamic properties of these compounds. Data on whether some potentially toxic compounds are absorbed in doses sufficient to cause adverse health effects are often not available. In this situation of inadequate information, a more pragmatic approach may be appropriate, and advice has to be based on judgment rather than fact.

In most cases, the incidence of adverse health effects associated with herbal remedies is unknown. It is commonly accepted that there is underreporting of drug adverse effects; this also applies to herbal remedies. First, health care professionals may not identify adverse effects or may not realise that such effects should be reported. Second, there is evidence that consumers are less likely to inform their health care professionals of any unwanted health effects of herbal remedies.[106] Despite this, studies of those inquiries that have been made to poison control centres in the United Kingdom and United States (by medical professionals and consumers) have so far shown that herbal remedies are relatively safe.[107,108]

As stated previously, any suspected adverse health effects from herbal remedies should be reported to the appropriate monitoring system. However, attribution of a health problem to the use of herbal remedies should not be used as the easy option when no obvious medical condition or cause can be identified. Because of the complexities involved with herbal products and the associated issues of misidentification and adulteration, many adverse reactions that have been attributed to herbs in the current literature need to be critically evaluated. This is one of the main objectives of this book.

REFERENCES

1. Edwards IR, Aronson JK: Adverse drug reactions: definitions, diagnosis and management, *Lancet* 356:1255-1259, 2000.
2. Slifman NR: Contamination of botanical dietary supplements by *Digitalis lanata*, *N Engl J Med* 339:806-811, 1998.
3. Zhu M, Phillipson JD: Hong Kong samples of Chinese medicine "Fang ji" contain aristolochic acid, *Int J Pharmacognosy* 34:283-289, 1996.
4. Blumenthal M: Kava: the peaceful herb of the south pacific, *Natural Pharmacy* April:12-15, 1997.
5. Farah MH, Edwards R, Lindquist M, et al: International reporting of adverse health effects associated with herbal medicines, *Pharmacoepidemiol Drug Saf* 9:105-112, 2000.
6. Farah MH: Personal communication, 2003.
7. IPCS International Programme on Chemical Safety: *Environmental health criteria 80—pyrrolizidine alkaloids*, Geneva, 1988, WHO.
8. Mattocks AR: *Chemistry and toxicology of pyrrolizidine alkaloids*, New York, 1986, Academic Press.
9. Winship KA: Toxicity of comfrey, *Adverse Drug React Toxicol Rev* 10:47-59, 1991.
10. Weston CFM, Cooper BT, Davies JD, et al: Venoocclusive disease of the liver secondary to the ingestion of comfrey, *BMJ* 295:183, 1987.
11. Awang DVC: Comfrey, *Can Pharm J* 120:100-104, 1987.
12. Roberts DJ: Pyrrolizidine alkaloids, *Nat Prod Rep* 12:413-418, 1995.
13. Larrey D, Vial T, Pauwels A, et al: Hepatitis after germander (*Teucrium chamaedrys*) administration: another instance of herbal medicine hepatotoxicity, *Ann Intern Med* 117:129-132, 1992.
14. Loeper J, Descatoire V, Letteron P, et al: Hepatotoxicity of germander in mice, *Gastroenterology* 106:464-472, 1994.
15. De Smet PAGM: Health risks of herbal remedies, *Drug Saf* 13:81-93, 1995.
16. Benninger J, Schneider HT, Schuppan D, et al: Acute hepatitis induced by greater celandine (*Chelidonium majus*), *Gastroenterology* 117:1234-1237, 1999.
17. Nadir A, Sangeeta A, King, P, Marshall JB: Acute hepatitis associated with the use of a Chinese herbal product, Ma-Huang, *Am J Gastroenterol* 91:1436-1438, 1996.
18. Borum ML: Fulminant exacerbation of autoimmune hepatitis after the use of ma-huang, *Am J Gastroenterol* 96:1654-1655, 2001.
19. Pillans PI: *Herbal medicine and toxic hepatitis*, N Z Med J 107:432-433, 1994.
20. Kane JA, Kane SP, Jain S: Hepatitis induced by traditional Chinese herbs; possible toxic components, *Gut* 36:146-147, 1995.
21. Perharic L, Shaw D, Leon C, De Smet PA, Murray VS: Possible association of liver damage with the use of Chinese herbal medicine for skin disease, *Vet Hum Toxicol* 37:562-566, 1995.
22. Vautier G, Spiller RC: Safety of complementary medicines should be monitored, *BMJ* 311:633, 1995.
23. McRae CA, Agarwal K, Mutimer D, Bassendine MF: Hepatitis associated with Chinese herbs, *Eur J Gastroenterol Hepatol* 14:559-562, 2002.
24. Melchart D, Linde K, Hager S, et al: Monitoring of liver enzymes in patients treated with traditional Chinese drugs, *Complement Ther Med* 7:208-216, 1999.
25. Al-Khafaji M: Monitoring of liver enzymes in patients on Chinese medicine, *JCM* 62:6-10, 2000.
26. But PH, Choi KL: Jin bu huan anodyne tablets, a mislabeled and misclassified medicine, *J Hong Kong Med Assoc* 46:302-305, 1994.
27. Horowitz RS, Feldhaus K, Dart RC, Stermitz FR, Beck JJ: The clinical spectrum of jin bu huan toxicity, *Arch Intern Med* 156:899-903, 1996.
28. Gaw A, Cowan RA, O'Reilly D, et al: *Clinical biochemistry*, ed 2, Edinburgh, 1999, Churchill Livingstone.
29. Vanherweghem JL, Depierreux M, Tielemans C, et al: Rapidly progressive interstitial renal fibrosis in young women; association with slimming regimen including Chinese herbs, *Lancet* 341:387-391, 1993.
30. Nortier JL, Muniz Martinez M-C, Schmeiser HH: Urothelial carcinoma associated with the use of a Chinese herb (*Aristolochia fangchi*), *N Engl J Med* 342:1686-1692, 2000.
31. Lord G, Tagore R, Cook T, et al: Nephropathy caused by Chinese herbs in the UK, *Lancet* 354:481-482, 1999.
32. Pena JM, Borras M, Ramos J, et al: Rapidly progressive interstitial renal fibrosis due to a chronic intake of a herb (*Aristolochia pistolochia*) infusion, *Nephrol Dial Transplant* 11:1359-1360, 1996.
33. Tanaka, A, Shinkai, S, Kasuno K, et al: Chinese herbs nephropathy in the Kansai area: a warning report, *Jpn J Nephrol* 39:438-440, 1997.
34. Zhang M, Zhang D: Kidney nourishing and blood activating therapy for aristolochic acid nephropathy in 65 cases, *Shanghai J Trad Chin Med* 37:30-32, 2003.
35. Stengel B, Jones E: Insuffisance renale terminale associee a la consommation d'herbs chinoises en France, *Nephrologie* 19:15-20, 1998.
36. Cosyns JP: Aristolochic acid and "Chinese herbs nephropathy," *Drug Saf* 26:33-48, 2003.
37. Reginster F, Jadoul M, van Ypersele de Strihou C: Chinese herbs nephropathy presentation, natural history and fate after transplantation, *Nephrol Dial Transplant* 12:81-86, 1997.
38. Vanherweghem JL, Abramowicz D, Tielemans C, et al: Effects of steroids on the progression of renal failure in

chronic interstitial renal fibrosis: a pilot study in Chinese herbs nephropathy, *Am J Kidney Dis* 27:209-215, 1996.

39. Lord G, Cook T, Arlt VM, Schmeiser H, Williams G, Pusey CD: Urothelial malignant disease and Chinese herbal nephropathy, *Lancet* 358:1515-1516, 2001.

40. Nortier JL, Schmeiser HH, Muniz Martinez M-C, et al: Invasive urothelial carcinoma after exposure to Chinese herbal medicine containing aristolochic acid may occur without severe renal failure, *Nephrol Dial Transplant* 18:426-428, 2003.

41. Arlt VM, Pfohl-Leszkowicz A, Cosyns J, Schmeiser HH: Analysis of DNA adducts formed by ochratoxin A and aristolochic acid in patients with Chinese herbs nephropathy, *Mutat Res* 494:143-150, 2001.

42. Cosyns JP, Jadoul M, Squifflet JP, Wese FX, van Ypersele de Strihou C: Urothelial lesions in Chinese-herb nephropathy, *Am J Kidney Dis* 33:1011-1017, 1999.

43. Martinez MC, Nortier J, Vereerstraeten P, Vanherweghem JL: Progression rate of Chinese herb nephropathy: impact of Aristolochia fangchi ingested dose, *Nephrol Dial Transplant* 17:408-412, 2002.

44. Tanaka A, Nishida R, Maeda K, Sugawara A, Kuwahara T: Chinese herb nephropathy in Japan presents adult onset Fanconi syndrome: could different components of aristolochic acids cause a different type of Chinese herb nephropathy? *Clin Nephrol* 53:301-306, 2000.

45. Tanaka A, Nishida R, Yoshida T, Koshikawa M, Goto M, Kuwahara T: Outbreak of Chinese herb nephropathy in Japan: are there any differences from Belgium? *Intern Med* 40:296-300, 2001.

46. Krumme B, Endmeir R, Vanhaelen M, Walb D: Reversible Fanconi syndrome after ingestion of a Chinese herbal "remedy" containing aristolochic acid, *Nephrol Dial Transplant* 16:400-402, 2001.

47. Zhang M-Z, Zhang D-N: Kidney nourishing and blood activating therapy for aristolochic acid nephropathy in 65 cases, *Shanghai J Trad Chin Med* 37:30-32, 2003.

48. Sanz P, Reig R: Clinical and pathological findings in fatal plant oxalosis. A review, *Am J Forensic Med Pathol* 13:342-345, 1992.

49. Reig R, Sanz P, Blanche C, et al: Fatal poisoning by Rumex crispus (curled dock): pathological findings and application of scanning electron microscopy, *Vet Hum Toxicol* 32:468-470, 1991.

50. De Stefani E, Fierro L, Mendilaharsu M, et al: Meat intake, "mate" drinking and renal cell cancer in Uruguay: a case-control study, *Br J Cancer* 78:1239-1243, 1998.

51. Pharmacopoeia Commission of the PRC: *Pharmacopoeia of the People's Republic of China, English edition*, Beijing, 1992, Guangdong Science and Technology Press.

52. Leung AY, Foster S: *Encyclopedia of common natural ingredients used in food, drugs and cosmetics*, ed 2, New York, 1996, John Wiley & Sons.

53. Tai YT: Adverse effects from traditional Chinese medicine, *Lancet* 341:892, 1993.

54. Kolev ST, Leman P, Kite GC, et al: Toxicity following accidental ingestion of Aconitum containing Chinese remedy, *Hum Exp Toxicol* 15:839-842, 1996.

55. But PP-H, Tai Y-T, Young K: Three fatal cases of herbal aconite poisoning, *Vet Hum Toxicol* 36:212-215, 1994.

56. Tai Y-T, But P, Young K, et al: Cardiotoxicity after accidental herb-induced aconite poisoning, *Lancet* 340:1254-1256, 1992.

57. Chen HC, Hsieh MT, Change SS, et al: Long-term reno-cardiovascular effects of orally administered aconite tuber in humans, *Am J Chin Med* 18:25-33, 1990.

58. Foster S, Chongxi Y: *Herbal emissaries*, Vermont, 1992, Healing Arts Press.

59. Miwa H, Iijima M, Tanaka S, et al: Generalised convulsions after consuming a large amount of ginkgo nuts, *Epilepsia* 42:280-281, 2001.

60. Kajiyama Y, Fujii K, Takeuchi H, et al: Ginkgo seed poisoning, *Pediatrics* 109:325-327, 2002.

61. Chan K, Cheung L: *Interactions between Chinese herbal medicinal products and orthodox drug*, Amserdam, Neth, 2000, Harwood Academic Press.

62. Upton R, editor: *American herbal pharmacopoeia and therapeutic compendium dang gui root; Angelica sinensis (Oliv.) diels*, Santa Cruz, 2003, AHP.

63. Engelsen J, Nielsen JD, Hansen KF: [Effect of coenzyme Q10 and Ginkgo biloba on warfarin dosage in patients on long-term warfarin treatment], *Ugeskr Laeger* 165:1868-1871, 2003.

64. Gilbert GJ: Ginkgo biloba, *Neurology* 48:1137, 1997.

65. Rowin J, Lewis SL: Spontaneous bilateral subdural hematomas with chronic Ginkgo biloba ingestion, *Neurology* 46:1775-1776, 1996.

66. Vale S: Subarachnoid haemorrhage associated with Ginkgo biloba, *Lancet* 352:36, 1998.

67. Rosenblatt M, Mindel J: Spontaneous hyphema associated with ingestion of Ginkgo biloba extract, *N Engl J Med* 336:1108, 1997.

68. Matthews MK: Association of Ginkgo biloba with intracerebral hemorrhage, *Neurology* 50:1934, 1998.

69. Mills S, Bone K: *Principles and practice of phytotherapy: modern herbal medicine*, Edinburgh, 2000, Churchill Livingstone.

70. Medicines Control Agency: Psoralea corylifolia fruit in traditional Chinese medicines causing severe skin reaction, *Curr Prob Pharmacovigilance* 27:12-13, 2001.

71. Boffa MJ, Gilmour E, Ead RD: Celery soup causing severe phototoxicity during PUVA therapy, *Br J Dermatol* 135:334, 1996.

72. Brockmoller J, Reum T, Bauer S, et al: Hypericin and pseudohypericin; pharmacokinetics and effects on photosensitivity in humans, *Pharmapsychiatry* 30(suppl 2):94-101, 1997.

73. British Herbal Medicine's Association Scientific Committee: *British herbal pharmacopoeia*, Cowling, 1983, BHMA.

74. Segelman AB, Segelman FP, Karliner, J Sofia RD: Sassafras and herb tea: potential health hazards, *JAMA* 236:477, 1976.

75. Opdyke DLJ: Safrole, *Food Cosmet Toxicol* 12:983-986, 1974.

76. McPherson FJ, Bridges JW, Parke DV: The effects of benzopyrene and safrole on biphenyl 2-hydroxylase and

other drug metabolizing enzymes, *Biochem J* 154:773-780, 1976.

77. Duke JA: *Handbook of medicinal herbs*, Boca Raton: 1985, CRC.

78. Luo G, Guenthner TM: Metabolism of allylbensene 2′,3′-oxide and estragole 2′,3′-oxide in the isolated perfused rat liver, *J Pharmacol Exp Ther* 272:588-596, 1995.

79. Miller JA, Miller EC: The metabolic activation and nucleic acid adducts of naturally-occurring carcinogens: recent results with ethyl carbamate and the spice flavors safrole and estragole, *Br J Cancer* 48:1-15, 1983.

80. Bruneton J: *Pharmacognosy, phytochemistry, medicinal plants*, Andover, UK, 1995, Intercept Ltd.

81. McGuffin M, Hobbs C, Upton R, Goldberg A, editors: *Botanical safety handbook*, Boca Raton, 1997, CRC Press.

82. Wichtl M, Bisset N, editors: *Herbal drugs and phytopharmaceuticals*, Stuttgart, 1994, Medpharm GmbH Scientific Publishers.

83. Opdyke DJL: Calamus oil, *Food Cosmet Toxicol* 15:623-626, 1977.

84. Corrigan D: Juniperus species. In De Smet et al, editors: *Adverse effects of herbal drugs*, vol 2, Berlin, 1993, Springer-Verlag.

85. Tisserand R, Balacs T: *Essential oil safety*, Edinburgh, 1995, Churchill Livingstone.

86. Heil BM, Schilcher H: Juniper berries oil: the fate of a traditional diuretic, 24th International Symposium on Essential Oils, Technische Universitat, Berlin, July 21-24, 1993, Poster 38.

87. Lewis WH, Smith PR: Pokeroot herbal tea poisoning, *JAMA* 242:2759-2760, 1979.

88. Roberge R, Brader E, Martin ML, et al: The root of evil—pokeweed intoxication, *Ann Emerg Med* 15:470-473, 1986.

89. Barker BE, Farnes P, LaMarche PH: Peripheral blood plasmacytosis following systemic exposure to *Phytolacca americana* (Pokeweed), *Paediatrics* 38:490-493, 1966.

90. Barker BE, Farnes P, LaMarche PH: Haematological effects of pokeweed, *Lancet* i:437, 1967.

91. Lewis WH, Smith PR: Pokeroot herbal tea poisoning, *JAMA* 242:2759-2760, 1979.

92. Coeugniet EG, Elek E: Immunomodulation with Viscum album and Echinacea purpurea extracts, *Onkologie* 10(supp 3):27-33, 1987.

93. Evans MR, Preece AW: *Viscum album*—a possible treatment for cancer? *Bristol Med Chir J* 88:17-20, 1973.

94. Anderson LA, Phillipson JD: Mistletoe—the magic herb, *Pharm J* 229:437-439, 1982.

95. Hall AH, Spoerke DG, Rumack BH: Assessing mistletoe toxicity, *Ann Emerg Med* 15:1320-1323, 1986.

96. Bruneton J: *Toxic plants. Dangerous to humans and animals*, Andover, UK, 1999, Intercept Ltd.

97. Hsu H-Y: *Oriental materia medica*, Long Beach, Cal, 1986, Oriental Healing Arts Institute.

98. Upton R, editor: *American herbal pharmacopoeia and therapeutic compendium: willow bark salix spp. Analytical, quality control and therapeutic monographs*, Santa Cruz, 1999, AHP.

99. Scientific Committee of ESCOP (European Scientific Cooperative on Phytotherapy): ESCOP monographs: Salicis cortex. European Scientific Cooperative on Phytotherapy, ESCOP Secretariat, UK, July 1997.

100. Chandler RF, Anderson LA, Phillipson JDl: Laetrile in perspective, *Can Pharm J* 117:517-520, 1984.

101. Chandler RF, Anderson LA, Phillipson JD: Controversial laetrile, *Pharm J* 232:330-332, 1984.

102. De Smet PAGM, editor: *Adverse effects of herbal drugs 2*, New York, 1993, Springer-Verlag.

103. Shekelle PG, Hardy ML, Morton SC, et al: Efficacy and safety of ephedra and ephedrine for weight loss and athletic performance—a meta analysis, *JAMA* 280:1537-1545, 2003.

104. Anderson IB, Mullen WH, Meeker JE, et al: Pennyroyal toxicity: measurement of toxic metabolites in two cases and review of the literature, *Ann Intern Med* 124:726-734, 1996.

105. Bakerink JA, Gosper SM, Dimand RJ, Eldridge MW: Multiple organ failure after ingestion of pennyroyal oil from tea in two infants, *Pediatrics* 98:944-947, 1996.

106. Barnes J, Mills SY, Abbott NC, Willoughby M, Ernst E: Different standards for reporting ADRs to herbal remedies and conventional OTC medicines face to face interviews with 515 users of herbal remedies, *Br J Clin Pharmacol* 45:496-500, 1998.

107. Palmer ME, Haller C, McKinney PE, et al: Adverse events associated with dietary supplements, *Lancet* 361:101-106, 2003.

108. Shaw D, Leon C, Kolev S, Murray V: Traditional remedies and food supplements; a five year toxicological study (1991-1995), *Drug Saf* 17:342-356, 1997.

3

THE ADVERSE PLACEBO EFFECT AND TRANSIENT TREATMENT REACTIONS

Simon Mills

There are important confounding factors in the assessment of herbal safety or that of any other medication. A proportion of the adverse effects reported to physicians or other health practitioners for a medicine are likely not to be caused by any innate property of that agent. There are two main types of adverse reaction that may owe more to the characteristics of the person at the time of consumption than to the properties of the medicine itself. These are the nocebo effect and transient adverse therapeutic reactions.

THE NOCEBO EFFECT

During recent years the full impact of the positive effect of placebo, the nontreatment control in many clinical studies, has become apparent. It was part of medical folklore that approximately 30% of patients would get better through suggestion alone or in response to a dummy treatment.[1] In fact the evidence is more intriguing. Placebo benefits can occur in any proportion of a treatment group, from almost none to almost all in any test group,

depending on the condition and circumstances.[2,3] Contrary to earlier medical prejudices, it is difficult to characterise "placebo reactors" as such,[4] although some unexpected trends may be detected. For example, in controlled trials for the treatment of depression, men were more responsive than women to placebo (29.8% vs. 24.3%); married patients were more responsive (38.15%) than widowed/separated/divorced (21.9%) or single (16.7%) patients; and patients aged more than 60 years were more susceptible than younger patients. Educational level achieved and duration of illness were not predictive. Severity of illness proved most noteworthy, with the placebo response rate higher in more mildly affected patients (40.8% vs. 23.4%).[5] However, placebo responses are particularly strong also in surgery,[6] and contrary to many assumptions, they also can occur in animals.[7] In preventing coughing the placebo response may be approximately 85%.[8] In the case of duodenal ulcers, placebo benefit was linked to frequency of dosing.[9] Placebos have time-effect curves and peak, cumulative, and carryover effects similar to those of active medications.[3] It is usually assumed that placebo responses are somehow imaginary or at least transient. However, this is not borne out by the evidence,[10,11] and placebos can lead to long-term benefits, including in such conditions as benign prostatic hyperplasia,[12] parkinsonism,[13] multiple sclerosis,[14] ulcerative colitis,[15] duodenal ulceration,[9] and schizophrenia.[16] Investigations into the mechanisms of placebo response have involved powerful neural signalling mechanisms, such as endorphin, norepinephrine, and nitric oxide,[17] and in the case of analgesic effects, inhibition of cholecystokinin.[18]

With such apparent potency it is not surprising that placebos can also generate significant levels of adverse effects. This is referred to as the nocebo phenomenon. In one review of trials involving 1228 healthy volunteers, adverse placebo responses were reported at 19% (increasing to 28% on repeated dosing of placebo).[19] Overall the most frequent adverse events reported were headache (7%), drowsiness (5%), and asthenia (4%).

In many ways placebos resemble the drugs with which they are being compared. In a review of a range of randomised, placebo-controlled, multicentre studies of five different medications in the areas of cardiology, neurology/psychiatry, metabolism, and gastroenterology, it was shown that the placebo side effect profile was largely similar to the side effect profile of the active treatment.[20] A number of interactions between placebos and medications have also been reported; in the case of placebos these tend to resemble the effects of drugs that they are matching.[21] Other research demonstrates that the placebo response is bidirectional (i.e., analgesic and algesic).[18]

The nocebo effect may intrude on some of the most critical measures of side effects of drugs or herbs. One of the standard tests applied to monitor these are liver function tests (see also Chapter 12); therefore, it is sobering to note that at least one, alanine transaminase (ALT), is subject to adverse placebo effects. In a review of 13 phase I trials of new drugs (i.e., on healthy volunteers) it was found that more than 1 in 5 of the 93 subjects on placebo showed at least one ALT value above the upper limit of the normal range

when taking placebo, and 7.5% had at least one value twice this limit.[22]

Implications of Nocebo

The impact of the placebo effect on the assessment of efficacy in any treatment is dramatic and has been discussed by this author elsewhere.[23] There are pointers in the literature of placebo and spontaneous remission to the potency of self-healing functions within the living body, functions which it appears need little extra stimulation to be mobilised, perhaps most effectively associated with the event having more meaning to the patient.[24-27] Interpretation of the nocebo effect in this light raises interesting theoretical questions. If the placebo effect is the nudging of self-healing (i.e., a small impact riding a larger wave), what is the tide that nocebo rides?

One important study suggests that the nocebo effect reflects the power of adverse suggestibility. Several factors were found to be associated with the reporting of nonspecific side effects while taking active medication:

1) the patient's expectations of adverse effects at the outset of treatment;

2) a process of conditioning in which the patient learns from previous experiences to associate medication taking with somatic symptoms;

3) certain psychological characteristics, such as anxiety, depression, and the tendency to somatise; and

4) situational and contextual factors.[28]

The implication of these findings is that there are patients and situations in which nocebo effects are most likely to be reported and that many could be reduced by having a quiet reassuring word with patients. Whether this would actually reduce the incidence of the adverse effects or simply make the patient more likely to tolerate them and less likely to report them is arguable, especially given the wider placebo literature that strongly suggests that placebo responders are not predictable. However, avoiding the nocebo effect of negative or thoughtless statements to a patient is a skill that some physicians apparently lack. Too much honesty can sometimes impair a patient's hope and morale, and it often profits the clinical encounter to combine medical conviction with an appreciation of the patient's belief system and aspirations.[29]

It is becoming clearer that the nonspecific effects in treatment can affect conclusions drawn about efficacy and safety of any agent. In any review of the safety of herbal medicine the potential of nonspecific side effects should be identified. However, as another review has suggested, the risk-benefit of placebo in clinical trials may overall be positive![30]

TRANSIENT THERAPEUTIC ADVERSE EFFECTS OF HERBAL TREATMENT

The extent of nonspecific adverse reactions to treatment may contribute in part to a common experience in the consulting room. Minor adverse events to herbal treatment are probably common, especially at the beginning of a course of treatment.

In earlier times herbal treatments were often robust and even unpleasant. A consistent feature of traditional therapeutics was the importance of inducing vomiting and catharsis as a first step for the management of acute infective or inflammatory conditions (one underlying rationale might have been the quick removal from the body of bile, a potentially useful measure). In other cases the need was to reduce worm infestations or manage other severe acute conditions with robust measures. Such treatments were understood to be debilitating and were best recommended only for patients with the most robust constitutions. In modern times they have almost completely been replaced by new synthetic prescription medicines, and herbal practice has taken on a more gentle and supportive role.

Therefore, the majority of adverse events in a modern herbal treatment are transient and minor. Practitioners may have reports from patients that include the following:
- Diuresis
- Exacerbation of skin inflammations
- Changes in bowel performance (e.g., constipation, diarrhoea, or irregularity)
- Change in patterns of presenting headaches, including exacerbation
- Increased (productive) coughing in bronchopulmonary conditions
- Heartburn or dyspeptic symptoms
- Exacerbation of menstrual symptoms
- Fatigue

Many of these events are likely to be innate to the disease processes. Even positive changes to a diseased steady state may lead to discomfitures. Homoeopaths have long recognised the phenomena as a prelude to repair in their term the "healing crisis." Exacerbations are also noted in the naturopathic experience: overenthusiastic fasts have long been associated with skin eruptions. In neither situation can there be a conventional adverse drug reaction.

Neither can the nocebo effect account for all such cases. An adverse development can be a feature of the course of the illness or a change in the sick state. Some conditions are notable for their predisposition to exacerbation. Managing an inflammatory skin disease without flare-up can be a challenge. Readjusting disturbed menstrual functions usually involves unfamiliar transitionary patterns that may be uncomfortable. Managing a migrainous constitution requires nimble therapeutic footwork to avoid occasional severe exacerbations. An inflamed or sensitive stomach can be difficult to settle smoothly with oral herbal preparations.

On the Hippocratic principle *primum non nocere*—first do no harm—good practitioners have sought to avoid healing crises and longer-term exacerbations. Nevertheless passing discomforts can happen. Technically they are adverse reactions and in some cases could even be reported as such. If they do turn out to be inevitable it is the role of the practitioner to make sure that they quickly lead to improvements.

REFERENCES

1. de Craen AJ, Kaptchuk TJ, Tijssen JG, Kleijnen J: Placebos and placebo effects in medicine: historical overview, *J R Soc Med* 92:511-515, 1999.
2. McQuay H, Carroll D, Moore A: Variation in the placebo effect in randomised controlled trials of analgesics: all is as blind as it seems, *Pain* 64:331-335, 1996.
3. Turner JA, Deyo RA, Loeser JD, Von Korff M, Fordyce WE: The importance of placebo effects in pain treatment and research, *JAMA* 271:1609-1614, 1994.
4. Kamien JB, Bickel WK, Oliveto AH, et al: Placebo-effects contribute to differences in the acquisition of drug discrimination by humans: a retrospective analysis, *Behav Pharmacol* 6:187-194, 1995.

5. Wilcox CS, Cohn JB, Linden RD, et al: Predictors of placebo response: a retrospective analysis, *Psychopharmacol Bull* 28:157-162, 1992.

6. Freeman TB, Vawter DE, Leaverton PE, et al: Use of placebo surgery in controlled trials of a cellular-based therapy for Parkinson's disease, *N Engl J Med* 341:988-992, 1999.

7. McMillan FD: The placebo effect in animals, *J Am Vet Med Assoc* 215:992-999, 1999.

8. Eccles R: The powerful placebo in cough studies? *Pulm Pharmacol Ther* 15:303-308, 2002.

9. de Craen AJ, Moerman DE, Heisterkamp SH, et al: Placebo effect in the treatment of duodenal ulcer, *Br J Clin Pharmacol* 48:853-860, 1999.

10. Fine PG, Roberts WJ, Gillette RG, Child TR: Slowly developing placebo responses confound tests of intravenous phentolamine to determine mechanisms underlying idiopathic chronic low back pain, *Pain* 56:235-242, 1994.

11. Spiller RC: Problems and challenges in the design of irritable bowel syndrome clinical trials: experience from published trials, *Am J Med* 107:91-97, 1999.

12. Hansen BJ, Meyhoff HH, Nordling J, Mensink HJA, Mogensen P, Larsen EH: Placebo effects in the pharmacological treatment of uncomplicated benign prostatic hyperplasia, *Scand J Urol Nephrol* 30:373-377, 1996.

13. Shetty N, Friedman JH, Kieburtz K, et al: The placebo response in Parkinson's disease. Parkinson study group. *Clin Neuropharmacol* 22:207-212, 1999.

14. La Mantia L, Eoli M, Salmaggi A, Milanese C: Does a placebo-effect exist in clinical trials on multiple sclerosis? Review of the literature, *Ital J Neurol Sci* 17:135-139, 1996.

15. Ilnyckyj A, Shanahan F, Anton PA, Cheang M, Bernstein CN: Quantification of the placebo response in ulcerative colitis, *Gastroenterology* 112:1854-1858, 1997.

16. Lewander T: Placebo response in schizophrenia, *Eur Psychiatry* 9:119-120, 1994.

17. Stefano GB, Fricchione GL, Slingsby BT, Benson H: The placebo effect and relaxation response: neural processes and their coupling to constitutive nitric oxide, *Brain Res Brain Res Rev* 35:1-19, 2001.

18. Benedetti F, Amanzio M: The neurobiology of placebo analgesia: from endogenous opioids to cholecystokinin, *Prog Neurobiol* 52:109-125, 1997.

19. Rosenzweig P, Brohier S, Zipfel A: The placebo effect in healthy volunteers: influence of experimental conditions on the adverse events profile during phase I studies, *Clin Pharmacol Ther* 54:578-583, 1993.

20. Weihrauch TR, Gauler TC: Placebo-efficacy and adverse effects in controlled clinical trials, *Arzneimittelforschung* 49:385-393, 1999.

21. Kleijnen J, De Craen AJM, Van Everdingen J, Krol L: Placebo effect in double-blind clinical trials: a review of interactions with medications, *Lancet* 344:1347-1349, 1994.

22. Rosenzweig P, Miget N, Brohier S: Transaminase elevation on placebo during phase I trials: prevalence and significance, *Br J Clin Pharmacol* 48:19-23, 1999.

23. Mills S, Bone K: *Principles and practice of phytotherapy: modern herbal medicine*, London, 2000, Churchill Livingstone.

24. Moerman DE, Jonas WB: Deconstructing the placebo effect and finding the meaning response, *Ann Intern Med* 136:471-476, 2002.

25. Kaptchuk TJ: The placebo effect in alternative medicine: can the performance of a healing ritual have clinical significance? *Ann Intern Med* 136:817-825, 2002.

26. Slingsby B: The prozac boom and its placebogenic counterpart—a culturally fashioned phenomenon, *Med Sci Monit* 8:389-393, 2002.

27. Thompson WG: Placebos: a review of the placebo response, *Am J Gastroenterol* 95:1637-1643, 2000.

28. Barsky AJ, Saintfort R, Rogers MP, Borus JF: Nonspecific medication side effects and the nocebo phenomenon, *JAMA* 287:622-627, 2002.

29. Spiegel H: Nocebo: the power of suggestibility, *Prev Med* 26:616-621, 1997.

30. Ernst E: Towards a risk-benefit evaluation of placebos, *Wien Med Wochenschr* 148:461-463, 1998.

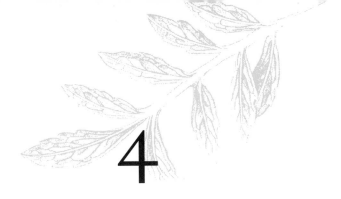

4

Idiosyncratic Drug Reactions

Simon Mills

INTRODUCTION

It has been a general assumption among practitioners and adherents of herbal medicine that their remedies are essentially safer than conventional synthetic drugs. Until relatively recently toxicologic issues were seen not to apply much to everyday herbal practice. As will be seen elsewhere in this text much of this assumption is borne out. Most of the herbs used in herbal practice do have a safer profile than even the mildest synthetic drug. However, there is new awareness that complacency is unwise. There are infrequent but occasionally severe harmful reactions to herbal medicines, and literal toxicity is probably not the main issue in most of these cases. As will be seen in the discussion on kava (see Chapter 12), a herb that is probably not inherently toxic has been effectively removed from therapeutic use across the world because modern surveillance procedures have detected rare but serious consequences of its consumption.

Not all harm caused by conventional drugs is because of their inherent toxicity. Up to 5% of all hospital admissions are the result of adverse drug reactions (ADRs).[1] It has been estimated that approximately 25% of these ADRs do not result from purely pharmacologic mechanisms.[2] There are four types of adverse effects

sometimes used in the toxicologic literature: type A, type B, type C, and type D.

Type A effects are those effects that are related to the pharmacologic effects of the drug and are dosage related. Type B effects are those effects that are often allergic or idiosyncratic reactions, characteristically occurring in only a minority of patients and usually unrelated to dosage, and that are serious, unexpected, and unpredictable. Type C effects are those effects related to problems associated with long-term use of a drug. Type D effects are delayed effects, such as carcinogenicity or teratogenicity (see also Chapter 2).

It is important to note that any of these reactions may be rare enough to be easily missed. Current practice by the Food and Drug Administration in the United States is to approve a drug for general release after an average of 1500 human exposures. However, many drugs have toxic effects in 1 in 10,000 individuals or fewer. A statistical "law of three" suggests that to have a 95% chance of seeing one adverse reaction one would need to see three times as many encounters as indicated by its probability of causing harm (i.e., 30,000 patients under the same treatment in the above case)! Therefore, the only likelihood that any pattern of adverse effects will be seen is when a large community of prescribers and patients are involved in coordinated data recording. This is even more likely to be the case with idiosyncratic reactions.

TYPES OF UNPREDICTABLE (TYPE B) ADVERSE REACTION

Subcategories of individual adverse reactions have sometimes also been identified.

Intolerance

Intolerance is the least severe level of unpredictable adverse reaction and is an exaggeration of pharmacologic or toxic effects of the drug among vulnerable subsets of patients.

Allergic/hypersensitivity Reactions

Allergic and hypersensitivity reactions are mediated by a number of mechanisms, including the development of drug-specific immunoglobulin (Ig) E antibodies, serum sickness–like reactions in response to drug-antibody complexes, direct release of inflammatory mediators, or involvement of the immune system by other mechanisms.[3] The term can be confusing. For example the term "allergic" is sometimes used to describe idiosyncratic reactions that are immune related, especially when toxicity appears after several asymptomatic administrations of the compound (sensitisation period; see Chapter 10 for more discussion of this phenomenon).

Idiosyncratic Drug Reactions

Idiosyncratic drug reactions (IDRs) include anaphylaxis, blood dyscrasias, hepatotoxicity, and severe cutaneous reactions. Severe reactions are often characterised by fever, joint pain, and internal organ involvement and can be marked by eosinophilia (increased levels of eosinophil cells in the blood). It is currently believed that the majority of these reactions are immune mediated and are caused by antigenic conjugates formed from the combination of a reactive metabolite of a drug with cellular proteins.[4,5] In particular, drug-induced lupus is an autoimmune syndrome.

The prediction of IDRs has been made difficult because there are no suitable experimental models to determine this type of drug behaviour. Even epidemiologic evidence is unreliable because of the lack of consensus regarding definition of these syndromes.[6] However, with the following new insights into the mechanisms it may become possible to identify patterns and susceptibilities.

It appears that the initiation of an idiosyncratic reaction involves two steps:

1) Drug activation to reactive metabolites; and

2) Adduct formation and immune stimulation.

Drug Activation

It is likely that most idiosyncratic reactions are not caused by the drug itself but by a reactive metabolite. In the majority of cases, members of the cytochrome P450 family of enzymes form reactive intermediates (see Chapter 5). These products are usually formed at low quantities. However, genetic disposition (e.g., enhanced expression of the catalysing enzyme or deficiency of protective factors such as glutathione) or certain external conditions (e.g., co-medication with inducers of cytochrome P450 metabolism) may lead to toxic intermediates being available at dangerous quantities.

The incidence and nature of adverse reactions associated with a given drug are probably determined in large part by the location of metabolite formation. Most reactive metabolites have a short biological half-life, and although small amounts may escape the organ where they are formed, these metabolites are unlikely to reach sufficient concentrations to cause toxicity in other organs. Also in view of the reactive nature of the metabolites involved, in most cases it is likely that the metabolite is formed in the organ where toxicity occurs. The liver is the major site of drug metabolism, and it is a common target for idiosyncratic drug reactions. The consequences are elaborated below.

Of the extrahepatic sources of reactive drug metabolites, neutrophils and leucocytes have received the most attention because of their vast numbers and robust oxidising machinery.[7] In this case the enzyme system most likely responsible for the formation of reactive metabolites is the NADPH oxidase/myeloperoxidase system. Many drugs associated with autoimmunity are susceptible to oxidative transformation by myeloperoxidase. The oxidised drug metabolites may have increased immunologic effects leading to blood dyscrasias, agranulocytosis, aplastic anaemia, and the generalised inflammatory disturbances seen in rheumatic or lupus reactions.[8]

In other tissues low in cytochrome P450 activity, prostaglandin H synthase may also be responsible for bioactivation (e.g., in the kidney paracetamol [acetaminophen] toxicity is thought to result from activation via this enzyme). The phase II or conjugation enzymes may also be important in the ultimate bioactivation of some drug molecules.[9]

Certain functional groups, which are readily oxidised to reactive metabolites by in vitro cultures, are associated with a high incidence of adverse reactions.[7] Risks are particularly high if biotransformation yields products with chemical substructures such as quinones, phenols, acyl halides, and aromatic and hydroxyl amines.[10]

Some reactive metabolites, such as acyl glucuronides (notably produced by nonsteroidal antiinflammatory drugs [NSAIDs][11]), circulate freely, possibly binding ("forming adducts") with plasma proteins and hepatocellular proteins, thus leading to adverse reactions in almost any organ.

Adduct Formation and Immune Stimulation

It is likely that the first step in the mechanism of drug-induced autoimmunity is that the reactive metabolite (occasionally the drug itself) must irreversibly bind to some structure—it forms covalent "adducts" with one or other protein molecule. This new complex then assumes different antigenic properties that can initiate an immunologic response.

Once an antibody reaction has occurred to a new metabolite-protein complex, the reactive metabolite itself may then also become a *hapten*, a compound not intrinsically antigenic that can hereafter elicit an effective immune response even when combined with another protein. This means that antibodies or T lymphocytes are formed that are able to recognise drug-derived haptens and that are responsible for the clinical manifestations of the reaction.[12] Penicillin is well known as liable to form haptens, and there is increasing evidence for the role of T lymphocytes in severe skin reactions to drugs.[13] Rechallenge means increased new hapten levels, which in this case are sufficient to induce T-lymphocyte cytolysis.[14] A feature of hapten formation is that it cannot be mimicked or predicted in in vitro studies.

However, in many other cases, the mechanism appears to be more complex. In some cases, true *autoantibodies* are produced that do not require the presence of the drug, and furthermore, the antibodies produced often are the same as those induced by other stimuli, such as viruses. This suggests either molecular mimicry or a common alteration in the processing and presentation of antigens.[15]

GENERAL CLINICAL FEATURES

Allowing for the wide variety of pathophysiologic pathways the clinical features of IDRs are:

1) low frequency;
2) independence of dose;
3) typical immune system manifestations such as fever and eosinophilia;
4) delay between the initiation of treatment and onset of the reaction;
5) a shortened delay on rechallenge; and
6) occasional presence of autoantibodies in the serum of patients.[14]

IDIOSYNCRATIC REACTIONS INVOLVING THE LIVER

The adverse reactions associated with kava mainly involved liver damage, and as already seen the liver remains the most vulnerable locus for these events despite several protective mechanisms in liver cells (e.g., epoxide hydrolases and conjugation with glutathione). Everything known about the kava reactions suggests that they are idiosyncratic, but being definitive about any form of liver damage is notoriously difficult. Idiosyncratic hepatic reactions may mimic almost any kind of liver disease or toxic reaction. In many cases the main clinical problem is to distinguish drug-induced hepatic disease from that caused by viral hepatitis; in others the lesion produced is a more chronic one and may resemble chronic aggressive hepatitis or cirrhosis.

Hepatic idiosyncratic reactions fall within these two categories: those that are the consequence of an unusual metabolism of the drug (metabolic idiosyncrasy), and those resulting from an immune-mediated cell injury to hepatocytes that have been in contact with the drug previously (allergic hepatitis).[12,14]

Suspicion of immunologically based drug sensitivity most frequently occurs after manifestations of hypersensitivity, such as fever, skin rashes, arthritis, and eosinophilia, or from liver biopsy. However, the symptoms may be confined to and confused with those of hepatitis. Skin testing with the drug is usually negative, as are tests for a specific antibody to the drug or in vitro evidence of delayed hypersensitivity, such as lymphocyte transformation. It is likely that many drugs involved in hypersensitivity reactions are haptens, and this makes in vitro testing difficult.

The differences between toxic and idiosyncratic hepatic injury are summarised in Table 4-1.

EXAMPLES OF DRUGS INITIATING IDRS

Antiepileptic drugs are among the most likely to cause IDRs, and much of the general research into the mechanisms involved has been in connection with this group of drugs.

Antidepressant drugs are associated with a range of idiosyncratic reactions affecting particularly the liver, skin, and the haematologic and central nervous systems. These reactions seem to be mediated by chemically reactive metabolites formed by the cytochrome P450 enzyme system, the toxicity occurring either directly or indirectly via an immune mechanism.[16]

Urticaria and angioedema may be elicited by a considerable number of drugs, particularly *NSAIDs, angiotensin-converting enzyme (ACE) inhibitors*, radiocontrast media, and *antibiotics*. Pathogenic mechanisms involved include pseudoallergy, idiosyncrasy, IgE-mediated hypersensitivity, and IgG-mediated immunologic mechanisms.[17]

The hepatic reactions associated with *herbal remedies* have not always been well characterized. In the case of kava the damage has included hepatocellular necrosis with cholestasis (see Chapter 2). A genetic deficiency in the cytochrome P450 CYP2D6 was identified in at least one case (see Chapter 5).

Germander was associated with its adverse reactions with fulminant hepatitis. The metabolic activation by cytochrome P450 of its diterpenoids into hepatotoxic epoxides is believed to cause toxicity (see Chapter 2).[18]

Pyrrolizidine alkaloids are genuinely hepatotoxic and lead to venoocclusive disease, which results in ischaemic damage and centrilobular necrosis.

RISK FACTORS

Among the known risk factors for idiosyncratic reactions are increasing age, polypharmacy, and liver and renal disease. Female patients have a

Table **4-1**   **Comparison of Toxic and Idiosyncratic Causes of Liver Damage**

	Hepatotoxins	IDRs
Mechanisms	Direct cytoplasmic poisons	Sensitisation
Pathology	Zonal necrosis, fatty infiltration, venoocclusive disease	Cholestasis, hepatitis-like granulomata
Susceptibility	All individuals	<1%
Animal models	Yes	No
Dose relationship	Direct	None
Latent period	1-2 days	Variable
Associated features	Renal failure	Fever, rash, arthralgia, eosinophilia

1.5- to 1.7-fold greater risk of developing an IDR, including adverse skin reactions, compared with male patients. Women generally have a lower lean body mass, a reduced hepatic clearance, and differences in activity of cytochrome P450 enzymes (40% increase in CYP3A4 and varied decrease in CYP2D6, CYP2C19, and CYP1A2) and metabolise drugs at different rates compared with men.[1]

In children cytochrome P450-catalysed metabolism is increased.[19] Other age-related changes are the consequence of a number of individual factors (e.g., morbidity associated with polypharmacy, decrease in renal or liver function in the elderly population, hypoalbuminaemia, and reduced body weight).[2]

Susceptibility to liver reactions may be caused by either *genetic factors* (e.g., changed levels of cytochrome P450 isoenzymes or defects in protective mechanisms, such as epoxide hydrolase, glutathione metabolism, and acetylation) or *acquired factors* (e.g., malnutrition or chronic intake of alcohol or other microsomal enzyme inducers).

RISK ASSESSMENT

Most drugs can probably form reactive metabolites, but a simple comparison of covalent binding in vitro is unlikely to provide an accurate indication of the relative risk of a drug causing an idiosyncratic reaction because it does not provide an indication of how efficiently the metabolite is detoxified in vivo. Laboratory tests are also unable to predict hapten formation. There are also few adequate animal models and few ways to replicate the mechanisms in any model.

In the absence of a better understanding of the mechanisms of idiosyncratic reactions, there are a few screening procedures that could reduce the probability that a drug will be associated with IDRs. One method may be to screen subjects for the formation of reactive metabolites and halt use or development of drugs that form significant amounts of such metabolites. However, such metabolites are not easy to screen for. Another variable risk factor would be the ability of the reactive metabolite to cause cell damage.

In the case of IDRs to antiepileptic drugs, four inexpensive, simple methods of identifying high-risk patients have been proposed.

Patients liable to IDRs from valproic acid compared with age-matched control subjects have
• Deficient erythrocyte glutathione peroxidase activity
• Low plasma selenium concentrations
• Low calculated oxidative protection ratios
Patients with felbamate-associated aplastic anaemia also have
• Deficient erythrocyte glutathione peroxidase
• Low erythrocyte superoxide dismutase (SOD)
• Low glutathione reductase activities[20]
A possible "at-risk" clinical profile for antiepileptic drugs has been proposed:
• Identification of biomarkers that measure the formation of a toxic metabolite
• Identification of biomarkers indicating deficient detoxification abilities
• Identification of at-risk genetic markers[20]
There is evidence to suggest that an IDR is more likely if there is some "danger signal." Thus drugs that cause some degree of cell stress or damage may be more likely to lead to a high incidence of IDRs.[21] However, the exact nature of the putative danger signals is unknown. It should be possible to develop in vitro systems to assess the potential of drugs to bind to critical proteins either directly or indirectly after metabolic activation to protein-reactive metabolites (bioactivation).[22]

Paradoxically more potent drugs may decrease the incidence of IDRs: it appears that drugs given at a dose of 10 mg/day or less are associated with a low incidence of IDRs, although there are some notable exceptions.[23] This suggests a possible benefit in using herbal remedies with multiple constituents—the individual concentrations of active constituents in a dose will usually be far less.

CONCLUSIONS AND RECOMMENDATIONS

The herbal sector is advised to become more proactive in understanding and anticipating idiosyncratic reactions. The unfortunate case of kava has provided the necessary alert. Improved pharmacovigilance by regulators across the world (see Chapter 11) will mean that there will be more IDRs identified for herbal remedies. What constructively can be done to minimise these problems in the future?

By definition IDRs are unpredictable, and there is no likelihood that a model will be found to change this. However, more is becoming known about the circumstances in which idiosyncratic reactions are more likely to occur. It is probable that these will be better understood. It is possible that if another kava case were to occur, identifying risk situations could lead to agreement on effective labelled warnings and professional advice rather than blanket banning. However, this will require some coordinated information gathering and political consensus.

Idiosyncratic reactions involve interaction between the substance and the person who takes it. Liability to an unfortunate encounter is likely to involve identifiable characteristics on both sides.

In the case of patients some significant vulnerabilities are already identifiable:

- Polypharmacy particularly involving drugs with enzyme-inducing properties
- Reduced renal or liver function
- Malnutrition
- Chronic intake of alcohol

Investigations may identify general risks:
- Reduced body weight
- Hypoalbuminaemia

With increasing use of more advanced metabolic profiling, more specific enzyme deficiencies may be identified:

- Epoxide hydrolase
- Glutathione peroxidase and reductase
- SOD
- Other antioxidant mechanisms (including low selenium levels)

New mapping technologies may also in the future identify those with particular disturbances in cytochrome P450 or other drug-metabolising activity.

Clearer identification of at-risk individuals may lead to the use of labelled warnings as a future policy in the event of a future kava incident. Such policies are likely to be led by the pharmaceutical sector in the case of notorious generators of IDRs, such as antiepileptic and antidepressant drugs. The herbal sector could usefully monitor and apply developments in these areas.

In the case of the herbal remedy itself it will be possible to screen in vitro for the products of biotransformation. Plant products that showed the ability to yield reactive molecules, such as acyl glucuronides and halides, quinones, or amines, and importantly, produced these at high levels, may sustain closer scrutiny. Conversely, many familiar herbal remedies could be effectively vetted by such screening. The herbal sector could take the initiative in grading remedies by liability to causing idiosyncratic reactions.

REFERENCES

1. Rademaker M: Do women have more adverse drug reactions? *Am J Clin Dermatol* 2:349-351, 2001.
2. Hoigne R, Lawson DH, Weber E: Risk factors for adverse drug reactions—epidemiological approaches, *Eur J Clin Pharmacol* 39:321-325, 1990.
3. Rieder MJ: Mechanisms of unpredictable adverse drug reactions, *Drug Saf* 11:196-212, 1994.
4. Ju C, Uetrecht JP: Mechanism of idiosyncratic drug reactions: reactive metabolite formation, protein binding and the regulation of the immune system, *Curr Drug Metab* 3: 367-377, 2002.
5. Leeder JS: Mechanisms of idiosyncratic hypersensitivity reactions to antiepileptic drugs, *Epilepsia* 39(suppl): S8-16, 1998.
6. Knowles SR, Uetrecht J, Shear NH: Idiosyncratic drug reactions: the reactive metabolite syndromes, *Lancet* 356:1587-1591, 2000.
7. Uetrecht JP: The role of leukocyte-generated reactive metabolites in the pathogenesis of idiosyncratic drug reactions, *Drug Metab Rev* 24:299-366, 1992.
8. Rubin RL, Kretz-Rommel A: Phagocyte-mediated oxidation in idiosyncratic adverse drug reactions, *Curr Opin Hematol* 8:34-40, 2001.
9. Pirmohamed M, Madden S, Park BK: Idiosyncratic drug reactions. Metabolic bioactivation as a pathogenic mechanism, *Clin Pharmacokinet* 31:215-230, 1996.
10. Petersen KU: From toxic precursors to safe drugs. Mechanisms and relevance of idiosyncratic drug reactions, *Arzneimittelforschung* 52:423-429, 2002.
11. Boelsterli UA, Zimmerman HJ, Kretz-Rommel A: Idiosyncratic liver toxicity of nonsteroidal antiinflammatory drugs: molecular mechanisms and pathology, *Crit Rev Toxicol* 25:207-235, 1995.
12. Castell JV: Allergic hepatitis: a drug-mediated organ-specific immune reaction, *Clin Exp Allergy* 28(suppl):13-19, 1998.
13. Park BK, Kitteringham NR, Powell H, Pirmohamed M: Advances in molecular toxicology-towards understanding idiosyncratic drug toxicity, *Toxicology* 153:39-60, 2000.

14. Dansette PM, Bonierbale E, Minoletti C, Beaune PH, Pessayre D, Mansuy D: Drug-induced immunotoxicity, *Eur J Drug Metab Pharmacokinet* 23:443-451, 1998.

15. Uetrecht JP: Current trends in drug-induced autoimmunity, *Toxicology* 119:37-43, 1997.

16. Pirmohamed M, Kitteringham NR, Park BK: Idiosyncratic reactions to antidepressants: a review of the possible mechanisms and predisposing factors, *Pharmacol Ther* 53:105-125, 1992.

17. Bircher AJ: Drug-induced urticaria and angioedema caused by non-IgE mediated pathomechanisms, *Eur J Dermatol* 9:657-663, 1999.

18. Lekehal M, Pessayre D, Lereau JM, Moulis C, Fouraste I, Fau D: Hepatotoxicity of the herbal medicine germander: metabolic activation of its furano diterpenoids by cytochrome P450 3A depletes cytoskeleton-associated protein thiols and forms plasma membrane blebs in rat hepatocytes, *Hepatology* 24:212-218, 1996.

19. Anderson GD: Children versus adults: pharmacokinetic and adverse-effect differences, *Epilepsia* 43:53-59, 2002.

20. Glauser TA: Idiosyncratic reactions: new methods of identifying high-risk patients, *Epilepsia* 41(suppl):S16-29, 2000.

21. Uetrecht JP: Is it possible to more accurately predict which drug candidates will cause idiosyncratic drug reactions? *Curr Drug Metab* 1:133-141, 2000.

22. Park BK, Naisbitt DJ, Gordon SF, Kitteringham NR, Pirmohamed M: Metabolic activation in drug allergies, *Toxicology* 158:11-23, 2001.

23. Uetrecht J: Prediction of a new drug's potential to cause idiosyncratic reactions, *Curr Opin Drug Discov Devel* 4:55-59, 2001.

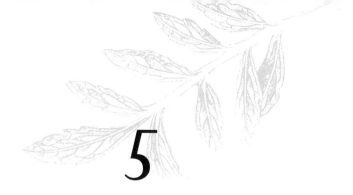

5

HUMAN-PLANT INTERACTIONS

Simon Mills

A view of many of those who use or prescribe herbal remedies is that the natural environment is essentially benign and that human industrial and technologic activity has provided a new hazard to healthy living: natural things are essentially safe, and synthetic chemicals and drugs are toxic by default. Like all worldviews it is not entirely without foundation—the safety risk of herbal remedies is generally lower than most modern drugs. However, any rigorous assessment of natural ecologies shows that the romantic assumption is fundamentally flawed.

Close scrutiny of the physiology of living organisms confirms that there is a balance in their relationships with other organisms in their ecosystems from accommodation and symbiosis on one hand to vigorous defensiveness on the other. The obvious fact is that not all in the garden is lovely, that by definition organisms differ in their metabolic requirements, that each secretion and excretion changes the environment, and that there may be many territorial or predator-prey competitions to justify more aggressive chemical postures. In each organism's environment much, if not most, of the material encountered may be potentially harmful.

In his seminal textbook, *Introduction to Ecological Biochemistry*, Harborne[1] demonstrates that the evolution of species, particularly of plant species, is accompanied by the production of a wealth of secondary metabolites, some involved in regulatory functions and others involved in defence activities, that may not be welcome additions to the diet of animals feeding on them. These chemicals do not fit smoothly in the primary metabolising processes in the animal body. Whereas undergraduate medical biochemistry concentrates largely on the human body's mechanisms for metabolising primary nutrients, like carbohydrates, proteins, fats, and vitamins, there is little attention to the mechanisms required for dealing with the infinite variety of these secondary materials.

It is only recently that the subtlety and power of the mechanisms in the body for dealing with secondary material in the environment have been appreciated. The term "xenobiotic" has been coined as an appropriate descriptive for the often challenging substances encountered by the body, and the risks involved in addressing them are now better understood. Most importantly in medicine has been the realisation that in addition to obvious challenges to the body's metabolic machinery posed by synthetic drugs and chemical adulterants of the environment, many constituents of natural products, food, and herbal medicines are xenobiotics, which are equally challenging.

The body needs to use complex enzymatic machinery to deal with all foreign materials whether synthetic or natural. As will be discussed, this means that there is a possibility of interaction between the different foreign materials as well.

The rosy view of natural health care needs to be amended. The body is in a state of alert even for constituents of the most natural materials it encounters. Under most circumstances the mechanisms for dealing with environmental stressors are effective, and the risks of perturbations and interactions are low. Nevertheless hypersensitivities to natural xenobiotics sometimes occur and may be the basis for some overt allergies (e.g., shellfish and peanuts). More significantly the modern use of powerful drugs with a narrow therapeutic window (in which the effective dose is close to the dangerous dose) raises new concerns about the potential for metabolic interactions between natural and synthetic constituents. This means that the most benign natural material can significantly affect the outcome of disease.

To understand these issues better it is necessary first to consider the nature of the main metabolic machinery for diverse foreign materials in the environment. By far the most prominent of these, although not the only mechanism, is the group of enzymes known as cytochromes P450 (CYP450s).

CYTOCHROME P450 ENZYME SYSTEM

The CYP450 enzyme system is a uniquely complex hierarchy of 14 enzyme families and many more subfamilies located in most organs and tissues of the body. It involves more than 500 *P450* genes.[2] Together, these proteins metabolise an extraordinary diversity of substrates, ranging from small molecules such as methanol (molecular weight, 42) to large molecules such as cyclosporin (molecular weight, 1203), planar molecules like dioxin, and globular molecules such as phenobarbitone. This versatility directly reflects the variety of enzyme structures (isoforms) in the system.

The CYP450 system metabolises a wide range of endogenous metabolites in the liver,

kidney, lungs, skin, digestive tract, and other tissues. The system also appears to be the prominent mechanism in the living organism for processing ingested exogenous chemicals, the xenobiotics. Xenobiotic metabolism occurs in two phases: phase I involves oxidation, reduction, and hydrolysis, and phase II involves synthesis and conjugation. The CYP450 isoenzymes are involved in phase I oxidative reactions. Therefore, the CYP450 system provides an effective first-pass system for the elimination of foreign molecules entering by way of the digestive tract, lungs, or skin.[3] However, this beneficial effect may be an inconvenience for the administration of medicines, especially because interindividual variation makes CYP450 effects on ingested drugs difficult to predict. In the heart, for example, CYP450 enzymes have been linked with the metabolism and variable activity of verapamil on that organ.[4]

Although overall CYP450 composition is genetically determined, the day-to-day detailed outcomes of CYP450 metabolism appear to be closely tied to environmental and ingested influences and lifestyle factors.[5] These can have significant outcomes and cause potential problems.

An immediate further difficulty is that two different molecules subjected to the same metabolising CYP450 enzyme may competitively interact with one another. These CYP450 interactions generally result from one of two processes: inhibition and induction. *Induction* means that a substance stimulates the synthesis of the enzyme, and its metabolic capacity is increased. *Inhibition* means competitive binding at an enzyme's binding site(s). A drug with a high affinity for an enzyme will slow the metabolism of any low affinity drug. It is thus very possible that one xenobiotic or drug will radically affect the CYP450 breakdown of another (see later and Table 5-1). A large number of specific influences on various CYP450s have been identified. Recently these have included the herb St. John's wort *(Hypericum perforatum)*, implicated as a potentially significant new influence on the use of several prescription medicines.[6] A review of the evidence in the case of St. John's wort will be discussed. However, in light of the questions that have arisen around this issue, it may be useful to consider the context into which this new xenobiotic perturbation should be placed. It is likely that St. John's wort is not unique or even unusual in its potential to interact with the body's metabolising enzymes.

Other potential difficulties may arise. Most CYP450 metabolism is a process of detoxication, leading to the generation of inactive polar molecules for elimination in urine or bile. In some cases, however, CYP450 metabolites are reactive and can lead to carcinogenicity, immunotoxicity, cell necrosis, and other harmful consequences. It has long been realised that there are also pronounced interindividual differences in drug-metabolising activity, leading to marked differences in plasma levels of drugs after the same therapeutic dose.

THE XENOBIOTIC LOAD

The body daily consumes a diversity of molecules that are not processed by the primary metabolic pathways. Many, perhaps most, even allowing for industrial pollutants in the modern world, are likely to be from natural sources. Plants synthesise a wide variety of secondary metabolites in addition to those necessary for their structure and core metabolic functions. The obvious questions about the fate of secondary plant metabolites when ingested by animals and humans were addressed in one of the earliest reviews of the concept of xenobiotics.[7] Their roles remain poorly understood in most cases but are likely to include the regulation of growth and development, attraction of pollinators, other reproductive functions, and particularly defence against fungi, viruses, and insects.[1]

Therefore, almost by definition such molecules have the potential for significant impact on metabolic pathways. It is arguable that humans and other animals have evolved with complex enzyme defences themselves specifically to neutralise the potential disruptive effects of a huge diversity of natural xenobiotics.

The irony of an uneasy relationship in the natural world between various species and their defences is obvious to the herbal practitioner. Chemical defences in plants include many

pharmacologically interesting constituents that underpin traditional herbal medicine.[1]

Nitrogenous Secondary Metabolites

- Nonprotein amino acids
- Cyanogenic glycosides
- Glucosinolates
- Alkaloids
- Peptides

Nonnitrogenous Secondary Metabolites

- Iridoids
- Sesquiterpene lactones
- Cardiac glycosides
- Saponins
- Furanocoumarins
- Isoflavonoids
- Quinones
- Polyacetylenes

One could note that potentially the most potent xenobiotics are specifically those plant constituents that are seen as most important in plant remedies!

XENOBIOTIC INTERACTIONS WITH CYP450S

The conventional drug literature has increasingly demonstrated evidence of interactions between drugs and CYP450s and thus with other drugs. It is possible to collate some of these in respect of the individual enzyme families. They help practitioners to modify prescription of the relevant medicines and to consider the way in which they may affect each other's availability and activity in the body. What is also becoming clear is that such tables should include natural products, foods, and herbal medicines as well. Table 5-1 includes some of the known experimental interactions.

In Table 5-1 *Substrates* are agents on which the enzyme family concerned acts. *Inhibitors* reduce that action and thus increase the half-life of the substrate and its impact on the organism. Inhibition means competitive binding at an enzyme's binding site(s). A drug with a high affinity for an enzyme will slow the metabolism of any low affinity drug. In other words, drugs that are substrates may also competitively inhibit any other substrate. This is

Table **5-1**   **Potential Involvement of Natural Products in CYP450 Drug Metabolism**[*]

P450 Enzyme family	Substrates	Inhibitors	Inducers
CYP1A1 Metabolises polycyclic hydrocarbons; genetic polymorphism of the gene may play a role in the predisposition to cancer		**Galangin**[8] **Vitamin A**[10]	**Brassicas**[9] Dioxins Lansoprazole **Low calcium diet**[11] Omeprazole Smoking
CYP1A2 May activate procarcinogens, such as heterocyclic amines and aryl amines; high activity may increase the risk of spontaneous abortion	Acetaminophen Amitriptyline Aromatic amines **Caffeine**[16] Clozapine[17] Cyclobenzaprine Imipramine **Melatonin** Mexillitene Naproxen Phenacetin Propranolol Riluzole Tacrine Theophylline	Cimetidine Diltiazem **Flavones**[13,14] Fluoroquinolone antibiotics Fluvoxamine Furafylline **Quercetin**[18] Tacrine Ticlopidine Verapamil	**Brassicas**[9] **Charcoal-grilled beef**[12] Cigarette smoke[15] Omeprazole Phenobarbital Phenytoin
CYP2A6 Metabolises a number of drugs, activates a variety of precarcinogens, and is the predominant enzyme for the metabolism of nicotine to cotinine; activity affected more by environmental influences than genetics[19]	Butadiene Coumarin **Nicotine**[21]	8-Methoxypsoralen **Grapefruit**[20] Tranylcypromine	Barbiturates
CYP2C9 CYP2Cs are a major group accounting for 20% of drug metabolism including most NSAIDs and COX-2 inhibitors; amino acid polymorphisms (more common in whites and Hispanics than in Asians and Africans) can dangerously impair metabolism of warfarin	Celecoxib Naproxen Phenytoin S-warfarin Sildenafil (Viagra) Sulfamethoxazole Tamoxifen Tolbutamide Torsemide Angiotensin II blockers NSAID drugs Oral hypoglycaemics (e.g., tolbutamide, glipizide)	Amiodarone Fluconazole Isoniazid Sulfaphenazole Sulfinpyrazone Ticlopidine	Barbiturates Rifampin

Table **5-1   Potential Involvement of Natural Products in CYP450 Drug Metabolism**[*]**—cont'd**

P450 Enzyme family	Substrates	Inhibitors	Inducers
CYP2C19 Involved in the metabolism of proton pump inhibitors, antiepileptics, cardiovascular drugs, antimalarial drugs, oral contraceptives, and tricyclic antidepressants; absent in 20-30% of Asians. Mutations in the CYP2C19 gene common to most major ethnic groups can result in the clinically important poor metabolizer (PM) phenotype	Amitriptyline Citalopram Clomipramine Cyclophosphamide Diazepam Hexobarbital Imipramine Omeprazole Phenytoin Proguanil Progesterone Propranolol	Fluoxetine Fluvoxamine Ketoconazole Lansoprazole Omeprazole Ticlopidine Tranylcypromine **Ginkgo**[22] **Kava**[22] **St. John's wort**[22]	Barbiturates Rifampin
CYP2D6 Localises to the endoplasmic reticulum; is known to metabolise up to 20% of commonly prescribed drugs; 8% of whites have reduced metabolising capacity, whereas 30% of East Africans have increased capacity; critical determinant in the success of anti-depressant drug treatment	Codeine Dextromethorphan Ethylmorphine Flecainide Neuroleptics **Nicotine** Ondansetron Tramadol Antiarrhythmics Antidepressants (e.g., amitriptyline, clomipramine, desipramine, and imipramine) Antipsychotics (e.g., haloperidol, risperidone, and thioridazine) β-Blockers	Ajmalicine Amiodarone Chinidin Chlorpheniramine Cimetidine Clomipramine Fluoxetine Haloperidol Mibefradil Methadone Paroxetine Quinidine Ritonavir	
CYP2E1 Induced in hepatocytes by heavy consumption of ethanol and certain other drugs, is a potent generator of superoxide, and may mediate alcoholic hepatotoxicity	Acetaminophen **Caffeine** Chlorzoxazone Dapsone Enflurane **Theophylline** Alcohols	Dimethyl sulphoxide Disulfiram **Dandelion**[25]	Chlormethiazole **Diallyl sulphide**[23] **in garlic**[24] **Ethanol**[26] Isoniazid **Isothiocyanates in brassicas** **Low carbohydrate diet**[27,28]

(Continued)

Table **5-1   Potential involvement of natural products in CYP450 drug metabolism[*]—cont'd**

P450 Enzyme family	Substrates	Inhibitors	Inducers
CYP3A4[30]			
The most abundant cytochrome P450 in human liver, comprising ~30% of the total liver P450 content; also found in the gut; an important role in endogenous processes, most notably steroid catabolism, and also plays a fundamental role in the metabolism of >50% of currently prescribed drugs; majority of CYP3A substrates are also capable of inducing CYP3A activity, mainly through transcriptional activation; this implies competitive metabolism of any drug substrate in this table[31]	Acetaminophen Buspirone[32] Carbamazepine Cyclosporin[33,34] Digitoxin Diazepam[35] Fluoxetine Haloperidol Methadone Quinidine Sildenafil (Viagra) Trazodone Warfarin[38]	Amiodarone Cimetidine Clarithromycin Clotrimazole Erythromycin Fluoxetine Fluvoxamine **Garlic[36]** Ketoconazole Mibefradil Nefazodone **Red wine[37]** Ritonavir Troleandomycin	Carbamazepine Dexamethasone Phenobarbital Phenytoin Rifabutin Rifampin **St. John's wort** Troglitazone Troleandomycin
	Antihistamines (e.g., chlorpheniramine) Calcium channel blockers (e.g., verapamil, nifedipine, and felodipine)[48] HIV protease inhibitors (e.g., indinavir)[49,50] HMG CoA reductase inhibitors (e.g., lovastatin)[51,52] Macrolide antibiotics (e.g., erythromycin)[54] Steroids (e.g., cortisol)	*Citrus* **spp. (e.g., grapefruit)[39-47]** HIV protease inhibitors **Umbelliferous herbs** **Various herbs[53]**	

Natural products or derivatives in bold.
[*]*With acknowledgement to Dr. David Flockhart from the Clinical Pharmacology Division, Indiana University of Department of Medicine (http://medicine.iupui.edu/flockhart/).*

likely to be particularly significant in polypharmacy, in which taking several substrates will have an additive mutually inhibitory effect. *Inducers* increase CYP450 metabolism of the substrate, and this reduces its half-life and efficacy. Any inducer or inhibitor can affect any substrate listed for each enzyme family.

Many of the synthetic drug entries in Table 5-1 are drawn from an exhaustive list published by Dr. David Flockhart from the Clinical Pharmacology Division, Indiana University of Department of Medicine (http://medicine. iupui.edu/flockhart/). Importantly in a rapidly changing field, this is continually updated.

It is important to note that in the majority of cases the evidence for these reactions follows laboratory work, in vitro studies, and investigations of the effects of agents in rats (notably Sprague-Dawley rats). Many of the molecules studied are unlikely to reach the body's tissues after oral consumption and digestion and liver metabolism. Some may not be absorbed, whereas others may reach the liver in the first pass effect from the portal system. Therefore, such observations only raise the possibility of interactions and activities in real life. Nevertheless, based on such interactions, since 1998 the Food and Drug Administration has removed or restricted terfenadine, mibefradil, astemizole, grepafloxacin, and, notably, cisapride. The good health care practitioner should start to consider such prospects as well.

As Table 5-1 suggests, a major focus of interest has been the impact of natural products on the CYP450 3A4 (CYP3A4) enzyme. In one study 21 commercial ethanolic herbal extracts and tinctures and 13 related pure plant compounds were analysed for their in vitro inhibitory capability on CYP3A4 metabolite formation. Approximately 75% of the commercial products and 50% of the pure compounds showed significant inhibition in this laboratory context. The most powerful inhibitors were *Hydrastis canadensis* (goldenseal), *H. perforatum* (St. John's wort), and *Uncaria tomentosa* (cat's claw). This group was followed by *Echinacea angustifolia* roots, *Matricaria chamomilla* (chamomile), and *Glycyrrhiza glabra* (licorice). Hypericin and naringenin were among the most powerful in vitro inhibitors of the pure plant compounds.[53]

MISCELLANEOUS EFFECTS OF NATURAL PRODUCTS ON CYP450S

In addition to the specific activities in Table 5-1, a wider dossier of effects on CYP450 metabolism by natural products and their constituents is accumulating. These are often mixed or incomplete observations and again are largely from laboratory studies rather than clinical situations, but they point to a wider potential for interaction between foods, herbs, and synthetic drugs.

A reduced impact of herbal remedies in normal dosage alone is suggested in studies of the effects on CYP450 activities of the flavonolignans of *Silybum marianum* (milk thistle). The authors detected significant inhibition of CYP2D6, CYP2E1, and CYP3A4 but only at doses higher than would be achievable in therapeutic doses.[55]

Cruciferous Herbs and Brassica Vegetables[56]

Effects on warfarin[57] and caffeine[58] metabolism have been observed. Active constituents include indoles such as glucobrassin, indole-3-carbinol (CYP1A1 and CYP1A2), indole-3-carbonitrile,[59] phenethyl isothiacyanate (CYP2B1 and CYP2E1),[60] sulforaphane, and phenethylisothiocyanate (CYP2E1).

Garlic and Other Members of the Onion Family

A number of studies have demonstrated effects.[61-63] Active constituents include diallyl sulphide, diallyl disulphide (CYP1A2 and CYP2E1), allyl methyl sulphide, and allyl mercapten (CYP2E1).

Spices[64]

Activity has been seen in piperine from peppers,[65] myristicine from nutmeg, eugenol from cloves,[66] and capsaicin from chilli peppers (CYP2E1).[67]

Other Herbal Remedies

Effects have been noted for ginseng,[68] rosemary,[69] and Chinese species of *Gentiana* and *Scutellaria*.[70] Various other Chinese herbal medicines have been shown to interact with drug metabolism, in many cases through a CYP450 mechanism.[22,71-75]

Common medicinal plant constituents have been shown to affect CYP450 metabolism:
- Furanocoumarins in grapefruit[76] (e.g., 6,7,-dihydroxybergamottin) and the Umbelliferae[77] (e.g., species of *Angelica*)[78]
- Flavones[79] (CYP1A1, CYP1A2, and CYP2B)
- Terpenoids, especially camphor (CYP2B), citral, and linalool (CYP4A1)[80]

- Planar anthraquinone (anthraflavic acid; CYP1A1 and CYP1A2)[81]

ST. JOHN'S WORT AND CYP450 ACTIVITY

During the early 1990s consumption of St. John's wort in Germany and then other Western countries increased dramatically as its effect for the management of mild to moderate depressive conditions became understood. Industry sources suggest that there were approximately 106 million daily doses taken in Germany in 1992, and there was a huge growth in the use of the herb in the United States later in that decade. With such sudden modern human exposure it was not surprising that latent problems of interaction with other medicines became apparent for the first time. These have been covered elsewhere in this text (see Chapter 6), and it has also become clear that an impact on CYP450 metabolism is a key component of these interactions.

Effects of St. John's wort on CYP450 enzymes have been induced from case reports.

In a randomised single-blind placebo-controlled cross-over study, 10 healthy young men received an 11-day treatment of either St. John's wort or placebo with a single 12-mg dose of phenprocoumon. Compared with placebo the St. John's wort treatment arm led to a significant decrease in the proportion of free phenprocoumon. An effect on CYP450 metabolism was proposed as a possible explanation.[82]

In a single-blinded placebo-controlled parallel-grouped study 12 volunteers received digoxin with placebo and 13 received digoxin with St. John's wort extract LI160 (Lichtwer Pharma, Berlin, Germany). Compared with the placebo group those volunteers taking St. John's wort showed a significant decrease in the blood levels of digoxin. An effect on CYP450 metabolism was proposed.[83]

Based on a case report suggesting an effect of St. John's wort intake in reducing theophylline blood levels in an otherwise stable prescription regimen, investigators demonstrated in vitro induction effects of hypericin on a relevant gene sequence known as xenobiotic response element present in the gene promotors of the CYP450 enzymes. The authors suggested that the isozyme CYP1A2 responsible for metabolising theophylline was involved.[84]

There have been other more direct demonstrations of the effects of St. John's wort on CYP450 activity.

In an observation reflecting possible induction of CYP3A4, urinary excretion of 6β-hydroxycortisol was increased significantly by 300 mg St. John's wort solid extract in 50 healthy subjects.[85] In a similar study 6β-hydroxycortisol clearance increased in 13 subjects taking St. John's wort at 300 mg (0.3% hypericin) three times a day for 14 days.[86]

Negative findings of St. John's wort effects on CYP3A4 and CYP2D6 were reported in a study of 16 healthy subjects coadministered dextromethorphan and caffeine as probes.[87] However, the same team reported positive effects of St. John's wort on CYP1A2 activity as measured by urinary metabolites of caffeine in 16 subjects.[88]

In a study of seven healthy volunteers, oral administration of St. John's wort had no significant effect on the metabolism of probes dextromethorphan and alprazolam, suggesting no effect on CYP2D6 and CYP3A4 activity, respectively.[89]

Together, the aforementioned evidence suggests that St. John's wort may induce CYP450 isoenzyme CYP3A4 and possibly CYP1A2 and CYP2C9. As will be discussed,[53] hypericin may be one of the most active constituents in this respect.

Although St. John's wort has clearly become the most notable case in which a herbal remedy has demonstrated effects on CYP450 activity and drug metabolism, it is arguable in this review that it will not prove to be unique.

POSITIVE INFLUENCE ON CYP450 METABOLISM

Not all interactions between xenobiotics and CYP450s need be harmful. It is possible that some phytochemicals, such as isothiocyanates from vegetables of the cabbage family,[90] diosmin from citrus fruits, pungent principles in spices,[91] and resveratrol from grapes, may enhance detoxification processes by their induction of CYP450s and thereby have antimutagenic,[92] anticarcinogenetic,[93,94] and cardioprotective properties.[95]

It is also possible that constituents of cruciferous vegetables, by potently inhibiting CYP2E1, may also protect the liver against the effects of excessive alcohol consumption.[96]

DIETARY IMPACT ON CYP450 METABOLISM

It is already apparent that many food constituents are xenobiotic, and Table 5-1 indicates that they could have appreciable effects on drug metabolism. This has led to the realisation that diet can play a major part in effective prescription management.[5] This is also likely to be the case for dietary supplements with vitamin E,[97] fish oil,[63,98] propolis,[99] and carotenoids,[100] all showing effects on CYP450 metabolism. There are recent reports on interactions between cranberry juice and warfarin,[101] which underline this point.

Members of the CYP450 supergene family are responsible for the majority of activations of procarcinogens to ultimate carcinogens in the body. The extent of such activations is itself affected by everyday influences: different isoforms of CYP450 are regulated differently by ethanol, diet, and environmental inducers and have different substrate specificities and different propensity to be inhibited or activated by dietary components.[102]

STRUCTURE-ACTIVITY RELATIONSHIPS FOR CYP INDUCTION

There have been efforts toward understanding the mechanisms of P450 regulation.[103,104] In the case of CYP1 group, planar molecules are essential for induction[105]; in the case of CYP2, it takes an intact allyl group.[106] However, like most research in this field these mechanisms are still poorly understood.

CONCLUSIONS

It is clear from this review that there is enormous prospect of interaction between modern drugs and natural products, especially in food, but also including herbal medicines. These are likely to be an essential feature of the coevolution of plants and animals but may only become clinically hazardous with the recent introduction of powerful drugs with a narrow dose range between efficacy and toxicity.[107]

Therefore, it will be important to develop practical strategies to take advantage of these new findings when advising patients prescribed drugs with a narrow therapeutic index (see Chapter 6). Herbal practitioners have long been cautious to use remedies when patients are also taking anticoagulants, digoxin, insulin, antiepileptic drugs, and other powerful medication. This review may lead to an even greater awareness of the risks involved when patients are taking such critical medication. However, such cautions should extend much more widely than the prescription of herbal remedies. It is also clear that the main risk of interactions, simply because of the quantities involved, is with the diet.

Understanding of CYP450s has emerged only in the past two decades, and most discoveries of the xenobiotic influences on these enzymes have been recent. It is most likely that as investigative techniques become more sophisticated there will be many additions to the current list of products, including natural products, that will be shown to affect CYP450 metabolism and thus by implication, the metabolism of some prescription drugs.

Future cases like St. John's wort, in which a herb is targeted as an apparent risk, may more effectively be put into a wider context. Many, perhaps most, natural products can interact with prescribed drugs. The problem is with the management of these prescriptions, especially in dietary advice, rather than in the consumption of natural products themselves.

REFERENCES

1. Harborne JB: *Introduction to ecological biochemistry*, ed 3, London, 1988, Academic Press.
2. Danielson PB: The cytochrome P450 superfamily: biochemistry, evolution and drug metabolism in humans, *Curr Drug Metab* 3:561-597.
3. Park BK: Cytochrome P450 enzymes in the heart, *Lancet* 355:945-946, 2000.
4. Thum T, Borlak J: Gene expression in distinct regions of the heart, *Lancet* 355:979-983, 2000.

5. Ioannides C: Effect of diet and nutrition on the expression of cytochromes P450, *Xenobiotica* 29:109-154, 1999.

6. Ernst E: Second thoughts about safety of St. John's wort, *Lancet* 354:2014-2015, 1999.

7. Milburn P: Biotransformation of xenobiotics by animals. In Harborne JB, editor: *Biochemical aspects of plant and animal coevolution*, London, 1978, Academic Press.

8. Ciolino HP, Yeh GC: The flavonoid galangin is an inhibitor of CYP1A1 activity and an agonist/antagonist of the aryl hydrocarbon receptor, *Br J Cancer* 79:1340-1346, 1999.

9. Vang O, Jensen H, Autrup H: Induction of cytochrome P-4501A1, 1A2, 11B1, 11B2 and 11E1 by broccoli in rat liver and colon, *Chem Biol Interact* 78:85-96, 1991.

10. Inouye K, Mae T, Kondo S, Ohkawa H: Inhibitory effects of vitamin A and vitamin K on rat cytochrome P4501A1-dependent monooxygenase activity, *Biochem Biophys Res Commun* 262:565-569, 1999.

11. Armbrecht HJ, Hodam TL, Boltz MA, Kumar VB: Capacity of a low calcium diet to induce the renal vitamin D 1a-hydroxylase is decreased in adult rats, *Biochem Biophys Res Commun* 255:731-734, 1999.

12. Fontana RJ, Lown KS, Paine MF, et al: Effects of a chargrilled meat diet on expression of CYP3A, CYP1A, and P-glycoprotein levels in healthy volunteers, *Gastroenterology* 117:89-98, 1999.

13. Dai R, Zhai S, Wei X, Pincus MR, Vestal RE, Friedman FK: Inhibition of human cytochrome P450 1A2 by flavones: a molecular modeling study, *J Protein Chem* 17:643-650, 1998.

14. Obermeier MT, White RE, Yang CS: Effects of bioflavonoids on hepatic P450 activities, *Xenobiotica* 25:575-584, 1995.

15. Vistisen K, Loft S, Poulsen HE: Cytochrome P450 1A2 activity in man measured by caffeine metabolism: effect of smoking, broccoli and exercise, *Adv Exp Med Biol* 283:407-411, 1991.

16. Nordmark A, Lundgren S, Cnattingius S, Rane A: Dietary caffeine as a probe agent for assessment of cytochrome P4501A2 activity in random urine samples, *Br J Clin Pharmacol* 47:397-402, 1999.

17. Carrillo JA, Herraiz AG, Ramos SI, Benítez J: Effects of caffeine withdrawal from the diet on the metabolism of clozapine in schizophrenic patients, *J Clin Psychopharmacol* 18:311-316, 1998.

18. Rodgers EH, Grant MH: The effect of the flavonoids, quercetin, myricetin and epicatechin on the growth and enzyme activities of MCF7 human breast cancer cells, *Chem Biol Interact* 27:213-228, 1998.

19. Aklillu E, Herrlin K, Gustafsson LL, Bertilsson L, Ingelman-Sundberg M: Evidence for environmental influence on CYP2D6-catalysed debrisoquine hydroxylation as demonstrated by phenotyping and genotyping of Ethiopians living in Ethiopia or in Sweden, *Pharmacogenetics* 12:375-383, 2002.

20. Merkel U, Sigusch H, Hoffmann A: Grapefruit juice inhibits 7-hydroxylation of coumarin in healthy volunteers, *Eur J Clin Pharmacol* 46:175-177, 1994.

21. Sellers EM, Kaplan HL, Tyndale RF: Inhibition of cytochrome P450 2A6 increases nicotine's oral bioavailability and decreases smoking, *Clin Pharmacol Ther* 68:35-43, 2000.

22. Zou L, Harkey MR, Henderson GL: Effects of herbal components on cDNA-expressed cytochrome P450 enzyme catalytic activity, *Life Sci* 71:1579-1589, 2002.

23. Loizou GD, Cocker J: The effects of alcohol and diallyl sulphide on CYP2E1 activity in humans: a phenotyping study using chlorzoxazone, *Hum Exp Toxicol* 20:321-327, 2001.

24. Park KA, Kweon S, Choi H: Anticarcinogenic effect and modification of cytochrome P450 2E1 by dietary garlic powder in diethylnitrosamine-initiated rat hepatocarcinogenesis, *J Biochem Mol Biol* 35:615-622, 2002.

25. Maliakal PP, Wanwimolruk S: Effect of herbal teas on hepatic drug metabolizing enzymes in rats, *J Pharm Pharmacol* 53:1323-1329, 2001.

26. Djordjevic D, Nikolic J, Stefanovic V: Ethanol interactions with other cytochrome P450 substrates including drugs, xenobiotics, and carcinogens, *Pathol Biol (Paris)* 46:760-770, 1998.

27. Korourian S, Hakkak R, Ronis MJ, et al: Diet and risk of ethanol-induced hepatotoxicity: carbohydrate-fat relationships in rats, *Toxicol Sci* 47:110-117, 1999.

28. Tsukada H, Wang PY, Kaneko T, Wang Y, Nakano M, Sato A: Dietary carbohydrate intake plays an important role in preventing alcoholic fatty liver in the rat, *J Hepatol* 29:715-724, 1998.

29. Dresser GK, Spence JD, Bailey DG: Pharmacokinetic-pharmacodynamic consequences and clinical relevance of cytochrome P450 3A4 inhibition, *Clin Pharmacokinet* 38:41-57, 2000.

30. Ghosh SS, Basu AK, Ghosh S, et al: Renal and hepatic family 3A cytochromes P450 (CYP3A) in spontaneously hypertensive rats, *Biochem Pharmacol* 50:49-54, 1995.

31. Plant NJ, Gibson GG: Evaluation of the toxicological relevance of CYP3A4 induction, *Curr Opin Drug Discov Devel* 6:50-56, 2003.

32. Lilja JJ, Kivisto KT, Backman JT, et al: Grapefruit juice substantially increases plasma concentrations of buspirone, *Clin Pharmacol Ther* 64:655-660, 1998.

33. Min DI, Ku YM, Perry PJ, et al: Effect of grapefruit juice on cyclosporine pharmacokinetics in renal transplant patients, *Transplantation* 62:123-125, 1996.

34. Mangano NG, Cutuli VM, Caruso A, De Bernardis E, Amico-Roxas M: Grapefruit juice effects on the bioavailability of cyclosporin-A in rats, *Eur Rev Med Pharmacol Sci* 5:1-6, 2001.

35. Ozdemir M, Aktan Y, Boydag BS, et al: Interaction between grapefruit juice and diazepam in humans, *Eur J Drug Metab Pharmacokinet* 23:55-59, 1998.

36. Foster BC, Foster MS, Vandenhoek S, et al: An in vitro evaluation of human cytochrome P450 3A4 and P-glycoprotein inhibition by garlic, *J Pharm Pharm Sci* 4:176-184, 2001.

37. Offman EM, Freeman DJ, Dresser GK, Munoz C, Bend JR, Bailey DG: Red wine-cisapride interaction:

comparison with grapefruit juice, *Clin Pharmacol Ther* 70:17-23, 2001.

38. Runkel M, Bourian M, Tegtmeier M, Legrum W: The character of inhibition of the metabolism of 1,2-benzopyrone (coumarin) by grapefruit juice in human, *Eur J Clin Pharmacol* 53:265-269, 1997.

39. Tassaneeyakul W, Guo LQ, Fukuda K, Ohta T, Yamazoe Y: Inhibition selectivity of grapefruit juice components on human cytochromes P450, *Arch Biochem Biophys* 378:356-363, 2000.

40. Ohta T, Nagahashi M, Hosoi S, Tsukamoto S: Dihydroxy-bergamottin caproate as a potent and stable CYP3A4 inhibitor, *Bioorg Med Chem* 10:969-973, 2002.

41. Bailey DG, Malcolm J, Arnold O, Spence JD: Grapefruit juice-drug interactions, *Br J Clin Pharmacol* 46:101-110, 1998.

42. Edwards DJ, Fitzsimmons ME, Schuetz EG, et al: 6′,7′-Dihydroxybergamottin in grapefruit juice and Seville orange juice: effects on cyclosporine disposition, entero-cyte CYP3A4, and P-glycoprotein, *Clin Pharmacol Ther* 65:237-244, 1999.

43. Gross AS, Goh YD, Addison RS, et al: Influence of grape-fruit juice on cisapride pharmacokinetics, *Clin Pharmacol Ther* 65:395-401, 1999.

44. Hollander AA, van Rooij J, Lentjes GW, et al: The effect of grapefruit juice on cyclosporine and prednisone metabolism in transplant patients, *Clin Pharmacol Ther* 57:318-324, 1995.

45. Hukkinen SK, Varhe A, Olkkola KT, et al: Plasma concen-trations of triazolam are increased by concomitant ingestion of grapefruit juice, *Clin Pharmacol Ther* 58:127-131, 1995.

46. Guo LQ, Taniguchi M, Xiao YQ, Baba K, Ohta T, Yamazoe Y: Inhibitory effect of natural furanocoumarins on human microsomal cytochrome P450 3A activity, *Jpn J Pharmacol* 82:122-129, 2000.

47. He K, Iyer KR, Hayes RN, et al: Inactivation of cytochrome P450 3A4 by bergamottin, a component of grapefruit juice, *Chem Res Toxicol* 1:252-259, 1998.

48. Lown KS, Bailey DG, Fontana RJ, et al: Grapefruit juice increases felodipine oral availability in humans by decreasing intestinal CYP3A protein expression, *J Clin Invest* 99:2545-2553, 1997.

49. Pisciteill S, Buratair AH, Chairt D, et al: Indinavir con-centrations and St. John's wort, *Lancet* 355:547-549, 2000.

50. Penzak SR, Acosta EP, Turner M, et al: Effect of Seville orange juice and grapefruit juice on indinavir pharmaco-kinetics, *J Clin Pharmacol* 42:1165-1170, 2002.

51. Kantola T, Kivisto KT, Neuvonen PJ: Grapefruit juice greatly increases serum concentrations of lovastatin acid, *Clin Pharmacol Ther* 63:397-402, 1998.

52. Ubeaud G, Hagenbach J, Vandenschrieck S, et al: In vitro inhibition of simvastatin metabolism in rat and human liver by naringenin, *Life Sci* 65:1403-1412, 1999.

53. Budzinski JW, Foster BC, Vandenhoek S, Arnason JT: An in vitro evaluation of human cytochrome P450 3A4 inhi-bition by selected commercial herbal extracts and tinc-tures, *Phytomedicine* 7:273-282, 2000.

54. Kanazawa S, Ohkubo T, Sugawara K: The effects of grape-fruit juice on the pharmacokinetics of erythromycin, *Eur J Clin Pharmacol* 56:799-803, 2001.

55. Zuber R, Modriansky M, Dvorak Z, et al: Effect of silybin and its congeners on human liver microsomal cytochrome P450 activities, *Phytother Res* 16:632-638, 2002.

56. Kall MA, Vang O, Clausen J: Effects of dietary broccoli on human drug metabolising activity, *Cancer Lett* 114:169-170, 1997.

57. Ovesen L, Lyduch S, Idorn ML: The effect of a diet rich in brussels sprouts on warfarin pharmacokinetics, *Eur J Clin Pharmacol* 34:521-523, 1988.

58. McDanell RE, Henderson LA, Russell K, McLean AEM: The effect of brassica vegetable consumption on caffeine metab-olism in humans, *Human Exp Toxicol* 11:167-172, 1992.

59. Vang O, Frandsen H, Hansen KT, et al: Modulation of drug-metabolising enzyme expression by condensation products of indole-3-ylcarbinole, an inducer in crucifer-ous vegetables, *Pharmacol Toxicol* 84:59-65, 1999.

60. Staack R, Kingston S, Wallig MA, et al: A comparison of the individual and collective effects of four glucosinolate breakdown products from brussels sprouts on induction of detoxification enzymes, *Toxicol Appl Pharmacol* 149:17-23, 1998.

61. Wu CC, Sheen LY, Chen HW, Kuo WW, Tsai SJ, Lii CK: Differential effects of garlic oil and its three major organosulfur components on the hepatic detoxification system in rats, *J Agric Food Chem* 50:378-383, 2002.

62. Guyonnet D, Belloir C, Suschetet M, Siess MH, Le Bon AM: Antimutagenic activity of organosulfur compounds from Allium is associated with phase II enzyme induction, *Mutat Res* 495:135-145, 2001.

63. Chen HW, Tsai CW, Yang JJ, Liu CT, Kuo WW, Lii CK: The combined effects of garlic oil and fish oil on the hepatic antioxidant and drug-metabolizing enzymes of rats, *Br J Nutr* 89:189-200, 2003.

64. Wickramasinghe RH, Muller G, Norpoth K: Spectral evi-dence of interaction of spice constituents with hepatic microsomal cytochrome P-450, *Cytobios* 29:25-27, 1980.

65. Koul S, Koul JL, Taneja SC, et al: Structure-activity rela-tionship of piperine and its synthetic analogues for their inhibitory potentials of rat hepatic microsomal constitu-tive and inducible cytochrome P450 activities, *Bioorg Med Chem* 8:251-268, 2000.

66. Rompelberg CJ, Vogels JT, de Vogel N, et al: Effect of short-term dietary administration of eugenol in humans, *Hum Exp Toxicol* 15:129-135, 1996.

67. Surh Y: Molecular mechanisms of chemopreventive effects of selected dietary and medicinal phenolic sub-stances, *Mutat Res* 428:305-327, 1999.

68. Henderson GL, Harkey MR, Gershwin ME, et al: Effects of ginseng components on c-DNA-expressed cytochrome P450 enzyme catalytic activity, *Life Sci* 65:209-214, 1999.

69. Offord EA, Mace K, Avanti O, Pfeifer AM: Mechanisms involved in the chemoprotective effects of rosemary extract studied in human liver and bronchial cells, *Cancer Lett* 114:275-281, 1997.

70. Kang JJ, Chen YC, Kuo WC, et al: Modulation of microsomal cytochrome P450 by Scutellariae Radix and Gentianae scabrae Radix in rat liver, *Am J Chin Med* 24:19-29, 1996.

71. Lin SY, Hou SJ, Perng RI, et al: Effect of traditional Chinese herbal medicines on the pharmacokinetics of western drugs in Sprague-Dawley rats of different ages (11): aminophylline-huan shao tan and aminophylline-pu chung yi chi tang, *Mech Ageing Dev* 66:93-106, 1992.

72. Liu GT: Effects of some compounds isolated from Chinese medicinal herbs on hepatic microsomal cytochrome P-450 and their potential biological consequences, *Drug Metab Rev* 23:439-465, 1991.

73. Obnishi T, Yoneyama H, Hamamoto T, et al: Induction of cytochrome P-450-linked monooxygenase system in rat liver microsomes by xiao-chaihu-tang, *Am J Chin Med* 24:143-151, 1996.

74. Wong BY, Lau BH, Yamasaki T, Teel RW: Inhibition of dexamethasone-induced cytochrome P450-mediated mutagenicity and metabolism of aflatoxin B1 by Chinese medicinal herbs, *Eur J Cancer Prev* 2:351-356, 1993.

75. Yin J, Wennberg RP, Miller M: Induction of hepatic bilirubin and drug metabolizing enzymes by individual herbs present in the traditional Chinese medicine, yin zhi huang, *Dev Pharmacol Ther* 20:186-194, 1993.

76. Fuhr U: Drug interactions with grapefruit juice. Extent, probable mechanism and clinical relevance, *Drug Saf* 18:251-272, 1998.

77. Guo L-Q, Taniguchi M, Chen Q-Y, Baba K, Yamazoe Y: Inhibitory potential of herbal medicines on human cytochrome P450-mediated oxidation: properties of *Umbelliferous* or *Citrus* crude drugs and their relative prescriptions, *Jpn J Pharmacol* 85:399-408, 2001.

78. Ishihara K, Kushida H, Yuzurihara M, et al: Interactions of drugs and Chinese herbs: pharmacokinetic changes of tolbutamide and diazepam caused by extract of Angelica dahurica, *J Pharm Pharmacol* 52:1023-1029, 2000.

79. Dai R, Jacobson KA, Robinson RC, et al: Differential effects of flavonoids on testosterone-metabolizing cytochrome P450s, *Life Sci* 61:75-80, 1997.

80. Roffey SJ, Walker R, Gibson GG: Hepatic peroxisomal and microsomal enzyme induction by citral and linalool in rats, *Food Chem Toxicol* 28:403-408, 1990.

81. Ayrton AD, Ioannides C, Walker R: Induction of rat hepatic cytochrome P-450 I proteins by the antimutagen anthraflavic acid, *Food Chem Toxicol* 26:909-915, 1988.

82. Maurer A, Johne A, Brockmoller J, et al: Interaction of St. John's wort extract with phenprocoumon, *Jahreskongreb fur Klinische Pharmakologie* June:79, 1999.

83. Johne A, Brockmoller J, Bauer S, et al: Interaction of St. John's wort extract with digoxin, *Jahreskongreb fur Klinische Pharmakologie* June:80, 1999.

84. Nebel A, Schneider BJ, Baker RK, Kroll DJ: Potential metabolic interaction between St. John's wort and theophylline, *Ann Pharmacother* 33:502, 1999.

85. Kerb R, Bauer S, Brockmolier J, Roots I: Urinary 6 B-hydrocortisol excretion rate is affected by treatment with hypericum extract, *Eur J Clin Pharmacol* 52:A186, 1997.

86. Roby CA, Kantor E, Anderson GD, Burstein AH: St. John's wort impact on CYP3A4 activity, New Clinical Drug Evaluation Unit Program 39th Annual Meeting, Boca Raton, June 1-4, 1999, Poster 129.

87. Ereshefsky B, Gewertz N, Francis Lamb YW, et al: Determination of SJW differential metabolism at CYP2D6 and CYP3A4, using dextromethorphan probe methodology, New Clinical Drug Evaluation Unit Program 39th Annual Meeting, Boca Raton, June 1-4, 1999, Poster 130.

88. Gewertz N, Ereshefsky B, Francis Lamb YW, et al: Determination of the differential effects of St. John's wort on the CYP1A2 and NAT2 metabolic pathways using caffeine probe methodology, New Clinical Drug Evaluation Unit Program 39th Annual Meeting, Boca Raton, June 1-4, 1999, Poster 131.

89. Markovitz JS, DeVane CL, Carson SW, et al: Effect of St. John's wort on cytochrome (CYP) P-450 activity in healthy volunteers, *J Eur Coll Neuropsychopharmacol* 9:S367, 1999.

90. Paolini M: Brussels sprouts: an exceptionally rich source of ambiguity for anticancer strategies, *Toxicol Appl Pharmacol* 152:293-294, 1998.

91. Surh YJ, Lee E, Lee JM: Chemoprotective properties of some pungent ingredients present in red pepper and ginger, *Mutat Res* 402:259-267, 1998.

92. Surh YJ: More than spice: capsaicin in hot chili peppers makes tumor cells commit suicide, *J Natl Cancer Inst* 94:1263-1265, 2002.

93. Teel RW, Huynh H: Modulation by phytochemicals of cytochrome P450-linked enzyme activity, *Cancer Lett* 133:135-141, 1998.

94. Wattenberg LW: Chemoprevention of carcinogenesis by minor non-nutrient constituents of the diet. In Parke DV, Ioannides C, Walker R, editors: *Food, nutrition and chemical toxicity*, 1993.

95. Nanjee MN, Verhagen H, van Poppel G, Rompelberg CJ, van Bladeren PJ, Miller NE: Do dietary phytochemicals with cytochrome P-450 enzyme-inducing activity increase high-density-lipoprotein concentrations in humans? *Am J Clin Nutr* 64:706-711, 1996.

96. McCarty MF: Inhibition of CYP2E1 with natural agents may be a feasible strategy for minimizing the hepatotoxicity of ethanol, *Med Hypotheses* 56:8-11, 2001.

97. Chen HW, Lii CK, Sung WC, Ko YJ: Effect of vitamin E on rat hepatic cytochrome P-450 activity, *Nutr Cancer* 313:178-183, 1998.

98. Lutz M, Bonilla S, Concha J, Alvarado J, Barraza P: Effect of dietary oils, cholesterol and antioxidant vitamin supplementation on liver microsomal fluidity and xenobiotic-metabolizing enzymes in rats, *Ann Nutr Metab* 42:350-359, 1998.

99. Lin SC, Chung CY, Chiang CL, Hsu SH: The influence of propolis ethanol extract on liver microsomal enzymes and glutathione after chronic alcohol administration, *Am J Chin Med* 27:83-93, 1999.

100. Jewell C, O'Brien NM: Effect of dietary supplementation with carotenoids on xenobiotic metabolizing enzymes in

the liver, lung, kidney and small intestine of the rat, *Br J Nutr* 81:235-242, 1999.

101. http://medicines.mhra.gov.uk/ourwork/monitor-safetqualmed/currentproblems/ cpsept2003.pdf

102. Warner M, Hellmold H, Magnusson M, Rylander T, Hedlund E, Gustafsson JA: Extrahepatic cytochrome P450: role in in situ toxicity and cell-specific hormone sensitivity, *Arch Toxicol Suppl* 20:455-463, 1998.

103. Lewis DF, Jacobs MN, Dickins M, Lake BG: Quantitative structure-activity relationships for inducers of cytochromes P450 and nuclear receptor ligands involved in P450 regulation within the CYP1, CYP2, CYP3 and CYP4 families, *Toxicology* 176:51-57, 2002.

104. Lewis DF, Ioannides C, Parke DV, Schulte-Hermann R: Quantitative structure-activity relationships in a series of

endogenous and synthetic steroids exhibiting induction of CYP3A activity and hepatomegaly associated with increased DNA synthesis, *J Steroid Biochem Mol Biol* 74:179-185, 2000.

105. Tassaneeyakul W, Birkett DJ, Veronese ME, et al: Specificity of substrate and inhibitor probes for human cytochromes P450 1A1 and 1A2, *J Pharmacol Exp Ther* 265:401-407, 1993.

106. Reicks MM, Crankshaw DL: Modulation of rat hepatic cytochrome P-450 activity by garlic organosulfur compounds, *Nutr Cancer* 25:241-248, 1996.

107. Dresser GK, Bailey DG: A basic conceptual and practical overview of interactions with highly prescribed drugs, *Can J Clin Pharmacol* 9:191-198, 2002.

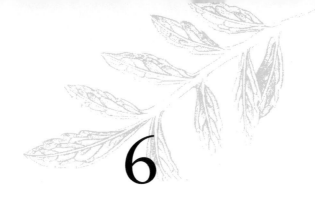

6

ADVERSE HERB-DRUG INTERACTIONS

Kerry Bone, Simon Mills, Michelle Morgan, and Berris Burgoyne

INFORMATION AND MISINFORMATION

The possibility of interactions between herbal and conventional medicines has undoubtedly become one of the prominent expressed views on the part of the health professional and, in terms of Western media coverage, a common alarm call for the public as well. No substantial text on herbs can now afford to be without its list of possible interactions, and there are many versions available. Along the way, however, the story has become extremely confused. In the absence of much hard data, speculation in one source has tended to become an accepted statement in the next, a biblical fact in a subsequent magazine article, only to be quoted back in the next professional conference. Glaring technical inconsistencies have also appeared and have assumed their own mythological status. In the midst of this confusion, the real cautions are lost or diminished.

It is time for the Augeian stables to be cleaned. In this chapter we will scrutinise the most commonly accepted wisdoms about herb-drug interactions (HDIs), challenge those without adequate rationale, and more clearly order those interactions that are left into theoretically possible and established.

However, this review will need to be rigorous. In the previous chapter the theoretical case is made that all consumed materials that are not primary metabolites for the body can compete in the complex secondary metabolising machinery (e.g., the cytochrome P450 [CYP450] enzyme system). The plant world contains innumerable "xenobiotics" that rely on the same processing mechanisms as synthetic drugs: induction or inhibition of one by the other is proving to be commonplace. In the case of powerful modern drugs with a narrow therapeutic window, this base level of interaction can be critical (although this is more likely to be a problem with foods than with lower doses of herbs). If any natural material, food or remedy, can interfere with the availability of warfarin or digoxin, then prescription of such powerful drugs needs to be accompanied by better dietary instructions and more frequent monitoring. The potential disruptive role of any particular herb can then be understood in context, and perhaps that herb will not be unduly restricted.

There is also a need of critical discretion for another reason. The case of St. John's wort is salutary. Monographs on this important remedy until the mid-1990s stated clearly that no interactions were to be expected. In a short time the interaction file for this medicine was the largest for any herb. Those who use herbs need to be alert to the possibility of more St. John's wort interactions. Therefore, all the more reason to clear the decks of confusing clutter and to adopt sound, consistent policies for reducing the risk of interactions and recognising them quickly when they occur.

For these reasons the interaction tables in this chapter are smaller than many, even than one the authors have previously published.[1] We hope this will be the most rational basis to proceed in this area.

HYPERCAUTIONS AND MISINFORMATION

There are increasingly alarming reports of dangers that may follow HDIs. An article in the August 2000 edition of *Alternative and Complementary Therapies*[2] indicated a basic lack of knowledge of phytochemistry and phytotherapy when it was suggested that St. John's wort and other immunostimulant herbs can interact with immunosuppressive drugs and photosensitisers, that ginseng and other herbs "that contain cardiac glycosides" will interact with digoxin, and that black cohosh, chamomile, feverfew, and other "tannin-containing herbs" will interact with iron supplements.

According to an article published in the *British Medical Journal*, valerian interacts with barbiturates, and echinacea interacts with anabolic steroids, among many other equally unlikely assertions.[3]

Even the herbal profession can be affected by paroxysms of hypercaution: despite massive consumption in the Middle East and elsewhere, an article in a newsletter of the National Institute of Medical Herbalists (U.K.) claimed that parsley was contraindicated with warfarin, along with garlic and celery among others. As has been seen in the previous chapter, the risk of interactions with warfarin is something to watch closely in each patient; however, to deny entire cultures the chance to use warfarin safely could perhaps be described as "overkill".

Some of the misinformation appears to be derived from an article by pharmacist Lucinda Miller in the journal *Archives of Internal Medicine* in 1998.[4] The title of the study is "Herbal medicinals, selected clinical considerations focusing on known or potential drug-herb interactions". Unfortunately many who have quoted the article have overlooked the critical qualifier "potential".

Some examples from this source follow, showing how unfounded scare stories have become accepted. About the herb chamomile it is stated:

> Chamomile contains coumarin which is reported to exert an antispasmodic effect. However, this effect has not yet translated into any coagulation disorders despite widespread human use. Because chamomile's effects on the coagulation system have not yet been studied, it is unknown if a clinically significant drug-herb interaction exists with known anticoagulants such as warfarin.[4]

One of the many misunderstandings made by pharmacists not well trained in phytochemistry (the chemistry of plants) is confusion about the word coumarin. The herb sweet clover *(Melilotus officinalis)* contains coumarin. "Sweet clover disease" was a bleeding disorder first noted in cattle fed spoiled sweet clover. Although it was described in the 1920s, it was not until 1941 that the causative factor was identified as dicoumarol.[5] Dicoumarol, formed from coumarin by bacterial action in damaged hay, was subsequently developed as the first oral anticoagulant. However, its anticoagulant action is slow in onset and difficult to terminate, and this led to the use of synthetic analogues, the most widely used of which is warfarin. Properly dried sweet clover does not contain dicoumarol and has no anticoagulant activity under normal circumstances. Coumarin has an anticoagulant activity that is 1000 times less than dicoumarol because it lacks a 4-hydroxy group in its chemical structure. A double-blind, comparative study of 41 patients with chronic venous insufficiency found that an oral coumarin/troxerutin preparation given for 6 weeks did not cause anticoagulant effects.[6] There were no significant changes in coagulation, clotting factors, or fibrinolysis during the treatment period.

Therefore, to the phytochemist the term "coumarin" means plant chemicals based on the coumarin structure. However, to pharmacists the term coumarin means anticoagulant drugs derived from or related to phytochemicals in the coumarin group. As confirmed in the aforementioned study, there is no evidence that normal coumarins found in common plants (and not altered by bacteria, and so on) have any anticoagulant activity.

Secondly, chamomile does not contain coumarin as such, but the coumarin derivates herniarin and umbelliferone.[7] Feeding massive amounts of chamomile to rats (more chamomile tea than could be drunk in 1 year) produced no toxic effects.[8] The rats certainly did not bleed to death, as they would if fed dicoumarol, a rat poison.

Therefore, chamomile tea drinkers should have no fear of warfarin (other than the normal respect for this highly dangerous drug).

Dr. Miller writes about echinacea:

Since hepatotoxic effects may be associated with persistent use, it should not be taken with other known hepatotoxic drugs (e.g. anabolic steroids, amiodarone, methotrexate, or ketoconazole). However, the magnitude of this hepatotoxicity has been questioned since Echinacea lacks the 1,2 unsaturated necrine ring system associated with hepatotoxicity of pyrrolizidine alkaloids.[4]

Pyrrolizidine alkaloids that lack the unsaturated necrine ring can never be hepatotoxic under any circumstances.[9] In other words the magnitude of the hepatotoxicity of echinacea on current credible knowledge is zero.

About feverfew the following statement is made:

Feverfew has been shown to inhibit platelet activity. Hence, it is advised to avoid use of feverfew in patients receiving warfarin or other anticoagulants.[4]

However, the antiplatelet activity of feverfew has been shown only in test tube research at concentrations that are not reached when patients take oral doses of the herb. Furthermore, the platelets of patients taking feverfew aggregated normally to adenosine diphosphate and thrombin, indicating that normal aggregating mechanisms are intact.[10]

The daily dose of feverfew leaves recommended for migraine is usually <200 mg. No constituent in feverfew is found at more than a few per cent. Even assuming the constituents with antiplatelet activity total 5%, this means that for feverfew to have significant antiplatelet activity, these compounds would need to be active at a daily dose of 10 mg. They would be much more potent than aspirin, and drug companies would have patented them as novel antiplatelet drugs decades ago.

Dr. Miller states in connection with valerian:

Furthermore, valerian has been shown to prolong thiopental- and pentobarbital-induced sleep. Hence, valerian should not be used with barbiturates.[4]

Of the three references quoted, one is about a completely different species of valerian, and another mentions valerian in commentary. For the one valid source supporting this hypothesis, valerian was given in very high doses in an animal study. There is no clinical support for this caution.

Although Dr. Miller is probably the writer most popularly quoted in sensationalist articles and press releases, others have made similar mistakes. Even in a generally well-written text on this topic, the author falls for the phytochemistry and coumarin trap when he writes that horsechestnut may enhance the effects of coumarin-based anticoagulants, "due to the antithrombin activity of aesculin", a phytochemical coumarin.[11] This error is further compounded by the fact that horsechestnut seeds are the commonly used part, and aesculin is only found in high levels in the bark of this plant.

Facts and Comparisons, a popular natural products review newsletter published in the United States by "experts in the field", has issued two tables on HDIs.[12,13] These contain many inaccuracies that barely merit refutation, such as:

- Herbal diuretics may increase the toxicity of NSAIDs;
- Bayberry has "corticosteroid activity" so it will interact in many ways because of this property;
- Herbs with "active principles which have sedative effects" such as nettle,

ground ivy, sage, and borage will possibly "increase the risk of seizure" when taken with anticonvulsants; and

- Herbs containing sympathomimetic amines such as "agnus castus alkaloids" will increase the risk of hypertensive crisis with monoamine oxidase (MAO) inhibitors.

Case reports may be quoted inaccurately or out of context. For example, one case report was as follows:

> An elderly patient was found to have elevated blood pressure and treatment with a thiazide diuretic was started. She then started taking ginkgo biloba. After a week, the patient's blood pressure was found to have increased further, and this elevation was maintained for a few weeks. Blood pressure returned to pre-treatment levels when both the diuretic and the ginkgo were stopped. Due to the severity of the response there was no rechallenge. Ginkgo biloba is a peripheral vasodilator, and there have been no reports of increased blood pressure from clinical trials.[14]

This may have been an adverse reaction to ginkgo, the diuretic drug acting on its own, or a combination of the two. No follow-up evaluation has been conducted, but the assertion that ginkgo will interact with thiazide diuretics has now been perpetuated in the literature.[15]

POTENTIAL, PROBABLE, AND ACTUAL

Much of the confusion in the literature involves the loose use of risk descriptors. The term "potential" encompasses a wide range of probabilities. For example, in physics it is potentially possible that a billiard ball will fall through a table to the floor, but this potential event is unlikely to happen within the lifetime of our universe. Rather more probable is the potential risk that the next plane flight will crash. However, this catastrophic probability is insufficient to greatly affect the willingness of people to fly. A "potential" risk needs underpinning with something quantifiable and then should be put into the wider context of benefit and risk. If the potential risk is merely spec-

ulative and poorly founded, then it barely affects the gains that may follow.

Therefore, with any potential risk the likely benefits should be weighted as well. If the risk is high, then the benefits must be great. However, if the risk is low or speculative, then proof of benefit may also be unnecessary.

In reality the best information about HDIs will come from case observations and scientific studies, as was the case with St. John's wort. In other words important HDIs will be found by discovery, not by speculation and extrapolation. A proposal for rational use of language is made in Box 6-1.

ADOPTING A RATIONAL PERSPECTIVE

In a review of the scientific literature on HDIs it was reported that:

> This systematic review summarizes the indirect published evidence on this topic. Its results show that numerous suggestions about such interactions exist. Serious doubts, however, remain as to the reliability of this information.... Therefore, more rigorous research is urgently required.[16]

Can the concerned healthcare professional find reliable sources on HDIs? The answer is that although there is no infallible source, some reviews are helpful because they largely report what is reasonable and known and do not speculate excessively (and especially not from a poor knowledge base of phytochemistry or herbal pharmacology).

Recent reviews are recommended: a two-part article in *HerbalGram* (number 49) by Mark Blumenthal,[17] the review in *The Lancet* by Adriane Fugh-Berman that largely reports on known consequences,[18] and the review in *American Family Physician* by Melanie Johns-Cupp.[19]

Tables 6-1 and 6-2 are HDI and drug-herb interaction (DHI) reference tables respectively. The tables are designed to be accurate and responsible and are based on a critical assessment of the available information. In addition, the latter part of this chapter and the various relevant monographs contain a more complete discussion of some of the issues summarised in these tables.

Box **6-1** ❧ A Rational Classification of Potential HDIs

1. **Confirmed** from clinical observation and studies (e.g., St. John's wort and digoxin)
2. **Attributed** from clinical reports
   - Probable
   - Possible
   - Unlikely
3. **Speculated** from the pharmacology of the herb and the drug
   - Probable: based on confirmed pharmacological properties of the herb in humans (e.g., licorice)
   - Possible: based on possible pharmacological effects of the herb in humans
   - Speculative: based on pharmacological effects from animal research involving oral doses that reflect human doses
   - Highly speculative: based on pharmacological properties of the herb or its constituents identified by:
   In vitro research
   Animal research given by injection
   Animal research involving large oral doses
4. **Inaccurate or misleading**
   - Based on mistaken assumptions about the herb, its phytochemistry, the plant part used, or its pharmacological effects

---

As well as referring to reliable sources, much can be gained by observing some simple rules and cautions. These are discussed below.

1. If someone is taking any drug and wishes to take herbs as well, it is best they seek the advice of a professional trained in herbal therapy. Practitioners should ask patients to bring all the drugs they are taking, rather than relying on their anecdotal recall of what drugs they are taking.

2. Some drugs have a narrow therapeutic window: they can become dangerously toxic or ineffective with only relatively small changes in their blood concentrations. They include digoxin, warfarin, antirejection drugs, many anti-HIV drugs, phenytoin, and phenobarbital. The practitioner should exercise great caution when prescribing herbs for patients on these drugs. Even foods can cause trouble: soy milk has been reported as lowering international normalised ratio (INR) values in a patient taking warfarin.[20]

3. If heart, liver, or kidney function is impaired, in the elderly population, pregnant women, or those who have received an organ transplant, or in those with a genetic disorder that disturbs normal biochemical functions, the practitioner should exercise particularly great caution when prescribing herbs for patients taking the aforementioned drugs or any other drugs. Care should also be exercised with patients who exhibit long-term use of laxative herbs or potassium-losing diuretics.

4. It should be recommended that critical drugs be taken at different times of day from herbs (and food) to reduce chemical or pharmacokinetic interactions. They should be separated by at least 1 hour, preferably more.

5. All herbs should be stopped approximately 1 week before surgery (although St. Mary's thistle (milk thistle) may help reduce the toxic aftereffects of anaesthetic drugs).[21]

6. Using reliable sources for HDIs (those that differentiate the known from the speculative), practitioners should apply critical research faculties to understanding the herbal remedies they wish to use or recommend.

Text continued on pg. 82.

Table 6-1　**Potential Herb-Drug Interactions For Common Herbs**

Herb	Drug	Potential interaction	Basis of concern	Recommended action
Andrographis (*Andrographis paniculata*)	Warfarin	May potentiate effect of drug	Clinical study: ex vivo inhibition of platelet aggregation[1]	Monitor (low level of risk)
Astragalus (*Astragalus membranaceus*)	Cyclophosphamide	May reduce effectiveness of drug	Theoretical concern based on in vivo animal studies[2,3]	Monitor (low level of risk)
Berberine-containing herbs (e.g., barberry [*Berberis vulgaris*], Indian barberry [*B. aristata*], golden seal [*Hydrastis canadensis*], Oregon grape [*Mahonia aquifolium*])	Drugs that displace the protein binding of bilirubin (e.g., phenylbutazone)	May potentiate effect of drug on displacing bilirubin	Theoretical concern based on in vivo animal study with berberine (10-20 mg/kg, intraperitoneally)[4]	Monitor (low level of risk)
Betel nut* (see also Tannin-containing herbs)	Neuroleptics	May cause EPS	Case report,[5] although a more recent cross-sectional study found chewing betel did not increase EPS[6]	Monitor (very low level of risk)
Bilberry (*Vaccinium myrtillus*)	Warfarin	Potentiation of bleeding possible at high bilberry doses	Antiplatelet activity observed ex vivo in blood from healthy volunteers after high doses of bilberry (173 mg/day anthocyanins)[7]	Monitor at high doses (>100 mg/day anthocyanins, low level of risk)
Bladderwrack (*Fucus vesiculosus*)	Hyperthyroid medication (e.g., carbimazole)	May decrease effectiveness of drug because of natural iodine content[8]	Theoretical concern, no cases reported	Contraindicated unless under close supervision
	Lithium carbonate	May potentiate effect of drug	Theoretical concern based on iodine content[8]; case reports have linked lithium carbonate alone to hyperthyroidism[9]	Monitor (very low level of risk)

(Continued)

Table 6-1 **Potential Herb-Drug Interactions For Common Herbs—cont'd**

Herb	Drug	Potential interaction	Basis of concern	Recommended action
	Thyroid replacement therapies (e.g., thyroxine)	May add to effect of drug	Theoretical concern linked to a case report in which "kelp" caused hyperthyroidism in a person not taking thyroxine[10]	Monitor (low level of risk)
Bugleweed (*Lycopus virginicus, L. europaeus*)	Radioactive iodine	May interfere with administration of diagnostic procedures using radioactive isotopes[11]	Case report	Contraindicated
	Thyroid hormones	Should not be administered concurrently with preparations containing thyroid hormone[12]	Theoretical concern based on deliberations of German Commission E	Contraindicated
Caffeine-containing herbs (e.g., guarana, cola, maté)	Aspirin	May potentiate effect of drug	Clinical study (caffeine citrate, 120 mg)[13]	Monitor (low level of risk)
	Benzothiadiazines (e.g., diazoxide)	Enhances the plasma renin response to drug	Clinical study (caffeine, 750 mg/day)[14]	Monitor (very low level of risk)
	Carbamazepine	May decrease bioavailability of drug	Clinical study (caffeine, 300 mg)[15]	Monitor (low level of risk)
	Certain quinolone antibiotics (e.g., norfloxacin, ciprofloxacin, enoxacin, clinafloxacin)	May alter the kinetics of drug; plasma concentration of caffeine may increase	Clinical studies[16-20] (caffeine, 100 mg,[16] 220-230 mg[20])	Monitor (very low level of risk)
	Clozapine	Decreased clearance of drug	Clinical trial (caffeine, 400-1000 mg)[21]	Monitor (very low level of risk)
	Disulfiram (alcohol deterrent)	Plasma concentration of caffeine may increase	Clinical study (caffeine)[22]	Monitor (very low level of risk)
	Idrocilamide (muscle relaxant)	Plasma concentration of caffeine may increase	Clinical study (caffeine)[23]	Monitor (very low level of risk)
	Oestrogen-containing oral contraceptive (long-term use)	Plasma concentration of caffeine may increase	Clinical study (caffeine, 162 mg)[24]	Monitor (very low level of risk)
	SSRI (e.g., fluvoxamine)	Plasma concentration of caffeine may increase	Clinical study (caffeine, 200 mg)[25]	Monitor (very low level of risk)
	Theophylline	May reduce metabolism of drug	Clinical study[26] (2-7 cups instant coffee)	Monitor (low level of risk)

Herb	Drug	Effect	Basis	Recommendation
Cardioactive glycoside-containing herbs (e.g., lily of the valley [*Convallaria majalis*], squill [*Urginea maritima*], pheasant's eye [*Adonis vernalis*])	Calcium, quinidine, glucocorticoids (long term), laxatives, saluretics	May potentiate effect of drug and induce side effects	Theoretical concern based on the deliberations of German Commission E (pharmacology of constituents)[12]	Monitor (low level of risk)
Cayenne (*Capsicum* spp.)	ACE inhibitor	Cough induced by topical capsaicin[27]	Theoretical concern because capsaicin depletes substance P	Monitor (very low level of risk)
	Theophylline	Increased absorption and bioavailability[28]	Clinical study	Monitor (low level of risk)
Celery seed (*Apium graveolens*)	Thyroxine	Reduced serum levels of thyroxine[29]	Case reports	Monitor (very low level of risk)
Coleus (*Coleus forskohlii*)	Antiplatelet medication	May potentiate effects of drug	Theoretical concern based on in vivo animal study of standardised Coleus extract and the active constituent forskolin[30]	Monitor (low level of risk)
	Hypotensive medication	May potentiate effects of drug	Theoretical concern based on ability of forskolin to lower blood pressure in vivo[31]	Monitor (low level of risk)
	Prescribed medication	May potentiate effects of drug	Theoretical concern based on ability of forskolin to activate increased intracellular cyclic AMP in vitro[32]	Monitor (low level of risk)
Cranberry (*Vaccinium macrocarpon*)	Warfarin	May potentiate effect of drug	Case reports[33]	Monitor (low level of risk)
Dan shen (*Salvia miltiorrhiza*)	Warfarin	May potentiate effect of drug: increased INR,[34-36] prolonged APTT	Case reports	Contraindicated
Devil's claw (*Harpagophytum procumbens*)	Warfarin	Purpura[37] possibly caused by increased bleeding tendency	One case report with few details; unlikely to occur	Monitor (very low level of risk)

(Continued)

Table 6-1 **Potential Herb-Drug Interactions For Common Herbs—cont'd**

Herb	Drug	Potential interaction	Basis of concern	Recommended action
Diuretic herbs (e.g., horsetail, juniper, corn silk, buchu, uva ursi)	Lithium	May potentiate effect of drug increasing the risk of lithium toxicity	Case study[38]	Monitor (very low level of risk)
Dong quai (*Angelica sinensis*)	Warfarin	May potentiate effect of drug; increased INR and PT;[39] increased INR and widespread bruising[40]	Case reports	Monitor (low level of risk)
Echinacea (*Echinacea angustifolia*, *E. purpurea*, *E. pallida*)	Immunosuppressant medication	May decrease effectiveness of drug[41,42]	Theoretical concern based on immune-enhancing activity; no adverse events reported	Contraindicated
Ephedra (*Ephedra* spp.)	α- and β-adrenergic agonists	Reinforcement of effect	MIMS recommendation[43]	Monitor (medium level of risk)
	Antihypertensive drugs	May negate effect	MIMS recommendation[43]	Monitor (medium level of risk)
	Cardiac glycosides	May cause heart rhythm disturbances	German Commission E recommendation[12]	Monitor (medium level of risk)
	CNS stimulants (e.g., caffeine, amphetamines)	Reinforcement of effect	Theoretical concern	Monitor (low level of risk)
	Ergot alkaloid derivatives and oxytocin	May increase the risk of hypertension	German Commission E recommendation[12]	Monitor (low level of risk)
	Guanethidine	May negate antihypertensive effect	German Commission E and MIMS recommendation[12,43]	Monitor (low level of risk)
	Halothane or cyclopropane	May cause heart rhythm disturbances	German Commission E and MIMS recommendation[12,43]	Monitor (medium level of risk)
	MAO inhibitors	May increase the risk of hypertension	German Commission E and MIMS recommendation[12,43]	Contraindicated
	SSRIs	Potentiation effects possible in regard to serotonin levels	Case report (paroxetine + ephedrine-containing OTC)[44]	Monitor (low level of risk)

Herb	Drug	Effect	Evidence	Recommendation
Fenugreek (*Trigonella foenum-graecum*, see also hypoglycaemic herbs)	Iron	Inhibition of iron absorption	Epidemiological study of preschool children in Ethiopia (plant part and quantity ingested undefined)[45]	In anaemia and when iron supplementation is required, do not take simultaneously with meals or iron supplements
Fibre-containing herbs (e.g., psyllium [*Plantago ovata*, *P. ispaghula*, *P. psyllium*], marshmallow [*Althaea officinalis*], slippery elm [*Ulmus rubra*], combined marshmallow, slippery elm, and psyllium)	Carbamazepine	Decreases plasma concentration of drug	Clinical study (psyllium)[46]	Take at least 2 hr away from medication
	Iron	Slight but significant inhibition of nonhaem iron absorption	Clinical studies[47,48] (*Plantago* spp., 5 g)[47]	In anaemia and when iron supplementation is required, do not take simultaneously with meals or iron supplements
	Lithium	May decrease absorption of drug	Case report (psyllium)[49]; Hydrophilic psyllium may prevent lithium from ionising	Take at least 2 hr away from medication
	Prescribed medication†	May slow or reduce absorption of drugs	Theoretical concern based on absorbent properties of fibre-containing herbs	Take at least 2 hr away from medication
	Riboflavin (vitamin B2)	May decrease absorption of vitamin	Clinical studies (psyllium)[50]	Take at least 2 hr away from medication
Garlic (*Allium sativum*)	Aspirin	Could increase bleeding time[51]	Case reports of increased bleeding tendency with high garlic intake[52-54]	Monitor at doses equivalent to >5 g/day fresh garlic
	HIV protease inhibitors (e.g., saquinavir)	Decreased serum levels of saquinavir[55]	Clinical study	Monitor (medium level of risk)
	Paracetamol	Alteration of metabolism of drug (slight increase in sulphate conjugation); consequences unknown	Clinical study[56]	Monitor (low level of risk)
	Warfarin	May potentiate effect of drug: increased INR observed[57]; large doses could increase bleeding tendency	Case reports of possible interaction[57] and increased bleeding tendency[52-54]	Contraindicated for doses equivalent to >5 g/day fresh garlic unless under close supervision
Ginger (*Zingiber officinale*)	Antacids	May decrease effectiveness of drug	Theoretical concern because ginger increases gastric secretory activity[41]	Monitor (low level of risk)
	Warfarin	Increased risk of spontaneous bleeding	Inhibits platelet aggregation and thromboxane after high doses (5 g/day) in volunteers (no effect at 2 g/day); mechanism reportedly involves inhibition of platelet cyclooxygenase[41]; no cases of adverse interactions reported[58]	Monitor at doses <4 g/day dried ginger; contraindicated unless under close supervision at doses >4 g/day dried ginger

(Continued)

Table 6-1 **Potential Herb-Drug Interactions For Common Herbs—cont'd**

Herb	Drug	Potential interaction	Basis of concern	Recommended action
Ginkgo (*Ginkgo biloba*)	Anticonvulsant medication (e.g., sodium valproate, carbamazepine)	May decrease the effectiveness of drug	Theoretical concern based on in vivo animal studies[59]; two case reports[60]	Monitor (medium level of risk)
	Antiplatelet and anticoagulant drugs (e.g., aspirin, warfarin)	Increased bleeding tendency; ginkgo extract could have clinical antiplatelet activity	Rare case reports of spontaneous bleeding, including concomitant intake of aspirin or warfarin[61-63]; interactions with warfarin and aspirin are not supported by clinical studies[64,65]	Aspirin, monitor (low level of risk); Warfarin, monitor (medium level of risk)
	Haloperidol	May potentiate the efficiency of haloperidol in patients with schizophrenia[66]	Randomised, controlled trial	Prescribe cautiously; reduce drug if necessary in conjunction with prescribing physician
	Rofecoxib	Increased bleeding tendency	Case report[67]	Monitor (low level of risk)
	SSRI (e.g., trazodone)	May increase the function of GABA receptor leading to sedation	Case report in a patient with Alzheimer's disease[68]	Monitor (very low level of risk)
	Thiazide diuretic	May elevate blood pressure	Dubious case report[37]	Monitor (very low level of risk)
Green tea (*Camellia sinensis*, see also Polyphenol- and Tannin-containing herbs)	Warfarin	May decrease effectiveness of drug	One case reported of decreased INR[69]; epidemiological studies have not reported this issue	Monitor (low level of risk)
Guggul (*Commiphora mukul*)	Antiplatelet and anticoagulant drugs (e.g., aspirin, warfarin)	May potentiate effect of drug	Theoretical concern based on possible anticoagulant activity in a clinical trial[70]	Monitor (low level of risk)
	Diltiazem	May reduce plasma concentration of drug	Pharmacokinetic study with ethyl acetate fraction of guggul[71]	Monitor (low level of risk)
	Hyperthyroid medication (e.g., carbimazole)	May reduce the effectiveness of drug	Theoretical based on an in vivo animal study with guggulsterones[72]	Monitor (low level of risk)
	Propranolol	May reduce plasma concentration of drug	Pharmacokinetic study with ethyl acetate fraction of guggul[71]	Monitor (low level of risk)

Herb	Drug	Effect	Comment	Recommendation
Hawthorn (*Crataegus monogyna, C. laevigata, C. oxyacantha*)	β-blockers and other hypotensive drugs	May increase effectiveness of drug	Clinical studies demonstrate hawthorn causes a slight reduction in blood pressure in patients with heart conditions[41]	Monitor (low level of risk)
	Digitalis glycosides	May increase effectiveness of drug	Clinical studies indicate a (beneficial) synergistic effect[73,74]	Monitor (low level of risk)
Hibiscus (*Hibiscus sabdarifa*)	Chloroquine	May decrease bioavailability	Clinical study[75]	Monitor (low level of risk)
Hypoglycaemic herbs (e.g., *Gymnema sylvestre*, goat's rue [*Galega officinalis*], fenugreek [*Trigonella foenum-graecum*])	Hypoglycaemic drugs and insulin	Enhanced reduction of blood glucose	Theoretical concern, no documented case histories	Prescribe cautiously and monitor blood sugar regularly; warn patient about possible hypoglycaemia; reduce drug if necessary in conjunction with prescribing physician
Kava (*Piper methysticum*)	CNS depressants (e.g., alcohol, barbiturates, benzodiazepines)	Potentiation of drug effects	Theoretical concern based on deliberations of German Commission E[12] and the anxiolytic activity of kava[41]; two apparent case reports (kava + benzodiazepines)[76,77]	Monitor (low level of risk)
	L-dopa and other Parkinson's disease treatments	Possible dopamine antagonist effects	Cases suggestive of dopamine antagonism reported[78]	Contraindicated unless under close supervision
Korean ginseng (*Panax ginseng*)	Antihypertensive medications	May decrease effectiveness of drug	Theoretical concern because hypertension is a feature of GAS; clinical significance unclear[41]	Monitor (very low level of risk)
	CNS stimulants	May potentiate effects of drug[41]	Theoretical concern because CNS stimulation is a feature of GAS; clinical significance unclear	Monitor (low level of risk)
	Hypoglycaemics	May potentiate hypoglycaemic activity of drug[42]	Theoretical concern based on clinically observed hypoglycaemic activity of ginseng[79]; clinical significance unclear	Monitor (very low level of risk)
	MAO inhibitors (e.g., phenelzine)	Headache and tremor, mania	Case reports[80,81]	Contraindicated

(Continued)

Table 6-1   **Potential Herb-Drug Interactions For Common Herbs—cont'd**

Herb	Drug	Potential interaction	Basis of concern	Recommended action
	Sildenafil	Potentiation of drug possible	Theoretical concern based on in vitro studies that show ginseng increases nitric oxide release from corpus cavernosum tissue[82,83]	Monitor (very low level of risk)
	Warfarin	May decrease effectiveness of drug: decreased INR reported[84]	One case reported,[84] but clinical significance unclear	Monitor (low level of risk)
Laxative (anthraquinone-containing) herbs (e.g., aloe resin [*Aloe barbadensis*], cascara [*Rhamnus purshiana*], senna [*Cassia* spp.], yellow dock [*Rumex crispus*])	Antiarrhythmic agents	May affect activity if potassium deficiency resulting from long-term laxative abuse is present	German Commission E and ESCOP recommendation[12,85]	Avoid excessive doses of laxatives; maintain patients on a high potassium diet
	Cardiac glycosides	May potentiate activity if potassium deficiency resulting from long-term laxative abuse is present	German Commission E and ESCOP recommendation[12,85]	Monitor (low level of risk at normal doses)
	Potassium depleting agents (e.g., thiazide diuretics, licorice root [*Glycyrrhiza glabra*]	May increase potassium depletion	German Commission E and ESCOP recommendation[12,85]	Avoid excessive doses of laxatives; maintain patients on a high potassium diet
	Prescribed medication	May decrease gastrointestinal transit time and absorption of coadministered agents	Theoretical concern[12,85]	Monitor (very low level of risk at normal doses)
Licorice (*Glycyrrhiza glabra*)	Antihypertensive medications	May decrease effectiveness of drug when consumed in high doses; licorice can cause pseudoaldosteronism, which includes oedema and high blood pressure[41]	Theoretical concern based on case reports of hypertension after intake of licorice-containing confectionery[41]	Avoid long-term use at doses >100 mg/day glycyrrhizin unless under close supervision; place patients on a high potassium diet
	Cortisol	Potentiation of drug possible by inhibition of drug metabolism	Theoretical concern based on pharmacological studies and one early clinical study with the constituent (glycyrrhizin); no observed cases[41]	Monitor (low level of risk)

Herb	Drug/substance	Effect	Evidence	Recommendation
	Digoxin	Excessive licorice intake causes hypokalaemia, which can potentiate the toxicity of the drug[12]	Clinical studies of active constituents and case reports of hypokalaemia from confectionery intake (large doses)[41]; one case report of ingestion of herbal laxative containing licorice (1.2 g/day) and rhubarb (4.8 g/day)[86]	Avoid long-term use at doses >100 mg/day glycyrrhizin unless under close supervision; place patients on a high potassium diet
	Prednisolone	Increases levels of drug by decreasing drug metabolism[41]	Theoretical concern based on clinical studies of oral administration of active constituent glycyrrhizin[87,88]	Monitor (low level of risk)
	Thiazide diuretics and other potassium-depleting drugs	The combined effect of licorice and the drug could result in excessive potassium loss[12]	Clinical studies of active constituents and case reports from confectionery intake (large doses)[41]	Avoid long-term use at doses >100 mg/day glycyrrhizin; place patients on a high potassium diet
Lycium (*Lycium barbarum*)	Warfarin	May potentiate effect of drug, increased INR	Case report[89]	Contraindicated
Meadowsweet (*Filipendula ulmaria*, see also Tannin-containing herbs)	Warfarin	May potentiate effects of drug	Theoretical concern based on in vivo animal studies demonstrating anticoagulant activity[90]	Monitor (low level of risk)
Pau d'Arco (*Tabebuia avellanedae*)	Anticoagulants	May potentiate effect of drug	Theoretical based on prolonged prothrombin time observed in clinical trial of lapachol (>2 g/day); no toxicity seen at doses <1.5 g[91]	Monitor (low level of risk)
Piperine-containing herbs (e.g., long pepper [*Piper longum*], black pepper [*Piper nigrum*])	Prescribed medication	May enhance bioavailability of drug	Clinical studies (piperine, 20 mg)[92,93]	Monitor (low level of risk)
Polyphenolic‡ and flavonoid-containing herbs, especially peppermint (*Mentha x piperita*), pennyroyal	Iron	Inhibition of nonhaem iron§ absorption	Clinical studies[94-98] (polyphenols per serving, ~30 mg[95] and 50-200 mg[94]); results for green tea have been conflicting[99-101]	In anaemia and when iron supplementation is required, do not take simultaneously with meals or iron supplements

(Continued)

Table 6-1   Potential Herb-Drug Interactions For Common Herbs—cont'd

Herb	Drug	Potential interaction	Basis of concern	Recommended action
(Mentha pulegium), vervain (Verbena officinalis), lime flower (Tilia cordata), chamomile (Matricaria recutita), green tea (Camellia sinensis), rosemary (Rosmarinus officinalis); see also Tannin-containing herbs				
Poke root (Phytolacca decandra)	Immunosuppressant medication	May decrease effectiveness of drug	Theoretical concern based on immune-enhancing activity; no adverse events reported	Contraindicated
Saw palmetto (Serenoa spp.)	Warfarin	May potentiate effect of drug: increased INR	Case report[102]	Monitor (low level of risk)
Schisandra (Schisandra chinensis)	Prescribed medication	May accelerate clearance from body	Theoretical concern based on in vivo studies demonstrating enhanced phase I/II hepatic metabolism[103,104]	Monitor (medium level of risk)
Scotch broom (Cytisus scoparius)	MAO inhibitors	May cause an increase in blood pressure	Theoretical based on presence of tyramine[12]	Monitor (very low level of risk)
Siberian ginseng (Eleutherococcus senticosus)	Digoxin	Apparently raised serum concentrations[105]	Herb probably interfered with digoxin assay (patient had unchanged ECG despite apparent digoxin concentration of 5.2 nmol/L)	Monitor (very low level of risk)
St. John's wort (Hypericum perforatum)	Amitriptyline	Decreases drug levels[106]	Clinical study	Monitor (medium level of risk)
	Anticonvulsants (e.g., phenytoin, carbamazepine, phenobarbitone)	May decrease drug levels via CYP induction[107-109]	Theoretical concern; an open clinical trial demonstrated no effect on carbamazepine pharmacokinetics in healthy volunteers[110]	Monitor (low level of risk)

(*Continued*)

Antihistamine (e.g., fexofenadine)	Decreases drug levels[111]	Clinical study	Monitor (medium level of risk)
Benzodiazepines (e.g., midazolam)	Decreases drug levels[112]	Clinical study	Monitor (medium level of risk)
Chemotherapeutic drugs (e.g., irinotecan)	Decreases drug levels[113,114]	Clinical studies	Contraindicated
Combined oral contraceptives	Breakthrough bleeding reported which was attributed to increased metabolism of drug[115,116]	Clinical significance unclear; cases of unwanted pregnancies have been reported[117,118]	Monitor (low level of risk)
Digoxin	Decreases drug levels[119-121] but is dependent on dose of herb[120]	Clinical studies	Contraindicated at doses >1 g/day dried herb
HIV nonnucleoside transcriptase inhibitors (e.g., nevirapine)	Decreases drug levels[122]	Case report	Contraindicated
Immunosuppressives (e.g., cyclosporin)	Decreases drug levels	Case reports[115,123-130] and case series[131,132]	Contraindicated
Other HIV protease inhibitors (e.g., indinavir)	Decreases drug levels[133]	Clinical study	Contraindicated
Phenprocoumon	Decreases plasma drug levels[134]	Clinical study	Contraindicated
Photosensitising agents (e.g., δ-aminolaevulinic acid)‖	Phototoxic reaction (occurred at subphototoxic threshold)	Clinical study (1 case)[135]	Monitor (low level of risk)
Simvastatin¶	Decreases drug levels[136]	Clinical study	Monitor (medium level of risk)
SSRIs (e.g., paroxetine, trazodone, sertraline, and other serotonergic agents, e.g., nefazodone, venlafaxine)	Potentiation effects possible in regard to serotonin levels[137-142]	Clinical significance of case reports unclear	Monitor (very low level of risk)
Theophylline	Decreases drug levels[143]	Case report	Monitor (low level of risk)
Warfarin	Decreases drug levels and INR[116]	Case reports	Contraindicated

Table 6-1   **Potential Herb-Drug Interactions For Common Herbs—cont'd**

Herb	Drug	Potential interaction	Basis of concern	Recommended action
Sweet clover (*Melilotus officinalis*)	Aspirin	Increased bleeding tendency	Theoretical concern because it contains coumarin[144]	Monitor (very low level of risk)
	Warfarin	Increased bleeding tendency	Theoretical concern because it contains coumarin[144]	Monitor (very low level of risk)
Tannin-‡ or OPC-containing herbs (e.g., cranesbill root [*Geranium maculatum*], grape seed extract [*Vitis vinifera*], green tea [*Camellia sinensis*], #St. John's wort [*Hypericum perforatum*], meadowsweet [*Filpendula ulmaria*], hawthorn [*Crataegus* spp.], raspberry leaf [*Rubus idaeus*], peppermint [*Mentha x piperita*], uva ursi [*Arctostaphylos uva-ursi*], willow herb [*Epilobium parviflorum*], willow bark [*Salix* spp.]; see also Polyphenol-containing herbs)	Alkaloids and other alkaline drugs	May reduce absorption	Theoretical concern[12] and based on use as antidotes in cases of alkaloid poisoning[145] and the ability of tannins to precipitate alkaloids	Take at least 2 hr away from medication
	Minerals, especially iron	May reduce absorption of nonhaem iron from food	Clinical studies[94,146-150] (black tea, 2.5 g/150 mL)[146]; cases of iron deficiency/reduced iron absorption: heavy black tea drinkers[151,152] and those ingesting sorghum (0.15% tannins)[153,**]; in a clinical study tea consumption showed a small, nonsignificant adverse effect on zinc bioavailability[154]	Take at least 2 hr away from medication
	Thiamine	May reduce absorption from food	Diet survey[155] and clinical studies,[156,157] tea drinking, tea chewing, betel nut chewing	Take at least 2 hr away from medication

Herb	Drug	Effect	Evidence	Recommendation
Tropane alkaloid-containing herbs (i.e., herbs containing hyoscyamine [atropine] and scopolamine [hyoscine]; e.g., belladonna [*Atropa belladonna*], henbane [*Hyoscyamus niger*], jimson weed [*Datura stramonium*], Scopolia [*Scopolia carniolica*])	Amantadine, quinidine, tricyclic antidepressants	May potentiate (anticholinergic) effect of drug and induce side effects	Theoretical concern based on pharmacology of constituents[12]	Contraindicated
Turmeric (*Curcuma longa*)	Antiplatelet or anticoagulant medications (e.g., aspirin and warfarin)	May potentiate effects of drug	Theoretical concern based on in vitro and in vivo studies mainly of the active constituent curcumin demonstrating antiplatelet activity[41]	Monitor (low level of risk at normal doses); contraindicated in high doses (>15 g/day dried tuber)
Valerian (*Valeriana officinalis*, *V. edulis*)	CNS depressants or alcohol	May potentiate effects of drug	Theoretical concern expressed by US Pharmacopeial Convention; however, a clinical study indicated no potentiation with alcohol[158]	Monitor (very low level of risk)
Willow bark (*Salix alba*, *S. daphnoides*, *S. purpurea*, *S. fragilis*; see also Tannin-containing herbs)	Warfarin	May potentiate effects of drug	Clinical study observed mild but significant antiplatelet activity[159]	Monitor (low level of risk)
Yohimbine-containing herbs (e.g., yohimbe [*Pausinystalia yohimbe*])	Clonidine	May antagonise analgesic effect of drug	Clinical study (yohimbine, 16 mg)[160]	Contraindicated
	Drugs that interfere with neuronal uptake or metabolism of noradrenalin	Increases plasma noradrenalin and produces a pressor response	Extrapolation from clinical study (yohimbine, 21.6 mg)[161]	Monitor (low level of risk)
	Naloxone	Synergistic effect	Clinical study (yohimbine hydrochloride, 15-30 mg)[162]	Contraindicated

(Continued)

Table 6-1 **Potential Herb-Drug Interactions For Common Herbs—cont'd**

Herb	Drug	Potential interaction	Basis of concern	Recommended action
	Tricyclic antidepressants (e.g., desipramine, clomipramine, amitriptyline)	May increase blood pressure and induce side effects	Clinical studies (>4 mg yohimbine)[163-166]	Contraindicated

CODE

Contraindicated: *Do not prescribe the indicated herb.*

Monitor: *Can prescribe the indicated herb but maintain close contact and review the patient's status on a regular basis. Note that where the risk is assessed as medium, self-prescription of the herb in conjunction with the drug is not advisable.*

This herb-drug interaction table covers a more comprehensive range of herbs than the drug-herb interaction table (Table 6-2). This chart contains information the authors believe to be reliable or that has received considerable attention as potential issues. However, many theoretical concerns expressed by other authors have not been included.

*This relates less to herbal medicine and more to lifestyle: betel nut is human's fourth most widely used drug after nicotine, ethanol, and caffeine. "Betel chewing" describes the practice of masticating a quid of ingredients, including the seed of the Areca catechu palm (betel nut), the leaf Piper betle, and lime.[6] Tobacco leaf may also be included.[155]

†Psyllium administration had no effect on digoxin levels in a clinical study.[167]

‡The word tannin has a long-established and extensive usage, although it is considered in more recent years to lack precision. Polyphenol is the preferred term when considering the properties at a molecular level. Plant polyphenols are broadly divisible into proanthocyanidins (condensed tannins) and polyesters based on gallic and/or hexahydroxydiphenic acid and their derivatives (hydrolysable tannins).[148]

§Haem iron is derived from haemoglobin and myoglobin mainly in meat products. Nonhaem iron is derived mainly from cereals, vegetables, and fruits.

∥Used in photodiagnosis and photodynamic therapy.

¶Plasma concentration of pravastatin not affected.

#Green tea did not inhibit iron absorption in two clinical trials involving anaemia patients.[168,169]

**Sorghum also contains phytate. Phytate and polyphenol inhibit nutrients such as iron.[170,171]

ACE, Angiotensin-converting enzyme; AMP, adenosine monophosphate; APTT, activated partial thromboplastin time; CNS, central nervous system; CYP, cytochrome P450; ECG, electrocardiogram/graph; EPS, extrapyramidal symptoms; GABA, γ-aminobutyric acid; GAS, Ginseng abuse syndrome; INR, international normalised ratio; MAO, monoamine oxidase; OTC, over-the-counter pharmaceutical preparation; PT, prothrombin time; SSRI, selective serotonin reuptake inhibitors.

Table 6-1 References

1. Zhang YZ, Tang JZ, Zhang YJ: Zhongguo Zhong Xi Yi Jie He Za Zhi 14:28-30, 34, 35, 1994.
2. Chu DT, Wong WL, Mavligit GM: J Clin Lab Immunol 25:125-129, 1988.
3. Chu DT, Sun Y, Lin JR: Zhong Xi Yi Jie He Za Zhi 9:326, 351-354, 1989.
4. Chan E: Biol Neonate 63:201-208, 1993.
5. Deahl M: Mov Disord 4:330-332, 1989.
6. Sullivan RJ, Allen JS, Otto C, et al: Micronesia, Br J Psychiatry 177:174-178, 2000.
7. Pulliero G, Montin S, Bettini V, et al: Fitoterapia 60:69-75, 1989.
8. de Smet PAGM, Keller K, Hansel R, et al, editors: Adverse effects of herbal drugs, vol 3, Berlin, 1997, Springer-Verlag.
9. Sadoul JL, Kezachian B, Freychet P: Ann Endocrinol (Paris) 54:353-358, 1994.
10. Miller LG: Arch Intern Med 158:2200-2211, 1998.
11. de Smet PAGM, Keller K, Hansel R, et al, editors: Adverse effects of herbal drugs, vol 2, Berlin, 1993, Springer-Verlag.
12. Blumenthal M, et al, editors: The complete German commission E monographs: therapeutic guide to herbal medicines, Austin, 1998, American Botanical Council.

13. *Yoovathaworn KC, Sriwatanakul K, Thithapandha A: Eur J Drug Metab Pharmacokinet 11:71-76, 1986.*
14. *Brown NJ, Porter J, Ryder D, et al: J Pharmacol Exp Ther 256:56-61, 1991.*
15. *Vaz J, Kulkarni C, David J, et al: Indian J Exp Biol 36:112-114, 1998.*
16. *Healy DP, Polk RE, Kanawati L, et al: Antimicrob Agents Chemother 33:474-478, 1989.*
17. *Carbo M, Segura J, de la Torre R, et al: Clin Pharmacol Ther 45:234-240, 1989.*
18. *Harder S, Fuhr U, Staib AH, et al: Am J Med 87:89S-91S, 1989.*
19. *Randinitis EJ, Alvey CW, Koup JR, et al: Antimicrob Agents Chemother 45:2543-2552, 2001.*
20. *Stille W, Harder S, Mieke S, et al: J Antimicrob Chemother 20:729-734, 1987.*
21. *Hagg S, Spigset O, Mjorndal T, et al: Br J Clin Pharmacol 49:59-63, 2000.*
22. *Beach CA, Mays DC, Guiler RC et al: Clin Pharmacol Ther 39:265-270, 1986.*
23. *Brazier JL, Descotes J, Lery N, et al: Eur J Clin Pharmacol 17:37-43, 1980.*
24. *Abernethy DR, Todd EL: Eur J Clin Pharmacol 28:425-428, 1985.*
25. *Jeppesen U, Loft S, Poulsen HE, et al: Pharmacogenetics 6:213-222, 1996.*
26. *Sato J, Nakata H, Owada E, et al: Eur J Clin Pharmacol 44:295-298, 1993.*
27. *Hakas JF Jr: Ann Allergy 65:322-323, 1990.*
28. *Bouraoui A, Toum A, Bouchoucha S, et al: Thérapie 41:467-471, 1986.*
29. *Moses G: Australian Prescriber 24:6, 2001.*
30. *de Souza NJ: J Ethnopharmacol 38:177-180, 1993.*
31. *de Souza NJ, Dohadwalla AN, Reden J: Med Res Rev 3:201-219, 1983.*
32. *Seamon KB, Daly JW: J Cyclic Nucleotide Res 7:201-224, 1981.*
33. *Committee on Safety of Medicines: Curr Prob Pharmacovigilance 29:8, 2003.*
34. *Tam LS, Chan TY, Leung WK, et al: Aust N Z J Med 25:258, 1995.*
35. *Yu CM, Chan JC, Sanderson JE: J Intern Med 241:337-339, 1997.*
36. *Izzat MB, Yim AP, El-Zufari MH: Ann Thorac Surg 66:941-942, 1998.*
37. *Shaw D, Leon C, Kolev S, et al: Drug Saf 17:342-356, 1997.*
38. *Mills S, Bone K: Principles and practice of phytotherapy: modern herbal medicine, Edinburgh, 2000, Churchill Livingstone.*
39. *Pyevich D, Bogenschutz MP: Am J Psychiatry 158:1329, 2001.*
40. *Page RL, Lawrence JD: Pharmacotherapy 19:870-876, 1999.*
41. *Ellis GR, Stephens MR: BMJ 319:650, 1999.*
42. *Newall CA, Anderson LA, Phillipson JD: Herbal medicines—a guide for health-care professionals, London, 1996, Pharmaceutical Press.*
43. *E-MIMS version 4.00.0457. St. Leonards, NSW, Australia, 2000, MIMS Australia Pty Ltd.*
44. *Skop BP, Finkelstein JA, Mareth TR, et al: Am J Emerg Med 12:642-644, 1994.*
45. *Adish AA, Esrey SA, Gyorkos TW, et al: Public Health Nutr 2:243-252, 1999.*
46. *Etman MA: Drug Dev Indust Pharm 21:1901-1906, 1995.*
47. *Rossander L: Scand J Gastroenterol Suppl 129:68-72, 1987.*
48. *Cook JD, Noble NL, Morck TA, et al: Gastroenterology 85:1354-1358, 1983.*
49. *Perlman BB: Lancet 335:416, 1990.*
50. *Roe DA, Kalkwarf H, Stevens J: J Am Diet Assoc 88:211-213, 1988.*
51. *Muller J, Clauson K: Drug Benef Trends 10:33-50, 1998.*
52. *Rose KD, Croissant PD, Parliament CF, et al: Neurosurgery 26:880-882, 1990.*
53. *Burnham BE: Plast Reconstr Surg 95:213, 1995.*
54. *German K, Kumar U, Blackford HN: Br J Urol 76:518, 1995.*

55. Piscitelli SC, Burstein AH, Welden N, et al: 8th Conference on Retroviruses and Opportunistic Infections, Chicago, February 4-7, 2000, abstract 734.
56. Gwilt PR, Lear CL, Tempero MA, et al: Cancer Epidemiol Biomarkers Prev 3:155-160, 1994.
57. Sunter W: Pharm J 246:722, 1991.
58. Vaes LP, Chyka PA: Ann Pharmacother 34:1478-1482, 2000.
59. Manocha A, Pillai KK, Husain SZ: Indian J Pharmacol 28:84-87, 1996.
60. Korth RM: MMW Fortschr Med 143:13, 2001.
61. Rosenblatt M, Mindel J: N Engl J Med 336:1108, 1997.
62. Fessenden JM, Wittenborn W, Clarke L: Am Surg 67:33-35, 2001.
63. Matthews MK Jr: Neurology 50:1933-1934, 1998.
64. Engelsen J, Nielsen JD, Winther K: Thromb Haemost 87:1075-1076, 2002.
65. DeLoughery TG, Kaye JA, Morris CD, et al: Blood 11:3809, 2002 (abstract).
66. Zhang XY, Zhou DF, Su JM, et al: J Clin Psychopharmacol 21:85-88, 2001.
67. Hoffman T: Hawaii Med J 60:290, 2001.
68. Galluzzi S, Zanetti O, Binetti G, et al: J Neurol Neurosurg Psychiatry 68:679-680, 2000.
69. Taylor JR, Wilt VM: Ann Pharmacother 33:426-428, 1999.
70. Satyavati GV: Guggulipid: a promising hypolipidaemic agent from gum guggul (Commiphora wightii). In Wagner H, FarnsWorth NR, editors: Economic and medicinal plant research, vol 5, London, 1991, Academic Press.
71. Dalvi SS, Nayak VK, Pohujani SM, et al: J Assoc Physicians India 42:454-455, 1994.
72. Tripathi SN, Gupta M, Sen SP, et al: Indian J Exp Biol 13:15-18, 1975.
73. Wolkerstorfer H: Munch Med Wochenschr 108:438-441, 1966.
74. Jaursch U, Lander E, Schmidt R, et al: Med Welt 27:1547-1552, 1969.
75. Mahmoud BM, Ali HM, Homeida MM, et al: J Antimicrob Chemother 33:1005-1009, 1994.
76. Almeida JC, Grimsley EW: Ann Intern Med 125:940-941, 1996.
77. Cartledge A, Rutherford J: Rapid response (electronic letter), BMJ Feb 2001. Available at: bmj.com/cgi/eletters/322/7279/139#12643. Assessed February 21, 2002.
78. Schelosky L, Raffauf C, Jendroska K, et al: J Neurol Neurosurg Psychiatry 58:639-640, 1995.
79. Sotaniemi EA, Haapakoski E, Rautio A: Diabetes Care 18:1373-1375, 1995.
80. Jones BD, Runikis AM: J Clin Psychopharmacol 7:201-202, 1987.
81. Shader RI, Greenblatt DJ: J Clin Psychopharmacol 8:235, 1988.
82. Gillis CN: Biochem Pharmacol 54:1-8, 1997.
83. Kim HJ, Woo DS, Lee G, et al: Br J Urol 82:744-748, 1998.
84. Janetzky K, Morreale AP: Am J Health Syst Pharm 54:692-693, 1997.
85. Scientific Committee of ESCOP (European Scientific Cooperative on Phytotherapy): ESCOP monographs (Aloe capensis, Rhamni purshiani cortex, Sennae folium, Sennae fructus acutifoliae, Sennae fructus angustifoliae), Devon, UK, 1997, European Scientific Cooperative on Phytotherapy.
86. Harada T, Ohtaki E, Misu K, et al: Cardiology 98:218, 2002.
87. Chen MF, Shimada F, Kato H, et al: Endocrinol Jpn 38:167-174, 1991.
88. Chen MF, Shimada F, Kato H, et al: Endocrinol Jpn 37:331-341, 1990.
89. Lam AY, Elmer GW, Mohutsky MA: Ann Pharmacother 35:1199-1201, 2001.
90. Liapina LA, Koval'chuk GA: Izv Akad Nauk Ser Biol Jul-Aug:625-628, 1993.
91. Block JB, Serpeck AA, Miller W, et al: Cancer Chemother Rep 2 4:27-28, 1974.
92. Bano G, Raina RK, Zutshi U, et al: Eur J Clin Pharmacol 41:615-617, 1991.
93. Shoba G, Joy D, Joseph T, et al: Planta Med 64:353-356, 1998.

94. Hurrell RF, Reddy M, Cook JD: Br J Nutr 81:289-295, 1999.
95. Samman S, Sandstrom B, Toft MB, et al: Am J Clin Nutr 73:607-612, 2001.
96. Tuntawiroon M, Sritongkul N, Brune M, et al: Am J Clin Nutr 53:554-557, 1991.
97. Cook JD, Reddy MB, Hurrell RF: Am J Clin Nutr 61:800-804, 1995.
98. Morck TA, Lynch SR, Cook JD: Am J Clin Nutr 37:416-420, 1983.
99. Prystai EA, Kies CV, Driskell JA: Nutr Res 19:167-177, 1999.
100. Kubota K, Sakurai T, Nakazato K, et al: Nippon Ronen Igakkai Zasshi 27:555-558, 1990.
101. Mitamura T, Kitazono M,Yoshimura O, et al: Nippon Sanka Fujinka Gakkai Zasshi 41:688-694, 1989.
102. Yue QY, Jansson K: J Am Geriatr Soc 49:838, 2001.
103. Ko KM, Ip SP, Poon MK, et al: Planta Med 61:134-137, 1995.
104. Lu H, Liu GT: Zhongguo Yao Li Xue Bao 11:331-335, 1990.
105. McRae S: CMAJ 155:293-295, 1996.
106. Johne A, Schmider J, Brockmoller J, et al: J Clin Psychopharmacol 22:46-54, 2002.
107. Australian Therapeutic Goods Administration. Media release, March 2000.
108. Breckenridge A: Message from Committee on Safety of Medicines, London, 2000, Medicines Control Agency.
109. Henney JE: JAMA 283:1679, 2000.
110. Burstein AH, Horton RL, Dunn T, et al: Clin Pharmacol Ther 68:605-612, 2000.
111. Wang Z, Hamman MA, Huang SM, et al: Clin Pharmacol Ther 71:414-420, 2002.
112. Wang Z, Gorski JC, Hamman MA, et al: Clin Pharmacol Ther 70:317-326, 2001.
113. Mathijssen RH,Verweij J, de Bruijn P, et al: J Natl Cancer Inst 94:1247-1249, 2002.
114. Mansky PJ, Straus SE: J Natl Cancer Inst 94:1187-1188, 2002.
115. Bon S, Hartmann K, Kuhn M: Schweiz Apoth 16:535-536, 1999.
116. Yue QY, Bergquist C, Gerden B: Lancet 355:576-577, 2000.
117. Information from the MPA (Medical Products Agency, Sweden) and the MCA (Medicines Control Agency, UK). Information on file MediHerb Pty Ltd,Warwick, Australia.
118. Schwarz UI, Buschel B, Kirch W: Br J Clin Pharmacol 55:112-113, 2003.
119. Johne A, Brockmoller J, Bauer S, et al: Clin Pharmacol Ther 66:338-345, 1999.
120. Uehleke B, Mueller SC, Uehleke B, et al: Phytomed 7(suppl 2):20, 2000.
121. Durr D, Stieger B, Kullak-Ublick GA, et al: Clin Pharmacol Ther 68:598-604, 2000.
122. de Maat MMR, Hoetelmans RMW, Mathot RAA, et al: AIDS 15:420-421, 2001.
123. Ahmed SM, Banner NR, Dubrey SW: J Heart Lung Transplant 20:795, 2001.
124. Ruschitzka F, Meier PJ, Turina M, et al: Lancet 355:548-549, 2000.
125. Mai I, Kruger H, Budde K, et al: Int J Clin Pharmacol Ther 38:500-502, 2000.
126. Karliova M, Treichel U, Malago M, et al: J Hepatol 33:853-855, 2000.
127. Rey JM,Walter G: Med J Aust 169:583-586, 1998.
128. Barone GW, Gurley BJ, Ketel BL, et al: Transplantation 71:239-241, 2001.
129. Barone GW, Gurley BJ, Ketel BL, et al: Ann Pharmacother 34:1013-1016, 2000.
130. Moschella C, Jaber BL: Am J Kidney Dis 38:1105-1107, 2001.
131. Beer AM, Ostermann T: Med Klin (Munich) 96:480-483, 2001.
132. Breidenbach T, Kliem V, Burg M, et al: Transplantation 69:2229-2230, 2000.
133. Piscitelli SC, Burstein AH, Chaitt D, et al: Lancet 355:547-548, 2000.

134. Maurer A, Johne A, Bauer S, et al: Eur J Clin Pharmacol 55:22, 1999 (abstract).
135. Ladner DP, Klein SD, Steiner RA, et al: Br J Dermatol 144:916-918, 2001.
136. Sugimoto K, Ohmori M, Tsuruoka S, et al: Clin Pharmacol Ther 70:518-524, 2001.
137. Gordon JB: Am Fam Physician 57:950, 953, 1998.
138. Demott K: Clin Psychiatry News 26:28, 1998.
139. Barbenel DM, Yasufi B, O'Shea D, et al: J Psychopharmacol 14:84-86, 2000.
140. Lantz MS, Buchalter E, Giambanco V: J Geriatr Psychiatry Neurol 12:7-10, 1999.
141. Prost N, Tichadou L, Rodor F, et al: Presse Med 29:1285-1286, 2000.
142. Waksman JC, Heard K, Jolliff H, et al: Clin Toxicol 38:521, 2000.
143. Nebel A, Schneider BJ, Baker RK, et al: Ann Pharmacother 33:502, 1999.
144. Harder S, Thurmann P: Clin Pharmacokinet 30:416-444, 1996.
145. Pharmaceutical Society of Great Britain: British Pharmaceutical Codex 1934, London, 1941, The Pharmaceutical Press.
146. Rossander L, Hallberg L, Bjorn-Rasmussen E: Am J Clin Nutr 32:2484-2489, 1979.
147. Disler PB, Lynch SR, Charlton RW, et al: Gut 16:193-200, 1975.
148. Haslam E, Lilley TH: Crit Rev Food Sci Nutr 27:1-40, 1988.
149. Derman D, Sayers M, Lynch SR, et al: Br J Nutr 38:261-269, 1977.
150. Merhav H, Amitai Y, Palti H, et al: Am J Clin Nutr 41:1210-1213, 1985.
151. Zijp IM, Korver O, Tijburg LB: Crit Rev Food Sci Nutr 40:371-398, 2000.
152. Gabrielli GB, De Sandre G: Haematologica 80:518-520, 1995.
153. Chung KT, Wong TY, Wei CI, et al: Crit Rev Food Sci Nutr 38:421-464, 1998.
154. Ganji V, Kies CV: Plant Foods Hum Nutr 46:267-276, 1994.
155. Vimokesant SL, Hilker DM, Nakornchai S, et al: Am J Clin Nutr 28:1458-1463, 1975.
156. Vimokesant SL, Nakornchai S, Dhanamitta S, et al: Nutr Rep Int 9:371-376, 1974.
157. Wang RS, Kies C: Plant Foods Hum Nutr 41:337-353, 1991.
158. Herberg KW: Therapiewoche 44:704-713, 1994.
159. Krivoy N, Pavlotzky E, Chrubasik S, et al: Planta Med 67:209-212, 2001.
160. Liu N, Bonnet F, Delaunay L, et al: Br J Anaesth 70:515-518, 1993.
161. Grossman E, Rosenthal T, Peleg E, et al: J Cardiovasc Pharmacol 22:22-26, 1993.
162. Charney DS, Heninger GR: Arch Gen Psychiatry 43:1037-1041, 1986.
163. Charney DS, Price LH, Heninger GR: Arch Gen Psychiatry 43:1155-1161, 1986.
164. Lacomblez L, Bensimon G, Isnard F, et al: Clin Pharmacol Ther 45:241-251, 1989.
165. Bagheri H, Picault P, Schmitt L, et al: Br J Clin Pharmacol 37:93-96, 1994.
166. Bagheri H, Schmitt L, Berlan M, et al: Br J Clin Pharmacol 34:555-558, 1992.
167. Nordstrom M, Melander A, Robertsson E, et al: Drug Nutr Interact 5:67-69, 1987.
168. Mitamura T, Kitazono M, Yoshimura O, et al: Nippon Sanka Fujinka Gakkai Zasshi 41:688-694, 1989.
169. Kubota K, Sakurai T, Nakazato K, et al: Nippon Ronen Igakkai Zasshi 27:555-558, 1990.
170. Lynch SR: Nutr Rev 55:102-110, 1997.
171. Gillooly M, Bothwell TH, Charlton RW, et al: Br J Nutr 51:37-46, 1984.

Table **6–2**   **Potential Drug-Herb Interactions For Common Medicines**

Drug	Herb	Potential interaction	Basis of concern	Recommended action
ANTICOAGULANTS				
Aspirin	Garlic (*Allium sativum*)	Could increase bleeding time[1]	Antiplatelet and fibrinolytic activities of garlic	Monitor at doses >5 g/day fresh garlic
	Ginkgo (*Ginkgo biloba*)	Antiplatelet activity caused by PAF antagonism[2]	Rare case report of spontaneous bleeding[3]	Monitor (low level of risk)
	Dan shen (*Salvia miltiorrhiza*)	Displaces salicylate-protein binding thus increasing free salicylate levels[4]	In vitro study	Monitor (low level of risk)
Phenprocoumon	St. John's wort (*Hypericum perforatum*)	Decrease in free levels of drug[5]	Clinical trial	Contraindicated
Warfarin	Bilberry (*Vaccinium myrtillus*)	Potentiation of effects of drug possible at high bilberry doses	Antiplatelet activity observed for high doses of bilberry in human volunteers[6]	Monitor at high doses (>100 mg/day anthocyanins, low level of risk)
	Dan shen (*Salvia miltiorrhiza*)	Increased INR, prolonged PT/PTT[7-9]	Decreased elimination of warfarin in vivo[10], cases reported[7-9]	Contraindicated
	Devil's claw (*Harpagophytum procumbens*)	Purpura[11]	One case history; unlikely to occur	Monitor (very low level of risk)
	Dong quai (*Angelica sinensis*)	Increased INR and widespread bruising	Case reports[12,13]	Contraindicated
	Garlic (*Allium sativum*)	Large doses could increase INR	Reports of possible interaction[14] and increased bleeding tendency[15-17]	Contraindicated for doses >5 g/day fresh garlic equivalent unless under close supervision
	Ginger (*Zingiber officinalis*)	Increased risk of spontaneous bleeding	Decreased platelet aggregation after high doses reported caused by inhibition of platelet cyclooxygenase products[18]; ginger also inhibits thromboxane synthetase in vitro[19]; no adverse interactions reported	Monitor at doses <4 g/day dried ginger; contraindicated unless under close supervision at doses >4 g/day dried ginger
	Ginkgo (*Ginkgo biloba*)	Increased risk of spontaneous bleeding	Case report[20]	Monitor (medium level of risk)

(Continued)

Table 6-2   **Potential Drug-Herb Interactions For Common Medicines—cont'd**

Drug	Herb	Potential interaction	Basis of concern	Recommended action
	Korean ginseng (*Panax ginseng*)	Decreased effects of drug possible,[1] decreased INR reported[21]	One case reported[21]; clinical significance unclear because of conflicting evidence[22]	Monitor (low level of risk)
	Pau d'Arco (*Tabebuia avellanedae*)	Potentiates anticoagulant effect as naphthoquinones have warfarin-like activity[1]	Theoretical concern, no case reports	Contraindicated unless under close supervision
	St. John's wort (*Hypericum perforatum*)	Decreases INR[23]	Case reports	Contraindicated
	Miscellaneous	Report of increased bleeding time with use of boldo-fenugreek mixture[24] and with a Chinese herb mixture[25]	Case report	Monitor (medium level of risk)
ANTICONVULSANTS/ ANTIEPILEPTICS	St. John's wort (*Hypericum perforatum*)	Decreases drug levels via CYP450 induction[26-28]	Theoretical concern, although an open trial found no effect on carbamazepine pharmacokinetics[29]	Monitor (low level of risk)
ANTIDEPRESSANTS				
Lithium	Psyllium (*Plantago ovata*)	Decreased lithium concentrations[30]	Case report; hydrophilic psyllium may prevent lithium from ionising	Take psyllium at least 2 hr away from medication
Monoamine oxidase inhibitors	Korean ginseng (*Panax ginseng*)	Headache and tremor, mania	Case reports[31,32]	Contraindicated
SSRIs and other serotonergic agents	St. John's wort (*Hypericum perforatum*)	Potentiation effects possible in regards to serotonin levels[33-38]	Theoretical concern; clinical significance of case reports unclear	Monitor (very low level of risk)

Drug	Herb	Effect	Comment	Recommendation
Tricyclic antidepressants	Yohimbe (*Pausinystalia yohimbe*)	Hypertension[39]	Yohimbine alone can cause hypertension (e.g., 15-21.6 mg),[40,41] but lower doses (>4 mg) cause hypertension when combined with tricyclic antidepressants[39,42-44]; hypotensive effect is stronger in hypertensive than normotensive individuals[45]	Contraindicated
ANTI-HIV DRUGS				
HIV nonnucleoside transcriptase inhibitors	St. John's wort (*Hypericum perforatum*)	Likely to decrease drug levels[46]	Case report	Contraindicated
Indinavir and other HIV protease inhibitors	St. John's wort (*Hypericum perforatum*)	Decreases drug levels[47]	Clinical study	Contraindicated
ANTIHYPERTENSIVES				
	Guarana (*Paullinia cupana*)	May decrease effectiveness of drug	CNS stimulant effects of caffeine; no cases reported	Monitor (low level of risk)
	Korean ginseng (*Panax ginseng*)	May decrease effectiveness of drug	Theoretical concern, clinical significance unclear[18]	Monitor (very low level of risk)
	Licorice (*Glycyrrhiza glabra*)	May decrease effectiveness of drug when used >4-6 weeks in high doses; can result in pseudoaldosteronism, oedema, inhibition of renin-angiotensin system → elevation in blood pressure[18]	Theoretical concern based on case reports of hypertension following intake of licorice-containing confectionery	Avoid long-term use (> 4-6 wk) at doses >100 mg/day glycyrrhizin unless under close supervision; place patients on a high potassium diet
ACE inhibitor	Cayenne (*Capsicum* spp.)	Cough induced by topical capsaicin[48]	Theoretical concern because capsaicin depletes substance P	Monitor (very low level of risk)

(Continued)

Table 6–2 **Potential Drug-Herb Interactions For Common Medicines—cont'd**

Drug	Herb	Potential interaction	Basis of concern	Recommended action
ANTIVIRALS				
Acyclovir	St. John's wort (*Hypericum perforatum*)	Effective dose lowered[49]	Case report (of uncertain relevance)	Monitor (low level of risk); be prepared to reduce dose or shorten treatment
CNS AGENTS				
Benzodiazepines and other CNS depressants	Kava (*Piper methysticum*)	Possible increase in tranquillising effects[50,51]	Two apparent case reports[50,52]	Monitor (low level of risk)
CNS stimulants	Korean ginseng (*Panax ginseng*)	May potentiate effects of drug if used at excessive doses[18]	Theoretical concern, clinical significance unclear	Monitor (low level of risk)
L-dopa and other Parkinson's disease treatments	Kava (*Piper methysticum*)	Possible dopamine antagonist effects	Cases suggestive of dopamine antagonism reported[53,54]	Contraindicated unless under close supervision
DIGOXIN				
	Siberian ginseng (*Eleutherococcus senticosus*)	Raised digoxin concentrations[55]	Herb probably interfered with digoxin assay (patient had unchanged ECG despite apparent digoxin concentration of 5.2 nmol/L)	Monitor (very low level of risk)
	Laxative herbs (e.g., senna, cascara, aloe resin)	Enhanced digoxin toxicity caused by potassium depletion possible if long-term laxative abuse is present	Theoretical concern, no documented case histories	Monitor (low level of risk at normal doses)
	Licorice (*Glycyrrhiza glabra*)	May increase patient's sensitivity to drug with long-term use >4-6 weeks at high doses because of hypokalaemic side effects	Case reports[18,56]	Avoid long-term use at doses >100 mg/day glycyrrhizin unless under close supervision; place patients on a high potassium diet.
	St. John's wort (*Hypericum perforatum*)	Decreases drug levels[57-59] but is dependent on dose of herb[58]	Clinical studies	Contraindicated at doses >1 g/day dried herb

	Herb	Effect	Evidence	Recommendation
DIURETICS				
Loop diuretics	Korean ginseng (*Panax ginseng*)	Hypertensive effects	Case report (possible causality at best)[60]	Monitor (very low level of risk)
Thiazide diuretics	Laxative herbs (e.g., senna, cascara, aloe resin)	Aggravated loss of potassium	Theoretical concern, no documented case histories	Avoid excessive doses of laxatives; maintain patients on a high potassium diet
	Licorice (*Glycyrrhiza glabra*)	Increases urinary excretion of potassium, increased risk of developing hypokalaemia[61]	Case reports from confectionery intake[18,62-64]	Avoid long-term use at doses >100 mg/day glycyrrhizin; place patients on a high potassium diet
IMMUNOSUPPRESSANTS				
	Echinacea (*Echinacea angustifolia, E. purpurea, E. pallida*)	May decrease effectiveness of drug[1,65]	Theoretical based on immune-enhancing activity of echinacea; no adverse cases reported	Contraindicated
Cyclosporin	St. John's wort (*Hypericum perforatum*)	Decreases serum levels via CYP450 induction[66] or P-glycoprotein	Case reports[66-74] and case series[75,76]	Contraindicated
IRON SUPPLEMENTS				
	Various herb teas containing polyphenolics, flavonoids, and tannins, especially coffee and black tea	Reduction in absorption of iron supplements and absorption of nonhaem iron from food	Clinical studies[77-88]	In anaemia and when iron supplementation is required, do not take simultaneously with meals or iron supplements
INSULIN/ HYPOGLYCAEMICS				
	High-fibre herbs (e.g., psyllium, isphagula, linseed [flaxseed])	May reduce need for insulin,[89,90] although the effect depends on the fibre ingested	Clinical trials	Monitor (low level of risk)
	Hypoglycaemic herbs (e.g., karela, Gymnema, goat's rue, fenugreek)	Enhanced reduction of blood glucose	Theoretical concern, no documented case histories	Prescribe cautiously and monitor blood sugar regularly; warn patient about possible hypoglycaemia; reduce drug if necessary in conjunction with prescribing physician

(Continued)

Table 6-2   **Potential Drug-Herb Interactions For Common Medicines—cont'd**

Drug	Herb	Potential interaction	Basis of concern	Recommended action
	Korean ginseng (*Panax ginseng*)	May potentiate hypoglycaemic effects[65]	Theoretical concern, clinical significance unclear	Monitor (very low level of risk)
ORAL CONTRACEPTIVES	St. John's wort (*Hypericum perforatum*)	Breakthrough bleeding reported in rare case reports[23,67]	Clinical significance unclear; cases of unwanted pregnancies have been reported[91,92]	Monitor (low level of risk)
SILDENAFIL	Korean ginseng (*Panax ginseng*)	Potentiation effects of drug possible	Theoretical concern; herb shown to increase NO release from corpus cavernosum[93-96]	Monitor (very low level of risk)
STEROIDS	Licorice (*Glycyrrhiza glabra*)	Increases levels of drug by decreasing plasma clearance[18]	Pharmacological studies in humans[97,98]	Monitor (low level of risk)
THEOPHYLLINE	Cayenne (*Capsicum spp.*)	Increased absorption and bioavailability[99]	Clinical study	Monitor (low level of risk)
	St. John's wort (*Hypericum perforatum*)	Decreases drug levels via CYP450 induction[100]	Case report	Monitor (low level of risk)
UV AND PSORALEN THERAPY	St. John's wort (*Hypericum perforatum*)	Possible increased sensitivity to UV light	Theoretical concern	Monitor (medium level of risk); avoid in high doses during UV treatment
	Umbelliferous plants rich in furanocoumarins (e.g., *Angelica spp.*, carrot)	Possible increased sensitivity to UV light	Theoretical concern	Monitor (low level of risk); avoid in high doses during UV treatment

ACE, Angiotensin-converting enzyme; CNS, central nervous system; CYP, cytochrome P450; ECG, electrocardiogram/graph; INR, international normalised ratio; PAF, platelet activating factor; PT, prothrombin time; PTT, partial thromboplastin time; SSRI, selective serotonin reuptake inhibitor.

Table 6-2 References

1. Muller J, Clauson K: Drug BenefTrends 10:33-50, 1998.

2. *Miller LG: Arch Intern Med 158:2200-2211, 1998.*
3. *Rosenblatt M, Mindel J: N Engl J Med 336:1108, 1997.*
4. *Gupta D, Jalali M, Wells A, et al: J Clin Lab Anal 16:290-294, 2002.*
5. *Maurer A, Johne A, Bauer S, et al: Eur J Clin Pharmacol 55:22, 1999 (abstract).*
6. *Pulliero G, Montin S, Bettini V, et al: Fitoterapia 60:69-75, 1989.*
7. *Tam LS, Chan TY, Leung WK, et al: Aust N Z J Med 25:258, 1995.*
8. *Yu CM, Chan JC, Sanderson JE: J Intern Med 241:337-339, 1997.*
9. *Izzat MB, Yim AP, El-Zufari MH: Ann Thorac Surg 66:941-942, 1998.*
10. *Chan K, Lo AC, Yeung JH, et al: J Pharm Pharmacol 47:402-406, 1995.*
11. *Shaw D, Leon C, Kolev S, et al: Drug Saf 17:342-356, 1997.*
12. *Pyevich D, Bogenschutz MP: Am J Psychiatry 158:1329, 2001.*
13. *Page RL, Lawrence JD: Pharmacotherapy 19:870-876, 1999.*
14. *Sunter W: Pharm J 246:722, 1991.*
15. *Rose KD, Croissant PD, Parliament CF, et al: Neurosurgery 26:880-882, 1990.*
16. *Burnham BE: Plast Reconstr Surg 95:213, 1995.*
17. *German K, Kumar U, Blackford HN: Br J Urol 76:518, 1995.*
18. *Ellis GR, Stephens MR: BMJ 319:650, 1999.*
19. *Srivastava KC: Biomed Biochim Acta 43:S335-346, 1984.*
20. *Matthews MK Jr: Neurology 50:1933-1934, 1998.*
21. *Janetzky K, Morreale AP: Am J Health Syst Pharm 54:692-693, 1997.*
22. *Coon JT, Ernst E: Drug Saf 25:323-344, 2002.*
23. *Yue QY, Bergquist C, Gerden B: Lancet 355:576-577, 2000.*
24. *Lambert JP, Cormier A: Pharmacotherapy 21:509-512, 2001.*
25. *Wong AL, Chan TY: Ann Pharmacother 37:836-838, 2003.*
26. *Australian Therapeutic Goods Administration. Media release, March 2000.*
27. *Breckenridge A: Message from Committee on Safety of Medicines, London, 2000, Medicines Control Agency.*
28. *Henney JE: JAMA 283:1679, 2000.*
29. *Burstein AH, Horton RL, Dunn T, et al: Clin Pharmacol Ther 68:605-612, 2000.*
30. *Perlman BB: Lancet 335:416, 1990.*
31. *Jones BD, Runikis AM: J Clin Psychopharmacol 7:201-202, 1987.*
32. *Shader RI, Greenblatt DJ: J Clin Psychopharmacol 8:235, 1988.*
33. *Gordon JB: Am Fam Physician 57:950, 953, 1998.*
34. *Demott K: Clin Psychiatry News 26:28, 1998.*
35. *Barbenel DM, Yusufi B, O'Shea D, et al: J Psychopharmacol 14:84-86, 2000.*
36. *Lantz MS, Buchalter E, Giambanco V: J Geriatr Psychiatry Neurol 12:7-10, 1999.*
37. *Prost N, Tichadou L, Rodor F, et al: Presse Med 29:1285-1286, 2000.*
38. *Waksman JC, Heard K, Jolliff H, et al: Clin Toxicol 38:521, 2000.*
39. *Lacomblez L, Bensimon G, Isnard F, et al: Clin Pharmacol Ther 45:241-251, 1989.*
40. *Lynch SR: Nutr Rev 55:102-110, 1997.*
41. *Charney DS, Heninger GR, Sternberg DE: Life Sci 30:2033-2041, 1982.*

42. Charney DS, Price LH, Heninger GR: Arch Gen Psychiatry 43:1155-1161, 1986.
43. Bagheri H, Picault P, Schmitt L, et al: Br J Clin Pharmacol 37:93-96, 1994.
44. Bagheri H, Schmitt L, Berlan M, et al: Br J Clin Pharmacol 34:555-558, 1992.
45. de Smet PAGM, Keller K, Hansel R, et al, editors: Adverse effects of herbal drugs, vol 3, Berlin, 1997, Springer-Verlag.
46. de Maat MMR, Hoetelmans RMW, Mathot RAA, et al: AIDS 15:420-421, 2001.
47. Piscitelli SC, Burstein AH, Chaitt D, et al: Lancet 355:547-548, 2000.
48. Hakas JF Jr: Ann Allergy 65:322-323, 1990.
49. Report from German Bundesinstitut für Arzneimittel und Medizinprodukte (BfArM).
50. Almeida JC, Grimsley EW: Ann Intern Med 125:940-941, 1996.
51. Herberg KW, Winter U: 2nd International Congress on Phytomedicine, Munich, September 11-14, 1996, P-77.
52. Cartledge A, Rutherford J: Rapid response (electronic letter), BMJ Feb 2001. Available at: bmj.com/cgi/eletters/322/7279/139#12643. Assessed February 21, 2002.
53. Schelosky L, Raffauf C, Jendroska K, et al: J Neurol Neurosurg Psychiatry 58:639-640, 1995.
54. Izzo AA, Ernst E: Drugs 61:2163-2175, 2001.
55. McRae S: CMAJ 155:293-295, 1996.
56. Harada T, Ohtaki E, Misu K, et al: Cardiology 98:218, 2002.
57. Johne A, Brockmoller J, Bauer S, et al: Clin Pharmacol Ther 66:338-345, 1999.
58. Uehleke B, Mueller SC, Uehleke B, et al: Phytomed 7(suppl 2):20, 2000.
59. Durr D, Stieger B, Kullak-Ublick GA, et al: Clin Pharmacol Ther 68:598-604, 2000.
60. Becker BN, Greene J, Evanson J, et al: JAMA 276:606-607, 1996.
61. Blumenthal M, et al, editors: The complete German commission E monographs: therapeutic guide to herbal medicines, Austin, 1998, American Botanical Council.
62. Heidemann HT, Kreuzfelder E: Klin Wochenschr 61:303-305, 1983.
63. Chataway SJ, Mumford CJ, Ironside JW: Postgrad Med J 73:593-594, 1997.
64. Folkersen L, Knudsen NA, Teglbjaerg PS: Ugeskr Laeger 158:7420-7421, 1996.
65. Newall CA, Anderson LA, Phillipson JD: Herbal medicines—a guide for health-care professionals, London, 1996, Pharmaceutical Press.
66. Ruschitzka F, Meier PJ, Turina M, et al: Lancet 355:548-549, 2000.
67. Bon S, Hartmann K, Kuhn M: Schweiz Apoth 16:535-536, 1999.
68. Ahmed SM, Banner NR, Dubrey SW: J Heart Lung Transplant 20:795, 2001.
69. Mai I, Kruger H, Budde K, et al: Int J Clin Pharmacol Ther 38:500-502, 2000.
70. Karliova M, Treichel U, Malago M, et al: J Hepatol 33:853-855, 2000.
71. Rey JM, Walter G: Med J Aust 169:583-586, 1998.
72. Barone GW, Gurley BJ, Ketel BL, et al: Transplantation 71:239-241, 2001.
73. Barone GW, Gurley BJ, Ketel BL, et al: Ann Pharmacother 34:1013-1016, 2000.
74. Moschella C, Jaber BL: Am J Kidney Dis 38:1105-1107, 2001.
75. Beer AM, Ostermann T: Med Klin (Munich) 96:480-483, 2001.
76. Breidenbach T, Kliem V, Burg M, et al: Transplantation 69:2229-2230, 2000.
77. Hurrell RF, Reddy M, Cook JD: Br J Nutr 81:289-295, 1999.
78. Samman S, Sandstrom B, Toft MB, et al: Am J Clin Nutr 73:607-612, 2001.
79. Tuntawiroon M, Sritongkul N, Brune M, et al: Am J Clin Nutr 53:554-557, 1991.
80. Cook JD, Reddy MB, Hurrell RF: Am J Clin Nutr 61:800-804, 1995.

81. *Morck TA, Lynch SR, Cook JD: Am J Clin Nutr 37:416-420, 1983.*

82. *Rossander L, Hallberg L, Bjorn-Rasmussen E: Am J Clin Nutr 32:2484-2489, 1979.*

83. *Disler PB, Lynch SR, Charlton RW, et al: Gut 16:193-200, 1975.*

84. *Haslam E, Lilley TH: Crit Rev Food Sci Nutr 27:1-40, 1988.*

85. *Derman D, Sayers M, Lynch SR, et al: Br J Nutr 38:261-269, 1977.*

86. *Merhav H, Amitai Y, Palti H, et al: Am J Clin Nutr 41:1210-1213, 1985.*

87. *Zijp IM, Korver O, Tijburg LB: Crit Rev Food Sci Nutr 40:371-398, 2000.*

88. *Gabrielli GB, De Sandre G: Haematologica 80:518-520, 1995.*

89. *Capani F, Consoli A, Del Pont A, et al: IRCS J Med Sci 8:661, 1980.*

90. *Vaaler S, Hanssen KF, Aagenaes O: Acta Med Scand 208:389-391, 1980.*

91. *Information from the MPA (Medical Products Agency, Sweden) and the MCA (Medicines Control Agency, UK). Information on file MediHerb Pty Ltd, Warwick, Australia.*

92. *Schwarz UI, Buschel B, Kirch W: Br J Clin Pharmacol 55:112-113, 2003.*

93. *Gillis CN: Biochem Pharmacol 54:1-8, 1997.*

94. *Kim HJ, Woo DS, Lee G, et al: Br J Urol 82:744-748, 1998.*

95. *Choi YD, Xin ZC, Choi HK: Int J Impot Res 10:37-43, 1998.*

96. *Choi HK, Seong DH, Rha KH: Int J Impot Res 7:181-186, 1995.*

97. *Chen MF, Shimada F, Kato H, et al: Endocrinol Jpn 38:167-174, 1991.*

98. *Chen MF, Shimada F, Kato H, et al: Endocrinol Jpn 37:331-341, 1990.*

99. *Bouraoui A, Toum A, Bouchoucha S, et al: Thérapie 41:467-471, 1986.*

100. *Nebel A, Schneider BJ, Baker RK, et al: Ann Pharmacother 33:502, 1999.*

7. Patients or clients should be asked to report any suspected HDIs to the practitioner, who should report these further (e.g., to PhytoNET at http://www.escop.com).

8. Some drugs (e.g., antihypertensives, antidiabetic drugs) require careful control for their effects to be maintained. Herbal remedies may make them more or less effective. In the ideal situation the dose of the drug could be adjusted.

9. The use of antioxidants (including herbs) in conjunction with chemotherapy and radiotherapy for cancer is controversial. Practitioners should be aware of the issues and make an informed recommendation to their patients.

10. HDIs will be dose related for the herb and the drug. This has recently been shown for St. John's wort and digoxin.

The way forward is to generate more reliable data. This can be achieved by:

- Better monitoring of HDIs in clinical practice;
- Better monitoring of HDIs in clinical trials;
- Conducting active research into HDIs (human studies are most reliable);
- Better understanding the effects of phytochemicals on absorption, metabolism, and distribution of drugs;
- Informing patients to watch for HDIs;
- Encouraging reliable reviews;
- Requiring manufacturers to report HDIs for their products (as is the case in the European Union); and
- Practitioners following the aforementioned guidelines and becoming well informed about HDIs.

It is in everyone's interests to obtain reliable information about HDIs.

HERB-DRUG INTERACTIONS: AN ASSESSMENT OF DOCUMENTED CASES FOR SOME COMMONLY USED HERBS

There is no doubt that in recent times there has been an increase in the number of reports in the medical literature about HDIs.

To be able to assess the relevance of case reports, basic information needs to be gathered, preferably at the time of the incident. The following questions need to be answered:

- Dosage of the herb?
- Dosage of the drug?
- How long was each of these medications taken?
- Was the dosage of either of these medications changed before the supposed interaction?
- What other prescription or nonprescription medicines were taken at the time of the supposed interaction?
- Was the dosage of any of these medications altered in any way?
- Were any new medications added just before the supposed interaction?
- What is the patient's medical history?
- Were there any significant changes in diet or lifestyle just before the supposed interaction?
- How valid is the conclusion that the herb was involved in an interaction with a drug?

One also needs information about the product that was taken. In particular:

- Has the herb been authenticated?
- Has the herb been checked for contaminants?

If these questions cannot be answered it leads to another that may be unanswerable: "what did the person actually take?" In some cases the necessary questions are asked, the appropriate testing is carried out on the product, and an educated conclusion can be reached. However, in many cases this information is not sought, and it is therefore difficult to assess with any real accuracy the validity of these reports.

An interaction between a herb and a drug can have a pharmacodynamic (i.e., similar or opposing effects) or a pharmacokinetic basis. Pharmacodynamic interactions are in theory predictable, although it is a fair observation that there is far more speculation concerning these interactions than actual reported cases. In contrast, pharmacokinetic interactions, in which the herb alters the pharmacokinetic profile of a drug making it more or less available to the body, are unpredictable and, by their very nature, of far greater cause for concern. This is an emerging field of enquiry, and the best example to date is the findings for St. John's wort.

A number of documented HDIs for some key herbs are described. For more information on interactions for these and other herbs, see the individual monographs in this text.

St. John's Wort *(Hypericum perforatum)*

In late 1999 and early 2000 a number of possible drug interactions with St. John's wort were reported in the medical and scientific literature. As a result of these reports, concern about the safety of St. John's wort has been questioned, and stiff warnings about interactions with medications have been introduced on labels across the world.

It is postulated that St. John's wort induces CYP450 enzymes and/or P-glycoprotein, thus decreasing the bioavailability of many drugs. These are thought to be the underlying mechanisms behind many of the St. John's wort–drug interactions that have been reported (see the monograph on St. John's wort, p. 585).

Interaction with Anticoagulant Medications

Many anticoagulants, including warfarin, are metabolised via CYP450 enzymes, and because alterations in their concentrations can be life threatening it is important that patients

are aware of dietary and lifestyle factors and other medications that may influence their effectiveness. If St. John's wort does significantly induce CYP450 enzymes there is a possibility, when taken concurrently with these drugs, that the desired anticoagulant activity of the drugs could be decreased.

The reports listed below concern possible interactions between St. John's wort and phenprocoumon (clinical study) and warfarin. The latter consists of seven cases reported to the Medical Products Agency in Sweden since 1998. These are listed in Table 6-3 because information is unfortunately limited.[22]

Phenprocoumon

Researchers conducted a single-blind, placebo-controlled study with 10 healthy men (aged 18 to 50 years) to investigate the interaction of St. John's wort and phenprocoumon (anticoagulant). Volunteers received either placebo or 900 mg/day St. John's wort extract (LI 160) for 11 days. On day 11 they were given a dose of phenprocoumon (12 mg). The serum levels of the drug were lower in the St. John's wort group than in the placebo group.[23]

Warfarin

For details regarding warfarin, see Table 6-3.

Table **6-3**   **Potential Interactions Recorded Between St. John's Wort and Anticoagulant Drugs**

Patients (sex/age)	INR before St. John's wort	INR during St. John's wort	Duration of warfarin treatment	INR levels
F, 61 yr	N/A	1.2	Years	INR increased after stopping St. John's wort
F, 84 yr	2.9-3.6	1.5	Stable for 6 mo	INR returned to target range without St. John's wort
F, 56 yr	2.6	1.5	Unknown	INR returned to previous value after St. John's wort
M, 85 yr	2.1-4.1	1.5	Long time	INR decreased and dose increased while taking St. John's wort
F, 79 yr	2.5-3.8	1.7	2.5 yr	Increased from 18.5 to 21.25 mg/wk
M, 65 yr	2.4-3.6	2.0-2.1	4 yr	Increased from 37.5 to 40 mg/wk
M, 76 yr	2.3	1.1	10 days	Increased

F, Female; INR, international normalised ratio; M, male.

Interaction with Digoxin

The only report to date concerning an interaction between St. John's wort and digoxin came from a clinical study. There have been no credible reports in the literature concerning actual cases.

In a single-blind, placebo-controlled study, researchers looked at the interaction of digoxin with St. John's wort. Twenty-five healthy volunteers received 0.25 mg digoxin twice daily for 5 days until a steady state for digoxin was reached. They were then divided into two groups and given 0.25 mg digoxin once a day with either placebo or 900 mg/day of St. John's wort for 10 days. At the end of these 10 days the digoxin level was 25% lower in the St. John's wort-treated group when compared with the placebo-treated group.[24]

Interaction with HIV-1 Medication

The clinical trial presented below examined the possibility of St. John's wort reducing the serum levels, and thus the effectiveness, of indinavir (a protease inhibitor). Although this study demonstrated a reduction in serum indinavir levels in the participants, there have been no reports of actual clinical cases. In assessing this research we need to consider that this was a small study group with healthy volunteers. It is apparent that we need information on actual cases or, at the very least, larger clinical studies.

Six healthy male volunteers took part in a study to determine the effects of St. John's wort extract on serum levels of indinavir. On day 1 they were given 800 mg indinavir orally in the morning on an empty stomach. They were given two more doses throughout the day at 8-hour intervals. Another 800-mg dose was administered on the morning of day 2, and blood samples were taken at 0.5, 1, 2, 3, 4, and 5 hours after dosing.

On day 3 they were given St. John's wort 300 mg (0.3% hypericin) three times a day for 14 days. At days 16 and 17 (days 14 and 15 of St. John's wort administration) they were again given indinavir in the same manner as days 1 and 2. Blood samples were again taken and compared with those taken before St. John's wort administration was commenced.

The results of the second blood samples demonstrated that St. John's wort caused a decrease in indinavir levels ranging from 49% to 99% (mean range, 57%) during the 5-hour period. Extrapolated 8-hour indinavir levels were decreased by 81%.[25]

In light of this study and the fact that low plasma concentrations of protease inhibitors are a cause of antiretroviral resistance and treatment failure, and that indinavir and many other types of HIV medications are metabolised via CYP450 enzymes, it would be prudent to avoid the use of St. John's wort in patients with HIV receiving drug therapy until more information is available.

Interaction with Cyclosporin

Cyclosporin is an immunosuppressive drug given to patients who have undergone organ transplant to prevent rejection of the transplanted body part. Two cases of acute heart transplant rejection were reported in the February 2000 issue of *The Lancet*. Both of these patients were examined at the same clinic within 1 week of each other for a routine procedure.

In the first case a 61-year-old man was admitted to hospital to undergo elective endomyocardial biopsy 11 months after heart transplantation. His immunosuppressive regimen consisted of cyclosporin (125 mg twice daily), azathioprine (100 mg daily), and low-dose corticosteroids (7.5 mg daily), and he had experienced an event-free course since the transplant procedure. Three weeks before admission he had started taking St. John's wort 300 mg three times daily for mild depression.

On admission tests revealed cyclosporin plasma levels were decreased, although he was feeling well apart from nonspecific fatigue. Biopsy revealed acute transplant rejection. Cyclosporin was increased, and other drug treatment instigated to manage the rejection. The rejection episode was resolved, and cyclosporin levels returned to therapeutic range after stopping St. John's wort treatment. There were no further episodes of rejection.

The second case was a 63-year-old woman also admitted to hospital for elective endomyocardial biopsy. Her heart transplantation had been performed 20 months earlier. As with the previously described case, she had had an event-free course and was maintained on immunosuppressive therapy of cyclosporin, azathioprine, and corticosteroids. She had been prescribed St. John's wort 300 mg three times a day by a psychiatrist for anxiety and depression. Cyclosporin levels were found to be low, and biopsy showed acute rejection. Once St. John's wort treatment was stopped, cyclosporin returned to therapeutic values.

The authors concluded that the induction of CYP450 enzymes by St. John's wort was responsible for the decreased serum levels of cyclosporin. It has also been suggested by other researchers that St. John's wort may induce intestinal P-glycoprotein drug transporter, which could contribute to decreased absorption of the cyclosporin.[26]

An earlier case report of a possible cyclosporin/St. John's wort interaction was published in the *Medical Journal of Australia* in 1998. This case involved a woman in her mid-20s whose cyclosporin levels decreased to 25% of previous levels. No other details are available.[27]

In light of the aforementioned case reports and until further studies are carried out, it would be advisable not to prescribe St. John's wort to patients who are taking cyclosporin, especially for those in whom the decrease of serum cyclosporin could be life threatening as in organ transplant recipients.

Interactions with Antidepressant Medications

Serotonin syndrome is an adverse drug effect characterised by altered mental status, autonomic dysfunction, and neuromuscular abnormalities. It is most frequently caused by the use of selective serotonin reuptake inhibitors (SSRIs) and MAO inhibitors. A case of suspected serotonin syndrome has been reported. The woman aged 50 years had stopped taking paroxetine (an SSRI) 10 days before commencing St. John's wort therapy. After this short time, she restarted the paroxetine to assist her sleep. The following day she experienced lethargy and grogginess. The author postulated that an adverse reaction occurred between the SSRI and *Hypericum*.[28] However, the evidence for this conclusion was not strong. More recently a report has appeared that documented five cases of serotonin syndrome in elderly people (who are most susceptible to this problem).[29]

It may follow that people (especially elderly people) taking conventional antidepressant drugs are more susceptible to serotonin syndrome if they also take St. John's wort. However, it should also be considered that these drugs are capable of causing this syndrome on their own. Therefore, a link with St. John's wort intake may only be coincidental.

Interaction with Anaesthetics

The American Society of Anesthesiologists issued a warning in 1999 against taking St. John's wort just before surgery because of a dangerous interaction with anaesthetic agents. A brief article warning of these dangers has also been published.[30]

The Society based their conclusions on the fact that St. John's wort is a strong inhibitor of MAO. However, it is now acknowledged that St. John's wort is a clinically insignificant inhibitor of MAO.[31]

Ginkgo biloba

In the cases discussed here it is assumed that ginkgo may have potentiated the anticoagulant effect of aspirin and warfarin. It is interesting to note that despite the extensive use of ginkgo, predominantly among the elderly population, and the tendency for elderly people to have spontaneous bleeds, these are the only two cases to date that report such interactions despite millions of orthodox ginkgo prescriptions in continental Europe and a mandatory adverse drug reporting scheme for physicians there. However, because of the individuality of patients and the sensitivity of warfarin, caution should be exercised when prescribing ginkgo to patients taking anticoagulant medication, especially warfarin.

Interaction with Aspirin

A 70-year-old man with no history of eye trauma, ischaemia, or vascular occlusion experienced spontaneous bleeding from the iris into the anterior chamber of the eye. He had been taking 325 mg/day of aspirin for 3 years and had started taking ginkgo 1 week before the bleeding (40 mg concentrated extract twice/day). He stopped the ginkgo but continued the aspirin. There was no recurrence of the bleeding during the next 3-month follow-up period.[32]

Interaction with Warfarin

A 78-year-old woman, who had been stable with warfarin therapy for 5 years after a coronary artery bypass, had an intracranial haemorrhage 2 months after starting *Ginkgo biloba* (dose unknown). She also had hypertension, a previous myocardial infarction, atrial fibrillation, and sick sinus syndrome.[33]

Garlic (*Allium sativum*)

High doses of garlic, as food or medicine, are not advisable for patients with a history of bleeding disorders or for those taking anticoagulant medication and should be stopped before surgery.

Interaction with Warfarin

Two cases of possible interaction between garlic and warfarin were reported in 1991. Both patients had been stable with warfarin therapy, and both experienced an increase in INR after ingesting garlic tablets or pearls. No other changes in habits or medication had occurred in either case.[34]

Ginseng (*Panax ginseng*)

In a recent systematic review of the safety of ginseng, the authors conclude that most reports are inconclusive as to the role of ginseng itself rather than other factors and conclude that ginseng is rarely associated with adverse events and interactions.[35] The following are among the cases reported.

Interaction with Warfarin

Ingestion of *P. ginseng* is suspected of antagonising the effect of warfarin in a 47-year-old man who had been taking warfarin for 4 to 5 years. His other medications included diltiazem hydrochloride, nitroglycerin, and salsalate. His INR ranged from 3.0 to 4.0 with a warfarin dose of 5 mg/day (7.5 mg on Tuesdays). Two weeks after he started taking ginseng capsules his INR had decreased to 2.5. He stopped taking the ginseng, and 2 weeks later his INR was 3.3. The patient denied changing any of his medications or taking any other over-the-counter supplements.[36]

A study to examine the influences of ginseng on the pharmacokinetics and pharmacodynamics of warfarin in rats was carried out to find a possible mode of action after the aforementioned case report. The researchers could find no link between ginseng and the decreased activity of warfarin. Their data demonstrate that the absorption, distribution, metabolism, and elimination of warfarin and the pharmacological effect of warfarin were not altered by the presence of ginseng. There were no detectable levels of vitamin K in the ginseng extract.

However, the authors advise not to overinterpret these data because of the possible limitations of extrapolating animal data to humans.[37] However, in view of this study and the lack of other reported case histories, it seems unlikely that ginseng interacts with warfarin.

Interaction with Phenelzine

Two cases of possible interactions between *P. ginseng* and phenelzine (Parnate), an MAO inhibitor, have been reported.

In the first case, a 64-year-old woman had experienced insomnia, headache, and tremulousness when she started taking a product called "Natrol High" along with her phenelzine. One of the components of Natrol High is ginseng. Later she drank ginseng tea while still taking phenelzine and experienced the same symptoms. She had used the same ginseng tea before starting the phenelzine without any adverse effects.[38]

The second is the case of a 42-year-old woman experiencing irritability, tension headaches, and occasional vague visual hallucinations while she was taking ginseng and bee pollen concurrently with phenelzine. She discontinued the antidepressant medication but subsequently began to become depressed again. The phenelzine was recommended without the ginseng and bee pollen, and the only side effect seemed to be episodes of headaches.[39]

Interaction with Alcohol

P. ginseng increases the rate of alcohol clearance. Forty minutes after ingestion of 72 g of ethanol/65 kg body weight, blood alcohol levels were 35.2% lower in the ginseng-treated group than in the placebo group, although there were variations in different individuals. The dose of ginseng used was 3 g extract/65 kg body weight.[40]

Kava *(Piper methysticum)*

Interaction with alprazolam

In a letter entitled "Coma from the Health Food Store", the author reports the case of a 54-year-old man who was hospitalised in a lethargic and disoriented state. He was taking alprazolam (Xanax), cimetidine (Tagamet), and terazosin (Hytrin). His vital signs and laboratory tests were normal. His blood alcohol levels were negative, and a drug screen was positive for benzodiazepines. He had been taking kava for 3 days and denied an overdose of kava or alprazolam. The dose of kava is not stated.[41]

The title "Coma from the Health Food Store" seems a little sensationalistic. The dose of kava was not listed in this report and probably was not known by the authors. There is also the possibility that this patient may have had an overdose of alprazolam. This type of scenario is much more likely to occur with the self-prescription of kava than if a patient is treated by a competent clinician. Nonetheless, excessive doses of kava should be avoided in those taking sedative medication or antidepressants.

REFERENCES

1. Mills S, Bone K: *Principles and practice of phytotherapy: modern herbal medicine*, Edinburgh, 2000, Churchill Livingstone, pp 104-107.
2. Horowitz S: Combining supplements and prescription drugs. What your patients need to know, *Altern Comp Ther* 6:177-183, 2000.
3. Vickers A, Zollman C: ABC of complementary medicine: herbal medicine, *BMJ* 319:1050-1053, 1999.
4. Miller LG: Herbal medicinals: selected clinical considerations focusing on known or potential drug-herb interactions, *Arch Intern Med* 158:2200-2211, 1998.
5. Stahmann MA, Huebner CF, Link KP: Studies of the hemorrhagic sweet clover disease, *J Biol Chem* 138:513-527, 1941.
6. Kostering VH, Bandura B, Merten HA, et al: The behavior of blood clotting and its inhibitors under long term treatment with 5,6-benzo-alpha-pyrone (coumarin). Double blind study, *Arzneimittelforschung* 35:1303-1306, 1985.
7. Mills S, Bone K: *Principles and practice of phytotherapy: modern herbal medicine*, Edinburgh, 2000, Churchill Livingstone, p 320.
8. Mills S, Bone K: *Principles and practice of phytotherapy: modern herbal medicine*, Edinburgh, 2000, Churchill Livingstone, p 324.
9. De Smet PAGM, Keller K, Hansel R, Chandler RF, editors: *Adverse effects of herbal drugs 1*, Berlin Heidelberg, 1992, Springer-Verlag, pp 193-195.
10. Mills S, Bone K: *Principles and practice of phytotherapy: modern herbal medicine*, Edinburgh, 2000, Edinburgh, p 387.
11. Brinker F. Interactions of pharmaceutical and botanical medicines, *J Naturopathic Med* 7:14-20, 1997.
12. Facts and Comparisons. Potential herb-drug interactions. *Review of Natural Products*, 1-5, December 1998.
13. Facts and Comparisons. Specific herb-drug interactions. *Review of Natural Products*, 1-8, December 1998.
14. Shaw D, Leon C, Kolev S, et al: Traditional remedies and food supplements. A 5-year toxicological study (1991-1995), *Drug Saf* 17:342-356, 1997.
15. Ko R: Adverse reactions to watch for in patients using herbal remedies, *West J Med* 171:181-186, 1999.
16. Ernst E: Possible interactions between synthetic and herbal medicinal products. Part 1: a systematic review of the indirect evidence, *Perfusion* 13:4-15, 2000.
17. Blumenthal M: Selected herb-drug interactions, *HerbalGram* 49:58-63, 2000.
18. Fugh-Berman A: Herb-drug interactions, *Lancet* 355:134-138, 2000.
19. Johns-Cupp M: Herbal remedies: adverse effects and drug interactions, *Am Fam Physician* 59:1239-1244, 1999.
20. Cambria-Kiely JA: Effect of soy milk on warfarin efficacy, *Ann Pharmacother* 36:1893-1896, 2002.
21. Mills S, Bone K: *Principles and practice of phytotherapy: modern herbal medicine*, Edinburgh, 2000, Churchill Livingstone, pp 553-562.
22. Yue QY, Bergquist C, Gerden B: Safety of St John's wort (Hypericum perforatum), *Lancet* 355:576-577, 2000.
23. Mauer A, Johne A, Bauer S, et al: Interaction of St. John's wort extract with phenprocoumon, *Eur J Clin Pharmacol* 55:A22, 1999.
24. Johne A, Brockmuller J, Bauer S, et al: Pharmacokinetic interaction of digoxin with an herbal extract from St John's wort (*Hypericum perforatum*), *Clin Pharmacol Ther* 66:338-345, 1999.
25. Piscitelli SC, Burstein AH, Chaitt D, et al: Indinavir concentrations and St. John's wort, *Lancet* 355:547-548, 2000.
26. Ruschitzka F, Meier PJ, Turina M, et al: Acute heart transplant rejection due to Saint John's wort, *Lancet* 355:548-549, 2000.
27. Rey JM, Walter G: Hypericum perforatum (St. John's wort) in depression: pest or blessing? *Med J Aust* 169:583-586, 1998.
28. Gordon JB: SSRIs and St. John's wort: possible toxicity? *Am Fam Physician* 57:950, 953, 1998.
29. Lantz MS, Buchalter E, Giambanco V: St. John's wort and antidepressant drug interactions in the elderly, *J Geriatr Psychiatry Neurol* 12:7-10, 1999.
30. Ciordia R: Beware "St. John's wort," potential herbal danger, *J Clin Monit Comput* 14:215, 1998.
31. Mills S, Bone K: *Principles and practice of phytotherapy: modern herbal medicine*, Edinburgh, 2000, Churchill Livingstone, pp 542-552.

32. Rosenblatt M, Mindel J: Spontaneous hyphema associated with ingestion of Ginkgo biloba extract, *N Engl J Med* 336:1108, 1997.

33. Matthews MK Jr: Association of Ginkgo biloba with intracerebral hemorrhage, *Neurology* 50:1933-1934, 1998.

34. D'Arcy PF, McElnay JC, Welling PG, editors: *Mechanisms of drug interactions*, Berlin, 1996, Springer-Verlag, pp 340-341.

35. Coon JT, Ernst E: Panax ginseng: a systematic review of adverse effects and drug interactions, *Drug Saf* 25:323-344, 2002.

36. Janetzky K, Morreale AP: Probable interaction between warfarin and ginseng, *Am J Health Syst Pharm* 54:692-693, 1997.

37. Zhu M, Chan KW, Ng LS, et al: Possible influences of ginseng on the pharmacokinetics and pharmacodynamics of warfarin in rats, *J Pharm Pharmacol* 51:175-180, 1999.

38. Shader RI, Greenblatt DJ: Phenelzine and the dream machine—ramblings and reflections, *J Clin Psychopharmacol* 5:65, 1985.

39. Jones BD, Runikis AM: Interaction of ginseng with phenelzine, *J Clin Psychopharmacol* 7:201-202, 1987.

40. Lee FC, Ko JH, Park JK, et al: Effects of Panax ginseng on blood alcohol clearance in man, *Clin Exp Pharmacl Physiol* 14:543-546, 1987.

41. Almeida JC, Grimsley EW: Coma from the health food store: interaction between kava and alprazolam, *Ann Intern Med* 125:940-941, 1996.

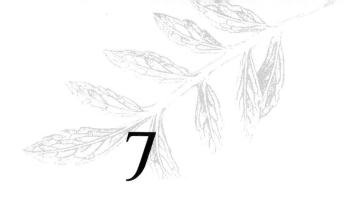

7

Safety Considerations During Pregnancy and Lactation

Kerry Bone

PREGNANCY

Background and Perspective

The following risks could potentially be associated with the use of a herb during pregnancy:

- Toxicity to the mother, which may also indirectly impair the health or development of the child;
- Toxicity to the child (i.e., foetotoxicity);
- Developmental malformations (i.e., teratogenesis);
- Increased risk of miscarriage; and
- Health effects on the child, both short term and long term (e.g., increased risk of chronic health problems later in life, such as cancer).

There is currently no consensus regarding the safety considerations surrounding the use of herbs during pregnancy. On one hand, some regulatory authorities appear to be adopting the policy that if there is no clear evidence of safety from controlled clinical trials, then a herb should not be recommended during pregnancy. This is well illustrated by deliberations of the Complementary Medicines Evaluation Committee (CMEC) of the Australian Therapeutic Goods Administration (TGA). CMEC assessed the safe use of over-the-counter (OTC) products containing kava *(Piper methysticum)* and came to the conclusion, despite the lack of evidence for harm from kava during pregnancy (and well before any link between kava and hepatotoxicity was suggested), that kava products should carry the following warning: "Not for prolonged use. If symptoms persist seek advice from a health care practitioner. Those who are pregnant or nursing are not recommended to use Kava." The American Herbal Products Association also suggests that professional advice should be sought before using kava during pregnancy.[1]

Some scientists with little clinical experience in prescribing herbs have speculated about harmful effects that may ensue from the use of herbs during pregnancy. They appear to adopt the stance that even if a negative effect from a herb is only remotely possible, then that herb should not be taken during pregnancy. The unspoken assumption here is that herbs are only marginally efficacious, if at all, so even the remotest risk during pregnancy is unacceptable. This approach is exemplified by the list provided in the book by Newall et al.[2]

Conversely, there are many professional herbalists and other clinicians who routinely prescribe a wide range of herbs during pregnancy. In addition self-prescription of herbs by pregnant women is already widespread and appears to be increasing.[3] There are few case reports attributing harmful effects to the use of herbs during pregnancy, especially when cases of intentional overdose are excluded.

Although few would disagree that this lack of consensus is unsatisfactory and that more information is essential, the paucity of human safety data for conventional pharmaceuticals demonstrates that this problem is not just confined to herbal products. This was well illustrated by a recent survey of the use of prescription drugs in France during pregnancy, which is discussed below.[4]

A survey of the records of the French Health Insurance Service of drug prescriptions during pregnancy for 1000 women living in southwest France showed that 99% of the women received a prescription for at least one drug during pregnancy. The US Food and Drug Administration (FDA) risk classification system was used to categorise the medicines given (Table 7-1).[5] The mean number of prescriptions was a staggering 13.6 medications per woman with 1.6% of the women receiving one or more drugs from the FDA category X (foetal risk outweighs benefits). Underlining the lack of positive human safety data for many prescription drugs were the observations that almost 90% of the women received drugs from the C category (no controlled studies in pregnant women and adverse or no animal data) and that 59.3% were prescribed drugs from the D category (adverse effects from controlled studies in pregnant women).

The implied hierarchy of risk in the FDA A, B, C, D, and X classification can be misleading.[6] When the FDA approves a medication for marketing in the United States, the pregnancy section of the label is based on preclinical studies and perhaps a few inadvertent human exposures occurring during clinical trials. Given the information available at approval, most med-

ications are assigned to pregnancy category C. This designation indicates that human data are lacking and animal studies showed no harm or were not done. With no requirements for systematic review and label updates, 66% of all medications with a pregnancy category are now in category C. Only a handful of medications are labelled pregnancy category X, including not only frank human teratogens such as thalidomide but also nonteratogens that provide no known benefit to pregnant women. Similarly, less than 1% of medications have the pregnancy category A rating because this degree of safety needs to be documented by well-controlled human studies.[7]

According to a press article issued by Lauran Neergaard of the Associated Press on December 18, 2000, the FDA plans to develop new rules that will require drug manufacturers to update their drug labels annually with any pregnancy safety data, such as independent research or case reports. The article adds that most drug companies avoid studying pregnant women and typically just reveal the results of animal studies. It quotes Dr. Sandra Kweder from the FDA, who asserted that: "If most pregnant women knew how little information there is . . . they would be greatly surprised."

The article also draws attention to concerns over the use of OTC medications during pregnancy, including drugs, vitamins, and herbal products. Regarding OTC drugs, several of these have been linked to adverse effects on the foetus, including birth defects.[8] A superficial scan of the safety literature for prescription and OTC drugs revealed a link between anticonvulsant drugs and birth defects[9] and nonsteroidal antiinflammatory drugs and increased risk of miscarriage.[10]

Inconsistencies and Misinformation

Various texts list herbs that should be avoided during pregnancy. However, there is often not good agreement between these sources, as can be seen in Table 7-2. This table compares pregnancy information from five herbal texts for eight common herbs. A tick indicates that the author(s) considers the particular herb safe to take during pregnancy; a cross indicates the opposite. A tick and a cross indicate a qualified yes for pregnancy.

Table **7-1**   **FDA Classification of Medications Used During Pregnancy and Lactation**

The FDA classifies drugs in one of five categories based on their teratogenic potential	
Category A	Controlled studies in pregnant women demonstrate no foetal risk (e.g., folic acid and levothyroxine).
Category B	Controlled animal studies have not shown a foetal risk, but there are no studies done on women OR controlled studies in animals have shown a foetal risk that was not reproduced in controlled human studies (e.g., amoxicillin and ceftriaxone).
Category C	Controlled animal studies have demonstrated adverse foetal effects, and there are no human studies or there are no controlled studies in humans or animals (e.g., nifedipine and omeprazole).
Category D	Controlled studies in humans demonstrate adverse foetal effects, but the benefits of using the drug are greater than the risks (e.g., propylthiouracil).
Category X	Controlled studies in animals and humans have demonstrated adverse foetal effects, or there is evidence of foetal risk based on human experience. The risk of using these drugs outweighs any possible benefit. The drug is absolutely contraindicated in pregnancy (e.g., misoprostol, warfarin, and isotretinoin).

From Larimore WL: Medications used in pregnancy and lactation. Online coverage from the 50th Annual Meeting of the American Academy of Family Physicians Scientific Assembly, September 16-20, 1998. Available at: http://medscape.com/Medscape/CNO/1998/AFFP/09.18.../AAFP.18.559.Lari.html.
Most drugs prescribed for pregnant women are category B or C. Category A drugs are uncommon because controlled studies in pregnant women are rare.

Table **7-2**   **Herb Use During Pregnancy: A Comparison of Advice from Several Texts**

	Mills and Bone[11]	Brinker[12]	AHPA Safety Book[1]	Commission E[13]	Newell et al[2]
Ginger	✓	✓✗	✗	✗	✓✗
St. John's wort	✓	✗	✓	✓	✗
Echinacea	✓	✓	✓	✓	✓
Fennel	✓	✗	✓	✓	–
Senna	✓	✓✗	✗	✗	✓✗
Licorice	✓	✗	✗	✗	✗
Chamomile	✓	✗	✓	✓	✗
Raspberry leaves	–	✗	✓	–	✗

✓, Indicates that the particular herb is safe to take during pregnancy; ✗, indicates that the particular herb is unsafe to take during pregnancy; ✓✗, indicates a qualified yes for pregnancy.

Referring specifically to the information in Table 7-2, the only herb for which there is a consensus is echinacea. Most authors have doubts about the use of senna *(Senna alexandrina)* and licorice *(Glycyrrhiza glabra)* during pregnancy, although their safety has been established by clinical trials (see later in this chapter). Ginger is widely used by pregnant women for nausea, although again the majority of authors have concerns about its use.

A published survey of the popular literature found there was no consensus about whether certain herbs were safe for use during pregnancy.[14] Sixteen sources (12%) cited the use of ginger and 11 (15%) noted the use of raspberry leaf as unsafe during pregnancy.

Why do these disagreements exist? It could be argued that they are because of a lack of safety data; however, in the case of senna, which is a widely used OTC medication, this is clearly not the case. The stance taken by some authors is highly conservative. Any animal or in vitro study of a plant or its phytochemical constituents that may be remotely construed to have a negative effect during pregnancy is taken as evidence for contraindication during pregnancy. In addition, some authors believe that any herb with suggested oestrogenic activity is unsafe during pregnancy.

Using the same criteria, intake of soya, linseeds, potatoes, and black pepper by pregnant women would be contraindicated. Soya and linseeds are oestrogenic; potatoes contain glycoalkaloids, which are teratogenic in animal experiments; and piperine from black pepper disrupts pregnancy in mice.[15]

A number of commonly accepted "truths" are open to question. For example, old pharmacopoeias carry warnings about the use of aloe resin, an anthraquinone-based laxative, during pregnancy. It was said to cause miscarriage. However, a well-documented case history of a woman who consumed a large quantity of aloe revealed that it resulted in little more than slight vaginal bleeding.[16]

What the inconsistencies accurately reflect is the need for an adequate classification system: one that specifically categorises the existing pregnancy information for each herb, as is currently the case for conventional drugs. Such a system is proposed later in this chapter and has been adopted for the safety monographs in this book.

Misinformation and misunderstandings of the use of herbs in pregnancy are also expressed by health care professionals and found in the literature. One gynaecologist in Perth, Australia instructs his patients not to consume slippery elm (Ulmus rubra) powder during pregnancy. Slippery elm is a mucilaginous herb that swells when mixed with water and is used for its demulcent and bulk laxative properties. Vaginal insertion of whole slippery elm bark has been used to procure abortion. Similar in principle to the use of the laminaria

tent,[17] the bark swells and dilates the cervix. Clearly there is no relationship between this use and the oral intake of the powdered bark.

Other misinformation stems from a confusion of phytochemistry. For example, it is often stated in texts that celery (Apium graveolens) fruit (seeds) is contraindicated during pregnancy because it contains significant amounts of apiol, when in fact this is not the case. Parsley (Petroselinum crispum, formerly Apium petroselinum) is rich in apiol. However, pregnant women are not typically instructed to avoid parsley salads during pregnancy. Similarly, it is often written that buchu (Agathosma betulina) is contraindicated during pregnancy, presumably because it contains significant levels of pulegone, when in fact this particular species of Agathosma does not.[18]

Sometimes substitution of a herb makes it unsafe during pregnancy. For example, germander (Teucrium spp.) substituted for skullcap (Scutellaria lateriflora) would be a safety concern. Buchu also is often listed as unsafe during pregnancy as mentioned previously. At doses less than 2 g/day this is not so, provided that the species used is Agathosma betulina. Only other species of Agathosma that are used as substitutes contain high levels of the potentially toxic compound pulegone in their essential oil.

Classifying Herbs in Terms of Available Pregnancy Data

The classification of herbs as permitted or prohibited during pregnancy is limited in the information it provides and, as has been shown in this chapter, leads to inconsistencies in the literature. A descriptive risk classification, similar to that used for conventional drugs, would be more informative. In addition it would allow for the application of professional judgement in terms of assessing the known risk versus the perceived benefit for the individual patient. It is proposed that the classification system recommended for drugs by the Australian TGA is particularly appropriate for herbs (Table 7-3).

This system allows for individual perspectives to be accommodated. For example, the highly conservative clinician may only ever wish to recommend herbs in category A. A risk-averse clinician may choose to only prescribe herbs in categories A and B1 or categories A,

Table **7-3**   **The Australian Therapeutic Goods Administration Classification for Drugs in Pregnancy**

Category A	Drugs that have been taken by many pregnant women and women of child-bearing age without any proven increase in the frequency of malformations or other direct or indirect harmful effects on the foetus having been observed.
Category B1	Drugs that have been taken by only a limited number of pregnant women and women of child-bearing age without an increase in the frequency of malformation or other direct or indirect harmful effects on the human foetus having been observed. Studies in animals have not shown evidence of an increased occurrence of foetal damage.
Category B2	Drugs that have been taken by only a limited number of pregnant women and women of child-bearing age, without an increase in the frequency of malformation or other direct or indirect harmful effects on the human foetus having been observed. Studies in animals are inadequate or may be lacking, but available data show no evidence of an increased occurrence of foetal damage.
Category B3	Drugs that have been taken by only a limited number of pregnant women and women of child-bearing age, without an increase in the malformation or other direct or indirect harmful effects on the human foetus having been observed. Studies in animals have shown evidence of an increased occurrence of foetal damage, the significance of which is considered uncertain in humans.
Category C	Drugs that, owing to their pharmacological effects, have caused or may be suspected of causing, harmful effects on the human foetus or neonate without causing malformations. These effects may be reversible.
Category D	Drugs that have caused, are suspected to have caused, or may be expected to cause an increased incidence of human foetal malformations or irreversible damage. These drugs also have adverse pharmacological effects.
Category X	Drugs that have such a high risk of causing permanent damage to the foetus that they should not be used in pregnancy or when there is a possibility of pregnancy.

For drugs in B1, B2, or B3 categories, human data are lacking or inadequate, and subcategorisation is based on available animal data. **The allocation of a B category does NOT imply greater safety than the C category.** *Drugs in category D are not absolutely contraindicated in pregnancy (e.g., anticonvulsants). Moreover, in some cases, the D category has been assigned based on suspicion.*
From Prescribing medicines in pregnancy: an Australian categorisation of risk of drug use in pregnancy, *Therapeutic Goods Administration, Australian Drug Evaluation Committee, 1999.*

B1, and B2. Other clinicians may see benefit in occasionally prescribing herbs in category C, but herbs in categories C and D should generally be avoided, especially during the first trimester. Examples of suggested categories for various herbs are provided in Table 7-4.

General Guidelines for Recommending Herbs During Pregnancy

Although in general it is often safe to prescribe certain herbs during pregnancy, this should only be done if there is a worthwhile need. All medication should especially be kept to a minimum during the first 3 months of pregnancy, but it is acceptable to judiciously use herbs to manage morning sickness and threatened

miscarriage during this period. Appropriate care should also be exercised if a patient is attempting to become pregnant.

Caution with the use of herbs should be particularly exercised when there is a history of miscarriage or difficult conception. A recent history of low back pain with bearing-down abdominal pain or vaginal discharge or bleeding should be regarded as a potential miscarriage and managed cautiously.

Known toxic or poisonous plants (e.g., those with a poison classification) should be avoided. These include bryony *(Bryonia)*, aconite *(Aconitum)*, bloodroot *(Sanguinaria)*, Ephedra, and poke root *(Phytolacca)*. Some herbs, such as lobelia and gelsemium, may be used

Table **7-4   Examples of Herbs Classified for Use in Pregnancy**

Category A	Raspberry leaf, ginger, senna, echinacea, chamomile (apart from allergy), *Panax ginseng*, bilberry, and turmeric
Category B1	*Astragalus*, valerian, ginkgo, St. John's wort, and bupleurum
Category B2	Buchu and black cohosh
Category B3	*Andrographis*
Category C	Bearberry and golden seal
Category D	Rue, *Adhatoda*, pau d'arco, and poke root
Category X	*Aristolochia*, *Senecio*, and boldo

during childbirth. See Table 7-5 for the list of potentially toxic herbs, which also should not be used during pregnancy.

Pure herbal volatile (essential) oils should not be taken internally during pregnancy. This is because volatile oils are a highly concentrated dosage form, and the risk of excessive doses is accordingly much greater. For example, chamomile *(Matricaria)* contains approximately 0.5% volatile oil; therefore, the pure oil is 200 times stronger than the dried herb. The exception here is intake of low quantities of oils used in flavouring, such as spearmint, peppermint, aniseed, and orange oil.

Laxative herbs containing anthraquinones should be avoided in high doses, although as noted previously these are probably safe even in high amounts. They include aloe resin *(Aloe barbadensis)*, cascara *(Rhamnus purshiana)*, senna *(Senna* spp.), and rhubarb *(Rheum officinale)*. The Commission E (an expert German government committee) believes that all these herbs containing anthraquinone-type laxative compounds are contraindicated during pregnancy.

Documented Use of Herbs During Pregnancy

Controlled studies of the use of Western herbs during pregnancy are relatively few. Two hundred and six women who used echinacea products during their pregnancy were followed in a prospective controlled study.[19] Of these, 112 women used the herb during the first trimester. There was no difference in pregnancy outcomes for the echinacea group and the control group in terms of live births, spon-

taneous abortions, and major malformations. The authors concluded that this first prospective study suggests that gestational use of echinacea during organogenesis is not associated with an increased risk of major malformations.

Consumption of licorice (as confectionery) and specifically glycyrrhizin intake was linked to slightly premature birth (2.5 days for ≥500 mg/week glycyrrhizin, which was classified as heavy intake).[20] Babies with heavy exposure to glycyrrhizin were not significantly lighter at birth, but they were significantly more likely to be born earlier. This heavy level of glycyrrhizin intake, which reflects typical Western herbal doses (15 to 20 g/week of licorice root), did not influence maternal blood pressure.

A review of 10 clinical studies involving 937 pregnant women treated with various senna preparations during periods ranging from 2 weeks to 9 months found good laxative effects.[21] There were no side effects relevant to pregnancy, even in high-risk patients with a tendency to premature labour or with bleeding during late pregnancy.

A controlled, retrospective study found that oral intake of evening primrose oil (1500 mg/day for 1 week and then 500 mg thereafter) from the 37th week until birth did not shorten gestation or decrease overall length of labour.[22] Evening primrose oil use may have prolonged labour in a percentage of users, although the dosage used was less than the typically recommended 3 to 4 g/day.

A retrospective, observational controlled study found that raspberry leaf can shorten labour with no identified side effects for the

Table **7-5**   **Toxic or Potentially Toxic Herbs Not To Be Taken During Pregnancy***

Abrus precatorius seed and root	Jequirity	*Lithospermum* (all or any species)	
Aconitum spp.	Aconite	Lobelia	
Acorus calamus	Sweet flag	Mandragora	Mandrake
Adonis vernalis		*Menispermum canadense*	Yellow parilla
Ammi visnaga		*Mentha pulegium*	Pennyroyal
Apocynum		Oleander	
Aristolochia (all or any species)	Snakeroot, birthwort	*Opuntia cylindrica*	San Pedro cactus
Arnica (all or any species) other than for external use	Arnica	*Papaver somniferum*	Opium poppy
Arum maculatum	Cuckoopint, lords and ladies	*Peganum harmala*	Wild rue
Belladonna	Deadly nightshade	*Petasites* (all or any species)	Butterbur
Brugmansia		*Peumus boldus*	Boldo
Brunfelsia uniflora	Manaca, mercury	*Phytolacca decandra* (*P. americana*)	Poke root, pokeweed
Calotropis		Podophyllum resin	
Catha edulis	Khat	*Pteridium aquilinum*	Bracken fern
Chenopodium ambrosioides	Wormseed oil	Rauwolfia	
Cicuta virosa	Cowbane	*Ricinus communis,* other than the fixed oil of the seed	Castor tree
Cinchona	Quinine bark	*Robinia pseudoacacia,* other than the leaf and flower	False acacia
Colchicum		*Schoenocaulon officinale* (*Sabadilla officinarum, Veratrum officinale*)	Sabadilla
Convallaria	Lily of the valley	*Scopolia carniolica*	
Coronilla		*Semecarpus anacardium* (*Anacardium orientale*), other than the seed	Marking nut tree
Crotalaria (all or any species)		*Senecio* (all or any species)	

Categories D or X: see Table 7-3 for explanation of categories.

(*Continued*)

Table **7-5**   **Toxic or Potentially Toxic Herbs Not To Be Taken During Pregnancy*—cont'd**

Croton (all or any species)	Cascarilla, Croton	*Solanum* (all or any species) except stems of *Solanum dulcamara* (bittersweet) and potatoes	
Cynoglossum officinale	Hound's tongue	*Sophora secundiflora*	Mescal bean
Daphne mezereum	Mezereum	*Spigelia marilandica*	Pink root, worm grass
Datura	Jimson weed	Staphisagria	
Digitalis	Foxgloves	Strophanthus	
Dryopteris filix-mas	Male fern	Strychnos	Nux vomica
Duboisia		*Strychnos gaulthieriana*	
Echium vulgare	Viper's bugloss	*Strychnos ignatii* (*Ignatia amara*)	Ignatious bean
Erysimum		*Symphytum* (all or any species)	Comfrey
Euonymus europaeus	European spindle tree	*Tamus communis* fruit and root	Black bryony
Galanthus	Snowdrop	*Tanacetum vulgare* (except in preparations containing 0.8% or less of oil of tansy)	Tansy
Gelsemium		*Teucrium* (all or any species)	Germander
Heliotropium (all or any species)	Heliotrope	Thevetia	
Helleborus (all or any species)	Hellebore	*Toxicodendron radicans* (*Rhus toxicodendron*)	Poison ivy
Hyoscyamus	Henbane	*Tussilago farfara*	Coltsfoot
Lantana camara	Lantana	*Virola sebifera*	Cuajo negro, camaticaro
Lathyrus sativus, other than the cooked seed	Grass pea	Yohimbe (yohimbine)	

*Categories D or X: see Table 7-3 for explanation of categories.

women or their babies.[23] Ingestion of raspberry leaf may also decrease the likelihood of preterm and postterm labour, evidenced by the smaller spread of gestation period among the raspberry leaf group. An unexpected finding appears to indicate that women who ingest raspberry leaf may be less likely to require artificial rupture of their membranes, caesarean section, forceps delivery, or vacuum birth than the women in the control group.

A follow-up trial of randomised, double-blind, placebo-controlled design was conducted by the same research team and involved 192 women treated from 32 weeks of pregnancy to labour.[24] The women in the treatment group were given 1.2 g raspberry leaf twice daily. There were no adverse effects, but there also was no shortening of the first stage of labour. The second stage was shortened by 9.6 minutes. A lower rate of forceps delivery was observed in the raspberry leaf group (19.3% vs. 30.4% for control participants). The authors suggested that earlier intervention and a higher dose should be studied.

Ginger is widely used to manage morning sickness, and fresh ginger is used in this way in traditional Chinese medicine. Despite the many clinical trials of ginger therapy for motion sickness, until recently there was only one small, short-term (4 days) pregnancy trial for hyperemesis gravidarum (30 patients, crossover design).[25] There was no evidence of any adverse outcomes caused by ginger use.

Recently results from two new trials have been released. A small Thai study that used a 4 × 250 mg dose of dried ginger powder for 4 days found a significant reduction in nausea ($P = 0.014$) and vomiting ($P < 0.001$) compared with placebo (28 patients received ginger; 35 received placebo).[26] No important side effects or adverse effects of ginger on pregnancy outcome were noted. Scientists at the University of New South Wales studied 120 pregnant women (vitamin B6 nonresponders) who were given 4 × 125 mg ginger extract (a high dose) or placebo for 4 days. Relief rates were 76% for the ginger group compared with 46% for placebo.[27]

Although these controlled studies of ginger therapy during pregnancy revealed no adverse effects, the period of use of the ginger was relatively short at 4 days. Because nausea during pregnancy can extend for several months, studies with longer treatment periods are needed.

A case-control study in Papua New Guinea demonstrated that a group of 315 women who chewed betel nut (*Areca catechu* nut mixed with *Piper betel* and slaked lime) during pregnancy had a lower frequency of anaemia than those who did not.[28] No adverse effects on the mother or foetus were observed from the betel nut consumption.

Apart from the studies on raspberry leaf and ginger noted previously, there are relatively few clinical studies on Western herbs. Most of the herbal clinical trials for health problems during pregnancy are from China. For example, in a Hong Kong study of 88 patients taking *Panax ginseng* during their pregnancy, only one had preeclampsia compared with eight in a control group ($P < 0.02$).[29]

Maternal foetal blood group incompatibility (105 cases of ABO type and 21 cases of Rh

type) treatment with a traditional Chinese medicine formula (Chinese motherwort, Banksia rose, white peony, dong quai, and ligusticum) significantly reduced perinatal mortality from 50% (control) to 7.7% (treated).[30] Twenty-eight patients with intrauterine growth retardation at weeks 31 to 34 were treated with ginseng saponin tablets. There was a strong tendency to normalise growth.[31] Low-dose rhubarb treatment (0.75 g/day) or placebo was given from week 28 onward to women at risk of pregnancy-induced hypertension (PIH). Only 5.7% of the treated group developed PIH compared with 20.8% of the control group.[32]

In countries where traditional Chinese medicine is practised, neonatal jaundice in infants with glucose-6-phosphate dehydrogenase (G6PD) deficiency has been attributed to the general use of herbs by the mother during pregnancy.[33] However, the assumption that Chinese herbs can act as haemolytic agents in G6PD-deficient infants has been questioned. In a cohort of 1008 mother-infant pairs there was no association between maternal herb consumption during pregnancy and the incidence or severity of neonatal jaundice in the offspring, including those who were deficient in G6PD.[34] However, there is a potential safety issue concerning the administration of Chinese herbs to manage existing neonatal jaundice (see Chapter 9).

A few surveys involving pregnant women or recommendations by health care professionals have been published. For example, a survey of 150 pregnant women attending an academic medical centre found 20 (13%) had used dietary supplements during pregnancy.[35] The most commonly used products were echinacea (6.9%), pregnancy tea that contained a variety of herbs (8.9%), and ginger (6.7%). Most patients informed their primary care provider of their use of supplements.

A survey of physicians and naturopaths and their respective students found that the most popular product recommended by medical doctors and naturopaths was echinacea, followed by St. John's wort.[36] Only one physician recommended a herbal product to a pregnant patient compared with 49% of the naturopaths who were comfortable doing so. Herbal products commonly recommended by naturopaths were echinacea (24%), raspberry leaf (24%), and nettle leaf (8%).

In a survey of North Carolina certified nurse-midwives, it was found that 73% recommended herbal therapy to their pregnant patients.[37] Herbs commonly recommended included ginger, peppermint, raspberry leaf, chamomile, evening primrose oil, black cohosh, and blue cohosh.

Use of Herbs Late in Pregnancy

A national survey of nurse-midwives in the United States found that approximately 50% suggested the use of herbs for labour stimulation.[38] Treatments commonly used were black cohosh, blue cohosh, raspberry leaf, castor oil, and evening primrose oil. The use of herbs near term to facilitate labour is common to many cultures. However, in some cases this has been linked to adverse events. Zoapatle (*Montanoa tomentosa*) is used as an oxytocic treatment in Mexico. Eight cases were reported in which pregnant women drank infusions of the herb during labour, and their newborn children subsequently exhibited dangerous cardiorespiratory depression.[39] A retrospective survey of patients attending a South African hospital found a higher incidence of meconium-stained fluid and caesarean section rates in the group of women reporting ingestion of herbs compared with a control group.[40]

The use of Western herbs, such as raspberry leaf and evening primrose oil, to induce or facilitate labour appears in general to be safe, although more controlled studies are needed. However, concerns have been raised about the safety of blue cohosh.

Several adverse events have been associated with maternal ingestion of blue cohosh (*Caulophyllum thalictroides*) or products containing blue cohosh. A midwife attempted induction of labour using a combination of blue and black cohosh given orally at approximately 42 weeks gestation.[41] After normal labour, the female baby was not able to breathe spontaneously and was administered cardiac massage and oxygen. The child sustained central nervous system hypoxic-ischaemic damage, which may have been related to myocardial toxicity.[42]

In their discussion of possible mechanisms behind this adverse reaction, the authors offered extrapolations and generalisations from animal studies.[41] The relevance of these extrapolations was appropriately challenged, particularly those pertaining to black cohosh (*Cimicifuga racemosa*).[43]

Profound neonatal congestive heart failure was linked to maternal consumption of blue cohosh tablets.[44] Beginning approximately 1 month before delivery, the mother took three tablets per day, even though she was advised to take only one per day. The infant exhibited signs of severe cardiac injury and was hospitalised for 31 days. At follow-up evaluation at age 2 years the child was doing well but remained on digoxin therapy. Cardiomegaly and mildly reduced left ventricular function were evident.

The FDA's Special Nutritionals Adverse Event Monitoring System database (which lists adverse events but is not subject to preconditions, analysis, or peer review) also contains two cases possibly associated with blue cohosh, including stroke in an infant.[45]

Attempts have been made to understand these adverse events in terms of the phytochemical content of blue cohosh.[46] Four known alkaloids, including anagyrine, were newly identified in blue cohosh, and a novel alkaloid thalictroidine was discovered. The alkaloids in blue cohosh belong to several phytochemical classes but are predominantly from the quinolizidine class. These alkaloids were tested in an in vitro rat embryo culture. Taspine showed high embryotoxicity, and N-methylcytisine was found to be teratogenic. The authors caution that more experiments are needed to substantiate their outcomes and examine possible consequences for the human foetus.

Anagyrine is responsible for the congenital deformity crooked calf disease.[46] The disease is not believed to occur in humans, although one case report linked a similar human congenital deformity to maternal consumption of anagyrine-contaminated goat's milk during early pregnancy.[47] Anagyrine did not demonstrate teratogenic properties in a rat embryo study.[48] However, these teratogenic and embryotoxic effects are more relevant to the use of blue cohosh in early pregnancy, which is generally avoided.

Blue cohosh was traditionally used to alleviate dysmenorrhoea and pain of childbirth and to promote delivery.[49] It was also used for amenorrhoea, rheumatic pain, and epilepsy. More recently it has been included in a clinically researched proprietary formula (Mastodynon) for the alleviation of premenstrual syndrome and mastalgia.[50] Given the widespread usage of blue cohosh by nurse-midwives noted previously, why have more adverse events not been reported?

It is generally acknowledged that blue cohosh is contraindicated during pregnancy except near term, although this restriction is not always promoted or observed. However, toxicity from short-term use of blue cohosh to induce labour (as in the first case history) is unlikely to explain the serious adverse effects observed. Perhaps the blue cohosh was used for longer periods than stated or maybe the adverse effects were idiosyncratic rather than toxic.

The presence of quinolizidine alkaloids, including sparteine in blue cohosh, could explain its oxytocic activity and its occasional toxicity. Sparteine was once widely used as an oxytocic drug, but it fell out of favour because of the uterine spasm that occurred in women who were unable to metabolise it effectively. Approximately 5% of male and female subjects studied were unable to metabolise sparteine by N-oxidation,[51] and this defect appears to have a genetic basis.[52]

N-methylcytisine, the proposed teratogenic compound in blue cohosh, is a quinolizidine alkaloid with a structure closely related to sparteine. Perhaps, like sparteine, a percentage of women are unable to efficiently metabolise this alkaloid (and others in blue cohosh), resulting in the observed adverse effects.

In an article published in the *Journal of Nurse-Midwifery*, Belew, drawing on information gained from personal communications, makes the following points about the historical and current use of blue cohosh[53]:

- Blue cohosh was used by the Native Americans to prevent miscarriages and induce labour;
- Herbalist Moore notes that physicians of the 19th century did not use blue cohosh

routinely, but rather used it for only the most difficult labours;
- A number of midwives have stopped using blue cohosh because they noted increased incidence of meconium-stained fluid, foetal tachycardia or foetal distress, and a high-pitched or inconsolable neonatal cry associated with the use of blue cohosh; and
- Some contemporary herbalists teach "this is not a benign herb" and caution against any use during pregnancy and childbirth.

Given the aforementioned recent findings concerning the blue cohosh alkaloids and the possible association with serious adverse reactions, caution should prevail with its use to promote delivery.

The Concept of Herbal Emmenagogues and its Relevance to Pregnancy

In herbal therapy, the term emmenagogue is often used to describe herbs reputed to "bring on the menses" or "stimulate menstrual flow". It is no coincidence that many clinicians consider emmenagogue herbs to also be abortifacients. In other words, emmenagogues were used to "bring on the menses" when they were delayed by pregnancy. The term was a convenient euphemism for times not as liberal as these. However, it does not necessarily follow that emmenagogues are abortifacients.

The concept of emmenagogue has created a mindset among some clinicians that the greatest risk of prescribing herbs during pregnancy is that of miscarriage. This contrasts with conventional drugs for which, probably as a result of the thalidomide tragedy, the focus of concern is more on foetotoxicity and teratogenicity. However, there is little evidence to suggest that commonly used Western herbal remedies are uniquely more prone to cause miscarriage.

Some writers have extrapolated possible mechanisms behind the abortifacient activity of emmenagogues by suggesting that they stimulate uterine contractions. However, this is the least likely explanation for how an agent may initiate menstrual flow in a nonpregnant woman. Subtle hormonal effects are a far more likely explanation for this phenomenon.

Research has demonstrated that there are plants that can stimulate uterine contraction (e.g., *Leonurus artemisia*).[54] Abortifacient activity has also been shown for plants, with the most powerful active components being identified as proteins, such as trichosanthin from *Trichosanthes kirilowii*.[55,56] An extract of neem seeds *(Azadirachta indica)* can induce abortion, but the mechanism of action is thought to be immune mediated, not stimulation of uterine contraction per se.[57,58] Needles of the lodgepole pine *(Pinus contorta)* and juniper *(Juniperus communis)* contain high levels of the fatty acid isocupressic acid, which exhibits pronounced abortifacient activity by causing decreased uterine blood flow.[59,60]

Several herbs that contain essential oils are thought to be emmenagogues and abortifacients. These include parsley *(Petroselinum crispum)*, tansy *(Tanacetum vulgare)*, rue *(Ruta graveolens)*, and pennyroyal *(Mentha pulegium)*. In reviewing the available case reports concerning the use of these essential oils (usually at doses that would be virtually impossible to achieve using the whole herbal extract), Tisserand and Balacs[61] concluded that with the exception of apiol-rich oils (parsley) and sabinyl-acetate–rich oils (Spanish sage), there appears to be no clear evidence that any essential oils present an abortifacient risk.

Many of the commonly used emmenagogue herbs may be excluded from use during pregnancy because of potential toxicity, undesirable hormonal effects, or other possible detrimental effects. However, abortifacient activity is probably the least likely reason for any safety concerns regarding their use during pregnancy.

Phytooestrogens

Many plants contain substances that are weakly oestrogenic, known as phytooestrogens. The phytooestrogens can be divided into five main chemical classes: flavonoids, especially isoflavonoids; lignans; saponins; sterols; and some essential oils (e.g., fennel and clary sage oils).

The medical world still lives in fear of another diethylstilbestrol (DES). This was a potent synthetic nonsteroidal oestrogen, liberally used from 1940 to 1960 to manage threatened abortion, toxaemia of pregnancy, and gestational diabetes. In the 1970s there was a noticeable increase in the incidence of a rare clear cell adenocarcinoma of the vagina. These tumours were found to occur in women whose mothers had been treated with DES during pregnancy. The female embryos were exposed to DES during organogenesis. Other anomalies of the female reproductive tract have been reported.

There is a concern in some circles that phytooestrogens may act like DES and cause toxic effects on the female tract in utero. However, the important consideration is that phytooestrogens are weakly oestrogenic, whereas DES is so powerful that it depresses serum gonadotropin levels and induces uterine growth in relatively small doses. A sheep living on clover *(Trifolium* spp., which contain isoflavonoid phytooestrogens) may show these effects, but they do not occur with normal human consumption of phytooestrogens from either food or herbal medicine.

Moreover, one of the richest sources of phytooestrogens is the soya bean. If phytooestrogen intake did represent a real risk during pregnancy, then problems similar to those caused by DES should be higher in countries in which soya is a staple. These have not been reliably observed.

Moreover, animal experiments involving the intake of the isoflavone genistein (found in soya) at normal dietary levels during pregnancy have not demonstrated adverse effects.[62,63] A survey of seven young healthy Japanese women and their babies at delivery found high levels of isoflavonoid phytooestrogens in the healthy infants, indicating transfer of isoflavonoids from the maternal to foetal compartment.[64] Rather than suggesting harm from this phenomenon, the authors postulated that this could reflect on a reduced risk of hormone-dependent cancers later in life.

As part of the Avon Longitudinal Study of Pregnancy and Childhood (ALSPAC) Study, the association between maternal diet, particularly vegetarianism and consumption of phytooestrogens, and the incidence of hypospadias in male infants was investigated.[65] Of 7928 boys born to mothers taking part in the study, 51 cases of hypospadias were identified. Mothers who were vegetarian during their pregnancy had an adjusted odds ratio of 4.99 (95% confidence interval, 2.10 to 11.88) of giving birth to a boy with hypospadias. However, whether this association is reflected elsewhere or is linked to the maternal consumption of phytooestrogens remains to be investigated.

Teratogenicity and Foetotoxicity

Knowledge about the teratogenic effects of leaves, bark, and fruits of plants has come from the observation of grazing animals. It should be kept in mind that in these circumstances the intake of the herb by the animal can be large and that the animals are consuming parts of the plant that may not be used by humans. Several of these plants are known poisons, and human intake is specifically avoided. Based on these observations and resultant experiments, three categories have been assigned[48,66,67]:

- Known teratogens in known teratogenic plants: *Lupinus, Veratrum, Conium,* and *Solanum* spp.;
- Known teratogenic plants with unidentified teratogens: *Astragalus* (not the species used in herbal therapy), *Nicotiana, Ferula,* and *Trachymene* spp.; and
- Suspected teratogenic plants: *Datura, Prunus, Sorghum,* and *Senecio* spp.

Information about the potential teratogenicity or foetotoxicity of medicines is generated from animal studies under controlled experimental conditions. Relatively few herbs have been studied in such models. Some examples of such studies are described here; others are provided in the various safety monographs in the second half of the book.

The teratogenicity of Baical skullcap (*Scutellaria baicalensis*) was studied in rats. Three dosages were used: 0.25 g/kg (group 1), 12.49 g/kg (group 2), and 24.98 g/kg (group 3). An increase in the incidence of skeletal variations (lumbar rib) was observed, which was only marked for groups 2 and 3. There was also a dose-dependent increase in dilation of the ureter. No significant differences for the other parameters tested were detected.[68] The normal human dose for Baical skullcap is approximately 0.05 g/kg. Given the aforementioned results it would be prudent not to use Baical skullcap for extended periods during early pregnancy; however, more studies are needed to draw definitive conclusions about any teratogenic activity of Baical skullcap. Therefore, it has been assigned the pregnancy classification B3.

In a randomised, placebo-controlled study, mice exposed antenatally to St. John's wort were subjected to behavioural testing.[69] No deficits on selected behavioural tasks by developing mice were observed. Maternal administration of St. John's wort before and throughout gestation did not affect long-term growth and physical maturation of the offspring of exposed mice.[70]

An extract of boldo (*Peumus boldus*) and the constituent boldine showed abortive and teratogenic activity in rats.[71] Several species of plants used in herbal therapy contain pyrrolizidine alkaloids that have been shown to act as teratogens.[72] These include comfrey (*Symphytum officinale*) and coltsfoot (*Tussilago farfara*). Valepotriates from valerian induced some alterations after administration by the intraperitoneal route, but doses given orally were innocuous to pregnant rats and their offspring.[73]

Teratogenesis attributed to herb use by humans has occasionally been reported. The Chinese herb thundergod vine (*Tripterygium wilfordii*) is attracting attention as a therapy for rheumatoid arthritis. However, an infant was delivered normally at 38 weeks with a huge cystic mass protruding from the occiput, which was diagnosed as occipital meningoencephalocele and cerebellar agenesis.[74] His mother had taken the herb for rheumatoid arthritis early in her pregnancy.

Podophyllum resin (American mandrake) was applied five times for 4 hours from the 23rd to the 29th week of pregnancy. At birth, a simian crease on the left hand and a preauricular skin tag were noted in the infant.[75]

A woman who allegedly took *Eleutherococcus senticosus* during her pregnancy gave birth to a baby with neonatal androgenisation, the so-called hairy baby syndrome.[76] It was later suggested that the mother had consumed the Chinese herb *Periploca sepium*, which had been substituted for the *E. senticosus*.[77]

LACTATION

Although the majority of herbs are probably safe to use for the nursing mother, there is little known about how secondary plant metabolites may pass into the breast milk and possibly affect the infant. Obviously toxic and poisonous herbs should be avoided (see Table 7-5). As during pregnancy, oral doses of pure essential oils should be avoided during breast-feeding. High doses of herbal medicines that contain potentially toxic essential oils, such as wormwood and tansy, should also be avoided.

The German Commission E and ESCOP monographs on bearberry (Arctostaphylos uva-ursi) recommend against its use during lactation. One report suggests that dong quai (Angelica sinensis) may have caused hypertension in a woman and her breast-fed infant.[78]

Many herbs have traditionally been used to promote breast milk and are described in the literature as galactagogues. However, there is little clinical research on their effects. Chaste tree demonstrated a favourable effect on milk production in 80% of 125 subjects in a case observation study.[79] In an open, controlled trial of 817 patients, a significant effect was observed from chaste tree treatment with average milk production approximately three times that of controls after 20 days of treatment.[80] However, the recent discovery of the dopaminergic activity of chaste tree suggests that it could have the opposite effect on breast milk production, particularly at higher doses.[81,82]

Although concerns have been expressed about the use of anthraquinone-containing laxative herbs during breast-feeding, this is not supported by the current clinical evidence. The excretion of rhein, a weakly active laxative metabolite of sennosides, was investigated in 100 breast milk samples of 20 postpartum women after intake of a standardised senna laxative.[83] After daily doses of 5 g of the senna laxative containing 15 mg sennosides for 3 days, the rhein concentration in milk samples from every lactation during 24 hours postdose varied between 0 and 27 ng/mL, with values <10 ng/mL in 94%. Based on median values, 0.007% of the sennoside intake (calculated as rhein) was excreted in breast milk. None of the breast-fed infants had an abnormal stool consistency.

However, animal experiments have found that active metabolites of plants can potentially be transferred to the offspring at pharmacologically active levels. For example, the possible transfer of the active principle(s) of mace (aril of the plant Myristica fragrans) through the transmammary route and its ability to modulate hepatic xenobiotic metabolising enzymes in the progeny of mice were studied.[84] An aqueous suspension of mace at the dose levels of 0.025 or 0.1 g/animal/day was administered by oral gavage from day 1 of lactation and continued daily for 14 or 21 days. Dams receiving mace treatment and their pups showed significantly elevated hepatic sulphhydryl content, glutathione S-transferase and glutathione reductase activities, and cytochrome b5 content. Hepatic cytochrome P450 content decreased in dams ($P < 0.05$) receiving the lower mace dose for 21 days and the pups ($P < 0.001$), but it increased in dams receiving the higher dose for both time periods ($P < 0.001$) and the lower dose for 14 days ($P < 0.05$). Only the 14-day-old pups of dams receiving either mace dose showed significantly elevated ($P < 0.001$) levels of hepatic glutathione peroxidase.

The American Academy of Pediatrics published guidelines and a classification system for drugs used in lactating women.[85] The classification is as follows:

ND: No data available

C: Compatible with breast-feeding

CC: Compatible with breast-feeding but use caution

SD: Strongly discouraged in breast-feeding

X: Contraindicated in breast-feeding

These classifications are based on controlled studies in animals or humans and on data gathered from using the drugs in pregnant women. Most medications fall into the category ND.

The aforementioned classification will be used throughout this text in the herbal safety monographs. Clearly, as for conventional drugs, many herbs are in the ND category. When herbs have a recorded traditional use as galactagogues, they have been classified as C, compatible with breast-feeding.

CONCLUSIONS AND RECOMMENDATIONS

Throughout the world many pregnant women consume a great variety of herbs. Although it is reasonable to state that the safety of herbs during pregnancy and lactation is not well documented in humans, the same observation can also be made for conventional drugs, which are also widely used during pregnancy.

Rather than classifying herbs simply as safe or unsafe during pregnancy, it is suggested that a classification system be adopted that provides the degree of safety information that is available for each individual herb. Such a classification would provide a more realistic basis for a risk-benefit analysis. Some professionals or patients may choose to not prescribe or take any herbs during pregnancy or perhaps only the few herbs in category A. Others may see a possible benefit in prescribing or taking herbs with a B or C classification. However, it is recommended that herbs with a C or D classification are only used during pregnancy under close and highly trained supervision.

REFERENCES

1. McGuffin M, Hobbs C, Upton R, Goldberg A, editors: *American Herbal Products Association's botanical safety handbook,* Boca Raton, 1997, CRC Press.
2. Newall CA, Anderson LA, Phillipson JD: *Herbal medicines: a guide for health-care professionals*, London, 1996, Pharmaceutical Press.
3. Gibson PS, Powrie R, Star J: Herbal and alternative medicine use during pregnancy: a cross-sectional survey, *Obstet Gynecol* 97(suppl 1):S44-S45, 2001.
4. Lacroix I, Damase-Michel C, Lapeyre-Mestre M, et al: Prescription of drugs during pregnancy in France, *Lancet* 356:1735-1736, 2000.
5. Larimore WL: Medications used in pregnancy and lactation. Online coverage from the 50th Annual Meeting of the American Academy of Family Physicians Scientific Assembly, September 16-20, 1998. Available at: http://medscape.com/Medscape/CNO/1998/AFFP/0 9.18.../AAFP.18.559.Lari.htm.
6. Weiss SR: Prescription medication use in pregnancy, *Medscape Pharmacother*, 2000. Available at: http://www. medscape.com/pharmacology/journal/2000/v02.n06.../pnt-mp7387.weis.htm.
7. Hamilton H: Presentation to the Pregnancy Labeling Subcommittee of the Advisory Committee for Reproductive Health Drugs. Gaithersburg, Maryland. March 29, 2000. Cited in Weiss SR: Prescription medication use in pregnancy, *Medscape Pharmacother*, 2000. Available at: http://www.medscape.com/pharmacology/journal/2000/v02.n06.../pnt-mp7387.weis.htm.
8. Kacew S: Effect of over-the-counter drugs on the unborn child: what is known and how should this influence prescribing? *Paediatr Drugs* 1:75-80, 1999.
9. Holmes LB, Harvey EA, Coull BA, et al: The teratogenicity of anticonvulsant drugs, *N Engl J Med* 344:1132-1138, 2001.
10. Nielsen GL, Sorensen HT, Larsen H, et al: Risk of adverse birth outcome and miscarriage in pregnant users of non-steroidal anti-inflammatory drugs: population based observational study and case-control study, *BMJ* 322:266-270, 2001.
11. Mills S, Bone K: *Principles and practice of phytotherapy: modern herbal medicine*, Edinburgh, 2000, Churchill Livingstone.
12. Brinker F: *Herb contraindications and drug interactions*, ed 2, Sandy, 1998, Eclectic Medical Publications.
13. Blumenthal M, et al, editors: *The complete German Commission E monographs: therapeutic guide to herbal medicines*, Austin, 1998, American Botanical Council.
14. Wilkinson JM: What do we know about herbal morning sickness treatments? A literature survey, *Midwifery* 16:224-228, 2000.
15. Daware MB, Mujumdar AM, Ghaskadbi S: Reproductive toxicity of piperine in Swiss albino mice, *Planta Med* 66:231-236, 2000.
16. Vago O: Toxic and caustic complications through use of so-called abortifacients, *Z Geburtshilfe Perinatol* 170:272-277, 1969.
17. Stubblefield PG, Naftolin F, Frigoletto F, et al: Laminaria augmentation of intro-amniotic PGF2 for midtrimester pregnancy termination, *Prostaglandins* 10:413-422, 1975.
18. Lehmann R: Personal communication, 1999.
19. Gallo M, Sarkar M, Au W, et al: Pregnancy outcome following gestational exposure to Echinacea; a prospective controlled study, *Arch Intern Med* 160:3141-3143, 2000.
20. Strandberg TE, Jarvenpaa AL, Vanhanen H, et al: Birth outcome in relation to licorice consumption during pregnancy, *Am J Epidemiol* 153:1085-1088, 2001.
21. Leng-Peschlow E: Risk assessment for senna during pregnancy, *Pharmacology* 44(suppl 1):20-22, 1992.
22. Dove D, Johnson P: Oral evening primrose oil: its effect on length of pregnancy and selected intrapartum outcomes in low-risk nulliparous women, *J Nurse-Midwifery* 44:320-324, 1999.
23. Parsons M, Simpson, Ponton T: Raspberry leaf and its effect on labour: safety and efficacy, *J Aust Coll Midwives* 12:20-25, 1999.
24. Simpson M, Parson M, Greenwood J, et al: Raspberry leaf in pregnancy: its safety and efficacy in labor, *J Midwifery Womens Health* 46:51-59, 2001.
25. Fischer-Rasmussen W, Kjaer SK, Dahl C, et al: Ginger treatment of hyperemesis gravidarum, *Eur J Obstet Gynecol Reprod Biol* 38:19-24, 1990.
26. Vutyavanich T, Kraisarin T, Ruangsri R: Ginger for nausea and vomiting in pregnancy: randomized, double-masked, placebo-controlled trial, *Obstet Gynecol* 97:577-582, 2001.
27. Eden J: Ginger caps relieve morning sickness, *Medical Observer* July 21, 2000.
28. Taufa T: Betel-nut chewing and pregnancy, *Papua New Guinea Med J* 31:229-233, 1988.
29. Chin RK: Ginseng and common pregnancy disorders, *Asia Oceania J Obstet Gynaecol* 17:379-380, 1991.
30. Bian X, Xu Y, Zhu L, et al: Prevention of maternal-fetal blood group incompatibility with traditional Chinese herbal medicine, *Chin Med J (Engl)* 111:585-587, 1998.

31. Zhang WY, Teng H, Zheng Y: [Ginseng saponin treatment for intrauterine growth retardation], Zhonghua Yi Xue Za Zhi 74:608-610, 646, 1994.

32. Zhang ZJ, Cheng WW, Yang YM: [Low-dose of processed rhubarb in preventing pregnancy induced hypertension], Zhonghua Fu Chan Ke Za Zhi 29:463-464, 509, 1994.

33. Wong HB: Effects of herbs and drugs during pregnancy and lactation, J Singapore Paediatr Soc 21:169-178, 1979.

34. Fok TF: Neonatal jaundice–traditional Chinese medicine approach, J Perinatol 21:S98-S100, 2001.

35. Tsui B, Dennehy CE, Tsourounis C: A survey of dietary supplement use during pregnancy at an academic medical center, Am J Obstet Gynecol 185:433-437, 2001.

36. Einarson A, Lawrimore T, Brand P, et al: Attitudes and practices of physicians and naturopaths toward herbal products, including use during pregnancy and lactation, Can J Clin Pharmacol 7:45-49, 2000.

37. Allaire AD, Moos MK, Wells SR: Complementary and alternative medicine in pregnancy: a survey of North Carolina certified nurse-midwives, Obstet Gynecol 95:19-23, 2000.

38. McFarlin BL, Gisbon MH, O'Rear J, et al: A national survey of herbal preparation use by nurse-midwives for labor stimulation, J Nurse-Midwifery 44:205-216, 1999.

39. Montoya-Cabrera MA, Simental-Toba A, Sanchez-Rodriguez S, et al: [Cardiorespiratory depression in 8 newborn infants whose mothers took "yucuyahui" (Zoapatle-Montanoa tomentosa) during labor], Gac Med Mex 134:611-615, 1998.

40. Mabina MH, Pitsoe SB, Moodley J: The effect of traditional herbal medicines on pregnancy outcome. The King Edward VIII Hospital experience, S Afr Med J 87:1008-1010, 1997.

41. Gunn TR, Wright IM: The use of black and blue cohosh in labour, N Z Med J 109:410-411, 1996.

42. Wright IMR: Neonatal effects of maternal consumption of blue cohosh, J Pediatr 134:384-385, 1999.

43. Baillie N, Rasmussen P: Black and blue cohosh in labour, N Z Med J 110:20-21, 1997.

44. Jones TK, Lawson BM: Profound neonatal congestive heart failure caused by maternal consumption of blue cohosh herbal medication, J Pediatr 132:550-552, 1998.

45. US Food and Drug Administration Center for Food Safety and Applied Nutrition Office of Special Nutritionals: The Special Nutritionals Adverse Event Monitoring System. Available at: http://vm.cfsan.fda.gov/~dms/aems.html.

46. Kennelly EJ, Flynn TJ, Mazzola EP, et al: Detecting potential teratogenic alkaloids from blue cohosh rhizomes using an in vitro rat embryo culture, J Nat Prod 62:1385-1389, 1999.

47. Ortega JA, Lazerson J: Anagyrine-induced red cell aplasia, vascular anomaly, and skeletal dysplasia, J Pediatr 111:93-99, 1987.

48. Keller RF: Teratogens in plants, J Animal Sci 58:1029-1039, 1984.

49. Felter HW, Lloyd JU: King's American dispensatory, vol 1, ed 18, revision 3, 1905; reprinted Portland, 1983, Eclectic Medical Publications, pp 468-472.

50. Kubista E, Muller G, Spona J: [Treatment of mastopathies with cyclic mastodynia. Clinical results and hormonal profiles], Rev Fr Gynecol Obstet 82:221-227, 1987.

51. Eichelbaum M, Spannbrucker N, Steincke B, et al: Defective N-oxidation of sparteine in man: a new pharmacogenetic defect, Eur J Clin Pharmacol 16:183-187, 1979.

52. Vinks A, Inaba T, Otton SV, et al: Sparteine metabolism in Canadian Caucasians, Clin Pharmacol Ther 31:23-29, 1982.

53. Belew C: Herbs and the childbearing woman: guidelines for midwives, J Nurse-Midwifery 44:231-252, 1999.

54. Chan WC, Wong YC, Kong YC, et al: Clinical observation on the uterotonic effect of I-mu Ts'ao (Leonurus artemisia), Am J Chin Med 11:77-83, 1983.

55. Yeung HW, Feng Z, Li WW, et al: Abortifacient activity in leaves, roots and seeds of Phytolacca acinosa, J Ethnopharmacol 21:31-35, 1987.

56. Maraganore JM, Joseph M, Bailey MC: Purification and characterization of trichosanthin. Homology to the ricin A chain and implications as to mechanism of abortifacient activity, J Biol Chem 262:11628-11633, 1987.

57. Mukherjee S, Garg S, Talwar GP: Early post implantation contraceptive effects of a purified fraction of neem (Azadirachta indica) seeds, given orally in rats: possible mechanisms involved, J Ethnopharmacol 67:287-296, 1999.

58. Mukherjee S, Talwar GP: Termination of pregnancy in rodents by oral administration of praneem, a purified neem seed extract, Am J Reprod Immunol 35:51-56, 1996.

59. Gardner DR, Panter KE, James LF, et al: Abortifacient effects of lodgepole pine (Pinus contorta) and common juniper (Juniperus communis) on cattle, Vet Hum Toxicol 40:260-263, 1998.

60. Ford SP, Rosazza JP, Al-Mahmoud MS, et al: Abortifacient effects of a unique class of vasoactive lipids from Pinus ponderosa needles, J Anim Sci 77:2187-2193, 1999.

61. Tisserand R, Balacs T: Essential oil safety, Edinburgh, 1995, Churchill Livingstone.

62. Flynn KM, Ferguson SA, Delclos KB, et al: Effects of genistein exposure on sexually dimorphic behaviors in rats, Toxicol Sci 55:311-319, 2000.

63. Casanova M, You L, Archibeque-Engle S, et al: Effects of dietary genistein on reproductive development of Sprague-Dawley rats, Toxicologist 48:375, 1999.

64. Adlercreutz H, Yamada T, Wahala K, et al: Maternal and neonatal phytoestrogens in Japanese women during birth, Am J Obstet Gynecol 180:737-743, 1999.

65. North K, Golding J: A maternal vegetarian diet in pregnancy is associated with hypospadias. The ALSPAC Study Team. Avon Longitudinal Study of Pregnancy and Childhood, BJU Int 85:107-113, 2000.

66. Shlosberg A, Egyed MN: Examples of poisonous plants in Israel of importance to animals and man, Arch Toxicol Suppl 6:194-196, 1983.

67. Beier RC: Natural pesticides and bioactive components in foods, Rev Environ Contam Toxicol 113:47-137, 1990.

68. Kim SH, Kim YH, Han SS, et al: Teratogenicity study of Scutellariae Radix in rats, Reprod Toxicol 7:73-79, 1993.

69. Rayburn WF, Christensen HD, Gonzalez CL: Effect of antenatal exposure to Saint John's wort (Hypericum) on

neurobehavior of developing mice, *Am J Obstet Gynecol* 183:1225-1231, 2000.

70. Rayburn WF, Gonzalez CL, Christensen HD, et al: Effect of prenatally administered hypericum (St John's wort) on growth and physical maturation of mouse offspring, *Am J Obstet Gynecol* 184:191-195, 2001.

71. Almeida ER, Melo AM, Xavier H: Toxicological evaluation of the hydro-alcohol extract of the dry leaves of Peumus boldus and boldine in rats, *Phytother Res* 14:99-102, 2000.

72. Prakash AS, Pereira TN, Reilly PE, et al: Pyrrolizidine alkaloids in human diet, *Mutat Res* 443:53-67, 1999.

73. Tufik S, Fujita K, Seabra MD, et al: Effects of a prolonged administration of valepotriates in rats on the mothers and their offspring, *J Ethnopharmacol* 41:39-44, 1994.

74. Takei A, Nagashima G, Suzuki R, et al: Meningoencephalocele associated with Tripterygium wilfordii treatment, *Pediatr Neurosurg* 27:45-48, 1997.

75. Karol MD, Conner CS, Watanabe AS, et al: Podophyllum: suspected teratogenicity from topical application, *Clin Toxicol* 16:283-286, 1980.

76. Koren G, Randor S, Martin S, et al: Maternal ginseng use associated with neonatal androgenization, *JAMA* 264;2866, 1990.

77. Awang DV: Maternal use of ginseng and neonatal androgenization, *JAMA* 266:363, 1991.

78. Nambiar S, Schwartz RH, Constantino A: Hypertension in mother and baby linked to ingestion of Chinese herbal medicine, *West J Med* 171:152, 1999.

79. Noack M: Unsere erfahrungen mit agnus castus oligoplex bei der laktations steigerung, *Dtsch Med Wschr* 9:204-206, 1943.

80. Mohr W: Gedanken zur forderung des stillens durch medikamente, *Hippokrates* 28:586-591, 1957.

81. Sliutz G, Speiser P, Schultz AM, et al: Agnus castus extracts inhibit prolactin secretion of rat pituitary cells, *Horm Metab Res* 25:253-255, 1993.

82. Winterhoff H: 212th American Chemical Society National Meeting, Orlando, August 25-29, 1996. Abstract No. 105.

83. Faber P, Strenge-Hesse A: Relevance of rhein excretion into breast milk, *Pharmacology* 36(suppl 1):212-220, 1988.

84. Chhabra SK, Rao AR: Transmammary modulation of xenobiotic metabolizing enzymes in liver of mouse pups by mace (Myristica fragrans Houtt.), *J Ethnopharmacol* 42:169-177, 1994.

85. American Academy of Pediatrics Committee on Drugs: The transfer of drugs and other chemicals into human milk, *Pediatrics* 93:137-150, 1994.

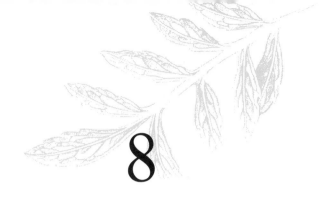

8

The Impact of Quality Issues on the Safety of Herbal Products

Kerry Bone

Probably the most commonly documented reason for toxic or adverse reactions to herbal products is the presence of adulterants. In this context the term "adulterants" can be defined as the intentional or unintentional presence of undeclared ingredients that impact adversely on the safety of the product. This adulteration may be caused by:

- Unintentional or intentional substitution of one or more herbal ingredients with toxic species;
- Intentional addition of a conventional chemical drug, either of natural or synthetic origin;
- Environmental contamination of the herb with a chemical or pathogen; and
- Intentional addition of a "natural" active component that is responsible for the adverse reaction, such as a microorganism, mineral, or nutrient.

These problems can generally be overcome with responsible manufacture, adequate testing, and, above all, a commitment to pharma-

ceutical level good manufacturing practice (GMP).

GMP at the pharmaceutical level is legally required for the manufacture of herbal products in many countries, such as Australia, Japan, Canada, and Germany. Pharmaceutical GMP is a specialised system of quality assurance that is extremely exacting and comprehensive. Its objective is to ensure the quality of the finished product. Manufacturers operating under pharmaceutical GMP must comply with a code of practice. There are many such codes in effect throughout the world, but they generally share common similarities. Companies that manufacture herbal products are regularly inspected against the code operating in their country, which is typically the same code applied to manufacturers of pharmaceutical drugs. Procedures and observances under GMP include:

- Validation of equipment and processes;
- Documented standard operating procedures covering every aspect of manufacture;

- Documented cleaning and calibration logs for equipment;
- Control of the manufacturing environment, air, and water;
- Quarantine and unique identification and testing of raw materials, labels, and packaging;
- In the case of herbal ingredients, identification must be confirmed by comparison with a verified reference material for that particular plant part and species;
- Discrete batch identification for products;
- Comprehensive batch record documentation;
- Reconciliation of raw materials, product, packaging, and labels;
- Quarantine and testing of finished products;
- Documented release-for-sale procedures;
- Testing of stability of finished products; and
- Documentation of customer complaints and recall procedures.

In addition to the aforementioned procedures, special requirements also exist for herbal products such as testing for microbiological quality and screening for contaminants such as pesticides, heavy metals, and radioactivity. Herbs are biological entities and hence not only run the risk of being misidentified but also carry a history that may have resulted in the presence of undesirable contaminants.

However, it must be stressed that GMP is only a code of practice. A manufacturer's level of compliance with GMP must be high to avoid some of the pitfalls described here.

ADULTERATION WITH TOXIC HERBS

The intentional or unintentional substitution of herbal ingredients with other plant species is the most fundamental, and currently most relevant, quality issue for herbal products. At best it will compromise the efficacy of the herbal product. At worst it has resulted in most serious health consequences.

There are several examples in the literature, but the most infamous and tragic example is that commonly referred to (perhaps incorrectly) as Chinese herb nephropathy (CHN). In

Belgium, a group of medical doctors running a slimming program decided to include herbs in their treatment. One of the herbs they wanted to include was *Stephania tetrandra,* but many patients in fact received *Aristolochia fangchi*, which contains aristolochic acid.[1,2] This substitution is relatively common and has been attributed to the herbs having the same PinYin name: Fang Ji.[3] Many women developed renal failure and required dialysis. One theory put forward was that a diuretic drug that the women received potentiated the nephrotoxicity of the aristolochic acid. The drug was acetazolamide, a sulfonamide drug that can cause metabolic acidosis, anorexia, and weight loss and can be nephrotoxic. However, aristolochic acid has been known as a nephrotoxin for decades, and cases not linked to the concurrent use of drugs have also been reported (to be discussed).[4]

In 1997 it was reported that two women involved in this tragedy subsequently developed urothelial cancer caused by the genotoxicity of aristolochic acid.[5] An article published in June 1999 reported further cases of urothelial cancer. Cosyns et al[6] tested 10 patients with CHN *(A. fangchi)*. Four (40%) were found to have urothelial carcinoma, and abnormal cells were found in all of the 10 patients. Nortier et al[7] (June 2000) concluded that the incidence of urothelial cancer among patients with CHN is high and that the risk was related to the cumulative dose of the herb. They report treating 105 patients with CHN of whom 43 had been admitted with end-stage renal failure. Thirty-nine of these patients were tested for urothelial carcinoma. Eighteen cases were found, and mild-to-moderate dysplasia was found in a further 19 patients.

Cases of CHN have also been reported in France, Spain, Japan, the United Kingdom, and Taiwan, where cases of urothelial carcinoma have also been detected.[7] *Aristolochia* spp. can also be used as substitutes for several other Chinese herbs,[8] and Chinese herbal products found to contain aristolochic acid have been recalled in several countries (e.g., Australia[9] and the United States[10]).

Other examples of toxic herb substitution are detailed here. A letter to the *British Medical Journal* in 1996 asserted that podophyllum poisoning had developed into a miniepidemic in Hong Kong.[11] The poisoning was caused by ingestion of the herb known in Cantonese as Gwai Kou, which is derived from the roots and rhizomes of *Podophyllum hexandrum* (also known as *P. emodi*). The herb appeared in Hong Kong in 1989 as an adulterant of Lung Dam Cho (*Gentiana* spp.) and led to two cases of neuropathy and encephalopathy. Around the same period, this herb was found in Taipei and Kuala Lumpur as an adulterant of another herb, Wai Ling Sin, which is the root of *Clematis* spp. Nine cases of neuropathy have been reported in Hong Kong. Approximately 10% of 234 samples of Wai Ling Sin taken from Hong Kong outlets were found to be podophyllum.

Herb substitution with toxic consequences has also occurred in the Western world. One that is relatively common is the substitution of the hepatotoxic herb germander (*Teucrium* spp.) for skullcap (*Scutellaria lateriflora*). This is discussed in detail in the skullcap monograph in this text. One case of hepatotoxicity in the United Kingdom, which was supposedly associated with skullcap, was verified to have resulted from the intake of the substitute herb *Teucrium canadense*, which has the common name pink skullcap.[12]

A case was described in the early 1990s of a woman who gave birth to a baby with excessive body hair after reportedly consuming herbal tablets containing Siberian ginseng (*Eleutherococcus senticosus*) during her pregnancy.[13] However, tests revealed that the woman had taken Chinese silk vine (*Periploca sepium*), apparently a common substitute for *E. senticosus*.[14] Intake of *E. senticosus* has been associated with falsely elevated digoxin levels, possibly because of an interaction with the digoxin assay.[15] However, it has also been suggested that this phenomenon may also be caused by substitution of *Periploca* because this herb contains cardiac glycosides.[16]

There have been several accounts of commercial herbal tea products adulterated with plant parts of *Atropa belladonna*. This can lead to symptoms of atropine poisoning, such as tachycardia, rapid or stertorous respiration, hyperpyrexia, restlessness, confusion, and hallucinations passing into delirium. Examples include burdock root tea (contaminated with belladonna root),[17,18] stinging nettle tea (contaminated with belladonna leaf),[19] and comfrey leaf tea (contaminated with belladonna leaf).[20,21]

Sometimes unintentional adulteration can occur when harvesting a herb from the wild for personal use. Venoocclusive disease of the liver was diagnosed in an 18-month-old boy who had regularly consumed a herbal tea mixture.[22] The tea contained peppermint and what the mother thought was coltsfoot (*Tussilago farfara*). However, macroscopic and microscopic analysis of the leaf material indicated that the parents had erroneously gathered alpendost (*Adenostyles alliariae*) instead of coltsfoot. The two plants can be confused, especially after the flowering period. This may also explain why coltsfoot has developed a reputation as a toxic herb in some quarters.

Four cases of poisoning associated with consumption of herbal teas mistakenly made with poisonous plants were reported in the United States.[23] Two cases were in Arizona where infants were fed large amounts of a tea prepared supposedly from gordolobo (*Gnaphalium* spp.) but which instead contained *Senecio longilobus* (a species also known as gordolobo, which contains hepatotoxic pyrrolizidine alkaloids). One of the children died. The two other cases from Washington, both fatal, involved an elderly couple who mistakenly harvested foxgloves (*Digitalis* spp.) instead of comfrey (*Symphytum* spp.). The two plants resemble each other in the stage before flowering.

In some instances the substituted herb is the same plant part and species but is a more toxic preparation or chemotype. A good example of this is the Chinese herb aconite (*Aconitum carmichaelii* or *Aconitum kusnezoffii*). In traditional Chinese medicine aconite root is cured to reduce its toxicity. If this is not done or is performed improperly, the root will be highly toxic. Processing (curing) can reduce the toxicity by as much as 90%.[24] Most reported cases of poisoning (many of which were fatal) appear to be caused by the cured root,[24-26] although inadequate processing or inappropriate preparation by the patient have also been implicated.[24,25]

ADULTERATION WITH SYNTHETIC DRUGS

Perhaps the most reprehensible form of adulteration of herbal products is the intentional addition of a conventional drug that is not declared on the label. Most of the documented cases occur for products made in Asia, but successful prosecutions have also occurred in Australia under the Therapeutics Goods Act. This problem has been consistently reported in the literature since the 1970s, and a number of recent examples indicate that it is still current.

Cow's Head brand Tung Shueh is a product promoted for problems of the "heart, liver and kidney" and other problems such as spasms, rheumatism, and poor circulation. Analysis found 3.86 mg of indomethacin, 16 mg of mefenamic acid, 7.94 mg of diclofenac, and 0.73 mg of diazepam per pill.[27] At the recommended dose of 12 pills a day, a consumer would unknowingly ingest 10 mg of diazepam and be at risk of side effects from the antiinflammatory agents.

Jin Bu Huan anodyne tablets for sale in health food shops in Denver contained 36% tetrahydropalmatine (THP). THP is a potent compound that is found in the Chinese herbs Stephania root and corydalis but at much lower levels. Jin bu huan has been associated with hepatitis[28] and poisoning in children.[29]

A case of Stevens-Johnson syndrome was attributed to ginseng *(Panax ginseng)* intake.[30] However, the authors correctly caution that the ginseng tablets used by the patient may have contained undeclared drugs. Because the product was not analysed, this adverse reaction cannot be conclusively attributed to the herb.

Other examples of the adulteration of Chinese herbal medicines with synthetic drugs are provided in two recent reviews[31,32] and also in Chapter 9. A wide variety of agents, including corticosteroids, nonsteroidal antiinflammatory drugs, analgesics, benzodiazepines, anticonvulsants, and hypoglycaemic drugs, have been found. Some recent cases not reviewed in these sources are described here.

Cases of adrenal suppression have been linked to the intake of Chinese herbal products. A Taiwanese study found that 8 of 13 patients with severe illness and low cortisol levels reported using herbal products.[33] However, only two of these eight patients failed the corticotropin stimulation test, suggestive of true adrenocortical insufficiency. The contents of the herbal products consumed by the patients were not tested. Two cases of adrenal suppression were reported in

New Zealand and attributed to the intake of the Chinese herbal product Shen Loon.[34] The product was later found to contain the corticosteroid betamethasone, although the authors suggested other factors could be involved as well.

Undeclared codeine was detected in a Chinese antiasthmatic proprietary product.[35] A recent phenomenon that has fortunately received a high degree of media attention is the adulteration of Chinese weight-loss products with banned weight-loss drugs such as fenfluramine. This has led to toxic reactions or fatalities in the United Kingdom, Singapore, Japan, and China.[36-39] The US Food and Drug Administration (FDA) also issued a warning about these products.[40] As a response to this publicity (and presumably pressure from the Japanese government) it was announced in 2002 that China had launched a nationwide crackdown on the illegal practices of adding pharmaceutical drugs to slimming pills.[41] It is hoped this concern will extend to the many other products adulterated with synthetic drugs.

One area that deserves noting is the potential for herbal products adulterated with synthetic drugs to cause failures of random drug tests. Some athletes have already offered this as an explanation for testing positive to banned substances. The chemical androstenedione is used in popular muscle-building nutrition and herbal supplements in the United States.[42] Whether regular use of this agent will lead to failure of drug tests is unclear. One curious case was that of a patient who tested positive for a cocaine metabolite in her urine but denied abuse.[43] This was traced to a mugwort *(Artemisia vulgaris)* tea that had somehow been contaminated with cocaine.

ADULTERATION WITH SYNTHETIC DRUGS: THE CAUTIONARY TALE OF PC-SPES

PC-SPES was a herbal formulation specifically targeted for the management of prostate cancer (hence PC) developed and patented in the early 1990s by a research chemist.[44] It contained seven Chinese herbs and one American herb (saw palmetto, *Serenoa repens*). The product was successful in the US marketplace, and there were consistent anecdotal accounts of its efficacy, especially for controlling prostate-specific antigen levels. In particular, naturopathic physicians and holistic medical doctors prescribed the product to many patients. Being a US-sponsored product they had no reason to believe it was anything other than a herbal product even though it was manufactured in China.

PC-SPES soon began to attract the interest of well-respected research scientists, including those at Johns Hopkins School of Medicine, Harvard Medical School, and the National Center for Complementary and Alternative Medicine.[44] In 2002 three reviews of the use of PC-SPES were published, which surveyed the major publications on its pharmacology and clinical activity.[45-47] By early 2002 there were 116 published clinical and laboratory-based studies of PC-SPES.[48]

The reviews highlighted the significant in vitro and in vivo activities of PC-SPES in prostate cancer models and noted the small number of positive but preliminary clinical trials.[45-47] Oestrogenic activity was confirmed for the product, which was consistent with some of the side effects exhibited by patients taking the formulation, including gynaecomastia, loss of libido, decrease in body hair, and superficial thrombosis. However, there was also another worrying and paradoxical side effect of PC-SPES: it was linked to severe bleeding in one case[49] and suspected of potentiating the effects of warfarin in another.[50]

Another perspective on PC-SPES began to emerge in 2002 at about the same time the aforementioned reviews were published. In early April a group of scientists presented their findings to the 93rd Meeting of the American Association for Cancer Research that PC-SPES samples from 1996 to 2001 contained the oestrogenic drug diethylstilbestrol (DES) and warfarin and indomethacin.[51,52] Their comprehensive results were published in September.[53] Earlier in February the FDA alerted consumers to stop taking PC-SPES because the California Department of Health Services had detected the presence of warfarin. Another product called SPES from the same corporation had been found to contain the antianxiety drug alprazolam.[54] The manufacturer undertook a voluntary recall, and PC-SPES was subsequently withdrawn from the market.[44]

The inventor of PC-SPES has claimed that none of the contaminant drugs were present in therapeutic amounts and that batches of the product without DES were still clinically effective.[55] However, analysis has shown that nine capsules of PC-SPES per day (the recommended dose) could deliver a dose of up to 0.5 mg of DES, which is considered to be a therapeutic dose.[53] The source and motives behind the adulterants in PC-SPES remain a mystery, but charges have been laid against some of the parties involved.

HEAVY METALS

Heavy metals in herbal products can be present as unwanted contaminants or they can be added intentionally. In the traditional Chinese and Indian systems of medicine, minerals containing heavy metals are sometimes added to formulations to obtain a desired therapeutic effect. For the case of Chinese herbal products, examples of both instances are extensively discussed in Chapter 9 and also in a recent systematic review.[56]

In Ayurveda and Unani, the traditional medical systems of the Indian subcontinent, the use of herbal formulations containing intentionally high levels of heavy metals is considered an important aspect of the therapeutic armamentarium. It is argued that if such products are carefully formulated and skilfully prescribed, they do not result in toxic effects. Nonetheless, toxic effects have been reported.

A recent review discussed 15 case reports of lead (the most number of cases), arsenic, and mercury poisoning from traditional Indian remedies consumed in the United Kingdom, United States, Canada, Australia, India, and Italy.[57] The authors also noted the worrying finding that several surveys of traditional Indian herbal products revealed high levels of lead, mercury, arsenic, and cadmium in many products. Other studies reported in the review found elevated blood lead levels in consistent users of Indian herbal products. Additional cases of lead poisoning caused by Indian herbal products have been published since this review (e.g., one from Australia[58] and another from Holland[59]).

The issue of the potential contamination of herbal products with heavy metals from the environment is far more subtle and complex. Levels of safe exposure for elements such as cadmium, lead, mercury, and inorganic arsenic have been set by health authorities such as the World Health Organisation (WHO) in terms of provisional tolerable weekly intake (PTWI) values (Table 8-1).[60]

Assuming an average body weight of 60 kg, de Smet has provided a formula to calculate the theoretical maximally tolerable level in mg/kg for a crude herb. Note that in this formula PTWI is expressed as mg/kg, whereas the unit μg/kg is used in Table 8-1. The formula is as follows:

Theoretically maximally tolerable level (mg/kg)

$$= \frac{PTWI\ (mg/kg) \times 60 \times extraction\ factor}{Average\ weekly\ herb\ consumption\ (kg) \times 100}$$

The extraction factor is the fraction of heavy metals that can be extracted from the crude herb. Therefore for a finished product this value should be assumed to be 1. For the preparation of herbal teas and ethanolic extracts, the extraction factor could be expected to be <1, and in some cases it could be low.

Surveys have found unacceptable levels of heavy metals in some herbal raw materials and products. A survey of 34 samples of some common Indian herbs found that the concentrations of lead and cadmium were beyond the permissible WHO limits for most of the samples studied.[61] In contrast, an analysis of 21 over-the-counter ginseng *(Panax ginseng)* products revealed cadmium and lead levels within acceptable limits.[62]

The cadmium and lead concentrations of some herbs, herbal infusions, and herbal preparations used by children and adults were meas-

Table **8-1   Provisional Tolerable Weekly Intake (PTWI) Values for Toxic Metals, as Established by FAO and WHO**[60]

Metal	PTWI value (μg/kg/wk)
Lead	50
Cadmium	7
Mercury	5
Arsenic (inorganic)	15

FAO, Food and Agriculture Organization of the United Nations; WHO, World Health Organization.

ured in a Polish study.[63] Unacceptable levels of cadmium and lead were found in many of the products. A product containing nettle *(Urtica dioica)* was recalled in the United States in 2002 because it contained "excessive" levels of lead.[64]

A survey of heavy metals in crude herbs that included data for >12,000 samples supplied by a number of herbal supply companies in Germany concluded that although cadmium appears to have a propensity to accumulate in some herbs, contamination with mercury is not a problem.[65] The authors suggested that limits of 10 mg/kg for lead and 0.5 mg/kg for cadmium were rational and achievable, with the notable exception of a few herbs that appear to accumulate these metals and for which slightly higher limits should apply.

Adverse reactions have perhaps erroneously been attributed to the intake of herbs contaminated with heavy metals. A Croatian case of drug-induced nephritis in a child was linked to the intake of herbs contaminated with cadmium.[66] The patient had been treated with a homemade herbal mixture; however, the levels of cadmium found in these herbs did not appear to be unacceptably high. The herb bladderwrack *(Fucus vesiculosus)* and also other seaweeds naturally accumulate arsenic. However, much of this arsenic is organically bound, as for many sea foods, and not considered to be toxic.[67] Nonetheless, a case of nephrotoxicity was attributed to bladderwrack intake based on its arsenic content.[68] See the monograph on bladderwrack in this text for more details on this issue.

MICROBIAL CONTAMINATION AND MYCOTOXINS

Herbs are biological substances and hence will naturally contain large numbers of a variety of microorganisms. Acceptable levels for the microbial contamination of herbs and herbal products have been designated in the British Pharmacopoeia (BP) and are outlined in Table 8-2. The processing of herbs, particularly extraction with ethanol-water mixtures (as in the preparation of tinctures and liquid extracts) or processing with boiling water to make an infusion or decoction, will result in a substantial reduction in the microbiological burden.

Table 8-2 **Limits for Microbiological Quality of Pharmaceutical Preparations According to the British Pharmacopoeia[69]**

Total viable aerobic count	Enterobacteria and other Gram-negative bacteria	Absence of *Pseudomonas aeruginosa*	Absence of *Staphylococcus aureus*	Absence of *Escherichia coli*	Absence of *Salmonella*
CATEGORY 2					
Preparations for topical use and for use in the respiratory tract except when required to be sterile and transdermal patches (including the adhesive and backing layer)					
Not more than 10^2 microorganisms (aerobic bacteria plus fungi) per g, per mL, or per patch	*Transdermal patches* Absence of enterobacteria and certain other Gram-negative bacteria, determined on one patch *Other preparations* Not more than 10^1 enterobacteria and certain other Gram-negative bacteria per g or per mL	Determined on 1 g, 1 mL, or 1 patch	Determined on 1 g, 1 mL, or 1 patch	—	—
CATEGORY 3					
Preparations for oral and rectal administration					
Not more than 10^3 aerobic bacteria and not more than 10^2 fungi per g or per mL	—	—	—	In 1 g or 1 mL	—

Preparations for oral administration containing raw materials of natural origin (animal, vegetable, or mineral) for which antimicrobial pretreatment is not feasible and for which the competent authority accepts a microbial contamination of the raw material exceeding 10^3 viable microorganism per g or per mL; herbal remedies described in Category 4 are excluded

Not more than 10^4 aerobic bacteria and not more than 10^2 fungi per g or per mL	Not more than 10^2 enterobacteria and certain other Gram-negative bacteria per g or per mL	In 1 g or 1 mL	In 1 g or 1 mL	In 10 g or 10 mL
CATEGORY 4				
Herbal medicinal products consisting solely of one or more herbal drugs (whole, reduced, or powdered)				
Herbal medicinal products to which boiling water is added before use				
Not more than 10^7 aerobic bacteria and not more than 10^5 fungi per g or per mL	—	Not more than 10^2 per g or per mL using suitable dilutions	—	—
Herbal medicinal products to which boiling water is not added before use				
Not more than 10^5 aerobic bacteria and not more than 10^4 fungi per g or per mL	Not more than 10^3 enterobacteria and certain other Gram-negative bacteria per g or per mL	1 g or 1 mL	—	10 g or 10 mL

Not surprisingly, surveys of crude medicinal herbs have found high levels of total aerobic organisms, Enterobacteriaceae and coliform organisms, and yeasts and moulds.[70,71] A survey of 138 medicinal herbs found that although none of the samples contained enterohaemorrhagic *Escherichia coli*, Salmonellae, *Pseudomonas aeruginosa*, Listeriae, *Staphylococcus aureus*, or *Candida albicans*, four samples were positive for *E. coli*, two samples were presumptively positive for *Campylobacter jejuni*, and nine herbs contained a potentially aflatoxigenic mould.[72]

It is expected that the manufacturing processes will target a substantial reduction in the bioburden (e.g., by extracting with ethanol-water mixtures as mentioned previously); therefore, what is more relevant are the levels in finished products. A survey of 425 licensed herbal products by the UK Medicines Control Agency found that the majority of products complied with European Pharmacopoeia (EP) standards.[73] However, some products, especially the solid oral dosage forms, were found to contain undesirable organisms, such as *Enterobacter* spp. (31% of all samples), *Enterococcus faecalis* or *faecium* (23%), and *Clostridium perfringens* (6%). Twenty-two percent also exceeded the EP standard for total aerobic bacterial count. However, adverse effects caused by the consumption of microbially contaminated herbal products appear to be rare and are likely to mainly occur in individuals with compromised immunity.

Mycotoxins are toxic metabolites produced by fungi. Aflatoxins, which are produced by toxigenic strains of certain *Aspergillus* spp., are toxic, carcinogenic, and teratogenic. Most surveys of medicinal herbs for aflatoxins have not found excessive levels.[74,75] However, researchers in India and Egypt have found significant levels of contamination in some herb samples.[76,77] This might be expected because the higher heat and humidity in tropical regions could favour the development of fungal growth if inadequate drying procedures are used. A follow-up study by the Indian group detected aflatoxins in seed samples of two different Indian herbs.[78] Seeds usually contain appreciable levels of fixed oil (fat), which would encourage fungal growth.

Seventy-nine prepackaged samples of 12 different types of spice powders (5 cardamom, 5 cayenne pepper, 8 chilli, 5 cloves, 7 cumin, 5 curry powder, 5 ginger, 5 mustard, 10 nutmeg, 12 paprika, 5 saffron, and 7 white pepper) were selected from supermarkets and ethnic shops in Lisbon (Portugal) for estimation of aflatoxins by immunoaffinity column clean-up followed by high-performance liquid chromatography. Aflatoxin B_1 (AFB_1) was detected in 34 samples of prepackaged spices (43.0%). All of the cayenne pepper samples were contaminated with levels ranging from 2 to 32 µg AFB_1/kg. Three nutmeg samples contained levels ranging from 1 to 5 µg/kg; three samples had levels ranging from 6 to 20 µg/kg; and there were two with 54 µg/kg and 58 µg/kg. Paprika contained levels of AFB_1 ranging from 1 to 20 µg/kg. Chilli, cumin, curry powder, saffron, and white pepper samples had levels ranging from 1 to 5 µg/kg. Aflatoxins were not detected in cardamom, cloves, ginger, and mustard. None of the samples analysed contained aflatoxins B_2, G_1, and G_2.[79] The peanut industry sets a safety standard for peanuts of 15 µg/kg, and for all other foods the maximum level must not exceed 5 µg/kg.[80]

Ochratoxins are a group of fungal toxins produced by certain strains of *Aspergillus* and *Penicillium*. Ochratoxin A is the most toxic. Of 126 samples of four spices purchased from shops, ochratoxin A was found to exceed 10 µg/kg in 14 of 26 black pepper samples, 20 of 50 coriander samples, 2 of 25 ginger samples, and 9 of 25 turmeric samples. A higher frequency of contamination was found in the seed spices.[81]

PESTICIDES AND HERBICIDES

There is an obvious preference by consumers in several countries for herbs that have been organically grown (and are certified as such). Nonetheless, many medicinal herbs are harvested from the wild and may be contaminated with pesticides and herbicides from nearby agricultural activities or could be collected from areas where the soil is contaminated. Many commercial herb crops also are grown with the assistance of these agents.

Acceptable levels for a wide variety of pesticides have been defined in the EP. These are provided in Table 8-3. The German government

Table **8-3**   **Limits for Pesticide Residues in Crude Herbs and in Herbal Products as Defined in the BP[85]**

Substance	Limit (mg/kg)
Alachlor	0.02
Aldrin and dieldrin (sum of)	0.05
Azinphos-methyl	1.0
Bromopropylate	3.0
Chlordane (sum of *cis*, *trans*-, and oxychlordane)	0.05
Chlorfenvinphos	0.5
Chlorpyrifos	0.2
Chlorpyrifos-methyl	0.1
Cypermethrin (and isomers)	1.0
DDT (sum of p,p'-DDT, o,p'-DDT, p,p'-DDE and p,p'-TDE)	1.0
Deltamethrin	0.5
Diazinon	0.5
Dichlorvos	1.0
Dithiocarbamates (as CS_2)	2.0
Endosulfan (sum of isomers and endosulfan sulphate)	3.0
Endrin	0.05
Ethion	2.0
Fenitrothion	0.5
Fenvalerate	1.5
Fonofos	0.05
Heptachlor (sum of heptachlor and heptachlor-epoxide)	0.05
Hexachlorobenzene	0.1
Hexachlorocyclohexane isomers (other than γ)	0.3
Lindane (γ-hexachlorocyclohexane)	0.6
Malathion	1.0
Methidathion	0.2
Parathion	0.5
Parathion-methyl	0.2
Permethrin	1.0

Table **8-3**   **Limits for Pesticide Residues in Crude Herbs and in Herbal Products as Defined in the BP[85]—cont'd**

Substance	Limit (mg/kg)
Phosalone	0.1
Piperonyl butoxide	3.0
Pirimiphos-methyl	4.0
Pyrethrins (sum of)	3.0
Quintozene (sum of quintozene, pentachloroanaline, and methyl pentachlorophenyl sulphide)	1.0

BP, British Pharmacopoeia; DDT, dichlorodiphenyltrichloroethane.

has set a food standard for nonmedicinal herbal teas. Surveys of crude herbs on the German market found that between 18% and 26% of tested samples did not pass the food standard for pesticide residues.[82-84]

A survey of organochlorine residues in common Indian spices found low levels of hexachlorocyclohexane, including lindane, and dichlorodiphenyltrichloroethane (DDT).[86] Low levels of organophosphorus pesticides were measured in samples of five spices collected from local markets in Egypt.[87] The highest levels of organophosphates were found in cumin.

CONCLUSIONS AND RECOMMENDATIONS

Herbal products should be purchased from manufacturers who comply with pharmaceutical GMP and who have adequate and active screening procedures in place for microbial contamination, heavy metals, pesticides, and aflatoxins.

Herbal products must be manufactured in a legal environment that does not permit the addition of undeclared ingredients such as synthetic drugs and where offenders are adequately prosecuted and the penalties are high. Products imported from countries that do not have such standards in place should at best not be permitted for general sale and at least should be screened for potential adulterants before they are allowed onto the market.

The correct identification of a medicinal herb in terms of botanical species and plant part is paramount to the safe use of herbal products. Manufacturers should be obliged to have adequate identification procedures in place. The collection of herbs from the wild by inexperienced harvesters should be discouraged.

REFERENCES

1. Vanherweghem JL, Depierreux M, Tielemans C, et al: Rapidly progressive interstitial renal fibrosis in young women: association with slimming regimen including Chinese herbs, *Lancet* 341:387-391, 1993.
2. Vanhaelen M, Vanhaelen-Fastre R, But P, et al: Identification of aristolochic acid in Chinese herbs, *Lancet* 343:174, 1994
3. Chen JK: Nephropathy associated with the use of Aristolochia, *Herbal Gram* 48:44-45, 2000.
4. De Smet PAGM, Keller K, Hansel R, et al, editors: *Adverse effects of herbal drugs, vol 1,* Berlin, 1992, Springer-Verlag, pp 79-89.
5. Reginster F, Jadoul M, van Ypersele de Strihou C: Chinese herbs nephropathy presentation, natural history and fate after transplantation, *Nephrol Dial Transplant* 12:81-86, 1997.
6. Cosyns JP, Jadoul M, Squifflet JP, et al: Urothelial lesions in Chinese-herb nephropathy, *Am J Kidney Dis* 33:1011-1017, 1999.
7. Nortier JL, Martinez MC, Schmeiser HH, et al: Urothelial carcinoma associated with the use of a Chinese herb (Aristolochia fangchi), *N Engl J Med* 342:1686-1692, 2000.
8. U.S. Food and Drug Administration: Listing of botanical ingredients of concern. U.S. Food and Drug Administration, Center for Food Safety and Applied Nutrition, Office of Nutritional Products, Labeling, and Dietary Supplements. Revised April 9, 2001. Available at: http://www.cfsan.fda.gov/~dms/supplmnt.htlm.
9. Therapeutic Goods Administration: Urgent medicine recall, reference R2001/549, December 6, 2001. Produced by Therapeutic Goods Administration, December 7, 2001. Available at: http://www.health.gov.au/tga/docs/html/-longdon.htm.
10. Associated Press: Contaminated Chinese herbs recalled. January 4, 2001. Available at: http://www.sfgate.com/cgi-bin/article.cgi%3Ffile%3D/news/archive/2001/01/04/national1049EST0555.DTL&type%3Dhealth. Accessed February 14, 2003.
11. But PP, Tomlinson B, Cheung KO, et al: Adulterants of herbal products can cause poisoning, *BMJ* 313:117, 1996.
12. De Smet PAGM: Health risks of herbal remedies, *Drug Saf* 13:81-93, 1995.
13. Koren G, Randor S, Martin S, et al: Maternal ginseng use associated with neonatal androgenization, *JAMA* 264:2866, 1990.
14. Awang DVC: Maternal use of ginseng and neonatal androgenization, *JAMA* 266:363, 1991.
15. McRae S: Elevated serum digoxin levels in a patient taking digoxin and Siberian ginseng, *CMAJ* 155:293-295, 1996.
16. Wong HCG: Probable false authentication of herbal plants: ginseng, *Arch Intern Med* 159:1142, 1999.
17. Bryson PD, Watanabe AS, Rumack BH, et al: Burdock root tea poisoning. Case report involving a commercial preparation, *JAMA* 239:2157, 1978.
18. Bryson PD: Burdock root tea poisoning, *JAMA* 240:1586, 1978.
19. Scholz H, Kascha S, Zingerle H: [Atropine poisoning from "health tea"], *Fortschr Med* 98:1525-1526, 1980.
20. Galizia EJ: Clinical curio: hallucinations in elderly tea drinkers, *BMJ* 287:979, 1983.
21. Routledge PA, Spriggs TLB: Atropine as possible contaminant of comfrey tea, *Lancet* 1:963-964, 1989.
22. Sperl W, Stuppner H, Gassner I, et al: Reversible hepatic veno-occlusive disease in an infant after consumption of pyrrolizidine-containing herbal tea, *Eur J Pediatr* 154:112-116, 1995.
23. Stillman AE, Huxtable RJ, Fox DW, et al: Poisoning associated with herbal teas—Arizona, Washington, *Morb Mortal Wkly Rep* 26:257-259, 1977.
24. Chan TYK, Tse LKK, Chan JCN, et al: Aconitine poisoning due to Chinese herbal medicines: a review, *Vet Human Toxicol* 36:452-455, 1994.
25. But PPH, Tai YT, Young K: Three fatal cases of herbal aconite poisoning, *Vet Human Toxicol* 36:212-215, 1994.
26. Chan TYK, Chan JCN, Tomlinson B, et al: Poisoning by Chinese herbal medicines in Hong Kong: a hospital-based study, *Vet Human Toxicol* 36:546-547, 1994.
27. Anderson LA: Concern regarding herbal toxicities: case reports and counseling tips, *Ann Pharmacother* 30:79-80, 1996.
28. McRae CA, Agarwal K, Mutimer D, et al: Hepatitis associated with Chinese herbs, *Eur J Gastroenterol Hepatol* 14:559-562, 2002.
29. Horowitz RS, Feldhaus K, Dart RC, et al: The clinical spectrum of *Jin Bu Huan* toxicity, *Arch Intern Med* 156:899-903, 1996.
30. Dega H, Laporte JL, Frances C, et al: Ginseng as a cause for Stevens-Johnson syndrome? *Lancet* 347:1344, 1996.
31. Ko RJ: Causes, epidemiology, and clinical evaluation of suspected herbal poisoning, *Clin Toxicol* 37:697-708, 1999.
32. Ernst E: Adulteration of Chinese herbal medicines with synthetic drugs: a systematic review, *J Intern Med* 252:107-113, 2002.
33. Chang SS, Liaw SJ, Bullard MJ, et al: Adrenal insufficiency in critically ill emergency department patients: a Taiwan preliminary study, *Acad Emerg Med* 8:761-764, 2001.
34. Florkowski CM, Elder PA, Lewis JG, et al: Two cases of adrenal suppression following a Chinese herbal remedy: a cause for concern? *N Z Med J* 115:223-224, 2002.
35. Liu SY, Woo SO, Holmes MJ, et al: LC and LC-MS-MS analyses of undeclared codeine in antiasthmatic Chinese proprietary medicine, *J Pharm Biomed Anal* 22:481-486, 2000.

36. Metcalfe K, Corns C, Fahie-Wilson M, et al: Chinese medicines for slimming still cause health problems, *BMJ* 324: 679, 2002.

37. Koo E: Chinese medicine appeal outweighs diet pill worry. Reuters August 29, 2002. Available at: http://www.manilatimes.net/national/2002/aug/29/opinion/20020829o pi6.html. Accessed September 2, 2002.

38. Shimbun Y: Chinese diet aids kill 1, sicken 11. *Daily Yomiuri Online* July 12, 2002. Available at: http:www.yomirui.co.jp/ newse/20020712wo21.htm. Accessed July 15, 2002.

39. Maria K: New diet pill blamed for at least 1 death in China, VOANews.com July 15, 2002. Accessed July 17, 2002.

40. U.S. Food and Drug Administration: FDA warns public about Chinese diet pills containing fenfluramine. Available at: http://www.fda.gov/bbs/topics/NEWS/2002/ NEW00826.html. August 13, 2002.

41. Xinhua News Agency: Illegal slimming pills, fake Viagra face crackdown. Xinhuanet 2002-07-30. Available at: http://news.xinhuanet.com/english/2002-07/30/content_504528.htm. Accessed August 5, 2002.

42. Haber G: Tampa, Fla., law firm sues over "muscle-building" supplements. Available at: http://www.newsalert.com/ bin/story?StoryId=Cpudjqaicve0TrfjvrW&Print=1&& Nav=research-.Accessed August 5, 2002.

43. Hickey K, Seliem R, Shields J, et al: A positive drug test in the pain management patient: deception or herbal cross-reactivity? *Clin Chem* 48:958-960, 2002.

44. Ochs R: Going to bat for prostate cancer herbs. Newsday.com October 8, 2002. Available at: http://www.newsday.com/templates/misc/printstory.jsp?slug= ny%2Ddsbelow2956740oct08&sec. Accessed October 10, 2002.

45. Oh WK, Small EJ: PC-SPES and prostate cancer, *Urol Clin North Am* 29:59-66, 2002.

46. Thomson JO, Dzubak P, Hajduch M: Prostate cancer and the food supplement, PC-SPES, *Neoplasma* 49:69-74, 2002.

47. Marks LS, DiPaola RS, Nelson P, et al: PC-SPES: herbal formulation for prostate cancer, *Urology* 60:369-377, 2002.

48. Pandha HS, Kirby RS: PC-SPES: phytotherapy for prostate cancer, *Lancet* 359:2213-2215, 2002.

49. Weinrobe MC, Montgomery B: Acquired bleeding diathesis in a patient taking PC-SPES, *N Engl J Med* 345:1213-1214, 2001.

50. Davis NB, Nahlik L, Vogelzang NJ: Does PC-SPES interact with warfarin? *J Urol* 167:1793, 2002.

51. BW HealthWire: Chemical analysis confirms PC-SPES contains DES, indomethacin and warfarin; results presented at AACR late breaking session. April 9, 2002. Available at: http://www.newsalert.com/bin/ story?StoryId=CpljNqbKbyta0nJm&Print. Accessed April 11, 2002.

52. Arnold K: Tests of three herbal therapies yield disappointing results, *J Natl Cancer Inst* 94:649, 2002.

53. Sovak M, Seligson AL, Konas M, et al: Herbal composition PC-SPES for management of prostate cancer: identification of active principles, *J Natl Cancer Inst* 94:1275-1281, 2002.

54. Reuters Health: Prostate herbals contain prescription drugs: FDA. February 8, 2002. Available at: http://abc-news.go.com/wire/Living/reuters20020208_458.html. Accessed February 14, 2002.

55. Reynolds T: Contamination of PC-SPES remains a mystery, *J Natl Cancer Inst* 94:1266-1268, 2002.

56. Ernst E, Coon JT: Heavy metals in traditional Chinese medicines: a systematic review, *Clin Pharmacol Ther* 70:497-504, 2001.

57. Ernst E: Heavy metals in traditional Indian remedies, *Eur J Clin Pharmacol* 57:891-896, 2002.

58. Tait PA, Vora A, James S, et al: Severe congenital lead poisoning in a preterm infant due to a herbal remedy, *Med J Aust* 177:193-195, 2002.

59. van Vonderen MGA, Klinkenberg-Knol EC, Craanen ME, et al: Severe gastrointestinal symptoms due to lead poisoning from Indian traditional medicine, *Am J Gastroenterol* 95:1591-1592, 2000.

60. de Smet PAGM, Keller K, Hansel R, et al, editors: *Adverse Effects of Herbal Drugs, vol 1,* Berlin, 1992, Springer-Verlag, p 39.

61. Rai V, Kakkar P, Khatoon S, et al: Heavy metal accumulation in some herbal drugs, *Pharm Biol* 39:384-387, 2001.

62. Khan IA, Allgood J, Walker LA, et al: Determination of heavy metals and pesiticides in ginseng products, *J AOAC Int* 84:936-939, 2001.

63. Bloniarz J, Zareba S, Rahnama M: [Cadmium and lead content in some herbs, herbal preparation and herbal infusions used by children and adults], *Przegl Lek* 58(suppl 7):39-43, 2001.

64. Associated Press: Supplement recalled after lead found. June 28, 2002. Available at: http://www.ci.berkeley.ca.us/ news/2002/07jul/070202natureswayrecall.html. Accessed July 1, 2002.

65. Kabelitz L: Heavy metals in herbal drugs, *Eur J Herbal Med (Phytotherapy)* 4:25-33, 1998.

66. Subat-Dezulovic M, Slavic I, Rozmanic V, et al: Drug-induced acute tubulointerstitial nephritis: a case with elevated urinary cadmium, *Pediatr Nephrol* 17:382-385, 2002.

67. Storelli MM, Marcotrigiano GO: Organic and inorganic arsenic and lead in fish from the South Adriatic Sea, Italy, *Food Addit Contam* 17:763-768, 2000.

68. Conz PA, La Greca G, Benedetti P, et al: Fucus vesiculosus: a nephrotoxic alga? *Nephrol Dial Transplant* 13:526-527, 1998.

69. British Pharmacopoeia: 2002 CD-ROM, Crown Copyright, 2002, A324 Appendix XVI D.

70. Kneifel W, Czech E, Kopp B: Microbial contamination of medicinal plants—a review, *Planta Med* 68:5-15, 2002.

71. Martins HM, Martins ML, Dias MI, et al: Evaluation of microbiological quality of medicinal plants used in natural infusions, *Int J Food Microbiol* 68:149-153, 2001.

72. Czech C, Kneifel W, Kopp B: Microbiological status of commercially available medicinal herbal drugs—a screening study, *Planta Med* 67:263-269, 2001.

73. Alexander RG, Wilson DA, Davidson AG: Medicines Control Agency investigation of the microbial quality of herbal products, *Pharm J* 259:259-261, 1997.

74. Hirokoto H, Moroxumi S, Wauke T, et al: Fungal contamination and mycotoxin detection of powdered herbal drugs, *Appl Environ Microbiol* 36:252-256, 1978.

75. Leimbeck R: Teedrogen—Wie steht es mit der mikrobiologischen Qualität, *Dtsch Apoth Ztg* 127:1221-1226, 1987.

76. Roy AK, Prasad MM, Kumari N, et al: Studies on association of mycoflora with drug-plants and aflatoxin producing potentiality of *Aspergillus flavus*, *Ind Phytopathol* 41:261-262, 1988.

77. Hilal SH, Soliman FM, Mahmoud II, et al: Quantitative study of the mutagenic activity of folkloric Egyptian herbs. II. Lecture presented at the 47th International Congress of Pharmaceutical Sciences of the Federation Internationale Pharmacetique, Amsterdam, August 31 to September 4, 1987.

78. Kumari V, Chourasia HK, Roy AK: Aflatoxin contamination in seeds of medicinal value, *Curr Sci* 58:512-513, 1989.

79. Martins ML, Martins HM, Bernardo F: Aflatoxins in spices marketed in Portugal, *Food Addit Contam* 18:315-319, 2001.

80. Health Protection Service Food Survey Report 1998-99: Quality of peanut products. ACT Department of Health, Housing and Community Care. Available at: http://www.health.act.gov.au/publications/foodsurvey/1998-99/peanuts98.html. Accessed February 25, 2003.

81. Thirumala-Devi K, Mayo MA, Reddy G, et al: Occurrence of ochratoxin A in black pepper, coriander, ginger and turmeric in India, *Food Addit Contam* 18:830-835, 2001.

82. Schilcher H: [Residues and impurities in medicinal plants and drug preparations (author's transl)], *Planta Med* 44:65-77, 1982.

83. Ali SL: Bestimmung der pestiziden Rückstände und anderer bedenklicher Veruntreinigungen—wie toxische Metallspuren—in Arzneipflanzen. I. Mitt: Pestizid-Rückstände in Arzneidrogen. *Pharm Ind* 45:1154-1156, 1983.

84. Ali SL: Bestimmung der Pestizidrückstände und toxischen Schwermetallspuren in Arzneidrogen und deren Teeaufgüssen, *Pharm Ztg* 132:633-638, 1987.

85. British Pharmacopoeia: 2002 CD-ROM, Crown Copyright, 2002, A232 Appendix XI L.

86. Srivastava LP, Budhwar R, Raizada RB: Organochlorine pesticide residues in Indian spices, *Bull Environ Contam Toxicol* 67:856-862, 2001.

87. Ahmed MT, Loutfy N, Yousef Y: Contamination of medicinal herbs with organophosphorus insecticides, *Bull Environ Contam Toxicol* 66:421-426, 2001.

9

SAFETY CONCERNS INVOLVING CHINESE HERBAL MEDICINE

Trina Ward

Herbal medicine is particularly well established and widespread in China, and there is considerable information about the effects of these remedies from a part of the world that includes up to one-third of the human population. From this vast experience it is likely that overt acute toxicity for traditional remedies will have been identified fairly well. However, it is also certain that low-level or long-term adverse events, or those adverse events that occur rarely, will only be identified by systematic modern communications and coordinated record keeping. This inevitably means that the full story on the safety of traditional remedies lags far behind their positive reputation. Such processes are increasingly international and will involve bodies like the World Health Organization (WHO) Collaborating Centre for International Drug Monitoring in Uppsala, Sweden. However, there are particular methodologic difficulties in collecting reliable data on adverse effects from a traditional medical system: the reporting behaviour differs between orthodox practitioners and traditional Chinese medicine (TCM) practitioners,[1] and users of herbal medicines are less likely to report adverse events associated with their

herbal use than with their use of pharmaceutical medications.[2] Therefore it is reasonable to expect the problem to have a greater magnitude than existing reports suggest.

Herbal medicines are considered a major cause of concern because of problems with their adverse effects, improper use, and quality control.[3] Adverse reactions can be associated with a herb's intrinsic toxicity, its improper use such as when used to intentionally overdose, herb-herb or herb-drug interactions (HDIs), or idiosyncratic reactions. Quality control problems can give rise to adverse events after adulteration, misidentification or intentional substitution, contamination or poor processing or preparation, inappropriate labelling or advertisement of a product, and improper dosage.

Although Chinese herbal medicine (CHM) safety issues have involved all of the aforementioned causes, the hepatotoxicity of herbal medicines is considered a particular concern,[4] and there are also grave quality control-related issues, such as misidentification of the intended herb and presence of adulterants including Western pharmaceuticals and heavy metals.[5-8] Such cases and others that involve the herb prescribed at the wrong dose or not prescribed according to the TCM theories highlight the need for regulation.[8,9] Medical professionals, aware of the complexities of CHM, have also warned of the need for prescribing by trained practitioners.[10,11]

ACUTE TOXICITY

It is claimed that combining herbs according to the theory of TCM counteracts the toxicity of herbs such as guang fang ji 广防己 *(Aristolochia fangchi)*.[12] Although this remains untested, there is considerable evidence that preparation methods can influence a herb's toxicity. It is acknowledged that the more serious direct poisonings caused by Chinese herbs involve products containing aconitine, podophyllin, or anticholinergics.[13] It has been estimated that approximately 70% of severe poisonings caused by CHMs are caused by chuan wu 川乌 *(Aconitum carmichaeli)* and cao wu 草乌 *(Aconitum kusnezoffii)* alone.[14] There are many cases reported with fatal outcomes from taking aconite roots. In Hong Kong two men died after taking herbal medicines including aconite for minor musculoskeletal pain. The doses were far in excess of that recommended in the pharmacopoeia of the People's Republic of China (PRC).[15] A further 2 deaths and 15 near-fatal poisonings are described as accidental poisonings attributed to aconites.[16] The principal component of *Aconitum* remedies is the alkaloid aconitine, a neurotoxin that may induce severe neurologic symptoms and cardiovascular collapse. The amounts and components of alkaloids in the herbs determine the severity of the clinical features of poisoning. The roots are prepared by soaking and boiling in water, resulting in the hydrolysis of aconite alkaloids into the less toxic benzylaconine derivatives; because this herb is directly toxic, the dose and preparation method are crucial to its toxicity.[17]

Hepatotoxicity

The hepatotoxicity of CHMs repeatedly reported in the literature[18-20] has resulted in two deaths in the United Kingdom.[18] The vast majority of cases of conventional drug-induced liver disease would be classified as unpredictable idiosyncratic drug reactions.[21] A review of the hepatotoxicity of botanicals concluded that they also follow an idiosyncratic pattern because they do not seem to lead to toxic effects in everyone taking them and that they commonly lack a strict dose-dependency pattern.[22] This also appears to be the case with Chinese herb-induced liver disease. In light of recent incidence data transient changes and idiosyncratic reactions do appear to occur.[23,24] However, this does not stop statements being made in reputable journals, such as the *British Medical Journal*, in which McCarthy and Wilkinson[25] wrote that plant extracts from *Dictamnus dasycarpus*, bai xian pi 白鲜皮, and *Paeonia* spp., mu dan pi 牡丹皮, bai shao 白芍, or chi shao 赤芍, were found to be hepatotoxic. Such a statement was based on one reference that had been incorrectly interpreted.[26] This has subsequently been cited in journals, at seminars, and in the media without close reference to the original source material, which did not come to this conclusion but simply stated that these two plants were the only common ingredients in that case series of only two cases. Although it was hypothesised that these two plants could be the toxic components, no further evidence supported this. The Traditional Remedies Surveillance Team (TRST) of the Medical Toxicology Unit has repeatedly stated that no single ingredient has been implicated in the cases of hepatic reactions to herbs that they have investigated:

> "...no known hepatotoxic herbs have been identified, and a comparison of all the prescriptions has shown no common herbal ingredient."[27]

> "The plant material varied so no single ingredient could account for liver injury in this case series."[18]

There is still a lack of incidence data to fully define this problem, which is not unique to CHM (see Chapter 12).

HEAVY METALS

Because CHM is not confined to the use of plants alone,[28] the WHO recognises this fact, and its definition of herbal medicine encompasses this[29]:

"A plant-derived material or preparation with therapeutic or other human health benefits which contains either raw or processed ingredients from one or more plants. In some traditions, materials of inorganic or animal origin may also be present."

Although the overlap between herbal traditions is immense, certain safety aspects do not apply to all traditions. The presence of heavy metals is one example of a safety issue specific to certain traditional systems, including the Chinese one, and such use of nonplant materials has given added concerns (see Chapter 8).[28]

Heavy metals found in Chinese herbal products include mercury, cadmium, lead, arsenic, copper, manganese, and thallium. There are reports documenting the high numbers of products contaminated with heavy metals.[30,31] In Singapore of 99 samples, 28 contained levels of mercury above the legal limit for mercury of 0.5 μ/g set by the government of Singapore. Such levels suggest that mercury was added rather than a contaminant. Whereas for lead, four products were found to exceed the legal limits of 20 μ/g but at levels where contamination was a possible source of the metal. Three products contained copper >150 μ/g; one was high enough to be considered an intentional addition.[31] The Californian Department of Health Services, Food and Drug Branch conducted a similar survey and found of 251 products analysed, 35 contained mercury, 24 contained lead, and 36 contained arsenic in ranges from just below the legal limit to thousands of times above it.[30] In the United States, 32 herbal balls were tested, and all contained mercury, as cinnabar, with quantities varying between 80.7 and 621.3 mg/ball. Arsenic levels of between 3.21 and 36.6 mg/ball were also found.[32]

Authors have presumed that when pharmaceutical drugs are present in herbal products they are added intentionally, whereas when heavy metals are present this results unintentionally.[33] From reviewing reports and traditional texts it is clear that the presence of heavy metals is often intended. Although contamination may account for some cases, after the identification of mercury in watermelon frost spray, xi gua shuang 西瓜霜, the authors

tested various batches of the same product, and they were all negative, suggesting that in this case contamination occurred during the production or packaging process.[34]

It was established, while testing plant specimens for pollutants, that only cadmium and lead were potential problems through environmental contamination and that mercury was not a problem for herbal drugs.[35] CHM uses minerals and animal products, and these may influence such levels of contamination; it was found that the average values found for lead, cadmium, arsenic, cobalt, and manganese in drugs of mineral origin are higher than those derived from plants and animals. Copper levels were higher in drugs of animal origin.[36]

In the text *Pharmacopoeia of the People's Republic of China* (1988 English edition), which is an official reference to the manufacture of Chinese herbal products in the PRC, of 168 formulae 31 contain mercuric salts. In the most recent (2000) English language edition, of 459 formulae 46 contain mercuric salts.

Three sources of the same formula of Tian Wang Bu Xin Wan 天王补心丸 were tested in the United Kingdom. The products originated from three different manufacturers: two from the PRC and one from Taiwan. The product was chosen specifically because it would have traditionally contained mercury as an added ingredient; however, mercury was unlabelled in English or Chinese. On testing it was found that the product manufactured by Beijing Tong Ren Tang (PRC manufacturer) contained a weekly intake at the recommended dose range of 406 to 812 mg mercuric salts. The product manufactured by Kaifeng factory (PRC manufacturer) contained a weekly intake at the recommended dose of 19.6 mg mercuric salts, and the product manufactured by Sheng Chang (Taiwan manufacturer) had no mercuric salts present.[37] These tests resulted in the removal of the adulterated products from sale. It was claimed that the Beijing Tong Ren Tang product was a fake and not produced by that factory at all, revealing a further quality control problem found with Chinese herbal products.

The levels in the two products containing mercury far exceed the WHO provisional tolerable weekly intake of mercury for a 70-kg adult of 350 μg (0.35 mg).[38] Mercury levels found are in keeping with it being an additive rather than a contaminant. The maximum foodstuff allowance is 0.03 to 0.05 mg/kg. In the United Kingdom there are no limits on acceptable levels of mercury contamination for imported products. The Medicines Control Agency (MCA) state on their web site that it is illegal for mercury to be present in herbal products.

Mercury in CHM is present as mercuric salts: cinnabar or red mercuric sulphide, known as zhu sha 朱砂, and calomel or mercurous chloride, known as qing fen 轻粉. Less commonly Hong Yang Hua Gong 红氧化汞 (Hydrargyri oxydum rubrum) is also used. These are assigned the properties and actions, according to traditional theories, of being slightly cold, sweet, and toxic. They enter the heart channel, quiet the spirit, calm fright, brighten the eyes, and relieve toxins.[39] Formulae containing mercuric salts were traditionally called dan 丹. The function was to calm mania, manage palpitations caused by fright, calm agitation, and relieve insomnia, dizziness, and clouded vision. Mercuric salts were also used to relieve toxic swellings as an external application at a daily dose of 20 to 35 mg.

The possibility that buffering of the toxic potential of mercuric salts occurs within a Chinese herbal formula has not been explored in the literature. Cases reported indicate this is not always an effective mechanism if it exists at all. The scale of the problem is difficult reliably to estimate from individual case reports; the incidence and prevalence are not known.

The belief that, as there is an historical precedent for the use of mercury, it must be safe to use is not founded. The dangers of following tradition have been highlighted by a series of studies outside the field of herbal medicine. These studies demonstrated that neonatal tetanus infection, causing high rates of infant mortality, was linked to the application of ghee, warmed on fires using dung as fuel, to the umbilicus, believed to prevent infection. When this traditional North Pakistani practice was stopped, the infant mortality rate decreased greatly.[40]

The problem with mercury is that it accumulates in the body; although the half-life of absorbed mercury may be estimated at months, there will be a fraction that lasts up to 27 years.[41] A complicated interplay exists between mercury and other elements, including selenium, which could be responsible for the long half-life of a fraction of the mercury. Its half-life also depends on the tissues in which it is stored. Although more organic mercury is absorbed compared with inorganic mercury, it is eliminated more quickly, whereas inorganic mercury, such as cinnabar, is retained for many years. There is considerable variation in individuals' absorption rates, depending on, among other things, one's nutritional status, age, sex, and alcohol intake. Mercury accumulates in the brain, thyroid, pituitary, pancreas, liver, testes, ovaries, and prostate. The developing foetus has been reported to show neurologic disturbances and delayed development after a mother's excessive methylmercury intake.[42]

The kidney is the critical organ affected by ingestion of inorganic mercury. Poisonings have occurred through the use of skin-lightening creams applied only externally.[43] The kidney develops nephrotic syndrome, which is an immunotoxic response. Inorganic mercury (such as cinnabar) may induce autoimmune glomerulonephritis. The implications are that in immunologically sensitive individuals it is not possible to set a level for mercury below which mercury-related signs and symptoms will not occur. Mercury compounds may also affect the menstrual cycle and foetal development without any signs of mercury intoxication. The lowest observed adverse effect level in animal studies for the development of autoimmune glomerulonephritis is 0.05 mg/kg.[41] It has also been hypothesised that mercury deposits make antibiotics ineffective or provide a protective mechanism for Chlamydia trachomatis and herpes family viruses against antibiotic treatments.[44]

When mercury has been used in medicine in the past, its toxicity has been recognised and has now been largely replaced with less hazardous substances. When it is still used, this use is surrounded by concerns over its safety or is only used as a last resort.

Chinese-prepared products used externally only have resulted in a fatality.[45] A Chinese man sought treatment at a New York hospital for lethargy, decreased urinary output, black stools, and nausea. Despite treatment with dimercaprol he died from kidney failure 6 days after admission. He had used herbal dressings containing calomel for a 2-month period for a broken arm. The same hospital saw another fatality despite treatment with dimercaprol: a 50-year-old Chinese woman, who had taken five pills, one per day from seven prescribed, for an inflamed hip. These contained 12 g of calomel; renal injury was among the causes of death. A 4-year-old child was examined for a 3-month history of neurologic symptoms, including deterioration of gait, drooling, and dysphagia. All his tests were normal, and he was discharged without diagnosis. Later at another hospital, questioning revealed that his mother had given him a Chinese preparation containing calomel for respiratory problems; on analysis arsenic was also found to be present. He was treated with dimercaprol, but 11 months later still showed residual abnormal movements and learning difficulties.

Analysis of prepared products taken by a U.K. patient with AIDS showed that she was prescribed pills containing a daily intake of cinnabar of 706 mg; arsenic and lead were also present.[46] The products were An Gong Niu Huang Wan 安宫牛黄丸 and Zhu Sha An Shen Wan 硃砂安神丸. Such products are commonly sold over the counter in the United Kingdom via high street herbal outlets for anyone with minor complaints such as insomnia and as such could be taken long term. An Gong Niu Huang Wan 安宫牛黄丸 was removed from the marketplace by the MCA, and all registered herbalists were alerted to the dangers of the product after the aforementioned case was recognised.

One of the major U.K. importers was taken to court by the MCA in 2000. The importer Mayway U.K. had supplied Niu Huang Jie Du Wan 牛黄解毒丸 to a TCM practitioner in Bristol, but the product was subsequently found to contain quantities of arsenic and was withdrawn from sale. The Magistrate fined the company £5000, the maximum penalty for an offence tried in the Magistrate Court.

Long-term mercury exposure may result in neurologic deficits that persist. After 3 months of a Chinese herbal preparation a patient developed generalised paralysis of all limbs, which persisted 2 years later.[47]

Thallium poisoning has also been reported after using Chinese herbs; however, this case is less clear because other batches of the product Nutrien were all clear. These two cases may be the result of contamination of a particular batch of the product at some stage during manufacture. However, the authors hypothesise that there may be more undiagnosed cases.[48]

Several reports have involved children. Several of the products listed in the *Pharmacopoeia of the People's Republic of China* (2000 edition), with heavy metals as intended ingredients, are designed for use with children specifically. Lead poisoning from the product Po Ying Tan (Bao Ying Dan) 保嬰丹 has been described in a 4-month-old baby.[5] This product has also been shown to contain mercury.[45] In the case of a 2-month-old baby, the herbal powder applied to the buccal mucosa contained 23.3% lead by weight.[49] Mercury poisoning presented as tics in a 5-year-old boy given herbs sprayed onto mouth ulcers.[50] The resistance to change in the light of such reports is highlighted by a Taiwanese report in which, despite cases annually and one fatality, the public and Chinese medicine practitioners still use the product Ba-Pao-Neu-Hwang-San 八宝牛黄散.[51] Children may be given higher dose/kg body weight than is usual for adults and may also consume additional herbs through a mother's diet via breast milk.

Manganese poisoning is less commonly reported, but a case presenting as severe chorea in a patient taking Chien Pu Wan 车普丸 has been described.[52]

In all these cases, diagnosis was delayed. Awareness of the potential hazards of CHM is poor among the public and medical profession. Reports, such as those discussed previously and others,[46] are made in the medical literature to bring the subject to the attention of the medical profession, but such information may bypass herbal practitioners and the general public. The need for medical practitioners to take a full case history including details of herbal medicines and supplements used by the patient is a recurring message.[53,54]

ADULTERATION WITH CONVENTIONAL DRUGS

The scale of the problem of pharmaceutical drug additives is outlined by surveys that found undeclared pharmaceutical drugs in 7%

of 243 Asian patent medicines, and 5% of 260 Asian patent medicines contained labelled pharmaceutical ingredients.[30] In an analysis of intentional poisonings with Chinese patent medicines (CPM), products containing paracetamol caused the most serious events.[6] Some of the pharmaceutical drugs included may be highly dangerous; CPMs were found adulterated with Western drugs that have been banned because of their toxicity.[55] In the United Kingdom several cases of herbal creams adulterated with dexamethasone and other corticosteroids have been established (see Chapter 8).[56,57]

Chuei-Fong-Tou-Geu-Wan 追风透骨丸 has been banned in Hong Kong because it has been found to contain many pharmaceutical drugs.[55] Undeclared mefenamic acid in Tung Shueh 通血丸 pills indicated for arthralgia resulted in dialysis-dependent acute renal failure.[58] Herbal products sold for arthralgia have also been reported as containing prescription drugs, including steroids and nonsteroidal antiinflammatory drugs.[59] A study in Taiwan investigated unrecognised adrenal dysfunction in critically ill emergency department patients. The results indicate that adrenal dysfunction is common among a group of critically ill patients seen in this Taiwanese emergency department and that the use of herbal drugs was high in the patients with low serum cortisols. The authors suggest that further studies are required to confirm these findings and clarify whether a number of herbal medications contain corticosteroids.[60]

Medical records of five patients with complications resulting from Chinese herbal pills were reviewed, and the pills were analysed. All contained mefenamic acid and diazepam. Complications related to the presence of these substances included massive gastrointestinal bleeding.[61] The first case of adulteration with anticonvulsants was reported. Phenytoin was found in a CPM, which resulted in the patient admitted to hospital in a coma. As with so many of these reports the ingredient was not labelled.[62]

The adulteration of herbal medicines with pharmaceutical drugs when unlabelled is clearly not only dangerous but also unethical. The practice here has been described as "unscrupulous."[63] However, when the pharmaceutical additive is labelled the ethics need to be reviewed. In the PRC the concept of using Chinese medicines with pharmaceutical drugs to maximise the benefits of both is well established. There are many reports of using the two systems simultaneously.[64-66] Hence although illegal in the United Kingdom, the intentions are not always as unscrupulous as first appears. When the labelling includes all ingredients but is only in Chinese the dangers are as if unlabelled. In one survey of 28 products found to contain mercury, only 2 were labelled,[31] and 32% of 260 products contained undeclared pharmaceuticals or heavy metals.[30]

HERB-DRUG INTERACTIONS AND ADVERSE REACTIONS

Cases of HDIs are appearing in the literature. Interactions are potentially the most dangerous when a drug's dosage has a narrow therapeutic range, such as with warfarin.[67] Such drugs can be highly toxic with potential adverse effects if blood levels fall outside the therapeutic range. They have the potential to be quickly and acutely affected by concomitant herbal drugs. Several Chinese medicines are known to interact with warfarin, including *Salvia miltiorrhiza* (dan shen 丹参)[68,69] and *Zingiber officinale* Roscoe (sheng jiang 生姜).[70] The reports printed frequently provide incomplete information, reflecting the emerging nature of this knowledge. Argento et al.,[71] for example, in a review of interactions with anticoagulants rightly or wrongly included passionflower, juniper, *Verbena officinalis*, *Ganoderma japonicum*, papaw, *S. miltiorrhiza*, ginseng, devil's claw, garlic, quinine, ginkgo, ginger, red clover, and horse chestnut but ignored *Angelica sinensis* (dang gui 当归; see Chapter 6).

A variety of individual reports highlight the need for continued collection of safety data on CHM. A finding in 1990 challenged traditional theories.[72] *Coptis chinensis* (huang lian 黄连), which is widely given to newborn infants by Chinese mothers to clear toxic products of pregnancy, was found to displace bilirubin from its serum-binding site.[73] *Artemisia scoparia* (Yin Chen 茵陈) is used in Chinese paediatric hospitals to manage neonatal jaundice. It has also been found to displace bilirubin from its protein-binding site.[74] On one hand the results will support herbalists' observations that those treated would become less jaundiced; however, this increased amount of free bilirubin would greatly increase the risk of brain damage, in much the same way as the antibiotic Gantrisin does.

The potent hormonal effects of some Chinese herbs are reflected in two worrying reports. One involved foetal androgenisation resulting from a mother's intake of herbs; the other involved the development of gynaecomastia after the intake of *Angelica sinensis* (dang gui 当 归). Both would be described as improper use by a herbalist.[75] The identification of the herbs in the neonatal case has also been questioned.[76] A possible association has been reported between *A. sinensis* and hypertension in a mother and breast-fed baby.[77]

The long-term effects of Chinese herbs are difficult to assess. Laboratory and animal studies indicate that certain herbs may have a mutagenic potential.[78,79] Delayed effects of herbal medicines are difficult to ascertain; the need for better information on the embryotoxic and foetotoxic risks is needed because lack of adverse reports does not exclude the possible risks.

THE WAY FORWARD

The future of CHM clearly rests on overcoming the vast array of quality control problems that exist. In the United Kingdom these problems are being tackled by the Chinese Medicine Association of Suppliers, which is planning a tracking procedure from field to pharmacy and the establishment of a kitemark system. The organisation has had to build bridges between different cultures and rival companies to achieve its goals. The kitemark process will be circular starting from the source (i.e., the growers). The scheme will be implemented following agreement over criteria and procedures and policies with the profession and relevant government agencies. All the data throughout the kitemark scheme for each batch will be recorded in a database that can be used for monitoring purposes. A third authoritative body will conduct the audit and monitoring to ensure neutrality. The soil will be tested for pollutants, heavy metals, and fertilising agents to

ensure that international requirements are met. The seeds and the seedlings will also be authenticated. Harvesting, drying, processing, and treatment of herbs will follow agreed procedures and policies. Biodiversity monitoring will also be carried out to ensure that batches are compliant with the Convention on International Trade in Endangered Species of Wild Fauna and Flora (CITES). Packaging will conform to the agreed policy and procedure, and further authentication will take place before products are packed and sealed before storage in warehouses ready for export. The warehouses will meet with health and safety regulations to ensure the products are appropriately stored. When the goods arrive into the U.K. port, random samples will be laboratory tested. These tests will be carried out by laboratories on the MCA-approved list. The laboratory will then issue a certificate if the results data match the accompanying certificates for the batch. The goods will then be registered, and a kitemark serial number will be issued for that batch ready for sale to the public. The authoritative body will carry out an annual unannounced inspection or audit of the members' warehouses.

A compulsory policy for Register of Chinese Herbal Medicine members to reduce the risk of idiosyncratic hepatic reactions is in place, involving providing verbal and written information on recognising such an event.

The legal status of herbs is in a state of transition, and state registration of the profession is also planned, which will serve to raise educational standards and place safety at the forefront of practice.

REFERENCES

1. Bensoussan A, Myers SP, Carlton AL: Risks associated with the practice of traditional Chinese medicine: an Australian study, *Arch Fam Med* 9:1071-1078, 2000.
2. Barnes J, Abbott NC, Willoughby M, Ernst E: Different standards for reporting ADRS to herbal remedies & conventional OTC medicines: interviews with 515 users of herbal remedies, *FACT* 2:185, 1997.
3. Joshi BS, Kaul PN: Alternative medicine: herbal drugs and their critical appraisal—part I, *Prog Drug Res* 56:1-76, 2001.
4. Pillans PI: Toxicity of herbal products, *N Z Med J* 108:469-471, 1995.

5. Chan H, Yeh YY, Billmeier GJ, et al: Lead poisoning from ingestion of Chinese herbal medicine, *Clin Toxicol* 10:273-281, 1977.

6. Chan TY, Chan KK, Chan AY, Critchley JA: Poisoning due to Chinese proprietary medicines, *Hum Exp Toxicol* 14:434-436, 1995.

7. Chan TH, Wong KC, Chan JCN: Severe salicylate poisoning associated with the intake of Chinese medicinal oil ("red flower oil"), *Aust N Z J Med* 25:57, 1995.

8. Vanherweghem J, Depierreux M, Tielemans C, et al: Rapidly progressive interstitial renal fibrosis in young women: association with slimming regimen including Chinese herbs, *Lancet* 341:387-391, 1997.

9. Tai Y-T, But PP-H, Lau C-P, Young K: Cardiotoxicity after accidental herb-induced aconite poisoning, *Lancet* 340:1254-1256, 1992.

10. Tai Y-T, But PP-H, Young K, Lau C-P: Adverse effects from traditional Chinese medicine, *Lancet* 341:892, 1993.

11. Atherton DJ, Brostoff J, Rustin MHA: Need for correct identification of herbs in herbal poisoning, *Lancet* 341:637-638, 1993.

12. But PP: Need for correct identification of herbs in herbal poisoning, *Lancet* 341:637, 1993.

13. Chan TY, Critchley JA: Usage and adverse effects of Chinese herbal medicines, *Hum Exp Toxicol* 15:5-12, 1996.

14. Chan TY, Tomlinson B, Tse LK, Chan JC, Chan WW, Critchley JA: Aconitine poisoning due to Chinese herbal medicines: a review, *Vet Hum Toxicol* 36:452-455, 1994.

15. Dickens P, Tai YT, But PP, Tomlinson B, Ng HK, Yan KW: Fatal accidental aconitine poisoning following ingestion of Chinese herbal medicine: a report of two cases, *Forensic Sci Int* 67:55-58, 1994.

16. Tai YT, But PP, Young K, Lau CP: Cardiotoxicity after accidental herb-induced aconite poisoning, *Lancet* 340:1254-1256, 1992.

17. Chang HM, But PPH: *Pharmacology and applications of Chinese materia medica,* Singapore, 1987, World Scientific Publishing Co Ltd.

18. Perharic L, Shaw D, Leon C, De Smet P, Murray V: Possible association of liver damage with the use of Chinese herbal medicine for skin disease, *Vet Human Toxicol* 37: 562-566, 1995.

19. Pillans PI: Herbal medicine and toxic hepatitis, *N Z Med J* 107:432-433, 1994.

20. Itoh S, Marutani K, Nishijima T, Matsuo S, Itabashi M: Liver injuries induced by herbal medicine, syo-saiko-to (xiao-chai-hu-tang), *Dig Dis Sci* 40:1845-1848, 1995.

21. Farrell GC: *Drug-induced liver disease*, Edinburgh, 1995, Churchill Livingstone.

22. Stickel F, Egerer G, Seitz HK: Hepatotoxicity of botanicals, *Public Health Nutr* 3:111, 2000.

23. Melchart D, Linde K, Weidenhammer W, Hager S, Shaw D, Bauer R: Liver enzyme elevations in patients treated with traditional Chinese medicine, *JAMA* 282:28-29, 1999.

24. Al-Khafaji M: Liver test results of patients on Chinese medicine, 1999.

25. McCarthy M, Wilkinson ML: Recent advances—hepatology. *BMJ* 318:1256-1259, 1999.

26. Kane JA, Kane SP, Jain S: Hepatitis induced by traditional Chinese herbs; possible toxic components, *Gut* 36:146-147, 1995.

27. Shaw D, Leon C, Kolev S, Murray V: *Toxicological problems resulting from exposure to traditional medicines and food supplements 1991–1997,* London, 1997, MAFF.

28. Zhu YP, Woerdenbag HJ: Traditional Chinese medicine, *Pharmacy World Sci* 17:103-112, 1995.

29. WHO: *Research guidelines for evaluating the safety and efficacy of herbal medicines,* Geneva, 1993, WHO.

30. Ko RJ: Adulterants in Asian patent medicines, *N Engl J Med* 339:847-848, 1998.

31. Wong MK, Koh LL: Mercury, lead and other heavy metals in Chinese medicines, *Biol Trace Elem Res* 10:91-97, 1986.

32. Espinoza EO, Mann MJ, Bleasdell B: Arsenic and mercury in traditional Chinese herbal balls, *N Engl J Med* 333:803-804, 1995.

33. Dreskin SC: A prescription drug packaged in China and sold as an ethnic remedy, *JAMA* 283:2393, 2000.

34. Li AM: Batch testing of Xi Gua Shuang, 2001.

35. Kabelitz K: Heavy metals in herbal drugs, *Eur J Herbal Med* 4:25-33.

36. Chuang IC, Chen KS, Huang YL, Lee PN, Lin TH: Determination of trace elements in some natural drugs by atomic absorption spectrometry, *Biol Trace Elem Res* 76:235-244, 2000.

37. Ward T: *Prospects for monitoring safety aspects within Chinese medicine, an iterative study,* University of Exeter, 2002.

38. De Smet P: Adverse effects of herbal drugs, 34-47, 1991.

39. Kun-Ying Y: *The illustrated Chinese materia medica crude and prepared,* Taipei, 1992, SMC Publishing Inc.

40. Bennett J, Ma C, Traverso H, Agha SB, Boring J: Neonatal tetanus associated with topical umbilical ghee: covert role of cow dung, *Int J Epidemiol* 28:1172-1175, 1999.

41. WHO: *Report no. 118: inorganic mercury,* Geneva, 1991, WHO.

42. Satoh H: Occupational and environmental toxicology of mercury and its compounds, *Ind Health* 38:153-164, 2000.

43. MAFF: Food surveillance paper no. 53: cadmium, mercury and other metals in food. London, 1998, MAFF.

44. Omura Y, Beckman SL: Role of mercury (Hg) in resistant infections & effective treatment of Chlamydia trachomatis and Herpes family viral infections (and potential treatment for cancer) by removing localized Hg deposits with Chinese parsley and delivering effective antibiotics using various drug uptake enhancement methods, *Acupunct Electrother Res* 20:195-229, 1995.

45. Kang-Yum K, Oransky SH: Chinese patent medicine as a potential source of mercury poisoning, *Vet Hum Toxicol* 34:235-238, 1992.

46. Shaw D, House I, Kolev S, Murray V: Should herbal medicines be licensed? *BMJ* 311:451-452, 1995.

47. Chu CC, Huang CC, Ryu SJ, Wu TN: Chronic inorganic mercury induced peripheral neuropathy, *Acta Neurol Scand* 98:461-465, 1998.

48. Schaumburg HH, Berger A: Alopecia and sensory polyneuropathy from thallium in a Chinese herbal medication, *JAMA* 268:3430-3431, 1992.

49. Yu ECL, Yeung CY: Lead encephalopathy due to herbal medicine, *Chin Med J* 100:915-917, 1987.

50. Li AM, Chan MH, Leung TF, Cheung RC, Lam CW, Fok TF: Mercury intoxication presenting with tics, *Arch Dis Child* 83:174-175, 2000.

51. Chi YW, Chen SL, Yang MH, Hwang RC, Chu ML: Heavy metals in traditional Chinese medicine: ba-pao-neu-hwang-san, *Zhonghua Min Guo Xiao Er Ke Yi Xue Hui Za Zhi* 34:181-190, 1993.

52. de Krom MC, Boreas AM, Hardy EL: [Manganese poisoning due to use of Chien Pu Wan tablets], *Ned Tijdschr Geneeskd* 138:2010-2012, 1994.

53. Tomlinson B, Chan TY, Chan JC, Critchley JA, But PP: Toxicity of complementary therapies: an eastern perspective, *J Clin Pharmacol* 40:451-456, 2000.

54. Chitturi S, Farrell GC: Herbal hepatotoxicity: an expanding but poorly defined problem, *J Gastroenterol Hepatol* 15:1093-1099, 2000.

55. Chan TY, Critchley JA: The spectrum of poisonings in Hong Kong: an overview, *Vet Human Toxicol* 36:135-137, 1994.

56. Ernst E: Adverse effects of herbal drugs in dermatology, *Br J Dermatol* 143:923-929, 2001.

57. Keane FM, Munn SE, Du Vivier AWP, Taylor NF, Higgins EM: Analysis of Chinese herbal creams prescribed for dermatological conditions, *BMJ* 318:563-564, 1999.

58. Diamond JR, Pallone TL: Acute interstitial nephritis following use of tung shueh pills, *Am J Kidney Dis* 24:219-221, 1994.

59. Goldman JA, Myerson G: Chinese herbal medicine: camouflaged prescription antiinflammatory drugs, corticosteroids, and lead, *Arthritis Rheumatism* 34:1207, 1991.

60. Chang SS, Liaw SJ, Bullard MJ, Chiu TF, Chen JC, Liao HC: Adrenal insufficiency in critically ill emergency department patients: a taiwan preliminary study, *Acad Emerg Med* 8:761-764, 2001.

61. Gertner E, Marshall PS, Filandrinos D, Potek A, Smith T: Complications resulting from the use of Chinese herbal medications containing undeclared prescription drugs, *Arthritis Rheumatism* 38:614-617, 1995.

62. Lau KK, Lai CK, Chan AW: Phenytoin poisoning after using Chinese proprietary medicines, *Hum Exp Toxicol* 19:385-386, 2000.

63. Strack M: Problems with herbal treatments, *N Z Med J* 107:515, 1994.

64. Cai R, Luo H, Xiao Y: [Clinical study of pulmonary encephalopathy with integrated traditional Chinese and Western medicine], *Zhongguo Zhong Xi Yi Jie He Za Zhi* 18:140-141, 1998.

65. Zhang X, Liu S, Liang Y: [Clinical study on treatment of moderate and advanced stage cancers by Bailong tablets combined with chemotherapy], *Zhongguo Zhong XiYi Jie He Za Zhi* 18:24-25, 1998.

66. Gao X, Rao H, Niu X, Hu J: An approach to the integration of acupuncture and drug, *J Tradit Chin Med* 21:45-49, 2001.

67. Miller LG: Herbal medicinals: selected clinical considerations focusing on known or potential drug-herb interactions, *Arch Intern Med* 158:2200-2211, 1998.

68. Tam LS, Chan TY, Leung WK, Critchley JA: Warfarin interactions with Chinese traditional medicines: danshen and methyl salicylate medicated oil, *Aust N Z J Med* 25:258, 1995.

69. Chan TY: Interaction between warfarin and danshen (Salvia miltiorrhiza), *Ann Pharmacother* 35:501-504, 2001.

70. Ko R: Adverse reactions to watch for in patients using herbal remedies, *West J Med* 171:181-186, 1999.

71. Argento A, Tiraferri E, Marzaloni M: Oral anticoagulants and medicinal plants. An emerging interaction, *Ann Ital Med Int* 15:139-143, 2000.

72. Yeung CY, Lee FT, Wong HN: Effect of a popular Chinese herb on neonatal bilirubin protein binding, *Biol Neonate* 58:98-103, 1990.

73. Yeung CY: Neonatal hyperbilirubinaemia in Chinese, *Trop Geog Med* 25:151-157, 1973.

74. Yeung CY, Leung CS, Chen YZ: An old traditional herbal remedy for neonatal jaundice with a newly identified risk, *J Paediatr Child Health* 29:292-294, 1993.

75. Koren G, Randor S, Martin S, Danneman D: Maternal ginseng use associated with neonatal androgenization, *JAMA* 264:2866, 1990.

76. Awang D: Maternal use of ginseng and neonatal androgenization, *JAMA* 265:1828, 1991.

77. Nambiar S, Schwartz RH, Constantino A, Vienna VA: Hypertension in mother and baby linked to ingestion of Chinese herbal medicine, *West J Med* 171:152, 1999.

78. Yin XJ, Liu DX, Wang HC, Zhou Y: A study on the mutagenicity of 102 raw pharmaceuticals used in Chinese traditional medicine, *Mutat Res* 260:73-82, 1991.

79. Huang NJ, Meng JH, Chen CM: Mutagenicity of 30 Chinese herbs and pharmaceuticals, *Prog Clin Biol Res* 340e:224, 1990.

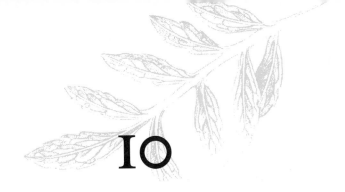

10

ALLERGIC REACTIONS TO HERBAL MEDICINES

Stephen Myers and Hans Wohlmuth

In theory, any pharmaceutical drug can induce an immune response; however, in practice some drugs are more likely to elicit clinically relevant immune responses than others. Some drugs are intrinsically immunogenic because of their molecular configuration, whereas other drugs with a molecular mass of <1000 D are incapable of inducing an immune response in their native state. For these smaller molecular weight substances to elicit an immune response, they need to undergo bioactivation by binding to a protein and forming an immune complex.[1] Similarly all herbal medicines can potentially induce an immune response. Given the complex chemical profile of herbal medicines, which contain a mixture of high and low molecular weight substances, the potential for immunogenic reactions is probably increased. Clinicians should remain alert to the potential for such responses to herbal medicines.

Adverse drug reactions (ADRs) are classified as predictable (type A) reactions and unpredictable (type B) reactions. Predictable reactions are those related to the pharmacological actions of the drug, such as direct toxicity, and are the most common form of ADRs (approximately 80%). In contrast, unpredictable reactions are not related to the pharmacological actions of the drug and are generally uncommon. Immune-mediated or allergic reactions are unpredictable and comprise between 6% and 10% of all ADRs to pharmaceutical drugs.[1] Comparative data for herbal medicines are currently unavailable. It has been assumed that herbal medicines follow this general trend: that allergic reactions do occur but that they are generally uncommon. Support for this assumption is derived from the widespread and long-standing use of herbal medicines by the international community, where the number of cases of allergic reactions cited in the literature is relatively small, considering the degree of community exposure. To confirm this observation, more rigorous investigation needs to be undertaken to clarify the extent of herbal medicine-induced allergic reactions.

Skin reactions to herbal medicines are common in individuals involved in the occupational handling of herbs. These reactions generally result in an irritant contact dermatitis, which is common in workers handling herbs from the buttercup (Ranunculaceae), spurge

(Euphorbiaceae), and daisy (Asteraceae, also known as Compositae) families.[2] These occupational reactions are not immune mediated and are caused by chemical irritants within the plants, including alkaloids, saponins, and anthraquinones. Other occupational skin reactions include mechanical irritation from spines, irritant hairs, or irritant crystals on the plant surface. Workers in the herbal medicine industry are also exposed to the potential for immune-mediated reactions. Allergic dermatitis,[3] urticaria,[4] and occupational asthma[5] have been reported. Although these occupational reactions are outside the scope of this review, it is important for health professionals to be aware that handling herbal materials can result in irritant and allergic reactions. Two cases of occupational asthma reported in the literature highlight the risk of allergic reactions in health professionals. The first was in a Korean pharmacist, who handled herbal materials as part of his profession and showed an early asthmatic response to dang gui (dong quai, *Angelica sinensis*) in a bronchoprovocation test.[6] The second case was a Canadian herbalist, who reported that her asthma symptoms were worse at work and showed an asthmatic response to licorice *(Glycyrrhiza glabra)* root powder on bronchoprovocation.[7]

A systematic review of all cases of allergic reactions to herbal medicines is beyond the scope of this chapter. The literature cited has been selected to provide examples of a wide range of clinical conditions and responses to a broad range of herbs. For the majority of cases described here, there are fairly strong reasons to suspect a causal relationship between the exposure and the allergic reaction. This is not always the case in clinical reports, in which the causality of the reactions has not always been effectively assessed, and the authors do not provide enough information for the readers to determine the nature of the association.

There are a number of ways that the material used in this review could have been classified. We considered that the most practical classification was one based on clinical presentation, with a discussion of individual herbs that have been reported to be associated with a specific presentation. The material could equally have been classified by plant species,

plant family, or by plant constituents. These various classifications can be found in the literature. However, we have toward the end of the chapter dedicated a short section to one constituent class with particularly high allergenic potential, the sesquiterpene lactones.

Allergic reactions in consumers of herbal products, either self-prescribed or prescribed by health professionals, range from allergic contact dermatitis to anaphylactic shock. Allergic reactions can be classified according to the Coombs and Gell classification system into (1) immediate-type hypersensitivity reactions (mediated by drug-specific immunoglobulin [Ig] E antibodies); (2) cytotoxic and immune complex reactions (mediated by drug-specific IgG or IgM antibodies); and (3) delayed-type hypersensitivity reactions (mediated by drug-specific T lymphocytes).[8] Gruchalla[1] points out that although these categories seem relatively straightforward, classifying reactions to pharmaceutical agents into these categories is challenging because of a lack of understanding of the mechanism underlying specific reactions. Here again the complexity of constituents in plants further compounds the difficulty of this exercise for herbs. This reinforces our choice of a clinical classification that outlines the reactions according to clinical presentation. Many of the issues and reactions described are also reflected in the appropriate safety monographs for individual herbs that are contained in this book.

SKIN REACTIONS

Allergic Contact Dermatitis

Allergic contact dermatitis occurs in individuals who have been previously sensitised to a plant or plant product. The mechanism involves plant molecules penetrating the epidermis and reacting with specific IgE bound mast cells, which results in the release of inflammatory mediators, including histamine, prostaglandins, and leukotrienes.[2] Investigation of allergic contact dermatitis is generally undertaken by patch testing. Further to the role of herbs in medicinal use, it is important to recognise that natural botanical extracts are becoming increasingly used by the cosmetics industry and that herbal and plant components of cosmetics may be responsible for allergic skin reactions.[9]

Arnica *(Arnica montana)* (Family Asteraceae)

The topical application of arnica, in the form of creams, ointments, or liniments, for sprains and bruises is a well-documented cause of allergic contact dermatitis, and numerous cases have been reported.[9,10] The allergenic and sensitising compounds in arnica are several sesquiterpene lactones, including helenalin.[10] Cross-reactivity to other sesquiterpene lactone-containing plants appears to be widespread, and therefore sensitivity to other Asteraceae species greatly increases the risk of an allergic response to arnica.[9,10]

German chamomile *(Matricaria recutita)* (Family Asteraceae)

A case from Spain reported a 26-year-old woman who used a topical preparation of chamomile tea and presented with acute facial eczema.[11] Four days before presentation the woman dyed her eyebrows, which immediately felt itchy. She immediately applied nitrofurazone and a topical application of chamomile tea. Patch testing to sesquiterpene lactones 0.1% was positive (3+). The authors describe patch testing to German chamomile tea and refer to a table for results, which are unfortunately not present. Given the title of the communication one presumes that the test was positive. However, the lack of data decreases the value of this case report. Ten control subjects were patch tested with the chamomile tea and gave a negative result. Patch testing was negative for Roman chamomile but was positive for yarrow *(Achillea millefolium)* 1% (2+) and feverfew *(Tanacetum vulgare)* 1% (3+), which might explain the reactivity to the sesquiterpene lactones. Fifteen days after the patch testing the woman developed an episode of oedema and itching of the oral mucosa and eczema of the arms and trunk and anal pruritus. She had consumed a cup of chamomile tea the day before. The authors considered this to be the first report of systemic contact dermatitis from German chamomile.

Roman chamomile *(Chamaemelum nobile,* syn. *Anthemis nobilis)* (Family Asteraceae)

Two cases reported allergic contact dermatitis of the nipple in breast-feeding mothers in the United Kingdom.[12] In the first case, a 32-year-old woman who had breast-fed her fifth child for 10 weeks, developed severe exudative eczema of both nipples and areolae. She had applied a commercial preparation containing 10.5% chamomile oil to manage cracked nipples. Patch testing showed a positive response (3+) for the ointment and the chamomile oil at 2 days and a negative reaction to other ingredients. Ten controls were negative to chamomile oil 0.1%. The second case was a 38-year-old woman who was breast-feeding her second child when she developed severe bilateral eczema of the nipples and areolae after the application of the same commercial chamomile preparation implicated in the first case. She had previously used the same preparation without problems. Patch testing showed a positive response (3+) for the chamomile oil at 2 days and a negative reaction to other ingredients.

Elecampane *(Inula helenium)* (Family Asteraceae)

From Italy, a case reported a 32-year-old woman who presented with a 1-month history of diffuse dermatitis after using a herbal massage preparation for 1 month.[13] The herbal preparation contained *Inula helenium, Achillea millefolium, Articum lappa,* and *Laurus nobilis.* The condition rapidly improved on avoidance of the preparation. Patch testing was positive (2+) to the preparation and a sesquiterpene lactone mix 0.1%. No control subjects were used to ensure that the commercial preparation was not irritant on patch testing. The sesquiterpene lactone mix contained equimolar amounts of alantolactone (an eudesmanolide derived from *Inula helenium*), costunolide (a germacranolide from costus oil), and dehydrocostus lactone (a guianolide from costus oil). The authors report that a careful history revealed that the patient had taken tablets containing *Inula helenium* extract for a genital infection 1 year previously and had experienced facial eczema while taking the tablets.

Garlic *(Allium sativum)* (Family Liliaceae)

A case reported a 58-year-old man who had a 35-year history of recurring cheiropompholyx (a vesicular pattern of eczema affecting the skin of the hands).[14] The episodes occurred once or twice a year and cleared within 2 to 3 weeks. Nine months before the presentation he commenced taking air-dried garlic tablets for hyperlipidemia. His hands had flared up severely and persisted for 8 months until he ran out of garlic tablets. Patch testing was positive (2+) to garlic. A double-blind oral provocation test to the garlic tablets was undertaken, causing a marked flare-up after taking the garlic tablet and no reaction with the placebo tablet.

Gotu kola *(Centella asiatica)* (Family Apiaceae)

A case reported a 39-year-old woman who was treated with a commercial *Centella* preparation in combination with a topical corticosteroid for the management of a skin lesion.[15] A red vesicular reaction, with exudation and intense itching, occurred on the abdomen after 20 days. A few days later it spread to the trunk and limbs. The condition responded to oral steroids and resolved in 1 week. Patch testing was positive (3+) to the commercial *Centella* preparation and *Centella* powder 1%. There was no reaction to the topical corticosteroid, fluocinolone acetonide 0.025%, or other components of corticosteroid preparation. Patch testing on 50 controls with *Centella* powder 1% was negative.

The sensitising capacity of *Centella asiatica* extract and its triterpenoid constituents asiaticoside, asiatic acid, and madecassic acid was studied in guinea pigs and in a 30-year-old woman who developed eczema on her left hand after using a commercial preparation of *Centella*.[16] The woman had a positive (3+) reaction to the commercial preparation at 1 and 3 days. The three triterpenic acids at 10% produced no response. In the sensitisation and challenge experiment, groups of 10 guinea pigs received a sensitisation injection of either the whole extract or a pure compound and were then rested for 11 days. Challenge with a 30% concentrate of the raw extract given as an epicutaneous injection gave only 1+ in a single

animal at the 24-hour and 40-hour readings. The three triterpenic acids were also weak sensitisers, with only madecassic acid showing a "crescendo" response over three readings; however, at no stage was a 2+ response obtained. The author concluded that the risk of acquiring contact sensitivity to this plant or its constituents is low.

Lavender *(Lavandula* spp.*)* oil (Family Lamiaceae)

Two cases reported facial dermatitis from the application of lavender essential oil to the pillow.[17] The first case was a 71-year-old woman who presented with a 4-day history of acute eczema predominantly on her left cheek and forehead. She had a history of reacting to commercial face creams and had since used fragrance-free cosmetics. She had a positive (2+) patch test to lavender. On examination she had denied using any perfumed products but revealed when questioned specifically about lavender use that she had commenced using lavender oil drops on her pillow. The condition resolved after 2 weeks with a combination of a new pillow, avoidance of lavender, and topical corticosteroids. The second case was a 76-year-old man who presented with an itchy eruption on his right cheek and forehead. Examination showed a unilateral right-sided facial dermatitis. He had a history of severe hemiplegia since a stroke. He denied using cosmetics; however, a bottle of lavender oil was found in the bedroom during a domiciliary consultation. Patch testing showed a positive reaction (2+) to lavender. The condition resolved by avoiding lavender oil.

Licorice *(Glycyrrhiza glabra)* (Family Fabaceae)

A Japanese case reported a 43-year-old woman who presented with an itchy reddish eruption on her face.[18] The eruption had been present for 1 month. Patch testing showed a positive reaction to a facial cream, foundation, and essence the patient had been using and to 33 allergens of a cosmetic series. Further tests with 7 ingredients from the three cosmetic products showed a positive (1+) reaction to oil-soluble licorice extracts at 2 and 3 days at

0.5%, 1%, and 5%. In 11 controls the results were negative for these three concentrations at 2 and 3 days. This case illustrates the potential for botanical extracts in cosmetics to be the cause of allergic skin reactions.

Myrrh *(Commiphora myrrha)* (Family Burseraceae)

A case reported a 45-year-old woman who received Chinese herbs from a bonesetter in Hong Kong.[19] The woman complained of sudden onset of itching, redness, and swelling of her sprained right wrist 5 days after applying the Chinese herbs. On examination there was a well-defined, bright red, oedematous patch with vesicles over her right wrist. The herbal mixture included 20 herbs, but the report does not indicate the dosage form. Patch testing of the mixture without myrrh and mastic was negative, as was mastic alone. Myrrh showed a positive (2+) reaction. The article also reports patch testing of 20 patients with contact dermatitis from causes other than bonesetter's herbs, and none showed any reaction to myrrh. An additional 20 patients with contact dermatitis to bonesetter's herbs were also tested: 12 were positive (11 patients 2+ and 1 patient 1+), representing 60% of the sample. The same authors reported two additional cases with myrrh sensitivity in a case series of a Chinese orthopaedic solution, Tieh Ta Yao Gin.[20] The first was of a 30-year-old woman with a left wrist sprain, who reported an itchy red rash on day 11 of using the solution. Patch testing was positive (2+) for the solution and myrrh and negative for the other ingredients. The second was a 29-year-old man with a left knee sprain who noticed itchiness and redness on day 7 of using the solution. Patch testing was positive (2+) for the solution, myrrh, and mastic and negative for other constituents. A control study of 10 patients with contact dermatitis to agents other than Chinese herbs showed no reaction to patch testing with either the solution or any of its constituents at either day 2 or day 4. A third case in the series showed sensitivity to mastic. Myrrh and mastic are gum resins widely used in traditional Chinese medicine to relieve pain and swelling caused by traumatic injury.

A case reported a 36-year-old man who applied myrrh extract to a surgical wound to promote healing after inguinal surgery in Saudi Arabia.[21] The type of extract was not stated. He developed erythema and itching over the surgical site, extending to the whole abdomen. He had applied the same material to a previous surgical wound without complications, and the authors considered this to be the sensitising incident. Patch testing was positive (3+) for the myrrh preparation. No control subjects were used to ensure that the preparation was not irritant on patch testing. The lesions responded to topical corticosteroids and resolved after 2 weeks.

Spearmint *(Mentha spicata)* (Family Lamiaceae)

A case of allergic contact dermatitis in a 64-year-old non-atopic woman has been reported from Italy.[22] She had previously had contact dermatitis from shoes and leather items and developed painful localised oedematous and vesicular lesions on her right knee after the repeated application of a compress made from fresh spearmint leaves. Patch testing was positive for an alcoholic spearmint extract, spearmint oil, and peppermint oil but was negative for menthol. Another spearmint oil constituent, L-carvone, has previously been implicated as the allergen involved in oral contact dermatitis to toothpaste.[23]

Vervain *(Verbena officinalis)* (Family Verbenaceae)

A case reported a 60-year-old woman who developed an erythematous, exudative eruption with intense itching on her chest 8 to 12 hours after applying a plaster of vervain.[24] The application consisted of an omelette made from egg white and the small lilac flowers of vervain, presumably cooked in oil or fat. She had used the treatment previously without any trouble. Patch testing was carried out on the parts (flower, leaf, and stem) of the fresh plant and aqueous and ether extracts of the whole plant. Positive (2+) reactions were elicited from the flower, leaf, and ether extract at 4 days. No reaction was observed with the stem or aqueous extract, suggesting that the allergen was lipid soluble. Patch testing with the fresh plant was negative in 10 controls. The authors consider that several circumstances may have conspired to cause dermatitis, including the sensitivity of the chest area, the prolonged contact, and the warm oily vehicle (the omelette).

Erythema Multiforme–Like Contact Dermatitis

Erythema multiforme is an acute, recurrent, inflammatory, hypersensitivity reaction affecting the skin and mucous membranes and is often associated with reactions to drugs or microorganisms. Superficial dermal oedema leads to the formation of vesicles and bullae, and characteristic "bull's eye" lesions occur on the skin surface. Histological features include lymphocytic infiltrate around the superficial dermal blood vessels, basement membrane, and keratinocytes.[25]

Cayenne *(Capsicum annuum)* (Family Solanaceae)

An Italian case reported a 65-year-old woman who presented with an eruption on her right knee 2 days after topical application of cayenne.[26] The woman applied a homemade alcoholic tincture of cayenne for its antirheumatic effects. She had erythematous plaques, vesicles, and small bullae with numerous target-like lesions on examination. Findings on biopsy were consistent with erythema multiforme. The condition responded to oral steroids. Patch testing 1 month after steroid withdrawal was positive. Twenty control subjects were negative.

Tea tree *(Melaleuca alternifolia)* oil (Family Myrtaceae)

A Canadian case reported a 46-year-old Chinese man who presented with an extensive erythema multiforme-like reaction.[27] Three weeks before presentation the man sustained a superficial abrasion on his left shin, which he treated with tea tree oil daily under an occlusive dressing. After 2 weeks of treatment the area became red and itchy. The tea tree oil was discontinued, but during the next 7 days the lesion spread. On examination an 8 × 20-cm scarlet, annular plaque with a purpuric margin was seen on the left shin. Numerous erythe-

matous papules and plaques, ranging in size from 0.5 to 3 cm, also were scattered on the trunk and extensor aspect of the extremities. Findings on biopsy were consistent with erythema multiforme. The man was treated with oral prednisone and hydroxyzine and topical betamethasone valerate cream, and the lesions cleared in 2 weeks. Five months later patch testing was performed using an oxidised sample of his original tea tree oil preparation and a fresh tea tree oil sample. At 96 hours the oxidised version showed a stronger reaction (3+) than the fresh sample (2+). These finding are consistent with data demonstrating that the oxidation products of tea tree oil have a sensitising capacity 3 times stronger than fresh tea tree oil. The authors note that erythema multiforme secondary to allergic contact dermatitis is a rare but well-characterised phenomenon.

Systemic Contact Dermatitis

This is a more generalised skin reaction that occurs in individuals after the oral administration of a substance to which topical sensitisation has previously occurred.

Echinacea (*Echinacea* spp.) (Family Asteraceae)

An Australian case reported a 48-year-old woman who developed a maculopapular rash on her abdomen and thighs within 2 days of taking unspecified echinacea tablets.[28] The rash was managed with topical steroids and resolved within 1 week. One week later the patient developed a similar but more severe and generalised pruritic rash within 2 days of again ingesting the same echinacea product. She was treated with oral steroids, and the rash gradually subsided during a 6-week period. Although the positive rechallenge is suggestive of a causal relationship between the echinacea product and the skin reaction, a skin prick test 5 months later with an echinacea preparation (not the one she had ingested) was negative.

Goldenrod *(Solidago virgaurea)* (Family Asteraceae)

A German case reported a 53-year-old man who presented with a 5-day history of generalised maculopapular eczema.[29] The skin lesions, which were itchy, occurred 6 days after oral treatment with a preparation containing goldenrod fluid extract, which he was taking for relapsing epididymitis and which resolved after a few days. The eczema responded to topical corticosteroids and resolved in 10 days. In addition to the skin condition he had cellulitis of the right foot, which required antibiotics. Patch testing was positive (3+) to goldenrod and negative to the other ingredients in the preparation. No controls were tested. The plant is known as a weak sensitiser.[30]

Kava *(Piper methysticum)* (Family Piperaceae)

A German case reported a 36-year-old woman who presented with a generalised rash and severe itching.[31] She had been taking a commercial preparation containing kava root extract (120 mg daily) for 3 weeks to manage anxiety. She presented 4 days after having stopped taking the preparation. On examination she had generalised erythema and papules, along with wheals on her trunk. The rash cleared rapidly with oral steroids and antihistamines; however, the itching persisted for several weeks. Patch testing 6 weeks after the condition resolved showed a positive reaction (2+) for the commercial kava preparation. Patch testing of the preparation in 10 controls was negative.

Papaya (paw-paw) *(Carica papaya)* (Family Caricaceae)

A case of systemic contact dermatitis after the ingestion of throat lozenges containing freeze-dried papaya juice concentrate was reported from Switzerland.[32] A 55-year-old woman developed a symmetric, maculopapular rash on her abdomen and upper arms approximately 2 days after consuming the lozenges. Patch testing was positive for papaya juice, but hypersensitivity to papain, the proteolytic enzyme present in papaya fruit, was not evident. Occupational allergy to papain of delayed and immediate type is known from workers involved in the production of the enzyme.

Urticaria

Urticaria is characterised by widespread itchy wheals or hives. It often occurs with angioedema, which is characterised by deep mucocutaneous

swelling. Acute urticaria is often IgE-mediated, and the most effective therapy is allergen avoidance.[33]

Garlic *(Allium sativum)* (Family Liliaceae)

An Italian case reported a 35-year-old woman with recurrent episodes of urticaria and angioedema.[34] She had experienced many episodes during the previous 2 years, all of which were associated with the ingestion of foods containing either raw or cooked garlic. Skin prick testing with a large panel of commercial food extracts was negative. A single strong reaction (4+) was induced by garlic extract. The woman later showed a positive reaction on skin prick testing to a commercial garlic preparation and to fresh garlic. Cases of garlic-induced erythematous reactions have been noted on direct skin exposure.[35] The failure to provide negative controls detracts from this case report.

Echinacea *(Echinacea* spp.) (Family Asteraceae)

Five cases of urticaria associated with echinacea have been reported from Australia, but no details of these cases are available (see Echinacea entry under "Anaphylactic Reactions").[36]

OCULAR REACTIONS

German chamomile *(Matricaria recutita)* (Family Asteraceae)

A German case reported a 37-year-old woman with a history of recurrent periorbital swelling.[37] The woman had experienced 3 episodes in 2 weeks with the swelling spreading to the cheeks and forehead. She was patch tested with her own cosmetics, and a cosmetic preparation containing 12.5% plant extracts showed a positive response (2+). Testing with individual ingredients showed a positive test at day 2 (1+) and day 4 (2+) to bisabolol alone. Bisabolol, a sesquiterpene alcohol, can constitute up to 50% of the essential oil of German chamomile. Patch tests in 30 controls were negative.

A Spanish case series reported seven hay fever patients with conjunctivitis.[38] Each of the individuals had conjunctivitis after eye washing with German chamomile tea. These reactions were immediate, and two of the individuals had lid angioedema. The patients (4 men and 3 women) were aged 21 to 51 years. Skin prick testing showed an immediate positive response to chamomile tea extract and *Matricaria* pollen in all seven patients. Conjunctival provocation tests with low concentrations of chamomile tea extract were also positive in all seven cases. All seven patients also had detectable IgE reactivity to chamomile tea extract as measured by an enzyme-linked immunosorbent assay (ELISA) technique. All seven patients tolerated oral provocation with chamomile tea. One hundred consecutive hay fever patients acted as control subjects. Eight of them showed a positive response to *Matricaria* pollen, and five of these had a positive reaction to chamomile tea. Only two of the five demonstrated a positive response to conjunctival provocation (2% of the total control population). These control data strongly suggest that nonirritant mechanisms mediated the conjunctival reactions of the seven hay fever patients and support the conclusion that chamomile tea can cause allergic conjunctivitis.

Witch hazel *(Hamamelis virginiana)* (Family Hamamelidaceae)

A Finnish case reported a 31-year-old woman with periorbital oedema.[39] The woman developed the oedema around both eyes within 1 week of commencing use of a new eye gel. She ceased the eye gel and started to use "alternative" remedies. The condition worsened and in subsequent days spread to the face and neck and developed into eczema. The dermatitis resolved with corticosteroids and avoidance of any cosmetics or alternative remedies. Patch testing showed a positive response to the eye gel (1+) and to its ingredients, witch hazel distillate (2+) and cucumber extract (1+). Five control patients patch tested negative to the eye gel. The reaction to cucumber extract was equivocal because the results of serial dilution were unconvincing.

ORAL REACTIONS

Peppermint *(Mentha × piperita)* (Family Lamiaceae)

A Scottish case series reported 12 patients with contact sensitivity to the flavouring agents men-

thol and peppermint oil.[40] Screening of 512 patients referred for an assessment of the possible role of contact sensitivity in their dental complaints between 1989 and 1992 produced 12 patients who were positive on patch testing to menthol 5% and peppermint oil 1%. Five patients with burning mouth syndrome demonstrated reactions to menthol and/or peppermint. One was strongly positive to both; 3 were positive to menthol only; and one was positive to peppermint only. Of 4 patients with recurrent oral ulceration, all were sensitive to both substances. Three patients with oral lichenoid reactions tested positive to menthol on patch testing; two of them were also sensitive to peppermint. Follow-up review of 9 of the 12 patients occurred 9 to 48 months after this assessment. Four reported clearance of their condition, and 2 reported substantial improvement based on the strategy of avoiding menthol and peppermint. A 62-year-old woman saw a 3-year history of burning mouth syndrome resolve in 3 days by avoiding her menthol-containing toothpaste and mouthwash. Another patient, a 31-year-old man, reported that an 8-year history of recurrent mouth ulcers ceased by changing to menthol-free toothpaste and avoiding a peppermint-flavoured mouthwash. A 48-year-old man requiring oral steroids to control chronic mouth ulceration, which had repeatedly occurred during the previous 6 months, ceased taking steroids and reported no ulceration during an 18-month steroid-free period by avoiding peppermint and menthol. A 32-year-old woman reported complete clearance of her intraoral lichenoid reactions after avoidance of menthol and peppermint and had no recurrences during a 2-year period. Of the three patients who did not show any improvement as a result of avoiding peppermint and menthol, one decided to tolerate the condition rather than change routine, whereas another improved on removal of old mercury-containing amalgam fillings.

ASTHMA

Echinacea *(Echinacea* spp.) (Family Asteraceae)

Two Australian cases of asthma induced by echinacea products have been published.[28] One concerned a 19-year-old woman with a history of allergic rhinitis but not asthma who experienced an acute asthma attack within 10 minutes of taking an unspecified echinacea tea, believed to be her first exposure to echinacea. She also developed itchy eyes and runny nose. A skin prick test 1 week later with an echinacea preparation (not the one she had ingested) produced a 3-mm wheal. The report emphasises that this patient had not previously been exposed to echinacea, thus implying that the reaction was the result of cross-reactivity. However, the use of echinacea-containing products is so widespread in Australia that previous (but unrecognised) exposure cannot be conclusively ruled out.

The second Australian case is that of a 56-year-old man, also with a history of allergic rhinitis but not asthma, who on three separate occasions developed severe breathing difficulties and coughing within 2 hours of taking unspecified echinacea tablets for an upper respiratory infection. The patient had not taken any other medication, and there was no known food or drug allergy. The symptoms resolved within a few days. A skin prick test with an echinacea preparation (different from the one he had ingested) was negative.

ANAPHYLACTIC REACTIONS

Anaphylaxis is a severe allergic reaction caused by the systemic release of histamine and other inflammatory mediators. It is characterised by laryngeal oedema, lower airway obstruction, and hypotension. The common causes are IgE-mediated sensitivity to food such as peanuts and shellfish. Management requires the prompt administration of adrenaline, which is repeated as necessary to reverse the actions of histamine.[33]

Chamomile (Family Asteraceae): German (*Matricaria recutita*) and Roman (*Chamaemelum nobile*, syn. *Anthemis nobilis*)

A case from the United States involving an unspecified chamomile species was published in 1973.[41] A 35-year-old woman with a history of hayfever caused by ragweed (*Ambrosia* spp.; family Asteraceae) developed abdominal cramps, swelling of the tongue and lips, throat tightness, and diffuse pruritus immediately after sipping chamomile tea. She was treated with an antihistamine and a steroid and recovered in a couple of hours. She subsequently produced a positive response to a scratch test with chamomile tea.

From Spain a case reported an 8-year old boy with a history of hay fever and asthma who experienced an anaphylactic reaction to chamomile tea.[42] A few minutes after taking the tea, the boy developed dyspnoea, coughing, wheezing, vomiting, and generalised pruritus. After arriving at hospital he lost consciousness and was treated with adrenaline, prednisolone, an antihistamine, and intravenous fluids before making a full recovery. Cross-reactivity between *Matricaria* and *Artemisia* pollen was demonstrated by ELISA technique, and the authors suggest that *Artemisia* pollen may have been the sensitising agent because the boy had never before been exposed to chamomile. Although this is plausible, it seems difficult to rule out previous exposure to a common herb like chamomile in a child.

A tragic case resulting in the death of a newborn was reported from Austria.[43] During labour, a healthy 35-year-old woman was given an enema containing glycerol and a proprietary chamomile flower extract (although not stated, we believe this product was most likely made from *Matricaria recutita*). She developed larynx oedema, urticaria, tachycardia, and hypotension and required emergency treatment. An emergency caesarean section was carried out, but the newborn showed severe asphyxia and died the following day. Chamomile-specific IgE was confirmed by radioallergosorbent test (RAST). Immunoblot tests revealed the presence in chamomile of a homologue of the birch pollen allergen Bet v 1. Homologues of this allergen are present in many taxonomically related and unrelated plants and may give rise to allergenic cross-reactivity.

Another case of anaphylaxis resulting from a chamomile enema was reported from Australia.[44] It involved a 69-year-old Ukrainian immigrant with a history of seasonal rhinitis who was administered the enema for constipation by his wife, who was a trained medical practitioner. Within minutes he developed dyspnoea, flushing, and an urticarial rash on the inside of his arms. He was given oral prednisolone immediately and subsequently received nebulised salbutamol. Skin prick testing was positive to the chamomile tea bag used to prepare the enema and ragweed.

A systematic case series from an allergy unit at an Austrian university detailed 10 cases, including the aforementioned case of the woman in labour, of anaphylactic reactions to chamomile.[45] The two most serious cases involved the administration of chamomile in the form of an enema. All 10 cases presented with rhinoconjunctivitis, dyspnoea, and wheezing and some also with urticaria, angioedema, hypotension, vomiting, or diarrhoea. Only two patients showed IgE binding to a Bet v 1 homologue, whereas the majority of the patients were sensitised to mugwort (*Artemisia vulgaris*; family Asteraceae).

The potential for cross-reactivity between chamomile and other common allergenic plants, considered with the fact that chamomile, in particular German chamomile, is widely used as a medicinal plant, likely means that allergic reactions, including anaphylactic reactions, are more likely to occur to chamomile than to most other medicinal plants. Particular caution is warranted in cases in which there is a history of sensitivity to other Asteraceae plants, such as mugwort.

Garlic *(Allium sativum)* (Family Liliaceae)

A case of anaphylaxis in a 23-year-old woman after the ingestion of raw young garlic has been reported from Spain.[46] The woman had a history of allergy to pollen and seeds, including peanuts, walnuts, hazelnuts, almonds, and sunflower seed, and had experienced three previous episodes of food-dependant, exercise-induced anaphylaxis when aged 19 to 20 years. In the present case she had ingested a meal consisting of eggs, shrimp, and young garlic. Within a few minutes of the meal and without exercise she developed generalised urticaria and facial angioedema. These symptoms were followed with a feeling of sickness, hypotension, and loss of consciousness. She was taken to an emergency department and treated with adrenaline, intravenous fluids, and hydrocortisone, and the symptoms resolved within 24 hours. Subsequent skin

prick tests gave positive results for various pollens. Raw young garlic produced a large wheal (23×14 mm), whereas heated young garlic and garlic clove produced much smaller wheals. Analysis indicated the presence of proteins in the fresh young garlic that were absent from stored garlic and garlic cloves. After her recovery, the patient again consumed eggs, shrimp, and garlic cloves on several occasions without any ill effects, but she did not eat raw young garlic again.

Echinacea (*Echinacea* spp.) (Family Asteraceae)

An Australian case reported a 37-year-old woman who presented with anaphylactic symptoms.[47] The woman had a history of taking complementary medicines, including echinacea, on an irregular basis for 2 to 3 years. On the morning of the anaphylactic reaction she ingested vitamins B1 and E, a herbal iron preparation, vitamin B complex, a multivitamin capsule, zinc, antioxidants, a garlic and onion preparation, and evening primrose oil. This was in a 5- to 10-minute period at 7:30 AM. At 7:45 AM the woman took 5 mL of a commercially prepared aqueous alcohol (40%) preparation of echinacea, which was diluted in blackcurrant juice. This represented an extract calculated to be produced from 3825 mg of whole plant extract of *Echinacea angustifolia* and 150 mg dry root of *Echinacea purpurea*. On taking the extract she experienced an unusual immediate burning of the mouth and throat. By 8:00 AM she developed tightness in the chest, generalised urticaria, and diarrhoea within a few minutes of eating a mouthful or two of rice cereal and soy milk. The patient was taken to hospital by ambulance after self-administering 75 mg of promethazine by mouth. She was observed in the emergency department for 2 hours, and her symptoms completely resolved without the need for further treatment.

Her intercurrent problems included mild wheezing precipitated by infection, allergic rhinitis, and "oral allergy syndrome". The latter manifested as oral pruritus caused by various raw fruit and vegetables. She was also allergic to banana with accidental exposure resulting in urticaria and/or angioedema. Physical findings were unremarkable. She had taken echinacea intermittently for an extended period (the case report was published in 1998 and notes her use had been from the early 1990s) without any reaction. Within weeks before this incident she had taken a dose from the same bottle.

Skin prick testing using commercially available glycerinated allergen extracts (10% wt/vol) showed a positive response to house dust mite (*Dermatophagoides pteronyssinus*, 10 mm), cat epithelium (5 mm), perennial rye grass (*Lolium perenne*, 10 mm), canary grass (*Phalaris canariensis*, 8 mm), birch tree pollen (*Betula* sp., 10 mm), and *Alternaria tenius* mould (3 mm). Histamine (10 mg/mL) was used as a positive control (10 mm), and 50% glycerine/saline was used as a negative control (0 mm). Testing with the aqueous echinacea mixture she ingested on the day of the incident gave a 3-mm flare alone. Testing with a glycerinated extract from the same manufacturer, which she had also previously taken, resulted in a 3-mm wheal and 5-mm surrounding flare. Similar results were obtained from using the same extracts in serial dilutions. RAST testing of the patient's serum confirmed the presence of echinacea-binding IgE. Negative reactions were observed to commercial extracts of rice and soy protein, the fruit juice in which the echinacea was diluted, and to crude extracts of the other supplements she was taking. Skin prick testing of 84 consecutive patients with asthma or allergic rhinitis demonstrated a positive response to the same extracts in 16 subjects (19%). Only two had previously consumed echinacea. Almost all of these patients had strong reactivity to grass pollens (94%). There also was positive response to house dust mite (56%), *Alternaria* mould (40%), cat epithelium (19%), and birch pollen (3%).

The report also provided data on responses to echinacea-binding IgE undertaken by RAST testing on randomly selected sera from atopic patients. Eleven of 15 cases were positive (8 weak, 2 moderate, and 1 strong). The author suggested that the presence of positive RAST and skin tests to echinacea in asymptomatic atopic individuals raises the possibility of cross-reactivity to structurally related proteins common to echinacea, areoallergens of a diverse nature, and perhaps even foods. He argued that if such cross-reactivity does occur, patients with atopy may be at particular risk of developing life-threatening reactions to complementary medicines with even their first exposure.

A response to this report[48] noted that the immediate pharyngeal irritation reported was most likely caused by the isobutyl amide constituent echinacein, which causes marked pharyngeal tingling and increased salivation.[49] Because there is a plausible alternative explanation for this symptom, the case for a causal association in this instance is weaker, raising the possibility that the reaction was caused by a food item consumed or one of the many dietary supplements taken. The gold standard for demonstrating a causal relationship in immune-mediated reactions is to rechallenge the individual with the suspected causative agent. This is obviously problematic and unethical in cases of anaphylaxis. In many such cases other, less reliable, tests are used to estimate the likelihood of a causal relationship. In such cases drug reaction-monitoring groups would rate the causality as probable, rather than certain, and would await additional cases to determine the extent of the problem.

This case report caused widespread community concern in Australia and resulted in many individuals ceasing to take echinacea preparations. This was evident by the significant decrease in the echinacea market following the media reports of this reaction. The primary reason for this response was the conjecture based on the RAST and skin prick testing that 20% were at risk of anaphylactic reactions due to the purported potential cross-reactivity. This might have provided protection to some individuals and thus could be considered a benefit. Conversely, one could consider that the reduction in echinacea use resulted in an increased frequency or severity of the conditions for which echinacea might provide some protection because of its immunomodulatory properties.[50] This could be considered a risk. Although it is not currently possible to carry out a risk-benefit analysis of this nature, this concept generally does not enter into discussions regarding the risks of herbal medicine. In this instance the plausibility of such a large number of individuals being at risk of anaphylactic reactions was challenged, especially because this was the first case report in the literature.[48] It was estimated that in 1998, 200 million tablets and liquid doses containing echinacea would be purchased by Australian consumers. This degree of usage should have given rise to at least 2000 cases of anaphylaxis in Australia during the past decade. This figure is based on the conservative estimate of a 1% reaction in the 20% of individuals with the potential cross-reactivity reported by Mullins in 1 million Australian consumers during the past decade. Again, conservatively, this should represent 20,000 international cases during the same period. Although it has been argued that ADRs to complementary medicine are underreported,[51] it is highly unlikely that thousands or even hundreds of anaphylactic reactions would have gone unnoticed. As such the conjecture, although theoretically plausible, is not supported by evidence.

An additional case of echinacea-associated anaphylaxis in a 31-year-old woman was reported in a case series of five patients with reactions to echinacea, which included the case outlined previously.[28] Within 20 minutes of taking an echinacea-containing preparation this woman developed generalised urticaria, facial and upper respiratory angioedema, difficulty swallowing, bronchospasm, dizziness, and disorientation. Symptoms resolved gradually in several hours. Before this incident she had taken echinacea tablets on 3 of the preceding 4 days. She had experienced headache and mild facial angioedema within 20 minutes of each administration and had no symptoms on the echinacea-free day. The patient had a known history of allergic reactions and perennial allergic rhinitis with seasonal aggravation. She had known allergy to latex and an urticarial reaction to sulphur-containing dried fruits. On one occasion she had experienced an episode of exercise-induced anaphylaxis; however, it was considered that rye, mushroom, or nonsteroidal antiinflammatory drugs might have been responsible. No further episodes occurred after avoidance of these substances. The patient was a health professional, and she could not identify any of her known allergy

triggers on the days in question, and she considered the consumption of echinacea the probable cause of the reaction. Skin prick testing 1 year later with the aqueous alcohol (40%) preparation of echinacea from the first case presented previously was negative. In this case, causality would be rated as probable; however, it cannot be considered to be certain.

Between July 1996 and November 1998 the Australian Adverse Drug Reactions Advisory Committee (ADRAC) received 21 reports of allergic-like effects associated with exposure to echinacea.[36] These cases, which may include the two cases detailed previously and the three cases described elsewhere in this chapter, involved individuals aged 3 to 58 years, with symptoms of bronchospasm (9), dyspnoea (8), urticaria (5), chest pain (4), and angioedema (3). Twelve patients of the 18 for whom a medical history was available had a history of asthma (7) or allergic rhinitis/conjunctivitis/hayfever (5). Unfortunately the brief report did not rate the cases in terms of the likelihood of a causal link between symptoms and echinacea exposure, but it was stated that echinacea was the "only suspected cause" in 19 of the 21 cases.

Given the available evidence, there appears to be little doubt that echinacea preparations can cause allergic reactions in susceptible individuals. In this respect the echinacea species are no different from any other plant species. The critical issue, from a public health and safety perspective, is how prevalent such allergic reactions are. Echinacea preparations are among the most commonly used herbal medicines in many industrialised countries. In Germany, general practitioners wrote >2.5 million prescriptions for echinacea-based medications in 1993,[50] and Australian consumers purchased an estimated 200 million doses of echinacea in 1998.[48] On the background of this intensive and widespread therapeutic use of echinacea for more than two decades, there is no evidence to suggest that allergic reactions to echinacea are more than rare and isolated events in susceptible individuals. Were the echinacea species highly allergenic plants, as has been suggested,[47] then surely far more cases of allergic reactions would have been reported.

Nevertheless a cautious approach is still prudent in the case of individuals with a known allergy to other members of the daisy family (Asteraceae).

Linseed *(Linum usitatissimum)* (Family Linaceae)

A case of anaphylaxis in a 40-year-old woman after ingestion of linseed oil has been reported from Spain.[52] She had no history of allergy or atopy but developed itchy and weeping eyes, palmar pruritus, generalised urticaria, nausea, and vomiting approximately 10 minutes after taking a spoonful of linseed oil. She was treated at an emergency department and recovered promptly. A subsequent skin prick test was positive to linseed, and the presence of IgE antibody was demonstrated. A 22-kD protein was identified as the likely causative allergen. The authors note that IgE-mediated occupational asthma has been described in workers involved in the processing of linseed oil.

Psyllium *(Plantago ovata)* (Family Plantaginaceae)

At least four cases of anaphylaxis after the ingestion of psyllium-based laxatives have been reported in the literature. In Finland, a 33-year-old female nurse experienced an anaphylactic reaction after taking a granulated psyllium laxative.[53] She developed a generalised urticarial rash within 1 hour of taking the preparation and sought treatment at a hospital. During the next hour her condition deteriorated markedly, as she developed profuse diarrhoea, hypotension, and slight dyspnoea before losing consciousness. She was treated with intravenous corticosteroids and plasma expanders and made a full recovery. The presence of serum IgE antibodies to psyllium and the laxative preparation was demonstrated by RAST.

Two similar cases, both involving nurses with a history of allergy, have been reported from Canada.[54] In the first case, a 39-year-old woman with a history of allergic symptoms resulting from occupational exposure to psyllium took a dose of prescribed psyllium for constipation. She quickly developed generalised urticaria, angioedema, laryngeal

oedema, flushing, tachycardia, and light-headedness and was hospitalised. She subsequently produced a strong positive response to psyllium in a skin prick test and also returned a positive result for IgE antibodies to psyllium in a RAST.

The second Canadian case concerned a 42-year-old female nurse with a history of allergic rhinitis and asthma, including allergic symptoms when dispensing pulverised psyllium to patients. She ingested a single dose of crystallised psyllium and within 1 hour developed generalised pruritus, urticaria, severe flushing, tachycardia, angioedema, vomiting, and light-headedness. She was successfully treated at an emergency department. Subsequent rechallenge at a hospital with the same psyllium product caused immediate anaphylaxis with dyspnoea and loss of consciousness. Subcutaneous adrenaline did not immediately resolve the situation, but she recovered after receiving intravenous corticosteroids for several hours.

A fourth case concerned a 40-year-old woman who had taken psyllium for several years before developing an urticarial rash involving the entire body except the face, swollen lips, and chest tightness.[55] After discontinuing the psyllium treatment for 1 week, the patient challenged herself with a dose of the psyllium preparation and within 15 minutes developed breathing difficulties and flaring of the rash. She recovered after adrenaline treatment. She had elevated total serum IgE and tested positive for psyllium-specific IgE in a modified RAST.

Anaphylaxis has also been reported in individuals who consumed a psyllium-containing cereal.[56,57] In addition, occupational asthma resulting from psyllium has been described, and occupational exposure to psyllium may be associated with high rates of sensitisation.[58,59]

Thyme *(Thymus vulgaris)* and Oregano *(Origanum vulgare)* (Family Lamiaceae)

A case of a 45-year-old man who experienced three anaphylactic reactions immediately after the consumption of foods flavoured with thyme (two occasions) and oregano (one occasion) has been reported from Spain.[60] He had a 25-year history of IgE-mediated rhinitis and asthma caused by grass pollen. Each anaphylactic episode was characterised by pruritus, swelling of the lips and tongue, dysphagia, dysphonia, progressive breathing difficulties, and facial oedema. On two occasions he also developed severe hypotension, nausea, and vomiting. Each time he was treated at an emergency department with adrenaline, corticosteroids, antihistamines, and fluid therapy. Subsequent ingestion of the offending foods, without the thyme or oregano flavourings, did not produce any symptoms. Skin prick tests showed positive reactions to thyme and oregano but also to six other Lamiaceae species tested, suggesting cross-sensitivity between different species in this family. The species tested were, apart from thyme and oregano, basil *(Ocimum basilicum)*, lavender *(Lavandula officinalis)*, hyssop *(Hyssopus officinalis)*, marjoram *(Origanum majorana)*, peppermint *(Mentha × piperita)*, and sage *(Salvia officinalis)*.

HERB CONSTITUENTS WITH HIGH ALLERGENICITY: SESQUITERPENE LACTONES

Although the classification used for this review has been based on clinical presentation rather than phytochemical constituents, there is one class of constituents that deserves a special mention because of its recognised allergenicity. These are the sesquiterpene lactones.

Sesquiterpene lactones are 15-carbon terpenoid compounds containing a lactone ring. They occur sporadically in a few plant families and lichens but are common in the daisy family Asteraceae (syn. Compositae). Sesquiterpene lactones are a well-documented cause of allergic contact dermatitis.[61,62] The presence of an exocyclic α-methylene group (i.e., a $C=CH_2$ group) appears to be important for the allergenicity of sesquiterpene lactones, although other factors must also be required because not all sesquiterpene lactones possessing an α-methylene group are allergenic.[10,62] Cross-reactivity occurs between different sesquiterpene lactones.[62]

Sesquiterpene lactones can induce the delayed type of hypersensitivity only when in direct contact with the skin, and when taken orally these compounds rarely produce aller-gic responses, although exacerbation of preexisting contact dermatitis and stomatitis and throat swelling have been reported in people with contact allergy to Asteraceae plants.[10] Therefore the oral administration of sesquiterpene lactone-containing medicinal plant preparations does not represent any particular risk in terms of allergic reactions except in individuals who are already sensitised, in which case caution is advisable. The use of topical preparations of plants such as arnica *(Arnica* spp.) and German chamomile *(Matricaria recutita)* is clearly contraindicated in such individuals.

The Asteraceae, or daisy, family is one of the largest of flowering plant families, comprising some 23,000 species or approximately 9% of all known plant species.[63] The family is divided into 2 subfamilies and 12 tribes. Most reported cases of contact dermatitis from daisy family members have involved species from only three tribes: Heliantheae, Astereae, and Anthemideae.[62] A number of medicinal plants used in Western herbal medicine have been implicated in sesquiterpene lactone-induced contact dermatitis (Box 10-1); most of these belong to the tribe Anthemideae. Species that are particularly well known for their potential to cause contact dermatitis include arnica *(Arnica* spp.), feverfew *(Tanacetum parthenium)*, and elecampane *(Inula helenium)*.[10]

CONCLUSIONS AND RECOMMENDATIONS

In this chapter, we have reviewed allergic reactions to herbs ranging from skin conditions to anaphylactic reactions. In most cases these reactions are unpredictable, and the clinician needs to be alert to the fact that any herbal medicine may give rise to these types of reactions. When prescribing herbal medicines to individuals with a history of plant allergy, the clinician should consider the potential for cross-reactivity between species belonging to the same plant family. Depending on the type of the previous reaction, the use of medicinal plants from the same family might be a relative or absolute contraindication, and caution should be exercised when prescribing herbal medicine for these patients. The prescribing of

---

Box **10-1** ❧❧ SESQUITERPENE LACTONE-CONTAINING MEDICINAL PLANTS OF THE FAMILY
ASTERACEAE

Achillea millefolium (yarrow)
Arnica spp. (arnica)
Artemisia vulgaris (mugwort)
Cichorium intybus (chicory)
Cnicus benedictus (blessed thistle)
Cynara scolymus (globe artichoke)
Inula helenium (elecampane)
Lactuca sativa (wild lettuce)
Matricaria recutita (German chamomile)
Tanacetum parthenium (feverfew)
Tanacetum vulgare (tansy)
Taraxacum officinale (dandelion)

From Warshaw EM, Zug KA: Sesquiterpene lactone allergy, *Am J Contact Dermat* 7:1-23, 1996; and
Hausen BM: Sesquiterpene lactones—general discussion, In De Smet PAGM, Keller K, Hänsel R, Chandler RF, editors:
Adverse effects of herbal drugs, vol 1, Berlin, 1991, Springer.

a medicinal plant from the same family as one that has caused a previous allergic reaction should be avoided when a safer alternative exists.

In every clinical encounter in which herbal medicines are prescribed, the potential for an allergic reaction exists. Although these reactions are generally rare, most herbal practitioners will encounter a number of allergic reactions in a practice lifetime. An awareness of the symptoms associated with the different types of allergic reactions coupled with an alertness to their presentation will enable these reactions to be identified quickly and treated appropriately. The clinical acumen of the herbal prescriber is an essential component to ensure the safe delivery of this traditional medicine.

REFERENCES

1. Gruchalla RS: Drug allergy, *J Allergy Clin Immunol* 111:S548-S559, 2003.
2. Mantle D, Gok MA, Lennard TW: Adverse and beneficial effects of plant extracts on skin and skin disorders, *Adverse Drug React Toxicol Rev* 20:89-103, 2001.
3. Hjorther AB, Christophersen C, Hausen BM, Menne T: Occupational allergic contact dermatitis from carnosol, a naturally-occurring compound present in rosemary, *Contact Dermatitis* 37:99-100, 1997.
4. Estrada JL, Gozalo F, Cecchini C, Casquete E: Contact urticaria from hops (Humulus lupulus) in a patient with previous urticaria-angioedema from peanut, chestnut and banana, *Contact Dermatitis* 46:127, 2002.
5. Vandenplas O, Depelchin S, Toussaint G, Delwiche JP, Weyer RV, Saintremy JM: Occupational asthma caused by sarsaparilla root dust, *J Allergy Clin Immunol* 97:1416-1418, 1996.
6. Lee SK, Cho HK, Cho SH, Kim SS, Nahm DH, Park HS: Occupational asthma and rhinitis caused by multiple herbal agents in a pharmacist, *Ann Allergy Asthma Immunol* 86:469-474, 2001.
7. Cartier A, Malo JL, Labrecque M: Occupational asthma due to liquorice roots, *Allergy* 57:863, 2002.
8. Coombs R, Gell PG: Classification of allergic reactions responsible for clinical hypersensitivity and disease. In Gell P, Coombs RR, Lachman PJ, editors: *Clinical aspects of immunology,* Oxford, 1975, Blackwell Scientific Publications.
9. Kiken DA, Cohen DE: Contact dermatitis to botanical extracts, *Am J Contact Dermat* 13:148-152, 2002.
10. Hausen BM: Sesquiterpene lactones—general discussion. In De Smet PAGM, Keller K, Hänsel R, Chandler RF, editors: *Adverse effects of herbal drugs, vol 1,* Berlin, 1991, Springer.
11. Rodriguez-Serna M, Sanchez-Motilla JM, Ramon R, Aliaga A: Allergic and systemic contact dermatitis from *Matricaria chamomilla* tea, *Contact Dermatitis* 39:192-193, 1998.
12. McGeorge BC, Steele MC: Allergic contact dermatitis of the nipple from Roman chamomile ointment, *Contact Dermatitis* 24:139-140, 1991.
13. Pazzaglia M, Venturo N, Borda G, Tosti A: Contact dermatitis due to a massage liniment containing Inula helenium extract, *Contact Dermatitis* 33:267, 1995.

14. Burden AD, Wilkinson SM, Beck MH, Chalmers RG: Garlic-induced systemic contact dermatitis, *Contact Dermatitis* 30:299-300, 1994.

15. Danese P, Carnevali C, Bertazzoni MG: Allergic contact dermatitis due to *Centella asiatica* extract, *Contact Dermatitis* 31:201, 1994.

16. Hausen BM: *Centella asiatica* (Indian pennywort), an effective therapeutic but a weak sensitizer, *Contact Dermatitis* 29:175-179, 1993.

17. Coulson IH, Khan AS: Facial "pillow" dermatitis due to lavender oil allergy, *Contact Dermatitis* 41:111, 1999.

18. Nishioka K, Seguchi T: Contact allergy due to oil-soluble licorice extracts in cosmetic products, *Contact Dermatitis* 40:56, 1999.

19. Lee TY, Lam TH: Myrrh is the putative allergen in bonesetter's herbs dermatitis, *Contact Dermatitis* 29:279, 1993.

20. Lee TY, Lam TH: Allergic contact dermatitis due to a Chinese orthopaedic solution tieh ta yao gin, *Contact Dermatitis* 28:89-90, 1993.

21. Al-Suwaidan SN, Gad el Rab MO, Al-Fakhiry S, Al Hoqail I, Al-Maziad A, Sherif AB: Allergic contact dermatitis from myrrh, a topical herbal medicine used to promote healing, *Contact Dermatitis* 39:137, 1998.

22. Bonamonte D, Mundo L, Daddabbo M, Foti C: Allergic contact dermatitis from Mentha spicata (spearmint), *Contact Dermatitis* 45:298, 2001.

23. Worm M, Jeep S, Sterry W, Zuberbier T: Perioral contact dermatitis caused by L-carvone in toothpaste, *Contact Dermatitis* 38:338, 1998.

24. Del Pozo MD, Gastaminza G, Navarro JA, et al: Allergic contact dermatitis from Verbena officinalis L, *Contact Dermatitis* 31:200-201, 1994.

25. McCance K, Huether SE: *Pathophysiology,* ed 4, St. Louis, 2002, Mosby.

26. Raccagni AA, Bardazzi F, Baldari U, Righini MG: Erythema-multiforme-like contact dermatitis due to capsicum, *Contact Dermatitis* 33:353-354, 1995.

27. Khanna M, Qasem K, Sasseville D: Allergic contact dermatitis to tea tree oil with erythema multiforme-like Id reaction, *Am J Contact Dermat* 11:238-242, 2000.

28. Mullins RJ, Heddle R: Adverse reactions associated with echinacea: the Australian experience, *Ann Allergy Asthma Immunol* 88:42-51, 2000.

29. Schätzle M, Agathos M, Breit R: Allergic contact dermatitis from goldenrod (Herba solidaginis) after systemic administration, *Contact Dermatitis* 39:271-272, 1998.

30. Zeller W, de Gols M, Hausen BM: The sensitizing capacity of Compositae plants. VI. Guinea pig sensitization experiments with ornamental plants and weeds using different methods, *Arch Dermatol Res* 277:28-35, 1985.

31. Schmidt P, Boehncke WH: Delayed-type hypersensitivity reaction to kava-kava extract, *Contact Dermatitis* 42:363-364, 2000.

32. Iliev D, Elsner P: Generalized drug reaction due to papaya juice in throat lozenges, *Dermatology* 194:364-366, 1997.

33. Kay AB: Allergy and allergic diseases. Second of two parts, *N Engl J Med* 344:109-113, 2001.

34. Asero R, Mistrello G, Roncarolo D, Antoniotti PL, Falagiani P: A case of garlic allergy, *J Allergy Clin Immunol* 101:427-428, 1998.

35. Rafaat M, Leung AK: Garlic burns, *Pediatr Dermatol* 17:475-476, 2000.

36. Allergic reactions with echinacea, *Aust Adverse Drug React Bull* 18:3, 1999.

37. Wilkinson SM, Hausen BM, Beck MH: Allergic contact dermatitis from plant extracts in a cosmetic, *Contact Dermatitis* 33:58-59, 1995.

38. Subiza J, Subiza JL, Alonso M, et al: Allergic conjunctivitis to chamomile tea, *Ann Allergy* 65:127-132, 1990.

39. Granlund H: Contact allergy to witch hazel, *Contact Dermatitis* 31:195, 1994.

40. Morton CA, Garioch J, Todd P, Lamey PJ, Forsyth A: Contact sensitivity to menthol and peppermint in patients with intra-oral symptoms, *Contact Dermatitis* 32:281-284, 1995.

41. Benner MH, Lee HJ: Anaphylactic reaction to chamomile tea, *J Allergy Clin Immunol* 52:307-308, 1973.

42. Subiza J, Subiza JL, Hinojosa M, et al: Anaphylactic reaction after the ingestion of chamomile tea: a study of cross-reactivity with other composite pollens, *J Allergy Clin Immunol* 84:353-358, 1989.

43. Jensen-Jarolim E, Reider N, Fritsch R, Breiteneder H: Fatal outcome of anaphylaxis to chamomile-containing enema during labor: a case study, *J Allergy Clin Immunol* 102:1041-1042, 1998.

44. Thien FC: Chamomile tea enema anaphylaxis, *Med J Aust* 175:54, 2001.

45. Reider N, Sepp N, Fritsch P, Weinlich G, Jensen-Jarolim E: Anaphylaxis to camomile: clinical features and allergen cross-reactivity, *Clin Exp Allergy* 30:1436-1443, 2000.

46. Perez-Pimiento AJ, Moneo I, Santaolalla M, de Paz S, Fernandez-Parra B, Dominguez-Lazaro AR: Anaphylactic reaction to young garlic, *Allergy* 54:626-629, 1999.

47. Mullins RJ: Echinacea-associated anaphylaxis, *Med J Aust* 168:170-171, 1998.

48. Myers SP, Wohlmuth H: Echinacea-associated anaphylaxis, *Med J Aust* 168:583-584, 1998.

49. Bauer R, Wagner H: Echinacea species as potential immunostimulatory drugs. In Wagner H, Farnsworth NR, editors: *Economic and medicinal plant research, vol 5,* London, 1991, Academic Press.

50. Melchart D, Linde K, Worku F, Bauer R, Wagner H: Immunomodulation with Echinacea—a systematic review of controlled clinical trials, *Phytomedicine* 1:245-254, 1994.

51. Drew AK, Myers SP: Safety issues in herbal medicine: implications for the health professions, *Med J Aust* 166:538-541, 1997.

52. Alonso L, Marcos ML, Blanco JG, et al: Anaphylaxis caused by linseed (flaxseed) intake, *J Allergy Clin Immunol* 98:469-470, 1996.

53. Suhonen R, Kantola I, Bjorksten F: Anaphylactic shock due to ingestion of psyllium laxative, *Allergy* 38:363-365, 1983.

54. Sussman GL, Dorian W: Psyllium anaphylaxis, *Allergy Proc* 11:241-242, 1990.

55. Freeman GL: Psyllium hypersensitivity, *Ann Allergy* 73:490-492, 1994.

56. Drake CL, Moses ES, Tandberg D: Systemic anaphylaxis after ingestion of a psyllium-containing breakfast cereal, *Am J Emerg Med* 9:449-451, 1991.

57. Lantner RR, Espiritu BR, Zumerchik P, Tobin MC: Anaphylaxis following ingestion of a psyllium-containing cereal, *JAMA* 264:2534-2536, 1990.

58. Kirby J, Bardy JD, Malo JL, et al: Prevalence of IgE sensitization to psyllium in two pharmaceutical companies, *J Allergy Clin Immunol* 77:134, 1986 (abstract).

59. Coransson K, Michaelson NG: Ispaghula powder: an allergen in the work environment, *South J Work Environ Health* 5:257-261, 1979.

60. Benito M, Jorro G, Morales C, Pelaez A, Fernandez A: Labiatae allergy: systemic reactions due to ingestion of oregano and thyme, *Ann Allergy Asthma Immunol* 76:416-418, 1996.

61. Gordon LA: Compositae dermatitis, *Australas J Dermatol* 40:123-128, 1999.

62. Warshaw EM, Zug KA: Sesquiterpene lactone allergy, *Am J Contact Dermat* 7:1-23, 1996.

63. Mabberley DJ: *The plant-book: a portable dictionary of the vascular plants,* Cambridge, 1997, Cambridge University Press.

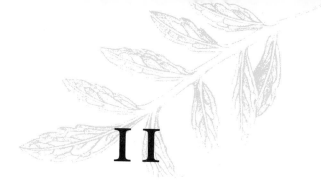

PHARMACOVIGILANCE OF HERBAL MEDICINES

Joanne Barnes

This chapter discusses issues in pharmacovigilance of herbal medicines and reviews the methods available to monitor the safety of herbal medicinal products (HMPs). Many of the examples used in this chapter are from the United Kingdom and Europe. The classification of herbal products as medicines in Europe may have advantages in developing more rigorous adverse drug reaction (ADR) monitoring for herbal medicines. However, the information gleaned in this medical context may usefully be applied to countries such as the United States, where herbs are classified as dietary supplements. The word "drug" appears throughout this chapter (e.g., in the phrase adverse drug reactions) but is used in its broadest sense (i.e., to include herbal medicines; also referred to here by their European term herbal medicinal products or HMPs).

WHAT IS PHARMACOVIGILANCE OF HERBAL MEDICINES?

Pharmacovigilance has been defined as "the study of the safety of marketed drugs under the practical conditions of clinical usage in large communities".[1] It is also referred to as "postmarketing surveillance" in recognition of the fact that not all safety concerns relating to a particular drug will be known when it is first marketed; therefore, continued monitoring is necessary. Its aims and activities include monitoring drug safety, identifying ADRs in humans, assessing benefits and risks, and responding to and communicating information on drug safety concerns. These apply equally to herbal medicines, and there is no need nor is it desirable to separate pharmacovigilance of "conventional" medicines and that of herbal medicines.[2] However, the current model of pharmacovigilance and its science and processes have developed in relation to conventional medicines, and applying the existing model and its tools to monitor the safety of herbal medicines presents additional challenges.

For those unfamiliar with the discipline of pharmacovigilance, explanations of selected key terms are given in Box 11-1. Formal definitions have been developed by several organisations concerned with pharmacovigilance, but there is not necessarily universal agreement on terminology.[3] In some cases, definitions adopted by different organisations and expert groups vary on fundamental criteria, such as causality.

Box 11-1 EXPLANATIONS OF SELECTED TERMS USED IN PHARMACOVIGILANCE[*]

Adverse drug reaction (ADR)

A harmful and unintended response to a drug when used at typical clinical doses. It includes drug interactions, but there is a lack of consensus whether it should include effects of drug misuse, such as overdose. There is at least an implication of a causal relationship with use of the drug. An *unexpected ADR* is one that is atypical for the drug based on its intended uses or known characteristics. A *serious ADR* includes one that is fatal, life threatening, disabling, incapacitating, results in or prolongs hospitalisation, a congenital abnormality, or is otherwise medically significant. A *suspected ADR* is one that *may* have a causal relationship with the drug. ADR is sometimes used synonymously with *adverse effect*.

Adverse event

Any harmful or unintended medical, clinical, or health outcome occurring during or after drug treatment, which is not necessarily related to use of the drug (e.g., broken leg during use of *Hypericum perforatum*).

Side effect

An unintended response to a drug when used at typical clinical doses and related to the pharmacologic effects of the drug. A side effect can be "positive" (i.e., beneficial) or "negative" (harmful).

Signal

Information relating to a possible new ADR but which requires further investigation and validation. A signal may relate to new information on an already-known association between a drug and an adverse effect. Signals can originate from a variety of sources, including spontaneous reports (yellow cards), formal studies (including clinical trials), scientific literature, unpublished data (e.g., from manufacturers), and patient reports. Increasingly, automated signal generation systems are being used to complement human evaluation.

Pharmacoepidemiology

The study of the effects (adverse or beneficial) of drugs in large numbers of people.

---

[*]These explanations are provided to assist readers with little or no knowledge of pharmacovigilance and should not be taken as definitions. Formal definitions of these and other pharmacovigilance terms have been developed and adopted by national centres participating in the World Health Organization (WHO) International Drug Monitoring Programme.[3,4]

Historical Background

Wide recognition of the need to assess and monitor the safety of medicines followed the thalidomide disaster of the 1950s and 1960s when up to 10,000 living children worldwide were born with phocomelia (congenital limb deformities) as a result of in utero exposure to the hypnotic and antiemetic drug thalidomide.[5] At the time, there was little formal drug regulation around the world. For the first 20 or so years afterward, changes and new initiatives in drug safety monitoring were introduced mainly as a result of further high-profile drug disasters.[6] By contrast, improvements during the past 20 years mainly have been proactive, often associated with advances in information technology. The science and processes of pharmacovigilance have developed in relation to conventional medicines, but there is an increasing awareness of the need to develop pharmacovigilance practices for herbal medicines; the World Health Organization (WHO) has produced draft guidelines on this.[7] At present, though, pharmacovigilance of herbal medicines is in the early stages of its development.

Legal Framework in Europe

The European Union (EU) Directive 2001/83/EC provides the legal framework for pharmacovigilance for licensed medicines.[8] This legislation requires pharmaceutical companies to demonstrate to the relevant competent authority for licensing medicines the quality, safety, and efficacy of their products before marketing. After assessment, the licensing authority may, or may not, grant a marketing authorisation (MA; product licence). Licensed products (including licensed HMPs) should comply with regulatory provisions on pharmacovigilance. In summary, these include requirements for MA holders (for their licensed products) to:

- Have constant access to an appropriately qualified person responsible for pharmacovigilance;
- Maintain detailed records of all suspected ADRs occurring worldwide;
- Record and report all suspected serious ADRs notified to them by a health care professional in the EU to the licensing authority within 15 calendar days (this is a two-way process, and the licensing authority is required to notify the MA holder within 15 calendar days of any such reports that it receives); and
- Include all other ADRs as part of periodic safety update reports submitted to the licensing authority.

In addition, there are practical initiatives aimed at achieving uniform global safety information to facilitate communication, reporting, and signal generation, with which MA holders were to have complied by January 2003. The most important of these are listed below.

- Implementing the use of Medical Dictionary for Regulatory Activities (MedDRA), a new international standard medical terminology, into pharmacovigilance activities.[9] At present, MA holders and regulatory authorities do not necessarily use the same medical coding dictionary for ADRs.
- Connection to and compliance with EudraVigilance, the new European pharmacovigilance system at the European Medicines Evaluation Agency. EudraVigilance is an electronic data-processing network to facilitate the exchange, processing, and evaluation of pharmacovigilance information

related to medicinal products authorised in the EU.[10]

At present, in the United Kingdom at least, most herbal medicines are marketed as herbal medicines exempt from licensing or as unlicensed food supplements[11]; therefore, their manufacturers are not required to demonstrate to the competent authority the quality, safety, and efficacy of these products before marketing nor for these products to comply with regulatory provisions on pharmacovigilance.

The situation is set to change if the new EU directive on traditional HMPs is implemented as planned by 2005.[12] The directive requires EU member states each to set up a new registration scheme for traditional HMPs. The schemes will require manufacturers to provide bibliographic data on the safety of their products and evidence that the herb has been used traditionally in the EU for at least 15 years and to manufacture products according to the principles of good manufacturing practice. MA holders for products registered under the directive will be required to comply with relevant existing pharmaceutical legislation, including the provisions on pharmacovigilance, summarised previously.

At present, the lack of regulation for many HMPs has important implications for pharmacovigilance.[2] For example, the range of possible regulatory actions that the licensing authority can take in response to a herbal safety concern is limited for unlicensed HMPs and, for some possible regulatory responses, requires the voluntary cooperation of herbal medicine manufacturers.

METHODS FOR PHARMACOVIGILANCE OF HERBAL MEDICINES

Pharmacovigilance for conventional medicines draws on several different methods for monitoring safety. Some methods are used to identify suspected ADRs and are described as "hypothesis generating", and others are used to confirm or refute the suspicion and are "hypothesis testing".[5] Whereas these methods are well established for investigating safety concerns with conventional medicines, they have important limitations with regard to their application to herbal medicines, and it is likely that modified, even novel, approaches are needed. This section focuses on spontaneous reporting of ADRs as the method that currently plays the most significant role in pharmacovigilance of herbal medicines.

Spontaneous Reporting Schemes for ADRs

At present the main method used to generate signals of possible safety concerns associated with herbal medicines is spontaneous reporting schemes. Such schemes appear to function reasonably effectively in countries such as Germany where HMPs are registered as medicines.[13] However, in countries where herbal medicines are (mainly) marketed as unlicensed products and mostly used for self-treatment without supervision from a health care professional, spontaneous reporting schemes are likely to be less effective.

Countries in Europe have established reporting schemes for suspected ADRs associated with all medicinal products, including HMPs. In the United Kingdom, for example, the competent authority for licensing medicines, the Medicines and Healthcare products Regulatory Agency (MHRA; formerly known as the MCA), runs, in conjunction with the U.K. Committee on Safety of Medicines (CSM), the "yellow card" scheme for suspected ADR reporting. The scheme, established in 1964, has always applied to licensed medicines, including licensed herbal medicines, although it was not well publicised with regard to herbal medicines until October 1996, when it was extended to include reporting by recognised reporters (at the time, doctors, dentists, and coroners only) for unlicensed herbal medicines.[14] This move came after a 5-year study of traditional remedies and food supplements, carried out by a U.K. medical toxicology unit, identified ADRs associated with these types of products.[15] Today, after further extensions, all pharmacists,[16] nurses, midwives, and health visitors are also recognised as reporters,[17] and a pilot scheme for patient reporting is underway.[18] Reporter groups are encouraged to report *suspected* ADRs associated with any therapeutic agent on yellow cards, which are available in standard reference texts such as the British National Formulary. In the United Kingdom, community pharmacists are asked by the MHRA to concentrate on areas of limited reporting by doctors, such as licensed and unlicensed HMPs.[16]

In some European countries, reporting of suspected ADRs is mandatory for health care professionals. Reporting is mandatory for MA holders for their licensed HMPs, but there is no such requirement for manufacturers of unlicensed medicines (see Legal framework in Europe).

Reports from the U.K. CSM/MHRA yellow card scheme and those from over 70 other countries with national spontaneous reporting schemes for ADRs are fed into the WHO's Collaborating Centre for International Drug Monitoring at Uppsala, Sweden (known as the Uppsala Monitoring Centre [UMC]). Some of the UMC's key activities are analysing and screening the data it receives on suspected ADRs, identifying signals, and communicating safety information to stakeholders. The UMC recognises the problems inherent in ADR reporting for herbal medicines and has established a traditional medicines project to stimulate reporting in this area and to standardise information on herbal medicines, particularly with regard to nomenclature.[19] For example, a special set of herbal anatomical-therapeutic-chemical (ATC) codes has been developed that is fully compatible with the regular ATC classification system for conventional medicines. The UMC database, established in 1968, now holds more than 3 million reports of suspected ADRs, of which approximately 9000 relate to herbal medicines.[19]

Data Collected

The information requested on the U.K. yellow card (i.e., *patient details*, *suspected drug* or *drugs*, *suspected reactions*, other drugs, additional information, and *reporter details*; items in italics are the minimum criteria required for a report) is typical of that collected by reporting schemes across Europe and other developed countries and is the same regardless of the type of "suspected drug" (herbal or conventional). The current design of the yellow card does not lend itself well to collecting information on nonconventional (e.g., herbal) medicines.[2] Some examples of this are given below.

- The brand name, if known, is requested for suspected drug(s), but unlicensed HMPs legally are not permitted to use brand names but rather only the common or botanical name.[11] It would be more appropriate to request the Latin binomial name together with the plant part and the name of the supplier and, for finished HMPs, the name of the manufacturer because the composition of herbal medicines varies between manufacturers as can the pharmaceutical quality of unlicensed HMPs.[20,21] This should be considered when assessing reports of suspected ADRs associated with unlicensed HMPs.

- Other relevant information not specifically requested includes the formulation of the product (e.g., tablets or tincture) and the method of processing the crude herbal material (e.g., type of extract).[13] These factors also are relevant to the precise chemical composition and therefore potential toxicity of a herbal preparation.

- Many formulated HMPs comprise combinations of several herbal ingredients, and herbal-medicine practitioners often prescribe several herbs supplied together as a tincture, one or more of which may be the suspected herb. Some products contain herbal and non-herbal (e.g., vitamins and minerals) ingredients. It is difficult to record and identify suspected ingredients clearly on the current yellow card.

Reporting Rates

In the United Kingdom, despite initiatives to stimulate reporting of suspected ADRs associated with herbal medicines, the number of reports received by the CSM/MHRA remains low.[2] From 1964 through 1995, 832 reports were received, and since 1996, when the scheme was extended to include reporting for unlicensed herbal medicines, through 2002, 467 reports were received.[2,22] Many of these reports relate to suspected interactions between St. John's wort (*Hypericum perforatum*) and certain prescription medicines; in 2000,

there were 140 reports, of which 82 (60%) related to suspected ADRs associated with St. John's wort, and approximately 25% of these described suspected interactions.

It is not clear whether the low number of reports received reflects a low frequency of adverse effects associated with herbal medicines or whether there are other explanations (e.g., substantial underreporting).[2] Typically, a year-on-year increase in the number of reports received could be expected, with further increases following the inclusion of new reporter groups and other initiatives aimed at stimulating reporting.

Some preliminary evidence to suggest that there may be substantial underreporting of suspected ADRs associated with herbal medicines comes from studies involving pharmacists in the United Kingdom. Data from a CSM/MHRA 1-year pilot study (1997 through 1998) of community pharmacist ADR reporting showed that pharmacists, compared with general practitioners, submitted a higher proportion of reports of suspected ADRs associated with HMPs.[23] However, the total number of reports associated with HMPs submitted by both groups was low. Around the same time, a cross-sectional survey of more than 1300 community pharmacists not involved in the CSM/MHRA pilot scheme for pharmacist ADR reporting found that during the previous 12 months 11% had identified or received reports from the public/patients of suspected ADRs associated with "complementary medicines", approximately one-half of which related to herbal medicines. The same study found that almost 50% of pharmacist respondents were not aware that the yellow card scheme applies to herbal medicines.[24] It is recognised that pharmacists could make an important contribution to ADR reporting for HMPs, but it is likely that greater vigilance on the part of the pharmacist and initiatives to encourage herbal ADR reporting by pharmacists are required.

Signal Detection and Assessment

In the United Kingdom, because of the relatively small number of yellow card reports of suspected ADRs associated with HMPs, reports can be considered on a case-by-case basis. Signals are detected simply by numbers of reports, and causality assessment can be carried out using defined criteria (such as those adopted by the WHO[3]).

When large numbers of reports of suspected ADRs are held, automated screening methods are used increasingly for signal detection. For example, the MHRA uses proportional reporting ratios (PRRs; Box 11-2). This statistical approach involves calculating the proportion of the suspected reaction of interest occurring with the drug of interest against the background of all other reported suspected ADRs in the database.[25] It may be possible to obtain PRRs for some suspected ADRs associated with herbal medicines, such as St. John's wort, for which there are a reasonable number of ADR reports in the database.[2]

Once a signal has been confirmed, the next steps are to quantify the risk (determine its frequency), consider its implications for public health (i.e., severity and seriousness of the ADR, and benefit-risk analysis), and to discern whether there are opportunities to prevent the ADR (e.g., identification of at-risk groups). For prescription medicines, formal studies may also be carried out using the hypothesis-testing methods described here (see Other pharmacoepidemiologic studies), although as will be discussed, these methods have little, if any, application at present for herbal medicines.

At an appropriate moment, a judgement must be made about appropriate regulatory action, if any, to be taken. This could range from relatively simple amendments, such as dose reduction or information on coprescription of drugs and monitoring, to extreme action, such as immediate withdrawal of the product from the market.

Advantages and Limitations

Spontaneous reporting schemes have recognised advantages; for example, they monitor all medicines, all the time, and for all consumers and patients. However, they also have well-known limitations, and several of these may be even more important with regard to herbal medicines. In particular, underreporting is likely to be greater for herbal medicines than for conventional medicines for several reasons—because of the belief that herbal medicines are natural and therefore "safe", users may not associate ADRs with their use of such products,[13] and users of herbal medicines may be reluctant to report ADRs associated with these products to their doctor or pharmacist.[26] Even if suspected ADRs associated with herbal medicines are reported to health care professionals, there may be a lack of awareness among health care professionals that the yellow card scheme accepts reports for licensed and unlicensed HMPs.[24]

Another important limitation is that because herbal medicines are widely available from a range of outlets without the need for interaction with a health care professional, suspected ADRs associated with HMPs may be identified by or reported to an individual (e.g., herbalist) who is outside the formal system for ADR reporting.[2] Health food stores are a major outlet for HMPs, but it is not known whether staff in these outlets receive reports of suspected ADRs associated with such products or what action, if any, they take if they do.

Herbal Sector–Initiated Spontaneous Reporting Schemes

Several herbal practitioner and other organisations have initiated their own ADR reporting schemes.[2] Although this is a responsible and

---

Box **11-2** CALCULATION OF A PROPORTIONAL REPORTING RATIO (PRR)

	Drug of interest	All other drugs
Reaction of interest	a	b
All other reactions	c	d
PRR =	$(a \times d)/(b \times c)$	

potentially useful step forward when these schemes have developed a link with the licensing authority or WHO UMC, ad hoc schemes are not encouraged because there is a risk that numbers of reports are dispersed and signals may be missed. Furthermore, such schemes are also likely to be prone to limitations such as underreporting because practitioners may be reluctant to submit reports because of concerns over the consequences.

For example, the National Institute of Medical Herbalists (NIMH) in the United Kingdom accepts from its members reports of suspected ADRs associated with the herbal treatments they have prescribed. Reports are submitted on a modified yellow card. The NIMH sends an annual summary of reports received to the MHRA. From January 1994 to November 2001, the NIMH received 23 reports.[27] Most described suspected ADRs were associated with a combination of several herbs.

Prescription Event Monitoring

Prescription event monitoring (PEM) is a hypothesis-generating, noninterventional method used by the Drug Safety Research Unit (DSRU, a registered charity), Southampton, United Kingdom, to collect *adverse event* (*not* suspected ADR) data, currently only for newly marketed prescription drugs.[28] However, it is possible that modified PEM methodology could be applied to herbal medicines.

The standard method involves the DSRU deciding to monitor a particular newly licensed drug. The Prescription Pricing Authority (PPA), the organisation responsible for reimbursing pharmacists for prescriptions dispensed, is notified and identifies all prescriptions that have been dispensed for the drug of interest, together with details of the patient and the prescribing doctor. This information is sent to the DSRU, which then sends a "green form" for each patient to the prescriber, usually approximately 6 months after the initial prescription.[28] The form asks doctors to provide information (confidentially) on adverse events that have occurred since the patient was first prescribed the drug. The advantage in collecting adverse event data is

that it does not require the reporter (in this case, doctors) to have suspicions that symptoms or illnesses are drug related; data on *all* adverse health events occurring during or after treatment are recorded. Each study begins as soon as possible after the drug is first marketed and aims to collect data on at least 10,000 patients. Briefly, analysis of the data yields incidence densities for each adverse event reported, an estimate of the frequency.[28]

A protocol for modified PEM methodology has been developed by the DSRU in collaboration with the NIMH and other institutions. This approach involves using herbalists to provide adverse event data on green forms for patients treated with a specific herb (e.g., *Hypericum perforatum*). When patients give permission, a green form requesting adverse event data is also sent to their doctor. There are limitations to this method, such as whether sufficient patient numbers could be achieved and particularly that the herb of interest is not "newly marketed" so there may be preconceptions about its safety profile. Nevertheless, the protocol represents an innovative step forward in attempting to develop methods for herbal pharmacovigilance. Funding for a pilot study is being sought.

Another potential approach, based on PEM concepts, is to use community pharmacists to recruit all individuals (when consent is given) who purchase a specific HMP. Individuals, pharmacists, and doctors (when consent is given) could be followed up after an appropriate period and asked for data on adverse events. The feasibility of this approach has been demonstrated in a pilot study using a conventional over-the-counter medicine[29] but needs to be evaluated as a method for pharmacovigilance of HMPs.[2]

Other Pharmacoepidemiologic Studies

Once a signal has been confirmed, it is usual, at least for prescription medicines for which several options exist, for further investigation to be undertaken to gather more evidence and to strengthen or test a hypothesis. The methodology of the various available approaches is well established, and the characteristics, including limitations, of the various approaches are also well known.[30] In some cases, more than one approach may be used. However, most of the available methods and resources are limited in their application to exploring safety issues associated with herbal medicines.

Observational, Analytic Studies

Case-control studies involve identifying individuals with a particular disease and comparing them with individuals without the disease in terms of their previous use of (exposure to) the drug of interest. Therefore, case-control studies are always carried out retrospectively because they start with individuals who already have the health event of interest and explore backward to see whether the individual has used the drug(s) of interest. Cohort studies involve identifying individuals who have taken the drug of interest and following them for a time period to determine the outcome (e.g., a particular adverse health event). Thus, the direction of investigation with cohort studies is always prospective.

These types of studies each have recognised advantages and disadvantages.[30] For example, although case-control studies can explore exposures to one or more drugs and are relatively easy and inexpensive to conduct, their main problem lies in the selection of appropriate control subjects. Cohort studies can study one or more health outcomes, but the follow-up period can be long, depending on the outcome of interest, and they are expensive. Both methods are prone to various biases and confounding.

Some of the potential biases and difficulties involved with carrying out these types of studies may be enhanced when applied to investigating the safety of herbal medicines. For example, establishing and verifying exposure of cases and control subjects to the herbal medicine(s) of interest is problematic because in the United Kingdom herbal medicines are rarely prescribed and generally are not included on pharmacy patient records.[2] Also, consumers may change brands and be unable to recall which brand or manufacturer's product they used; therefore, defining exposure precisely will also be difficult.

Few such studies have been carried out for HMPs. One example investigated whether there was a relationship between colorectal cancer and abuse of preparations containing anthranoid laxatives.[13]

Computerised health record databases, such as the General Practice Research Database, can be used to carry out case-control and cohort studies.[31] However, such databases currently cannot be used to investigate herbal safety concerns because they are based on doctor's medical records, and very little information on nonprescribed medicines, including HMPs, is recorded.

Experimental Studies

Randomised clinical trials (RCTs) are the gold standard method for assessing whether an outcome is caused by an intervention (e.g., drug treatment). However, they are rarely, if ever, used with the primary aim of testing hypotheses relating to drug safety concerns, not least for ethical reasons. Clinical trials also include relatively small numbers of patients who usually take only the drug of interest and have only one specific illness. For these reasons, clinical trials have the statistical power only to detect common, acute adverse effects and do not evaluate the drug of interest as it is used in everyday clinical practice.

Systematic reviews and meta-analyses of adverse event data from several RCTs of specific herbal medicines have been carried out, but this approach is not without problems. Many existing RCTs of herbal medicines are of poor or limited methodologic quality, and systematic reviews/meta-analyses often ignore differences between different manufacturers' products containing the same herbal ingredient.[2]

COMMUNICATION OF HERBAL SAFETY CONCERNS

A key element of pharmacovigilance is the communication of information on drug safety concerns to all stakeholders. The timing, content, and delivery method for successful drug safety communications have been discussed extensively, although whether these need to be modified in any way for successful communication of herbal safety concerns is not known. The key characteristics of an effective drug safety communication are that it should be tailored to each specific recipient group (e.g., patients, health care professionals, and the media), understandable, open, informative, and balanced. However, communicating information on herbal safety concerns presents additional difficulties for several reasons:

- There is no statutory regulation for herbal-medicine practitioners and therefore no easily obtainable lists that can be used for communication of information;
- "Dear Doctor/Pharmacist" letters can be sent, but these health care professionals are unlikely to know which of their patients are using herbal medicines and therefore will be unable to pass on information to specific individuals;
- Many consumers/patients purchase herbal medicines from outlets where there is no health care professional present and without seeking professional advice; therefore, the popular media are often the only way of communicating information to such individuals; and
- Herbal safety concerns can be misunderstood, misinterpreted, and misreported, as can conventional drug safety concerns.[2]

In the United Kingdom, the competent authority has created a web site, aimed particularly at consumers and patients, devoted to providing early information on herbal safety concerns.[32]

THE FUTURE FOR HERBAL PHARMACOVIGILANCE

Improvements in basic pharmacovigilance for herbal medicines in Europe can be expected in the near future, assuming that the new EU directive for traditional HMPs is implemented as planned.[12] Manufacturers of HMPs registered under the directive will be required to adhere to quality standards, to provide bibliographic evidence of the safety of their products, and to comply with regulatory provisions on pharmacovigilance. At present, most research involving herbal medicines concentrates on establishing efficacy. The proposed traditional herbal medicinal products directive

may have the effect of shifting the emphasis of herbal-medicines research from efficacy to safety, thus potentially having a favourable impact on herbal pharmacovigilance. Although research into the safety of herbal medicines is to be welcomed, research into efficacy is also needed to develop products with good risk-benefit profiles.

Alongside improvements in pharmacovigilance for herbal medicines, the increasing use of these preparations, particularly by patients using conventional drugs and those with serious chronic illness, may result in the emergence of new safety concerns, such as signals of unexpected ADRs, those occurring with long-term use, and interactions with conventional medicines.[2] It is likely that tools to monitor the safety of such products will need to be developed for a more proactive approach to herbal pharmacovigilance. Such tools may be based on existing methodology—some ideas have been mentioned here—or may involve novel approaches.

In the long term, the future for ensuring the safety of herbal medicines may lie with pharmacogenetics and pharmacogenomics.[2] These relatively new fields of research are widely held to be central to the discovery of new drugs and to the future of therapeutics. It is reasonable to assume that individuals with a different genetic profile will have different responses to herbal medicines and to conventional drugs. However, optimising treatment, including reducing the potential for ADRs, based on a patient's genotype has barely been discussed in the context of herbal medicines.

REFERENCES

1. Mann RD, Andrews EB, editors: *Pharmacovigilance,* Chicester, 2002, Wiley.
2. Barnes J: Pharmacovigilance of herbal medicines. A UK perspective, *Drug Saf* 26:829-851, 2003.
3. Edwards RI, Biriell C: Harmonisation in pharmacovigilance, *Drug Saf* 10:93-102, 1994.
4. World Health Organisation (WHO) Collaborating Centre for International Drug Monitoring: Definitions. Available at: http://www.who-umc.org/defs.html. Accessed September 29, 2003.
5. Mann RD: Monitoring the safety of medicines. In *Clinical research manual,* Haslemere, UK, 1998, Euromed Communications.

6. Edwards RI: *Pharmacovigilance—beyond 2000. Opinion & evidence: drug safety,* ed 2, Auckland, 2001, Adis International Ltd.

7. World Health Organization: *Draft WHO guidelines on safety monitoring and pharmacovigilance of herbal medicines,* Geneva, 2003, World Health Organization.

8. Commission of the European Communities: *Directive 2001/83/EC,* Brussels, 2001, European Commission.

9. Brown EG: Effects of coding dictionary on signal generation. A consideration of use of MedDRA compared with WHO-ART, *Drug Saf* 25:445-452, 2002.

10. Barnes J: Eudravigilance, *Reactions* 907:3-4, 2002.

11. Barnes J, Anderson LA, Phillipson JD: *Herbal medicines. A guide for healthcare professionals,* ed 2, London, 2002, Pharmaceutical Press.

12. Commission of the European Communities: Directive 2004/24/EC of the European Parliament and of the Council of 31 March 2004 amending, as regards traditional herbal medicinal products, Directive 2001/83/EC on the Community code relating to medicinal products for human use, Brussels.

13. De Smet PAGM: An introduction to herbal pharmacovigilance. In De Smet PAGM, Keller K, Hänsel R, Chandler RF, editors: *Adverse effects of herbal drugs, vol 3,* Berlin, 1997, Springer-Verlag.

14. Anon: Extension of the yellow card scheme to unlicensed herbal remedies, *Curr Prob Pharmacovigilance* 22:10, 1996.

15. Shaw D, Leon C, Kolev S, Murray V: Traditional remedies and food supplements. A 5-year toxicological study (1991-1995), *Drug Saf* 17:342-356, 1997.

16. Anon: Extension of the yellow card scheme to pharmacists, *Curr Prob Pharmacovigilance* 23:3, 1997.

17. Committee on Safety of Medicines and Medicines and Healthcare Products Regulatory Agency: The yellow card scheme. Extension of the yellow card scheme to nurse reporters. Available at: *http://medicines.mhra.gov.uk/aboutagency/regframework/csm/csmhome.htm.* Accessed July 25, 2003.

18. Anon: Patients able to report ADRs via NHS Direct, *Pharm J* 270:608, 2003.

19. Farah MH, Edward R, Lindquist M, Leon C, Shaw D: International monitoring of adverse health effects associated with herbal medicines, *Pharmacoepidemiol Drug Saf* 9:105-112, 2000.

20. De Los Reyes GC, Koda RT: Determining hyperforin and hypericin content in eight brands of St. John's wort, *Am J Health Syst Pharm* 59:545-547, 2002.

21. Kressman S, Muller WE, Blume HH: Pharmaceutical quality of different Ginkgo biloba brands, *J Pharm Pharmacol* 54:661-669, 2002.

22. Medicines and Healthcare Products Regulatory Agency: *Adverse Drug Reaction On-line Information Tracking (ADROIT) system,* July 25, 2003.

23. Coulson R, Davis S: Community pharmacist reporting of suspected ADRs: (1) the first year of the yellow card demonstration scheme, *Pharm J* 263:786-788, 1999.

24. Barnes J: *An examination of the role of the pharmacist in the safe, effective and appropriate use of complementary medicines,* PhD thesis, London, 2001, University of London.

25. Evans S: Statistical methods of signal detection. In Mann RD, Andrews EB, editors: *Pharmacovigilance,* Chicester, 2002, Wiley.

26. Barnes J, Mills SY, Abbot NC, Willoughby M, Ernst E: Different standards for reporting ADRs to herbal remedies and conventional OTC medicines: face-to-face interviews with 515 users of herbal remedies, *Br J Clin Pharmacol* 45:496-500, 1998.

27. Broughton A: Yellow card reporting scheme, *Eur J Herb Med* Dec:3-6, 2001.

28. Shakir SAW: PEM in the UK. In Mann RD, Andrews EB, editors: *Pharmacovigilance,* Chicester, 2002, Wiley.

29. Sinclair HK, Bond CM, Hannaford PC: Pharmacovigilance of over-the-counter products based in community pharmacy: a feasible option? *Pharmacoepidemiol Drug Saf* 8:479-491, 1999.

30. Strom BL: How should one perform pharmacoepidemiology studies? Choosing among the available alternatives. In Strom BL, editor: *Pharmacoepidemiology,* ed 3, Chicester, 2000, Wiley.

31. General Practice Research Database: Available at: *http://www.gprd.com.* Accessed September 29, 2003.

32. Medicines and Healthcare products Regulatory Agency: Available at: http://www.mhra.gov.uk/ourwork/licensingmeds/ herbalmeds/herbalsafety.htm. Accessed September 29, 2003.

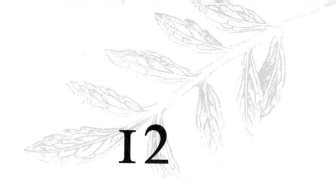

12

KAVA: A RISK-BENEFIT ASSESSMENT

Mathias Schmidt, Michelle Morgan, Kerry Bone, and Janice McMillan

In November 2001 the German Health Authority (BfArM; see Appendix 1 for abbreviations used) announced that it was intending to ban the use of kava (*Piper methysticum*) because of reported cases linking kava consumption with hepatotoxicity. Despite submissions from manufacturers, therapeutic use of kava was banned altogether in Germany in 2002 and several other countries such as Japan, France, and Canada followed suit. Late in 2002 it was announced that the Medicines Control Agency (MCA) in the United Kingdom would also be banning kava; in February 2003 Swissmedic (formerly IKS) in Switzerland followed. At the time of writing, the Australian government is currently considering whether availability of therapeutic goods containing kava should be restricted.

Since the action of the German authorities, government health administrations throughout the world have examined their databases for evidence of hepatotoxicity from kava use. Not surprisingly, more cases have come to light, but many of them are tenuous or inadequately reported. This chapter will review all known reported cases as of February 2003, with a view to arriving at an assessment as to whether the

actions by the various health authorities have been justified. Much depends on the risk to benefit perspective. How much risk is acceptable for a herbal product? How good does the evidence need to be to arrive at a favourable risk-benefit assessment? The question must also be asked whether the interests of the consumer have been served by the complete banning of a herb that offered a viable alternative to conventional anxiolytic drugs, which are well known to have many risks associated with their use.

SUMMARY AND CRITIQUE OF CASE REPORTS

A number of case reports of hepatotoxic effects possibly attributed to kava have been documented by various health authorities around the world. These are provided in tabular form in Appendix 2.

The table in Appendix 2 contains the case numbers used by relevant regulatory bodies (BfArM, MCA, European Agency for the Evaluation of Medicinal Products [EMEA], Food and Drug Administration (United States) [FDA], IKS, and Therapeutic Goods Administration (Australia) [TGA]) and other relevant information including literature and press sources. The case number assigned in the first column will be used throughout this document to enable easy reference to the case reports. Variation in the MCA numbers occurs in other documents, but that variation is not reported here.

Information provided in Appendix 2 was obtained from the following sources:

- The Committee on Safety of Medicines (CSM, part of MCA) analysis of case reports received worldwide to 10 July 2002 (68 case reports; listed as #1 to #68).[1]

- A literature review by Schmidt from the University of Muenster dated May 2003, which analysed 82 case reports dating from 1990 to 2003 (including #1 to #68) and details from the Adverse Reaction Monitoring System of the U.S. FDA (which provided an additional 12 case reports [#69 to #80]). Most of the FDA kava reports were provided by the American Herbal Products Association in a spreadsheet entitled "FDA kava reports, 1994-2002: Initial organization of 51 cases". Of the 51 cases provided in this FDA spreadsheet (last entry dated 25 February 2002), 31 did not describe hepatic adverse events. Recent case reports, one each from BfArM and the FDA, subsequent to the data listed here were obtained from the Schmidt review (#81, #82). The information listed in Appendix 2 for #81 did not appear in the official BfArM line listing (24 May 2002) and was obtained from the literature.[2] (There is no BfArM line listing available for #82, so it has not been included in Appendix 2.) Information for case #71 obtained from two sources (literature and the FDA) has been included for comparison.

- Australian TGA with details obtained from the adverse drug reactions system (1 case report, listed as #83).

The case details obtained from the MCA analysis are presented as provided. However, they do not list all the known information, and additional details are provided in the individual case discussions below. Additional details of those U.S. cases listed by the MCA (#51 to #63) can also be found in the FDA spreadsheet provided for the Waller analysis.[3]

Of these 83 case reports three have been identified as possible or definite duplicates (#26 and #28, #29 and #30, and #31 and #33).

Appendix 2 does not contain the three cases of hepatitis possibly associated with kava use in New Zealand, reported in the CSM *Risk–benefit analysis of Kava-kava*, 12 February 2002,[4] as sufficient details were not available.

A detailed analysis of the 83 cases follows. In addition to the information initially provided via spreadsheets from government regulatory bodies, additional case details have been obtained from the Schmidt, MCA, and Waller reviews and the FDA spreadsheet of 51 cases. The Schmidt review obtained additional information from the following sources:

- additional details provided by the BfArM with the ban of kava products dated 14 June 2002;

- additional details provided by an expert report from the BfArM for a law suit against the German authorities filed by some German producers;

- additional details from the producers of the implicated kava medications;

- detailed background data from the Swiss IKS forwarded to the producers of kava products in the process of the drug safety protocol of 2000;

- additional information obtained from the FDA; and

- case reports from the literature.

Botanical names have been noted here to assist the reader in recognising the herbs listed in the products allegedly consumed in the case reports. It should not imply that the botanical identity of these ingredients was verified either by the product label or by analysis.

Case #1

Case also identified as: MCA #1, MCA Case Report, EMEA #1

The 40-year-old man drank six bottles of wine per week, which may have caused or contributed to the abnormal liver function tests. This, combined with the symptoms of sore throat and nose bleeds, may indicate preexisting pathology unrelated to kava use. Although the outcome is recorded as recovery after stopping kava, no details are supplied regarding the cessation of alcohol intake.[5] If alcohol intake had continued, one possible explanation is that kava may have acted synergistically.

Assessment: Unlikely; case involved a large intake of alcohol.

Case #2
Case also identified as: MCA #2, MCA Case Report, EMEA #2

The female patient of unknown age was taking Prozac (fluoxetine) in addition to kava. At the time the data were compiled, the case was ongoing with a biopsy pending. The outcome is listed as "reaction continues," with no explanation of whether the kava intake had ceased. Fluoxetine is known to cause hepatotoxicity.[6]

Assessment: Unlikely; probably connected to concomitant medication.

Case #3
Case also identified as: MCA #3, MCA Case Report #3

The 48-year-old man with raised liver enzymes is listed as recovering after withdrawal of kava. The case report indicates he was also taking bendrofluazide (a thiazide diuretic). Liver damage is listed as a side-effect of this drug,[7] and it should be used with caution in hepatic insufficiency, which may be unpredictably aggravated.[8] The patient stopped taking kava after 8 years of occasional use for air sickness, during which he had stable but increased liver enzymes. The liver appeared to take time to recover.

Assessment: Possible, but connection to kava is not proven as the effect of concomitant medication and a preexisting problem cannot be ruled out.

Case #4
Case also identified as: MCA #4, BfArM #93/0351, EMEA #3
Reported by Schwabe GmbH & Co

Further details supplied by Schwabe, the company that reported this case, indicate that the 68-year-old woman displayed elevated liver enzymes prior to ingesting the kava product

(210 mg/day of kava lactones) and the enzyme values did not worsen during the kava treatment.[9]

Assessment: Unlikely, no connection to kava and should not have been listed as an adverse reaction.

Case #5
Case also identified as: MCA #5, EMEA #4
Lit: Strahl et al, 1998

This is a reasonably well-documented case[10] in which a 39-year-old woman had her elevated liver enzyme (glutamic-pyruvic transaminase [GPT]) level return to normal after cessation of the kava and other medications (below). The enzyme level rose after she resumed intake of the kava product (the other medications were not resumed). Although not defined in the literature, the kava product (providing 60 mg/day of kava lactones) is understood to have been an ethanol extract. Liver biopsy revealed acute necrotising hepatitis. Viral, autoimmune, and metabolic causes of the hepatitis were excluded. The patient was also taking paroxetine (antidepressant, 20 mg/day), a contraceptive (0.15 mg desogestrel + 0.02 mg ethinyl oestradiol per day, for 6 years) and occasionally St. John's wort (*Hypericum perforatum*, no product details). Paroxetine has caused abnormal liver function tests and severe liver toxicity.[8,11] Liver function may also be impaired by contraceptive use.[8,11,12]

Further testing[13] of this patient indicated that she was a poor metaboliser of debrisoquine (indicating a cytochrome P450 CYP2D6 deficiency). (Cytochrome P450 2D6, which is responsible for the metabolism of several antidepressants and neuroleptics, is constitutionally deficient in up to 10% of the population.[14])

By differential diagnosis an autoimmune aetiology was ruled out and a lymphocyte transformation test was not conducted after the positive rechallenge to kava. However, the shortened latency period points to an immunological sensitisation on initial intake.[11]

Assessment: Probable, due to genetic deficiency in detoxifying enzyme (CYP2D6) causing an idiosyncratic-immunologic hepatitis and perhaps exacerbated by concomitant medications.

Case #6

Case also identified as: MCA #6, EMEA #5

Lit: Kraft et al, 2001

A 60-year-old woman was admitted to hospital and was transferred to an intensive care unit with progressive liver failure, concomitant renal failure, and progressive encephalopathy. Biochemical tests revealed acute liver failure (hepatocellular necrosis with intrahepatic cholestasis) and serological tests ruled out viral hepatitis, metabolic, or autoimmune causes of liver failure. The patient received a liver transplant.[15]

The patient had suffered from pulmonary embolism 11 years earlier, with cardiopulmonary resuscitation, and had undergone an ovariectomy and cholecystectomy 21 years previously. For 8 years she had suffered depression.[16]

Concomitant medications included piretanide (a diuretic) which, according to the authors of the report,[15] could not be ruled out as contributing to the liver failure. Piretanide may cause cholangitis with intrahepatic cholestasis and increased transaminases.[17] The dosage of kava taken exceeded the recommended daily dosage regularly (4 tablets). Information from a relative revealed that the patient took extra kava doses ad libitum in addition to the already excessive regimen. Some statements indicated the use of up to 10 tablets per day.[16] The daily recommended dosage of this preparation when first released was 1 to 2 tablets per day but was recently reduced to 1 tablet per day (120 mg/day of kava lactones).

Assessment: Possible, but if so, due to excessive dosage of kava and probably connected to concomitant medication.

Case #7

Case also identified as: MCA #7, IKS #1999-2596, EMEA #6

As well as taking a kava product (an acetone extract providing 140 mg/day of kava lactones), the 46-year-old woman was also taking propranolol (80 mg) and an antihypertensive tablet containing valsartan (angiotensin II receptor antagonist) and hydrochlorothiazide (a thiazide diuretic) for 4.5 and 5.5 months, respectively. Elevated liver enzyme values and hepatitis are known possible side-effects of propranolol, valsartan can also cause elevation of liver enzyme levels, and thiazides can produce occasional cases of cholecystitis or icterus.[18]

Assessment: Possible, but may not be due to kava alone.

Case #8

Case also identified as: MCA #8, IKS #2000-0014, EMEA #7

The case of a 33-year-old woman who developed cholestatic hepatitis with icterus (jaundice) has also been described in the literature.[13,19] In addition to kava, she had taken a homoeopathic combination product for a period of 15 days about 1 month after beginning the kava.[20] The liver parameters were still deteriorating even 10 days after discontinuing medication. Values normalised within 8 weeks of discontinuation of kava. The finding of slightly higher IgM against Epstein–Barr virus (EBV) in this patient was not significant, since histology and serology results did not support evidence of EBV hepatitis. A lymphocyte transformation test performed after recovery indicated strong and concentration-dependent T-cell reactivity to the kava product, but not to the homoeopathic product.[13,21]

The patient consumed a massive amount of alcohol about 1 week before symptoms resulted in her hospitalisation. Pain medication was taken the day after the alcohol intake and consisted of a tablet containing propyphenazone, dihydroergotamine mesylate, and caffeine, and another tablet containing paracetamol, propyphenazone, and caffeine. Obstruction of the bile ducts and autoimmune disease was excluded, and liver biopsy suggested drug-induced hepatitis, not due to alcohol intake.[20]

Phenotyping of cytochrome P450 CYP2D6 activity with debrisoquine showed that the patient was a poor metaboliser.[13]

Assessment: Probable due to genetic deficiency in detoxifying enzyme (CYP2D6) causing an idiosyncratic immune-mediated hepatitis.

Case #9

Case also identified as: MCA #9, IKS #2000-2330, EMEA #8

The 59-year-old patient was diagnosed with painless jaundice with elevation of liver enzymes. Two weeks after discontinuing intake of a kava product, the liver values improved. The patient had also been taking celecoxib (a nonsteroidal antiinflammatory drug [NSAID], cyclooxygenase-2 [COX-2] inhibitor), which is known to cause raised liver function values, liver impairment, and hepatitis.[8,22] It is not known whether the celecoxib was also discontinued.

Assessment: Possible, but may be connected to concomitant medication.

Case #10

Case also identified as: MCA #10, IKS #2000-3502, EMEA #9

This Swiss case involving a 50-year-old man was also reported in the literature.[19,23] He presented with jaundice and very high liver enzyme values. Liver failure with rapid decline and encephalopathy developed. Obstruction of the bile ducts and a viral aetiology were excluded. He received a liver transplant. Histology of his liver showed extensive necrosis and infiltration of lymphocytes and eosinophils. Paracetamol was taken while in hospital after the onset of symptoms. Despite the case information listed in Appendix 2, the literature reports that he did not consume alcohol. He was also taking evening primrose oil (*Oenonthera biennis*).

The patient had been consuming the kava product above the maximum recommended therapeutic dosage (400 mg of extract [containing 280 mg/day of kava lactones] versus the recommended dose of 300 mg of extract).

Assessment: Probable, but dosage of kava was exceeded.

Case #11

Case also identified as: MCA #11, BfArM #90003882, EMEA #10

The 69-year-old woman developed cholestatic hepatitis, and was taking a preparation containing synthetic kavain (a kava lactone) and the following drugs: acetylsalicylic acid (unknown dosage), dehydrosanol (a diuretic combination containing bemetizide and triamterene) and pentoxifylline. Each of the orthodox medications is documented as causing an increase in liver enzymes and/or liver function impairment and jaundice.[24]

Assessment: Unlikely, probably connected to concomitant medication.

Case #12

Case also identified as: MCA #12, BfArM #92901203, EMEA #11

The case details of a 35-year-old man who suffered cholestatic hepatitis after ingesting a product containing synthetic kavain are inadequate for analysis. Duration of usage, concomitant medication and preexisting medical conditions are unknown.[25]

Assessment: Unassessable due to insufficient information.

Case #13

Case also identified as: MCA #13, IKS #93/0274, BfArM #93015209, EMEA #12

The symptoms of the 39-year-old woman, which included jaundice, started 12 weeks after intake of a kava product (210 mg/day of kava lactones). Alcohol was excluded as a cause but viral hepatitis was not excluded. Concomitant medications included L-thyroxine (taken for 3 months), diazepam (for 6 months), and a contraceptive containing ethinyloestradiol and levonorgestrel (for 16 years). Cholestatic jaundice has been reported in users of this contraceptive, as has cholelithiasis and hepatitis.[8] The BfArM excluded the causality of the contraceptive agent on the basis that abnormal liver function did not develop during its long-term use, which does not, however, prove that such an adverse event did not occur. Very rare cases of jaundice and increase in transaminases can occur from diazepam intake.[8] BfArM denied the ingestion of diazepam as it was not recorded in the physician's report from the hospital. The intake of diazepam, albeit irregular, was confirmed by the patient's general practitioner. BfArM further indicated that since ingestion was irregular it could not have been the cause, despite the fact that it was ingested prior to the onset of symptoms. The hospital physician indicated that viral hepatitis could not be excluded.[26]

Assessment: Possible, but connection to concomitant medication or an alternative aetiology is also possible.

Case #14

Case also identified as: MCA #14, BfArM #94006568, IKS #94/0259, EMEA #13

In this case of a 68-year-old woman, jaundice and cholestatic hepatitis were reported as side effects. In addition to kava, her other medications included a St. John's wort preparation (*Hypericum perforatum*, taken for 1 year) and an antacid (Maaloxan, aluminium–magnesium hydroxide, taken when needed). Liver biopsy indicated severe toxic–cholestatic liver damage and was consistent with an immunologically triggered hypersensitivity reaction, which led to an idiosyncratic damage of liver tissue. Drug-induced toxicity was not confirmed and an autoimmune process was not excluded. Normally the latency period for drug-induced idiosyncratic toxic hepatitis is 50 to 90 days. The two herbal products were taken for much longer than this before the adverse reaction occurred.[27]

Assessment: Possible, but an immunologically triggered hypersensitivity reaction not associated with kava cannot be ruled out.

Case #15

Case also identified as: MCA #15, BfArM #94901308, IKS#94/0117), EMEA #14

Adverse events for a 50-year-old woman were recorded as liver damage, hepatitis, jaundice, and elevated liver enzymes. In addition to kava (210 mg/day of kava lactones, taken for 2–3 months), her other medication included a diuretic containing furosemide and triamterene (unknown duration), atenolol (beta-

blocker, 5 to 6 years) and terfenadine (antihistamine, 12 years). A biopsy suggested drug-induced hepatitis, and alcohol was eliminated as a cause. Histological results indicated previous infection with hepatitis A, although liver function was not abnormal prior to the advent of the adverse effect. Although specific autoimmune antibodies could not be detected, there were signs of autoimmune hepatitis. Histological investigation also indicated that the liver reaction had begun prior to the first intake of the kava product. Prior to the adverse event, the patient had suffered viral infections, including hepatitis A, EBV, cytomegalovirus (CMV), and herpes simplex virus (HSV), all of which can have liver involvement. Three weeks after discontinuation of the kava product, a renewed increase of the transaminase levels occurred, which is not typical of drug-induced liver problems.[28]

Despite the fact that furosemide is documented as causing adverse effects on the liver,[8] BfArM denied the existence of such adverse effects. Although individual cases of severe liver damage occur for atenolol ingestion, a rechallenge with this drug during the patient's hospital stay had no effect on her liver function. The terfenadine was considered to be not implicated by BfArM as it had been taken for over 12 years, but this does not eliminate the possibility of an idiosyncratic immunological reaction. Hepatic side effects are documented for this drug,[28] which was being ingested at a higher dosage (300 mg/day) than is normally recommended (60 to 120 mg/day).

Assessment: Unlikely to be connected to kava, more likely to be caused by concomitant medication or autoimmune hepatitis.

Case #16

Case also identified as: MCA #16, BfArM #97002825; probable duplicate case with BfArM #97003551 (not listed here), EMEA #15

In this poorly documented case (or cases) a woman over 70 years of age presented with jaundice, liver damage, and cholestatic hepatitis. The ingested herbal product contained ginseng (*Panax ginseng*), kava (ethanol extract), devil's claw (*Harpagophytum procumbens*), hawthorn leaf and flower (*Crataegus monogyna*), pancreatin, bromelain, and papain. Other medications were a vitamin supplement named Eunova and prednisone; the latter was taken (although not originally listed) reportedly for a long time. The composition of the vitamin supplement was unclear: alpha-tocopherol 400 mg or 4000 IU vitamin A plus vitamins B_1, B_2, B_6, B_{12}, C, D_3, and E; nicotinamide, calcium pantothenate, biotin, rutoside, iron, copper, magnesium, potassium and manganese sulphate, zinc oxide, sodium molybdate, and dibasic calcium phosphate. This could indicate the vitamin supplement was a multivitamin and mineral mixture or a vitamin E preparation. The dosages of the herbal product and the vitamin supplement are unknown. The recommended dosage for the vitamin supplement Eunova is 2 tablets per day which would provide 8000 IE of vitamin A, an amount that can potentially cause hepatotoxic reactions.[27]

Assessment: Unassessable due to insufficient information.

Case #17
Case also identified as: MCA #17, BfArM #98004297, EMEA #16

The outcome of an 81-year-old woman who presented with jaundice, liver failure, and acute cholestatic hepatitis was death. The patient had been taking a kava product (120 mg/day of kava lactones) for over 10 months, a product containing hawthorn (*Crataegus monogyna*) extract and homoeopathics (8 months), hydrochlorothiazide (antihypertensive, 3 months) and a nitrendipine-containing product (antihypertensive, discontinued 5 months previously). Autopsy revealed acute hepatic dystrophy with histological signs of toxic hepatitis, with damage by alcohol not excluded. Histological data also showed cirrhotic transformation of the liver, which probably started at least 1.5 years prior to her death (long before the first administration of kava). One of BfArM's listings of this case contained a reference to alcohol abuse, but this appears to have been ignored in the official BfArM assessment. Rare cases of jaundice and

liver impairment are known to occur from hydrochlorothiazide and drugs of similar structure to nitrendipine. Alcoholic liver disease was worsened by intake of the latter.[29]

In addition, 3 months prior to the adverse reaction the patient was reportedly enrolled into the placebo group of the SCOPE study (Study on Cognition and Prognosis in the Elderly), which was designed to assess the effect of angiotensin II type 1 receptor blockers on major cardiovascular events in elderly patients with mild hypertension. BfArM suggested that inclusion into the study group would not have taken place if any irregularities of liver function had been noted.[29] However, this does not explain the histological data suggesting an earlier onset of reaction.

Assessment: Unlikely; connection to alcohol abuse likely.

Case #18
Case also identified as: MCA #18, BfArM #99500453, EMEA #17

The case involved a 59-year-old woman with hepatic cellular damage. She was taking hyoscine butylbromide (butylscopolammonium bromide) as needed and had been doing so for 15 years. According to the case report, sporadic notifications of hepatic side effects have occurred from intake of this drug.

There is some debate as to whether this patient took the kava product (ethanol extract providing 240 mg/day of kava lactones) listed in Appendix 2.[30] No data regarding preexisting medical conditions, laboratory or diagnostic tests, or alcohol consumption are available.

Assessment: Unassessable due to insufficient information.

Case #19
Case also identified as: MCA #19, BfArM #99062501, EMEA #18

This case of a 37-year-old woman originated from Brazil. Hepatitis was reported. Apart from the kava product (140 mg/day of kava lactones), concomitant medication included diclofenac (single treatment prior to the advent of the adverse reaction) and the contraceptive Microdiol (desogestrel + ethinyloestradiol, for 6 years). A rechallenge was negative for all three medications (kava, diclofenac, contraceptive), which excludes the possibility of an immunological aetiology.[31]

Diclofenac, a NSAID, has known hepatic side effects: elevation of serum aminotransferase enzymes (up to 2%), hepatitis with or without jaundice (<1%), fulminant hepatitis (isolated cases).[8] Hepatitis caused by a NSAID does not necessarily lead to a renewed hepatitis on rechallenge.[31,32]

Assessment : Unlikely, connection to concomitant medication likely.

Case #20
Case also identified as: MCA #20, BfArM #99003911, EMEA #19

A 62-year-old woman was hospitalised for jaundice, and a report of liver cell impairment was made. She had been taking a kava preparation for an unknown duration. Concomitant medication existed, but was not specified. She reputedly recovered after discontinuation of all medication. There was supposedly a rechallenge to the kava product, with recurrence of symptoms, but details were not provided by the treating physicians. Further diagnostic information and information concerning alcohol consumption were unavailable.[33]

Assessment : Unassessable due to insufficient information.

Case #21
Case also identified as: MCA #21, BfArM #99006005, EMEA #20

A 33-year-old woman was hospitalised with symptoms of acute hepatitis. Concomitant medication included cisapride taken for 4 months. A kava product (180 mg/day of kava lactones) had also been ingested for 4 months. Alcohol was ruled out as a cause, but antibodies were detected and she was treated for autoimmune hepatitis. The product manufacturer indicated that an alleged positive rechallenge occurred, resulting in toxic hepatitis, but further details could not be obtained from the treating physicians. Cisapride has caused reversible liver function impairment.[6,34]

Assessment : Possible, but further information required and concomitant medication cannot be ruled out as the cause.

Case #22
Case also identified as: MCA #22, BfArM #00003608, EMEA #21

A 21-year-old woman made a full recovery after treatment for jaundice, hepatitis and elevated liver enzymes, and other nonhepatic symptoms. The kava product that she had been taking for 7 months contained synthetic kavain in addition to standardised kava ethanol extract (total kavain per tablet equalled 50 mg). It was taken in much higher doses than normally recommended (up to 10 tablets per day, i.e. 500 mg/day of kava lactones, which is more than four times the maximum dose recommended by the Commission E). The recommended dosage was a maximum of 6 tablets per day.[35] Recorded concomitant medications included metoclopramide, paracetamol (prior to the adverse event, dosage unknown), pantoprazole (prior to adverse event, dosage unknown), a homoeopathic product containing celandine and a basil extract. There was also suspected use of the illegal drug Ecstasy within the same time frame. Complications of Ecstasy use (active component: methylenedioxymethamphetamine [MDMA]) include liver failure.[36] Her relatives caused postponement of a drug screening test at the time. Paracetamol, although a known hepatotoxin, had not been consumed long term. Metoclopramide is documented as causing raised liver enzymes, and pantoprazole and Ecstasy as causing liver failure. It is possible that the three medications may have acted synergistically. Histological investigations 4 months after the date of adverse reaction state an unchanged clinical picture of an autoimmune hepatitis.[37]

Assessment : Unlikely, concomitant medication, possible Ecstasy abuse, and/or autoimmune aetiology more likely.

Case #23

Case also identified as: MCA #23, BfArM
#00005994, EMEA #22

Lit: Sass et al, 2001

The case of a 50-year-old woman diagnosed with fulminant liver failure was also reported in the medical literature.[38] Signs and symptoms included jaundice, elevated liver enzymes, general poor health, hepatic encephalopathy, and coma. She had been taking a kava preparation (60 mg/day of kava lactones for 6 to 7 months) and several orthodox medications: Amaryl (glimepiride, a sulphonylurea, for 7 months), metformin (a biguanide, unknown period), an oral contraceptive containing oestradiol valerate + levonorgestrel (unknown period) and St. John's wort (*Hypericum perforatum*, 6 months).[39]

Liver biopsy indicated progressive necrosis of hepatic cells and she received a liver transplant. Contraceptive combinations are known to cause cholestasis, hepatitis, and cholestatic jaundice. Hepatic adverse effects are documented for both metformin and glimepiride. A known adverse reaction of metformin is lactic acidosis, the beginnings of which may have been present in this patient, which can lead to coma.[39]

Assessment : Possible, but concomitant medication cannot be ruled out as the cause.

Case #24

Case also identified as: MCA #24, BfArM
#00008627, EMEA #23

Lit: Brauer et al, 2001

Controversy surrounded the case of a 22-year-old woman, with some dubious reporting in the German media. Details of the case were reported in the scientific literature.[40] She had been taking a kava product for 4 months (240 mg kava lactones per day). Concomitant medications included rizatriptan (as needed), pain relief (possibly NSAID, as needed) and contraceptives (norgestimate + ethinyloestradiol; ethinyloestradiol + dienogest).[41]

The patient presented to the hospital because of persisting fatigue and nausea. She had very elevated serum bilirubin and increased liver enzymes. Medications were stopped but she developed fulminant liver failure. Liver biopsy

was negative for viral hepatitis and alcohol was eliminated as a cause. Necrosis of hepatic tissue and damage to the parenchyma was observed. She received a liver transplant, but a CMV infection and intrahepatic arterial stenosis occurred postsurgically. She then developed an *Aspergillus* infection (not viral hepatitis as stated by BfArM) due to immunosuppression, which finally led to her death.[41]

Contraceptive combinations are associated with cholestasis and jaundice. The other medications are unlikely to have contributed significantly. An investigation with the treating physician revealed that the patient had a hepatic incident over 3 years preceding this event. A drug-related aetiology was suspected, but the cause was not identified. The patient was an employee in a pharmacy and would have had relatively easy access to potential hepatotoxic medications. This lends weight to the drug-related aetiology.[41] Confirmation of the patient's employment was documented in the newspaper article.[42]

Assessment : Possible, but connection to kava is not proven as a preexisting hepatic problem cannot be ruled out.

Case #25

Case also identified as: MCA #25, BfArM
#01003089, EMEA #24

This case involved a 34-year-old woman who had been taking L-thyroxine (duration unknown, probably long term) and a kava product (120 mg/day of kava lactones for 3 months). Hepatitis and elevated liver enzymes were recorded as side effects. Use of alcohol and differential diagnostic information were not provided. Hepatotoxicity associated with L-thyroxine has occurred rarely.[43]

Assessment : Possible, but not enough data available.

Case #26

Case also identified as: MCA #26, BfArM #01004110
(EMEA #25); duplicate case BfArM #99006200,
EMEA #27

A female patient (aged 34 or 35) recovered fully from jaundice, elevated liver enzymes, and hepatitis upon discontinuation of medication which included paracetamol (as needed), a St. John's wort product (*Hypericum perforatum*) and a kava product (120 mg/day of kava lactones, duration unknown). Information received from the manufacturer of the kava product indicated that the patient suffered from multiple sclerosis. The patient's physician did not provide any information regarding treatment for the multiple sclerosis.[44]

Assessment: Unassessable due to insufficient information regarding concomitant medication for the treatment of multiple sclerosis.

Case #27

Case also identified as: MCA #27, BfArM #99005139, EMEA #26

In a 47-year-old woman, a transient increase in liver enzyme levels was recorded with concomitant use of fish oil (high dosage) and a kava product. Despite the information listed in Appendix 2 by BfArM, the liver values returned to normal without discontinuation of kava. Elevated liver enzymes can be a rare occurrence following a high dosage of fish oil.[45]

Assessment: Unlikely, no connection to kava.

Case #28

Case also identified as: MCA #28, BfArM #99006200, EMEA #27; duplicate case BfArM #01004110, EMEA #25

This was recognised by the MCA as a duplicate of case #26 (above).

Assessment: Unassessable due to insufficient information regarding concomitant medication for the treatment of multiple sclerosis.

Case #29

Case also identified as: MCA #29, BfArM #01001228, EMEA #28; duplicate case #01001924, EMEA #29 (see Case #30 below) and also BfArM #01001928 (not listed here)

A man aged 38 or 39 was reported to experience liver cell damage and hepatitis. Duplicate entries by BfArM appear to have occurred for this case, in which penicillin (intake for 1 day)

and "no other drugs" were listed in the concomitant medication field. The kava product (70 mg/day of kava lactones) was taken for 1 to 2 weeks. It is unclear why the patient took the antibiotic for 1 day. Either the adverse effect occurred after the ingestion of the antibiotic or, despite the usual recommendation, the entire course of antibiotics was not taken. No other details regarding differential diagnosis or alcohol intake are available. Although the incidence of hepatic adverse effects caused by penicillin are rare, hypersensitivity may occur on one intake, with hepatic side effects occurring with second intake.[46]

Assessment: Unlikely, difficult to assess with inadequate information, and a link to concomitant medication is possible.

Case #30

Case also identified as: MCA #30, BfArM #01001924, EMEA #29; duplicate case (see case #29 above)

This was recognised by BfArM and the MCA as a duplicate of case #29 (above).

Assessment: Unlikely, difficult to assess with inadequate information, and a link to medication is possible.

Case #31

Case also identified as: MCA #31, BfArM #01003950, EMEA #30; duplicate case BfArM #01003951, EMEA #32

This case refers to the same patient as in Case #33. Following a hepatitis incident in 2001, the female patient filed a self-report of a former supposed drug-induced hepatitis in 1993, which the patient said was due to the intake of Kavain Harras or Kava-ratiopharm (both ethanolic extracts). However, both products were commercially unavailable in 1993 and, according to the physician's records, no causative agent could be identified to explain the 1993 incident. In addition, there was no record with the BfArM in 1993 concerning a hepatitis connected to kava intake.[47,48]

In 2001, the then 56-year-old patient suffered from a slight increase in liver enzymes following oral administration of either Kavain

Harras N or Kava-ratiopharm. The product involved was not confirmed by the hospital's physicians, who filed the event as a transaminitis of unclear origin, possibly drug-related. Based on the supposed yet unconfirmed incident in 1993, BfArM lists a positive rechallenge to kava.

Concomitant to the kava intake in 2001, the following medications were taken: omeprazole (Antra MUPS, as needed), candesartan cilexetil (antihypertensive, intake for 2 months but discontinued 5 months before the onset of the hepatitis), losartan-potassium + hydrochlorothiazide (Lozaar plus, antihypertensive, taken since the discontinuation of candesartan cilexetil), oestradiol valerate (Estragest TTS, transdermally, long-term treatment), L-thyroxine (long-term treatment of Hashimoto thyroiditis), acetylcysteine (unknown duration) and several common cold remedies unlikely to have any impact on the liver. Each of these medications (excluding the cold remedies) has documented hepatic side effects: L-thyroxine (hepatotoxicity, rarely), transdermal oestradiol (asymptomatic impaired hepatic function, cholestatic jaundice; rarely), candesartan cilexetil and losartan (raised liver enzymes), hydrochlorothiazide (jaundice, cholecystitis; rare), omeprazole (hepatitis, liver failure, and hepatic-related encephalopathy). The combination of these drugs would have increased the chance of an hepatic side effect.[48]

The MCA analysis of this case indicates that the patient restarted kava while also taking her other medications,[1] although this information was not provided by BfArM.

Assessment: Unassessable on the basis of confusion in the listings and insufficient information; cause by concomitant medications quite possible.

Case #32
Case also identified as: MCA #32, BfArM #01006229, EMEA #31

A 32-year-old man received a liver transplant after a range of liver symptoms including elevated liver enzymes and liver necrosis necessitated such action. The patient had been taking a kava preparation for about 3 months (240 mg/day of kava lactones) and a valerian prepa-

ration occasionally. Viral and autoimmune hepatitis were excluded. Although no other concomitant medications, including drugs, are listed, it is not clear that this was the case.[49]

Assessment: Possible but further information required, including verification of no other concomitant medications.

Case #33
Case also identified as: MCA #33, BfArM #01003951, EMEA #32; duplicate case BfArM #01003950, EMEA #30

This case is a duplicate of case #31 (above).

Assessment: Unassessable on the basis of confusion in the listings and insufficient information; cause by concomitant medications quite possible.

Case #34
Case also identified as: MCA #34, BfArM #01006939, EMEA #33

A 36-year-old man with liver damage had no previous history of liver disorders. A viral or autoimmune hepatitis could be excluded. Further details of this case are scant except that a kava preparation (70 mg/day kava lactones) was taken over 6 weeks. The existence of this case report became known only after the ban on kava products was instigated (and not when it occurred in August 2000). The timing of the reporting of the case casts doubt on its validity.[50]

Assessment: Unassessable due to insufficient information and poor protocol of reporting.

Case #35
Case also identified as: MCA #35, BfArM #01008989, EMEA #34

A 39-year-old man reported a tendency to bleeding and hepatitis. He was taking a kava preparation (120 mg/day of kava lactones for over 7 months) and interferon beta-1a (intramuscularly, for over 5 years until less than 1 month prior to the adverse reaction). Interferon beta-1a is associated with abnormal liver function, hepatitis, and changes in blood cell composition, and doctors are advised to monitor the liver function of patients taking this medication. The hepatic adverse reaction occurred within a reasonable time period of the last injection.[51]

Assessment: Unlikely, probably connected to concomitant medication.

Case #36
Case also identified as: MCA #36, BfArM #01009681, EMEA #35

A 45-year-old man taking a kava ethanol extract (120 mg/day of kava lactones for 3 months) experienced elevated liver enzymes. No more information is available.[52]

Assessment: Unassessable due to insufficient information.

Case #37
Case also identified as: MCA #37, BfArM #01010222, EMEA #36

A 55-year-old man receiving hypoglycaemic medication (glibenclamide, presumably taken long-term) experienced elevated liver enzymes. He had also been taking a kava and valerian product for about 1 month (30 mg of kava lactones per day). No other information is available.[53] Increased hepatic enzymes, abnormal hepatic function, cholestasis, and cholestatic hepatitis are reported side effects of sulphonylureas.[8]

Assessment: Unlikely, difficult to assess with inadequate information, and causation by concomitant medication is possible.

Case #38
Case also identified as: MCA #38, BfArM #01010536, EMEA #37

A 45-year-old slightly obese woman complained of fatigue, abdominal pains, discoloured faeces, and dark urine when admitted to hospital. She had been taking an ethanol extract of kava (45 mg of kava lactones per day for 4 months), extract of globe artichoke (*Cynara scolymus*, occasionally) and St. John's wort (*Hypericum perforatum*) prior to administration of kava. She had elevated liver enzymes and serum bilirubin and low serum pro-

tein. C-reactive protein, creatinine, and urea were within the normal range. Alcohol abuse was excluded, blood tests for infections were negative. Ultrasound examination ruled out focal lesions, hepatomegaly, portal vessel thrombosis, and blocked bile ducts. There were signs of an ascites. A biopsy was not performed. She discontinued the kava and no other treatment was administered. The patient subsequently participated in an Internet discussion involving her case to which she added that she stated she had toxic effects on the kidneys and hair loss, which were not mentioned in the hospital report.[54]

Causes of ascites include cirrhosis of the liver and protein–calorie malnutrition. The use of globe artichoke by the patient suggests she may have been self-medicating a preexisting condition such as hyperlipidaemia or poor bile flow. It is unlikely that the globe artichoke would cause the above side effects or mask a major liver problem.

Assessment: Possible, but further information required and a preexisting condition cannot be ruled out.

Case #39
Case also identified as: MCA #39, EMEA #38

A 54-year-old woman experienced gall bladder pain. She had been consuming a kava preparation over an unknown period of time. Concomitant medications taken for an unknown period of time included triamterene (diuretic), L-thyroxine, and benalapril (enalapril, angiotensin-converting enzyme [ACE] inhibitor). No further information is available regarding preexisting medical conditions or examinations of the patient. Gall bladder pain does not indicate an adverse effect on the liver, especially hepatotoxicity.[55]

Assessment: Unlikely, further information required and should not have been listed as an adverse reaction of suspected hepatotoxicity.

Case #40
Case also identified as: MCA #40, BfArM #02000370, EMEA #39

A 46-year-old woman was hospitalised with the early stages of cirrhosis of the liver. She had been taking an ethanol extract of kava for 3.5 months (providing 240 mg/day of kava lactones), contraceptives (ethinyloestradiol valerate + levonorgestrel) and cyclandelate (vasodilator). Viral and autoimmune hepatitis were eliminated. After discontinuation of all medications the patient's condition slowly improved. Hepatic adverse effects are known for contraceptive use. According to the manufacturer, the patient was occupationally exposed to mercury. The time frame of kava intake (3.5 months) is of quite a short duration for it to be responsible for liver cirrhosis. Further biochemical and histological information is required.[56]

Assessment: Unassessable due to insufficient information, occupational exposure to hepatotoxin is more likely.

Case #41
Case also identified as: MCA #41, BfArM #02001135/#02002378, EMEA #40

A 61-year-old woman died as a result of necrotic liver failure. Apart from the medications she was taking there are no other details of preexisting medical conditions or further details of the liver pathology. She was taking the following medications: a kava product (ethanol extract providing 120 mg/day of kava lactones over 3 months); multivitamin and mineral product, Ginkgo product (12.5 mg/day ginkgo flavonoids, 3 mg/day terpene lactones, for 13 months), dehydrosanol (a diuretic combination containing bemetizide and triamterene, taken for 7 days), hymecromone (spasmolytic, choleretic, taken for 10 years) and omeprazole (3 years).[57]

The diuretic combination is known to have caused rare cases of jaundice. Hepatitis and hepatic failure are documented adverse effects of omeprazole, the incidence of hepatic side effects is calculated as 2.1 cases per 100,000.[8] Omeprazole had been ingested for 3 years, long enough for an adverse event to occur. BfArM discarded omeprazole as a possible cause on the basis that an adverse event had not occurred previously during the treatment period.[57]

Assessment: Possible, but connection to concomitant medication is more likely.

Case #42
Case also identified as: MCA #42, BfArM #02001414, EMEA #41

The 46-year-old woman experienced elevated liver enzymes and jaundice. She had taken a kava product (ethanol extract providing 360 mg/day for 1 month) (this exceeds the recommended dosage). No concomitant medications were listed. Viral hepatitis and infection with EBV could be excluded, but a CMV infection could not be excluded. According to the kava manufacturer, the patient was not assessed by a gastroenterologist and the case was poorly documented.[58]

Assessment: Unassessable due to insufficient information.

Case #43
Case also identified as: MCA #43, BfArM #02001776, EMEA #42

A 27-year-old man had been taking several anti-HIV medications for an unknown time period (nevirapine, stavudine, and lamivudine) and a kava preparation (ethanol extract providing 120 mg/day of kava lactones), also for an unknown period. Reported adverse effects included discoloured faeces and urine but no overt liver symptoms. No other information, including results of laboratory analyses, is available for this case report.[59]

Even if hepatic adverse effects had been reported, these could be explained by the intake of anti-HIV medications, as each of these drugs has documented hepatic adverse events associated with their use (e.g. hepatotoxicity [nevirapine], elevated serum transaminases, hepatitis, liver failure [stavudine], and elevated liver enzymes [lamivudine]).[8] The other symptoms reported by this patient, anxiety and sweating, are also side effects associated with use of stavudine.[59]

Assessment: Unlikely, concomitant medication more likely, and uncertain if the patient suffered hepatotoxicity.

Case #44
Case also identified as: MCA #44

Information received from MCA spreadsheet

This case report of a woman of unknown age from Germany was obtained from the MCA. She consumed a kava product for a period of 1 year. The adverse reaction is listed as increased liver enzymes. No other details are recorded.

It is understood that she was anorexic and taking fluoxetine, a drug known to produce liver toxicity.[60] The timing of the kava and fluoxetine intake are unknown.

Assessment: Unassessable due to insufficient information.

Case #45
Case also identified as: MCA #45, BfArM #02002732, EMEA #44

A 24-year-old woman is reported to have experienced elevated liver enzymes and jaundice. She had taken an ethanol extract of kava (120 mg/day of kava lactones) for a period of 3 months. No other medications were listed. No other details are recorded.[61]

Assessment: Unassessable due to insufficient information.

Case #46
Case also identified as: MCA #46, BfArM #02002090/#02002836, EMEA #45

Elevated liver enzymes were found as a result of a routine check-up in response to gastrointestinal complaints by a 26-year-old obese woman. Medications other than a kava product (see below) included sulfasalazine (for 5 months), diclofenac + colestyramine (5 months), hyoscine butylbromide, contraceptive (medroxyprogesterone acetate, by injection, long-term treatment) and omeprazole (40 mg/day; probably long term) (Table 12-1).[62]

Some of the conventional drugs the patient was taking have adverse effects associated with the liver, particularly omeprazole (elevated liver enzymes, hepatitis, liver failure, and hepatic-related encephalopathy), diclofenac (elevated liver enzymes, hepatitis [including

isolated cases of fulminant hepatitis]) and sulfasalazine (hepatitis).[8,32,62,63] The dose of omeprazole as maintenance treatment in the long term (>8 weeks) is normally 20 mg/day; this patient was taking 40 mg/day.

The kava product was taken for 1 week only. The reaction is more likely to be due to omeprazole and/or diclofenac, which had been ingested over a longer period of time. Although liver parameters were normal in February 2002, diclofenac had only been resumed for 2 weeks and an adverse reaction to this drug cannot be ruled out.

Assessment: Unlikely, connection to concomitant medication is more likely.

Case #47
Case also identified as: MCA #47, BfArM #02003010, EMEA #46

BfArM received a report on 30 December 2002 of a 47-year-old woman with a range of symptoms including bilirubinaemia, elevated liver enzymes, jaundice, and liver failure. Eventually a liver transplant was scheduled. She was taking a range of products, many of which were not listed in the BfArM case report, and included: a liquid mineral supplement, amino acid complex, silymarin (constituent group of St. Mary's thistle [*Silybum marianum*]), kava, and an antirheumatic homoeopathic remedy. Despite taking this range of products for the treatment of the liver and rheumatic complaints, BfArM indicated that the patient was in perfect health prior to the reported adverse event.[64]

Results of laboratory tests were negative for hepatitis A, B, and C and there were no autoimmune antibodies present. Liver biopsy indicated fibrosis and liver cell necrosis, which may have been drug induced. Magnetic resonance imaging suggested a long-existing sclerotic transformation of liver tissue, which had started prior to the ingestion of kava.[64]

The reporting of the kava dosage varied as shown in Table 12-2.[64]

Assessment: Unlikely, more likely due to preexisting liver damage.

Table **12-1   Case #46 Medication History**

June 2001	• Diagnosed with ankylosing spondylitis
	• Started sulfasalazine + diclofenac
Oct 2001	• No deviation in liver parameters
	• Part of ongoing monitoring re: sulfasalazine therapy
End Nov 2001	• Stress with pending exam
	• Ingestion of 4-6 capsules of kava product over a 1 week period (50 mg kava lactones per capsule; ethanol extract)
2 Dec 2001	• Went to hospital and complained of unspecified abdominal pain
	• Elevated serum GPT (80 U/L); normal value: <23 U/L
4 Dec 2001	• Liver parameters reanalysed and found to be elevated:
	– Serum GPT (572 U/L)
	– Serum GOT (220; normal value: <19 U/L)
	– Serum GGT (174; normal range: 6–28 U/L)
6 Dec 2001	• Admitted to hospital with suspected toxic hepatitis
	• All medications discontinued
	• Liver parameter results:
	– Serum GPT (306 U/L)
	– Serum GOT (within normal range)
	– Serum GGT (72 U/L)
	• Laboratory tests showed negative for viral hepatitis, including EBV and CMV; autoimmune antibodies not detected
21 Dec 2001	• Discharged from hospital with normal liver parameters
25 Jan 2002	• Antirheumatic medication not taken due to upcoming exam on 25/1/02
After the exam dated 25 Jan 2002	• Sulfasalazine and diclofenac restarted
	• New gastrointestinal complaints occurred
11 Feb 2002	• Liver function parameters analysed and found to be in normal range
	• Omeprazole restarted
13 Feb 2002	• Case reported to BfArM

Case #48

Case also identified as: MCA #48, BfArM #02003278, EMEA #47

The case of a 50-year-old man with increased liver enzymes was reported to BfArM. No information is available regarding preexisting medical conditions, concomitant medication, or the reported liver disorder. He is recorded as taking an acetone extract of kava (140 mg/day of kava lactones) for 3 months.[65]

Assessment: Unassessable due to insufficient information.

Table 12-2   **Reports Showing Varied Kava Dosages**

21 Jan 2002 (phone call from GP to the manufacturer)	1 capsule per day (50 mg/day of kava lactones) for 3 months
28 Jan 2002 (phone call from GP to the manufacturer)	17 capsules per day (850 mg/day of kava lactones) for an unknown period of time
Report to BfArM by GP	2 capsules (100 mg of kava lactones) taken twice per week for approximately 4 months just prior to the adverse event report
Report to the hospital by GP	16 tablets per day, time period not specified
Report when patient admitted to the transplant centre	Up to 10 capsules per day, time period not specified

Case #49

Case also identified as: MCA #49, BfArM #02003559, EMEA #48

A similar lack of detail is available for the case of another 50-year-old man with jaundice. He had been taking an ethanol extract of kava (120 mg/day of kava lactones) for over 6 months.[66]

Assessment: Unassessable due to insufficient information.

Case #50

Case also identified as: MCA #50, BfArM #02004364, EMEA #49

A 32-year-old woman is reported to have experienced elevated liver enzymes and hepatitis. In addition to an ethanol extract of kava (240 mg/day of kava lactones for over 1 month) she had been taking a contraceptive (desogestrel + ethinyloestradiol) for an unknown period of time. Liver function may be impaired by this type of contraception. However, there is insufficient information to determine causality.[67]

Assessment: Unassessable due to insufficient information.

Case #51

Case also identified as: MCA #51, FDA #14538, EMEA #50

A 60-year-old woman experienced fatigue, urinary tract infection, and an increase in liver enzymes. She had been taking the following medications for unknown duration and in unknown dosage: a kava product, a licorice product, chaparral leaf (*Larrea tridentata*), capecitabine and fluorouracil combined (antineoplastic and immune suppressant), docusate (laxative), piperazine oestrone sulphate, and an analgesic containing paracetamol and oxycodone. The patient had a locally advanced rectal cancer and was being treated with irradiation and chemotherapy. (The Waller analysis referred to metastatic rectal cancer.) Former surgical intervention included a thoracotomy 22 years previously and a lumbar disk surgery.[3,68]

In addition to fatigue, capecitabine can cause cholestatic hepatitis, hepatitis, and hepatic fibrosis.[8] All of the conventional medications are metabolized by the liver and can be associated with liver damage. The adverse reaction report indicated only that the patient's liver function tests revealed an increase in serum bilirubin and enzymes during the course of her treatment for cancer, but the liver appeared normal by ultrasound. The patient recovered after cessation of all medications. Although the reported resumption of two of the three chemotherapy drugs resulted in no further increase in liver enzyme values, there is no indication if the dose was adjusted or if other medications were also continued.[3]

The herb chaparral is known to cause hepatotoxicity in humans. A review of 18 case reports of adverse events associated with the ingestion of chaparral reported to the FDA between 1992 and 1994 found there was evidence of hepatotoxicity in 13 cases. Jaundice with a marked increase in serum liver enzymes occurred 3 to 52 weeks after the ingestion of chaparral.[69]

Assessment: Unlikely, more likely due to concomitant medication.

Case #52

Case also identified as: MCA #52, FDA #14723, EMEA #51

A 44-year-old woman suddenly suffered from chest and back pain during a medical checkup following an aortic dissection and a descending thoracic aneurysm resection. The routine laboratory examination showed an increase of lipase and LFTs and neutropenia. The treating physicians diagnosed the liver incident as a consequence of the recent surgical interventions which led to a focal ischaemia in the liver (also known as shock liver). Blood work also indicated signs of a possible viral hepatitis. The neutropenia was discussed as possibly drug-related; however, it was stated that such effects might occur with ingestion of virtually any drug. A connection to kava was not established.

However, when the report was filed by the pharmacist, the event was described as a symptom-free neutropenia, possibly connected to the intake of kava and B vitamins, whereas warfarin, celecoxib, oxycodon, citalopram, and an oestrogen patch were indicated as co-medication. Increases of liver enzyme activity are labelled for the antidepressant citalopram, the anticoagulant warfarin, and the antiinflammatory drug celecoxib.[3,70]

Assessment: Unrelated, diagnosed as a surgery-related ischaemic hepatitis (shock liver).

Case #53

Case also identified as: MCA #53, FDA #14810, EMEA #52

A 33-year-old woman is listed with several adverse effects including jaundiced skin, nausea, diarrhoea, and easy bruising. She was prepared for possible liver transplant. She had received chemotherapy for lymphoma 1 month prior to admission. Her medications included: unnamed chemotherapy, ranitidine

hydrochloride, echinacea/golden seal, an energy product containing ginseng, B100 (vitamin B?) and guarana; TUMS (calcium supplement?), a contraceptive (norethindrone acetate + ethinyloestradiol), women's vitamins and juices. The first case report also mentioned the intake of nizatidine. After detailed analysis of the labels of the products taken by the patient, the original report was corrected: there was no intake of nizatidine, kava was not a component of the herbal medicines taken by the patient, which in fact were a combination of golden seal (*Hydrastis canadensis*) and echinacea (*Echinacea* spp.), and a combination of ginseng, guarana (*Paullinia cupana*), and B vitamins. Hepatic adverse effects are known for ranitidine and are likely for the unknown chemotherapy.[71]

Assessment: Unrelated as no kava was ingested.

Case #54

Case also identified as: MCA #54, FDA #15035/ #15274, EMEA #53

A 45-year-old woman reported jaundice, pruritus, and cholestatic hepatitis, and successfully received a liver transplant. She had been taking a herbal extract containing kava, hops (*Humulus lupulus*), German chamomile (*Matricaria chamomilla*), and passionflower (*Passiflora incarnata*) for between 2 and 4 months with no intake on weekends. The daily dose of kava lactones corresponded to 150 mg. Concomitant medication included rabeprazole (proton pump inhibitor, structurally similar to omeprazole) taken for four consecutive days, only days before the onset of the incident. Pre-existing medical conditions included reflux and she indicated she had no allergies to food or drugs.

The patient consumed a very small amount of alcohol on rare occasions. Results were negative for viral hepatitis (A, B, C). Adverse effects on the liver are known for omeprazole and a case of liver failure has been documented for a patient taking rabeprazole and an antifungal medication (terbinafine).[63,72] The FDA was reported to be particularly concerned about this case, which was also investigated by the U.S. Centers for Disease Control and

Prevention (CDC).[73] The CDC investigation suggested that the rabeprazole was prescribed after the patient presented with nausea and weakness (and possible liver damage from her herbal preparation) and was only continued for 4 days.

The identity of the herbal components of the suspected medication was not analytically confirmed, even though a potential adulteration was discussed by the toxicologists. The FDA obtained a sample of the product for chemical analysis but the results are not known.[3] In the course of the follow-up, only kava was discussed as a possible cause, based on the current discussion of potential hepatic effects. The effects of the other herbal components and of rabeprazol were not considered.

Additional follow-up information was obtained for this case but it raises further questions, because of discrepancies between the physician's original report and information obtained in the follow-up. The discrepancies mainly concern the duration of a preexisting condition and the dosage and duration of kava intake (half the recommended dose for 8 weeks versus 2 tablets for about 4 months [as indicated above]).

Assessment: Possible, but concomitant medication cannot be ruled out as a cause.

Case #55
Case also identified as: MCA #55, FDA #15250, EMEA #54

A female obese patient (225 lb/102 kg) of unknown age herself reported to the FDA that high liver enzymes and a fatty liver occurred as adverse effects, detected by routine laboratory work and subsequent examination. The patient had taken a kava product with 30 mg kava lactones per day over a period of 2 years. Concomitant medication included a multivitamin preparation. Preexisting issues included environmental allergies, allergy-related asthma, excess weight, and moderate alcohol consumption.

A connection of the fatty liver and, as a consequence, elevated LFTs with kava is highly questionable. Obesity in middle-aged women is recognised as an infrequent, but major, cause

of subsequent nondrug-induced liver failure. In addition, neither the discussed liver cases within this review nor the observations from traditional medicine indicate that kava intake might lead to fatty liver, which, however, would have to be expected in obesity.[74]

Assessment: Unassessable due to insufficient information.

Case #56
Case also identified as: MCA #56, FDA #15281, EMEA #55

The case report of a 27-year-old woman includes a range of symptoms: jaundice, nausea, vomiting, ascites, abdominal pain, and elevated liver enzymes with possibly stage 3 hepatic encephalopathy. Her medications included two kava products (taken for 6 months), psyllium (*Plantago ovata*), vitamins B_6 and E, St. John's wort (*Hypericum perforatum*) extract and a phyto-oestrogen containing Mexican yam (species undefined), black cohosh (*Cimicifuga racemosa*) and dong quai (*Angelica sinensis*, taken for 4 months). The case details from the FDA indicate that "other aetiologies [were] excluded"; however, no further details are provided. An abdominal hysterectomy is listed as a preexisting medical condition. The MCA assessment indicates that alcohol had not been consumed in over 5 years.[75] Apparently, no analysis of the components of the "Sleepy tea" herbal mixture and the kava monopreparation were made.

Assessment: Possible, but connection to kava is not proven due to insufficient information and unknown composition of the concomitantly ingested product, and a preexisting problem cannot be ruled out.

Case #57
Case also identified as: MCA #57, FDA #15317, EMEA #56

Hepatitis was listed as an adverse effect in the case report of a 38-year-old man who ingested kava (product details unknown, duration unknown) in a binge once or twice per month. Eight capsules of 250 mg (presumably of kava extract) were taken. He also used St. John's wort extract. He drank alcohol regularly (three to four glasses of wine per week). No other medications or preexisting medical conditions were described. Within the case documentation of the FDA, liver infection was documented as the cause of the hepatitis, even though, according to the line-listing of the MCA, but not to the case documentation of the FDA, negative results were obtained for hepatitis A, B, and C.[1,76] The information provided is unclear: Did a liver infection occur at the time of reporting or did it exist as an earlier event?

Assessment: Unassessable due to insufficient information.

Case #58
Case also identified as: MCA #58, FDA #15319, EMEA #57

A 63-year-old man experienced nausea, haematemesis, hepatitis C, and hepatocellular liver injury. He had been taking a product which contained kava, magnesium orotate, and additional herbs for a period of 6 weeks. Hypertension was listed as a pre-existing medical condition and he had been taking enalapril maleate (ACE inhibitor) and hydrochlorothiazide (a thiazide diuretic) which was started 5 months prior to the kava intake.[77]

Thiazides can produce occasional cases of cholecystitis or icterus and ACE inhibitors can cause hepatotoxicity. The likely cause, however, was hepatitis C.[77]

Assessment: Unlikely, more likely due to preexisting medical conditions.

Case #59
Case also identified as: MCA #59, FDA #15466, EMEA #58

A 39-year-old woman experienced fatigue, influenza-like symptoms, jaundice, and hepatitis. She had been taking a kava product (which contained 70 mg of kava lactones per unit) and drinking a tea containing kava with 36 mg kava lactones per day, which totals 106 mg kava lactones per day for 6 months. Her liver function

parameters returned to normal within 4 weeks. Preexisting medical conditions included asthma and allergies to dust and animal dander. Concomitant medications included a contraceptive (undefined), tetracycline (2 times, including once right before the adverse effects), salbutamol (as needed), diphenhydramine, and undefined over-the-counter (OTC) drugs. Tetracycline is known to cause hepatic adverse effects and as the adverse reaction occurred right after the second intake, it may have been responsible. As information regarding the hepatitis, history of alcohol intake, and concomitant medications is lacking, an association to kava intake cannot be made.[78]

Assessment: Unlikely, more likely due to concomitant medication.

Case #60
Case also identified as: MCA #60, FDA #14951, EMEA #59

A 51-year-old woman was reported with elevated liver enzymes. She had been taking an undefined kava product for a period of 4 months. Other medications included: vitamin D, fish oil, multivitamin and mineral supplement, omega-3 and ginkgo extract. The patient had also complained of foot cramping. The symptoms reportedly ceased upon discontinuation of the kava product. No further information was provided regarding the dosage of the other medications or regarding her liver.[79]

Assessment: Unassessable due to insufficient information.

Case #61
Case also identified as: MCA #61, FDA #14995, EMEA #60

A 37-year-old woman experienced jaundice and fatty infiltration of the liver. She had taken a kava product (150 mg/day of kava lactones) at more than 2.5 times the recommended dosage for a period of 3–4 weeks. Other medications included: two homoeopathic remedies, various multivitamin, mineral and herbal products, bovine colostrum (to counter underweight and malabsorption syndrome), and a four-product "suite" with fish oil, additional minerals, vitamins, enzymes, and diverse herbal extracts (mountain mahogany leaves [*Cerocarpus montanus*], ragweed [*Ambrosia artemisifolia*], golden seal [*Hydrastis canadensis*], quince seed [*Cydonia oblonga*], boldo leaves [*Peumus boldus*], spearmint leaves, rose hips [*Rosa canina*], sete sangrias [*Cuphea* spp.], red beet [*Beta vulgaris*], and cha de bugre [*Cordia salicifolia*]) for 6 weeks until 1 week prior to the adverse event. She was underweight. Given this range of products it is likely that there are more preexisting conditions than were recorded. Alcohol intake was denied.[80]

None of the herbal extracts ingested in this case is known to cause adverse liver effects. However, several of the ingested plants are uncommon as medicinal plants, therefore the lack of data concerning hepatic effects does not automatically imply that they are harmless. Vitamin A was ingested in a dosage of approximately 7500 IU/day, which surpasses the U.S. Recommended Dietary Allowance (RDA) by 150% and is in a dosage range with potential adverse liver effects.

Assessment: Unassessable due to insufficient information.

Case #62
Case also identified as: MCA #62, FDA #15252, EMEA #61

A female of unknown age reported the following adverse effects to the FDA: fatigue, nausea, vomiting, and extremely elevated liver function parameters. She took a kava product (150 to 225 mg/day of kava lactones) for a period of 3 months. Other medications included a green tea formula containing green tea (*Camellia sinensis*), bitter orange peel (*Citrus aurantium*), Siberian ginseng (*Eleutherococcus senticosus*), fenugreek (*Trigonella foenum-graecum*), guarana (*Paullinia cupana*), kola (*Cola nitida*), ginger (*Zingiber officinale*), licorice (*Glycyrrhiza glabra*), additional caffeine, vanadium amino acid chelate, and chromium dinicotinate glycinate; coenzyme Q10 and a product called Snorease (containing bitter orange, coenzyme

Q10 and bromelain). There was no previous medical history of liver problems, alcohol intake was denied. According to the labelling, fatigue and nausea are also observed with the intake of coenzyme Q10 products, and nausea and vomiting with the intake of bromelain.

There is no information regarding the self-reported "extremely elevated LFTs", virus serology, or other preexisting medical conditions or intake of orthodox drugs.[1,81]

Assessment: Unassessable due to insufficient information.

Case #63
Case also identified as: MCA #63, FDA #15267, EMEA #62

This adverse reaction report involved a 51-year-old woman who experienced elevated liver enzymes, which reportedly returned to normal after ceasing intake of kava, ginkgo (*Ginkgo biloba*) extract, ginseng extract, St. John's wort (*Hypericum perforatum*) extract, vitamins A, D, and E, a calcium/magnesium complex and MSM (methylsulphonylmethane, a supplement generally used to treat arthritis). The duration of use of kava was listed as 2 months. There is no additional information regarding alcohol intake, dosage of these products (especially vitamin A which may effect the liver in high doses), virus serology, and preexisting medical conditions (did she have, for example, an arthritic condition which was, or had been, treated with conventional drugs?).[3,82]

Assessment: Unassessable due to insufficient information.

Case #64
Case also identified as: MCA #64, EMEA #63

Nausea and elevated serum gamma-glutamyl transpeptidase (GGT) was experienced by a 60-year-old woman who had been taking a kava product for at least 1 year at an unknown dosage. The patient recovered after stopping kava. No concomitant medications were stated.[83] Without further information regarding preexisting and previous medical conditions, as well as concomitant medications, it is not possible to associate kava with the cause of the adverse reaction.

Assessment: Unassessable due to insufficient information. Moreover, elevated GGT has been recorded after kava intake, but is not necessarily indicative of hepatotoxicity.

Case #65
Case also identified as: MCA #65, EMEA #64

A 39-year-old woman experienced increased transaminases. She had taken a kava product for a period of 2 months. Concomitant medication was not specified but "may cause hepatotoxicity".[84]

Assessment: Unlikely, more likely due to concomitant medication and/or preexisting medical condition.

Case #66
Case also identified as: MCA #66, EMEA #65

A female of unknown age experienced abnormal hepatic function. She had taken a kava product in the long term. Concomitant medication and outcome are unknown.

Assessment: Unassessable due to insufficient information.

Case #67
Case also identified as: MCA #67, EMEA #66

Abnormal liver function test results and jaundice were recorded as adverse effects in a 53-year-old woman. She had taken a kava product, St. John's wort (*Hypericum perforatum*), and multivitamins for an unknown period of time. The patient recovered after ceasing intake of "kava and other herbal preparations". The patient had a history of inflammation of the liver and at the time she had been drinking 6 beers per day. She stated that she has not been drinking since then. There is no further information regarding viral or autoimmune aetiologies.[85]

Assessment: Unassessable due to insufficient information.

Case #68
Case also identified as: MCA #68, EMEA #67

A 38-year-old man reported increased transaminases and hepatitis. There is no information regarding preexisting medical conditions, concomitant medication, or other medical information regarding his liver function and histology. According to the MCA, no other drugs were taken. He had been taking a kava product in the very low dose of 24 drops/day for a period of 2 weeks.[86]

Assessment: Unassessable due to insufficient information, but unlikely, due to the low dose taken and short duration of intake.

Case #69
Case also identified as: BfArM #02005178

Liver cell damage and liver damage was experienced by a woman of unknown age. She had taken a kava product (70 mg/day of kava lactones) for over 2 months. No other information is available.[87]

Assessment: Unassessable due to insufficient information.

Case #70
Case also identified as: BfArM #02002541

A 52-year-old woman experienced elevated transaminases. She had been taking a kava product (60 mg/day of kava lactones) for 3.5 months. No other information is provided.[88]

Assessment: Unassessable due to insufficient information.

Case #71
Case also identified as: FDA #14627
Lit: Humbertston et al, 2001

A 14-year-old girl was admitted to hospital with fulminant hepatic failure and received a liver transplant. Biopsy indicated necrosis consistent with drug-induced hepatitis. The LFTs were markedly elevated. Alternative causes of liver failure were negative. She had taken a herbal tea with vitamin C, vitamin B$_6$, vitamin B$_{12}$, a blend of Siberian ginseng root (*Eleutherococcus senticosus*), chamomile (*Matricaria chamomilla*), and kava root (equivalent to 60 mg of kava extract, standardised to 30% kava lactones), plus a mixture of peppermint leaves (*Mentha piperita*), cinnamon (*Cinnamomum zeylanicum*), lemon grass (*Cymbopogon* spp.), ginger root (*Zingiber officinalis*), licorice root (*Glycyrrhiza glabra*), natural lemon flavour and other natural flavours, roasted chicory root (*Cichorium intybus*) and catnip leaves (*Nepeta cataria*). Ingestion was stated as 2 tea bags per day (the FDA actually speaks of tablets, which is impossible as both stated brands are exclusively marketed in the form of tea bags), corresponding to 36 mg of kava lactones per day for seven consecutive days in August 2000. Between September and December 2000, she took another brand of herbal tea containing a blend of chamomile flowers (*Matricaria chamomilla*), Tilia estrella flowers (*Ternstroemia pringlei*), valerian root (*Valeriana officinalis*) and kava root, plus spearmint leaves, lemon grass (*Cymbopogon* spp.), hawthorn berries (*Crataegus monogyna*), and orange blossoms (*Citrus* spp.). This product was ingested in a dosage of two tea bags per day for a period of 44 days in total. The nature of the kava preparation in the tea (extract or powder, standardisation?) is not known.[89] As a concomitant medication, the occasional use of ibuprofen was stated (which has been linked to hepatotoxic reactions[8]). The intake of alcohol was denied. Virus serology and testing for autoantibodies were negative.

The FDA was reported to be particularly concerned about this case, which probably explains why the CDC also investigated this case further.[73] The CDC reported that the patient was in fact taking capsule versions of these products (which is definitively wrong), but that the other product ingredients (other than kava) were unknown to them.

According to the published case report, the causality of kava is supported by the circumstances. However, the products ingested had further components, which were not taken into consideration as potential causative agents. In addition, ibuprofen can also induce adverse hepatic effects as a class reaction to NSAIDs.[90]

Assessment : Possible, but the potential causative role of ibuprofen and the other herbal product components require further investigation.

Case #72
Lit: Stuckhard P., 2002

The case of a 43-year-old woman requiring a liver transplant was reported to a German newspaper.[91] It was apparently not reported to BfArM. She had supposedly taken a kava product at the recommended dosage for 6 weeks. Concomitant medication included St. John's wort (*Hypericum perforatum*), an iodine compound for the thyroid, and a beta-blocker.[92] See Table 12-3 for full chronological details of this patient's case.

The patient reported in a newspaper report that she was not sure whether the liver function test was indeed conducted in January 2001. The surgery she underwent earlier may have contributed, due to the use of anaesthesia which can cause liver problems. There is insufficient information to link this case to kava ingestion. Kava was not even taken before the first symptoms were presented. The original treating physician and physicians at three different hospitals were unable to find the cause.[92]

Assessment : Unlikely, more likely due to preexisting medical conditions.

Case #73
Lit: Hinzpeter W., 2002

The case of a 60-year-old woman was reported to the German media.[42] It was apparently not reported to BfArM. Liver failure with subsequent liver transplant were the reported adverse effects. She had reportedly taken a kava product at the recommended dosage for 3 months. There is no other information available.[93]

Assessment : Unassessable due to insufficient information.

Case #74
Case also identified as: FDA #10257

A 70-year-old woman with a long history of coronary heart disease was hospitalised for stroke and a prolapsed mitral value. During the course of her stay it was noted that some of her liver function parameters (GOT and GGT) were elevated by a factor of 2 to 3. She had been taking a multicompound preparation containing

Table **12-3   Details of Case #72**

End of 2000	• Patient underwent surgery for unknown reasons
	• Patient stated she never really recovered from the surgery in that she suffered fatigue and depression
Jan 2001	• Her physician conducted a urine and blood test (which reportedly included liver parameters)
	• Thyroid gland examined
	• Physician gave her sample packets of kava and St. John's wort
12 Jan 2001	• Patient presented complaining of fatigue
	• Reportedly her physician confirmed that the liver values were normal
	• Her physician prescribed the iodine preparation at a dosage of 1 tablet/week as a preventive measure, although the results of the thyroid tests were not yet available
20 Feb 2001	• Patient's health worsened, even after the first dose of the thyroid tablet she reported nausea, increased heart rate and erythema on her breast
	• Physician told her to discontinue the iodine preparation and prescribed a beta-blocker
22 Feb 2001	• Patient's health state worsened, she passed discoloured urine, her eyes were yellow
	• According to the patient this time the liver values "were really examined" and showed abnormality
	• Physician assumed a viral hepatitis
Several days later	• Patient visited a different physician and after a liver function test was admitted to hospital
	• Cause unknown but viral hepatitis was excluded
13 Mar 2001	• Patient scheduled for liver transplant

kava for an undisclosed time period: Herbalife K8 with "kava kava 40 mg " and "Biokawa 20 mg " containing 14.3% kavain, 15 mg DL-phenylalanine, 30 mg L-tryptophan, unknown amounts of extracts from alfalfa (*Medicago sativa*), ginger (*Zingiber officinale*), hops (*Humulus lupulus*), valerian (*Valeriana officinalis*), vervain (*Verbena officinalis*), and Yerba santa (*Eriodictyon californicum*). Concomitant medication included: propranolol (long term), aspirin (long term), fish oil and several vitamins (she described herself as a "vitamin freak"). When the patient was admitted, warfarin and lisinopril were prescribed to counter blood thickening (this was after the onset of the increased transaminases).

The case was filed as an adverse drug effect because the patient was thought to have suffered a blood thickening effect caused by ingestion of a vitamin K product. The ingested product later turned out not to contain vitamin K, but the above-mentioned mixture of herbs. The elevated transaminases were detected by routine laboratory analyses.

Elevated liver values and hepatitis are known and recorded for propranolol. Aspirin is known to produce increase of transaminases and is documented as causing impaired liver function in individual cases. Elevated transaminases are considered a class reaction of NSAIDs and are usually transient without treatment.

The herbs presumedly ingested are unlikely to cause adverse liver reactions, whereas the ingestion of high doses of fish oil is known to produce transient elevations of the liver enzymes as a nonpathological reaction pattern. During her hospitalisation her serum GOT fluctuated and increased despite the discontinuation of the herbal product.[94]

There is no information regarding possible exclusion of virus, autoimmune, or alcohol-induced hepatitis. It is unclear when the elevated liver enzymes occurred.

Assessment: Unassessable due to insufficient information.

Case #75
Case also identified as: FDA #11444

A 24-year-old man was hospitalised with hepatic encephalopathy and fulminant hepatic failure, and subsequently died. The patient, who was a body builder, denied the intake of steroidal hormones. He was taking a product "suite" with more than 121 components (which included vitamins, minerals, diverse herbals, enzymes, "vitaminoids" and basic nutrients, amongst which kava was part of a herbal blend [quality, form, and amount unknown]) until 3 weeks prior to the hospital admission. However, the symptoms were already present 3 weeks before the discontinuation of the products. According to the hospital's physician, the first symptoms of illness started after 2 months of exposure to the medication, with a 6-week history of feeling malaised and tired. Hepatitis A and B could be excluded. Hepatitis C testing was negative, but not entirely excluded. Blood chemistry showed elevated liver function parameters.[95]

The product HG1, for which ma huang (Herba Ephedrae) was indicated on the label, was analysed for ephedrine content. The tablets contained 3.3 mg of ephedrine per tablet. The OTC medications and formulas were reviewed by medical toxicologists; however, they were unable to find any specific aetiology for the liver failure. According to the evaluation, none of the ingredients of the formulas and OTC medications were suspected of causing fulminant liver failure, with the exception of an unconfirmed case of hepatotoxicity by ma huang (Herba Ephedrae). This, however, is only correct for the ingredients of the products within their single dosage as indicated on the labels. It should have been taken into account that the same ingredients were found in several of the products. The recommended U.S. RDAs were, in several cases, exceeded by the factor of several 100%, thus changing the overall picture, especially for trace minerals such as chromium. The evaluation of heavy metal toxicity by the hospital's toxicologists was aimed at typical liver toxins (arsenic, bismuth, mercury). As could be expected, this analysis yielded a negative result. However, it was not directed on the ingredients of the formulas, especially the grossly overdosed ones. The determination of chromium might have given another result.

Among the minerals taken, manganese overdosage (taken in a dosage of 21 mg/day, surpassing the U.S. recommendation by the factor of 10) might have contributed to the liver failure according to the literature. Vanadium, taken in a dosage of 34 mg/day clearly surpassed the dosage range considered as safe. In addition, chromium intake in a dosage scheme of 1.3 mg/day extremely surpassed the recommended safe upper limit of 250 μg. Hepatitis and abnormal liver function parameters are known as a reaction to the intake of corresponding amounts of chromium.

Among the vitamins, the intake of niacin in a dosage scheme corresponding 1000% of the U.S. RDA (200 mg/day) might also have contributed to the incident, as highly dosed niacin may cause hepatitis. The same is true for vitamin A, which was taken in a dosage scheme of 20,000 IU per day, surpassing the RDA by 400%.

The herbal drugs ingested included white willow (*Salix alba*), lettuce (*Lactuca sativa*), hawthorn (*Crataegus* spp.), peppermint (*Mentha piperita*), guarana, cayenne (*Capsicum frutescens, C. annuum*), raspberry (*Rubus idaeus*), rosemary (*Rosmarinus officinalis*), chamomile (*Matricaria chamomilla*), Chinese yam (*Dioscorea batatas*), ginseng (*Panax ginseng*), passionflower (*Passiflora incarnata*), aloe (*Aloe vera*), rose hips (*Rosa canina*), horsetail (*Equisetum arvense*), ginkgo (*Ginkgo biloba*), garlic (*Allium sativum*), borage oil (*Borago officinalis*), wheat grass (*Triticum* spp.), barley grass (*Hordeum* spp.), bilberry (*Vaccinium myrtillus*), green tea (*Camellia sinensis*), golden seal (*Hydrastis canadensis*), Echinacea (*Echinacea* spp.), parsley (*Petroselinum crispum*), valerian (*Valeriana officinalis*) and spirulina, which are not known to cause liver problems. Samsara (*Bidens ferulifolia*) and saussurea (*Saussurea* spp.) do not seem to be well investigated.

One case of jaundice induced by *p*-aminobenzoic acid was published in 1967,[95] and a 1986 review of 390 patients indicated that acute hepatic reaction to potassium *p*-aminobenzoate is at least uncommon if not rare.[96]

This incident was filed as a liver failure with unknown aetiology, possibly caused by hepatis C virus infection. However, a closer examination also shows other possible causes, among these iron in combination with a possible hepatitis C, chromium, vanadium, vitamin A, niacin, ephedra and *p*-aminobenzoic acid qualify at least as suspicious factors. A causality of kava was never proposed and, under the given circumstances, would be rather questionable.

Assessment: Unlikely, probably caused by chromium/vanadium or niacin toxicity.

Case #76
Case also identified as: FDA #13198

This adverse reaction report involved a 52-year-old woman who was hospitalised for treatment of congestive heart failure, acute renal failure, anasarca (generalised oedema) with weight gain, hyperkalaemia, and metabolic alkalosis. A biopsy confirmed liver cirrhosis. She had taken a kava preparation occasionally. Concomitant medication included regular intake of MSM (methylsulphonylmethane), a "green" product with spirulina, dry wheat grass juice (*Triticum* spp.), sprouted barley juice (*Hordeum* spp.), flaxseed/linseed oil (*Linum usitatissimum*), chlorella, bee pollen, ginseng (*Panax ginseng*), garlic (*Allium sativum*), Echinacea (*Echinacea* spp.), St. Mary's thistle (*Silybum marianum*), golden seal (*Hydrastis canadensis*), ginger root (*Zingiber officinalis*), ginkgo (*Ginkgo biloba*), cayenne (*Capsicum frutescens*), vitamins (unknown kind and amounts), minerals (unknown kind and amounts), bioflavonoids, enzymes, a multiglandular product, alfalfa and an amino acid/vitamins/mineral complex.

Occasional intake of a nettle (*Urtica dioica*) extract, an OTC product with grapefruit extract, glucomannan, vitamin B_6, lecithin, kelp, cider vinegar, uva ursi (*Arctostaphylos uva-ursi*) extract and L-phenylalanine, a St. Mary's thistle (*Silybum marianum*) seed extract, herbal sleeping tablets with valerian (*Valeriana* spp.) extract, passionflower (*Passiflora incarnata*),

celery seed (*Apium graveolens*), catnip (*Nepeta cataria*), hops (*Humulus lupulus*) and dried orange peel (*Citrus aurantium*), a coenzyme Q10 product with bioperine, "water pills" with buchu (*Agathosma betulina*), uva-ursi (*Arctostaphylos uva-ursi*), parsley (*Petroselinum crispum*), juniper berries (*Juniperus communis*) and potassium 120 mg, a lactobacillus/bifidobacterium combination product, an immune stimulating product with additional vitamins, minerals, gland extracts, enzymes and herbs, four different "antiallergic" homoeopathic multicomponent products, guaifenesin, and sodium cromoglycate. The patient had a history of hyperthyroidism and exposure to hepatitis C. Her alcohol intake was 1 to 2 drinks per day with binge drinking on weekends.[97]

Hepatitis A and B antibodies were negative. The products ingested point to a number of otherwise unknown preexisting medical conditions, among others allergies, liver problems, and a recent cold.

On closer inspection, none of the ingredients of the range of formulas would seem sufficiently suspicious as a causative agent in liver disease. Kava was never suspected by the FDA; in addition, the frequency of intake of the kava product was only indicated as "occasionally". With regard to the general health status, the hepatitis C infection, and the binge drinking of alcohol there is a high probability that kava had no part in the evolution of this liver failure.

Assessment: Unlikely, more likely due to alcohol intake with possible involvement of preexisting medical conditions.

Case #77
Case also identified as: FDA #15465; possible duplicate case FDA #15476 (listed together)

A 48-year-old man experienced what was described as liver pain. He had taken an undefined kava product for a period of 1 to 2 days at a dosage of 1 to 2 units (capsules/tablets not defined). A preexisting liver dysfunction was noted, which was later specified as hepatitis C.[98] The patient already had elevated liver function parameters prior to taking kava due to the hepatitis C, and after the kava ingestion the LFTs were not checked. From the nature and paucity of the information presented on this case it is a wonder it was ever recorded as an adverse reaction associated with kava.

Assessment: Unlikely, more likely due to preexisting medical condition (hepatitis C).

Case #78
Case also identified as: FDA #15556

A 72-year-old man himself reported to the FDA that he believed kava had aggravated a preexisting liver problem. He had taken a kava product for 2 weeks. Previous medical history included liver damage by hepatitis C. Concomitant medication included valerian.[99] This also should not have been recorded as an adverse reaction to kava when liver damage was already known.

Assessment: Unlikely, more likely due to preexisting medical conditions.

Case #79
Case also identified as: FDA #15249

A 53-year-old man himself reported to the FDA that he had experienced pain in the liver area. He indicated episodical kava ingestion for several years. He filed the report as he had heard of the investigation of the FDA regarding liver effects of kava. He had taken a kava product for 2 days, once on the day the adverse reaction occurred and again on an unknown occasion. In both cases he stated a "distinct painful sensation in the liver area". Following this incident, the patient took kava products of other manufacturers without any problem. Preexisting medical conditions included allergies and no concomitant medication was stated.[100]

Assessment: Should not have been included as there is no evidence of liver damage.

Case #80
Case also identified as: FDA #15320

Acute liver failure was experienced in a 41-year-old woman on 9 May 1999, which led to a liver transplant 11 days later. She had been taking an ethanol extract of kava for an unknown period of time at unknown dosage. Concomitant medications included: loratadine (antihistamine, taken for 3 months prior to the adverse event), St. John's wort powder (*Hypericum perforatum*, taken from 21 January 1999 until the day of the event), contraceptive containing ethinyloestradiol and an infusion of hypericin dissolved in 0.9% sodium chloride for phototherapy. In March 1999, the patient started loratadine for the treatment of an allergic reaction to the intravenous application of hypericin, taking a total of 160 mg loratadine over a 6-day period. After this allergic episode, the patient orally ingested St. John's wort until the day of the hepatic diagnosis.

There are case reports of hepatic adverse reactions to loratadine.[101] However, the intake occurred only for 6 days, 3 months prior to the incident. Contraceptives containing ethinyloestradiol are associated with hepatic adverse events, including hepatitis.[12] There is a lack of information regarding the liver failure and alcohol intake.

The effect of the administration of intravenous hypericin and oral St. John's wort extract on this patient's liver is not known. Phototoxic (skin) reactions to hypericin (a constituent of St. John's wort) have been noted in humans, usually from injection of hypericin or oral administration of high quantities of hypericin. Mild reversible liver enzyme elevations were recorded in some patients receiving St. John's wort extract. (Refer to the St. John's wort safety monograph.)

Assessment: Possible, but may not be due to kava alone, intravenous administration of hypericin may have contributed.

Case #81
Case also identified as: BfArM #02007130

A 38-year-old woman showed symptoms of an acute liver failure, but recovered. She had taken an ethanolic kava extract with 120 mg kava lactones per day over a period of at least 4 weeks for the treatment of anxiety. There was no co-medication stated. Nothing is known on preexisting medical conditions, virus serology, alcohol intake, or other relevant risk factors of liver disease.

Assessment : Unassessable due to insufficient information.

Case #82
Case also identified as: FDA #15564

An overweight patient (231 lb, 96 kg) of unknown age experienced hepatitis and liver cirrhosis, and ultimately died from fulminant liver failure. The patient did not smoke, and the relatives denied alcohol intake. His medication consisted of about 25 dietary supplements including herbals and minerals, among others magnesium (regularly taken every 2 hours), valerian (*Valeriana officinalis*), and saw palmetto (*Sabal serrulata*). In addition, an occasional intake of kava (exact preparation unknown) with 50 to 100 tablets over 1 year was stated. As preexisting medical conditions, polycythema rubra vera, arthralgia, and anxiety were mentioned. According to the relatives, the patient did not use steroid-type drugs.

Liver biopsy showed micronodular cirrhosis. No further information is available, especially on concomitant medication and further examinations such as virus serology or autoimmune antibody screening. The patient himself suggested the causality of kava, as during the hospitalisation he found references to the kava discussion on the Internet.

Assessment : Unassessable due to insufficient information.

Case #83
Case also identified as: ADRS #177303

A 56-year-old woman experienced symptoms of fatigue, jaundice, and hepatic necrosis. She died as a result of complications of liver failure during a liver transplant operation. She had been taking five separate complementary medicines for a period of 4 months: vitamin E; a vitamin B/mineral complex with chromium, B-group vitamins, calcium, magnesium, zinc and manganese; vitamin C, selenium; a combination of amino acids, vitamins and minerals; and a product labelled to contain kava with 60 mg kava lactones per tablet, passionflower (*Passiflora incarnata*), and supposedly skullcap (*Scutellaria lateriflora*).[60] Daily dosage unknown,

duration of intake for all mentioned drugs was approximately 3 to 4 months. Prior to taking these she had been taking several other complementary medicines (details of which were not disclosed by the Australian TGA) for about 3 months. She had not been taking any prescribed medicines, and drank only a minimal amount of alcohol. On admission, she had markedly abnormal liver function tests, with highly elevated transaminases, and elevations of bilirubin, alkaline phosphatase, and GGT. Liver biopsy showed a severe acute hepatitis with confluent necrosis, consistent with a viral or drug aetiology.[102]

According to the information in the ADRS line listing, the patient had a past infection or had been immunised with hepatitis A antigen. The case was subsequently reported in the *Medical Journal of Australia*. Assays for acute hepatitis A, B, and C viruses, Epstein–Barr virus, and cytomegalovirus were all negative. She had been previously well, except for a history of benign monoclonal gammopathy which had been diagnosed 12 months previously.[103] Monoclonal gammopathy is not connected to the occurrence of fulminant liver failure; however, heteroclonal gammopathy is. The correct diagnosis in this case has to be taken for granted.

Testing by the TGA of the suspected kava product confirmed the presence of kava and passionflower, but *Scutellaria lateriflora* was not detected. The identity of the third ingredient remains to be established. The presence of some other herbs reported to be hepatotoxic has been excluded.[102] Two independent analyses[104,105] of three batch samples of this product indicated that *Scutellaria lateriflora* was not present; however, the nature of the adulterants could not be established to date. Skullcap was possibly exchanged for the hepatotoxic *Teucrium* species (e.g. *T. chamaedrys*, one of the species commonly known as germander). This is an accidental adulteration frequently observed for this plant. Given the unknown composition of the kava-containing product, it is not possible to conclusively associate kava with the causality.

Chromium was also ingested amongst the complementary medicines she had been taking. Chromium may have contributed to hepatotoxicity.[106,107]

Assessment : Possible, but link to kava not established due to an unknown constituent of the kava-containing product. Previous medical conditions need closer examination given the mention of gammopathy, hepatitis A, and the apparent lack of information regarding other pathogens.

CRITICAL OVERVIEW OF THE EVIDENCE SUPPORTING AN HEPATOTOXIC REACTION FROM KAVA

Ideally, the investigation of an adverse drug reaction should result in some attribution of causality. Many schemes for classification of causality have been proposed in different countries. Table 12-4 outlines a recent scheme that is gaining popularity.[108]

Using this assessment, the CSM determined the classification of the 68 cases included in their analysis (#1 to #68), as described in Table 12-5.[1,4]

The above criteria for assessment were not universally applied. A comparative assessment of causality by three different government regulatory bodies of 16 (German and Swiss) cases, as described in Table 12-6, illustrates the differing assessments made. Note that many cases described as probable by the BfArM were rated as only possible or even given lower ratings (such as not assessable) by other authorities.[109]

In the Schmidt review shown in Table 12-7 the causal assessments were assigned for 80 cases (duplicates excluded).

In other words, only three cases could be attributed to kava with a high probability.

Table **12-4** **A Scheme Defining Causality Assessment of Suspected Adverse Drug Reactions**

Criteria	Assessment
Certain	• A clinical event, including a laboratory test abnormality, that occurs in a plausible time relation to drug administration, and which cannot be explained by concurrent disease or other drugs or chemicals
	• The response to withdrawal of the drug (dechallenge) should be clinically plausible
	• The event must be definitive pharmacologically or phenomenologically, using a satisfactory rechallenge procedure if necessary
Probable/likely	• A clinical event, including a laboratory test abnormality, with a reasonable time relation to administration of the drug, unlikely to be attributed to concurrent disease or other drugs or chemicals, and which follows a clinically reasonable response on withdrawal (dechallenge)
	• Rechallenge information is not required to fulfil this definition
Possible	• A clinical event, including a laboratory test abnormality, with a reasonable time relation to administration of the drug, but which could also be explained by concurrent disease or other drugs or chemicals
	• Information on drug withdrawal may be lacking or unclear
Unlikely	• A clinical event, including a laboratory test abnormality, with a temporal relation to administration of the drug, which makes a causal relation improbable, and in which other drugs, chemicals, or underlying disease provide plausible explanations
Conditional/unclassified	• A clinical event, including a laboratory test abnormality, reported as an adverse reaction, about which more data are essential for a proper assessment or the additional data are being examined
Unassessable/unclassifiable	• A report suggesting an adverse reaction that cannot be judged, because information is insufficient or contradictory and cannot be supplemented or verified

Table **12-5** **Assessment of 68 Cases by the MCA**

Classification	Number of reports	Case #
Probable	14	5, 8, 10, 20, 30*, 31*, 32, 54, 55, 56, 57, 60, 62, 68
Possible	30	1, 2, 3, 6, 7, 9, 12, 13, 14, 15, 16, 18, 19, 21, 22, 23, 24, 25, 26*, 28, 29*, 41, 52, 53, 59, 61, 63, 64, 65, 67
Unassessable	19	11, 33*, 34, 35, 36, 37, 38, 39, 40, 42, 43, 44, 45, 46, 47, 48, 49, 50, 66
Unlikely	5	4, 17, 27, 51, 58

Duplicate cases: 26/28, 29/30, 31/33.

In a report prepared by Dr. Waller for the American Herbal Products Association, the Professor of Pharmacology and Toxicology assessed the 30 German and Swiss case reports ("Data provided by BfArM" and a translation of the preliminary and the still incomplete Schmidt review) (Table 12-8).[3] Dr. Waller accepted the duplications indicated by Schmidt, and so reviewed 28 cases. Duplicate cases are indicated in brackets.

Waller suggested that there are only a few of these cases in which kava might be directly associated with liver damage, although more complete information is required for a scientific conclusion. These cases may have been hypersensitivity or idiosyncratic responses.

Table 12-9 is an assessment of 30 German and Swiss cases (with overlap of two) by the Traditional Medicines Evaluation Committee (TMEC), a subcommittee of the European

Table **12-6** **Evaluations of Identical Case Data by Different Authorities (Criteria Unknown)**

Case #	BfArM	MCA	EMEA
6	Probable	Possible	Possible
13	Probable	Possible	Possible
14	Possible	Possible	Possible
15	Probable	Not assessable	Possible
17	Probable	Unlikely	Unlikely
21	Probable	Not assessable	Possible
24	Probable	Possible	Possible
26/28	Probable	Possible	Possible
31/33	Certain	Probable	Probable/not assessable
32	Probable	Not assessable	Probable
34	Probable		Not assessable
38	Probable		Not assessable
40	Probable		Not assessable
42	Probable		Not assessable
46	Probable		Not assessable
47	Possible		Not assessable

Table 12-7   **Analysis of Cases by Schmidt**

Classification	Number of reports	Case #
Unrelated to kava	20	1, 4, 15, 17, 27, 39, 47, 52, 53, 55, 57, 58, 59, 72, 75, 76, 77, 78, 79, 80
Probably connected to concomitant medication	20	2, 6, 7, 9, 11, 13, 19, 21, 22, 23, 29, 31, 35, 37, 41, 43, 46, 51, 54, 74
Connection to kava doubtful	6	14, 16, 24, 56, 64, 67
Connection to kava not assessable due to insufficient documentation	31	3, 12, 18, 20, 25, 26, 32, 34, 36, 38, 40, 42, 44, 45, 48, 49, 50, 60, 61, 62, 63, 65, 66, 68, 69, 70, 71, 73, 81, 82, 83
Possible connection to kava with Commission E monograph-conforming dosage	1	5
Possible connection to kava with overdosing	2	8, 10

Herbal Practitioners' Association (EHPA). The classification contains some overlap, with cases appearing in more than one group.

Waller also reviewed 26 FDA cases provided to him at the time by the AHPA and considered only five to identify a liver-related symptom or problem in persons who were reported to be consuming kava. (The spreadsheet detailing the FDA information on these 26 cases is appended in his report. It is not known how these 26 cases were selected for analysis.) These five are reviewed below (#51, #52, #54, #63, and #76). In reviewing the non–liver-related adverse reaction cases he notes that there are two cases of chronic and high-dose consumption of kava that were not associated with any significant liver damage, which provides evidence that kava is not a direct hepatotoxin, even in extremely high concentrations. He concludes with the opinion that there is no scientifically supported association of liver disease with the use of kava which can be found using the FDA adverse reaction case reports. Overall, considering the evidence in the European and U.S. cases, and based on currently available information, kava, when taken in appropriate doses for reasonable periods of time, has no scientifically established potential for causing liver damage.[3]

Table 12-8   **Analysis of German and Swiss Case Reports by Dr. Waller**

Classification	Number of reports	Case #
Cases not attributable to kava	4	4, 17, 19, 27
Cases involving concomitant medication usage with known hepatic toxicity	10	7, 9, 11, 13, 15, 21, 22, 23, 29 (30), 33 (31)
Insufficient information to conclusively identify or fully eliminate kava as a potential causal agent, which include:	14	
• those with vastly inadequate information	6	12, 18, 20, 25, 26 (28), 32
• those with additional or confounding factors	5	8, 14, 16, 24, 28 (27)
• those with less inadequate information	3	5, 6, 10

Table **12-9**   **Assessment by TMEC January to April 2002**[110]

Classification	Number of reports	Case #
Cases of most concern, assessed as probable	5	5, 8, 10, 20, 31/33
Cases associated with taking synthetic kavain (a kava lactone)	4	11, 12, 22, 31/33
Patients taking oral contraceptive pills or hormone replacement therapy together with drugs that can be associated with liver damage	6	5, 13, 19, 23, 24, 31/33
Patients who were taking drugs that can be associated with liver damage	10	6, 7, 9, 11, 15, 17, 21, 22, 26/28, 29/30
Cases in which drugs not associated with liver damage, herbal medicines, or dietary supplements or kavain alone were taken	8	12, 14, 16, 18, 20, 25, 26/28, 27
Cases associated with an overdose of alcohol	2	8, 17
Cases not associated with other drug usage	2	10, 32

Overall, the quality of the data provided in these case reports was poor in most circumstances, there was little proof by rechallenge, and assessment of causality to kava was made, in most instances, without due consideration of concomitant medication. Investigation of preexisting medical conditions was also poor.

The assessments provided in "Summary and Critique of Case Reports" rate 3 cases as probable, 18 cases as possible (as defined in Table 12-4), 26 cases as unlikely, 33 cases as unassessable, 2 as unrelated to kava, and 1 which should not have been included.

Our extensive assessment of the data provided in "Summary and Critique of Case Reports" rates only three probable cases associated with kava use. For two of these three cases the kava was extracted with acetone (information is not available for the third case). Given the extensive time frame for gathering of data (e.g., #11 BfArM date October 1990) and the widespread use of kava (70 million daily doses in Germany per year at the time of its restriction), the incidence of a hepatic adverse reaction to kava is likely to be very rare. These data support the frequencies suggested in "Predicted Frequency of Response" (p.186).

THE PRODUCT INVOLVED IN THE AUSTRALIAN CASE REPORT

The product involved in the single Australian case report of hepatotoxicity linked to kava ingestion was labelled as containing kava, skullcap (*Scutellaria lateriflora*), and passionflower (*Passiflora incarnata*). Following reports from the TGA that the product did not contain skullcap, two current batches of the product were tested by an Australian company for the presence of kava, skullcap, passionflower, and two species of germander. Samples were run under three different high-performance liquid chromatography (HPLC) methods.[111] Germander (*Teucrium* spp., specifically *T. chamaedrys* and *T. canadensis*) was included in the analysis because species of *Teucrium* have been implicated in cases of hepatotoxicity and have been documented as substitutes for skullcap. In fact, the description given for dried skullcap in the *British Herbal Pharmacopoeia* 1983 is actually a description of a species of germander, and adulterations of *Scutellaria* with *Teucrium* species are reported rather frequently in the literature.

The assay of the two batches of the product could not confirm the presence of *Scutellaria lateriflora*, a second *Scutellaria* species (specifically *Scutellaria baicalensis*), or *Passiflora incarnata*. The presence of two selected species of germander could also not be confirmed, but this does not rule out germander substitution, since another species could be involved.

It is possible that the product contained another species of *Scutellaria*. However, this is not very likely since both batches of the product contained extremely low levels of flavonoids and *Scutellaria* species are known phytochemically to accumulate a considerable amount of flavonoids. In fact, levels of flavonoids found in the batches were more consistent with the levels corresponding to germander species.

Analysis of a third batch of the product performed by a German research group, using thin-layer chromatography (TLC) and HPLC methods, yielded similar results: the presence of kava and the absence of both *Scutellaria lateriflora* and *Passiflora incarnata*.[105] Subsequent analysis of the *Passiflora* raw material used in the product showed that it was indeed this herb, but was a poor-quality extract. This explains why its presence in the product was difficult to confirm.[111]

The issue of germander substitution for skullcap and resultant hepatotoxicity could be highly relevant to the current Australian market. A recent publication in the *Medical Journal of Australia*[112] reported six cases of hepatotoxicity attributed to use of herbal products. Of the six products involved, three supposedly contained skullcap (at least according to their labels). Given this news, linking hepatotoxicity to other Australian products labelled as containing skullcap, it is reasonable to suggest that an association with kava for the single Australian case must be seriously questioned.

In addition, chromium may have contributed to the hepatotoxicity.[106,107]

IS KAVA INHERENTLY HEPATOTOXIC?

Kava and its isolated constituents have not to date demonstrated toxic effects on liver parameters in standard experimental models (in vitro and in vivo). Some of the most relevant studies have not been published.[113,114]

A letter describing one of the Swiss cases mentioned above provides strong evidence that the hepatotoxicity was immune-mediated.[13] Also a deficiency of the drug-metabolising enzyme CYP2D6 (which occurs in 9% of the population) could be a predisposing factor.[13]

An Australian study of kava use in Aboriginal communities appears to support the contention that kava is inherently hepatotoxic.[115] However, concurrent use of alcohol is often widespread in such communities and any observed liver damage could be readily accounted for by this. Studies in Australia have shown that kava drinkers have markedly elevated levels of the liver enzyme GGT, and this has been construed as further proof of the inherent hepatotoxicity of kava.[116] However, while a survey of heavy kava drinkers in New Caledonia (8 g of kava lactones per week) did find evidence of raised GGT in about one-third, there were no signs of liver damage. The authors concluded that the probable explanation for the elevated GGT is enzymatic induction (as occurs with phenobarbital users), not hepatotoxicity. They concluded that cases of hepatotoxicity linked to kava are due to a rare immunoallergic mechanism.[117]

In a letter to the *Medical Journal of Australia* on 5 May 2003, two field researchers advised that the previously reported liver enzyme levels of Aboriginal kava users do not suggest acute inflammation and are not consistent with herb-induced hepatotoxicity. Clinical surveillance in the Northern Territory over 20 years has not documented any cases of fulminant hepatic failure attributable to kava use. This is despite the ingestion of doses estimated to be 10 to 50 times the recommended therapeutic doses for herbal products.[118]

PREDICTED FREQUENCY OF RESPONSE

Kava

The annual use of kava products, based on sales figures, has been estimated by one group at over 70 million daily doses in Germany and over 100 million daily doses in Europe.[119] According to the conservative sales figures of the German Institute of Medicinal Statistics, approximately 250 million daily doses of kava (ethanol extract) were sold during the past 10 years in German-speaking countries.[120] The sales of the acetone extract would have to be added to that number.

It has been suggested that 12 cases of probable liver toxicity have been reported to date in Germany and Switzerland (probably late 2001), for a calculated incidence of 0.23 cases per 1 million daily doses. This number does not allow for differentiation between products extracted with ethanol and acetone.[121]

According to the manufacturing company, a total of 80 million daily doses of the leading ethanol-based kava product Antares were taken from its introduction in 1992 up to the end of 1999. Only one single suspicious case was reported in that time (case #5, see above).[122]

On the basis of our assessment of the German and Swiss case reports (#4 to #50, #69, #70, #72, #73, and #81) only three cases of hepatotoxicity are probably associated with kava intake (#5, #8, and #10, and in the latter cases the dose exceeded the recommended dose). These data were gathered from 1990 to mid-2002. Using the following information the incidence can be estimated:

- a total of 80 million daily doses of the leading ethanol-based kava product (Antares) in Germany for 8 years (1992 to end of 1999);
- a total of 10 million capsules (corresponding to 5 million daily doses) of the ethanol-based kava product Kavasedon worldwide in the same time frame;
- 70 million daily doses in Germany per subsequent year (each year for 2000 to 2002);

- $85 + (70 \times 3) = 295$ million daily doses of kava;
- 3 cases of probable hepatotoxicity;
- incidence = 0.01 per million daily doses.

However, assuming a worst case scenario that every German and Swiss case (around 50) was probably associated with kava ingestion, and that data were only credibly gathered over 3 years, this gives an upper level of frequency of 0.24 cases per million daily doses. This frequency is still well below those documented for benzodiazepine drugs (see below), for which kava is considered by many as a credible and safer alternative.

Benzodiazepines/antianxiety/tranquillisers/psychotropics

The frequencies shown in Table 12-10 were calculated from cases of (suspected) hepatotoxicity reported to BfArM and corresponding drug sales in Germany for the period from September 1999 to August 2000. On the same basis, kava was estimated at causing 0.89 cases of hepatotoxicity per million daily doses.[121] In comparison to other treatments with potential for hepatotoxicity, this incidence has to be accepted as an extremely low figure.[121] So, while the frequency for kava given below is higher than those numbers arrived at elsewhere and above, it is still at the lower end of the hepatotoxicity incidences calculated for benzodiazepines.

In a randomised, placebo-controlled, multicentre trial, potentially serious reactions to alprazolam occurred in 10 of 263 subjects who received the drug (mean daily dose 5.7 mg). These included three cases of acute intoxication and two cases of hepatitis (i.e. frequency

Table **12-10**   **Relative Incidence of Suspected Hepatotoxic Reactions for Common Benzodiazepine Drugs and Kava**

	Incidence (*n*/Million Daily Doses)
Bromazepam	0.90
Oxazepam	1.23
Diazepam	2.12
Kava (ethanol and acetone extracts)	0.89

of hepatic adverse events equalled a very high 0.8%). This drug is commonly prescribed.[123]

Hepatotoxicity of psychotropic drugs occurs in a variable but small proportion of users and therefore can be considered unpredictable or idiosyncratic. When these uncommon adverse events occur in association with rash, eosinophilia, and/or a rapid positive rechallenge, sufficient circumstantial evidence exists to ascribe the medication to an immune-mediated hypersensitivity reaction. Acute overt reactions to drugs tend to have clinicopathological features of hepatitis, cholestasis, or both.[124]

Other Drugs

Antipsychotics

There is a high incidence of liver test abnormalities (>20%) with phenothiazine use, and a lower incidence of overt liver disease (0.1% to 1%). Features of hypersensitivity are seen in about half of the cases, including positive rechallenge.[125–128]

A survey of prescriptions in the UK from 1985 to 1991 revealed an overall incidence of chlorpromazine jaundice of 0.16%, increasing to 0.3% over age 70, more than 10 times higher than in those below age 50.[128]

A mild, transient increase in serum GPT occurred in 37% of recipients of clozapine.[129]

Antidepressants

Monoamine-oxidase inhibitors are all potential hepatotoxins. Overt hepatitis occurred in 1% of patients treated with iproniazid, with case fatalities approaching 20%.[130] The drug was withdrawn.

Hepatotoxic reactions, such as abnormal hepatic function, hepatitis (including cholestasis), hepatic failure, or necrosis and aggravation of hepatic damage, to the serotonin reuptake inhibitor fluoxetine have been reported, but are very rare (<0.01% of patients). Hepatitis and jaundice have been reported in less than 0.1% of patients using paroxetine. Hepatic failure, hepatitis, and jaundice have been reported in 0.01% to 0.1% of recipients of sertraline.[8] These incidences of hepatotoxicity are substantially higher than for kava.

Nefazodone (serotonin receptor blocker) has been associated with three cases of fulminant hepatic failure within 14 to 28 weeks of starting the drug. Liver transplantation was necessary in two cases, one of these patients died.[131]

Elevated transaminase and alkaline phosphatase levels are common (1% to 10%) in patients using the tricyclic antidepressants imipramine and clomipramine. Hepatitis with or without jaundice, acute hepatitis, and hepatic necrosis have been reported in less than 0.01% of patients using imipramine or clomipramine.[8]

The incidence of liver injury for the commonly used antidepressant amitriptyline is disturbingly high at 0.5% to 1%.[124]

NSAIDs

NSAID-induced liver injury results in 2.2 hospitalisations per 100,000 population per year.[132] While the incidence of NSAID-related jaundice may be as low as 0.1%, 0.01%, or even lower among recipients, plasma levels of transaminases may be abnormal in 5% to 15% of patients.[133]

The adjusted odds ratio for hepatotoxicity with sundilac has been estimated at almost twice that of indomethacin (5.0 vs. 2.6, respectively) despite their being in the same chemical class.[134] At least 25 individual cases of sundilac-associated jaundice have been reported in the literature.[133] About 20% of cases had hepatocellular injury, with about 5% of cases of jaundice ending in death.[135]

Significant hepatotoxicity occurs in approximately 1 to 5 per 100,000 diclofenac-exposed patients.[136] Abnormal aminotransferase plasma levels develop in about 15% of patients taking this drug. It has been implicated in at least 50 published reports of hepatocellular damage.[133] Massive necrosis with fulminant hepatic failure and death have been noted in about 10% of icteric cases.[137]

Estimates of clinically manifested hepatic toxicity associated with diclofenac, naproxen, or piroxicam range from 0.05 to 0.001%.[138] The incidence of liver damage (overt "hepatitis") induced by phenylbutazone was cited as 0.25% in one study.[139]

Piroxicam is one of the most widely used NSAIDs worldwide. Piroxicam caused a 1% to 2% incidence of elevated aminotransferase levels in early studies.[140] Instances of hepatic injury have been described, several of which involved fatal hepatic necrosis. Others showed severe cholestatic or mixed jaundice.[133]

Ibufenac was withdrawn when adverse liver reactions were observed in approximately 5% of individuals.[141,142] Ibufenac led to elevated aminotransferase levels in over 30% and jaundice in approximately 5% of individuals.[133]

Other Drugs

For most drugs, the risk of hepatotoxicity is 1 to 10 cases per 100,000 individuals exposed.[136] Kava would be below the lower end of this frequency, even if all reported cases were assumed to be linked.

In the United States, drugs and toxins account for as many as one-third of the cases of fulminant hepatic failure. The prognosis for drug-induced hepatitis is somewhat worse than that for viral hepatitis, with fatality rates approaching 10%.[136]

The Acute Liver Failure Study Group started in 1998 and collects data from 14 sites around the United States. The registry had enrolled 150 patients by the year 2000. Preliminary analysis suggests that 50% are related to drug hepatotoxicity (paracetamol toxicity in 32% and idiosyncratic reactions in 18%).[143]

Beard et al identified 12 hospitalisations for liver disorders judged possibly or probably attributable to use of outpatient medications other than anticancer drugs among 280,000 members of a managed care organisation during a 5-year period from 1977 through 1981.[144] This corresponds to an incidence of approximately one per 10^5 person-years (py) of exposure within the organisation. Walker and Cavanaugh found three cases of new-onset cases of liver disease of uncertain cause during the year 1989 among 71,000 adult members of a managed care organisation, yielding incidences of $4/10^5$ py and $24/10^5$ py, respectively.[145]

The incidence of liver function abnormalities in the general population of Massachusetts, in a study using computerised data files from a health maintenance organisation, found that drug-associated abnormalities were the most common. The incidence was 40.6 persons per 100,000 persons per year, with a 95% confidence interval of 29.3 to 51.8, based on a total of 50 cases. The study evaluated only outpatient use of prescription drugs, including NSAIDs, lipid-lowering agents, isoniazid, methotrexate, oral erythro-mycin, sulpha drugs, and chemotherapeutic drugs.[146]

Serum alanine aminotransferase exceeds the upper limit of normal in about 50% of recipients of tacrine. In 25%, the value is more than three times the upper limit, and in 2%, it is increased 20-fold.[147]

Troglitazone, a thiazolidinedione diabetic agent, produced severe and unpredictable hepatotoxicity and 61 related deaths.[148] The incidence of troglitazone-induced acute liver failure is estimated to be 1 in 8000 to 1 in 20,000 patients treated.[149] It took more than 3 years and 100 deaths or transplanted patients before the drug was withdrawn from the U.S. market.[150,151] It produced alanine aminotransferase elevations greater than three times upper limit of normal in 1 in 50 patients in clinical trials.[143] Abnormal liver function tests have not been recorded in any patients receiving kava in clinical trials (see "Efficacy of Kava" [p. 193]).

Toxic hepatitis developed in 1 of 127 peptic ulcer patients treated with cimetidine. Hepatocyte microsomal oxidase function noticeably declined in 1 in 8 patients subjected to the continuous 5-week treatment and in 1 in 5 patients given the treatment for a longer time.[152]

Hepatitis and cholestatic jaundice (occasionally severe) have been reported with a frequency of about 1 in 15,000 exposures of flucloxacillin.[8]

Dicloxacillin (a penicillin) has been associated with cholestatic hepatotoxicity and jaundice. The patterns of liver function test results and biopsy histology are similar to those with flucloxacillin. Information collected by the Swedish Adverse Drug Reaction Advisory Committee (SADRAC) over the period 1981 to 1994 provides 20 reports of liver damage possibly or probably caused by dicloxacillin. Over this period a total of 10.7 million defined daily doses (DDD) of dicloxacillin were prescribed in Sweden, giving a frequency of 1.8 reactions per million DDD. Over the period there were 127 reports of liver damage possibly or probably caused by flucloxacillin, at a frequency of 4.3 reactions per million DDD. Although there are obvious limitations of retrospective data reliant upon spontaneous doctor reporting, the SADRAC figures suggest that adverse hepatic events occur, or at least are reported, less frequently with dicloxacillin than flucloxacillin.[8]

CONFOUNDING FACTORS

One possibility that deserves consideration is the apparent higher prevalence of reaction for the acetone extract of kava. This could be due to the market leadership of this extract in Switzerland, but could also reflect on the particular phytochemical balance of an acetone-based extract. On the other hand, some of the reported cases involved ethanolic kava extracts. But the use of ethanolic extracts has not been confirmed in any of the cases rated as probable by us (and use of ethanolic extracts was definitively reported in only a few of the cases rated as possible).

If mode of preparation of kava is not an issue, and this remains to be established, the kava plant part used might be. In Europe, kava preparations are often manufactured from the root peelings or kava stumps (let alone the aerial peelings), which represent a cheap source of kava lactones. (In the South Pacific the kava root is often peeled and the locals drink this pale yellow root and export the darker peelings.) Kava preparations made from the whole peeled root, as used traditionally, could be less likely to cause hepatotoxicity (given the lack of reports of liver damage from Fiji and Vanuatu). In light of recent in vitro research (see below) this difference may be very important.

It is this factor, rather than the fact that traditional preparations of kava are water-based, which could explain the apparent lack of hepatotoxicity from kava use in the Pacific Islands (see "Indigenous Use of Kava and Safety" [p.192]). Indigenous use of kava in these regions can result in a chronic overdosage syndrome known as kava dermopathy, so it can hardly be suggested that the use of water-based preparations results in a lower exposure to kava phytochemicals. One reason for this is that the kava is often consumed as the finely ground root powder suspended in water, so in fact the whole root is being consumed. (However, one cannot rule out that there may be something protective missing from ethanolic or acetone extracts of kava which is present in water-based preparations.)

A new piperidine alkaloid ($3\alpha,4\alpha$-epoxy-5β-pipermethystine) has been isolated from the stem peelings (from the basal stem 0 to 20 cm above the ground) of one cultivar originating from Papua New Guinea (called Isa, and known in Hawaii as PNG). This constituent was present at a concentration of 0.93%, and was absent from the 10 other cultivars tested. Traditionally Isa has been used only occasionally for drinking purposes, since it causes prolonged nausea. However, as a pharmaceutical source it has recently gained popularity. In Hawaii, it is the only cultivar currently known to be less affected by the devastating viral disease known as kava dieback.[153] The safety implications of this discovery remain to be understood.

It is speculated that two potentially hepatotoxic 7,8-epoxidised kava lactones (based on in vitro tests) can be isolated from the hexane fraction of an acetone extract of kava root. The concentration of these epoxides in the Vanuatu kava root were very low (total of both amounting to 4 mg/kg). (The production of epoxides is a phase I metabolic reaction, which may have hepatotoxic consequences.) Incubation of six kava lactones with P450 enzymes and oxygen failed to produce kava lactone epoxides, but chemical oxidation of desmethoxyyangonin and 5,6-dihydromethysticin produced the kava lactone epoxides. Kavain and methysticin (which contain a double bond at C7–C8) combined with P450 enzymes produce desmethoxyyangonin and 5,6-dihydromethysticin respectively. Dihydrokavain and dihydromethysticin (lacking a double bond at C7–C8) could not be converted into desmethoxyyangonin and 5,6-dihydromethysticin. The authors hypothesised that the concomitant use of alcohol and/or prescription drugs in some patients may have primed the liver for hepatotoxicity by inducing the formation of P450 isoforms that were capable of transforming unsaturated kava lactones into 7,8-kavalactone epoxides.[154]

As a specific example of the issue of plant part, some kava extracts are a bright yellow colour indicating the presence of flavokavains. These are often lacking from European extracts (presumably prepared from peelings and stumps), as evidenced by their grey or brownish coloration, and are even intentionally removed for unknown reasons in the preparation of the acetone-based extract. The flavokavains, and perhaps other antioxidant compounds, from whole peeled kava root could provide a level of protection against hepatotoxic activity, as per the discussion below.

Chaparral is a herb suspected of causing hepatotoxicity. Linseed (also known as flaxseed [*Linum usitatissimum*]) and chaparral (*Larrea tridentata*) contain chemical components from the lignan group. A paper by scientists at the United States Food and Drug Administration described the development of methods to measure the specific lignans in these two herbs, and speculated on possible toxicity problems associated with their use.[155]

Linseeds contain the glucoside of the lignan secoisolariciresinol. Upon ingestion, this glucoside is hydrolysed enzymatically to the aglycone and transformed by intestinal microflora into the phyto-oestrogens enterodiol and enterolactone (Figure 12-1). While the authors concede that no adverse effects have been reported from the consumption of linseed products, they hypothesise that these phyto-oestrogens may have the potential to cause hepatotoxicity through mechanisms similar to those of hormonal oestrogens.

In contrast, chaparral contains nordihydroguaiaretic acid (NDGA) and other related lignans, and the use of this herb has been connected to hepatotoxicity. The authors provide an interesting theory to explain possible occasional hepatotoxicity from chaparral ingestion. They suggest that, under certain conditions, antioxidant compounds such as NDGA can become oxidant and generate free radicals. Moreover, if hepatic detoxification mechanisms are compromised, these compounds can also have toxic effects. (Every antioxidant compound exists in a reduced and an oxidised form, and if the oxidised form predominates, that compound will then act as a pro-oxidant.) Chemical studies of chaparral extracts indicate the presence of a number of reactive free-radical species and also the potentially toxic pro-oxidant compound guaiaretic acid diquinone (see Figure 12-1).

It is conceivable that under certain circumstances highly reactive pro-oxidant compounds may be produced from the kava lactones (Figure 12-2), which could result in haptenisation and immune-mediated hepatotoxicity.

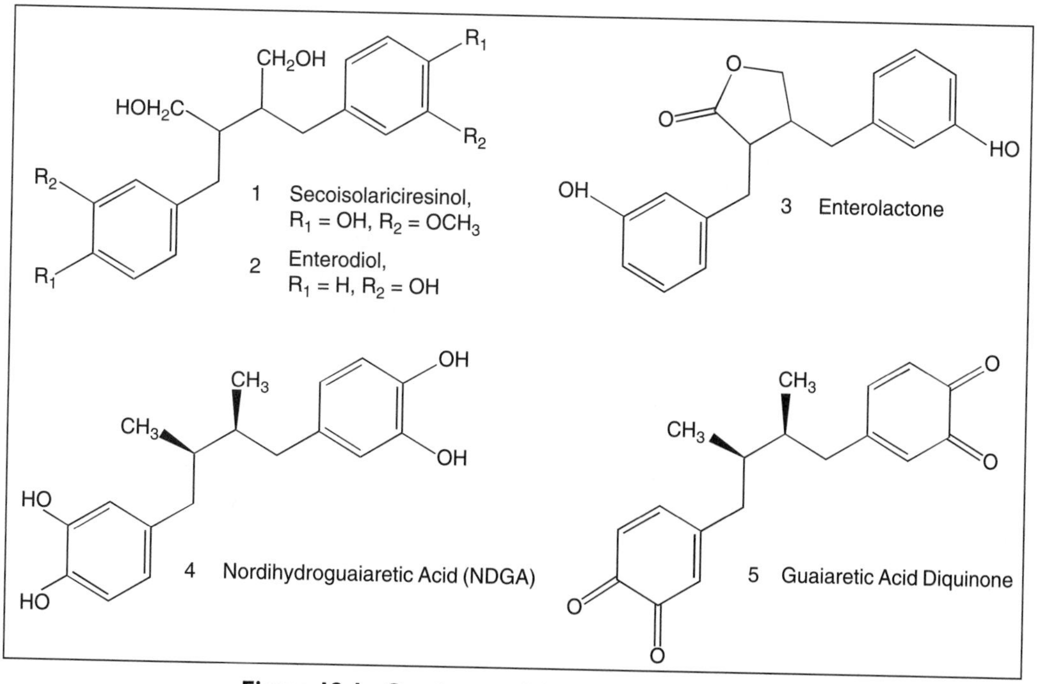

Figure 12-1. Constituents of chaparral (*Larrea tridentata*).

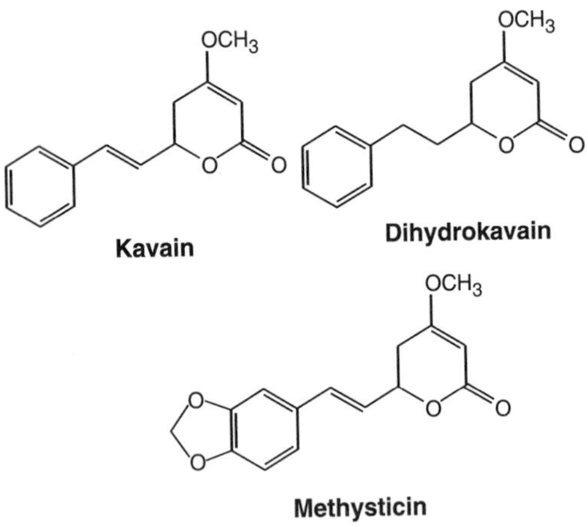

Figure 12-2. Constituents of kava (*Piper methysticum*).

Use of the whole root may help to prevent against this, because antioxidant phytochemicals are also coextracted. However, immunological reactions to kava do not seem to occur frequently. The number of suspect cases does not surpass the average allergic reaction occurring with virtually any otherwise unsuspect medication or food component.

INDIGENOUS USE OF KAVA AND SAFETY

Kava has a long history of safe use in the Pacific Islands and cases of hepatotoxicity have not been noted. An extensive review of the ethnobotany, history, and chemistry of kava, focusing on the Pacific Islands, published in 1993, makes no mention of adverse effects on the liver from even excessive use of kava.[156] Kava is, or was, consumed in a wide range of Pacific Ocean societies, from coastal areas on the large Melanesian island of New Guinea in the west to isolated Polynesian Hawaii, 7000 km distant to the north-east.

Kava became an integral part of island religious, economic, political, and social life, and even today it is a regular activity for many islanders. Traditionally, islanders ingested the kava lactones by drinking cold water infusions of chewed, ground, pounded, or otherwise macerated kava stumps and roots. In addition to its ceremonial and social function, kava was also used medicinally.

The principal author of the above review recently indicated that he drinks traditionally prepared kava every day and his regular annual medical check-up confirms that his liver is in good condition.[157] According to Singh and Singh,[158] in the South Pacific only men drink kava, often habitually and in much larger amounts than used in the West, yet their incidence of liver toxicity is low and similar to that of island women who do not take kava.

Is long-term consumption of kava generally safe? While more studies are needed, a recent epidemiological study found a substantially *lower* incidence of cancer among kava users, which contrasts strongly with the use of alcohol and tobacco.[159]

An Australian GP recalls that he spent 2 years living in Vanuatu, observing the regular, and occasionally heavy, kava consumption. Clinical evaluation revealed occasional cases of kava-related dermopathy and presumptive kava-related cerebral damage. At no time during his 2-year stay did he encounter any case of unexplained hepatitis, despite his vigilance, since 20% of the population were hepatitis B carriers.[160] A GP working in Auckland with the Pacific Island community reported a similar lack of hepatotoxicity in frequent kava users.[161]

Various reasons have been proposed for this lack of observed hepatotoxicity in the Pacific Islands, including the mode of preparation of kava and the part used (see "Confounding Factors" [p. 190]). However, another reason could be the relatively low use of alcohol and modern drugs by these communities. It could be that many or most of the cases attributed to kava in the West were, in fact, due to concomitant alcohol or drug consumption. There might even be the situation where the kava acted synergistically with these agents.

Aboriginal people living mostly in Arnhem Land began using kava in the early 1980s. They purchased imported powdered kava as an alcohol substitute.[156] As described above, the Australian study of kava use in Aboriginal communities does not support the inherent hepatotoxicity of kava.[115]

The Northern Territory government enacted legislation (Kava Management Act and Regulations) 11 May 1998. The legislation was introduced as part of a comprehensive package to minimise the harmful effects of kava use and to penalise illegal kava traders. The legislation was enacted in response to concerns about potential harmful effects of kava outlined in the report from the Menzies School of Health Research (referred to above).[116] A kava licensing system was proposed to assist communities to control the amount of kava consumed, reduce health damage through overuse, and diminish black market kava sales.[162] Presumably, the Northern Territory government would not have instigated legal use of kava if they had substantial concerns about its potential for hepatotoxicity.

This is supported by scientists investigating kava use within Aboriginal communities.[118] The abnormal but reversible GGT and alkaline phosphatase levels seen there in heavy kava drinkers does not appear to reflect a hepatotoxic process. Recommendations include monitoring of potential adverse effects of kava use in Aboriginal communities and Pacific countries, in addition to initiatives encouraging moderation in consumption. These field researchers working in the Northern Territory have suggested that the lack of hepatotoxicity observed there could be due to the fact that Western herbal products often involve different methods of extraction to those used traditionally (and in the Aboriginal communities).

EFFICACY OF KAVA

Recent Clinical Trials and Reviews

Standardised kava extract was significantly superior to placebo in the treatment of anxiety disorders of nonpsychotic origin in a randomised, double-blind trial lasting 5 weeks and involving 40 patients who had previously been treated with benzodiazepines. During the first treatment week, the dosage of kava extract was increased from 50 to 300 mg/day in the test group. Pretreatment with benzodiazepines was tapered off over 2 weeks. These dosage adjustments were followed by 3 weeks of treatment with kava extract or placebo. The authors concluded that further symptom reduction was shown after the change-over

from benzodiazepine treatment. Kava extract was well tolerated.[163]

In an open, observational, multicentre study involving 52 outpatients suffering from anxiety of nonpsychotic origin, 81% of patients rated the treatment as "very good" or "good" on a global improvement scale. Symptoms of anxiety, restlessness, and tension showed a pronounced decrease from baseline on a physician-rated scale. Patients received 200 to 600 mg of standardised kava extract per day (corresponding to 100 to 300 mg/day of kava lactones) for a mean treatment duration of 51 days. Adverse events were rare and mild.[164]

Fifty-four healthy volunteers underwent a standardised mental stress task and were then randomised to treatment with either kava extract (120 mg/day) or valerian extract (120 mg/day) or to a nonplacebo control group. After 1 week they repeated the task. The kava and valerian groups reported feeling under less pressure and their systolic blood pressure (BP) was significantly reduced compared to results a week earlier. Heart rate (HR) was reduced in the valerian group but not the kava group, and diastolic BP did not change in either group. There were no significant differences in BP, HR, or subjective reports of pressure in the control group.[165]

A meta-analysis[166] assessing seven randomised, double-blind, placebo-controlled trials found that kava extract significantly reduced anxiety (compared to placebo). The dosage of standardised kava extract prescribed varied and contained 60 to 240 mg/day of kava lactones. The duration of treatment ranged from 1 to 24 weeks. One trial[167] investigated the reduction in anxiety for preoperative patients who received kava extract the night before and 1 hour prior to surgery. This meta-analysis has also been published by the Cochrane Collaboration in 2002.[168] The authors of one of the trials[169] included in the meta-analysis concluded that the efficacy and tolerability of standardised kava extract recommend it as an alternative to tricyclic antidepressants and benzodiazepines for the treatment of anxiety.

Kava has also been shown to have therapeutic benefit in cases of situational anxiety. In a randomised, double-blind, placebo-controlled trial, standardised kava extract taken for 1 week significantly reduced anxiety compared to placebo in patients awaiting the results of medical diagnostic tests for suspected breast carcinoma. Fatigue, introverted behaviour, excitability, and depression were decreased and alertness was increased in patients receiving kava extract. The administered daily dose of kava contained 150 mg of kava lactones and corresponded to approximately 2.5 g of dried root.[170]

Preliminary findings suggest a beneficial effect of kava on baroreflex control of heart rate (BRC). Significantly more patients with generalised anxiety disorder exhibited improved BRC following treatment with kava compared to a placebo. There was no effect on respiratory sinus arrhythmia, a measure of the heart rate changes occurring with respiration. Patients in the study were a subgroup of a larger randomised, double-blind trial and received standardised kava extract or placebo for 4 weeks.[171]

In a pilot study, patients suffering from stress-induced insomnia were treated in each phase for 6 weeks with kava, then valerian, then a combination of kava and valerian, with washout periods between each treatment phase of 2 weeks. Total stress severity was significantly relieved by the kava and valerian single treatments (stress was measured in three areas: social, personal, and life events). Insomnia was significantly relieved by the combination of kava and valerian.[172]

Kava plus hormone replacement therapy significantly reduced menopausal anxiety compared to hormone replacement therapy alone in a controlled trial.[173]

Earlier Studies

The following information is an excerpt from *Principles and Practice of Phytotherapy: Modern Herbal Medicine* which reviewed the clinical trial information available on kava to 1998.[174]

Anxiety

Earlier trials used purified kavain at a dose of 400 mg/day. In a placebo-controlled, double-blind study of 84 patients with anxiety symptoms, kavain improved vigilance, memory, and reaction time.[175] In comparison with an antianxiety drug (oxazepam) in a placebo-controlled, double-blind trial of 38 patients with anxiety associated with neurotic disturbances, kavain demonstrated equivalent activity.[176] The substances proved to be equivalent in the nature and the potency of their anxiolytic action. Both treatments caused progressive improvement in two different anxiety scores over a 4-week period.

In a randomised, placebo-controlled double-blind study of 58 patients with anxiety not caused by psychotic disorders, a standardised kava extract significantly improved measures of anxiety and depression.[177,178] Patients received standardised kava extract (300 mg/day, containing 210 mg kava lactones) or placebo over a 4-week period. For patients receiving the kava extract, there was a significant reduction of anxiety, as measured by the Hamilton anxiety rating scale (HAM-A) (total score, $P < 0.02$). The difference in anxiety between kava and placebo began in the first week and increased during the course of treatment. No adverse effects were reported for the kava extract.

A standardised extract of kava was compared to the benzodiazepine drugs bromazepam and oxazepam in a randomised, controlled, double-blind study. One hundred and seventy-six outpatients were divided into three approximately equal groups. One group received kava extract equivalent to 210 mg of kava lactones per day, the second group received 15 mg of oxazepam per day and the third group received 9 mg of bromazepam. The total HAM-A score was reduced from 27.3 to 15.6 after 6 weeks of kava treatment, compared to 27.3 down to 13.4 for bromazepam and 27.7 down to 16.6 for oxazepam. Statistical analysis showed that kava treatment was equivalent to the benzodiazepine drugs. Side effects were higher in the conventional drug groups.[179]

Although there have been positive outcomes for the use of kava demonstrated in the above controlled trials, none of the trials lasted for more than 6 weeks, the inclusion criteria were insufficiently defined, and patient numbers were relatively small. These issues were addressed in a subsequent study. In a randomised, placebo-controlled, double-blind, multicentre study, 100 patients presenting with nervous anxiety, tension, and restlessness of nonpsychotic origin (DSM-III-R) were followed over a period of 6 months. Patients were randomised to receive either 300 mg/day of a concentrated kava extract containing 210 mg of kava lactones (equivalent to about 4 g of dried root) or placebo. Assessment was based on changes in the cumulative HAM-A score in addition to other assessments. Comparison of the pre- and post-therapy HAM-A scores revealed a significant ($P = 0.0015$) superiority of the kava treatment as against placebo. The difference between the two treatment groups was even apparent at 8 weeks ($P = 0.055$). Kava treatment led to a marked reduction in the symptoms of anxiety, together with its physical and psychic manifestations. In addition, the accompanying depressive component was positively influenced by kava. During the study, six adverse events in five patients were reported in the kava group. Four of these were rated by the investigator as not being related to the treatment, two (in both cases stomach upset) were rated as "possibly related". Fifteen adverse events from nine patients were reported in the placebo group. Seven patients dropped out under placebo and three under kava (two of these three were due to improvement of symptoms). There was no significant change in biochemical parameters during the study period and the overall tolerability of kava was rated as excellent. The authors concluded that their results support kava as a treatment alternative to tricyclic antidepressants and benzodiazepines in anxiety, with proven long-term efficacy and none of the tolerance problems associated with these drugs.[169,180]

Other Conditions

Past and recent clinical trials indicate kava extract and kava pyrones (especially dihydromethysticin) are not suitable for the treatment of epilepsy. Although effective in grand mal seizures, the trials were abandoned due to incidence of side effects (mainly skin problems) when used long term and in high doses. No efficacy was observed with petit mal.[181,182]

In a randomised, placebo-controlled, double-blind trial of 40 patients with neurovegetative symptoms associated with menopause, standardised kava extract (210 mg kava lactones per day for 8 weeks) produced a significant reduction in anxiety ($P < 0.01$), depression, severity of symptoms, and menopausal symptoms. The subjective well-being of patients improved with kava and the treatment was well tolerated.[183]

RISK–BENEFIT ANALYSIS AND THE OPINIONS OF EXPERT COMMITTEES

The Complementary Medicines Evaluation Committee (CMEC) of the Australian TGA considered the safety of kava-containing medicines on 8 and 12 August 2002. The Committee recommended to the TGA that it impose a strong warning statement on the label of all kava-containing medicines. It recommended that the warning statement indicate to consumers that kava-containing medicines:

- have been implicated in serious liver damage;
- be taken only under the supervision of a health care practitioner; and
- be used only for short periods of time, not exceeding 6 weeks.

Clearly CMEC is of the view that a risk-benefit assessment of kava indicates that it still should be available, but under more controlled conditions of use. This could involve the registration (as opposed to listing) of appropriate kava products and their sale through professional channels only.

In contrast, according to the Australian Adverse Drug Reactions Committee (ADRAC), which represents a more orthodox perspective, the risks associated with kava exceed the benefits and it should be completely withdrawn from the market in Australia.

At the meeting of the ADRAC held on 9 August 2002, the Committee considered the details of the adverse drug reaction report surrounding the death of the Australian woman after taking a number of complementary medicines, including one containing kava:

Members considered that with exclusion of other identifiable possible causes, kava was a plausible explanation for the patient's liver failure. . . . Members considered the potential benefits of kava for the indications in which it is used (anxiety, stress, restlessness). There are other agents of proven benefit for these indications. . . . The Committee considered that with this Australian case and the overseas reports of hepatotoxicity, the risks associated with kava exceed the benefits.

The Committee recommended that all manufactured products containing kava extracts be withdrawn from the market in Australia.

In a surprising move, the German Commission E, the expert committee on herbal medicines established by the German government, has published a strongly dissenting view from the BfArM.[184] It is signed by all the Commission E members (professors, scientists, and medical doctors). According to the Commission E they were taken aback by the precipitous action of the BfArM on kava and feel bypassed and that their scientific competence, and indeed role, has been questioned by this move. The members of the Commission E, all eminent experts in the field of herbal medicines, view the risk-benefit assessment for kava positively, provided certain precautions (appropriate for the German situation) are observed. One can only wonder at the motives of a government authority that appoints a committee with expertise in herbal matters and then bypasses its views and recommendations.

CONCLUSIONS AND RECOMMENDATIONS

It appears likely that certain types of kava products have the potential to cause a rare immune-mediated liver damage with an extremely low frequency of occurrence. The type of reaction that occurs appears to be typical of drug-induced liver damage, a phenomenon that can occur after the intake of many of the prescription and OTC drugs commonly available throughout the world. However, the frequency of hepatotoxicity for kava is, on current information, substantially lower than for these conventional drugs.

On the basis of the current information it can not be confirmed that all preparations of kava involving all types of raw materials will cause this hepatotoxic reaction. Probable cases, based on our assessment, have only been confirmed for the acetone extracts commonly used in Germany and Switzerland, with the exception of one case report (#5) from the intake of an ethanol-based extract, a case where the patient was shown to have an unusual metabolic enzyme pattern and at the same time developed an immunological reaction to kava intake (allergy). The absence of reported cases of hepatotoxicity in the Pacific Islands adds weight to this assertion.

The issue with kava raises a fundamental question for the regulation of herbal products. It is important that any outcomes for kava are credible to all stakeholders in this situation: regulators, industry, practitioners, and patients/customers. The question is: At what level of risk should a herbal product be completely restricted from use? It is quite likely that other popular herbs will be found to cause a low frequency of hepatotoxicity. Will they then be banned from use? Supplementary to this is the question: Can a mechanism be found to maintain the availability of kava which mitigates against the (low level) risk associated with its use?

If kava is made unavailable, then it is quite likely that, with modern communications, patients/consumers will source it for themselves through the Internet or via legal loopholes. This problem has already developed in Germany, where kava was totally banned.[185] So in the modern situation "banning" may in fact involve deregulation, not regulation of kava use.

As a way forward, it is recommended that kava products should carry warnings similar to those already recommended by the Australian CMEC in August 2002.

Also, kava is one of a growing number of herbal products which are probably best made available only on professional advice. That way its safe use can be monitored closely. It is suggested that companies selling kava through mass market and health food stores should reconsider this mode of distribution.

Finally, the issue of product liability insurance needs to be mentioned. Liability insurance is becoming more difficult to obtain in the dietary supplements area and many companies have already withdrawn kava from the U.S. market because of high insurance premiums or exclusion clauses listing kava (along with asbestos and thalidomide). The irony of this debate is that the insurance companies may have the final word on the risk-benefit assessment.

REFERENCES

In the references listed below Review 1 refers to the constantly updated document: Schmidt M: Is kava really hepatotoxic? An analysis of the known data on adverse effects of kava preparations on the liver, version 30/4/2003. Downloaded from www.uni-muenster.de/Chemie/PB/Kava/analyse.htm

1. Medicines Control Agency Assessment Report: *Kava-kava* (Piper methysticum) *and hepatotoxicity,* July 2002.
2. Loew D, Gaus W: Kava-kava: Tragedy of a wrong decision [in German], *Z Phytother* 23:267-281, 2002.
3. Waller DP: *Report on kava and liver damage,* February 15, 2002.
4. Medicines Control Agency: *Risk-benefit analysis of Kavakava,* February 12, 2002.
5. Review 1, Section 3.19
6. Review 1, Section 4.19
7. Olsson R: Liver damage due to antihypertensive drugs, *Acta Med Scand Suppl* 628:53-56, 1979.
8. E-MIMS. Version 4.00.0457. Havas MediMedia International, 2000.[electronic version]
9. Review 1, Section 3.3
10. Strahl S, Ehret V, Dahm HH, et al: Necrotizing hepatitis after taking herbal remedies [in German], *Dtsch Med Wschr* 123:1410-1414, 1998.
11. Review 1, Section 7.1
12. Review 1, Section 9.2
13. Russmann S, Lauterburg BH, Helbling A: Kava hepatotoxicity, *Ann Intern Med* 135:68-69, 2001.
14. Pollock BG, Mulsant BH, Sweet RA, et al: Prospective cytochrome P450 phenotyping for neuroleptic treatment in dementia, *Psychopharmacol Bull* 31:327-331, 1995.
15. Kraft M, Spahn TW, Menzel J, et al: Fulminant liver failure after administration of the herbal antidepressant Kava-Kava [in German], *Dtsch MedWschr* 126:970-972, 2001.
16. Review 1, Section 4.20
17. Bellaiche G, Lamouri N, Slama JL, et al: Cytolytic hepatic lesion associated with the ingestion of piretanide [in French], *Gastroenterol Clin Biol* 19:444-445, 1995.
18. Review 1, Section 4.8
19. Stoller R: Liver damage with kava extracts [in German], *Schweiz Arztezeit* 81:1335-1336, 2000.
20. Review 1, Section 8.1
21. Russmann S, Escher M, Stoller R, et al: Hepatotoxicity of Kava Kava (*Piper methysticum*) containing herbal drugs. Recent cases in Switzerland and investigations regarding the mechanism, *J Exp Klin Pharmakol Toxicol* 363:S40, 2001.
22. Review 1, Section 4.9
23. Escher M, Desmeules J, Giostra E, et al: Hepatitis associated with Kava, a herbal remedy for anxiety, *BMJ* 322:139, 2001.
24. Review 1, Section 4.1
25. Review 1, Section 6.1
26. Review 1, Section 4.2
27. Review 1, Section 5.1
28. Review 1, Section 3.4
29. Review 1, Section 3.1
30. Review 1, Section 6.3
31. Review 1, Section 4.10
32. Review 1, Section 9.4
33. Review 1, Section 6.2
34. Review 1, Section 4.3
35. Personal communication from the manufacturer of Kavain Harras Plus, October 22, 2002.
36. Pennings EJ, Konijn KZ, de Wolff FA: Clinical and toxicologic aspects of the use of Ecstasy [in Dutch], *Ned Tijdschr Geneeskd* 142:1942-1946, 1998.
37. Review 1, Section 4.4
38. Saß M, Schnabel S, Kröger J, Liebe S, et al: Acute liver failure from kava-kava – a rare indication for liver transplant [in German], *Z Gastroenterol* 39:491, 2000.
39. Review 1, Section 4.5
40. Brauer R-B, Pfab R, Becker K, et al: Fulminant liver failure after ingestion of the herbal medicine kava-kava [in German], *Z Gastroenterol* 39:491, 2000.
41. Review 1, Section 5.3
42. Hinzpeter W: Attack on the liver [in German], *Stern* May 29:23, 2002.
43. Review 1, Section 6.4
44. Review 1, Section 6.5
45. Review 1, Section 3.2
46. Review 1, Section 4.6
47. Review 1, Section 2.3
48. Review 1, Section 4.7
49. Review 1, Section 6.6
50. Review 1, Section 6.12
51. Review 1, Section 4.11
52. Review 1, Section 6.7
53. Review 1, Section 4.12
54. Review 1, Section 6.8
55. Review 1, Section 3.20
56. Review 1, Section 6.9
57. Review 1, Section 4.13
58. Review 1, Section 6.17
59. Review 1, Section 4.14
60. Review 1, Section 6.31
61. Review 1, Section 6.11
62. Review 1, Section 4.15

63. Review 1, Section 9.3

64. Review 1, Section 3.5

65. Review 1, Section 6.13

66. Review 1, Section 6.14

67. Review 1, Section 6.15

68. Review 1, Section 4.17

69. Sheikh NM, Philen RM, Love LA: Chaparral-associated hepatotoxicity, *Arch Intern Med* 157:913-919, 1997.

70. Review 1, Section 3.16

71. Review 1, Section 3.8

72. Review 1, Section 4.16

73. Centers for Disease Control and Prevention: Hepatic toxicity possibly associated with kava-containing products – United States, Germany and Switzerland, 1999-2002, *MMWR* 51:1065-1067, 2002. Available online: http://www.cdc.gov/mmwr/preview/mmwrhtml/mm5147a1.htm. Accessed 9 December 2002.

74. Review 1, Section 3.10

75. Review 1, Section 5.4

76. Review 1, Section 3.11

77. Review 1, Section 3.12

78. Review 1, Section 3.18

79. Review 1, Section 6.19

80. Review 1, Section 6.20

81. Review 1, Section 6.21

82. Review 1, Section 6.22

83. Review 1, Section 5.6

84. Review 1, Section 6.27

85. Review 1, Section 5.5

86. Review 1, Section 6.26

87. Review 1, Section 6.16

88. Review 1, Section 6.10

89. Humbertson CL, Akhtar J, Krenzelok EP: Acute hepatitis induced by kava kava, a herbal product derived from *Piper methysticum*, *J Toxicol* 39:549, 2001.

90. Review 1, Section 6.25

91. Stuckhard P: Poisoned liver after kava-kava [in German], *Neue Westfälische*, July 5, 2002.

92. Review 1, Section 3.6

93. Review 1, Section 6.18

94. Review 1, Section 4.18

95. Review 1, Section 3.15

96. Zarafonetis CJ, Dabich L, DeVol EB, et al: Potassium para-aminobenzoate and liver function test findings, *J Am Acad Dermatol* 15:144-149, 1986.

97. Review 1, Section 3.7

98. Review 1, Section 3.13

99. Review 1, Section 3.14

100. Review 1, Section 3.9

101. Review 1, Section 3.17

102. Therapeutic Goods Administration: *Information for sponsors: safety of kava-containing medicines. Guidance for sponsors of kava-containing medicines -August 2002*, August 28, 2002. Available online: http://www.health.gov.au:80/tga/docs/html/kavaspon.htm (accessed October 29, 2002).

103. Gow PJ, Connelly NJ, Hill RL, et al: Fatal fulminant hepatic failure induced by a natural therapy containing kava, *Med J Aust* 178:442-443, 2003.

104. Lehmann R, Penman K: Information on file, MediHerb Research Laboratory, University of Queensland, St. Lucia, Queensland 4072, Australia, 2002.

105. Schmidt M, Thomsen M: Poor quality in Australian kava product made responsible for hepatotoxicity: two out of three components not detectable on analysis, In-house report redinomedica AG, Munich, Germany, manuscript for publication in preparation.

106. Cerulli J, Grabe DW, Gauthier I, et al: Chromium picolinate toxicity, *Ann Pharmacother* 32:428-431, 1998.

107. Lanca S, Alves A, Vieira AI, et al: Chromium-induced toxic hepatitis, *Eur J Intern Med* 13:518-520, 2002.

108. Edwards IR, Aronson JK: Adverse drug reactions: definitions, diagnosis, and management, *Lancet* 356:1255-1259, 2000.

109. Review 1, Introduction section "Some background data—different evaluation"

110. Traditional Medicines Evaluation Committee: Response to concerns about *Piper methysticum* Forst. f., Kava, submission date January 11, 2002.

111. Lehmann R, Penman K: Private communication, MediHerb Pty Ltd, PO Box 713, Warwick Qld 4370, Australia.

112. Whiting PW, Clouston A, Kerlin P: Black cohosh and other herbal remedies associated with acute hepatitis, *Med J Aust* 177:432-435, 2002.

113. Sorrentino L: Toxicology Report/Kavapyron Complex (Kavasedon), Department of Experimental Pharmacology, University of Neapel, In-house report *Harras Pharma*, 1990.

114. Gebhardt R: Studies of the hepatotoxicity of Kava semi liquid extract in cultivated liver cells [in German], Internal report, *Harras Pharma Curarina*, 2001.

115. Mathews JD, Reiley MD, Fejo L, et al: Effects of the heavy usage of kava on physical health: summary of a pilot survey in an Aboriginal community, *Med J Aust* 148:548-555, 1988.

116. d'Abbs P, Burns C: Draft report on inquiry into the issue of kava regulation [prepared for the Sessional Committee on the Use and Abuse of Alcohol by the Community], Menzies School of Health Research, Darwin, September 1997.

117. Barguil Y: Kava and gamma-glutamyltransferase increase: hepatic enzymatic induction or liver function alteration. Electronic letter published http:/bmj.com March 21, 2001 in response to Escher M, Desmeules J, Giostra E, et al: Drug points: Hepatitis associated with kava, a herbal remedy for anxiety, *BMJ* 322:139, 2001.

118. Currie BJ, Clough AR: Kava hepatotoxicity with Western herbal products: does it occur with traditional kava use? *Med J Aust* 178:421-422, 2003.

119. Gruenwald J, Freder J: Kava – the present European situation, *Nutraceuticals World* Jan/Feb:22-24, 2002:

120. Schmidt M, Nahrstedt A: Is kava liver toxic? An analysis of the known facts regarding the liver risk of kava products [in German], *Dtsch Apoth Ztg* 142:1006-1011, 2002.

121. Schulze J, Meng G, Siegers CP: Safety assessment of kavalactone-containing herbal drugs in comparison to other psychotropics. Poster presentation, Annual Meeting of Swiss Society of Pharmacology, September 2001.

122. No authors listed. Adverse effects from kava-kava [in German], *Z Phytother* 21:188, 2000.

123. Noyes R, DuPont RL, Pecknold JC, et al: Alprazolam in panic disorder and agaraphobia: results from a multicenter trial. II. Patient acceptance, side effects and safety, *Arch Gen Psychiatry* 45:423-428, 1988.

124. Selim K, Kaplowitz N: Hepatotoxicity of psychotropic drugs, *Hepatology* 29:1347-1351, 1999.

125. Hollister L: Allergy to chlorpromazine manifested by jaundice, *Am J Med* 23:870-878, 1957. Cited in Selim K, Kaplowitz N: Hepatotoxicity of psychotropic drugs, *Hepatology* 29:1347-1351, 1999.

126. Zimmerman HJ: Update of hepatotoxicity due to classes of drugs in common clinical use: non-steroidal drugs, anti-inflammatory drugs, antibiotics, antihypertensives, and cardiac and psychotropic agents, *Semin Liver Dis* 10:322-338, 1990. Cited in Selim K, Kaplowitz N: Hepatotoxicity of psychotropic drugs, *Hepatology* 29:1347-1351, 1999.

127. Ishak KG, Irey NS: Hepatic injury associated with the phenothiazines, *Arch Pathol* 93:283-304, 1972. Cited in Selim K, Kaplowitz N: Hepatotoxicity of psychotropic drugs, *Hepatology* 29:1347-1351, 1999.

128. Derby L, Gutthann SP, Jick H, et al: Liver disorders in patients receiving chlorpromazine and isoniazid, *Pharmacotherapy* 13:354-358, 1993. Cited in Selim K, Kaplowitz N: Hepatotoxicity of psychotropic drugs, *Hepatology* 29(5):1347-1351, 1999.

129. Hummer M, Kurz M, Kurzthaler I, et al: Hepatotoxicity of clozapine, *J Clin Psychopharmacol* 17:314-317, 1997.

130. Rosenblum LE, Korn RJ, Zimmerman H: Hepatocellular jaundice as a complication of iproniazid therapy, *Arch Intern Med* 105:115-125, 1960. Cited in Selim K, Kaplowitz N: Hepatotoxicity of psychotropic drugs, *Hepatology* 29:1347-1351, 1999.

131. Aranda-Michel J, Koehler A, Bejarano B, et al: Nefazodone-induced liver failure: report of three cases, *Ann Intern Med* 130:285-288, 1999.

132. Carson JL, Strom BL, Duff A, et al: Safety of nonsteroidal anti-inflammatory drugs with respect to acute liver disease, *Arch Intern Med* 153:1331-1336, 1993.

133. Boelsterli UA, Zimmerman HJ, Kretz-Rommel A: Idiosyncratic liver toxicity of nonsteroidal antiinflammatory drugs: molecular mechanisms and pathology, *CRC Crit Rev Toxicol* 25:207-235, 1995.

134. Zimmerman HJ: Acetaminophen poisoning and NSAID toxicity, Presented at the American Association for the Study of Liver Diseases Postgraduate Course, Chicago Illinois, November 7, 1997: Cited in Tolman KG: Hepatotoxicity of non-narcotic analgesics, *Am J Med* 105:13S-19S, 1998.

135. Andrejak M, Davion T, Gineston JL, et al: Cross hepatotoxicity between non-steroidal anti-inflammatory drugs, *BMJ* 295:180-181, 1987. Cited in Boelsterli UA, Zimmerman HJ, Kretz-Rommel A: Idiosyncratic liver toxicity of nonsteroidal antiinflammatory drugs: molecular mechanisms and pathology, *CRC Crit Rev Toxicol* 25:207-235, 1995.

136. Tolman KG: Hepatotoxicity of non-narcotic analgesics, *Am J Med* 105(1B):13S-19S, 1998.

137. Banks T, Zimmerman HJ, Harter J, et al: Diclofenac-associated hepatic injury analysis of 181 cases, *Hepatology* (in press). Cited in Boelsterli UA, Zimmerman HJ, Kretz-Rommel A: Idiosyncratic liver toxicity of nonsteroidal antiinflammatory drugs: molecular mechanisms and pathology, *CRC Crit Rev Toxicol* 25:207-235, 1995.

138. Jick H, Derby LE, Rodriguez LAG, et al: Liver disease associated with diclofenac, naproxen, and piroxicam, *Pharmacotherapy* 12:207, 1992. Cited in Boelsterli UA, Zimmerman HJ, Kretz-Rommel A: Idiosyncratic liver toxicity of nonsteroidal antiinflammatory drugs: molecular mechanisms and pathology, *CRC Crit Rev Toxicol* 25:207-235, 1995.

139. Kuzell WC, Schaffarzick RW, Naugler WE: Phenylbutazone, further clinical evaluation, *Arch Intern Med* 92:603, 1953. Cited in Boelsterli UA, Zimmerman HJ, Kretz-Rommel A: Idiosyncratic liver toxicity of nonsteroidal antiinflammatory drugs: molecular mechanisms and pathology, *CRC Crit Rev Toxicol* 25:207-235, 1995.

140. Brogden RN, Heel RC, Speight TM, et al: Piroxicam. A reappraisal of its pharmacology and therapeutic efficacy, *Drugs* 28:292, 1984. Cited in Boelsterli UA, Zimmerman HJ, Kretz-Rommel A: Idiosyncratic liver toxicity of nonsteroidal antiinflammatory drugs: molecular mechanisms and pathology, *CRC Crit Rev Toxicol* 25:207-235, 1995.

141. Thompson M. Stephenson P, Percy JS: Ibufenac in the treatment of arthritis, *Ann Rheumat Dis* 23:397, 1964. Cited in Boelsterli UA, Zimmerman HJ, Kretz-Rommel A: Idiosyncratic liver toxicity of nonsteroidal antiinflammatory drugs: molecular mechanisms and pathology, *CRC Crit Rev Toxicol* 25:207-235, 1995.

142. Hart FD, Boardman PL: Ibufenac (4-isobutylphenyl acetic acid), *Ann Rheumat Dis* 24: 61, 1965. Cited in Boelsterli UA, Zimmerman HJ, Kretz-Rommel A: Idiosyncratic liver toxicity of nonsteroidal antiinflammatory drugs: molecular mechanisms and pathology, *CRC Crit Rev Toxicol* 25:207-235, 1995.

143. PhRMA/FDA/AASLD drug-induced hepatotoxicity white paper postmarketing considerations, November 2000.

144. Beard K, Belic L, Aselton P, et al: Outpatient drug-induced parenchymal liver disease requiring hospitalization, *J Clin Pharmacol* 26:633-637, 1986.

145. Walker AM, Cavanaugh RJ: The occurrence of new hepatic disorders in a defined population, *Post Marketing Surveillance* 1:107-117, 1992. Cited in PhRMA/FDA/AASLD drug-induced hepatotoxicity white paper postmarketing considerations, November 2000.

146. Duh MS, Walker AM, Kronlund KH: Descriptive epidemiology of acute liver enzyme abnormalities in the general population of central Massachusetts, *Pharmacoepidemiol Drug Saf* 8:275-283, 1999. Cited in PhRMA/FDA/AASLD drug-induced hepatotoxicity white paper postmarketing considerations, November 2000.

147. Watkins PB, Zimmerman HJ, Knapp MJ, et al: Hepatotoxic effects of tacrine administration in patients with Alzheimer's disease, *JAMA* 271:992-998, 1994.

148. Bailey CJ: The rise and fall of troglitazone, *Diabet Med* 17:414, 2000. Cited in O'Moore-Sullivan TM, Prins JB: Thiazolidinediones and type 2 diabetes: new drugs for an old disease, *Med J Aust* 176:381-386, 2002.

149. Lumpkin MM cited in O'Moore-Sullivan TM, Prins JB: Thiazolidinediones and type 2 diabetes: new drugs for an old disease, *Med J Aust* 176:381-386, 2002.

150. Gitlin N, Julie NL, Spurr CL, et al: Two cases of severe clinical and histologic hepatotoxicity associated with troglitazone, *Ann Intern Med* 129:36-38, 1998. Cited in Lee WM: Assessment causality in drug-induced liver injury, *J Hepatol* 33:1003-1005, 2000.

151. Neuschwander-Tetri BA, Isley WL, Oki JC, et al: Troglitazone-induced hepatic failure leading to liver transplantation. A case report, *Ann Intern Med* 129(1):38-41, 1998. Cited in Lee WM: Assessment causality in drug-induced liver injury, *J Hepatol* 33:1003-1005, 2000.

152. Geller LI, Bessonova GA, Griaznova MW: The effect of cimetidine and gastrozepin on liver function and the pharmacotherapy of "hepatogenous" gastroduodenal ulcers and erosions [in Russian], *Ter Arkh* 63:78-81, 1991.

153. Dragull K, Yoshida WY, Tang CS: Piperidine alkaloids from *Piper methysticum*, *Phytochem* 63:193-198, 2003.

154. Ono M, Chen S: Kava liver toxicity: possible causes and possible cures, 'Awa in 2002 a research update, University of Hawaii, Komohana Building, Hilo, 17 August 2002.

155. Obermeyer WR, Musser SM, Betz JM, et al: Chemical studies of phyto-oestrogens and related compounds in dietary supplements: flax and chaparral, *Proc Soc Exp Biol Med* 208:6-12, 1995.

156. Lebot V, Merlin M, Lindstrom L: *Kava—the Pacific elixir: the definitive guide to its ethnobotany, history and chemistry*, Yale University Press, 1992, New Haven.

157. Personal communication from Vincent Lebot, October 15, 2002.

158. Singh YN, Singh NN: Therapeutic potential of kava in the treatment of anxiety disorders, *CNS Drugs* 16:731-743, 2002.

159. Steiner GG: The correlation between cancer incidence and kava consumption, *Hawaii Med J* 59:420-422, 2000.

160. Personal communication from Graham Pinn, June 15, 2002.

161. Personal communication from Dr. Fiona McLean, October 15, 2002.

162. Northern Territory Treasury: Racing, Gaming and Licensing: Kava. Available online: http://www.nt.gov.au/ntt/licensing/kava/kava.htm (accessed October 29, 2002).

163. Malsch U, Kieser M: Efficacy of kava-kava in the treatment of non-psychotic anxiety, following pretreatment with benzodiazepines, *Psychopharmacology (Berl)* 157:277-283, 2001.

164. Scherer J: Kava-kava extract in anxiety disorders: An outpatient observational study, *Adv Ther* 15:261-269, 1998.

165. Cropley M, Cave Z, Ellis J, et al: Effect of kava and valerian on human physiological and psychological responses to mental stress assessed under laboratory conditions, *Phytother Res* 16:23-27, 2002.

166. Pittler MH, Ernst E: Efficacy of kava extract for treating anxiety: systematic review and meta-analysis, *J Clin Psychopharmacol* 20:84-89, 2000.

167. Mittmann U, Schmidt M, Vrastyakova J: Acute anxiolytic efficacy of kava semiliquid special extract and benzodiazepines as premedication in surgical interventions [in German], *J Pharmakol Ther* 9:99-108, 2000.

168. Pittler MH, Ernst E: Kava extract for treating anxiety, *Cochrane Database Syst Rev* 2:CD003383, 2002.

169. Volz HP, Kieser M: Kava-kava extract WS 1490 versus placebo in anxiety disorders – A randomized placebo-controlled 25-week outpatient trial, *Pharmacopsychiatry* 30:1-5, 1997.

170. Neuhaus W, Ghaemi Y, Schmidt T, et al: Treatment of perioperative anxiety in suspected breast carcinoma with a phytogenic tranquilizer [in German], *Zentralbl Gynakol* 122:561-565, 2000.

171. Watkins LL, Connor KM, Davidson JRT: Effect of kava extract on vagal cardiac control in generalized anxiety disorder: preliminary findings, *J Psychopharmacol* 15:283-286, 2001.

172. Wheatley D: Stress-induced insomnia treated with kava and valerian: singly and in combination, *Human Psychopharmacol* 16:353-356, 2001.

173. De Leo V, la Marca A, Morgante G, et al: Evaluation of combining kava extract with hormone replacement therapy in the treatment of postmenopausal anxiety, *Maturitas* 39:185-188, 2001.

174. Mills S, Bone K: *Principles and practice of phytotherapy: Modern herbal medicine*, Churchill Livingstone, Edinburgh, 2000, pp 460-462.

175. Scholing WE, Clausen HD: On the effect of d,l-kavain: experience with neuronika [in German], *Med Klin* 72:1301-1306, 1977.

176. Lindenberg D, Pitule-Schoedel H: D,L-kavain in comparison with oxazepam in anxiety disorders. A double-blind study of clinical effectiveness [in German], *Fortschr Med* 108:49-50, 53-54, 1990.

177. Kinzler E, Kromer J, Lehmann E: Effect of a special kava extract in patients with anxiety-, tension-, and excitation states of non-psychotic genesis. Double blind study with placebos over 4 weeks [in German], *Arzneim-Forsch* 41:584-588, 1991.

178. Lehmann E, Kinzler E, Friedemann J: Efficacy of a special Kava extract (*Piper methysticum*) in patients with states of anxiety, tension and excitedness of non-mental origin -A double-blind placebo-controlled study of four weeks treatment, *Phytomedicine* 3:113-119, 1996.

179. Woelk H, Kapoula O, Lehrl S, et al: A comparison of kava special extract WS 1490 and benzodiazepines in patients with anxiety [in German], *Z Allg Med* 69:271-277, 1993.

180. Volz HP: A randomized double-blind study on the anxiolytic effects of kava special extract WS 1490 in longterm

therapeutic use [in German], 6th Phytotherapy Conference, Berlin, October 5-7, 1995.

181. Kretzschmar R: Pharmacological examinations of the central nervous effects and the mechanism of action of kava (*Piper methysticum*) and its crystalline active substances [in German]. In Loew D, Rietbrock N (eds): *Herbal medicines in research and clinical application*, Steinkopff (Verlag), Darmstadt, 1995, pp 29-38.

182. Haensel R: Kava-kava (*Piper methysticum* G. Forster) in modern drug research: Portrait of a medicinal plant [in German], *Z Phytother* 17:180-195, 1996.

183. Warnecke G: Psychosomatic dysfunctions in the female climacteric. Clinical effectiveness and tolerance of Kava Extract WS 1490 [in German], *Fortschr Med* 109:119-122, 1991.

184. German Commission E: Kava-Kava: Declaration of the commission E [in German], *Z Phytother* 4:158, 2002.

185. Stafford N: Germans warned against kava products on Internet, Reuters Press Release, October 24, 2002.

186. Personal communication from M. Schmidt, August 2003.

Appendix 1   Abbreviations Used in Chapter 12

ACE	Angiotensin-converting enzyme
AdM	Agence du Médicament = French Medicines Agency
ADRAC	Adverse Drug Reactions Advisory Committee (TGA, Australia)
AFSSAPS	L'Agence française de sécurité sanitaire des produits de santé = French Health Products Safety Agency
AHPA	American Herbal Products Association
ARMS	Adverse Reaction Monitoring System of the FDA
BAH	Bundesverband der Arzneimittel-Hersteller e.V. = German Drug Manufacturer's Association
BfArM	Bundesinstitut für Arzneimittel und Medizinprodukte = German Federal Institute for Drugs and Medical Devices
BPI	Bundesverband der Pharmazeutischen Industrie e.V. = German Pharmaceutical Industry Assocn
CDC	Centers for Disease Control and Prevention (U.S.)
CIOMS	Council for International Organizations of Medical Sciences (WHO/UNESCO)
CMEC	Complementary Medicines Evaluation Committee (TGA, Australia)
CMV	Cytomegalovirus
COX-2	Cyclooxygenase-2
CSM	Committee on Safety of Medicines (U.K., part of MCA)
EBV	Epstein-Barr virus
EHPA	European Herbal Practitioners Association
EMEA	European Agency for the Evaluation of Medicinal Products
FDA	Food and Drug Administration (U.S.)
FSA	Food Safety Agency (U.K.)
GGT	Gamma-glutamyl transpeptidase
GOT	Glutamic-oxaloacetic transaminase (Also known as asparate aminotransferase [AST])
GP	General practitioner (medical doctor practising general medicine)
GPT	Glutamic-pyruvic transaminase (also known as alanine aminotransferase [ALT])
HAM-A	Hamilton anxiety rating scale
HPLC	High performance liquid chromatography
HSV	Herpes simplex virus
IKS	Interkantonale Kontrollstelle der Schweiz = Intercantonal Office for the Control of Medicines (Switzerland). Renamed Swissmedic in 2002
IMB	Irish Medicines Board
LFTs	Liver function tests
MCA	Medicines Control Agency (of U.K.)
MSM	Methylsulphonylmethane
NSAID	Nonsteroidal antiinflammatory drug
OICM	Office intercantonal de contrôle des médicaments

Appendix 1   Abbreviations Used in Chapter 12—Cont'd

PhVWP	Pharmacovigilance Working Party (of the EMEA, Europe)
RDA	Recommended dietary allowance
SADRAC	Swedish Adverse Drug Reaction Advisory Council
SSRI	Selective serotonin reuptake inhibitor
Swissmedic	Swiss Agency for Therapeutic Products (formerly IKS)
TGA	Therapeutic Goods Administration (Australia)
TLC	Thin layer chromatography
TMEC	Traditional Medicines Evaluation Committee (of the EHPA)

Appendix 2   **Data Relating to Case Reports of Suspected Hepatotoxicity Associated with Kava from Germany, Switzerland, the United States, Canada, France, and Australia**

NOTE: The information presented here is the officially distributed data as supplied, which is not necessarily complete or correct. Errors in this table are corrected in the discussion of these cases in the body of this article

#	Where reported	MCA #	Other case #	Age	Sex	Suspect product	Concomitant medication	Onset of reaction	Nature of reaction	Outcome	Further relevant information
1	UK	1	MCA Case Report; EMEA #1	40	m	Kava	None stated	3 months	Sore throat, nose bleeds, abnormal LFTs	Recovered after stopping Kava	Drinks approx. 6 bottles of wine a week
2	UK	2	MCA Case Report; EMEA #2	—	f	Kava (3 × 150 mg/day)	Prozac	2 months	Jaundice, increased LFTs	Reaction continues	Hospitalised for 7 weeks, biopsy pending
3	UK	3	MCA Case Report	48	m	Kava	Bendrofluazide	Approx. 8 years	Raised LFTs	Recovering after withdrawal of Kava	Patient stopped taking Kava due to the voluntary withdrawal, saw information on the website and after 8 years of stable, increased LFTs, the liver enzymes are returning to normal
4	Literature	4	Reported by Schwabe GmbH & Co; BfArM #93/0351; EMEA #3	68	f	3 × 70 mg/day (Laitan 100; acetone extract)			Increased liver enzymes		Hepatic problems prior to Kava treatment
5	Literature	5	Lit: Strahl et al., 1998; EMEA #4	39	f	60 mg/day?	Paroxetin, St. John's Wort PRN, hormonal ovulation inhibitors	6 months and 14 days after rechallenge	Severe hepatitis with confluent necrosis	Recovered on withdrawal of all drugs	Positive rechallenge with kava product. Hepatic side effects are described for hormonal ovulation inhibitors (been on them for 6 years)

#	Country	Ref	Citation	Age	Sex	Dose/extract	Concomitant medication	Duration	Diagnosis	Outcome	Comments
6	Literature	6	Lit: Kraft et al., 2001; EMEA #5	60	f	Up to 480 mg/day (Antares 120 mg; ethanol-extract)	Etilefrin-HCl, Piretanid	Approx. 1 year	Fulminant liver failure	Received liver transplant	Sporadic notifications of hepatic side effects under Piretanid. Patient taking 4× recommended dose
7	Switz.	7	IKS #1999-2596; EMEA #6	46	f	2 × 70 mg kava lactone	Propanolol, HCT, valsartan	4.5 months	Severe liver damage with icterus	Recovered after Kava stopped	Hepatic side effects also described for concomitant medication
8	Switz.	8	IKS #2000-0014; EMEA #7	33	f	3 × 70 mg/day (Laitan 100; acetone extract)	1 × approx. 60 g alcohol	2-3 months	Cholestatic hepatitis with icterus	Recovery after 6 weeks	Lab tests confirmed drug-induced hepatic damage and ruled out alcohol-induced damage despite single episode of high alcohol intake
9	Switz.	9	IKS #2000-2330; EMEA #8	60	f	70 mg/day (Laitan; acetone extract) 3 Wochen	Celecoxib	3 weeks	Increased bilirubin and transaminases, indolent icterus	Recovery after 2 weeks	Hepatic side effects also known for concomitant medication
10	Switz.	10	IKS #2000-3502; EMEA #9	50	m	3-4 × 70 mg (Laitan; acetone extract)	Alcohol moderately, 1-2 × paracetamol, evening primrose oil	Approx. 2 months	Acute necrotizing hepatitis, irreversible liver damage	Received liver transplant	Notifications of hepatic side effects under Paracetamol exist
11	Germany	11	BfArM #90003882; EMEA #10	69	f	2 × 200 mg (Neuronika; contains synthetic Kavain)	ASS, Dehydrosanol, Rentylin		Cholestatic hepatitis	Recovered	Hepatic side effects are described for all concomitant medication

(Continued)

Appendix 2   **Data Relating to Case Reports of Suspected Hepatotoxicity Associated with Kava from Germany, Switzerland, the United States, Canada, France, and Australia—cont'd**

#	Where reported	MCA #	Other case #	Age	Sex	Suspect product	Concomitant medication	Onset of reaction	Nature of reaction	Outcome	Further relevant information
12	Germany	12	BfArM #92901203; EMEA #11	35	m	2 × 200 mg (Neuronika; contains synthetic kavain)		Prolonged period	Cholestatic hepatitis	Recovery after discontinuation of kava product	
13	Germany	13	IKS #93/0274; BfArM #93015209; EMEA #12	39	f	3 × 70 mg/day (Laitan 100; acetone extract)	Diazepam, Gravistat, L-Thyroxine	Approx. 2 months	Upper abdominal pressure, nausea, vomiting, jaundice	Recovery after discontinuation of all medication	Hepatotoxicity also known for the concomitant medication
14	Germany	14	BfArM #94006568; IKS #94/0259; EMEA #13	68	f	3 × 70 mg/day (Laitan 100; acetone extract)	Neuroplant forte, Maaloxan if required	Approx. 2 years	Cholestatic hepatitis, jaundice. Diagnosed as immunological hypersensitivity reaction resulting in idiosyncratic hepatic damage	Recovered	Recovery after 97 days; sporadic notifications of increased liver parameters under Maaloxan
15	Germany	15	BfArM #94901308; IKS#94/0117; EMEA #14	50	f	3 × 70 mg/day (Laitan 100; acetone extract)	Teldane, Atenolol, Hydrotrix	Approx. 2 months	Increased liver enzymes, liver cell impairment, acute hepatitis with icterus		Hepatic side effects also described for concomitant medication
16	Germany	16	BfArM #97002825; probable duplicate with #97003551 (not listed here); EMEA #15	72 (75)	f	Phyto-Geriatrikum (with 25 mg dry extract with ethanol)	Eunova	Approx. 6 months (2 years for duplicate)	Jaundice, cholestatic hepatitis, hepatitis, liver cell impairment		No hepatic side effects known for concomitant medication

	Country	Reference	Age	Sex	Kava product/dose	Concomitant medication	Duration	Diagnosis	Outcome	Comments
17	Germany	BfArM #98004297; EMEA #16	81	f	2 × 60 mg (Kavatino; ethanol extract)	Hct Isis 12,5, Cralonin, Bayotensin (until 1/98)	Approx. 9 months	Toxic hepatitis with liver failure, acute yellow liver dystrophy	Died	Seldomly icterus under HCT, hepatic impairment by alcohol not excluded. Pathology showed that liver symptoms must have started at least 1.5 years prior to death. PMH -alcohol abuse
18	Germany	BfArM #99500453; EMEA #17	59	f	2 × 120 mg/day (Limbao 120)	Buscopan	Approx. 4 months	Liver cell impairment		Sporadic notifications of hepatic side effects under Buscopan, but not in SPC
19	Germany	BfArM #99062501; EMEA #18	37	f	2 × 70 mg/day (Laitan; acetone extract)	Microdiol since 5 years, 2 × Diclofenac im	2 months	Hepatitis	Recovered	Recovery after 3 months; hepatic side effects also known for concomitant medication. Negative rechallenge
20	Germany	BfArM #99003911; EMEA #19	62	f	(Kavatino; ethanol extract) 60 mg kava lactone	None denoted		Liver cell impairment	Recovered on withdrawal of all drugs	Positive rechallenge with kava product
21	Germany	BfArM #99006005; EMEA #20	33	f	(Kavatino; ethanol extract) 60 mg kava lactone	Cisapride	Approx. 4 months	Bilirubinaemia, hepatitis, increased liver enzymes, cirrhosis of the liver		Hepatic side effects also described for concomitant medication

(Continued)

Appendix 2   Data Relating to Case Reports of Suspected Hepatotoxicity Associated with Kava from Germany, Switzerland, the United States, Canada, France, and Australia—cont'd

#	Where reported	MCA #	Other case #	Age	Sex	Suspect product	Concomitant medication	Onset of reaction	Nature of reaction	Outcome	Further relevant information
22	Germany	22	BfArM #00003608; EMEA #21	21	f	8-10 × 50 mg (Kavain Harras plus)	Paspertin, Pantoprazol, Paracetamol, Basilikum-Tropfen	Approx. 6 months	Increased liver enzymes, jaundice, hepatitis		Patient was taking an excessive dose "overdose". Side effects also known for concomitant medication
23	Germany	23	BfArM #00005994; Lit: Sass et al. 2001; EMEA #22	50	f	60 mg/day (Kava-ratiopharm; ethanol extract)	Amaryl, Glucophage S, Gravistat followed by Klimonorm	Approx. 7 months	Fulminant liver failure	Received liver transplant	Hepatic side effects also known for concomitant medication
24	Germany	24	BfArM #00008627; Lit: Brauer et al. 2001; EMEA #23	22	f	2 × 120 mg (Antares; ethanol extract)	Maxalat if required, Pramino (beforehand Valette)	Approx. 3 months	Necrosis, complete destruction of the parenchyma, fulminant liver failure	Received liver transplant. Died	Hepatic side effects also known for Pramino
25	Germany	25	BfArM #01003089; EMEA #24	34	f	120 mg/day (Kava-ratiopharm; dry extract with ethanol)	Jodthyrox	Approx. 3 months	Hepatitis, increased liver enzymes	Recovery after discontinuation of the Kava medication	Sporadic notifications of hepatic side effects under Jodthrox
26	Germany	26	BfArM #01004110, EMEA #25; duplicate case #99006200; EMEA #27 (#28)	34	f	120 mg/day (Antares; ethanol extract)	St. John's wort	Approx. 3 month	Increased liver enzymes, jaundice, hepatitis	Recovered on withdrawal of Kava product	
27	Germany	27	BfArM #99005139; EMEA #26	47	f	(Antares 120; ethanol extract)	Fish oil capsules	Approx. 1 month	Increased liver enzymes	Recovered on withdrawal of all drugs	Kava product continued throughout

	Country	Case reference	Age	Sex	Product/dose	Concomitant medication	Duration	Diagnosis	Outcome	Remarks
28	Germany	BfArM #99006200, EMEA #27; duplicate case #01004110, EMEA #25 (see #26)	35	f	120 mg/day (Antares; ethanol extract)	Paracetamol	Approx. 1 month	Increased liver enzymes, jaundice, hepatitis	Recovered on withdrawal of Kava product	Notifications of hepatic side effects under paracetamol
29	Germany	BfArM #01001228, EMEA #28; duplicate case #01001924, EMEA #29 (see #30) and #01001928 (not listed here)	38	m	(Laitan 100; acetone extract)	Penicillin-V	Approx. 1 week	Liver cell impairment		
30	Germany	BfArM #01001924, EMEA #29; duplicate case (see above #29)	39	m	(Laitan 100; acetone extract)		Approx. 2 weeks	Liver cell impairment		No other drugs
31	Germany	BfArM #01003950, EMEA #30; duplicate case #01003951, EMEA #32 (see #33)	56	f	(Kavain by Fa. Harras and kava-ratiopharm)	L-Thyroxine, Lorzaar plus, Estragest patch, Antra MUPS		Hepatitis (1993 and 2001)		Positive rechallenge. Hepatic side effects also known for concomitant medication
32	Germany	BfArM #01006229; EMEA #31	32	m	240 mg/day (Antares 120 mg; ethanol extract)	Valerian (occasionally)	Approx. 3 months	Necrotizing hepatitis with insufficiency of the liver, metabolic-toxic-allergic drug damage	Received liver transplant	

(Continued)

Appendix 2 **Data Relating to Case Reports of Suspected Hepatotoxicity Associated with Kava from Germany, Switzerland, the United States, Canada, France, and Australia—cont'd**

#	Where reported	MCA #	Other case #	Age	Sex	Suspect product	Concomitant medication	Onset of reaction	Nature of reaction	Outcome	Further relevant information
33	Germany	33	BfArM #01003951, EMEA #32; duplicate case #01003950, EMEA #30 (see #31)	—	f	Kavain Harras	—	—	Hepatitis		
34	Germany	34	BfArM #01006939; EMEA #33	36	m	Laitan 100 (70 mg/day)	—	1 month	Hepatitis		
35	Germany	35	BfArM #01008989; EMEA #34	39	m	Kava (120 mg/day)	Avonex	7 months	Hepatitis and coagulation problems		
36	Germany	36	BfArM #01009681; EMEA #35	45	m	Kava (120 mg/day)	—	3 months	Increased liver enzymes		
37	Germany	37	BfArM #01010222; EMEA #36	55	m	Kava 3/day	Euglucon	1 month	Increased liver enzymes		
38	Germany	38	BfArM #01010536; EMEA #37	—	f	Maoni 1/day		—	Hepatitis, increased liver enzymes		
39	Germany	39	EMEA #38	54	f	Kava (120 mg/day)	Triamteren, thyroxine, benalapril	—	Gall bladder pain		
40	Germany	40	BfArM #02000370; EMEA #39	46	f	Antares 120 (240 mg/day)	Natil, Kilmonorm	4 months	Cirrhosis, unwell		
41	Germany	41	BfArM #02001135/ #02002378; EMEA #40	61	f	Kava (120 mg/day)	Omeprazol, Centrum, dehydrosanol	3 months	Hepatitis, jaundice, abdominal pressure, eczema, liver necrosis		Died

	Country		Report reference	Age	Sex	Product (dose)	Concomitant medication	Duration	Adverse event
42	Germany	42	BfArM #02001414; EMEA #41	46	f	Antares 120 (360 mg/day)	—	1 month	Increased liver enzymes, jaundice
43	Germany	43	BfArM #02001776; EMEA #42	27	m	Kava 2/day	Epivir, Viramune, Zerit	—	Discoloured faeces, abnormal urine, increased sweating, fear
44	Germany	44	Information received from MCA spreadsheet	—	f	Kava (120 mg/day)	—	1 year	Increased liver enzymes
45	Germany	45	BfArM #02002732; EMEA #44	24	f	Maoni forte (120 mg/day)	—	3 months	Increased liver enzymes, jaundice, abdominal pressure, generally unwell
46	Germany	46	BfArM #02002090/#02002836; EMEA #45	26	f	Kavasedon (50 mg for 6 days)	Azulfidine, Nervogastrol, Buscopan, MCP, Voltaren Resinat	—	Hepatitis*; increased liver enzymes
47	Germany	47	BfArM #02003010; EMEA #46	47	f	Kava 2/day	—	3 months	Increased liver enzymes, increased prothombin time, anorexia
48	Germany	48	BfArM #02003278; EMEA #47	50	m	Laitan 100 (2 × 70 mg/day)	—	3 months	Increased liver enzymes
49	Germany	49	BfArM #02003559; EMEA #48	50	m	Kava (120 mg/day)	—	5 months	Jaundice

*Incorrectly included in the line-listing as per advice from the notifier.[186]

(Continued)

Appendix 2 **Data Relating to Case Reports of Suspected Hepatotoxicity Associated with Kava from Germany, Switzerland, the United States, Canada, France, and Australia—cont'd**

#	Where reported	MCA #	Other case #	Age	Sex	Suspect product	Concomitant medication	Onset of reaction	Nature of reaction	Outcome	Further relevant information
50	Germany	50	BfArM #02004364; EMEA #49	32	f	Kava (240 mg/day)	Marvelon	1 month	Hepatitis, increased liver enzymes		
51	US	51	FDA #14538; EMEA #50	60	f	Kava, chaparral	Xeloda, Eniluracil, Perocet, 5-FU	Not known	Fatigue, increased LFTs	Recovered after stopping all medication	Preexisting medical conditions: advanced rectal cancer - possible metastases in liver. Restarted chemotherapy without any further increases in LFTs
52	US	52	FDA #14723; EMEA #51	44	f	Kava	OxyContin, Coumarin, Celexa, Celebrex, oestrogen patch	Not known	Neutropenia, increased LFTs	Neutropenia recovered after stopping medication. Outcome of hepatic problems not known	PMH -Marfan syndrome
53	US	53	FDA #14810; EMEA #52	33	f	Kava, Zantac	Echinacea/goldenseal, energy pack (ginseng, B100, guarana), Tums, LoEstrin, women's one a day.	Not known	Nausea, diarrhoea, jaundiced skin	Worked up for possible transplant	PMH -lymphoma with chemotherapy 1 month prior to admission
54	US	54	FDA #15035/ #15274; EMEA #53	45	f	Kava (1 tablet twice a day, but none at weekends,	Aciphex	4 months	Jaundice, puritus, cholestatic hepatitis	Received liver transplant	Hepatitis A-C = negative, low alcohol consumption on rare occasions

55	US	FDA #15250; EMEA #54	55	f	NutriZAC (50 mg Kava per tablet; 2 tablets/ day for 2 years) for about 4 months. Each tablet contains 75 mg kava lactones)	Multivitamins	2 years	Increased LFTs, fatty liver	Not known	Moderate alcohol consumption
56	US	FDA #15281; EMEA #55	27	f	Kava (Vitamin World; and 600 mg of kava in a tea 4/day for 6 months)	Psyllium, Vit B$_6$, Vit E, St. John's wort, phyto-oestrogen (Mexican yam, black cohosh, dong quai)	6 months	Nausea, vomiting, jaundice, increased LFTs, Stage 3 hepatic encephalopathy	Not known	Other aetiologies for liver disease excluded. No alcohol in 5 years. Preexisting medical condition: abdominal hysterectomy
57	US	FDA #15317; EMEA #56	38	m	Kava (product unknown), binge use described: 8 caps @ 250 mg 1-2 × per month	None stated	Not known	Liver infection, hepatitis	Recovered after stopping Kava	Repeated tests for viral causes of hepatitis all negative. 3-4 glasses of wine per week
58	US	FDA #15319; EMEA #57	63	m	Enalapril, Kava (50 mg/day for 1 month)	Vasotec (10 years)	1 month	Hepatocellular injury, nausea, haematemesis	Improving on stopping Kava and enalapril	PMH = hepatitis C

(Continued)

Appendix 2 **Data Relating to Case Reports of Suspected Hepatotoxicity Associated with Kava from Germany, Switzerland, the United States, Canada, France, and Australia—cont'd**

#	Where reported	MCA #	Other case #	Age	Sex	Suspect product	Concomitant medication	Onset of reaction	Nature of reaction	Outcome	Further relevant information
59	US	59	FDA #15466; EMEA #58	39	f	Kava (128 mg kava in 55% kava lactone extraction), Celestial Kava tea (60 mg kava in 30% kava lactone extraction)	Oral contraception, Albuterol, Benedryl, tetracycline	6 months	Tired, flu-like symptoms, jaundice	Recovered after Kava stopped	4 weeks for LFTs to return to normal
60	US	60	FDA #14951; EMEA #59	51	f	Kava (2 twice daily)	Vit D, Ginkgo, omega 3, multivitamins and minerals	4 months	Increased AST and ALT (1.5 times normal) and foot cramp	Recovered after stopping kava	
61	US	61	FDA #14995; EMEA #60	37	f	Kava Gold (acetone extract = 150 mg Kava lactones 5/day for 1 month)	None stated	3 weeks	Jaundice	Recovering after stopping Kava	Ultrasound showed fatty infiltration of liver. No PMH of alcohol abuse
62	US	62	FDA #15252; EMEA #61	62	f	Kava (200 mg, 1-3/day for about 3 months)	Green tea formula (2 weeks during the 3 month use of kava), CoQ10, Snorease	3 months	Fatigue, nausea, vomiting and increased LFTs	Improving on stopping Kava	Preexisting medical conditions: allergic to sulpha drugs

#	Country	Reference	Age	Sex	Product	Concomitant	Duration	Adverse effect	Outcome	Comments
63	US	FDA #15267; EMEA #62	51	f	Kava, Ginkgo, MSM	St. John's wort, ginseng, Vit A, D + E, flaxseed oil	2 months	Increased LFTs	Recovered after stopping Ginkgo, MSM and Kava	+ve rechallenge (but no details provided). Hepatitis A-C negative
64	France	EMEA #63	60	f	Kava	None stated	1 year	Nausea, GGT increased	Recovered after stopping Kava	
65	France	EMEA #64	39	f	Kava	Not specified, but may cause hepatotoxicity	2 months	Increased transaminases	Recovered after stopping Kava	
66	Canada	EMEA #65	–	f	Kava-kava	None stated	Long term	Hepatic function abnormal	Not known	
67	Canada	EMEA #66	53	f	Kava	St. John's wort, multivitamins		Jaundice, abnormal LFTs	Recovering after stopping Kava and other herbal preparations	History of inflammation of the liver while she was drinking 6 beers a day. She has not been drinking since then
68	Canada	EMEA #67	38	m	Kava-kava (may contain 30% kava root and 5% kava lactones). 12 gtts po twice daily.		2 weeks	Increased transaminases, hepatitis	Recovered after stopping kava	Does not drink alcohol
69	Germany	BfArM #02005178	–	f	Laitan (70 mg kava lactones, acetone extract), 70 mg per day over 2 months		2 months	Liver cell damage, liver failure		

(*Continued*)

Appendix 2　**Data Relating to Case Reports of Suspected Hepatotoxicity Associated with Kava from Germany, Switzerland, the United States, Canada, France, and Australia—cont'd**

#	Where reported	MCA # Other case #	Age	Sex	Suspect product	Concomitant medication	Onset of reaction	Nature of reaction	Outcome	Further relevant information
70	Germany	BfArM #02002541	52	f	Kava ratiopharm (60 mg kava lactones, ethanol extract), 60 mg per day over 3.5 months		3.5 months	Elevated transaminases		
71	US	FDA #14627	14	f	Celestial Seasonings Tension Tamer Extra and CSSleepytime Tea Extra (both tablets; both w/ kava); TT-2 tabs 1-5 ×/ week for 3-4 months; ST-2 tabs only 7 times at beginning of same period; taken from August to Dec 2000	None	3-4 months	Scleral icterus; hepatitis	Liver transplant	

(*Continued*)

#	Source	Reference	Age	Sex	Kava-containing product	Duration / concomitant medication	Event	Outcome	Comments
	Literature	Lit: Humbertston et al. 2001	14	f	Kava-containing product	6 months; had stopped taking for 1 month and resumed	Admitted to hospital with fulminant hepatic failure. Abnormal liver function tests	Required liver transplant	Liver biopsy showed hepatocellular necrosis consistent with chemical hepatitis. Alternative causes of liver failure were found to be negative
72	Literature (Press)	Lit: Stuckhard P. 2002.	43	f	Kava, recommended dosage	St. John's wort; iodine compound (for thyroid), betablocker	Liver failure with subsequent liver transplant	Elevated liver enzymes; liver transplantation	Viral hepatitis excluded. The patient had undergone surgery prior to taking kava
73	Literature (Press)	Lit: Hinzpeter W. 2002.	60	f	Kava, recommended dosage, for 3 months	3 months			
74	US	FDA #10257	70	f	K8 (Herbalife); ing. inc. "kava kava 40 mg" and "Biokawa 20 mg containing 14.3% kavain"; 3/day	Inderide and Aspirin (both for 15 years?); Coumadin and Zestril prescribed following event (?); fish oil; "several" vitamins (self-described "vitamin freak"); vitamin K (? Report is confusing -states Vit K but identifies K8 product as source, though states that label does not list this ingredient?)	Stroke; prolapsed mitral valve leading to prolonged (7 days?) hospitalisation; LFT elevated: GGT = 125-212, SGOT = 66-99, others normal range		Preexisting medical conditions: stroke 15 years earlier; self-described "chronic valve prolapse"; PCN allergy

Appendix 2 **Data Relating to Case Reports of Suspected Hepatotoxicity Associated with Kava from Germany, Switzerland, the United States, Canada, France, and Australia—cont'd**

#	Where reported	MCA # Other case #	Age	Sex	Suspect product	Concomitant medication	Onset of reaction	Nature of reaction	Outcome	Further relevant information
75	US	FDA #11444	24	m	7 product "suite" -Cybergenics (L&S Research), "Hard Gainers" 1-6 and Mega Weight Gain pwd; kava is listed as ing in HG6 (1st of 6 herbs, total = 200 mg); also: Vanadyl sulphate, multi-vit; vit C and chromium picc; discontinued 3-4 weeks prior to hospitalisation	None prior to treatment	3-4 weeks	Hospitalized w/ hepatic encephalopathy; fulminant hepatic failure; death		Preexisting medical conditions: none known
76	US	FDA #13198	52	f	Kava Kava (*Piper methysticum*) 300 mg (Puritan's Pride); dose N/A; used occasionally	4 DS taken regularly: MSM; "green" product; multi-glandular; alfalfa; 14 other DS taken occasionally or listed; 3 OTC listed		Hospitalized for treatment of congestive heart failure (right and left sides); acute renal failure; anasarca with 45 kg weight gain; hyperkalaemia and		Preexisting medical conditions: history of hyperthyroidism and exposure to hepatitis C; 1-2 alcoholic drinks per day with binge drinking weekends

					Kava product/dose	Concomitant medication	Duration	Symptoms	Preexisting conditions
77	US	FDA #15465; possible duplicate case FDA #15476 (listed together)	48	m	Kava; dose: 1 to 2 (?) per day; used for 5 days from 10 Dec to 15 Dec 2001	None stated	6 days	metabolic alkalosis; biopsy confirmed liver cirrhosis; Liver pain	Preexisting medical conditions: liver dysfunction
78	US	FDA #15556	72	m	Kava capsules (Hi-Health); 2 capsules, used for 2 weeks	Valerian	2 weeks	Felt ill; believed kava aggravated existing liver problems; self-report	Preexisting medical conditions: hepatitis C; liver damage
79	US	FDA #15249	53	m	NaturPharma Kava (Spring Valley); 2 caps each of 2 days; used the day the adverse reaction occurred and ?	None stated	1 day	Felt pain in liver area; self-report	Preexisting medical conditions: some allergies
80	US	FDA #15320	41	f	Kava (Limbao / BASF Generics); dose unknown; use dates not known	Lisino (loratadine), 10 mg, 18 February to 24 February 1999; St. John's wort (brand not stated) "powder" from 21 January 1999 to 9 May 1999; ethinyl oestradiol; "infusion of NaCl 0.9%"		Acute liver failure	Preexisting medical conditions: ?

(Continued)

Appendix 2 **Data Relating to Case Reports of Suspected Hepatotoxicity Associated with Kava from Germany, Switzerland, the United States, Canada, France, and Australia—cont'd**

#	Where reported	MCA # Other case #	Age	Sex	Suspect product	Concomitant medication	Onset of reaction	Nature of reaction	Outcome	Further relevant information
81	Germany	BfArM 02007130	38	f	Ethanolic kava extract, 1 × 120 mg daily	None	At least 4 weeks	Acute liver failure	Recovered	Intake of kava for treatment of anxiety
83	Australia	ADRS #177303	56	f	Kava 1800 Plus; 2 tablets daily (oral admin.)	From 25 March 2002 to 11 July 2002: alpha tocopherol, 670 mg daily; amino acids mos, 200 mg daily; ascorbic acid, 150 mg daily; magnesium amino acid chelate, 6.4 g daily	Date of onset: 29 July 2002; admitted to hospital 11 July 2002, operation 29 July 2002, date of death 29 July 2002	Jaundice, hepatic necrosis, fatigue	Death. Causality possible	Hepatitis A total detected - postinfection at immunisation for hepatitis A. Liver biopsy: severe acute hepatitis with confluent necrosis, appearance does not separate between a viral or drug reaction. Bilirubin: 209 (11/7/02), 396 (18/7/02), 534 (19/7/02), 551 (24/7/02); normal range = 18 mmol/L (?).SAP/ALP: 190 (11/7/02), 708 (18/7/02), 342 (19/7/02), 270 (24/7/02), normal range = 35 to 125 U/L. ALT/SGPT: 4539 (11/7/02), 1680 (18/7/02), 1651 (19/7/02),

640 (24/7/02), normal range = 55 U/L. GGT/SGGT/GGTF: 323 (11/7/02), 169 (18/7/02), 196 (19/7/02), 331 (24/7/02), normal range = 60 U/L. Prothrombin time: 25 (11/7/02), 44 (24/7/02). International normalised ratio: 2.3 (11/7/02), 4.2 (24/7/02). Minimal alcohol intake

PART

II

SAFETY MONOGRAPHS

Michelle Morgan, Kerry Bone, Simon Mills, and Janice McMillan

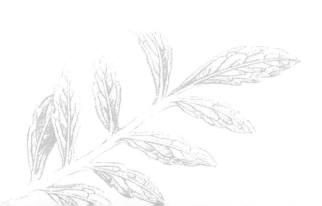

HOW TO USE THE MONOGRAPHS

The second part of the book contains 125 monographs presented in alphabetical order by common name. The aim of the monographs is to provide the reader with a summary of safety information relevant to modern clinical practice or to advise patients about their self-prescribed herbs.

The monographs are structured in the following way:

- Information that defines the herb by common names, botanical names, plant family and plant part used.
- A safety summary, which provides at a glance the authors' conclusions regarding the safety of the plant. This section includes pregnancy and lactation categories and relevant information for contraindications, warnings and precautions and adverse reactions and interactions.
- A brief outline of typical therapeutic use, actions and dosage of the herb.
- The remainder of the monograph reviews the safety information in more detail, including information from traditional sources, regulatory texts, and scientific research.

Common Name

Herb common names used throughout the monographs are presented in lower case.

Botanical Name

Linnaeus' system of nomenclature for all living things was first published in 1735 and is the classification system in current use. Nomenclature (naming) and taxonomy (classification) are continually changing scientific disciplines, so the botanical name (and its ranking) may change over time.

For example, the *Echinacea* species are currently being revised. A potential change includes[1]: *E. angustifolia* → *E. pallida* var. *angustifolia*. Changes which have been discovered but will not be enacted due to possible detriment to the pharmaceutical, herbal and agricultural industries include[2]:

- *E. purpurea* → *E. serotina*
- *E. laevigata* → *E. purpurea*

With the use of gene-sequencing techniques changes may increase in the future as a greater understanding of taxonomy at a genetic level develops. Of an estimated 5 million species (of living things), only about 1.5 million are documented at present and they are constantly being renamed and moved in the 20 or so categories of the Linnaean classification system. A new approach (phylogenetic nomenclature) which names groups of organisms that descend from a common ancestor is gaining popularity.[3]

Information about the botanical name and family has been sourced from the following (in order of preference):

- Mabberley DJ: *The plant book*, ed 2. Cambridge, 1997, Cambridge University Press. In the preparation of this book the author followed the system of Cronquist (1981) as modified by Kubitzki (1990) (pp ix-xiii).
- PLANTS database, United States Department of Agriculture (USDA).
- GRIN Taxonomy database, Agricultural Research Service, USDA.
- Global Plant Checklist, International Organization for Plant Information.

The Flora of China database provides additional information for certain plants not covered by the above sources.

The botanical name is usually a Latin binomial consisting of a generic name, which comes first followed by the specific epithet. Both components of the name are italicised. The generic name, which is capitalised, defines the genus to which the plant belongs. The authority, which follows the specific epithet, further defines the species. It indicates the scientist credited with naming the species (and hence the author of the name) and is often abbreviated (e.g., "Linnaeus" becomes "L"). The authority has been included in the initial identifying information in these monographs and, if necessary, in the Adulteration section, but is not retained throughout the remainder of the monograph (Table 1).

A botanical name may contain three Latin names when the species is further divided into subspecies or varieties (e.g. *Arnica chamissonis* subsp. *foliosa*,

Table 1 **Example of a Botanical Name**

Tilia cordata **Mill.**	
Generic name	Tilia
Specific epithet	cordata
Plant species	*Tilia cordata*
Authority	Mill. (short for Miller)

Viburnum opulus var. *americanum*). In the name *Tilia* x *vulgaris*, the x indicates that this is a hybrid (in this case *Tilia* x *vulgaris* is a cross of *T. cordata* and *T. platy-phyllos*).

After the first appearance in the text, the first Latin name may be abbreviated to its initial letter (e.g., *T. cordata*).

The botanical name presented first in the monographs is not necessarily the most recent name, but is the name most familiar to practitioners and consumers. Relevant botanical synonyms are listed in brackets after the preferred botanical name and may be more or less recent in terms of current nomenclature (Table 2).

Often more than one species (in the same genus) may be used therapeutically for the designated herb; these are called medicinally-interchangeable species. *Tilia cordata* is the preferred species for the uses described for lime flower, but *Tilia platyphyllos* can also be used for the same clinical applications and is therefore medicinally interchangeable. Medicinally-interchangeable species are listed after the first botanical name and separated by a comma (Table 3).

Information regarding medicinally-interchangeable species is obtained from authoritative texts and the various pharmacopoeias.

Table **2**   **Example of Botanical Synonyms**

Tilia cordata Mill. (*Tilia parvifolia* Ehrh., *Tilia ulmifolia* Scop.)	
Preferred botanical name	*Tilia cordata* Mill.
Botanical synonym	*Tilia parvifolia* Ehrh.
Botanical synonym	*Tilia ulmifolia* Scop.

Table **3**   **Example of Medicinally-Interchangeable Species**

Tilia cordata Mill. (*Tilia parvifolia* Ehrh., *Tilia ulmifolia* Scop.), *Tilia platyphyllos* Scop.	
Preferred botanical name	*Tilia cordata* Mill.
Botanical synonym	*Tilia parvifolia* Ehrh.
Botanical synonym	*Tilia ulmifolia* Scop.
Medicinally-interchangeable species	*Tilia platyphyllos* Scop

Family

Organisms are grouped into broader taxonomic categories, which are arranged in the following hierarchy:

Kingdom (plant or fungi) – Phylum – Class – Order – Family – Genus – Species

The family of a herb provides additional information of relevance to herbal use:
- Safety: plants of the Compositae or daisy family may cause contact allergy.
- Identification: some herbalists harvest or wildcraft herbs and the family provides additional information necessary for botanical identification.
- Potential therapeutic actions/applications: phytochemicals known to exist in a family may suggest a therapeutic action or application.

The texts and sources used for retrieval of the family are as defined above. Changes in taxonomy that have occurred after the publication of Mabberley (1997) are not necessarily represented here. Potential changes are still being debated in some cases, for example the Scrophulariaceae is undergoing revision, which may affect a number of herbs (including Rehmannia [listed in Gesneriaceae by some sources]), and there is debate as to whether *Hydrastis canadensis* should be in a family of its own rather than the Ranunculaceae (refer to AHP monograph for discussion[4]).

The authors have followed the convention of Mabberly in using what is often considered to be the "older" family names. However, according to the International Association of Botanical Nomenclature (St Louis Code, 1999), these as well as the "newer" alternative family names are valid (Table 4).

Plant Part Used

Lists the plant part(s) used for therapeutic purposes.

Typical Therapeutic Use, Actions

In order to assist the reader in understanding why their patients may be taking a herb, this section includes a brief outline of the therapeutic application of the herb from traditional systems, as well as prominent clinical trial information where available.

Table **4** **Examples of Alternative Naming for Plant Families**

Family Name	Alternative Family Name
Palmae	Arecaceae
Gramineae	Poaceae
Cruciferae	Brassicaceae
Leguminosae	Fabaceae
Guttiferae	Clusiaceae
Umbelliferae	Apiaceae
Labiatae	Lamiaceae
Compositae	Asteraceae

The main therapeutic actions of the herb are also provided.

Key Constituents

The Key constituents and Adulteration sections focus on constituents and species of importance to the therapeutic use of the herb and potential safety concerns.

A constituent may be of importance to the quality of the herb and its efficacy when prescribed. Where possible, key constituents have been quantified to assist the reader when considering the toxicology of that constituent.

Adulteration

Correct botanical species identification is both a quality and a potential safety issue. Administration of an incorrect species may lower the efficacy of the herb, but in some cases may cause an adverse reaction due to substitution with a toxic herb. This section also includes information regarding endangerment. Practitioners need to act to avert the potential loss of therapeutic plants, but this information is also relevant to safety because scarcity increases the cost of the herb and the potential for adverse reactions through substitution.

CITES (the Convention on International Trade in Endangered Species of Wild Fauna and Flora) currently provides the only international instrument for listing species whose numbers are considered to be sufficiently endangered to the extent that commercial trade must be monitored and controlled, or prohibited.[5]

Typical Dosage Forms & Dosage

Typical adult dosages have been supplied for the dried herb and a range of liquid extracts and tinctures. The information is obtained from authoritative traditional texts and authorities and reflects typical modern use. Doses above these levels might increase the risk of adverse reactions or toxicity (see Overdosage section).

The authoritative texts used mainly comprised the following:

- British Herbal Medicine Association's Scientific Committee: *British herbal pharmacopoeia.* Bournemouth, 1983, BHMA.
- British Herbal Medicine Association's Scientific Committee: *British herbal pharmacopoeia*, ed 4. Bournemouth, 1996, BHMA.
- Pharmacopoeia Commission of the People's Republic of China: *Pharmacopoeia of the People's Republic of China*, English ed. Beijing, 1997, Chemical Industry Press.
- Bensky D, Gamble A: *Chinese herbal medicine materia medica.* Seattle, 1986, Eastland Press.
- Scientific Committee of ESCOP (European Scientific Cooperative on Phytotherapy): *ESCOP monographs.* UK, March 1996 to October 1999, European Scientific Cooperative on Phytotherapy Secretariat.
- Blumenthal M, et al, eds: *The complete German Commission E monographs: therapeutic guide to herbal medicines.* Austin, 1998, American Botanical Council.
- Kapoor LD: *CRC handbook of Ayurvedic medicinal plants.* Boca Raton, 1990, CRC Press.
- Regional Research Laboratory and Indian Drug Manufacturers' Association: *Indian herbal pharmacopoeia.* Jammu-Tawi, 1998, Indian Drug Manufacturers' Association, Mumbai and Regional Research Laboratory.

In addition, dosages used in clinical trials were taken into account.

Contraindications

The information presented here is a critical review of traditional references, clinical trials and the modern understanding based on clinical practice. Often, contraindications are described for herbs in popular literature and medical articles, which have little realistic basis for recommendation. Contraindications listed in this section are done with a definite rationale and, where disagreement exists with other recognised references, the rationale is provided.

Use in Pregnancy

The following pregnancy categories are assigned on the basis of the available and relevant traditional and scientific information. Generally, traditional information about herbs with an emmenagogue action (bringing on menstruation) and in vitro studies demonstrating contraction of isolated uterine tissue are generally not included in the assessment. More reliable information is instead included, such as traditional pregnancy contraindications, animal models of the use of the herb or its constituents during pregnancy, as well as in vivo teratogenicity studies. It must be stressed that this categorisation is driven by the data and is designed, as much as possible, to remove the subjective element from assessing the safety of herbs in pregnancy. Therefore, to some readers there may be surprises as to how the various herbs have been assigned (Table 5).

(The pregnancy categories are adapted from the Australian publication *Medicines in pregnancy*, ed 4, 1999. See Chapter 7 for further information concerning the relevance of these categories.)

Category A has been assigned usually where the use of the herb in pregnancy is known to be widespread and there is at least one published study of its safe use in pregnancy. However, in some cases where the herb is widely used as a food, for example cranberry *(Vaccinium macrocarpon)*, then the requirement for a published study was not enforced.

Although the A to X classification provides a general guide to increasing safety concerns, it must be stressed again that these categories are assigned according to the data. Hence there are many herbs assigned to category B2. It is likely that the vast majority of these herbs are safe during pregnancy and in terms of risk deserve inclusion in category A (e.g., marshmallow). However, without documented studies of safe use during pregnancy, the category A assignment cannot be given to such herbs.

As stated earlier, this categorisation is designed to remove the subjectivity from assessing the safety information for herbs during pregnancy. The subjective element comes in when the reader interprets this information to guide the advice they give to their patients. For example, a highly cautious approach would be to use or advise herbs in category A only. It is up to each practitioner to use these

Table **5**   **Recommended Pregnancy Categories**

Category A	No proven increase in the frequency of malformation or other harmful effects on the foetus despite consumption by a large number of women
Category B1	No increase in frequency of malformation or other harmful effects on the foetus from limited use in women. No evidence of increased foetal damage in animal studies
Category B2	No increase in frequency of malformation or other harmful effects on the foetus from limited use in women. Animal studies are lacking
Category B3	No increase in frequency of malformation or other harmful effects on the foetus from limited use in women. Evidence of increased foetal damage in animal studies exists, although the relevance to humans is unknown
Category C	Has caused or is associated with a substantial risk of causing harmful effects on the foetus or neonate without causing malformations
Category D	Has caused or is associated with a substantial risk of causing foetal malformation or irreversible damage
Category X	High risk of damage to the foetus

data to conduct a risk–benefit analysis for each individual case, also taking into account the confidence and experience of the therapist in recommending herbs during pregnancy.

Use in Lactation

The lactation categories assigned are those advocated by the American Academy of Pediatrics in 1994 (Table 6) (see Chapter 7).

Table **6**   **Recommended Lactation Categories**

Category ND	No data available
Category C	Compatible with breastfeeding
Category CC	Compatible with breastfeeding but use caution
Category SD	Strongly discouraged in breastfeeding
Category X	Contraindicated in breastfeeding

Warnings & Precautions

Appropriate warnings and cautions are provided and may arise from consideration of data such as contraindications, clinical studies, case reports, the phytochemicals in the herb (if they are present in significant quantities) and its traditional uses.

Effect on Ability to Drive or Operate Machinery

In most cases there is very little pharmacological and clinical research to make a definite recommendation regarding effect on ability to drive or operate machinery. The recommendation is therefore presented on the basis of the knowledge of the herb, its constituents and traditional information.

Adverse Reactions

This section includes adverse reactions (ARs) documented in traditional texts, regulatory information, clinical trials and case reports. ARs caused by both topical and systemic administration are included.

Where multiple ARs are reported, they are often summarised in table form with relevant clinical details listed. The case reports are listed by year of publication, not the year of occurrence of the AR. Contentious ARs are discussed in greater detail. The listing of ARs does not automatically imply causality. In the majority of published ARs there is a deficiency of information, including identification of the plant material ingested (correct species, plant part) and dosage. There is rarely any verification that the product was not contaminated. Due consideration of concomitant drug ingestion is often not given.

Interactions

Herb–drug interactions are presented from reliable case reports, clinical studies and opinion of expert committees such as the German Commission E (see Regulatory status for explanation). In general a herb–drug interaction causing a possible beneficial effect, such as the herb increasing the effectiveness of an administered drug, is not included, particularly where it involves a known major action of the herb. A practitioner prescribing a herbal treatment to a patient concurrently taking a drug with a similar activity would be alert to such a possibility and should monitor the patient. However, the exception is where a positive reinforcement of the action of a drug by a herb might lead to harmful effects, such as with hypoglycaemic drugs and insulin. Concerns of this kind have been included.

In general, information about interactions between herb and drug derived from in vitro studies are not included, due to the unknown relevance of this work to oral administration in humans. Studies using experimental models (in vivo animal studies) are included since they may provide the basis for a possible interaction in humans.

Refer also to Chapter 6 and the table therein.

Safety in Children

Little specific scientific information about the safety of herbs in children exists. Recommendations are usually based on the knowledge of the herb, its constituents and traditional evidence of safe use in children.

Overdosage

Poisoning and adverse reactions resulting from overdosage (mostly in humans) are listed. Poisoning by parts of the plant other than the used part is sometimes included for clarification, since some texts assign such information to the herb without elaborating which plant part was involved.

Toxicology

This section provides the reader with information about the acute and chronic toxicology (including the lethal dose), mutagenicity and carcinogenicity for the herb and/or key herbal constituents. The route of administration is reported for both toxicological and teratogenicity data, since it affects the extrapolation to human use of the herb.

Abbreviations used throughout this section are found in Table 7.

LD_{50} Test

The LD_{50} test was introduced in 1927 for the biological standardisation of drugs.[6] With the mean lethal dose (LD_{50}) test, groups of experimental animals are treated with graduated doses of a test substance with the aim of obtaining a 50% or even higher mortality at the highest doses. The scientific significance of the classical LD_{50} test has been questioned on the basis of the relatively broad variability of the test results (more than 2-fold and up

Table **7**   **Abbreviations Used**

i.g.*	Intragastric
i.m.	Intramuscular
i.p.	Intraperitoneal
i.v.	Intravenous
LD_{50}	Lethal dose for 50% for the tested population
LOAEL	Lowest observed adverse effects level
MLD	Minimum lethal dose The highest dose of a chemical that does not alter the life span or severely affect the health of an animal
MOAEL	Minimum observed adverse effect level
MTD	Maximum tolerated dose
NOAEL	No observed adverse effect level The highest dosage administered that does not produce toxic effects
s.c.	Subcutaneous
TLV	Threshold limit value
TTL	Threshold toxic limit

In some cases "oral" has been used for "gavage" and "i.g." administration.

to 11-fold differences) and for animal welfare reasons.[7] Three recently developed alternative animal tests that significantly improve animal welfare – the fixed dose procedure, the acute toxic class method, and the up and down procedure – can now be used within a strategy of acute toxicity testing for all types of test substances and for regulatory and in-house purposes. In vitro cytotoxicity tests can be used as adjuncts to these alternative animal tests to improve dose level selection and reduce (at least modestly) the number of animals used. However, the total replacement of animal tests requires a considerable amount of further development[8] and such modern data are not yet currently available for most herbs.

The LD_{50} values can be grouped into toxicity levels,[9] as outlined in the Table 8 with examples.

In terms of categorising the acute toxicity of different herbs, assessments were based on dried herb equivalent quantities. In other words, an LD_{50} of 2000 mg/kg for a 5:1 extract would give a dried herb equivalent dosage of 10,000 mg/kg, indicating slight toxicity.

Ames Salmonella/Microsome Mutagenicity Assay (Salmonella Test; Ames Test)

This is a short-term bacterial reverse mutation assay specifically designed to detect a wide range of

Table **8**   **Interpreting LD_{50} Values**

Lethal Dose	Toxicity Level	Example
<1 mg/kg	Dangerously toxic	Dioxin: 0.045 mg/kg (oral, rat (female))
1-50 mg/kg	Extremely toxic	Indomethacin: 12.6 mg/kg (oral, rat) Dieldrin: 46 mg/kg (oral, rat)
50-500 mg/kg	Very toxic	Aristolochic acid: 55.9 mg/kg (oral, mouse (male)) Curare: 270 mg/kg (oral, rabbit) Paracetamol: 338 mg/kg (oral, mouse) Caffeine: 355 mg/kg (oral, rat (male))
500-5000 mg/kg	Moderately toxic	Atropine: 622 mg/kg (oral, rat) Aspirin: 1500 mg/kg (oral, rat) Baking soda: 4220 mg/kg (oral, rat)
5000-15000 mg/kg	Slightly toxic	Sodium cyanide: 6444 mg/kg (oral, rat) Monosodium succinate (food additive): >8 g/kg (oral, rat)
>15000 mg/kg	Practically nontoxic	Propylene glycol (cosmetics): 20000 mg/kg (oral, rat)

chemical substances that can produce genetic damage leading to gene mutations.[10] The test was developed by Ames and colleagues in the mid-1970s and became the most used test because of its initial promise of high qualitative (yes/no) predictivity for cancer in rodents and, by extension, in humans. The relationship between mutagenic potency prediction and quantitative carcinogenicity is, however, now known to be weak,[11] despite the fact that early studies with this assay indicated that greater than 90% of the known carcinogens tested were mutagenic and that 90% of the noncarcinogens tested were nonmutagenic. The power of this assay was derived from the use of a liver microsome fraction (S9 mix) containing the mixed function oxidase enzymes required to activate the test substance into precarcinogens (as might occur in the body after phase I metabolism by the liver). As the basis of the selection of chemicals for mutagenicity testing shifted to relative environmental importance, the sensitivity of the Salmonella assay for detecting carcinogens decreased. A negative result does not imply that the chemical will be noncarcinogenic. There are a large number of false-negatives produced (i.e., nongenotoxic carcinogens).[12]

Micronucleus Tests

This test involves induction and quantitative measurement of chromosomal damage leading to the formation of micronuclei in cells which have been exposed to genotoxic agents or ionising radiation.

SOS Chromotest

The SOS chromotest is a simple bacterial colorimetric assay for genotoxicity, which may be used as a primary screening tool or as part of a battery of short-term tests for carcinogens.

Regulatory Status

The regulatory status of the herb in Australia, China, Germany, the United Kingdom, and the United States is presented. This includes listings within the following official pharmacopoeias: *Pharmacopoeia of the People's Republic of China* 1997, *British Pharmacopoeia* 2002, *European Pharmacopoeia* 4.3 (01/2003) and *United States Pharmacopeia–National Formulary* (USP26-NF21, 2003). Other regulatory sources are defined in Table 9.

Table **9**   **Other Sources for Regulatory Information**

Australia	The Standard for the Uniform Scheduling of Drugs and Poisons (SUSDP) contains the decisions of the National Drugs and Poisons Schedule Committee (established under Section 52B of the Therapeutic Goods Act 1989), regarding the classification of drugs and poisons into Schedules for inclusion into the relevant legislation of the States and Territories. The SUSDP requires each State to adopt its recommendations by State law. State governments may regulate substances in addition to that recommended in the SUSDP. Legislation updated to SUSDP No. 17 Amendment No. 2, effective date 1st January 2003, was scrutinised for inclusions. Schedule 4 of the SUSDP (Prescription Only Medicine) lists substances which are available from a pharmacist on a prescription only basis (from a doctor or persons permitted by State or Territory legislation). Part 4 of Schedule 4 of the Therapeutic Goods Regulations specifies herbs which cannot be contained in any products listed on the Australian Register of Therapeutic Goods (ARTG), or which can only be present in minute doses or if other specified conditions are met. In other words, herbs on Part 4 of Schedule 4 are considered to be more toxic and cannot be included in over-the-counter herbal products without further safety evaluations (see below). Herbs on this list may be supplied as raw materials to practitioners provided they are not included in retail products. Products containing herbs on this list (except for those which are listed on SUSDP Appendix C or are restricted narcotics) can be registered on the ARTG after first passing evaluation for quality, safety and efficacy by a Therapeutic Goods Administration committee. Legislation updated to January 2003 was scrutinised for inclusions.

(Continued)

Table **9**   **Other Sources for Regulatory Information—cont'd**

UK & Europe	The General Sale List indicates the substances that can, with reasonable safety, be sold or otherwise supplied by or under the supervision of a pharmacist. Generally such products may be sold in retail outlets. Information is presented from the GSL updated in September 2002, and obtained from the Medicines Control Agency website. (The MCA merged with the Medicines Devices Agency on 1st April 2003 to form the Medicines and Healthcare products Regulatory Agency [www.mhra.gov.uk].) The GSL records substances often without a definitive common name or with a genus name only, and generally this convention is followed here. Maximum dose means the maximum quantity of the substance which can be delivered in a single dose (denoted as "maximum single dose" in the monographs). Maximum daily dose means the maximum quantity of the substance recommended in any period of 24 hours. Plants listed in Part II of the Medicines (Retail Sale or Supply of Herbal Remedies) Order 1977 SI 2130 can only be supplied following a one-to-one consultation with a practitioner, at the dosages and by the route of administration specified in Part III. The maximum dose, maximum daily dose or maximum percentage in a topical preparation are specified. Information current to March 2003 was scrutinised. The German Commission E was an expert committee of the German Federal Health Department set up in 1978. The committee reviewed the available scientific data and traditional information to assess the safety and efficacy of selected herbs. They published their findings as concise and unreferenced monographs—the supporting reference material is stored at the German Health Department. The Commission was discontinued in the early 1990s but much of the information remains valid. A positive Commission E monograph means that the indications are officially recognised by the German government, primarily for nonprescription and clinical applications. A negative Commission E monograph means that the German government does not advocate the use of the herb, either because of a lack of adequate scientific evidence for current or historical usage and/or because of potential or documented risks associated with its use.
US	GRAS (Part 582, US Code of Federal Regulations Title 21—Food and Drugs) is a listing of substances generally recognised as safe for their intended use, for example, for inclusion in food. The DSHEA legislation (Dietary Supplement Health and Education Act of 1994) has defined dietary supplements as "safe within a broad range of intake, and safety problems within the supplements are relatively rare". The intent of this legislation was to meet the concerns of consumers and manufacturers to help ensure that safe and appropriately-labelled products remain available to consumers. The provisions of DSHEA define dietary supplements and dietary ingredients, establish a new framework for assuring safety, outline guidelines for literature displayed where supplements are sold, provide for use of claims and nutritional support statements, regulate ingredient and nutrition labelling and grant the FDA (Food and Drug Administration) the authority to establish good manufacturing practice regulations.

REFERENCES

1. Binns SE, Baum BR, Arnason JT: *Syst Bot* 27(3):610-632, 2002.
2. Binns SE, Baum BR, Arnason JT: *Taxon* 50(4):1199-1200, 2001.
3. Milius S: *Science News* 156(17):268-270, 1999.
4. American Herbal Pharmacopoeia: *Goldenseal root – Hydrastis canadensis: analytical, quality control, and therapeutic monograph*, Santa Cruz, August 2001, American Herbal Pharmacopoeia.
5. Lewington A: *A review of the importation of medicinal plants and plant extracts into Europe*, Cambridge, 1993, TRAFFIC International, pp 31-32.
6. DePass LR: *Toxicol Lett* 49(2-3):159-170, 1989.
7. Schlede E, Mischke U, Roll R, et al: *Arch Toxicol* 66:455-470, 1992.
8. Botham PA: *ILAR J* 43(Suppl):S27-S30, 2002.
9. Munson PL, Mueller RA, Breese GR, eds: *Principles of pharmacology: basic concepts and clinical applications*, New York, 1995, Chapman & Hall, pp 1538-1543.
10. Mortelmans K, Zeiger E: *Mutat Res* 455(1-2):29-60, 2000.
11. Fetterman BA, Kim BS, Morgolin BH, et al: *Environ Mol Mutagen* 29(3):312-322, 1997.
12. Munson PL, Mueller RA, Breese GR, eds: *Principles of pharmacology: basic concepts and clinical applications*. New York, 1995, Chapman & Hall, pp 1602-1603.

ALOE

Other common names: Aloes, Barbados aloes[*], Cape aloes[*], Aloe vera gel
Botanical names: *Aloe* spp. including *A. vera* (L.) Burm. f. (*A. barbadensis* Mill.), and *A. ferox* Mill.
Family: Aloeaceae
Plant part used: Leaf latex or sap (aloe resin); mucilaginous gel from central part of leaf (aloe gel)

Safety Summary: Aloe Resin

Pregnancy category B3: No increase in frequency of malformation or other harmful effects on the foetus from limited use in women. Evidence of increased foetal damage in animal studies exists, although the relevance to humans is unknown.
Lactation category CC: Compatible with breast-feeding but use caution (due to the presence of anthraquinone glycosides).
Contraindications: Aloe products are contraindicated in those with known sensitivity. Stimulating laxatives are contraindicated in chronic constipation, intestinal obstruction, stenosis or atony, inflammatory bowel disease, abdominal pain of unknown origin, haemorrhoids, kidney disorders, severe dehydration states (with water and electrolyte depletion) and children under 10 years. Do not use during pregnancy or lactation without professional advice.
Warnings & precautions: Aloe products are best avoided during pregnancy and in those trying to conceive. Aloe resin should be used with caution during lactation. Stimulating laxatives should not be used for more than 2 weeks without professional advice and laxatives should not be given when any undiagnosed acute or persistent abdominal symptoms are present.
Adverse reactions: Abdominal pain and spasm, yellowish-brown or red discoloration of the urine, contact dermatitis
Interactions: Stimulating laxatives may decrease the gastrointestinal transit time and absorption of coadministered agents. Potassium deficiency (resulting from long-term laxative abuse) can potentiate the action of cardiac glycosides and may affect the action of antiarrhythmic agents. Potassium deficiency may be increased by concomitant use of thiazide diuretics, adrenocorticosteroids and licorice root.

[*]Barbados aloes = *Aloe barbadensis*; Cape aloes = various *Aloe* spp. including *A. ferox* and its hybrids.

Safety Summary: Aloe Gel

Pregnancy category B3: No increase in frequency of malformation or other harmful effects on the foetus from limited use in women. Evidence of increased foetal damage in animal studies exists, although the relevance to humans is unknown.
Lactation category ND: No data available.
Contraindications: Aloe products are contraindicated in those with known sensitivity. Do not use during pregnancy without professional advice.
Warnings & precautions: Aloe products are best avoided during pregnancy and in those trying to conceive.
Adverse reactions: Burning sensations and mild itching have been reported after topical use. Dermatitis has been reported after both oral and topical use.
Interactions: No precautions required on current evidence.

Typical Therapeutic Use

Aloe vera gel has demonstrated therapeutic benefit as a topical treatment for genital herpes[1,2] and psoriasis[3] in randomised, double-blind, placebo-controlled trials. In placebo-controlled trials, oral treatments with *A. vera* juice (10 mL/day)[4] and aloe gel[5] were of benefit to patients with hyperlipidaemia and aloe gel[5,6] aided glycaemic control in noninsulin-dependent diabetes mellitus. Aloe gel has been used traditionally in many countries for wound healing.[7] It has also been used in traditional Thai herbal medicine to treat peptic ulcers and as a topical treatment for burns and mouth ulcers.[8]

Aloe resin was traditionally used in Western herbal medicine as a laxative and as a topical treatment for burns, sunburn and mild abrasions.[9]

Actions

Aloe resin: Laxative, antiinflammatory.
Aloe gel: Immune enhancing, antiviral, vulnerary, antiinflammatory, antitumour, demulcent, emollient.

Key Constituents

Constituents of aloe leaf include anthraquinones and polysaccharides, such as acetylated glucomannans (also known as acemannan).[10] Aloe resin is a solid residue obtained from the latex or sap which exudes from the cut leaf. Its key constituents are anthraquinones, such as aloin A and B, aloinosides A and B and small amounts (0.5%) of aloe-emodin and chrysophanol.[11,12] Aloe gel is a mucilaginous material obtained mainly from the central part of the leaf. It is sometimes specifically prepared to be anthraquinone free and its key constituents are polysaccharides.[12]

Adulteration

Adulteration of individual *Aloe* species with others is very rare.[12] Solid aloe gel products can contain high proportions of carriers, such as guar gum and maltodextrin, despite claims they are concentrated pure gels.[13,14] *Aloe* spp. is listed on Appendix II of the Convention on International Trade in Endangered Species (CITES) as of May 2003, but *Aloe vera* (*A. barbadensis*) is exempted. In addition 21 species (not medicinal aloes) are listed in Appendix I.

Typical Dosage Forms & Dosage

Typical adult dosage ranges are:
- 25 to 100 mL/day of a 4.5:1 juice concentrate (predominantly the gel)
- 50 to 200 mg/day of powdered resin
- 1.5 to 4.5 mL/day of 1:10 tincture of the resin
- 2 to 8 mL/day of a 1:40 tincture of the resin

Contraindications

Aloe products are contraindicated in those with known sensitivity (see Adverse reactions).

Stimulating laxatives containing anthraquinones are contraindicated in chronic constipation, intestinal obstruction, stenosis or atony, inflammatory bowel disease, abdominal pain of unknown origin, severe dehydration states (with water and electrolyte depletion) and in children under 10 years. They are also contraindicated in patients with kidney disorders or haemorrhoids, as anthraquinones cause hyperaemia in the pelvic area, especially in high doses.[9,15-17]

Do not use aloe resin during pregnancy or lactation or aloe gel during pregnancy without professional advice.

Use in Pregnancy

Aloe products

Category B3: No increase in frequency of malformation or other harmful effects on the foetus from limited use in women. Evidence of increased foetal damage in animal studies exists, although the relevance to humans is unknown.

Aloe products are best avoided during pregnancy, especially in the first trimester, and in those trying to conceive.

Decoctions of *Aloe* spp. have been traditionally used by different African peoples to aid conception, promote health during pregnancy and assist labour.[18,19]

A. chabaudii (500 mg/kg i.p. and p.o.), *A. globuligemma* (500 mg/kg i.p.) and *A. cryptopoda* (500 mg/kg i.p.) were administered to pregnant mice and rats as aqueous leaf extracts on days 14 to 16 of pregnancy. No foetuses were expelled or resorbed, even at doses lethal to the dams. Surviving animals delivered normal sized litters of healthy pups at term.[20] A review of traditional Ayurvedic literature notes that *Aloe barbadensis* (form not defined) is listed as an abortifacient in four of the five sources checked. However, the definition of abortifacient was very broad and included emmenagogue, ecbolic (uterine contractor) and "antimetabolite".[21] Oral administration of leaf extracts of *A. vera* (100 to 500 mg/kg) from days 1 to 7 postcoitus in the rat showed some activity in preventing pregnancy in two studies, but extracts were inactive in another four studies.[22] *A. vera* leaf (125 mg/kg) prepared as an aqueous extract demonstrated abortifacient and teratogenic activity when it was orally administered to rats for 10 days after insemination.[23] Aqueous leaf extract exhibited in vitro stimulant activity in guinea pig uterine strips.[24] *A. chabaudii* leaf extract inhibited spontaneous contractions of the isolated rat uterus at a concentration of 1 mg/mL, but had no effect on the quiescent uterus.[25]

The Commission E and the *British Herbal Compendium* advise that aloe resin is contraindicated during pregnancy.[9,15] Concern exists that stimulating laxatives may cause reflex stimulation of the uterine muscles which may lead to miscarriage.[26,27] However, undesirable or damaging effects during pregnancy or on the foetus were not observed when aloe resin was used at the recommended dosage.[16] A woman who took an unspecified amount of aloes tincture in her second month of pregnancy experienced violent colic, tenesmus, watery diarrhoea and slight to moderate vaginal bleeding. Administration of spasmolytics stopped the bleeding and her pregnancy continued normally.[28]

Aloe resin extract (up to 1000 mg/kg) or aloin A (up to 200 mg/kg) did not demonstrate embryotoxic, teratogenic or foetotoxic activity after oral administration to rats.[16]

Use in Lactation

Aloe resin

Category CC: Compatible with breastfeeding but use caution.

Small amounts of anthraquinone metabolites may be excreted in the breast milk. One source stated that anthraquinone derivatives, such as cascara and danthron, have been reported to cause diarrhoea in the nursing infant but no references were provided.[29] Other sources, including the American Academy of Pediatrics, state that a laxative effect has not been observed in breastfeeding infants with anthraquinone-containing laxatives such as cascara and senna.[30-33]

Aloe resin was traditionally administered to breastfeeding mothers by the Eclectics to purge the nursing child.[34]

Aloe gel

Category ND: No data available.

Warnings & Precautions

Aloe products are best avoided during pregnancy, especially during the first trimester, and in those trying to conceive. Aloe resin should be used with caution during lactation.

Stimulating laxatives should not be used for more than 2 weeks without medical advice and laxatives should not be given when any undiagnosed acute or persistent abdominal symptoms are present (see Overdosage section).[15,16] Beware long-term laxative abuse and concomitant use of cardiac glycosides, antiarrythmic agents, thiazide diuretics, adrenocorticosteroids or licorice root (see Interactions).

Effect on Ability to Drive or Operate Machinery

No adverse effects expected.

Adverse Reactions

A 1999 review of clinical trials of topical and oral treatment with *A. vera* gel found that it was generally very well tolerated. Mild adverse reactions reported after topical treatment included burning sensations, contact dermatitis and mild itching.[35] Dermatitis has been reported after oral and topical use of aloe products in case reports, particularly the gel.[36-45] Cases involving a severe burning sensation and long-term erythema have been reported after topical application of aloe gel to skin that had been subjected to a chemical peel or dermabrasion.[46] However, in a controlled trial of acne patients who had undergone facial dermabrasion, areas treated with aloe gel healed more rapidly and completely than untreated zones. Burning sensations were noted in some cases.[47] A case of anaphylactic shock has been reported after injection of aloe.[48]

Abdominal pain and spasm can occur with use of aloe resin.[15,16] Yellowish-brown or red discoloration of the urine may also occur. This is due to the presence of anthraquinone metabolites and is not clinically significant.[15,16]

A 47-year-old man developed acute oliguric renal failure and liver dysfunction after ingestion of a herbal remedy. Analysis of the herbal remedy revealed the presence of Cape aloes.[49] Other herbs were probably involved.

Interactions

Stimulating laxatives may decrease the gastrointestinal transit time and absorption of co-administered agents. Potassium deficiency (resulting from long-term laxative abuse) can potentiate the action of cardiac glycosides and may affect the action of antiarrhythmic agents. Potassium deficiency can be increased by concomitant use of thiazide diuretics, corticosteroids and licorice root.[16,50] There is potential (but not established) interaction for the same reason with quinidine and licorice.

Oral administration of *A. vera* fresh leaf pulp extract (30 μL and 60 μL/day) for 14 days induced the phase II enzyme system in mice.[51]

Acemannan was found in one clinical trial to significantly decrease the bioavailability of zidovudine (antiretroviral), but caused no interaction in a further two trials.[52] In one of the later trials acemannan was administered at an oral dosage of 400 mg four times daily.[53]

Safety in Children

Aloe resin is generally listed as contraindicated in children.[15,16] The Eclectics traditionally used it as an enema for intestinal worms in children (650 mg in 85 mL of water). Also aloe resin administered to nursing mothers was said to purge breastfeeding infants.[34] This effect is probably only likely to occur at very large doses.

Overdosage

Long-term use or abuse of stimulating laxatives can cause dependence and a sluggish bowel with impaired function. It may also lead to disturbances of electrolyte balance (especially potassium deficiency), albuminuria and haematuria. Potassium deficiency can lead to disorders of heart function and muscular weakness, especially with concurrent use of cardiac glycosides, diuretics and corticosteroids. Chronic abuse of anthraquinone laxatives may cause pseudomelanosis coli (pigmentation of the colon) which is reversible[15,16] but has been associated with an increased risk of colorectal carcinoma.[54,55] However, the pseudomelanosis coli is probably a harmless state and any link to cancer may be more a reflection of anthraquinone exposure. For a complete discussion of this issue, refer to the senna (*Cassia* spp.) monograph.

Overdose with aloe resin causes griping pains and severe diarrhoea with accompanying fluid and electrolyte loss.[15,16] In serious cases this may lead to neuromuscular, cardiovascular and renal disturbances.[12,27] It has been alleged that fatal haemorrhagic gastroenteritis with renal irritation can occur

at doses of approximately 8 to 10 g and that doses of 1 g per day over several days are lethal.[12,56] However, this latter point seems overstated.

An analysis of the Johannesburg forensic database over the years 1991 to 1995 revealed two fatalities that were attributed to poisoning by aloe resin.[57] A patient with jaundice died after taking a preparation containing about 1 g of aloe, rhubarb, and senna combined. Autopsy revealed extensive liver damage and pathological changes in the kidneys, spleen, heart, and lungs.[58] However, other causes were not conclusively ruled out.

Toxicology

Table 1 lists LD_{50} data recorded for aloe extracts and aloin.[12,20,59,60]

Aloe resin and aloin A demonstrated low acute and subacute oral toxicity in rats and mice at effective laxative doses.[61-63] Mice orally administered aloe resin extract (up to 50 mg/kg/day) for 12 weeks or aloin (0.03% of diet) for 20 weeks did not demonstrate renal toxicity or significant change in serum electrolytes.[64,65] Inflammation of the colonic mucosa and an increase in sorbitol dehydrogenase levels were observed in the mice administered aloe resin extract.[64]

Freeze-dried aloe gel (up to 64 mg/kg, twice daily) given to rats and fresh or preserved aloe gel (up to 20 g/kg/day) in mice and rats did not exhibit toxic effects after oral administration. Chronic toxicity studies showed no toxic effect at doses of 5 g/kg/day for 45 days.[66,67] No significant toxic effects were observed when acemannan was orally admin-

Table 1   **LD$_{50}$ Data Recorded for Aloe Extracts and Aloin**

Substance	Route, Model	LD$_{50}$ Value (mg/kg)	Reference
Alcohol extract of A. vera leaf	Oral, mice	121	59
Extract of A. globuligemma	i.p., mice and rats	<250	20
Extract of A. chabaudii	i.p., mice and rats	250–500	20
Extract of A. cryptopoda	i.p., mice and rats	>1500	20
Alcohol extract of A. vera entire plant	i.p., mice	250	60
Aloin	i.v., mice	200	12

istered to rats as 5% of the diet for 14 days or at doses of up to 2 g/kg/day for 6 months. Similar results were observed in dogs at doses of up to 1.5 g/kg/day for 90 days.[68]

Life-long ingestion of freeze-dried *A. vera* gel (1% of diet) did not have toxic effects on rats and appeared to be associated with some beneficial effects on age-related disease.[69] Mice treated with *A. vera* leaf extract (100 mg/kg, oral) for 3 months had decreased red cell counts and exhibited sperm abnormalities. In the acute toxicity studies aloe (single oral doses 0.5 to 3 g/kg) exhibited no signs of toxicity.[70] Lyophilised aloe leaf demonstrated spermicidal activity against human sperm in vitro at concentrations of 7.5% and 10%.[71] A low molecular weight fraction from *A. vera* gel exhibited cytotoxicity in chicken and human cells in vitro.[72] Aloe leaf alcohol extract demonstrated toxicity in the brine shrimp assay at a concentration of 3.59 μg/mL.[59]

Even though in vitro, animal and human studies have shown a potential role for anthraquinones in both the initiation and promotion of tumorigenesis, the available information is still inconclusive.[54,55,73] Retrospective and prospective epidemiological studies found an increased risk of colon carcinoma in patients with a history of chronic abuse of anthraquinone-containing laxatives.[54,74] However, in a case control study with retrospective and prospective evaluation, no causal relationship between anthraquinoid laxative use and colorectal cancer could be detected.[75,76]

A large epidemiological study of lung cancer and smoking in Japan suggested that ingestion of aloe leaf juice prevented cancer in various organs.[77]

A. ferox aqueous extract demonstrated mutagenic activity in the rec-assay with *Bacillus subtilis*, but the methanol extract was not mutagenic. The aqueous and methanol extracts were not mutagenic in the Ames test with and without metabolic activation.[78] Aqueous-ethanolic extract of *A. vera* was shown to have antimutagenic activity in vitro.[79] Aloin and an aloe extract containing aloin (23%) and aloe-emodin (<0.07%) produced no mutagenic effects in bacterial and mammalian test systems in vitro.[15,80,81] Aloin (0.03% of diet) did not promote incidence and growth of colorectal adenomas and carcinomas in mice after 20 weeks.[65]

Although anthraquinones have been implicated in carcinogenesis, the available information is still inconclusive.[82] A senna-glycoside extract containing aloe-emodin (0.14%) in quantities similar to those in aloe resin preparations was not carcinogenic to rats after 2 years of oral administration.[83] Aloe-emodin demonstrated mutagenic and cell-transforming activity in in vitro tests[84-86] but failed to demonstrate mutagenic activity in a battery of in vivo tests.[84,86] It has also been shown to inhibit cell transformation[87] and to have antimutagenic activity[88] in vitro. Aloe-emodin exhibited phototoxic activity in vitro[89,90] and demonstrated carcinogenic activity in mice after topical application in the presence of UV light.[91] However, it has also demonstrated antitumour activity in vitro and in vivo[92,93] and aloe extract has suppressed UV mutagenesis in vitro.[94]

Chrysophanol is transformed, in a cytochrome P450-dependent oxidation, to aloe-emodin.[95] It may have tumour-promoting activity,[96] but has also exhibited cytotoxicity to cancer cell lines in vitro.[97] Chrysophanol failed to demonstrate mutagenic activity in in vitro tests, including the Ames test,[98-100] but demonstrated mutagenic activity in the Ames test with metabolic activation in other studies.[101,102]

Regulatory Status

See Table 2 for regulatory status in selected countries. A physician in the United States received a 46-month prison sentence for treating cancer patients with injections of *Aloe vera*.[103]

REFERENCES

1. Syed TA, Cheeema KM, Ashfaq A, et al: *J Eur Acad Dermatol Venereol* 7:294-295, 1996.
2. Syed TA, Afzal M, Ashfaq Ahmad S, et al: *J Dermatol Treat* 8:99-102, 1997.
3. Syed TA, Ahmad SA, Holt AH, et al: *Trop Med Int Health* 1:505-509, 1996.
4. Nasiff HA, Fajardo F, Velez F: *Rev Cuba Med Gen Integr* 9:43-51, 1993.
5. Yongchaiyudha S, Rungpitarangsi V, Bunyapraphatsara N, et al: *Phytomed* 3:241-243, 1996.
6. Bunyapraphatsara N, Yongchaiyudha S, Rungpitarangsi V, et al: *Phytomed* 3:245-248, 1996.
7. Grindlay D, Reynolds T: *J Ethnopharmacol* 16:117-151, 1986.

Table **2**   **Regulatory Status for Aloe in Selected Countries**

Australia	Aloe is not included in Part 4 of Schedule 4 of the Therapeutic Goods Regulations.
UK & Germany	Aloe resin (Barbados) is included on the General Sale List, with a maximum single dose of 50 mg. Aloe resin (Cape) is also included on the General Sale List, with a maximum single dose of 100 mg. Aloin can be administered in a maximum single dose of 20 mg. Aloe resin is covered by a positive Commission E monograph. Aloe resin is official in the *British Pharmacopoeia* 2002 and the *European Pharmacopoeia* 4.3.
US	Aloe latex is official in the *United States Pharmacopeia-National Formulary* (USP 26-NF 21, 2003). Aloe does not have generally recognised as safe (GRAS) status. It is freely available as a "dietary supplement" in the US under DSHEA legislation (Dietary Supplement Health and Education Act of 1994) but the resin must carry the following warning label: "This product contains *Aloe* spp. (Aloe). Read and follow directions carefully. Do not use if you have or develop diarrhea, loose stools, or abdominal pain. Consult your physician if you have frequent diarrhea. If you are pregnant, nursing, taking medication, or have a medical condition, consult your physician before using this product."*

The California Department of Health Services Food and Drug Branch issued an emergency regulation November 1, 1996, requiring that all herb teas and dietary supplements containing herbs with stimulant laxative activity carry a warning label. The herbs included in this regulation include aloe (Aloe ferox and other related species), buckthorn bark and berry (Rhamnus catharticus), cascara sagrada bark (Rhamnus purshiana), rhubarb root (Rheum palmatum), and senna leaf and pod (Cassia acutifolia, C. angustifolia, C. senna). The ruling exempts herb products made from aloe leaf gel, which normally does not contain significant natural levels of anthraquinones. The new ruling went into effect January 1, 1997.[104]

8. Farnsworth NR, Bunyapraphatsara N, eds: *Thai medicinal plants*, Bangkok, 1992, Medicinal Plant Information Center, 1992, p 35.
9. British Herbal Medicine Association: *British herbal compendium*, vol 1, Bournemouth, 1992, BHMA, pp 19-23.
10. Pelley RP: Aloe polysaccharides and their measurement. In *Inside aloe*, Texas, 1997, International Aloe Science Council, pp 4-7.
11. Wagner H, Bladt S: *Plant drug analysis: a thin layer chromatography atlas*, ed 2. Berlin, 1996, Springer-Verlag, p 56.
12. Blaschek W, Ebel S, Hackenthal E, et al: *HagerROM 2002: Hagers Handbuch der Drogen und Arzneistoffe*, Heidelberg: 2002, Springer.
13. Leung AY: *Drug Cosmet Ind* 120:34, 1977.
14. Kim KH, Lee JG, Kim DG, et al: *Arch Pharm Res* 21:514-520, 1998.
15. Blumenthal M et al., eds: *The complete German Commission E Monographs: therapeutic guide to herbal medicines*, Austin, 1998, American Botanical Council, pp 80-81.
16. Scientific Committee of ESCOP (European Scientific Cooperative on Phytotherapy): ESCOP Monographs: *Aloe capensis — Cape Aloes*, UK, 1997, European Scientific Cooperative on Phytotherapy, ESCOP Secretariat.
17. Hänsel R, Haas H: *Therapie mit phytopharmaka*, Berlin, 1983, Springer-Verlag, p 162.
18. Watt JM, Breyer-Brandwijk MG: *The medicinal and poisonous plants of southern and eastern Africa: being an account of their medicinal and other uses, chemical composition, pharmacological effects and toxicology in man and animal*, ed 2, Edinburgh, 1962, Livingstone, pp 680-684.
19. Veale DJ, Furman KI, Oliver DW: *J Ethnopharmacol* 36:185-191, 1992.
20. Parry O, Matambo C: *Cent Afr J Med* 38:409-414, 1992.
21. Casey RCD: *Indian J Med Sci* 14:590-600, 1960.
22. Kamboj VP, Dhawan BN: *J Ethnopharmacol* 6:191-226, 1982.
23. Nath D, Sethi N, Singh RK, et al: *J Ethnopharmacol* 36:147-154, 1992.
24. Saha JC, Savini EC, Kasinathan S: *Indian J Med Res* 49:130-151, 1961.
25. Parry O, Wenyika J: *Fitoterapia* 65:253-259, 1994.
26. Bisset NG, ed: *Herbal drugs and phytopharmaceuticals: a handbook for practice on a scientific basis*, Stuttgart, 1994, Medpharm Scientific Publishers, p 60.
27. Maiwald L: *Z Phytother* 7:153-156, 1986.
28. Vago O: *Z Geburtshilfe Perinatol* 170:272-277, 1969.
29. Busser J, Schultz J: *Frontiers Fetal Health* 3:11-22, 2001.
30. American Academy of Pediatrics: *Pediatrics* 108:776-789, 2001.
31. Faber P, Strenge-Hesse A: *Pharmacology* 36:212-220, 1988.
32. Tyson RM, Shrader EA: Perlman HH: *J Pediatr* 11:824-832, 1937.
33. Werthmann MW, Krees SV: *Med Ann Dist Columbia* 42:4-5, 1973.
34. Felter HW, Lloyd JU: *King's American dispensatory*, ed 18, 3rd rev, vol 1, first published 1905, reprinted Portland, 1983, Eclectic Medical Publications, pp 151-152.

35. Vogler BK, Ernst E: *Br J Gen Pract* 49:823-828, 1999.
36. Morrow DM, Rapaport MJ, Strick RA: *Arch Dermatol* 116:1064-1065, 1980.
37. Hogan DJ: *CMAJ* 138:336-338, 1988.
38. West I, Maibach HI: *Contact Dermatitis* 32:121, 1995.
39. Mitchell J, Rook A: *Botanical dermatology: plants and plant products injurious to the skin,* Vancouver, 1979, Greengrass, p 439.
40. Higashi N, Kume A, Ueda K: *HIFU* 38:576-580, 1996.
41. Nakamura T, Kotajima S: *Contact Dermatitis* 11:51, 1984.
42. Shoji A: *Contact Dermatitis* 8:164-167, 1982.
43. Savchak VI: *Vestn Dermatol Venereol* 12:44-45, 1977.
44. Diba SA: *Zh Ushn Nos Gorl Bolezn* 2:108, 1974.
45. Dominguez-Soto L: *Int J Dermatol* 31:372, 1992.
46. Hunter D, Frumkin A: *Cutis* 47:193-196, 1991.
47. Fulton JE: *J Dermatol Surg Oncol* 16:460-467, 1990.
48. Trakhtenberg SB: *Klin Med (Mosk)* 48:140-141, 1970.
49. Luyckx VA, Ballantine R, Claeys M, et al: *Am J Kidney Dis* 39:E13, 2002.
50. Blumenthal M. et al., eds: *The complete German Commission E Monographs: therapeutic guide to herbal medicines,* Austin, 1998, American Botanical Council, pp 80-81.
51. Singh RP, Dhanalakshmi S, Rao AR: *Phytomedicine* 7:209-219, 2000.
52. Robertson-Dallas S, Read SE, Bendayan R: *Pharmacotherapy* 17:1198-1209, 1997.
53. Montaner JS, Gill J, Singer J, et al: *J Acquir Immune Defic Syndr Hum Retrovirol* 12:153-157, 1996.
54. Siegers CP, von Hertzberg-Lottin E, Otte M, et al: *Gut* 34:1099-1101, 1993.
55. van Gorkom BA, de Vries EG, Karrenbeld A, et al: *Aliment Pharmacol Ther* 13:443-452, 1999.
56. Hänsel R, Haas H: *Therapie mit phytopharmaka,* Berlin, 1983, Springer-Verlag, p 166.
57. Stewart MJ, Moar JJ, Steenkamp P, et al: *Forensic Sci Int* 101:177-183, 1999.
58. Gerchow J: *Med Monatsschr* 5:328-330, 1951.
59. Lagarto Parra A, Silva Yhebra R, Guerra Sardinas I, et al: *Phytomedicine* 8:395-400, 2001.
60. Dhar ML, Dhar MM, Dhawan BN, et al: *Indian J Exp Biol* 6:232-247, 1968.
61. Bangel E, Pospisil M, Roetz E, et al: *Steiner-Informationdienst* 4:1-25, 1975.
62. Schmidt L: *Arch Exper Path Pharmakol* 226:207-218, 1955.
63. Nelemans FA: *Pharmacology* 14:73-77, 1976.
64. Siegers CP, Younes M, Herbst EW: *Z Phytother* 7:157-159, 1986.
65. Siegers CP, Siemers J, Baretton G: *Pharmacology* 47:205-208, 1993.
66. Watanasrisin J, cited in Yongchaiyudha S, Rungpitarangsi V, Bunyapraphatsara N, et al: *Phytomed* 3:241-243, 1996.
67. Jirakulchaiwong S, Wongkrajang Y, Bunyaprpphatsara N, et al., cited in Yongchaiyudha S, Rungpitarangsi V,

Bunyapraphatsara N, et al: *Phytomed* 3:241-243, 1996.
68. Fogleman RW, Shellenberger TE, Balmer MF, et al: *Vet Hum Toxicol* 34:144-147, 1992.
69. Ikeno Y, Hubbard GB, Lee S, et al: *Phytother Res* 16:712-718, 2002.
70. Shah AH, Qureshi S, Tariq M, et al: *Phytother Res* 3:25-29, 1989.
71. Fahim MS, Wang M: *Contraception* 53:231-236, 1996.
72. Avila H, Rivero J, Herrera F, et al: *Toxicon* 35:1423-1430, 1997.
73. Lee BM, Park KK: *Mut Res* 523-524:265-278, 2003.
74. Siegers CP: *TiPS* 13:229-231, 1992.
75. Loew D, Bergmann U, Schmidt M, et al: *Dtsch Apoth Ztg* 134:3180-3183, 1994.
76. Loew D: *Z Phytotherapie* 16:312-318, 1994.
77. Sakai R: *Jpn J Cancer Res* 80:513-520, 1989.
78. Morimoto I, Watanabe F, Osawa T, et al: *Mutat Res* 97:81-102, 1982.
79. Lee KH, Kang HG, Cho CH, et al: *Nat Prod Sci* 6:56-60, 2000.
80. Westendorf J: Anthranoid derivatives – *Aloe* species. In: de Smet PAGM, Keller K, Hansel R et al., eds: *Adverse Effects of Herbal Drugs,* vol 2, Berlin: Springer-Verlag, 1993, pp 121-122.
81. Brown JP: *Mutat Res* 75:243-277, 1980.
82. Lee BM, Park KK: *Mutat Res* 523-524:265-278, 2003.
83. Lyden-Sokolowski A, Nilsson A, Sjoberg P: *Pharmacology* 47:209-215, 1993.
84. Heidemann A, Miltenburger HG, Mengs U: *Pharmacology* 47:178-186, 1993.
85. Westendorf J, Marquardt H, Poginsky B, et al: *Mutat Res* 240:1-12, 1990.
86. Heidemann A, Volkner W, Mengs U: *Mutat Res* 367:123-133, 1996.
87. Woo SW, Nan JX, Lee SH, et al: *Pharmacol Toxicol* 90:193-198, 2002.
88. Nakasugi T, Nishida K, Komai K: *Mem Fac Agric Kinki Univ* 29:63-67, 1996.
89. Vath P, Wamer WG, Falvey DE: *Photochem Photobiol* 75:346-352, 2002.
90. Vargas F, Fraile G, Velasquez M, et al: *Pharmazie* 57:399-404, 2002.
91. Strickland FM, Muller HK, Stephens LC, et al: *Photochem Photobiol* 72:407-414, 2000.
92. Wasserman L, Avigad S, Beery E, et al: *Am J Dermatopathol* 24:17-22, 2002.
93. Pecere T, Gazzola MV, Mucignat C, et al: *Cancer Res* 60:2800-2804, 2000.
94. Ohtsuka AT, Nunoshiba K, Nakayama R, et al: *Mutat Res* 164:277-278, 1986.
95. Mueller SO, Stopper H, Dekant W: *Drug Metab Dispos* 26:540-546, 1998.
96. Wolfle D, Schmutte C, Westendorf J, et al: *Cancer Res* 50:6540-6544, 1990.
97. Nemeikaite-Ceniene A, Sergediene E, Nivinskas H, et al: *Z Naturforsch* [C] 57:822-827, 2002.

98. Mueller SO, Schmitt M, Dekant W, et al: *Food Chem Toxicol* 37:481-491, 1999.

99. Mengs U, Schuler D, Marshall RR: Mutat Res 492:69-72, 2001.

100. Stark AA, Townsend JM, Wogan GN, et al: *J Environ Pathol Toxicol* 2:313-324, 1978.

101. Tikkanen L, Matsushima T, Natori S: *Mutat Res* 116:297-304, 1983.

102. Liberman DF, Schaefer FL, Fink RC, et al: *Appl Environ Microbiol* 40:476-479, 1980.

103. FDA Office of Criminal Investigation: Conviction and sentencing in Aloe Vera case. Available from www.fda.gov/ora/about/enf_story/ch6/oci4.htm. Accessed July 2003.

104. Blumenthal M: *HerbalGram* 39: 26-27, 1997.

ANDROGRAPHIS

Other common names: Chuan Xin Lian, Kalmegh
Botanical names: *Andrographis paniculata* (Burm. f.)
Nees (*Justicia paniculata* Burm. f.)
Family: Acanthaceae
Plant part used: Aerial parts

Safety Summary

Pregnancy category B3: No increase in frequency of malformation or other harmful effects on the foetus from limited use in women. Evidence of increased foetal damage in animal studies exists, although the relevance to humans is unknown.
Lactation category ND: No data available.
Contraindications: Bitters are contraindicated in states of hyperacidity, especially duodenal ulcers. Bitters should be used with caution in oesophageal reflux. Do not use during pregnancy without professional advice.
Warnings & precautions: Andrographis is best avoided during early pregnancy.
Adverse reactions: Urticaria, headache and chest discomfort are side effects which occur with a low frequency and after oral use of the herb.
Interactions: Theoretically, long-term use in conjunction with immunosuppressive drugs is best avoided. Exercise caution in patients taking antiplatelet or anticoagulant medication.

Typical Therapeutic Use

Andrographis has demonstrated therapeutic benefit in the treatment and prevention of bacterial and viral respiratory tract infections in randomised, double-blind, placebo-controlled trials.[1-4] It is used to treat fever and dysentery in Ayurveda, traditional Thai and traditional Chinese medicine (TCM).[5-8] Andrographis is also indicated for respiratory infections in TCM.[7]

Actions

Bitter tonic, choleretic, immune enhancing, hepatoprotective, antipyretic, antiinflammatory, antiplatelet, antioxidant, anthelmintic.

Key Constituents

Constituents of andrographis aerial parts include diterpenoid lactones, which are collectively referred to as andrographolides and include andrographolide (0.1% to 2.6%), deoxyandrographolide and neoandrographolide.[9,10]

Adulteration

Andrographis echioides is an adulterant of *A. paniculata*.[10] Purchased extracts of *Andrographis paniculata* are often devoid of any andrographolide content.[11]

Typical Dosage Forms & Dosage

Typical adult dosage ranges are:
- 1.5 to 6 g/day of dried aerial parts
- 6 to 9 g/day of dried herb as an infusion
- 3 to 6 mL/day of a 1:2 liquid extract or equivalent in tablet or capsule form

Contraindications

Bitters are contraindicated in states of hyperacidity, especially duodenal ulcers. Bitters should be used with caution in oesophageal reflux. Do not use during pregnancy without professional advice.

Use in Pregnancy

Category B3: No increase in frequency of malformation or other harmful effects on the foetus from limited use in women. Evidence of increased foetal damage in animal studies exists, although the relevance to humans is unknown.

However, andrographis is best avoided during early pregnancy until more information is available regarding its antifertility activity. A product containing standardised extract of andrographis leaf has been used to treat the common cold in Scandinavia for over 20 years and no cases of pregnancy termination have been reported.[12] Results from experiments regarding possible antifertility effects in female animals are conflicting (see below).[13-17]

Female mice fed very high doses of andrographis powder (2 g/kg/day) for 6 weeks failed to conceive when mated with males of proven fertility in a controlled experiment.[13] Intraperitoneal injection of andrographis whole plant decoction prevented implantation in mice and caused abortion at different stages of gestation in mice and rabbits. The decoction also terminated early pregnancy when administered by oral, intravenous, subcutaneous, intramuscular and intrauterine routes in mice.[14] However, oral administration of andrographis extract to rats at doses less than 2 g/kg during the first 9 days of pregnancy failed to interrupt pregnancy, induce foetal resorption or alter the number of live offspring.[15] Andrographis stem powder (0.75% of diet) had no appreciable effect on fertility when fed to female mice for up to 4 weeks prior to mating.[16] Antifertility effects were not observed in mice fed the powdered leaf or root (1% of diet; approximately 2 g/kg/day) for 2 weeks prior to mating and for 3 weeks during mating.[16,17]

No teratogenic or toxic effects were observed when a suspension of andrographis leaf powder (200 and 400 mg/kg) was orally administered on alternate days for 4 weeks to mice in a controlled experiment.[18]

In vitro tests, which are of uncertain relevance to normal human use, have shown the following effects. Andrographis chloroform extract and andrographolide sodium succinate suppressed hormonal secretion and had a cytotoxic effect on cultured human placental chorionic trophoblastic tissue (aged between 6 and 8 weeks of pregnancy) in vitro.[19] Andrographis extract demonstrated uterine relaxant activity in vitro.[20]

Use in Lactation

Category ND: No data available.

Warnings & Precautions

Andrographis is best avoided during early pregnancy until more information is available regarding its antifertility activity (see Use in Pregnancy and Toxicology).

Effect on Ability to Drive or Operate Machinery

No adverse effects expected.

Adverse Reactions

Generally, andrographis has been well tolerated in clinical trials. One of 90 patients receiving andrographis extract reported unpleasant sensations in the chest and intensified headache,[1] and 2 of 50 patients reported urticaria,[2] in randomised, double-blind, placebo-controlled trials investigating respiratory infections. Andrographis extract was administered for 3 to 5 days at a dose of 1020 mg/day (containing 63 mg andrographolide and deoxyandrographolide).

A high incidence of adverse effects, including headache, fatigue, pruritis/rash, metallic/decreased taste and diarrhoea, was reported in a trial of pure andrographolide in HIV patients. One patient experienced an anaphylactic reaction.[21] The oral dose of andrographolide, 15 mg/kg/day for 3 weeks followed by 30 mg/kg/day for a further 3 weeks, was very high compared to the normal therapeutic dosages of andrographis extract. Cases of anaphylactic shock after injection of andrographis extract have been reported in China.[22]

Interactions

Antiplatelet activity was demonstrated ex vivo in the blood from patients with cardiac and cerebral vascular diseases taking andrographis extract.[23] This could possibly lead to an adverse interaction with antiplatelet and anticoagulant drugs.

Do not prescribe andrographis long term with immunosuppressant medication as it may decrease the effectiveness of the drug. This is a theoretical concern based on the immune-enhancing activity of andrographis. No case reports of this interaction have been published.

Safety in Children

Adverse events were not reported in a randomised, double-blind, placebo-controlled trial investigating the prevention of the common cold, in which healthy children were orally administered andrographis extract (200 mg/day), 5 days per week for 3 months.[3] Andrographis is traditionally used in Ayurvedic medicine to treat bowel complaints in infants and children.[5,6]

Overdosage

No incidents found in published literature. High doses may cause gastric discomfort, anorexia and vomiting.[22]

Toxicology

Table 1 lists LD_{50} data recorded for andrographis extract and its constituents.[22,24,25]

Table I   **LD$_{50}$ Data Recorded for Andrographis Extract and Its Constituents**

Substance	Route, Model	LD$_{50}$ Value (g/kg)	Reference
Andrographis methanol–aqueous (1:1) extract of whole plant	i.p., mice	>1.0	24
Andrographis alcohol extract (part not specified)	Oral, mice	>15	25
Andrographis alcohol extract (part not specified)	i.p., mice	14.98	25
Andrographis alcohol extract (part not specified)	s.c., mice	>15	25
Total lactones	Oral, mice	13.4	22
Andrographolide	Oral, mice	>40	22
Andrographolide sulfonate	i.v., mice	2.47-2.94	22
Deoxyandrographolide	Oral, mice	>20	22
Neoandrographolide	Oral, mice	>20	22

In acute toxicity studies, no toxic effects were observed in mice after oral administration of a suspension of andrographis leaf powder (2 g/kg), a suspension of leaf alcohol extract (2.4 g/kg) or andrographolide (3 g/kg).[18] Similarly, subcutaneous administration of andrographis leaf decoction (0.33 g/kg) to rabbits did not exhibit toxic effects.[26]

No toxic effects were observed in subacute oral toxicity tests when either a leaf powder suspension (200 and 400 mg/kg) or straight leaf powder (50 to 150 mg/kg) were administered on alternate days for 4 weeks to mice, or for 14 weeks to rats, respectively.[18] Also andrographolide (1 g/kg/day) administered to rats and rabbits for 7 days did not cause toxic effects.[22] Rats administered andrographis powder (part and route not specified) at dosages of 0.12, 1.2 and 2.4 g/kg/day for 6 months exhibited no abnormalities in growth rate, food consumption, clinical signs, serum biochemical parameters or histology.[25]

Oral administration of andrographolide (2 g/day) for 4 days caused a transient elevation of the liver enzyme serum glutamic pyruvic transaminase (SGPT) in healthy volunteers. Levels normalised upon discontinuation of andrographolide. Hepatic and renal functions were not impaired after doses of 0.9 g per day for 5 days.[22]

Effects of andrographis on male fertility show conflicting results. Reduced fertility and prolongation of gestation were observed in mice where the male was fed andrographis stem powder (0.75% of diet) prior to mating. As mating rates were not confirmed, these effects may have been due to a reduction in libido. Treated females mated with untreated males showed no appreciable change in fertility or gestational period.[16] In contrast, antifertility effects were not observed in mice fed the powdered leaf or root (1% of diet; approximately 2 g/kg/day) for 2 weeks prior to mating and for 3 weeks during mating.[16,17]

Oral administration of andrographis leaf powder (50 and 100 mg/kg/day) for 24 to 60 days to male rats resulted in the cessation of spermatogenesis and biochemical and degenerative changes in the testes and male accessory organs.[27,28] Decreased sperm counts, spermatozoa abnormalities, histopathological changes in the testes and lack of fertility were observed after oral administration of very high doses of andrographolide (25 and 50 mg/kg) for 48 days.[29] However, no significant differences were observed in reproductive organ weights, testicular histology or serum testosterone levels after oral administration of andrographis dried herb (5:1) ethanol extract (containing 5.6% andrographolide) at dosages of 20, 200 and 1000 mg/kg per day for 60 days. The authors concluded that the above variation in results might be due to differences in preparation of the plant material used.[30]

After nitrosation with nitrite under acidic conditions, an ethanol extract of andrographis became mutagenic to strains TA98 and TA100 (Salmonella/microsome test) either tested in the presence or absence of S9 mix.[31]

Regulatory Status

See Table 2 for regulatory status in selected countries.

Table **2**   **Regulatory Status for Andrographis in Selected Countries**

Australia	Andrographis is not included in Part 4 of Schedule 4 of the Therapeutic Goods Regulations.
China	Andrographis is official in the Pharmacopoeia of the People's Republic of China 1997. The usual adult dosage, usually administered in the form of a decoction, is listed as 6-9 g
UK & Germany	Andrographis is not included on the General Sale List. It was not included in the Commission E assessment.
US	Andrographis does not have generally recognised as safe (GRAS) status. However, it is freely available as a "dietary supplement" in the US under DSHEA legislation (Dietary Supplement Health and Education Act of 1994).

REFERENCES

1. Melchior J, Spasov AA, Ostrovskij OV, et al: *Phytomedicine* 7:341-350, 2000.
2. Melchior J, Palm S, Wikman G: *Phytomedicine* 3:315-318, 1996/7.
3. Caceres DD, Hancke JL, Burgos RA, et al: *Phytomedicine* 4:101-104, 1997.
4. Caceres DD, Hancke JL, Burgos RA, et al: *Phytomedicine* 6:217-223, 1999.
5. Chopra RN, Chopra IC, Handa KL, et al: *Chopra's indigenous drugs of India*, ed 2, Calcutta 1958, reprinted 1982, Academic Publishers, p 278.
6. Kapoor LD: *CRC Handbook of Ayurvedic medicinal plants*, Boca Raton, 1990, CRC Press, p 39.
7. Farnsworth NR, Bunyapraphatsara N, eds: *Thai medicinal plants*, Bangkok, 1992, Medicinal Plant Information Center, p 57.
8. Pharmacopoeia Commission of the People's Republic of China: *Pharmacopoeia of the People's Republic of China*, English ed, vol I, Beijing, 1997, Chemical Industry Press, pp 83-84.
9. Tang W, Eisenbrand G: *Chinese drugs of plant origin*, Berlin, 1992, Springer Verlag, pp 97-103.
10. Regional Research Laboratory and Indian Drug Manufacturers' Association: *Indian herbal pharmacopoeia*. Jammu-Tawi, 1998, Indian Drug Manufacturers' Association, Mumbai and Regional Research Laboratory, pp 18-29.
11. Lehmann R, Penman K: Information on file. St. Lucia, Queensland 4072, Australia, 2001, MediHerb Research Laboratory, University of Queensland,.
12. Panossian A, Kochikian A, Gabrielian E, et al: *Phytomedicine* 6:157-162, 1999.
13. Zoha MS, Hussain AH, Choudhury SA: *Bangladesh Med Res Counc Bull* 15:34-37, 1989.
14. But PPH: *Abst Chinese Med* 2:247-269, 1988.
15. Hancke J, 1997. Cited in Panossian A, Kochikian A, Gabrielian E, et al: *Phytomedicine* 6:157-162, 1999.
16. Shamsuzzoha M, Rahman MS, Ahmed MM: *Bangladesh Med Res Conc Bull* 5:14-18, 1979
17. Shamsuzzoha M, Shamsur RM, Mohiuddin AM, et al: *Lancet* 2:900, 1978.
18. Dhammaupakorn P, Chaichantipyuth C: *8th symposium, Faculty of Pharmacy*. Thailand, December 1989, Chulalongkorn University Bangkok.
19. Zhang X, Zhuang L, Li S, et al: *Acta Zool Sin* 31:52-58, 1985.
20. Burgos RA, Aguila MJ, Santiesteban ET, et al: *Phytother Res* 15:235-239, 2001.
21. Calabrese C, Berman SH, Babish JG, et al: *Phytother Res* 14:333-338, 2000.
22. Chang HM, But PP: *Pharmacology and applications of Chinese materia medica*, vol 2. Singapore, 1987, World Scientific, pp 918-928.
23. Zhang YZ, Tang JZ, Zhang YJ: *Zhongguo Zhong Xi Yi Jie He Za Zhi* 14:28-30,34,5, 1994.
24. Nakannishi K, Sasaki SI, Kiang AK, et al: *Chem Pharm Bull* 13:822, 1965.
25. Sithisomwongse N, Pengchata J, Cheewapatana S, et al: *Th J Pharm Sci* 14:109-117, 1989.
26. Dutta A, Sukul NC: *J Helminthol* 56:81-84, 1982.
27. Akbarsha MA, Manivannan B, Hamid KS, et al: *Indian J Exp Biol* 28:421-426, 1990.
28. Akbarsha MA, Manivannan B: *Indian J Comparative Animal Physiol* 11:103-108, 1993.
29. Akbarsha MA, Murugaian P: *Phytother Res* 14:432-435, 2000.
30. Burgos RA, Caballero EE, Sanchez NS, et al: *J Ethnopharmacol* 58:219-224, 1997.
31. Ieamworapong C, Kangsadalumpai K, Rojanapo W: *Environ Mol Mutagen* 14:93, 1989.

ARNICA

Botanical names: *Arnica montana* L., *A. chamissonis* Less. subsp. *foliosa* (Nutt.) Maguire
Family: Compositae
Plant part used: Flower

Safety Summary

Pregnancy category X: High risk of damage to the foetus when taken internally. For topical use only.
Lactation category X: Internal use is contraindicated in breastfeeding. For topical use only.
Contraindications: Not to be taken internally. Apply only to unbroken skin; withdraw on first sign of dermatitis. Contraindicated in those with known allergy to arnica.
Warnings & precautions: Not for prolonged external application. Individuals with known sensitivity to other members of the Compositae family should avoid use of arnica.
Adverse reactions: Allergic or irritant contact dermatitis.
Interactions: No precautions required on current evidence.

Typical Therapeutic Use

Topical application of arnica gel improved venous tone, oedema and the feeling of heaviness in the legs of patients with chronic venous insufficiency in a randomised, double-blind, placebo-controlled trial[1] and was more effective than a placebo gel for muscle ache in male volunteers.[2] Traditional use of arnica in Western herbal medicine includes topical treatment of bruises and strains.[3]

Actions

Topical use only: Antiinflammatory, antiecchymotic (against bruises), analgesic, antimicrobial.

Key Constituents

Constituents of arnica flower include sesquiterpene lactones of the pseudoguaianolide type (0.2% to 1.5%), such as helenalin, $11\alpha,13$-dihydrohelenalin and their esters; flavonoids,[4] an essential oil[5] and pyrrolizidine alkaloids.[6,7] The pyrrolizidine alkaloids in arnica have saturated necine bases, which indicates that they are nontoxic.[7]

Adulteration

Since *Arnica montana* is a protected species in many countries, it is liable to adulteration with various yellow flowering Compositae plants.[4,5,8,9] Arnica flower does not contain rutin and can therefore be easily distinguished from the most commonly occurring adulterant: *Heterotheca inuloides* (Mexican Arnica).[4,5] In addition to this species, the European Pharmacopoeia regards *Calendula officinalis* as an adulterant.

Shortage of *A. montana* has led to more widespread use of related species including *A. chamissonis*, *A. alpina*, *A. cordifolia*, *A. sororia*, *A. fulgens*, *A. longifolia* and *A. sachalinensis*. The latter three are particularly used for tinctures.[10,11] However, only *A. montana* is listed as official in the *British Herbal Pharmacopoeia*, *British Pharmacopoeia* and *European Pharmacopoeia*.[3,12,13] *A. chamissonis* subsp. *foliosa* is accepted by the German Commission E.[14]

Typical Dosage Forms & Dosage

Arnica is best not taken internally, unless in homoeopathic form. For external use, a 1:5 tincture is typically diluted 5 times with water and applied topically 2 to 3 times per day. Ointment contains 10% to 25% tincture or about 15% oil infusion of arnica (arnica flowers macerated in vegetable oil).

Contraindications

Not to be taken internally. Do not apply to broken skin or near the eyes or mouth. Withdraw on first sign of dermatitis. Contraindicated in those with known allergy to arnica.

Use in Pregnancy

Category X: High risk of damage to the foetus when taken internally. For topical use only (see Contraindications).

Miscarriage has been reported after overdose with ingested arnica tincture or infusion[9,15] (see Overdosage). Constituents of arnica have been shown to increase uterine tone and contraction, but arnica tincture has not demonstrated these actions. Arnifolin (1 to 5 mg/kg) increased the tone and strengthened periodical contractions of the rabbit uterus in situ and 6-O-acetyl-11,13-dihydrohelenalin contracted the isolated rat uterus.[9,16] Arnica tincture did not increase tone or contraction of iso-lated pregnant rabbit uteri.[9] Similar negative results were demonstrated in the cat after intravenous administration of 0.3 mL of fresh arnica extract.[17]

Use in Lactation

Category X: Internal use is contraindicated in breastfeeding.

For topical use only (see Contraindications). Do not apply near the nipple.

Warnings & Precautions

Not for prolonged external application. Individuals with known sensitivity to other members of the Compositae family (such as ragweed, daisies and chrysanthemums), or to plants from other families with sesquiterpene lactones which are chemically related to arnica (such as Lauraceae) should avoid use of arnica.[18]

Effect on Ability to Drive or Operate Machinery

No adverse effects expected.

Adverse Reactions

Cases of allergic or irritant contact dermatitis caused by topical application of arnica have been reported since 1844.[19] A review of the literature up to 1980 found more than 100 cases of contact dermatitis due to sensitisation with arnica. Most cases were induced by self-treatment with arnica tincture.[11] Reactions have also been reported after the use of other arnica preparations, including ointments, creams, soaps, lotions and shampoos.[18] Arnica ointments and plasters are considered to pose a much lower risk of reaction than other types of application.[10,20] Case reports of allergic contact dermatitis from the topical use of arnica, which have been proven by patch testing, have been published since the 1980 review.[21-23]

Arnica-sensitive individuals are known to cross-react with other Compositae and Lauraceae species.[18] Sesquiterpene lactone and epoxythymol-diester constituents have been proven to be both sensitising agents and to act as allergens.[11,24] It is likely that other constituents of arnica also contribute to the acquired hypersensitivity.[25] Sesquiterpene lactone-sensitive individuals tend to develop cross-reactions to chemically-related sesquiterpene lactones in other species.[26] The presence of an alpha-methylene-gamma-lactone group has been shown to be important for cross-reactivity between sesquiterpene lactones.[10]

A 1992 review reported that arnica contact allergy was recognised in 11% to 75% of patients at dermatology clinics.[18] However, a number of studies published since this review have reported much lower percentages, only up to 1.14%.[20,25,27,28]

The Commission E advises that prolonged treatment of damaged skin with arnica can cause oedematous dermatitis with the formation of pustules. Extended use may cause eczema. In treatment involving higher concentrations, primary toxic skin reactions with the formation of vesicles or even necrosis may occur.[14]

A case of leukaemia-related Sweet's syndrome, reportedly triggered by topical application of a cream containing 1.5% arnica, has been published. Pathergy (skin hyperreactivity) to arnica was suspected.[29]

Interactions

None required on current evidence.

Safety in Children

For topical use only.

Overdosage

The symptoms of overdose after oral ingestion of arnica include nausea, vomiting, diarrhoea, dizziness, trembling, increased heart rate, cardiac rhythm disturbances, difficulty with breathing and collapse.[8,15,30] Arnica poisoning has been observed to cause death due to circulatory paralysis with secondary respiratory arrest.[30]

A 19-year-old male mistakenly consumed an unknown amount of tea made from the leaves and flowers of arnica. Two hours later he experienced myalgia, headache and shaking chills and developed hyperthermia, tachycardia, hypotension and raised serum levels of creatinine, asparate aminotransferase and alanine aminotransferase. He was treated with fluids and dopamine and discharged 6 days later when his symptoms improved.[31] A man experienced stomach cramping and died within 36 hours of consuming 70 g of arnica tincture.[9]

Miscarriage has been reported after overdose with ingested arnica tincture or infusion.[9,15] A woman in the second month of pregnancy miscarried after a few days when she ingested an infusion of 20 g arnica flower. Ingestion of three tablespoons of self-prepared tincture of arnica flower led to miscarriage within 24 hours.[9] Multisystem failure has been reported due to ingestion of arnica with abortive intent.[32]

Toxicology

Table 1 lists LD$_{50}$ data recorded for arnica extract and its constituents.[9,33-36]

Aqueous alcohol extract of arnica did not demonstrate irritating, sensitising or phototoxic activity after topical application to the skin of rabbits or guinea pigs. Minimal irritant activity was observed when the 50% extract was instilled in the eyes of rabbits.[33] A short chain ether extract of arnica demonstrated strong dermal sensitising activity in guinea pigs.[37]

Arnica absolute (5% to 100%) induced slight patchy to moderate erythema in guinea pigs upon topical application. However, 75% absolute was not irritating or phototoxic to the skin of mice and 4% absolute was not irritating or sensitising to human volunteers in a maximisation study. Arnica absolute did not induce dermal sensitisation in guinea pigs.[33] (Arnica absolute is an alcohol extract of arnica concrete, which is obtained from the fresh flowers by an organic solvent extraction process.)

Arnica tincture was weakly mutagenic in the Ames test in vitro. The mutagenic activity was thought to be due to the flavonoid content, as it has been found to vary depending on plant origin and method of preparation.[38] Helenalin was inactive in this test.[39]

A single injection of helenalin (25 mg/kg) increased serum alanine aminotransferase, lactate dehydrogenase, urea nitrogen and sorbitol dehydrogenase within 6 hours in male mice. Intraperitoneal injection of helenalin (25 mg/kg/day) increased differential polymorphonuclear leukocyte counts and decreased lymphocyte counts and liver, thymus and spleen weights. Histological evaluation revealed substantial effects on lymphocytes of the thymus, spleen and mesenteric lymph nodes. Multiple helenalin exposures (25 mg/kg/day) also inhibited hepatic microsomal enzyme activities and decreased cytochrome P450 and cytochrome B5 contents.[35] Helenalin and helenalinacetate demonstrated dermal sensitising activity in guinea pigs at concentrations of 0.1% to 1%.[40]

The activity of helenalin has been attributed to its ability to alkylate sulphydryl groups.[41] In vitro and in vivo studies suggest that the cytotoxicity of helenalin is strongly dependent on hepatic glutathione levels, which helenalin rapidly depletes even at low concentrations.[42,43] Helenalin demonstrated chromosome-damaging activity in vitro in Chinese hamster ovarian cells.[9] The relevance of this result to the in vivo action of arnica has not been established.

Regulatory Status

See Table 2 for regulatory status in selected countries.

Table 1   **LD$_{50}$ Data Recorded for Arnica Extract and Its Constituents**

Substance	Route, Model	LD$_{50}$ Value	Reference
A. montana extract	Oral, mice	123 mg/kg	33
A. montana extract	Oral, rats	>5 g/kg	33
A. montana extract	i.p., mice	31 mg/kg	33
Sesquiterpene lactone enriched extract of *A. montana*	i.p., mice	280 mg/kg	9
Helenalin	Oral, mice	150 mg/kg	34
Helenalin	Oral, rats	125 mg/kg	34
Helenalin	Oral, hamsters	85 mg/kg	34
Helenalin	Oral, rabbits	90 mg/kg	34
Helenalin	Oral, sheep	100-125 mg/kg	34
Helenalin	i.p., mice	43 mg/kg	35
Helenalin	i.p., mice	9.86 mg/kg	36

Table **2**   **Regulatory Status for Arnica in Selected Countries**

Australia	Arnica for internal use is included in Part 4 of Schedule 4 of the Therapeutic Goods Act Regulations. It can be used for internal use if the recommended daily dose does not exceed the equivalent of 1 mg of the dry herbal material.
UK & Germany	Arnica for external use is listed on the General Sale List. It is covered by a positive Commission E monograph. Arnica is official in the *British Pharmacopoeia* 2002 and the *European Pharmacopoeia* 4.3.
US	Arnica does not have generally recognised as safe (GRAS) status. However, it is freely available as a "dietary supplement" in the US under DSHEA legislation (Dietary Supplement Health and Education Act of 1994).

REFERENCES

1. Quarz P, Landgrebe N, Wohling D, et al: *Z Phytother Abstractband* p 25, 1995.
2. Moog-Schulze JB: *Tijdschr Integr Geneeskunde* 9:105-112, 1993.
3. British Herbal Medicine Association's Scientific Committee: *British herbal pharmacopoeia,* Bournemouth, 1983, BHMA, pp. 30-31.
4. Wagner H, Bladt S. *Plant drug analysis: a thin layer chromatography atlas,* ed, 2, Berlin, 1996, Springer-Verlag, pp. 197, 214-215.
5. Bisset NG, ed (Wichtl M, ed, German edition): *Herbal drugs and phytopharmaceuticals,* Stuttgart, 1994, Medpharm Scientific Publishers, pp. 83-87.
6. Passreiter CM, Willuhn G, Roder E: *Planta Med* 58: 556-557, 1992.
7. Westendorf J: In De Smet PAGM, Keller K, Hansel R, et al., eds: *Adverse effects of herbal drugs,* vol. 1, Berlin, 1992, Springer-Verlag, p. 194.
8. Felter HW, Lloyd JU: *King's American dispensatory,* ed.18, rev. 3, vol. 1. First published 1905; reprinted Portland, 1983, Eclectic Medical Publications, pp. 278-281.
9. Blaschek W, Ebel S, Hackenthal E, et al: *HagerROM 2002: Hagers Handbuch der Drogen und Arzneistoffe,* Heidelberg, 2002, Springer.
10. Hausen BM, Herrmann HD, Willuhn G: *Contact Dermatitis* 4:3-10, 1978.
11. Hausen BM: *Hautarzt* 31(1):10-17, 1980.
12. *British pharmacopoeia 2002 CD-ROM,* Crown Copyright, 2002.
13. *European pharmacopoeia,* ed. 4(Suppl 4.3), Strasbourg, 2002, Council of Europe, pp. 672-674.
14. Blumenthal M, et al., eds: *The complete German Commission E monographs: therapeutic guide to herbal medicines,* Austin, 1998, American Botanical Council, pp. 83-84.
15. Merdinger O: *MMW* 85:1469-1470, 1938.
16. Rybalko KS, Trutneva EA, Kibal'chich PN: *Aptetschnoje Delo* 14:32-33, 1965.
17. Kreitmair H: *Mercks Jahresber* 50:106-107, 1936.
18. Hausen BM: In De Smet PAGM, Keller K, Hansel R, et al., eds: *Adverse effects of herbal drugs,* vol. 1, Springer-Verlag, Berlin, 1992, pp. 237-242.
19. Ochsenheimer J: *Osterr Med Wschr* pp 226-227, 1844.
20. Bruynzeel DP, van Ketel WG, Young E, et al: *Contact Dermatitis* 27:278-279, 1992.
21. Hormann HP, Korting HC: *Occup Environ Dermatoses* 42:246-249, 1994.
22. Hormann HP, Korting HC: *Phytomed* 4:315-317, 1995.
23. Pirker C, Moslinger T, Koller DY, et al: *Contact Dermatitis* 26:217-219, 1992.
24. Passreiter CM, Florack M, Willuhn G, et al: *Derm Ber Umwelt* 36:79-82, 1988.
25. Hausen BM: *Am J Contact Dermatitis* 7:94-99, 1996.
26. Hausen BM: In De Smet PAGM, Keller K, Hansel R, et al., eds: *Adverse effects of herbal drugs,* vol. 1., Berlin, 1992, Springer-Verlag, pp. 227-236.
27. Paulsen E, Andersen KE, Hausen BM: *Contact Dermatitis* 29:6-10, 1993.
28. Reider N, Komericki P, Hausen BM, et al: *Contact Dermatitis* 45:269-272, 2001.
29. Delmonte S, Brusati C, Parodi A, et al: *Dermatology* 197:195-196, 1998.
30. Hänsel R, Haas H: *Therapie mit Phytopharmaka,* Berlin, 1983, Springer-Verlag, p. 272.
31. Topliff A, Grande G: *J Toxicol Clin Toxicol* 38:518, 2000.
32. Ciganda C, Laborde A: *J Toxicol Clin Toxicol* 39:318-319, 2000.
33. [No authors listed]: *Int J Toxicol* 20:1-11, 2001.
34. Witzel DA, Ivie GW, Dollahite JW: *Am J Vet Res* 37:859-861, 1976.
35. Chapman DE, Roberts GB, Reynolds DJ, et al: *Fundam Appl Toxicol* 10:302-312, 1988.
36. Kim HL: *Res Commun Chem Pathol Pharmacol* 28:189-192, 1980.
37. Hausen BM: *Contact Dermatitis* 4:308, 1978.
38. Goggelmann W, Schimmer O: *Prog Clin Biol Res* 206:63-72, 1986.
39. MacGregor JT: *Food Cosmet Toxicol* 15:225-228, 1977.
40. Herrmann HD, Willuhn G, Hausen BM: *Planta Med* 34:299-304, 1978.
41. Willuhn G: In Lawson LD, Bauer R, eds: *Phytomedicines of Europe: chemistry and biological activity,* Washington DC, 1998, American Chemical Society, ACS Symposium Series 691, pp. 118-132.
42. Merrill J, Kim HL, Safe S: *Adv Exp Med Biol* 197:891-896, 1986.
43. Merrill JC, Kim HL, Safe S, et al: *J Toxicol Environ Health* 23:159-169, 1988.

ASTRAGALUS

Other common names: Milk-vetch root, Huangqi
Botanical names: *Astragalus membranaceus* (Fisch. ex Link) Bge. (*Phaca membranacea* Fisch. ex Link), *A. membranaceus* (Fisch.) Bge. var. *mongholicus* (Bge.) Hsiao
Family: Fabaceae
Plant part used: Root

Safety Summary

Pregnancy category B1: No increase in frequency of malformation or other harmful effects on the foetus from limited use in women. No evidence of increased foetal damage in animal studies.
Lactation category ND: No data available.
Contraindications: Not advisable in acute infections.
Warnings & precautions: None required on current evidence.
Adverse reactions: None found in published literature.
Interactions: May reduce the effectiveness of cyclophosphamide (an immunosuppressive agent).

Typical Therapeutic Use

Astragalus demonstrated therapeutic benefit in the treatment of leucopenia in a randomised trial,[1] ischaemic heart disease and angina pectoris in a controlled trial,[2] and prophylaxis of the common cold in an uncontrolled trial.[3] Traditional indications for astragalus in traditional Chinese medicine include fatigue with poor appetite and diarrhoea, prolapse of the uterus and rectum, abnormal uterine bleeding and spontaneous sweating.[3,4]

Actions

Immune enhancing, tonic, adaptogenic, cardiotonic, diuretic, hypotensive, antioxidant.

Key Constituents

Constituents of astragalus root include triterpenoid saponins (astragalosides), polysaccharides and flavonoids.[5] The levels of main constituents vary according to their origin and the age of the plant. The total astragaloside content from root samples was as follows[6]:

- *A. membranaceus* (cultivated sample from Heilongjiang), 2%
- *A. membranaceus* var. *mongholicus* (cultivated sample from Shanxi), 2.6%
- *A. membranaceus* var. *mongholicus* (non-cultivated sample from Shanxi), 3.6%.

Adulteration

Astragalus propinquus, *A. lepsensis*, *A. aksuensis*, *A. hoantchy*, *A. hoantchy* subsp. *dshimensis*, *A. lehmannianus*, *A. sieversianus* and *A. austrosibiricus* have been identified as adulterants of *Astragalus membranaceus*, whilst *Hedysarum polybotrys* is a substitute. Astragaloside IV is normally used as a marker for quality control. In the Japanese Pharmacopoeia 1996, substitutes including *A. chrysopterus*, *A. floridus* and *A. tongolensis* are officially permitted but these are not accepted in China.[6]

Typical Dosage Forms & Dosage

Typical adult dosage ranges are:
- 9 to 30 g/day of dried root by decoction
- 4.5 to 8.5 mL/day of a 1:2 liquid extract or equivalent in tablet or capsule form

Contraindications

Based on traditional considerations it is not advisable to prescribe astragalus in acute infections.

Use in Pregnancy

Category B1: No increase in frequency of malformation or other harmful effects on the foetus from limited use in women. No evidence of increased foetal damage in animal studies.

Some species of astragalus are known to induce locoism (a condition which can cause reproductive alterations), abortion, and occasional skeletal deformities in livestock.[7,8] *A. membranaceus* has not been identified as one of these species and swainsonine, the indolizidine alkaloid which is responsible for locoism,[9] has not been detected in *A. membranaceus*. It is unlikely that the astragalus species used medicinally are teratogenic, since the species that induce teratogenic effects are also known to be toxic. Moreover, a Chinese herbal formula (Man-Shen-Ling) which contains astragalus did not demonstrate teratogenic activity in animal models.[10]

Use in Lactation

Category ND: No data available.

Warnings & Precautions

None required.

Effect on Ability to Drive or Operate Machinery

No adverse effects expected.

Adverse Reactions

None known.

Interactions

In vivo studies suggest that astragalus may reduce the effectiveness of cyclophosphamide (an immunosuppressive agent).[11,12]

Safety in Children

No information available, but adverse effects are not expected.

Overdosage

No incidents found in published literature.

Toxicology

No adverse effects were observed within 48 hours after oral administration of astragalus at doses of 75 and 100 g/kg. The intraperitoneal LD_{50} of astragalus has been reported to be 40 g/kg in mice. However, intraperitoneal injection of 50 g/kg elicited no significant toxic reactions in mice in another study.[3] Aqueous extract of astragalus (1.25 mg/mL) modestly increased the incidence (16%) of aberrant cells in the Ames test in vitro.[13] In contrast, aqueous-methanolic extract of astragalus showed no mutagenic effects[14] and an aqueous extract demonstrated antimutagenic activity in vitro.[15] A Chinese herbal formula (Man-Shen-Ling) which contains astragalus did not exhibit toxic, mutagenic, teratogenic or carcinogenic effects in acute and chronic toxicity tests in animal models.[10]

Table I   **Regulatory Status for Astragalus in Selected Countries**

Australia	Astragalus is not included in Part 4 of Schedule 4 of the Therapeutic Goods Regulations.
China	Astragalus is official in the *Pharmacopoeia of the People's Republic of China* 1997. The usual adult dosage, usually administered in the form of a decoction, is listed as 9-30 g
UK & Germany	Astragalus is not included on the General Sale List. It was not included in the Commission E assessment.
US	Astragalus does not have generally recognised as safe (GRAS) status. However, it is freely available as a "dietary supplement" in the US under DSHEA legislation (Dietary Supplement Health and Education Act of 1994).

Regulatory Status

See Table I for regulatory status in selected countries.

REFERENCES

1. Weng XS: *Zhongguo Zhong Xi Yi Jie He Za Zhi* 15:462-464, 1995.
2. Li SQ, Yuan RX, Gao H: *Zhongguo Zhong Xi Yi Jie He Za Zhi* 15:77-80, 1995.
3. Chang H, But P: *Pharmacology and applications of Chinese materia medica*, vol 2, Singapore, 1987, World Scientific, pp 1041-1046.
4. Pharmacopoeia Commission of the People's Republic of China: *Pharmacopoeia of the People's Republic of China*, English ed, vol I, Beijing, 1997, Chemical Industry Press, pp 142-143.
5. Tang W, Eisenbrand G: *Chinese drugs of plant origin*, Berlin, 1992, Springer-Verlag, pp 191-197.
6. Ma XQ, Shi Q, Duan JA, et al: *J Agric Food Chem* 50:4861-4866, 2002.
7. James LF, Shupe JL, Binns W, et al: *Am J Vet Res* 28:1379-1388, 1967.
8. James LF, Keeler RF, Binns W: *Am J Vet Res* 30:377-380, 1969.
9. Molyneux RJ, James LF: *Science* 216:190-191, 1982.
10. Su ZZ, He YY, Chen G: *Zhongguo Zhong Xi Yi Jie He Za Zhi* 13(5):259-260, 269-272, 1993.
11. Chu DT, Wong WL, Mavligit GM: *J Clin Lab Immunol* 25:125-129, 1988.

12. Chu DT, Sun Y, Lin JR: *Zhong Xi Yi Jie He Za Zhi* 9:326, 351-354, 1989.

13. Tadaki S, Yamada S, Miyazawa N, et al: *Jap J Toxicol Environ Health* 41:463-469, 1995.

14. Yamamoto H, Mizutani T, Nomura H: *Yakugaku Zasshi* 102:596-601, 1982.

15. Wong BY, Lau BH, Tadi PP, et al: *Mutat Res* 279:209-216, 1992.

BACOPA

Other common name: Brahmi
Botanical names: *Bacopa monnieri* (L.) Pennell
(*Bacopa monniera* (L.) Pennell, *Herpestis monnieria*
Kunth, *Bramia monnieri* (L.) Pennell)
Family: Scrophulariaceae
Plant part used: Aerial parts

Safety Summary

Pregnancy category B2: No increase in frequency
of malformation or other harmful effects on the
foetus from limited use in women. Animal studies
are lacking.
Lactation category C: Compatible with breastfeeding.
Contraindications: None known.
Warnings & precautions: The use of herbs rich in
saponins is possibly inappropriate in coeliac disease,
fat malabsorption and vitamins A, D, E, and K deficiency, some upper digestive irritations and topically
to open wounds. Caution in patients with preexisting cholestasis.
Adverse reactions: Weakness, loss of concentration and dizziness have been reported for one
patient. Herbs rich in saponins may cause irritation
of the gastric mucous membranes and reflux.
Interactions: No precautions required on current
evidence.

Typical Therapeutic Use

Bacopa improved mental performance and memory in healthy adults in randomised, double-blind,
placebo-controlled trials[1,2] and demonstrated therapeutic benefit in patients with anxiety neurosis[3,4]
and epilepsy[5] in uncontrolled trials. Traditional indications for bacopa in Ayurvedic medicine include
nervous breakdown, epilepsy, insanity and debility.[6-8]

Actions

Cognition enhancing, nervine tonic, mild sedative,
mild anticonvulsant, anxiolytic, possibly adaptogenic.

Key Constituents

Constituents of bacopa include dammarane-type
(tetracyclic triterpenoid) saponins (bacosides),[9]
bacosine (a triterpene),[10] and flavonoids.[11]

Adulteration

Centella asiatica (gotu kola), which is also known as
Brahmi in India, is a relatively common adulterant.

Typical Dosage Forms & Dosage

Typical adult dosage ranges are:
- 5 to 10 g/day of dried aerial parts or by infusion
- 5 to 13 mL/day of a 1:2 liquid extract or equivalent in tablet or capsule form

Contraindications

None known.

Use in Pregnancy

Category B2: No increase in frequency of malformation or other harmful effects on the foetus from
limited use in women. Animal studies are lacking.
  Bacopa is recommended as a nervine tonic for
pregnant women in traditional Ayurvedic medicine.[12]

Use in Lactation

Category C: Compatible with breastfeeding.

Warnings & Precautions

The use of herbs rich in saponins is possibly inappropriate in coeliac disease, fat malabsorption and
vitamins A, D, E, and K deficiency, some upper digestive irritations, and topically to open wounds.
Saponin-containing herbs are best kept to a minimum in patients with preexisting cholestasis.

Effect on Ability to Drive or Operate Machinery

No adverse effects expected.

Adverse Reactions

One of 13 patients with epilepsy treated with a
defatted, ethanolic extract of bacopa (2 to 4
mg/kg/day) reported weakness, loss of concentration and dizziness during an uncontrolled trial. Blood
counts, haemoglobin and urine tests were normal
for all 13 patients.[5]

As with all herbs rich in saponins, oral use may cause irritation of the gastric mucous membranes and reflux.

Interactions

None known.

Safety in Children

Bacopa is used in children in Ayurvedic medicine[8] and has been used in clinical trials involving children.[5,13,14]

Overdosage

No incidents found in published literature.

Toxicology

Table 1 lists LD_{50} data recorded for bacopa extract.[15,16]

An ethanol extract of bacopa (10 to 200 mg/kg) produced no change in the behavioural response of mice.[15] Water extract of bacopa administered orally up to a dose of 5 g/kg did not demonstrate any toxicity in rats.[16]

A phase I, double-blind, placebo-controlled clinical trial investigated the safety of oral doses of bacosides in healthy male volunteers. The bacosides in single doses (20 to 300 mg) and multiple doses (100 and 200 mg) administered daily for 4 weeks were well tolerated and were devoid of adverse reactions.[17]

An ethanol extract of bacopa, a saponin-rich fraction, and bacoside A all demonstrated cytotoxic activity in the brine shrimp lethality assay in vitro.[18] However, saponins from bacopa did not demonstrate genotoxic activity in mice in vivo after intraperitoneal administration of 20, 40, or 80 mg/kg.[19]

Regulatory Status

See Table 2 for regulatory status in selected countries.

Table **2**   **Regulatory Status for Bacopa in Selected Countries**

Australia	Bacopa is not included in Part 4 of Schedule 4 of the Therapeutic Goods Regulations.
UK & Germany	Bacopa is not included on the General Sale List. It was not included in the Commission E assessment.
US	Bacopa does not have generally recognised as safe (GRAS) status. However, it is freely available as a "dietary supplement" in the US under DSHEA legislation (Dietary Supplement Health and Education Act of 1994).

Table **1**   **LD_{50} Data Recorded for Bacopa Extract**

Substance	Route, Model	LD_{50} Value	Reference
Bacopa ethanol extract	Route undefined, mice	520 mg/kg	15
Bacopa ethanol extract	Oral, rats	17 g/kg	16

REFERENCES

1. Stough C, Lloyd J, Clarke J, et al: *Psychopharmacology (Berl)* 156:481-484, 2001.
2. Roodenrys S, Booth D, Bulzomi S, et al: *Neuropsychopharmacology* 27: 279-281, 2002.
3. Udupa KN, Singh RH: *Clinical and experimental studies on Rasayana drugs and Pancakarma therapy*, ed 2, New Delhi, 1995, Central Council for Research in Ayurveda and Siddha, pp 29-30.
4. Singh RH, Singh L: *J Res Ayurveda Siddha* 1:133-148, 1980.
5. Mukherjee GD, Dey CD: *J Exp Med Sci* 11:82-85, 1968.
6. Chopra RN, Chopra IC, Handa KL, et al: *Chopra's indigenous drugs of India*, ed 2, 1958; reprinted Calcutta, 1982, Academic Publishers, pp 341-342.
7. Thakur RS, Puri HS, Husain A: *Major medicinal plants of India*. Lucknow, 1989, Central Institute of Medicinal and Aromatic Plants, pp 92-95.
8. Kapoor LD: *CRC handbook of Ayurvedic medicinal plants*. Boca Raton, 1990, CRC Press, p 61.
9. Chatterji N, Rastogi RP, Dhar ML: *Indian J Chem* 1:212-215, 1963.
10. Vohora SB, Khanna T, Athar M: *Fitoterapia* 68:361-365, 1997.
11. Proliac A, Chaboud A, Raynaud J: *Pharm Acta Helv* 66:153-154, 1991.

12. Sandu DV: *Indian therapeutics*, ed 2, Delhi, 1987, Sri Satguru Publications, p 24.

13. Kaur BR, Adhiraj J, Pandit PR, et al: *Indian Drugs* 35:200-203, 1998.

14. Sharma R, Chaturvedi C, Tewari PV: *J Res Educ Indian Med* 6:1-10, 1987.

15. Dar A, Channa S: *Phytother Res* 11:323-325, 1997.

16. Martis G, Rao A: *Fitoterapia* 63:399-404, 1992.

17. Singh HK, Dhawan BN: *Indian J Pharmacol* 29:S359-S365, 1997.

18. D'Souza P, Deepak M, Rani P, et al: *Phytother Res* 16:197-198, 2002.

19. Giri AK, Khan KA: *Cytologia (Tokyo)* 61:99-103, 1996.

BARBERRY & INDIAN BARBERRY

Botanical names: *Berberis vulgaris* L. (common names: barberry, Berberis), *Berberis aristata* DC. (common name: Indian barberry)
Family: Berberidaceae
Plant part used: Root and/or stem bark

Safety Summary

Pregnancy category C: Has caused or is associated with a substantial risk of causing harmful effects to the foetus or neonate without causing malformations (on the basis of the presence of berberine and related alkaloids and the implications for neonatal jaundice).
Lactation category SD: Strongly discouraged in breastfeeding (on the basis of the presence of berberine and related alkaloids).
Contraindications: Jaundiced neonates. Do not use during pregnancy or lactation without professional advice.
Warnings & precautions: Use cautiously in unconjugated hyperbilirubinaemia, acute or severe hepatocellular disease, septic cholecystitis, intestinal spasm or ileus, liver cancer.
Adverse reactions: None found in published literature.
Interactions: Drugs which displace the protein binding of bilirubin, such as phenylbutazone.

Typical Therapeutic Use

Traditional indications for barberry in Western herbal medicine include cholecystitis, cholelithiasis, jaundice and leishmaniasis.[1] Traditional indications for Indian barberry root bark in Ayurveda include intermittent fevers, jaundice, periodic neuralgia and dysentery.[2]

Actions

Antimicrobial, cholagogue, choleretic, antiemetic, mild laxative, bitter tonic (for both herbs).

Key Constituents

Key constituents of *Berberis vulgaris* root bark are alkaloids (up to 13%), including berberine (up to 6%), jatrorrhizine, palmatine with smaller amounts of oxyacanthine and magnoflorine.[3] The root bark is richest in alkaloids (12.8%), followed

by the stem bark (5.5%).[4] Indian barberry root bark also contains berberine (2.7% in powdered samples).[5]

Adulteration

A 1933 source indicates that *Berberis aristata* was often confused with other *Berberis* spp. (such as *B. lycium*, and *B. vulgaris*) in India.[6] Commercially available barberry root bark may contain branch and stem bark. Barberry sourced from India may not always be obtained from *B. vulgaris*.[7] *Berberis vulgaris* is a protected species in one or more regions of France.[8]

Typical Dosage Forms & Dosage

Typical adult dosage ranges for barberry:
- 3 to 6 g/day of dried bark or by decoction
- 6 to 9 mL/day of 1:1 liquid extract
- 3 to 6 mL/day of 1:2 liquid extract or equivalent in tablet or capsule form
- 6 to 12 mL/day of 1:10 tincture

Typical adult dosage ranges for Indian barberry:
- 2 oz, three times per day of decoction (6 oz:1 pint)
- 2 to 4.5 mL/day of 1:1 liquid extract

Contraindications

Barberry and Indian barberry: Although berberine-containing plants have been used in traditional Chinese medicine for the treatment of jaundiced neonates, berberine is thought to cause severe acute haemolysis and neonatal jaundice in babies with glucose-6-phosphate dehydrogenase deficiency.[9] However, a review published in 2001 questioned the causal relationship between the berberine-containing herb *Coptis chinensis* and haemolysis in glucose-6-phosphate dehydrogenase deficient infants (see Pregnancy section below).[10]

Additional information for Barberry: The *British Herbal Pharmacopoeia* 1983 advises that barberry is contraindicated in diarrhoea and early pregnancy.[1] The contraindication for diarrhoea may not be valid. Barberry bark was used by Eclectic practitioners for the treatment of chronic diarrhoea and dysentery,[11] and berberine has been administered in clinical trials for the treatment of diarrhoea.[12,13]

Do not use barberry or Indian barberry during pregnancy or lactation without professional advice.

Use in Pregnancy

Category C: Has caused or is associated with a substantial risk of causing harmful effects on the foetus or neonate without causing malformations (on the basis of the presence of berberine and related alkaloids and the implications for neonatal jaundice).

Berberine caused uterine contraction in both non-pregnant and pregnant experimental models.[14] In another study which investigated 10 berberine-containing plant extracts, stimulation or relaxation of isolated uterus occurred depending upon the extract tested. Results did not correlate with berberine content. This suggests that a berberine-containing herb will not necessarily produce uterine contractions merely because of the presence of berberine.[15] An alcohol extract of the bark of branches and stem of *Berberis vulgaris* enhanced the contractility of isolated uterus.[16]

The maternal LOAEL (lowest observed adverse effect level) for mated rats fed berberine chloride dihydrate from gestational day 6 to day 20 was measured at 531 mg/kg/day. Maternal NOAEL (no observed adverse effect level) was 282 mg/kg/day. The developmental LOAEL was 1313 mg/kg/day and the NOAEL was 531 mg/kg/day.[17] A follow-up study using the same protocol found similar results, but there was an absence of a significant effect for berberine on developmental toxicity. The developmental toxicity NOAEL can be raised to approximately 1100 mg/kg/day berberine.[18] This indicates that doses less than 1 g/kg berberine chloride dihydrate had no observable effect on offspring.

Berberine-containing plants are not recommended for use during pregnancy. The incidence of kernicterus in premature Chinese infants with neonatal jaundice has been reported to be in some cases associated with exposure to *Coptis chinensis* either by direct administration, transplacental absorption or via breast milk.[19] (Coptis contains 7% to 9% berberine.) This suggests that berberine-containing plants are best avoided during pregnancy and lactation.

Use in Lactation

Category SD: Strongly discouraged in breastfeeding (on the basis of the presence of berberine and related alkaloids).

Infants have been exposed to berberine via breast milk following maternal ingestion of berberine-containing plants.[19]

Warnings & Precautions

Choleretics and cholagogues should be used cautiously and may be inappropriate in the following:
- unconjugated hyperbilirubinaemia (jaundice following haemolytic diseases, hereditary disease like Gilbert's and Crigler-Najjar syndromes)
- acute or severe hepatocellular disease (e.g., following viral hepatitis, cirrhosis, adverse reactions to drugs e.g., anaesthetics, steroids, oestrogen, chlorpromazine)
- septic cholecystitis (where there is a risk of peritonitis)
- intestinal spasm or ileus
- liver cancer.

Effect on Ability to Drive or Operate Machinery

No adverse effects expected for either herb.

Adverse Reactions

None known for barberry and Indian barberry. Berberine is well tolerated up to 0.5 g.[20] Such doses of berberine are not reached using barberry or Indian barberry at the recommended dosage.

Interactions

Berberine demonstrated potent displacement of bilirubin in vitro and in vivo after chronic administration to rats (10 to 20 mg/kg i.p.). Berberine at this dosage range caused elevation in serum levels of bilirubin (since the binding of bilirubin to albumin decreased). However, at a dose of 2 mg/kg the displacement was not significant.[19] Hence berberine may reinforce the effects of other drugs that displace the protein binding of bilirubin.

Safety in Children

Berberine has been used to treat diarrhoea and giardiasis in children, which suggests that berberine-containing plants may be used. Treatment of newborns with neonatal jaundice is contraindicated.

Overdosage

Poisoning has been reported in 3 cases following ingestion of barberry leaf. Consumption of barberry berries has caused vomiting and diarrhoea.[7] The red berries, however, do not contain alkaloids and are used to prepare jams and beverages.[21] Only a trace amount of berberine is present in the leaves.[14,22]

The Commission E notes that no reports of poisoning with barberry are known, but that death from berberine poisoning has occurred. At doses higher than 0.5 g, berberine may cause dizziness, nose bleeds, dyspnoea, skin and eye irritation, gastrointestinal irritation, nausea, diarrhoea, nephritis and urinary tract disorders.[20] Such doses of berberine will not be reached from berberine-containing herbs used at the recommended therapeutic doses. In two clinical trials for acute diarrhoea due to enterotoxigenic *E. coli* and *Vibrio cholerae*, berberine was well tolerated in dosages of 0.8 to 1.2 g/day.[12,13]

Toxicology

Table 1 lists LD_{50} data recorded for barberry and Indian barberry extracts and their key constituents and implies low to moderate toxicity for the herbs.[15,23-26]

An investigation of 10 berberine-containing herbs (including *Berberis amuresis, B. thunbegii, Mahonia japonica, M. fortunei, Coptis japonica,* and *Hydrastis canadensis*) observed that the LD_{50} values (extracts, oral, mice) were not correlated with the berberine content.[15]

A single oral dose of berberine given to mice (4 mg/kg) one hour prior to the administration of a sublethal dose of strychnine enhanced the effect of strychnine causing 100% mortality. The authors suggest that the berberine had an inhibitory effect upon cytochrome P450 enzymes.[27]

Berberine has been found to partially insert into DNA in vitro.[28] Berberine hydrochloride was weakly mutagenic in *Salmonella typhimurium* strain TA98 in the absence of S9 mix, but was inactive towards strain TA100 under these conditions. In the presence of S9 mix (metabolic activation) it was nonmutagenic to both strains.[29] Berberine did not show genotoxic activity with or without metabolic activation in the SOS chromotest. It was inactive in treatments performed under nongrowth conditions, but showed mild mutagenic activity in dividing cells.[30]

An in vitro study demonstrated that berberine exhibits phosphorescence in ethanol. UVA irradiation of keratinocytes in the presence of berberine resulted in a decrease in cell viability and an increase in DNA damage.[31] The effect of the topical application of berberine or berberine-containing preparations and subsequent exposure to UVA irradiation or to natural light has not been studied.

Refer to the Oregon grape (*Mahonia aquifolium*) monograph for LD_{50} values of berbamine and oxyacanthine.

Regulatory Status

See Table 2 for regulatory status in selected countries.

Table **1** **LD_{50} Data Recorded for Barberry and Indian Barberry Extract and Constituents**

Substance	Route, Model	LD_{50} Value	Reference
Barberry root extract fraction*	Oral, mice	520 mg/kg	23
Barberry root extract fraction*	Oral, rats	1280 mg/kg	23
Indian barberry root ethanol extract	i.p., mice	200 mg/kg	24
Berberine	Oral, mice	329 mg/kg	15
Berberine	i.p., mice	23 mg/kg	25
Berberine sulfate	Oral, rats	>1 g/kg	26

*The fraction contained 80% berbamine and three unidentified isoquinoline alkaloids.

Table **2**   **Regulatory Status for Barberry and Indian Barberry in Selected Countries**

Australia	Barberry and Indian barberry are not included in Part 4 of Schedule 4 of the Therapeutic Goods Regulations.
UK & Germany	Barberry is included on the General Sale List (GSL). Indian barberry is not listed. Berberis (species undefined) is included on the GSL equivalent to a maximum single dose of 0.5 mg berberine. Barberry is covered by a negative Commission E monograph. Indian barberry was not included in the Commission E assessment.
US	Barberry and Indian barberry do not have generally recognised as safe (GRAS) status. However, both herbs are freely available as a "dietary supplement" in the US under DSHEA legislation (Dietary Supplement Health and Education Act of 1994).

REFERENCES

1. British Herbal Medicine Association's Scientific Committee: *British herbal pharmacopoeia*, Bournemouth, 1983, BHMA, pp 39-40.
2. Thakur RS, Puri HS, Husain A: *Major medicinal plants of India*, Lucknow, 1989, Central Institute of Medicinal and Aromatic Plants, pp 107-111.
3. Wagner H, Bladt S: *Plant drug analysis: a thin layer chromatography atlas*, ed 2, Berlin, 1996, Springer-Verlag, p 10.
4. Petcu P, Goina T: *Planta Med* 18:372-375, 1970.
5. Chauhan SK, Singh BP, Agrawal S: *Indian Drugs* 35:468-470, 1998.
6. Chopra RN, Chopra IC, Handa KL, et al: *Chopra's indigenous drugs of India*, ed 2, 1958; reprinted Calcutta, 1982, Academic Publishers, p 289.
7. Blaschek W, Ebel S, Hackenthal E, et al: *HagerROM 2002: Hagers Handbuch der Drogen und Arzneistoffe*. Heidelberg, 2002, Springer.
8. Lange D: *Europe's medicinal and aromatic plants: their use, trade and conservation*, Cambridge, 1998, TRAFFIC International, p IV.
9. Ho NK: *Singapore Med J* 37:645-651, 1996.
10. Fok TF: *J Perinatol* 21:S98-S100, 2001.
11. Felter HW, Lloyd JU: *King's American dispensatory*, ed 18, rev 3, vol 1. First published 1905; reprinted Portland, 1983, Eclectic Medical Publications, pp 345-346.
12. Rabbani GH, Butler T, Knight J, et al: *J Infect Dis* 155:979-984, 1987.
13. Khin-Maung U, Myo-Khin, Nyunt-Nyunt-Wai, et al: *J Diarrhoeal Dis Res* 5:184-187, 1987.
14. De Smet PAGM, Keller K, Hansel R, et al, eds: *Adverse effects of herbal drugs*, vol 1, Berlin, 1992, Springer-Verlag, pp 97-104.
15. Haginiwa J, Harada M: *Yakugaku Zasshi* 82:726-731, 1962.
16. Aliev RK, Yuzbashinskaya NA: *Doklady Akad Nauk Azerbaidzhan SSR* 9:231-237, 1953.
17. Price CJ, George JD, Marr MC, et al: *Teratology* 63:279, 2001.
18. NTP Study TER20102: *Final study report developmental toxicity evaluation for berberine chloride dihydrate (cas no. 5956-60-5) administered by gavage to Sprague-Dawley (CD®) rats on gestational days 6 through 19.* Available from the National Toxicology Program website: ntp-server.niehs.nih.gov. Accessed March 2003.
19. Chan E: *Biol Neonate* 63:201-208, 1993.
20. Blumenthal M et al, eds: *The complete German Commission E monographs: therapeutic guide to herbal medicines*, Austin, 1998, American Botanical Council, pp 309-310.
21. Frohne D, Pfander HJ: *A colour atlas of poisonous plants: a handbook for pharmacists, doctors, toxicologists, and biologists*, translated from the German ed 2 by Bisset NG: London, 1984, Wolfe Publishing, pp 70-71.
22. Hakim SAE, Mijovic V, Walker J: *Nature* 189:198-201, 1961.
23. Manolov P, Nikolov N, Markov M, et al: *Eksp Med Morfol* 24:41-45, 1985.
24. Dhar ML, Dhar MM, Dhawan BN, et al: Indian J Exp Biol 6:232-247, 1968.
25. Schmeller T, Latz-Bruning B, Wink M: *Phytochem* 44:257-266, 1997.
26. Kowalewski Z, Mrozikiewicz A, Bobkiewicz T, et al: *Acta Pol Pharm* 32:113-120, 1975.
27. Janbaz KH, Gilani AH: *Fitoterapia* 71:25-33, 2000.
28. Saran A, Srivastava S, Coutinho E, et al: *Indian J Biochem Biophys* 32:74-77, 1995.
29. Nozaka T, Watanabe F, Tadaki S, et al: *Mutat Res* 240:267-279, 1990.
30. Pasqual MS, Lauer CP, Moyna P, et al: *Mutat Res* 286:243-252, 1993.
31. Inbaraj JJ, Kukielczak BM, Bilski P, et al: *Chem Res Toxicol* 14:1529-1534, 2001.

BEARBERRY

Other common name: Uva ursi
Botanical name: *Arctostaphylos uva-ursi* (L.) Spreng
Family: Ericaceae
Plant part used: Leaf

Safety Summary

Pregnancy category C: Has caused or is associated with a substantial risk of causing harmful effects on the foetus or neonate without causing malformations. Theoretical foetotoxicity.
Lactation category SD: Strongly discouraged.
Contraindications: Kidney disease, pregnancy, lactation and children under 12 years old. In principle, the use of herbs containing high levels of tannins is contraindicated or at least inappropriate in constipation, iron deficiency anaemia and malnutrition.
Warnings & precautions: Because of the tannin content of this herb, long-term use should be avoided. Use cautiously in highly inflamed or ulcerated conditions of the gastrointestinal tract.
Adverse reactions: A potential adverse reaction due to the high tannin content is irritation of the mouth and gastrointestinal tract. Allergic contact dermatitis occurs occasionally from topical use.
Interactions: Take separately from oral thiamine, metal ion supplements or alkaloid-containing medications.

Typical Therapeutic Use

Traditional indications of bearberry leaf in Western herbal medicine include acute and recurrent infections of the lower urinary tract, such as cystitis and urethritis, where there are no other complications.[1]

Actions

Urinary antiseptic[2-4] (in vitro activity against *Citrobacter*, *Enterobacter*, *Escherischia*, *Klebsiella*, *Proteus*, *Pseudomonas* and *Staphylococcus*[5]), astringent, diuretic,[6] antiinflammatory.[7]

Key Constituents

Arbutin, which on glycolysis generates hydroquinone (normally between 6.3% to 9.16% – higher in autumn crops[8]), accompanied by variable amounts of methylarbutin (up to 4%) and by small quantities of the free aglycones hydroquinone and methylhydroquinone.[9] Bearberry also contains high levels of hydrolysable tannins (10% to 15%).[10]

Adulteration

Substitution with other species of Ericacea is not uncommon in commerce. *Vaccinium vitis-idaea* L., *V. uliginosum* L., *V. myrtillus* L. (bilberry), *Gaultheria procumbens* L. (wintergreen), *Arctostaphylos alpinus* (L.), *Buxus sempervirens* L. (common box) have all been detected in batches of "bearberry leaves". According to the German Pharmacopoeia, samples containing less than 6% arbutin should be considered as adulterated.

Arctostaphylos uva-ursi is protected and/or has restrictions for wildcrafting in several areas of Europe.[11]

Typical Dosage Forms & Dosage

Typical adult dosage ranges are:
- 3 to 12 g/day of dried leaf or by infusion
- 3 to 12 mL/day of a 1:1 liquid extract
- 4.5 to 8.5 mL/day of a 1:2 liquid extract or equivalent in tablet or capsule form
- 6 to 12 mL/day of a 1:5 tincture

Doses should deliver the equivalent of 400 to 800 mg arbutin per day, divided into 2 or 3 doses.

Contraindications

Various authorities have listed kidney disease,[10] pregnancy, lactation and in children under 12 years old.[12] No evidence to support these cautions is available; however, public caution is warranted.

In principle, the use of herbs with high levels of tannins is contraindicated or at least inappropriate in constipation, iron deficiency anaemia and malnutrition.

Use in Pregnancy

Category C: Has caused or is associated with a substantial risk of causing harmful effects on the foetus or neonate without causing malformations.

There is a theoretical risk to foetal development due to the uterotonic properties of arbutin in vivo.[13,14] Arbutin also occurs in food: wheat products (1 to 10 ppm), pears (4 to 15 ppm), and coffee and tea (0.1 ppm).[15]

Use in Lactation

Category SD: Bearberry leaf should be avoided during lactation due to the likely transfer of arbutin or hydroquinone to breast milk.[12]

Warnings & Precautions

Because of the tannin content of this herb, long-term use should be avoided (for both internal and topical use). Use cautiously in highly inflamed or ulcerated conditions of the gastrointestinal tract.

Effect on Ability to Drive or Operate Machinery

No adverse effects expected.

Adverse Reactions

Hydroquinone is a topical irritant and a hepatotoxin and the amount in bearberry leaf preparations should be controlled. Oral ingestion of 5 to 12 g has been fatal. Long-term external application of creams containing up to 10% of hydroquinone has caused skin colloid degeneration (see below).

Allergic contact dermatitis with skin colloid degeneration (ochronosis) or hyperpigmentation, has been reported after the topical use of creams containing hydroquinone up to 10%,[16] but not for preparations containing bearberry leaf. In fact the leaf inhibited melanin biosynthesis in vivo[17] through an inhibition of tyrosinase activity.[18,19]

High doses of tannins lead to excessive astringency on mucous membranes which has an irritating effect. Nausea and vomiting, cramping or constipation can occur due to stomach irritation from the high tannin content of bearberry leaf.

Interactions

Concomitant acidification of the urine (for instance by medicaments) may result in a reduction of efficacy.[20]

Tannins can bind metal ions, thiamine and alkaloids and reduce their absorption. Refer to the cranesbill root (Geranium maculatum) monograph for information regarding these interactions of tannins. Bearberry should be consumed at least 2 hours away from oral thiamine, mineral supplements such as iron, and alkaloid-containing drugs.

Topical use of bearberry has been observed to augment the topical antiinflammatory effects of prednisolone,[21] dexamethasone,[22] and indomethacin.[23]

Bearberry extract markedly potentiated the action of beta-lactam antibiotics against methicillin-resistant Staphylococcus aureus in vitro. The constituent corilagin (a polyphenol) was responsible for the activity.[24] However, whether this leads to a clinical urinary antiseptic effect is uncertain.

Safety in Children

Treatment is not recommended for children under the age of 12 years.[12]

Overdosage

Inflammation of the urinary mucosa and haematuria have been claimed as a consequence of high doses,[25] and there is a stated risk of liver damage.[26] Long-term use of high doses is to be avoided.

Toxicology

The oral LD_{50} of hydroquinone in 2% aqueous solution has been reported as between 320 and 550 mg/kg in various laboratory animals. In doses of 1 g, hydroquinone leads to tinnitus, emesis, delirium, convulsions and collapse.[27]

Arbutin and bearberry extracts are considerably less toxic than hydroquinone, as evidenced by the studies cited below.

In vivo, hydroquinone administered by intraperitoneal injection induced elevated micronucleus incidences. However, there was no induction of micronuclei in bone marrow when arbutin was administered orally (0.5 to 2.0 g/kg). Arbutin itself is not mutagenic, in concentrations up to 10^{-2} M in a gene mutation assay. An increase in mutation frequency was observed with concentrations of 10^{-3} M. Hydroquinone, used as a positive control, exhibited clear effects. However, any generated hydroquinone could exert its mutagenic potential.[28]

Refer to the cranesbill root (Geranium maculatum) monograph for information regarding interactions of tannins (see Interactions section).

Regulatory Status

See Table 1 for regulatory status in selected countries.

Table **1**   **Regulatory Status for Bearberry in Selected Countries**

Australia	Bearberry leaf is not included in Part 4 of Schedule 4 of the Therapeutic Goods Regulations.
UK & Germany	Bearberry is included on the General Sale List. It is covered by a positive Commission E monograph. Bearberry leaf is official in the *European Pharmacopoeia* 4.3.
US	Bearberry leaf does not have generally recognised as safe (GRAS) status. However, it is freely available as a "dietary supplement" in the US under DSHEA legislation (Dietary Supplement Health and Education Act of 1994).

REFERENCES

1. British Herbal Medicine Association's Scientific Committee: *British herbal pharmacopoeia*, Bournemouth, 1983, BHMA, pp 29-30.
2. Kedzia B, Kedzia B, Wrocinski T, et al: *Med Dosw Mikrobiol* 27:305-314, 1975.
3. Jahodar L, Leifertova I, Lisa M: *Pharmazie* 33:536-537, 1978.
4. Floresne-Vari H, Verzarne-Petri G, Kutasi M: *Acta Pharm Hung* 54:170-175, 1984.
5. Jahodar L, Jilek P, Patkova M, et al: *Cesk Farm* 34:174-178, 1985.
6. Beaux D, Fleurentin J, Mortier F: *Phytother Res* 13:222-225, 1999;
7. Kubo M, Ito M, Nakata H, et al: *Yakugaku Zasshi* 110:59-67, 1990.
8. Parejo I, Viladomat F, Bastida J, et al: *Phytochem Anal* 12:336-339, 2001.
9. Sticher O, Soldati F, Lehmann D: *Planta Med* 35:253-261, 1979.
10. British Herbal Medicine Association: *British herbal compendium*, vol 1, Bournemouth, 1992, BHMA, pp 211-213.
11. Lange D: *Europe's medicinal and aromatic plants: their use, trade and conservation*, Cambridge, 1998, TRAFFIC International, p III.
12. Blumenthal M, et al, eds: *The complete German commission E monographs: therapeutic guide to herbal medicines*, Austin, 1998, American Botanical Council, pp 224-225.
13. Shipochliev T: *Vet Med Nauki* 18:94-98, 1981.
14. Itabashi M, Aihara H, Inoue T, et al: *Iyakuhin Kenkyu* 19:282-297, 1988.
15. Deisinger PJ, Hill TS, English JC: *J Toxicol Environ Health* 47:31-46, 1996.
16. Howard KL, Ferner BB: *Cutis* 45:180-182, 1990.
17. Matsuda H, Higashino M, Nakai Y, et al: *Biol Pharm Bull* 19:153-156, 1996.
18. Matsuo K, Kobayashi M, Takuno Y, et al: *Yakugaku Zasshi* 117:1028-1032, 1997.
19. Matsuda H, Nakamura S, Shiomoto H, et al: *Yakugaku Zasshi* 112:276-282, 1992.
20. Frohne D: *Planta Med* 18:1-25, 1970.
21. Matsuda H, Nakata H, Tanaka T, et al: *Yakugaku Zasshi* 110:68-76, 1990.
22. Matsuda H, Nakamura S, Tanaka T, et al: *Yakugaku Zasshi* 112:673-677, 1992.
23. Matsuda H, Tanaka T, Kubo M: *Yakugaku Zasshi* 111:253-258, 1991.
24. Shimizu M, Shiota S, Mitzushima T, et al: *Antimicrob Agents Chemother* 45:3198-3201, 2001.
25. Stübler M, Krug E: *Leesers Lehrbuch der Homöopathie, Pflanzliche Arzneistoffe II*, Heidelberg, 1988, Haug-Verlag, pp 403–406.
26. Standardzulassung für Fertigarzneimittel: *Pharmazeutischer Verlag, deutscher Apotheker*, Frankfurt/Main, 1987/89, Verlag.
27. Woodard G, Hagan CE, Radomski JL: *Fed Proc* 8:348, 1949.
28. Mueller L, Kasper P: *Mutat Res* 360:291-292, 1996.

BILBERRY FRUIT

Botanical name: *Vaccinium myrtillus* L.
Family: Ericaceae
Plant part used: Fruit

Safety Summary

Pregnancy category A: No proven increase in the frequency of malformation or other harmful effects on the foetus despite consumption by a large number of women.
Lactation category C: Compatible with breastfeeding.
Contraindications: None required on current evidence.
Warnings & precautions: High doses (>100 mg/day anthocyanins) should be used cautiously in patients with haemorrhagic disorders and in those taking warfarin or antiplatelet drugs.
Adverse reactions: Mild side effects affecting the gastrointestinal, cutaneous or nervous systems.
Interactions: Caution with very high doses in patients taking warfarin or antiplatelet drugs.

Typical Therapeutic Use

A review of uncontrolled trials concluded that bilberry demonstrated therapeutic benefit in patients with venous insufficiency of the lower limbs.[1] Bilberry has also been found to be beneficial for various vision disorders in controlled and uncontrolled trials[2-6] and for vascular retinopathy in placebo-controlled trials.[7,8] Traditional indications for bilberry in Western herbal medicine include diarrhoea, scurvy and urinary complaints.[9]

Actions

Vasoprotective, antioedema, antioxidant, anti-inflammatory.

Key Constituents

Major constituents of bilberry fruit include anthocyanins (0.5%, also known as anthocyanosides: glycosides of delphinidin, malvidin, pelargonidin, cyanidin and petunidin)[10] and flavonoids. More recent chemical analysis indicates the presence of tannins to about 1.5%.[11]

Adulteration

Vaccinium uliginosum and *V. vitis-idaea* have been noted as adulterants.[12]

Typical Dosage Forms & Dosage

Typical adult dosage ranges are:
- 20 to 50 g/day of fresh fruit
- 3 to 6 mL/day of a 1:1 liquid extract
- extract standardised to contain 50 to 120 mg/day anthocyanins (equivalent to about 20 to 50 g of fresh fruit)

Contraindications

None known.

Use in Pregnancy

Category A: No proven increase in the frequency of malformation or other harmful effects on the foetus despite consumption by a large number of women.

A number of uncontrolled studies involving over 200 pregnant women have reported that bilberry extract is a safe and effective treatment for venous disorders, including haemorrhoids, with no adverse effects observed in mothers or infants. Doses of extract equivalent to 57 to 173 mg/day anthocyanins were administered for 60 to 102 days.[13-16]

Bilberry extract (standardised to 36% anthocyanins) did not demonstrate teratogenic activity or adversely influence fertility in rats.[17] Oral administration of anthocyanins (360 mg/kg) failed to demonstrate teratogenic activity in three successive generations of rats and rabbits.[18]

Use in Lactation

Category C: Compatible with breastfeeding.
Bilberry fruit is listed in one traditional Western herbal as an antigalactagogue.[9] However, no adverse effects are expected during lactation.[19]

Warnings & Precautions

High doses (>100 mg/day anthocyanins) should be used cautiously in patients with haemorrhagic disorders and in those taking warfarin or antiplatelet drugs. Platelet aggregation was inhibited ex vivo in blood from healthy volunteers after oral administration of a bilberry extract (equivalent to 173 mg/day anthocyanins) for 30 to 60 days.[20]

Effect on Ability to Drive or Operate Machinery

No adverse effects expected.

Adverse Reactions

A postmarketing surveillance study was conducted on 2295 patients with venous disorders and retinal microcirculation disorders who consumed Bilberry extract (standardised to 36% anthocyanins). Dosages ranged from the equivalent of 29 to 288 mg/day of anthocyanins for 14 to 60 days, with most patients (69.5%) consuming 115 mg/day of anthocyanins for 30 to 60 days. Ninety-four patients (4.1%) reported mild side effects affecting the gastrointestinal system (gastric pain, pyrosis and nausea in 3.3% of cases), skin (0.2%) or nervous system (0.2%).[21]

Ingestion of the whole fresh fruit (as opposed to extracts) may irritate the intestinal lining in sensitive individuals due to the presence of fruit fibre and acids.

Interactions

Possible interaction with warfarin and antiplatelet drugs, but only for very high doses (see Warnings & precautions).

Safety in Children

Concentrated bilberry powder (2.5:1 and 5:1) produced favourable results in infants with acute dyspepsia and was well tolerated.[22]

Overdosage

No incidents found in published literature.

Toxicology

Table 1 lists LD_{50} data recorded for bilberry extract and its constituents that indicate low oral toxicity.[17,18]

Oral administration of a single dose of bilberry extract (equivalent to 1.08 g/kg anthocyanins) to dogs did not result in adverse effects, apart from darkening of the urine and faeces, which was attributed to absorption of the extract.[17] No toxic effects were observed in chronic oral toxicity studies where anthocyanins (600 mg/day) were administered to rats for 90 days and to guinea pigs for 15 days,[18] or where bilberry extract was administered to rats and dogs for 6 months at doses equivalent to 45 to 180 mg/kg/day and 29 to 115 mg/kg/day anthocyanins, respectively.[17]

Weak mutagenic activity was observed in vitro for bilberry extract in the Ames test, probably due to the presence of the flavonoid quercetin.[23] However, bilberry extract (standardised to 36% anthocyanins) failed to demonstrate mutagenic activity in other in vitro studies with or without metabolic action, or in vivo after oral administration up to 5 g/kg to rats.[17,24]

Table 1   **LD_{50} Data Recorded for Bilberry Extract and Its Constituents**

Substance	Route, Model	LD_{50} Value	Reference
Bilberry extract (standardised to 36% anthocyanins)	Oral, rats and mice	>2 g (equivalent to 0.72 g/kg anthocyanins)	17
Anthocyanins	Oral, mice	>25 g/kg	18
Anthocyanins	Oral, rats	>20 g/kg	18
Anthocyanins	i.p., mice	4.11 g/kg	18
Anthocyanins	i.p., rats	2.35 g/kg	18
Anthocyanins	i.v., mice	84 mg/kg	18
Anthocyanins	i.v., rats	24 mg/kg	18

Regulatory Status

See Table 2 for regulatory status in selected countries. Bilberry fruit is consumed as a food, particularly as a jam in the United Kingdom.

Table **2   Regulatory Status for Bilberry in Selected Countries**

Australia	Bilberry is not included in Part 4 of Schedule 4 of the Therapeutic Goods Regulations.
UK & Germany	Bilberry is not included on the General Sale List. Bilberry fruit is covered by a positive Commission E monograph. Bilberry is official in the *British Pharmacopoeia* 2002 and the *European Pharmacopoeia* 4.3.
US	Bilberry does not have generally recognised as safe (GRAS) status. However, it is freely available as a "dietary supplement" in the US under DSHEA legislation (Dietary Supplement Health and Education Act of 1994).

REFERENCES

1. Berta V, Zucchi C: *Fitoterapia* 59:27, 1988.
2. Morazzoni P, Bombardelli E: *Fitoterapia* 67:3-29, 1996.
3. Fiorini G, Biancacci A, Graziano FM: *Ann Ottalmol Clin Ocul* 91:371-386, 1965.
4. Zavarise G: *Ann Ottalmol Clin Ocul* 94:209-214, 1968.
5. Jayle GE, Aubert L: *Therapie* 19:171-185, 1964.
6. Jayle GE, Aubury M, Gavini G, et al: *Ann Ocul* 198:556-562, 1965.
7. Repossi P, Malagola R, de Cadihac C: *Ann Ottalmol Clin Ocul* 113:357-361, 1987.
8. Perossini M, Guidi G, Chiellini S, et al: *Ann Ottalmol Clin Ocul* 113:1173-1190, 1987.
9. Grieve M: *A modern herbal*, vol I, New York, 1971, Dover Publications, pp 99-100.
10. Wagner H, Bladt S: *Plant drug analysis: a thin layer chromatography atlas*, ed 2, Berlin, 1996, Springer-Verlag, p 282.
11. Bisset NG, ed: *Herbal drugs and phytopharmaceuticals: a handbook for practice on a scientific basis*, Stuttgart, 1994, Medpharm Scientific Publishers, pp 351-352.
12. Blaschek W, Ebel S, Hackenthal E, et al: *HagerROM 2002: Hagers Handbuch der Drogen und Arzneistoffe*, Springer, Heidelberg, 2002.
13. Grismondi GL: *Minerva Gin* 33:221-230, 1981.
14. Teglio L, Tronconi R, Mazzanti C, et al: *Quad Clin Ostet Ginecol* 42:221-231, 1987.
15. Baisi F: Report on clinical trial of bilberry anthocyanosides in the treatment of venous insufficiency in pregnancy and of post-partum hemorrhoids [in Italian]. Livorno Hospital, 1987, Obstetrics and Gynecology Operating Unit.
16. Baudon J, Bruhat M, Plane C, et al: *Lyon Mediterr Med* 46, 1969.
17. Eandi M: Relazione dell'esperto sulla documentazione farmacologica e tossicologica relativa alla specialità Tegens®, 1987; cited in Morazzoni P, Bombardelli E: *Fitoterapia* 67(1):3-29, 1996.
18. Pourrat H, Bastide P, Dorier P, et al: *Chim Ther* 2:33-38, 1967.
19. Blumenthal M et al, eds: *The complete German commission E monographs: therapeutic guide to herbal medicines*, Austin, 1998, American Botanical Council, p 88.
20. Pulliero G, Montin S, Bettini V, et al: *Fitoterapia* 60:69-75, 1989.
21. Eandi M: Post marketing investigation on Tegens® preparation with respect to side effects, 1987; cited in Morazzoni P, Bombardelli E: *Fitoterapia* 67:3-29, 1996.
22. Tolan L, Barna V, Szigeti I, et al: *Pediatria* 18:375-379, 1969.
23. Schimmer O, Kruger A, Paulini H, et al: *Pharmazie* 49:448-451, 1994.
24. American Herbal Pharmacopoeia: *Bilberry fruit – Vaccinium myrtillus L.: standards of analysis, quality control and therapeutics*, Santa Cruz, 2001, American Herbal Pharmacopoeia.

BITTERSWEET

Other common name: Woody nightshade
Botanical name: *Solanum dulcamara* L.
Family: Solanaceae
Plant part used: Stem

Safety Summary

Pregnancy category B3: No increase in frequency of malformation or other harmful effects on the foetus from limited use in women. Evidence of increased foetal damage in animal studies exists (on the basis of studies on solasodine), although the relevance to humans is unknown.
Lactation category SD: Strongly discouraged in breastfeeding.
Contraindications: None required on current evidence. Do not use during pregnancy or lactation without professional advice.
Warnings & precautions: Caution is advised for women wishing to conceive. Depuratives can in many cases be provocative to skin disease. The use of herbs rich in saponins is possibly inappropriate in coeliac disease, fat malabsorption and vitamins A, D, E, and K deficiency, some upper digestive irritations and topically to open wounds. Caution in patients with preexisting cholestasis.
Adverse reactions: Herbs rich in saponins may cause irritation of the gastric mucous membranes and reflux.
Interactions: No precautions required on current evidence.

Typical Therapeutic Use

Traditional indications for bittersweet in Western herbal medicine include chronic and scaly skin disorders, catarrhal conditions, and rheumatism. Bittersweet is also used externally for skin disorders, ulcers, and tumours.[1]

In the late 1980s a cream containing a mixture of solasodine glycosides (including solamargine and solasonine) became available to Australian practitioners for the treatment of skin lesions (solar keratoses and basal cell carcinomas). It was found to be an effective treatment in uncontrolled clinical studies.[2] It was subsequently scheduled throughout Australia (indirectly via the scheduling of the component solasodine) and made available by prescription only. This product was made from a different species of Solanum, namely *S. sodomaeum*.

Actions

Depurative, diuretic, expectorant.

Key Constituents

Solanum dulcamara contains three main steroidal alkaloids: solasodine, tomatidenol and soladulcidine, which occur in varying proportions and mainly as glycoside derivatives (glycoalkaloids). The alkaloid content of the plant parts decreases in the following order: green berry, leaf, flower, stem, ripe berry. There are many chemotypes of *S. dulcamara*; the main two chemotypes contain predominantly tomatidenol and soladulcidine, respectively.[3,4] Bittersweet twig contains 0.07% to 0.4% steroidal alkaloid glycosides. Bittersweet stem also contains 1.8% steroidal saponins.[5]

The Commission E advises that medicinal bittersweet consists of dried, 2- to 3-year-old stems, harvested in spring prior to leafing or late autumn after leaves have dropped.[6] This may affect the level of active and potentially toxic constituents.

A number of references refer to bittersweet as a toxic plant on the basis of it containing the alkaloid "solanine". Early studies cite the presence of solanine in bittersweet stem; however, this has not been confirmed in more recent studies (above). If present, it is not one of the main alkaloids (and hence would be expected in an even lower amount). (Solanine is a general term originally used to describe the mixture of glycosidic alkaloids present in the potato (*S. tuberosum*) and consists mainly of α-solanine.) Early literature also indicated that the solanine alkaloids in *S. dulcamara* are associated with a small quantity of atropine-like alkaloid.[7] This has not been confirmed but see the Overdosage section below.

Adulteration

A number of species may be mistaken for *S. dulcamara* twig, including *Solanum nigrum*, *Lonicera xylostemum* and *L. caprifolium*.[5]

Typical Dosage Forms & Dosage

Typical adult dosage ranges are:

- 1 to 3 g/day of dried stem or by infusion
- 6 to 16 mL/day of a 1:1 liquid extract
- 2 to 4.5 mL/day of a 1:2 liquid extract or equivalent in tablet or capsule form

Contraindications

None known. Do not use during pregnancy or lactation without professional advice.

Use in Pregnancy

Category B3: No increase in frequency of malformation or other harmful effects on the foetus from limited use in women. Evidence of increased foetal damage in animal studies exists (on the basis of studies on solasodine), although the relevance to humans is unknown.

Bittersweet twig has demonstrated anovulatory activity in vivo.[8]

No gross abnormalities were detected in offspring of female rats fed solasodine (30 to 60 mg/day). There were three resorptions in one uterine horn of a rat fed solasodine at the higher dose. Solasodine does not satisfy the structural requirement of fused furan and piperidine rings, which occurs in the Veratrum teratogen cyclopamine (cyclopamine and solasodine were compared as they have similar chemical structures).[9] Solasodine produced deformities such as spina bifida, anencephaly and cranial bleb in 7% of newborn hamsters. Pregnant hamsters were administered high oral doses (1.2 to 1.6 g/kg).[10] At a dosage of 0.2 g/kg solasodine by gavage to hamsters, 10% of the litter from surviving dams presented deformations. However, no teratogenicity was observed following ingestion of a solasodine glycoside (0.5 g/kg).[11] Malformations were also induced in the offspring of hamsters administered high doses of bittersweet fruit.[12]

Use in Lactation

Category SD: Strongly discouraged in breastfeeding.

Because the alkaloids may pass into breast milk, use of bittersweet is not recommended during lactation.[5]

Warnings & Precautions

Caution is advised for women wishing to conceive.

Depuratives can in many cases be provocative to skin disease. Care needs to be taken to reduce the prospect of major exacerbations. The use of herbs rich in saponins is possibly inappropriate in coeliac disease, fat malabsorption and vitamins A, D, E, and K deficiency, some upper digestive irritations and topically to open wounds. Saponin-containing herbs are best kept to a minimum in patients with pre-existing cholestasis.

Effect on Ability to Drive or Operate Machinery

No adverse effects expected.

Adverse Reactions

As with all herbs rich in saponins, oral use may cause irritation of the gastric mucous membranes and reflux.

Interactions

None known.

Safety in Children

No information available regarding bittersweet stem.

Overdosage

In large doses, bittersweet is said to cause dryness and heat with stinging pain in the fauces (palate, base of tongue), accompanied with thirst, sickness in the stomach, vomiting, diarrhoea, prostration, or syncope (fainting), and spasmodic twitchings. With some people it depresses the action of the heart and arteries, and causes a moderate degree of lividity on the hands and face. The head usually feels heavy and dizzy, and a cutaneous erythema may develop.[1]

Toxic effects in humans are mainly caused by the fruits and result in gastrointestinal irritation and vomiting,[13] although a Dutch textbook indicates that excessive use of bittersweet stalk preparations has been associated with serious poisoning.[14] However, an authoritative text suggests that poisoning in humans by ingestion of bittersweet stem has not been observed.[5] Due to the small amount of alkaloids present and their low bioavailability, acute toxic doses are unlikely to be reached with therapeutic levels of the herb (at least 25 g would be needed for a toxic dose).[5]

Critical assessment of the fatal cases involving ingestion of bittersweet berries described in the literature (1964 to 1977) reveals a lack of definitive information, including the identity of the plant and the nature and amount of plant material ingested. In one reasonably well-researched fatality, 21 mg of solanine was isolated from the girl's liver and remnants of berries were found in her stomach. Bittersweet grew near her home.[15] A case of anticholinergic toxicity associated with ingestion of bittersweet berries has been reported. Analysis of the unripe berries of *S. dulcamara* (identified by a botanist via verbal description) revealed the presence of solasodine. However, such a reaction would normally be caused by the presence of atropine or hyoscyamine or similar alkaloids.[16] Topical application of mashed red berries and leaves of *Solanum dulcamara* on a child's lips and eyelids appears to have resulted in peripheral and mild central effects of atropinisation.[17]

One review of poisoning in children indicated that ingestion of bittersweet berries appears to be minimally toxic, with no association able to be made between symptoms and colour or quality of berry ingested.[18]

Toxicology

Occasional death in livestock has been historically attributed to this plant, although the part of the plant causing the death is not defined.[19]

Due to lack of definitive evidence for the presence of α-solanine in *Solanum dulcamara*, toxicity information for this compound is not included.

Eighty percent of hamsters died within 24 hours of receiving *S. dulcamara* decoction of green fruit and seeds (1.4 to 2.0 g) by gavage. The dried plant material contained 0.03% total alkaloids consisting of solasidine and soladulcidine glycoalkaloids.[20] This is in contrast to the low toxicity observed in hamsters administered 1.4 g/kg isolated solasidine by gavage.[11]

Regulatory Status

See Table 1 for regulatory status in selected countries.

Table 1 **Regulatory Status for Bittersweet in Selected Countries**

Australia	Bittersweet for internal use is included in Part 4 of Schedule 4 of the Therapeutic Goods Regulations. It can be used internally if the recommended daily dose does not exceed 10 mg of total steroidal alkaloids including solanine, solaneine and solanidine.
	The alkaloids and alkaloidal glycosides of plants of the genus Solanum are defined as restricted drugs in the Health (Drugs and Poisons) Amendment Regulation 1996 (enacted by the Queensland parliament).
UK & Germany	Bittersweet is not included on the General Sale List. It is covered by a positive Commission E monograph.
US	Bittersweet does not have generally recognised as safe (GRAS) status. However, it is freely available as a "dietary supplement" in the US under DSHEA legislation (Dietary Supplement Health and Education Act of 1994).

REFERENCES

1. Felter HW, Lloyd JU: *King's American dispensatory*, ed 18, rev 3, vol 1; first published 1905, reprinted Portland, 1983, Eclectic Medical Publications, pp 667-671.
2. Cham BE, Daunter B: *Drugs Today* 28:55-58, 1990.
3. Mathe I, Mathe I: Variation in alkaloids in *Solanum dulcamara* L. In Hawkes JG, Lester RN, Skelding AD, eds: *The biology and taxonomy of the Solanaceae*, Linnean Society Symposium Series Number 7, London, 1979, Academic Press, pp 211-222.
4. Mathe I, Mathe I: *Acta Bot* 19:441-451, 1973.
5. Blaschek W, Ebel S, Hackenthal E, et al: *HagerROM 2002: Hagers Handbuch der Drogen und Arzneistoffe*, Heidelberg, 2002, Springer.
6. Blumenthal M, et al, eds: *The complete German Commission E monographs: therapeutic guide to herbal medicines*, Austin, 1998, American Botanical Council, p 232.

7. Sollmann T: *A manual of pharmacology and its applications to therapeutics and toxicology*, ed 7, Philadelphia, 1948, WB Saunders, p 482.

8. Chaudhury RR: *Plants with possible antifertility activity*, Special Report Series No 55, New Delhi, 1966, Indian Council of Medical Research, pp 3-19.

9. Keeler RF: *Lancet* 1:1187-1188, 1973.

10. Keeler RF, Young S, Brown D: *Res Commum Chem Pathol Pharmacol* 13:723-730, 1976.

11. Keeler RF, Tu AT, eds: *Toxicology of plant and fungal compounds, handbook of natural toxins*, vol 6, New York, 1991, Marcel Dekker, pp 92-95.

12. Keeler RF, Baker DC, Gaffield W: *Toxicon* 28:873-884, 1990.

13. Frohne D: *Z Phytother* 14:337-342, 1993.

14. De Smet PAGM, Keller K, Hansel R, et al, eds: *Adverse effects of herbal drugs*, vol 2. Berlin, 1993, Springer-Verlag, p 78.

15. Frohne D, Pfander HJ: *A colour atlas of poisonous plants: a handbook for pharmacists, doctors, toxicologists, and biologists*, translated from the German ed 2 by Bisset NG, London, 1984, Wolfe Publishing, pp 215-216.

16. Ceha LJ, Presperin C, Young E, et al: *J Emerg Med* 15:65-69, 1997.

17. Rubinfeld RS, Currie JN: *J Clin Neuroophthalmol* 7:34-37, 1987.

18. Borys DJ, Herrick ME, Krenzelok EP, et al: *Vet Hum Toxicol* 34:351, 1992.

19. Kingsbury JM: *Poisonous plants for the United States and Canada*, Englewood Cliffs, 1964, Prentice Hall, p 289.

20. Baker DC, Keeler RF, Gaffield W: *Toxicon* 27:1331-1337, 1989.

BLACK COHOSH

Botanical names: *Cimicifuga racemosa* (L.) Nutt. (*Actaea racemosa* L.)
Family: Ranunculaceae
Plant part used: Root and rhizome

Safety Summary

Pregnancy category B2: No increase in frequency of malformation or other harmful effects on the foetus from limited use in women. Animal studies are lacking (see discussion below).
Lactation category SD: Strongly discouraged in breastfeeding.
Contraindications: Patients with oestrogen-dependent tumours, during pregnancy (except to assist with birth). Do not use during lactation without professional advice.
Warnings & precautions: The use of herbs rich in saponins is possibly inappropriate in coeliac disease, fat malabsorption and vitamins A, D, E, and K deficiency, some upper digestive irritations, and topically to open wounds. Caution in patients with preexisting cholestasis.
Adverse reactions: Mainly mild gastrointestinal upset. Possible rare hepatotoxic response. Herbs rich in saponins may also cause reflux.
Interactions: No precautions required on current evidence.

Typical Therapeutic Use

A review of the clinical data suggests that black cohosh demonstrates therapeutic efficacy for moderate to severe neurovegetative menopausal symptoms.[1] Traditional indications for black cohosh in Western herbal medicine include rheumatic pain, myalgia, and female reproductive disorders, including amenorrhoea and dysmenorrhoea.[2,3]

Actions

Antirheumatic, spasmolytic, oestrogen modulating, uterine tonic.

Key Constituents

Constituents of black cohosh root include triterpene glycosides (saponins) of the cycloartane type, including actein and cimicifugoside,[4] isoflavones (possibly), resins (cimicifugin), and caffeic and isoferulic acids.[5]

Adulteration

Other *Cimicifuga* species, particularly *C. americana*, have been unintentionally mixed with black cohosh, due to the similarity in above-ground appearance. Occasionally black cohosh is adulterated with the underground portions of baneberry (*Actaea pachypoda* and *A. rubra*).[6] In August 1998, Australian manufacturers were alerted to the possibility of substitution of black cohosh by other *Cimicifuga* spp. In May 2001 the Therapeutic Goods Administration Laboratories advised that 35% of the Australian products they tested indicated the presence of species other than *Cimicifuga racemosa*. Manufacturers were advised to verify their raw materials to ensure the correct *Cimicifuga* species is used. Other medicinal *Cimicifuga* spp. were implicated such as *C. foetida*, *C. dahurica*, *C. heracleifolia*, and *C. simplex*.[7]

Typical Dosage Forms & Dosage

Typical adult dosage ranges by Western herbalists are:

- 0.9 to 6 g/ day of dried root and rhizome or by decoction
- 0.9 to 6 mL/ day of a 1:1 liquid extract
- 1.5 to 3 mL/ day of a 1:2 liquid extract or equivalent in tablet or capsule form
- 6 to 12 mL/ day of a 1:10 tincture

However, herbalists typically now recommend doses at the lower end of these ranges. In addition, doses at the higher end have been linked to adverse reactions (see Overdosage section).

Typical adult dosage ranges used in most clinical trials of German products[66]:

- Standardised extract equivalent to 40 to 140 mg/day of dried root and rhizome and containing approximately 3% triterpene glycosides

Contraindications

Black cohosh is best avoided in patients with oestrogen-dependent tumours, such as breast cancer, until more information is available regarding possible oestrogenic activity.

In a recent in vivo study, oral administration of a standardised black cohosh extract (0.714, 7.14, or 71.4 mg/kg/day) did not stimulate cancerous growth in rats with oestrogen-dependent mammary gland tumours.[8]

Use in Pregnancy

Category B2: No increase in frequency of malformation or other harmful effects on the foetus from limited use in women. Animal studies are lacking.

The traditional position is generally that black cohosh should not be taken during pregnancy except to assist with birth. According to the British Herbal Compendium, black cohosh is contraindicated in pregnancy,[9] however, this restriction is not listed in the Commission E.[10] Black cohosh was widely used by the Eclectics in traditional Western herbal medicine as a partus praeparator, if taken in the last weeks of pregnancy.[3]

In a 1999 survey of certified nurse-midwives in the United States, black cohosh was used by 45% of the 90 respondents who used herbal medicine to stimulate labour. Adverse effects attributed to use of blue cohosh and black cohosh were not assigned separately and included nausea, increased meconium-stained fluid, and transient foetal tachycardia.[11]

After a normal labour, a female infant was not able to breathe spontaneously and sustained central nervous system (CNS) hypoxic-ischaemic damage. A midwife had attempted induction of labour using a combination of blue cohosh and black cohosh given orally (dosage undefined) at around 42 weeks' gestation.[12] It was not possible to identify the herbal preparation as the causative agent; however, this reaction may have been due to the blue cohosh (refer to the blue cohosh (Caulophyllum thalictroides) monograph).

A prospective, epidemiological study investigated the influence of first-trimester use of medications and vaccines in the 1950s on the occurrence of congenital malformations and foetal survival in approximately 3200 pregnancies. Black cohosh was used in 1 of 266 pregnancies where a malformation occurred and in 2 of 532 pregnancies from the comparison groups. The dose and duration of use of black cohosh and the nature of the malformation were not specified.[13] Black cohosh could not be identified as a causative agent.

Use in Lactation

Category SD: Strongly discouraged in breastfeeding. This consideration is based on a possible oestrogenic effect.

The British Herbal Compendium contraindicates black cohosh during lactation.[9] However, the Commission E does not list this restriction.[10]

Warnings & Precautions

The use of herbs rich in saponins is possibly inappropriate in coeliac disease, fat malabsorption and vitamins A, D, E, and K deficiency, some upper digestive irritations, and topically to open wounds. Saponin-containing herbs are best kept to a minimum in patients with preexisting cholestasis.

Effect on Ability to Drive or Operate Machinery

No adverse effects expected.

Adverse Reactions

A review published in 2000 found that mild gastrointestinal upset was the most frequent minor adverse event reported in clinical studies (average of 5.6% of patients across five studies). Other minor adverse events reported in clinical studies included headache, vertigo, weight gain, mastalgia, heavy feeling in the legs, and a stimulant effect. Vaginal bleeding has also been reported.[6] Traditional sources note that high doses cause a frontal headache with a dull, full, or bursting feeling.[3,14]

Two reviews published in 2003 confirm that adverse events with black cohosh are rare, mild, and reversible. Gastrointestinal upsets and rashes are the most common adverse events. A few serious adverse events have been recorded, including hepatic and circulatory conditions, but causality could not be determined.[15,16] Details of some of the case reports follow.

Use of black cohosh for 1 week by a 47-year-old woman for the symptoms of menopause was associated with jaundice, raised liver enzymes, and a raised international normalised ratio, resulting in liver transplantation. Histological examination of the liver revealed changes typically found as a result of a severe immunological reaction, rather than direct toxic injury.[17] A causal relationship between ingestion of black cohosh and acute hepatitis was not established, and viral causes were not definitely ruled out.[18]

A case was reported in 2001 of a woman diagnosed with grade 1 endometrioid adenocarcinoma of the endometrium "whose history was notable for extensive use of supplemental phytoestrogens". Herbs included chaste tree, dong quai, black cohosh, and licorice.[19] No causality was demonstrated.

A 45-year-old woman who had been taking separate bottled products of black cohosh, *Vitex agnus-castus* and evening primrose oil for 4 months had three nocturnal seizures within a 3-month period. The patient had also consumed one to two beers 24 to 48 hours prior to each incident.[20] It was not established whether the herbal preparations caused the seizures.

A 26-year-old woman presented at a hospital with chest pain. Her heart rate and blood pressure dropped temporarily during the course of monitoring. Her urine digoxin level was "elevated" at 0.9 ng/mL (but within the normal therapeutic range [0.5 to 2.0 ng/mL]). However, she was not taking digoxin. In addition to the contraceptive pill, she was taking a herbal preparation containing black cohosh, skullcap (*Scutellaria lateriflora*), lousewort (*Pedicularis canadensis*), hops (*Humulus lupulus*), valerian (*Valeriana officinalis*), and cayenne pepper (*Capsicum annuum*). The product was not available for analysis. The chest pain had started during her shift as a topless dancer, during which she had consumed four alcoholic drinks, but no illicit drugs.[21] This study inappropriately speculated on "digoxin-like factors" with cardiotonic activity, which were claimed to be "commonly" found in herbal teas. The source of the patient's symptoms remains a mystery, but factors that interfere with digoxin assays, yet are without cardiotonic activity, have been reported in some herbs (refer to the Siberian ginseng (*Eleutherococcus senticosus*) monograph by way of example).

As with all herbs rich in saponins, oral use may cause irritation of the gastric mucous membranes and reflux.

Interactions

Black cohosh extract augmented the antiproliferative action of tamoxifen on 17β-oestradiol-stimulated MCF-7 human breast cancer cells and antagonised the cell-proliferative effects of oestradiol in vitro.[22,23] A press release dated 7 April 2003 claimed that black cohosh appeared to increase the toxicity of the commonly used chemotherapy drugs doxorubicin and docetaxel, when tested on breast cancer cells in vitro.[24] Whether any of these interactions would also apply in vivo has not been established.

Safety in Children

No information is available on safety. However, black cohosh is noted in a traditional herbal medicine text as being of particular benefit to treat fever in children.[3]

Overdosage

According to early data, ingestion of 5 g of the herb or 12 g of the fluid extract can cause nausea, vomiting, violent headache, vertigo, joint pain, red eyes, and weak pulse. Visual and nervous disturbances have also been noted.[3,25-27] Some of these effects may have been due to the past adulteration of black cohosh with the poisonous plants red baneberry (*Actaea spicata*) and white cohosh or white baneberry (*A. panchypoda* [*A. alba*]).[28] However, in the absence of any further information, such doses of black cohosh are not recommended.

Toxicology

No toxic effects were observed from oral administration of standardised black cohosh extract (up to 5 g/kg/day) for 26 weeks in rats.[29] A constituent isolated from the chloroform fraction of black cohosh extract, likely to be actein, did not provoke acute toxicity when administered by intragastric and hypodermic routes to rabbits. The minimum lethal dose of this constituent was greater than 500 mg/kg (i.p.) in mice, 1000 mg/kg (oral) in rats, and 70 mg/kg (i.v.) in rabbits. In subchronic toxicity studies over 30 days, the minimum lethal dose was greater than 10 mg/kg (i.p.) in mice and 6 mg/kg (oral) in rabbits.[30]

Standardised black cohosh extract did not show mutagenic activity in the Ames test.[31] In July 2003 scientists from Duquesne University announced that the incidence of metastasis increased in sexually mature female transgenic (genetically engineered) mice fed a black cohosh extract (at amounts said to reflect the normal human dose) for 12 months. The incidence of mammary tumours was not increased.[32] This experimental model, in which female mice spontaneously develop mammary tumours through the activation of an oncogene common in human breast cancer, is still highly controversial in terms of providing reproducible and relevant results. The experimental conditions were highly artificial (for example feeding black cohosh to mice for 12 months is the equivalent of a woman taking it continuously for at least 30 years). To date (August 2003) details of the botanical and phytochemical content of the investigated extract are not available. The relevance of using a mouse model to assess the safety of a treatment that is already widely used in the community is questionable. Observational studies of women taking black cohosh are required.

Regulatory Status

See Table 1 for regulatory status in selected countries.

Table 1   **Regulatory Status for Black Cohosh in Selected Countries**

Australia	Black cohosh is not included in Part 4 of Schedule 4 of the Therapeutic Goods Regulations.
UK & Germany	Black cohosh is included on the General Sale list, with a maximum single dose of 200 mg. It is covered by a positive Commission E monograph.
US	Black cohosh does not have generally recognised as safe (GRAS) status. However, it is freely available as a "dietary supplement" in the US under DSHEA legislation (Dietary Supplement Health and Education Act of 1994).

REFERENCES

1. Liske E: *Adv Ther* 15:45-53, 1998.
2. British Herbal Medicine Association's Scientific Committee: *British herbal pharmacopoeia,* Bournemouth, 1983, BHMA, pp 65-66.
3. Felter HW, Lloyd JU: *King's American dispensatory,* ed 18, rev 3, vol 1, first published 1905, reprinted Portland, 1983, Eclectic Medical Publications, pp 528-533.
4. Hostettmann K, Marston A: *Chemistry & pharmacology of natural products: saponins,* Cambridge, 1995, Cambridge University Press, p 280.
5. Wagner H, Bladt S: *Plant drug analysis: A thin layer chromatography atlas,* ed 2, Berlin, 1996, Springer-Verlag, p 336.
6. American Herbal Pharmacopoeia: *Black cohosh rhizome: Actaea racemosa L. syn. Cimicifuga racemosa (L.) Nutt.: Analytical, quality control, and therapeutic monograph,* Santa Cruz, 2002, American Herbal Pharmacopoeia.
7. Information on file, MediHerb Pty Ltd, Warwick, Queensland 4072, Australia, 2003.
8. Freudenstein J, Dasenbrock C, Nisslein T: *Cancer Res* 62:3448-3452, 2002.
9. British Herbal Medicine Association: *British herbal compendium,* Bournemouth, 1992, BHMA, pp 34-36.
10. Blumenthal M, et al, eds: *The complete German Commission E monographs: Therapeutic guide to herbal medicines,* Austin, 1998, American Botanical Council, p 90.
11. McFarlin BL, Gibson MH, O'Rear J, et al: *J Nurse Midwifery* 44:205-216, 1999.
12. Gunn TR, Wright IM: *N Z Med J* 109:410-411, 1996.
13. Mellin GW: *Am J Obst Gynec* 90:1169-1180, 1964.
14. Felter HW: *The eclectic materia medica, pharmacology and therapeutics,* first published 1922, reprinted Portland, 1983, Eclectic Medical Publications, pp 466-469.
15. Dog TL, Powell KL, Weisman SM: *Menopause* 10:299-313, 2003.
16. Huntley A, Ernst E: *Menopause* 10:58-64, 2003.
17. Whiting PW, Clouston A, Kerlin P: *Med J Aust* 177:432-435, 2002.
18. Vitetta L, Thomsen M, Sali A: *Med J Aust* 178:411-412, 2003.
19. Johnson EB, Muto MC, Yanushpolsky EH, et al: *Obstet Gynecol* 98:947-950, 2001.
20. Shuster J: *Hosp Pharm* 31:1553-1554, 1996.
21. Scheinost ME: *J Am Osteopathic Assoc* 101:444-446, 2001.
22. German Patent DE 196 52 183 C1: Verwendung eines Extraktes aus Cimicifuga racemosa, Schaper & Brümmer Gmbh & Co. KG, 38259 Salzgitter, DE.
23. Freudenstein J, Bodinet C: *23rd International LOF-symposium on 'Phyto-oestrogens',* Belgium, 15 January 1999, Belgium, 1999, University of Gent, p 1.
24. Health-Reuters: Black cohosh may make breast cancer drug more toxic, Yahoo! News, 7 April 2003, available http://story.news.yahoo.com/news?tmpl=story&u=/nm/20030407/hl_nm/cancer_cohosh_dc_1 (accessed April 2003).
25. Mills SY: *The A-Z of modern herbalism,* London, 1989, Thorsons, p 39.
26. Grieve M: *A modern herbal,* vol 1, New York, 1971, Dover Publications, p 211.
27. Blaschek W, Ebel S, Hackenthal E, et al: *HagerROM 2002: Hagers Handbuch der Drogen und Arzneistoffe,* Heidelberg, 2002, Springer.
28. Grieve M: *A modern herbal,* vol 1, New York, 1971, Dover Publications, pp 81-82.
29. Korn WD: Six-month oral toxicity study with remifemin granulate in rats followed by an eight-week recovery period, International Bioresearch, Hannover, Germany, 1991.
30. Genazzani E, Sorrentino L: *Nature* 194:544-545, 1962.
31. Beuscher N: *Z Phytother* 16:301-310, 1995.
32. PRNewswire: Duquesne University research casts doubt on safety or black cohosh for women with breast cancer or at risk of developing breast cancer, NewsALERT 12 July 2003, available http://www.newsalert.com/bin/story?StoryId=CpW42qbWbrengmda4 (accessed July 2003).

BLACK HAW

Botanical name: *Viburnum prunifolium L.*
Family: Caprifoliaceae
Plant part used: Bark

Safety Summary

Pregnancy category B2: No increase in frequency of malformation or other harmful effects on the foetus from limited use in women. Animal studies are lacking.

Lactation category C: Compatible with breast-feeding.

Contraindications: None required on current evidence.

Warnings & precautions: The use of antispasmodics may be contraindicated, or at least inappropriate, in gastric and enteric poisoning incidents.

Adverse reactions: Nausea and vomiting may occur with large doses.

Interactions: No precautions required on current evidence.

Typical Therapeutic Use

Traditional indications for black haw in Western herbal medicine include dysmenorrhoea, false labour pains, threatened miscarriage, and asthma.[1]

Actions

Uterine sedative, bronchospasmolytic, antiasthmatic, hypotensive, astringent.

Key Constituents

Constituents of black haw bark include flavonoids (amentoflavone), iridoid glycosides, triterpenes and triterpenic acids, and coumarins (scopoletin).[2]

Adulteration

Cramp bark (*Viburnum opulus*) is the main adulterant of black haw.[3] The barks of other *Viburnum* spp. and of hawthorn (*Crataegus* spp.), *Acer spicatum, A. pennsylvanicum,* and *Cornus* spp. were also substituted in the early 20th century.[2,4] Of these, *V. rufidulum* continues to appear as an adulterant.[2]

Typical Dosage Forms & Dosage

Typical adult dosage ranges are:
- 7.5 to 15 g/day of dried bark or by infusion or decoction
- 12 to 24 mL/day of a 1:1 liquid extract
- 1.5 to 4.5 mL/day of a 1:2 liquid extract or equivalent in tablet or capsule form
- 15 to 30 mL/day of a 1:5 tincture

Contraindications

None known.

Use in Pregnancy

Category B2: No increase in frequency of malformation or other harmful effects on the foetus from limited use in women. Animal studies are lacking.

Early studies investigating the in vitro and in vivo uterine effects of black haw exhibited varying results, demonstrating no effect, contraction, or relaxation.[5-11] Reviews of these studies concluded that the findings were scientifically invalid due to significant design limitations.[12,13] The value of published research conducted prior to 1940 regarding *Viburnum* spp. should be questioned due to possible improper identification of the bark and possible adulteration with other species.[14] More recent studies have confirmed the uterine spasmolytic activity of black haw ethanolic extracts in vitro.[15-18]

Black haw has long been used in Western herbal medicine for false labour pains and threatened miscarriage.[1,2,19] Folk use as a contraceptive and for the treatment of morning sickness have also been recorded.[20]

Use in Lactation

Category C: Compatible with breastfeeding.

Warnings & Precautions

The use of antispasmodics may be contraindicated, or at least inappropriate, in gastric and enteric poisoning incidents.

According to the American Herbal Products Association,[21] those with a history of kidney stones are cautioned against using black haw due to the presence of oxalate/oxalic acid in the dried bark. Oxalate, as the potassium or calcium salt, is present in the cell sap of many plants and vegetables. Calcium oxalate is practically insoluble in water[22] and is unlikely to be present in aqueous ethanolic liquid extracts of black haw in sufficient quantities to justify this precaution.

Effect on Ability to Drive or Operate Machinery

No adverse effects expected.

Adverse Reactions

A traditional text claims that nausea and vomiting may occur with large doses.[19]

Interactions

As black haw contains scopoletin (a coumarin), there are suggestions that it may potentiate the effects of anticoagulant medications or cause haemorrhagic problems.[2] But there is no evidence to suggest anticoagulant activity in vivo,[23] and plant coumarins are unlikely to increase the risk of bleeding.[24]

Safety in Children

No information available, but adverse effects are not expected.

Overdosage

No incidents found in published literature, but see Adverse Reactions section above.

Toxicology

In acute toxicity studies in animals, black haw extract had a paralysing effect on the nervous system, and subcutaneous administration of 5 to 7 g of extract caused death by cardiac arrest.[25]

Black haw extract tested negative for mutagenic activity in the Ames test in vitro.[26]

Regulatory Status

See Table 1 for regulatory status in selected countries.

Table **1**   **Regulatory Status for Black Haw in Selected Countries**

Australia	Black haw is not included in Part 4 of Schedule 4 of the Therapeutic Goods Regulations.
UK & Germany	Black haw is included on the General Sale List. It was not included in the Commission E assessment.
US	Black haw does not have generally recognised as safe (GRAS) status. However, it is freely available as a "dietary supplement" in the US under DSHEA legislation (Dietary Supplement Health and Education Act of 1994).

REFERENCES

1. British Herbal Medicine Association's Scientific Committee: *British herbal pharmacopoeia*, Bournemouth, 1983, BHMA, p 231.
2. American Herbal Pharmacopoeia: *Black haw bark – Viburnum prunifolium: Analytical, quality control, and therapeutic monograph*: Santa Cruz, June 2000, American Herbal Pharmacopoeia.
3. Bisset NG, ed: *Herbal drugs and phytopharmaceuticals: A handbook for practice on a scientific basis*, Stuttgart, 1994, Medpharm Scientific Publishers, pp 525-526.
4. Lloyd JU: *Druggist Circ* 59:87-90, 1915.
5. Pilcher JD, Delzell WR, Burman GE: *Arch Intern Med* 18:557-583, 1916.
6. Pilcher JD, Delzell WR, Burman GE: *J Am Med Assoc* 67:490-492, 1916.
7. Pilcher JD: *Arch Int Med* 19:53-55, 1917.
8. Pilcher JD, Mauer RT: *Surgery Gynecol Obstet* 27:97-99, 1918.
9. Hager BH, Becht FC: *J Pharmacol Exp Ther* 13:61-70, 1919.
10. Munch JC: *J Am Pharm Assoc* 28: 886-887, 1939.
11. Munch JC, Pratt HJ: *Pharm Arch* 12:88-91, 1941.
12. Woodbury RA: *Drug Stand* 19:143-151, 1951.
13. Baldini L, Brambilla G, Parodi S: *Arch Ital Sci Farmacolog* 3:55-63, 1963.
14. American Herbal Pharmacopoeia: *Cramp bark – Viburnum opulus: Analytical, quality control, and therapeutic monograph*, Santa Cruz, February 2000, American Herbal Pharmacopoeia.
15. Balansard G, Chausse D, Boukef K, et al: *Med Plants Phytother* 17:123-132, 1983.
16. Jarboe CH, Schmidt CM, Nicholson JA, et al: *Nature* 212:837, 1966.
17. Jarboe CH, Zirvi KA, Nicholson JA, et al: *J Med Chem* 10:488-489, 1967.

18. Tomassini L, Cometa MF, Palmery M, et al: *Proceedings of the Societa Italiana di Fitochimica 9th National Congress. Societa Italiana di Fitochimica, Florence, 27-30 May,* 1988.

19. Felter HW, Lloyd JU: *King's American dispensatory,* ed 18, rev 3, vol 2, first published 1905, reprinted Portland, 1983, Eclectic Medical Publications, pp 2059-2062.

20. de Laszlo H, Henshaw PS: *Science* 119:626-631, 1954.

21. McGuffin M, Hobbs C, Upton R, Goldberg A eds: *American Herbal Products Association's botanical safety handbook,* Boca Raton, 1997, CRC Press, p 22.

22. Budavari S, et al, eds: *The Merck Index: An encyclopedia of chemicals, drugs and biologicals,* ed 12, Whitehouse Station, 1996, Merck & Co, p 275.

23. Patterson DSP, Roberts BA, O'Neill PA: *Vet Rec* 89:544-545, 1971.

24. Mills S, Bone K: *Principles and practice of phytotherapy: Modern herbal medicine,* Edinburgh, 2000, Churchill Livingstone, pp 51-52.

25. Blaschek W, Ebel S, Hackenthal E, et al: *HagerROM 2002: Hagers Handbuch der Drogen und Arzneistoffe.* Heidelberg, 2002, Springer.

26. Schimmer O, Kruger A, Paulini H, et al: *Pharmazie* 49:448-451, 1994.

BLACK WALNUT

Botanical name: *Juglans nigra* L.
Family: Juglandaceae
Plant part used: Green hull

Safety Summary

Pregnancy category B2: No increase in frequency of malformation or other harmful effects on the foetus from limited use in women. Animal studies are lacking.
Lactation category ND: No data available.
Contraindications: None required on current evidence.
Warnings & precautions: None required on current evidence.
Adverse reactions: None found in published literature.
Interactions: No precautions required on current evidence.

Typical Therapeutic Use

Traditional uses of black walnut (unripe) hulls in Western herbal medicine include worm infestation,[1] ringworm, diphtheria, and skin eruptions, especially herpes, eczema, and psoriasis.[2]

Actions

Anthelmintic, depurative.

Key Constituents

The unripe hulls of *Juglans nigra* contain 1,4-naphthoquinones, including juglone and plumbagin.[3] The juglone content in hulls varies with different cultivars and different months of growth.[4]

Adulteration

No adulterants known.

Typical Dosage Forms & Dosage

Typical adult dosage ranges are:
- 1.5 to 5.5 mL/ day of a 1:2 liquid extract or equivalent in tablet or capsule form

Contraindications

None known.

Use in Pregnancy

Category B2: No increase in frequency of malformation or other harmful effects on the foetus from limited use in women. Animal studies are lacking.

Use in Lactation

Category ND: No data available.

Warnings & Precautions

Due to the potential toxicity of naphthoquinones, excessive and prolonged dosing should be avoided.

Effect on Ability to Drive or Operate Machinery

No adverse effects expected.

Adverse Reactions

No adverse reactions in humans from the internal use of black walnut hulls have been documented. Contact dermatitis of the finger webs occurred in a man who had been picking black walnuts, and was likely to be due to contact with the juice of the nut. Reexposure to walnut hulls was negative.[5]

A well-documented adverse reaction, observed in horses exposed to the shavings or sawdust of the wood of black walnut, is laminitis (inflammation of the laminae of a horse's hoof). It is possible that compounds other than juglone, within the wood, are responsible for causing the symptoms.[6]

Interactions

None known.

Safety in Children

No information available.

Overdosage

No incidents found in published literature.

Toxicology

The LD_{50} of juglone in mice is 2.5 mg/kg,[7] with the route of administration likely to have been by intraperitoneal injection.[8] Histopathological changes in the lungs and liver of dogs administered juglone (5 mg/kg) intravenously indicated that juglone is toxic to the cell membrane, increasing capillary permeability.[9]

Juglone and plumbagin were mutagenic to *Salmonella typhimurium* strain TA2637 with metabolic activation.[10] However, juglone and plumbagin inhibited experimentally induced intestinal carcinogenesis in vivo. Rats were fed diets containing either juglone or plumbagin (0.02%) prior to carcinogen exposure.[11] The chemopreventative effect may be due to induction of phase II enzymes, as was demonstrated in rats after oral ingestion of juglone or plumbagin (approx. 2 to 20 mg/kg).[12]

Regulatory Status

See Table 1 for regulatory status in selected countries.

Table 1   Regulatory Status for Black Walnut in Selected Countries

Australia	Black walnut hulls are not listed in Part 4 of Schedule 4 of the Therapeutic Goods Regulations.
UK & Germany	Black walnut hulls are not included on the General Sale List. They were not included in the Commission E assessment.
US	Black walnut hulls do not have generally recognised as safe (GRAS) status. However, they are freely available as a "dietary supplement" in the US under DSHEA legislation (Dietary Supplement Health and Education Act of 1994).

REFERENCES

1. Felter HW, Lloyd JU: *King's American dispensatory*, ed 18, rev 3, vol 2, first published 1905, reprinted Portland, 1983, Eclectic Medical Publications, p 1090.
2. Culbreth DMR: *A manual of materia medica and pharmacology*, Naturopathic Medical Series, botanical vol 3, first published 1922, reprinted Portland, 1983, Eclectic Medical Publications, p 154.
3. Binder RG, Benson ME, Flath RA: *Phytochem* 28:2799-2801, 1989.
4. Lee KC, Campbell RW: *HortSci* 4:297-298, 1969.
5. Siegel JM: *Arch Dermatol Syph* 70:511-513, 1954.
6. Minnick PD, Brown CM: *Vet Hum Toxicol* 29:230-233, 1987.
7. Westfall BA, Russell RL, Auyong TK: *Science* 134:1617, 1961.
8. Auyong TK, Westfall BA, Russell RL: *Toxicon* 1:235-239, 1963.
9. Boelkins JN, Everson LK, Auyong TK: *Toxicon* 6:99-102, 1968.
10. Tikkanen L, Matusushima T, Natori S, et al: *Mutat Res* 124:25-34, 1983.
11. Sugie S, Okamoto K, Rahman KM, et al: *Cancer Lett* 127:177-183, 1998.
12. Munday R, Munday CM: *Planta Med* 66:399-402, 2000.

BLADDERWRACK

Other common name: Fucus. Often incorrectly referred to as kelp
Botanical name: *Fucus vesiculosus* L.
Family: Fucaceae
Plant part used: Thallus (plant body)

Safety Summary

Pregnancy category B2: No increase in frequency of malformation or other harmful effects on the foetus from limited use in women. Animal studies are lacking.
Lactation category CC: Compatible with breast-feeding but use caution.
Contraindications: Hyperthyroidism, cardiac problems associated with hyperthyroidism. Do not use during lactation without professional advice.
Warnings & precautions: Iodide sensitivity, underlying thyroid disorders other than conditions resulting from iodine deficiency or low thyroid function. Good quality products free of heavy metals should be administered. Long-term use (more than one month) should be closely monitored for evidence of thyroid overactivity. Caution during pregnancy and lactation.
Adverse reactions: Hyperthyroidism, hypothyroidism in patients with an underlying thyroid disease, raised thyroid stimulating hormone, acneiform eruptions. (In many of these cases it is uncertain that the seaweed treatment used was bladderwrack.)
Interactions: Thyroid replacement therapies (e.g., thyroxine), hyperthyroid medication (such as carbimazole), lithium carbonate and iodine-containing drugs (such as amiodarone, benziodarone).

Typical Therapeutic Use

Bladderwrack has been tested for the treatment of obesity, with varying results.[1,2] Traditional indications for bladderwrack in Western herbal medicine include obesity, underactive thyroid function, lymphadenoid goitre and rheumatoid arthritis.[3]

Actions

Weight reducing, thyroid stimulant, demulcent.

Key Constituents

Bladderwrack thallus contains trace minerals, particularly iodine (present as iodide—both free and protein bound). Other constituents include polysaccharides of several types (including alginic acid and fucans such as fucoidan), polyphenols, lipids and sterols.[4] The *European Pharmacopoeia* 4.3 designates that bladderwrack should contain 0.03% to 0.2% total iodine.[5]

Adulteration

Fucus serratus is considered an adulterant, but was official in the former Pharmacopoeia of the German Democratic Republic (*Arzneibuch der DDR*) 1985.[6] The *European Pharmacopoeia* lists *F. vesiculosus* L., *F. serratus* L. and *Ascophyllum nodosum* Le Jol (*Fucus nodosum* L.) as medicinal fucus.[5] The *British Herbal Pharmacopoeia* 1996 lists *Ascophyllum nodosum* (knotted wrack) in a separate monograph.[7] Analysis of *Fucus vesiculosus, F. serratus, F. spiralis* and *Ascophyllum nodosum* found that *A. nodosum* contained more iodine than the fucus species (0.07% vs 0.02% to 0.03%).[8] Deep sea kelp (*Laminaria* species) is also a potential adulterant for bladderwrack (which is an intertidal plant).

Typical Dosage Forms & Dosage

Typical adult dosage ranges are:
- 0.8 to 2 g/day of dried thallus
- 4.5 to 8.5 mL/day of a 1:1 liquid extract or equivalent in tablet or capsule form
- 4 to 10 mL/day of a 1:5 tincture

Contraindications

Hyperthyroidism and associated cardiac problems.[9] Do not use during lactation without professional advice.

Use in Pregnancy

Category B2: No increase in frequency of malformation or other harmful effects on the foetus from limited use in women. Animal studies are lacking.

Iodine can cross the placenta[10] and hence bladderwrack should not be taken in high and prolonged doses during pregnancy.

Use in Lactation

Category CC: Compatible with breastfeeding but use caution.

Iodides can be concentrated in breast milk[10] and hence bladderwrack should not be taken in high and prolonged doses during lactation.

Warnings & Precautions

Avoid in patients with known hypersensitivity to iodine and those with underlying thyroid disorders other than thyroid conditions resulting from iodine deficiency or low thyroid function. An American estimate in 1975 suggested that between 1% and 3% of the population are iodine sensitive.[11]

Seaweeds, including *Fucus vesiculosus*, take up heavy metals from their marine environment. It is important to use product manufactured from suitably grown plant material free of heavy metals. The *European Pharmacopoeia* recommends medicinal bladderwrack contains less than 10 ppm for the total content of cadmium, copper, iron, lead, nickel and zinc; less than 0.2 ppm of cadmium; and less than 1 ppm of arsenic.[5]

Caution during pregnancy and lactation.

Effect on Ability to Drive or Operate Machinery

No adverse effects expected.

Adverse Reactions

Bladderwrack is a shore-dwelling seaweed rich in iodine, much of which is organically bound. Organically-bound iodine is considerably more potent at stimulating the thyroid gland than mineral iodine. Marine organisms, including bladderwrack, naturally accumulate arsenic. However the arsenic is mainly organically bound and rapidly excreted. For this reason the World Health Organization has established a tolerable weekly intake for inorganic arsenic only, which is present in bladderwrack at considerably lower levels than the organic form. There are populations whose consumption of large quantities of fish results in organoarsenical intakes of about 0.05 mg/kg/day, with no reports of ill effects. The intake limits for iodine and arsenic are summarised in Table 1.[12,13]

Table 1   Recommended Tolerable Intakes of Iodine and Arsenic

Dietary allowance of iodine	0.10 to 0.14 mg/day (adult)
Provisional maximum tolerable daily intake of iodine	0.017 mg/kg
Maximum tolerable daily intake of inorganic arsenic	0.002 mg/kg
Provisional weekly tolerable intake of inorganic arsenic	0.015 mg/kg
Intake of organic arsenicals	Undefined

The Commission E advises that hyperthyroidism may be induced or made worse if iodine is ingested above the dosage of 0.15 mg/day (corresponding to around only 200 mg/day of bladderwrack). Allergic reactions are possible but rare.[14]

Case studies reporting adverse effects are listed in Table 2.[4,15-26] In these case studies the "kelp" tablets may include species other than *Fucus vesiculosus*. Most often the botanical species is undefined (as it was undefined on the product label). Information regarding iodine and arsenic content is provided where available. Many of these adverse events are more appropriately considered an overdosage and/or are due to contamination. Such adverse reactions may not result from use of good quality bladderwrack products consumed within the recommended dosage, although the traditional herbal doses do deliver relatively large amounts of iodine.

A study involving British vegan men found that ingestion of kelp (dose undefined) can be associated with raised levels of thyroid stimulating hormone.[27]

Hepatotoxicity was reported in a woman who took tablets that contained kelp, skullcap, mistletoe, wild lettuce and motherwort for several weeks on two separate occasions.[28] The presence of mistletoe in the product was later questioned, and it is possible that the skullcap was adulterated by germander.[29]

Interactions

Bladderwrack may interact with thyroid replacement therapies (such as thyroxine),[30] and with hyperthyroid medication e.g., carbimazole. It may decrease effectiveness of the drug due to natural iodine content.[10]

Table **2** **Case Studies Reporting Adverse Effects After Intake of Kelp or Bladderwrack**

Case Reports	Adverse Reaction	Ref
I case; kelp tablets (taken for 8 months)	Iodine-induced thyrotoxicosis	15
I case; 2 supplements containing kelp (more than I month; estimated intake of iodine including dietary sources: 2.4 mg/day)	Transient hyperthyroidism	4
I case; bladderwrack tablets (9 × 400 mg tablets/day) Analysis of tablets yielded the following: arsenic,*21 300 mg/g; cadmium, 0.3 ppm; mercury, 0.06 ppm; chromium, 4 ppm	Polyuria, polydipsia; possible nephropathy attributed to heavy metal ingestion	16
I case; mesotherapy† of at least 2 months duration	Subacute tubulointerstitial fibrosis, progressing to end-stage renal failure	17
I case; kelp tablets (3 × 550 mg tablets/day, for 6 weeks) Analysis of tablets yielded: arsenic, ‡1 300 mg/g (i.e., 2145 mg/day)	Severe dyserythropoiesis and autoimmune thrombocytopaenia	18
I case; kelp tablets (6 × 200 mg tablets/day, for 2 months)	Hyperthyroidism	19
I case; kelp tablets (4 to 6 tablets/day, containing 0.7 mg iodine (i.e., 2.4 to 4.2 mg), for at least 6 months)	Hyperthyroidism	20
2 cases, both with family history of goitre/hypothyroidism; • kelp powder (I spoonful/day containing approx. 10 mg iodine/day, for about I year) • dried kelp (added to bread dough, for some years)	Thyrotoxicosis	21
I case, preexisting thyroid disorder; kelp tablets (2 tablets/day)	Hypothyroidism and enlargement of goitre	22
2 cases; kelp tablets • 10 to 12 tablets/day, containing 15 mg iodine • tablets containing kelp, lecithin, vitamin B6 (dosage unknown)	Acneiform eruptions	23
2 cases; • several supplements including kelp tablets (dosage and period of ingestion unknown) • kelp tablets (several months)	Elevated arsenic excretion in both cases	24
I case, slightly abnormal thyroid gland; seaweed tablets (4 tablets/day, I to 2 mg/day iodine for 2 to 3 years)	Hyperthyroidism and goitre	25
I case, possible preexisting condition; seaweed tablets (sporadically for more than I year followed by 6 tablets/day regularly for I year; iodine content varied: 0.12 to 1.25 mg/tablet)	Hypothyroidism and goitre, chronic thyroiditis	26

* The method used suggests that this represents total arsenic.
†For this patient mesotherapy involved weekly intradermal injections of artichoke and euphyllin, and the following oral medications: fenfluramine, meprobamate, diethylpropion, acetazolamide, fucus extract, belladonna, cascara powder, laminaria powder, Stephania tetrandra, Magnolia officinalis and pancreas extract. It is possible that Aristolochia fangchi was administered instead of stephania. Acetazolamide, by causing urinary alkalinisation, may also have led to delayed excretion of a nephrotoxic agent.[17]
‡Method and hence type of arsenic measured is undefined.

Avoid prescribing in patients taking lithium carbonate (lithium carbonate potentiates the hypothyroid activity of iodide-containing products). Concomitant intake with other iodine-containing drugs (e.g., amiodarone, benziodarone) is not recommended. These drugs have a much larger risk of causing iodine-induced thyrotoxicosis than herbal medications.[10]

Safety in Children

No information available.

Overdosage

Inappropriate use of iodine-containing plants when consumed as a food or supplement can lead to toxic consequences including hyperthyroidism (especially in susceptible individuals), thyrotoxicosis, subclinical hypothyroidism and Hashimoto's thyroiditis.[10,27,31-33]

Based on the reviewed studies, it is concluded that an iodine intake of 1 mg/day or less is probably safe for the majority of the population, but will cause adverse effects for some individuals. Those who are most likely to respond adversely are those with other thyroid disorders or who are sensitive to iodine.[13]

Extrathyroidal effects may also occur in susceptible individuals as a result of iodine intake, such as oedema and dermatitis herpetiformis (doses up to 25 mg/day iodine; rare), iodide fever (50 to 500 mg/day iodine; rare), and iodine mumps (50 to 500 mg/day iodine).[10,34] However, iodine intake from iodine-rich foods and supplements are unlikely to reach even the lowest of these stated levels.[10]

Toxicology

No information is available for the toxicology of bladderwrack.

Regulatory Status

See Table 3 for regulatory status in selected countries.

Table **3** **Regulatory Status for Bladderwrack in Selected Countries**

Australia	Bladderwrack is not included in Part 4 of Schedule 4 of the Therapeutic Goods Regulations.
UK & Germany	Bladderwrack is included on the General Sale List. It is covered by a negative Commission E monograph. Bladderwrack is official in the *British Pharmacopoeia* 2002 and the *European Pharmacopoeia* 4.3.
US	Bladderwrack does not have generally recognised as safe (GRAS) status. However, it is freely available as a "dietary supplement" in the US under DSHEA legislation (Dietary Supplement Health and Education Act of 1994).

REFERENCES

1. Monego ET, Peixoto M do R, Jardim PC, et al: *Arq Bras Cardiol* 66:343-347, 1996.
2. Curro F, Amadeo A: *Arch Med Interna* 28:1343-1349, 1976.
3. British Herbal Medicine Association's Scientific Committee: *British herbal pharmacopoeia*, Bournemouth, 1983, BHMA, pp 94-95.
4. Eliason BC: *J Am Board Fam Pract* 11:478-480, 1998.
5. *European pharmacopoeia* ed 4, Suppl 4.3, Strasbourg, 2002, Council of Europe, pp 1227-1228.
6. Bisset NG, ed: *Herbal drugs and phytopharmaceuticals: a handbook for practice on a scientific basis*, Stuttgart, 1994, Medpharm Scientific Publishers, pp 212-213.
7. British Herbal Medicine Association's Scientific Committee: *British herbal pharmacopoeia*, ed 4, Bournemouth, 1996, BHMA, pp 28-29.
8. Muller D, Carnat A, Lamaison JL: *Plant Med Phytother* 5:194-201, 1991.
9. British Herbal Medicine Association: *British herbal compendium*, Bournemouth, 1992, BHMA, pp 37-39.
10. De Smet PAGM, Keller K, Hansel R, et al, eds: *Adverse effects of herbal drugs*, vol 3, Berlin, 1997, Springer-Verlag, pp 37-50.
11. No author listed: *JAMA* 233:9-10, 1975.
12. De Smet PAGM, Keller K, Hansel R, et al, eds: *Adverse effects of herbal drugs*, vol 1, Berlin, 1992, Springer-Verlag, pp 42-43.
13. No author listed: *Evaluation of certain food additives and contaminants. Thirty-third report of the joint FAO/WHO expert committee on food additives*, World Health Organization Technical Report Series 776, Geneva, 1989, World Health Organization, pp 27-28, 32-33.
14. Blumenthal M, et al, eds: *The complete German Commission E monographs: therapeutic guide to herbal medicines*, Austin, 1998, American Botanical Council, p 315.
15. Henzen C, Buess M, Brander L: *Schweiz Med Wochenschr* 129:658-664, 1999.
16. Conz PA, La Greca G, Bendetti P, et al: *Nephrol Dial Transplant* 13:526-527, 1998.
17. Farrell J, Campbell E, Walshe JJ: *Ren Fail* 17:759-764, 1995.
18. Pye KG, Kelsey SM, House IM, et al: *Lancet* 339:1540, 1992.
19. de Smet PA, Stricker BH, Wilderink F, et al: *Ned Tijdschr Geneeskd* 134:1058-1059, 1990.
20. Shilo S, Hirsch HJ: *Postgrad Med J* 62:661-662, 1986.
21. Skare S, Frey HM: *Acta Endocrinol* 94:332-336, 1980.
22. Leemhuis MP, Quaries van Ufford AC: *Ned Tijdschr Geneeskd* 124:1119, 1980.
23. Harrell BL, Rudolph AH: *Arch Dermatol* 112:560, 1976.
24. Walkiw O, Douglas DE: *Clin Toxicol* 8:325-331, 1975.
25. Liewendahl K, Gordin A: *Acta Med Scand* 196:237-239, 1974.
26. Liewendahl K, Turula M: *Acta Endocrinol* 71:289-296, 1972.

27. Key TJA, Thorogood M, Keenan J, et al: *J Hum Nutr Diet* 5:323-326, 1992.

28. Harvey J, Colin-Jones DG: *Br Med J* (Clin res ed) 282:186-187, 1981.

29. de Smet PAGM, Keller K, Hansel R, et al, eds: *Adverse effects of herbal drugs*, vol 2, Berlin, 1993, Springer-Verlag, pp 289-296.

30. Miller LG: *Arch Intern Med* 158:2200-2211, 1998.

31. Gessner O: *Gift-und Arzneipflanzen von Mitteleuropa*, ed 3, Heidelberg, 1974, Carl Winter Universitats verlag, pp 432-433.

32. Konno N, Makita H, Yuri K, et al: *J Clin Endocrinol Metab* 78:393-397, 1994.

33. Okamura K, Inoue K, Omae T: *Acta Endocrinol* 88:703-712, 1978.

34. Becker DV, Braverman LE, Dunn JT, et al: *JAMA* 252:659-661, 1984.

BLUE COHOSH

Botanical name: *Caulophyllum thalictroides* (L.) Michx.
Family: Berberidaceae
Plant part used: Root

Safety Summary

Pregnancy category D: Has caused or is associated with a substantial risk of causing foetal malformation or irreversible damage.
Lactation category X: Contraindicated in breast-feeding.
Contraindications: Women trying to conceive, early pregnancy, and lactation.
Warnings & precautions: Use in late pregnancy should only be undertaken by clinicians experienced with the use of blue cohosh for this application. The use of herbs rich in saponins is possibly inappropriate in coeliac disease, fat malabsorption, and vitamins A, D, E, and K deficiency, some upper digestive irritations, and topically to open wounds. Caution in patients with preexisting cholestasis.
Adverse reactions: Possible nausea in pregnant women and toxic effects to the foetus. Herbs rich in saponins may cause irritation of the gastric mucous membranes and reflux.
Interactions: No precautions required on current evidence.

Typical Therapeutic Use

Traditional indications for blue cohosh in Western herbal medicine include amenorrhoea, threatened miscarriage, false labour pains, dysmenorrhoea and rheumatic pains.[1]

Actions

Spasmolytic, uterine and ovarian tonic, emmenagogue, oxytocic.

Key Constituents

Constituents of blue cohosh root include quinolizidine alkaloids, such as N-methylcytisine (0.033% to 0.091%), anagyrine (0.012% to 0.029%), taspine (0.00013%), sparteine (amount unknown) and caulophyllumine (amount unknown),[2-6] and saponins, including caulosaponin (0.1%) and caulophyllosaponin.[7,8]

Adulteration

No adulterants reported.

Typical Dosage Forms & Dosage

Typical adult dosage ranges are:
- 0.9 to 3 g/day of dried root or by decoction
- 1.5 to 3 mL/day of a 1:1 liquid extract
- 1.5 to 3 mL/day of a 1:2 liquid extract or equivalent in tablet or capsule form

Contraindications

Due to possible teratogenic effects, blue cohosh is contraindicated in women wishing to conceive and in early pregnancy and lactation. Traditional texts such as the *British Herbal Pharmacopoeia* 1983 tend to support this by recommending that only small doses are advisable during the first trimester of pregnancy.[1] Use in late pregnancy has been linked to adverse events and should only be undertaken by clinicians experienced with the use of blue cohosh for this application.

Use in Pregnancy

Category D: Has caused or is associated with a substantial risk of causing foetal malformation or irreversible damage.

In a 1999 survey of certified nurse-midwives in the United States, blue cohosh was used by 64% of the 90 respondents who used herbal medicine to stimulate labour. Adverse effects attributed to the use of blue cohosh and black cohosh were nausea, increased meconium-stained fluid and transient foetal tachycardia.[9]

After a normal labour, a female infant was not able to breathe spontaneously and sustained CNS hypoxic–ischaemic damage. A midwife had attempted induction of labour using a combination of blue cohosh and black cohosh given orally (dosage undefined) at around 42 weeks gestation.[10] It was not possible to identify the herbal preparation as the causative agent.

Severe congestive heart failure and myocardial infarction in a newborn male were attributed to maternal consumption of blue cohosh tablets. The woman had been advised to take 1 tablet per day (dose not specified) but she took 3 tablets per day for 3 weeks prior to delivery. Cardiomegaly and mildly reduced left ventricular function were evident at 2 years of age.[11] The tablets were not analysed.

Stroke in an infant has been reported as a possible association with a blue cohosh-containing dietary supplement, in the FDA's Special Nutritionals Adverse Event Monitoring System database (which lists adverse events but is not subject to preconditions, analysis or peer review).[12]

Uterine stimulant effects have been observed for the liquid extract, hot water extract and saponin fraction of blue cohosh and isolated caulosaponin in vitro.[7,8,13] Intravenous administration of caulosaponin (5 to 10 mg/kg) increased uterine tone and rate of contraction in situ and in vivo in the rat.[8] An in vivo study in dogs indicated no effect on the uterus when blue cohosh was administered in high doses.[14]

The quinolizidine alkaloid sparteine has been used as an oxytocic drug in the past. It was found to cause uterine spasm in women who were unable to metabolise it effectively. This defect appears to have a genetic basis[15] and was present in about 5% of males and females in one study.[16]

High levels of the alkaloid anagyrine have been associated with a congenital deformity in cows called "crooked calf disease", which is caused by maternal ingestion of lupine plants during pregnancy.[17,18] Similar malformations in goats, dogs and a human infant have been reported in one case study. Maternal consumption of goat's milk contaminated with anagyrine was suspected to be the cause. The level of alkaloids in the milk was not measured.[19] The relevance of this report to the use of blue cohosh in pregnancy is unclear. It is thought that anagyrine may need to be metabolised by microflora in ruminants in order for it to exert a teratogenic effect.[3]

Anagyrine (500 μg/mL) did not demonstrate teratogenic effects in an in vitro rat embryo culture, but it did inhibit overall growth and development. This culture is not scored for skeletal development. N-methylcytisine (20 μg/mL) demonstrated teratogenic activity.[3] An ethyl acetate extract (250 μg/mL) and a butanol extract (500 μg/mL) of blue cohosh, and the constituents taspine (5 μg/mL) and caulophyllumine (5 μg/mL), demonstrated embryotoxicity in the same test.[3,6]

Use in Lactation

Category X: Contraindicated in breastfeeding (due to possible toxic effects reported above).

Warnings & Precautions

Use in late pregnancy should only be undertaken by clinicians experienced with the use of blue cohosh for this application.

The use of herbs rich in saponins is possibly inappropriate in coeliac disease, fat malabsorption, and vitamins A, D, E, and K deficiency, some upper digestive irritations, and topically to open wounds. Saponin-containing herbs are best kept to a minimum in patients with preexisting cholestasis.

Effect on Ability to Drive or Operate Machinery

No adverse effects expected.

Adverse Reactions

Refer to Use in pregnancy section above for adverse reactions in pregnancy.

Two adverse reaction reports possibly associated with blue cohosh-containing dietary supplements, including stroke in an infant as reported above, were lodged on the FDA's Special Nutritionals Adverse Event Monitoring System database.[12]

The powdered root of blue cohosh is noted as a mucous membrane irritant in a 19th century reference.[20]

As with all herbs rich in saponins, oral use may cause irritation of the gastric mucous membranes and reflux.

Interactions

None known.

Safety in Children

A number of sources warn about poisoning in children attracted to the blue fruits, but only one source states that toxicity has occurred and no references are provided.[21] Interestingly, the roasted seeds are reported to have been used as a coffee substitute.[22]

Table **1** **LD$_{50}$ Data Recorded for Blue Cohosh and Its Constituents**

Substance	Route, Model	LD$_{50}$ Value (mg/kg)	Reference
Methylcytisine	Oral, mice	>500	25
Methylcytisine	i.p., mice	51	25
Methylcytisine	i.v., mice	21	25
Caulosaponin	i.v., mice	11.8	8
Caulosaponin	i.v., rats	20.3	8

Overdosage

A 21-year-old female who was 6 weeks pregnant drank slippery elm tea (15 cups per day) and took blue cohosh tincture (cited as 10 to 20 doses per day) for 4 days in a failed attempt to induce abortion. She also used a douche containing parsley dipped in slippery elm tea. She experienced abdominal pain, vomiting, hyperthermia, hypertension, hyperventilation, diaphoresis, abdominal muscle fasciculations, muscular weakness and tachycardia.[23,24]

Toxicology

Table 1 lists LD$_{50}$ data recorded for blue cohosh and its constituents.[8,25]

Caulophyllosaponin and caulosaponin had a mild purgative action after a few hours in small cats when orally administered at a dose of 0.1 g.[26] In acute toxicity studies, intravenous administration of the higher doses of caulosaponin to mice (10 to 15 mg/kg) and rats (18 to 23 mg/kg) caused an increase in activity, ataxia and terminal clonic convulsions. Death appeared to be due to asphyxia. Chronic subcutaneous injection of caulosaponin (5 mg/kg/day) to rats for 60 days did not produce symptoms of toxicity or gross organ pathology. Microscopic examination revealed slight oedema of the renal tubuli epithelium and arterial wall thickening in the spleen. Caulosaponin (0.5% solution) produced irritant effects in rabbits when it was instilled in the eye and subcutaneously injected in the ear. Diastolic stoppage occurred in the rat heart in situ when doses of caulosaponin greater than 4 mg/kg were administered intravenously.[8]

Regulatory Status

See Table 2 for regulatory status in selected countries.

Table **2** **Regulatory Status for Blue Cohosh in Selected Countries**

Australia	Blue cohosh is not included in Part 4 of Schedule 4 of the Therapeutic Goods Regulations.
UK & Germany	Blue cohosh is included on the General Sale List, with a maximum single dose of 265 mg. It was not included in the Commission E assessment.
US	Blue cohosh does not have generally recognised as safe (GRAS) status. However, it is freely available as a "dietary supplement" in the US under DSHEA legislation (Dietary Supplement Health and Education Act of 1994).

REFERENCES

1. British Herbal Medicine Association's Scientific Committee: *British herbal pharmacopoeia*, Bournemouth, 1983, BHMA, pp 54-55.
2. Flom MS, Doskotch RW, Beal JL: *J Pharm Sci* 56:1515-1517, 1967.
3. Kennelly EJ, Flynn TJ, Mazzola EP, et al: *J Nat Prod* 62:1385-1389, 1999.
4. Betz JM, Andrzejewski D, Troy A, et al: *Phytochem Anal* 9:232-236, 1998.
5. Woldemariam TZ, Betz JM, Houghton PJ: *J Pharm Biomed Anal* 15:839-843, 1997.
6. Flynn TJ, Kennelly EJ, Mazzola EP, et al: *Teratology* 57:219, 1998.
7. Chandler F, ed: *Herbs: everyday reference for health professionals*. Ottawa, 2000, Canadian Pharmacists Association, pp 57-59.
8. Ferguson HC, Edwards LD: *J Am Pharm Assoc* 43:16-21, 1954.
9. McFarlin BL, Gibson MH, O'Rear J, et al: *J Nurse Midwifery* 44:205-216, 1999.
10. Gunn TR, Wright IM: *N Z Med J* 109:410-411, 1996.
11. Jones TK, Lawson BM: *J Pediatr* 132:550-552, 1998.

12. US Food and Drug Administration, Center for Food Safety and Applied Nutrition, Office of Special Nutritionals: The Special Nutritionals Adverse Event Monitoring System (database). http://vm.cfsan.fda.gov/~dms/aems.html

13. Pilcher JD, Delzell WR, Burman GE: *JAMA* 67:490-492, 1916.

14. Pilcher J, Maurer R: *Surg Gynecol Obstet* 27:97-99, 1918.

15. Vinks A, Inaba T, Otton SV, et al: *Clin Pharmacol Ther* 31:23-29, 1982.

16. Eichelbaum M, Spannbrucker N, Steincke B, et al: *Eur J Clin Pharmacol* 16:183-187, 1979.

17. Keeler RF: *Teratology* 7:23-30, 1973.

18. Keeler RF: *J Toxicol Environ Health* 1:887-898, 1976.

19. Ortega JA, Lazerson J: *J Pediatr* 111;87-89, 1987.

20. Mitchell J, Rook A: *Botanical dermatology: plants and plant products injurious to the skin*, Vancouver, 1979, Greengrass, p 434.

21. de Smet PAGM, Keller K, Hansel R, et al, eds: *Adverse effects of herbal drugs*, vol 2, Berlin, 1993, Springer-Verlag, pp 151-157.

22. Grieve M: *A modern herbal*, New York, 1971, Dover Publications, p 212.

23. Rao RB, Hoffman RS, Desiderio R, et al: *J Toxicol Clin Toxicol* 36:455, 1998.

24. Rao RB, Hoffman RS: *Vet Human Toxicol* 44:221-222, 2002.

25. Barlow RB, McLeod LJ: *Br J Pharmacol* 35:161-174, 1969.

26. Power FB, Salway AH: *J Chem Soc* 103:191-209, 1913.

BLUE FLAG

Botanical names: *Iris versicolor* L., *Iris caroliniana* Watson
Family: Iridaceae
Plant part used: Rhizome

Safety Summary

Pregnancy category B1: No increase in frequency of malformation or other harmful effects on the foetus from limited use in women. No evidence of increased foetal damage in animal studies.
Lactation category C: Compatible with breast-feeding.
Contraindications: None required on current evidence.
Warnings & precautions: Care needs to be taken to reduce the prospect of exacerbating chronic skin conditions.
Adverse reactions: May occur (particularly gastrointestinal upset) in sensitive individuals at or exceeding the high end of the recommended therapeutic dosage.
Interactions: No precautions required on current evidence.

Typical Therapeutic Use

Traditional indications for blue flag in Western herbal medicine include skin diseases, biliousness with constipation, and liver dysfunction.[1]

Actions

Depurative, laxative, cholagogue, lymphatic, diuretic.

Key Constituents

Blue flag contains triterpenoids (iridals), phenolic acids, a resin containing sterols and fatty acids, and an oleoresin. A very small amount of essential oil is present (0.025%), containing furfural.[2]

Adulteration

No adulterants known, although Eclectic texts indicate that care should be taken when sourcing the herb, in relation to the locality in which it is grown.[3] This probably relates more to quality than safety, with a lack of oleoresin being the issue.

Adulteration by other species of iris is common in commercial samples.[4] The required medicinal plant has a root with an internal pinkish colour[3,5] and material with a dark red-brown colour should be rejected.[3] It is also noted in Eclectic texts that the root resembles that of *Acorus calamus*.[3] *Iris versicolor* is listed as of concern in the German Federal Ordinance on the Conservation of European Wildlife and Natural Habitats, 1982.[6]

Typical Dosage Forms & Dosage

Typical adult dosage ranges are:
* 1.8 to 6 g/day of dried rhizome or by decoction
* 1.8 to 6 mL/day of a 1:1 liquid extract
* 3 to 6 mL/day of a 1:2 liquid extract or equivalent in tablet or capsule form
* 9 to 30 mL/day of a 1:5 tincture

Contraindications

None known.

Use in Pregnancy

Category B1: No increase in frequency of malformation or other harmful effects on the foetus from limited use in women. No evidence of increased foetal damage in animal studies.

Blue flag has been recommended for the treatment of vomiting of pregnancy (morning sickness), given in a low dosage.[2] A concentrated oleoresin preparation of blue flag (called iridin) given every night, followed by a saline cathartic in the morning, was also prescribed for morning sickness.[3] The term "iridin" used in this context should be distinguished from the isoflavone iridin present in other iris rhizomes and other plant species.

Use in Lactation

Category C: Compatible with breastfeeding.

Warnings & Precautions

Depuratives can in some cases be provocative to skin disease. Care needs to be taken to reduce the prospect of major exacerbations.

Effect on Ability to Drive or Operate Machinery

No adverse effects expected.

Adverse Reactions

Eclectic texts indicate that blue flag (most likely in large doses) can act violently on the gastrointestinal system causing vomiting, catharsis, with intestinal burning and severe colic. Large doses may cause nausea. Even at the high end of the therapeutic dose blue flag may cause abdominal pain and catharsis. Blue flag has caused neuralgia of the face, head and extremities when given in large doses. It was also historically used to produce salivation as part of a therapeutic process (although the prescribed dosage is not defined).[3,7] These Eclectic texts do not define whether the adverse effects are due to use of the fresh root, as another writer suggests.[8] Official texts such as the *British Herbal Pharmacopoeia* 1983 and the United States Dispensatory (ed 24, 1947) clearly indicate dried rhizome be only used medicinally.

Interactions

None reported.

Safety in Children

No information available, but adverse effects are not expected if an appropriate dosage is administered. Blue flag has been used to treat eczema in children.[3]

Overdosage

No incidents of human poisoning by blue flag rhizome have been found in the published literature. Blue flag has been mentioned as causing poisoning in humans and animals.[9] Poisoning in humans resulted from ingestion of *Iris versicolor* which had been eaten in mistake for *Acorus calamus*, owing to the close resemblance of the plants before reaching the flowering stage.[10] The plant juice can cause dermatitis in sensitive individuals. The rhizome of other iris species, such as *Iris pseudacorus* has been implicated in poisoning animals.[9] Cattle have been poisoned by eating iris plants (species undefined) down to and including some of the roots.[10]

Animals have died from ingestion of blue flag rhizome, with autopsy showing "marked congestion of the gastric and intestinal tissues".[3]

Toxicology

No information available on blue flag.

Furfural has the LD_{50} value of 127 mg/kg after oral administration in rats[11]; however, blue flag is only likely to contain traces of this component. (Traces of furfural also occur naturally in foods such as fruit, bread, tea and coffee.[12])

Regulatory Status

See Table 1 for regulatory status in selected countries.

Table **1**   **Regulatory Status for Blue Flag in Selected Countries**

Australia	Blue flag is not included in Part 4 of Schedule 4 of the Therapeutic Goods Regulations.
UK & Germany	Blue flag is included on the General Sale List, with a maximum daily dose of 600 mg. It was not included in the Commission E assessment.
US	Blue flag does not have generally recognised as safe (GRAS) status. However, it is freely available as a "dietary supplement" in the US under DSHEA legislation (Dietary Supplement Health and Education Act of 1994).

REFERENCES

1. British Herbal Medicine Association's Scientific Committee: *British herbal pharmacopoeia*, Bournemouth, 1983, BHMA, p 120.
2. British Herbal Medicine Association: *British herbal compendium*, vol 1, Bournemouth, 1992, BHMA, p 40.
3. Felter HW, Lloyd JU: *King's American dispensatory*, ed 18, rev 3, vol 2; first published 1905, reprinted Portland, 1983, Eclectic Medical Publications, pp 1077-1081.
4. Purbrick P: Information on file, MediHerb Pty Ltd, Warwick, Queensland 4072, Australia, 2003.
5. British Herbal Medicine Association's Scientific Committee: *British herbal pharmacopoeia*, ed 4, Bournemouth, 1996, BHMA, p 96.
6. Lange D: *Europe's medicinal and aromatic plants: their use, trade and conservation*, Cambridge, 1998, TRAFFIC International, p X.
7. Felter HW: *The Eclectic materia medica, pharmacology and therapeutics*, Naturopathic Medical Series, Botanical vol 1; first published 1922, reprinted

Portland, 1983, Eclectic Medical Publications, pp 435-436.

8. Grieve M: *A modern herbal*, vol 2, New York, 1971, Dover Publications, pp 439-440.

9. Munro DB: Canadian Poisonous Plants Information System, Ottawa, 1993, Centre for Land and Biological Resources Research. Electronic file, also available via http://sis.agr.gc.ca/pls/pp/poison?p_x=px within the Agriculture and Agri-Food Canada webpage.

10. Bruce EA: *J Am Vet Med Assoc* 56:72-74, 1919.

11. Jenner PM, Hagan EC, Taylor JM, et al: *Food Cosmet Toxicol* 2:327-343, 1964.

12. Fifty-first meeting of the Joint FAO/WHO Expert Committee on Food Additives (JECFA): *Safety evaluation of certain food additives*, Geneva, 1999, World Health Organization, WHO Food Additives Series 42.

BOLDO

Botanical name: *Peumus boldus* Mol.
Family: Monimiaceae
Plant part used: Leaf

Safety Summary

Pregnancy category X: High risk of damage to the foetus.
Lactation category X: Contraindicated in breast-feeding (on the basis of the toxicity of boldo essential oil).
Contraindications: Pregnancy and lactation.
Warnings & precautions: Do not exceed the recommended dosage. Avoid long-term use. Use cautiously in unconjugated hyperbilirubinaemia, acute or severe hepatocellular disease, septic cholecystitis, intestinal spasm or ileus, liver cancer.
Adverse reactions: None found in published literature.
Interactions: Possible interaction with warfarin leading to increased anticoagulant activity of the drug.

Typical Therapeutic Use

Traditional uses of boldo in Western herbal medicine include gallstones, pain in the liver or gallbladder, jaundice, gastric pain, cystitis, rheumatism, nervousness.[1,2] Therapeutic uses in Brazilian traditional medicine include liver and bowel dysfunction, and as a general tonic.[3] A placebo-controlled study involving healthy volunteers indicated that boldo extract prolonged intestinal transit time.[4]

Actions

Cholagogue, liver stimulant, sedative, diuretic, mild urinary demulcent, and antiseptic.

Key Constituents

Constituents of boldo leaf include isoquinoline alkaloids (0.2% to 0.5%) including boldine, essential oil, and small amounts of flavonoids.[5] The toxic constituent ascaridole is present in boldo essential oil.[6] Ascaridole is an anthelmintic agent.

The content of plant constituents is often dependent on where the plant is grown, and this is the case for boldo in terms of its essential oil and boldine contents.[7-9] Alpha- and beta-thujone are also present in some boldo essential oils.[9] The toxicity of boldo may be due to the presence of both ascaridole and the thujones.

Adulteration

Adulteration by the similar smelling and similarly distributed plant *Cryptocarya peumus* can occur.[10]

Typical Dosage Forms & Dosage

Typical adult dosage ranges are:
- 0.2 to 3 g/day of dried leaf or by infusion
- 0.3 to 0.9 mL/day of a 1:1 liquid extract
- 0.7 to 2 mL/day of a 1:2 liquid extract or equivalent in tablet or capsule form
- 1.5 to 6 mL/day of a 1:5 tincture
- 1.8 to 6 mL/day of a 1:10 tincture

Contraindications

Pregnancy and lactation.

Use in Pregnancy

Category X: High risk of damage to the foetus.

Oral treatment of pregnant rats with 800 mg/kg of boldo extract or boldine from day 1 to day 5 and from day 7 to day 12 resulted in anatomical alterations in the foetus. Incidents of blastocystotoxic-antizygotic action and several cases of abortive activity in both treated groups were observed. This suggests that boldo acts at the beginning of egg division and also during implantation. A dose of 500 mg/kg did not produce any toxicity to embryos.[11]

Use in Lactation

Category X: Contraindicated in breastfeeding (on the basis of the toxicity of boldo essential oil).

Warnings & Precautions

Given the toxicity of boldo essential oil, the recommended dosage should not be exceeded. Long-term therapy with boldo is probably not appropriate.

Choleretics and cholagogues should be used cautiously and may be inappropriate in the following:

- Unconjugated hyperbilirubinaemia (jaundice following haemolytic diseases, hereditary disease like Gilbert's and Crigler-Najjar syndromes)
- Acute or severe hepatocellular disease (e.g., following viral hepatitis, cirrhosis, adverse reactions to drugs such as anaesthetics, steroids, oestrogen, chlorpromazine)
- Septic cholecystitis (where there is a risk of peritonitis)
- Intestinal spasm or ileus
- Liver cancer

Effect on Ability to Drive or Operate Machinery

No adverse effects expected.

Adverse Reactions

None reported.

Interactions

A case has been reported indicating a probable interaction between warfarin and boldo and/or fenugreek (*Trigonella foenum-graecum*). A patient being treated with warfarin developed an increase in international normalised ratio (indicating decreased coagulation), which returned to normal after cessation of the herbs. This herb–drug interaction was observed a second time after both herbs were reintroduced a few days later.[12]

Safety in Children

No information available, but given the toxic properties of boldo, use in children is best avoided.

Overdosage

Emesis and spasms have been documented after very high doses.[13] In large doses, boldo paralyses the muscle fibres, causing death by arrest of respiration.[14]

Toxicology

Table 1 lists LD_{50} data recorded for boldo extract and its constituents.[15,16]

Oral doses as high as 3 g/kg of aqueous ethanolic extract of boldo did not produce acute toxicity in rats.[17] Convulsions were produced in rats by oral doses of 0.07 g/kg of boldo essential oil.[16]

Boldo extract and boldine administered orally for 90 days did not cause histological modification in the heart or kidney of rats. Low intensity alteration of hepatic tissue was observed.[11] The dose administered was not clearly defined.

Subcutaneous injection of 5 mg/kg total alkaloids of boldo produced vomiting, diarrhoea and epileptic symptoms in dogs. Lethal doses of boldine have been reported: 0.5 mg/kg (oral, mice), 1 g/kg (oral, guinea pigs), 0.25 mg/kg (s.c., mice), 0.5 g/kg (s.c., guinea pigs) and 25 mg/kg (i.v., cat).[18]

Boldine was not mutagenic in prokaryotic and eukaryotic organisms in vitro.[19] Boldine did not induce a statistically significant increase in the frequency of chromosome aberrations or sister-chromatid exchanges in vitro or in vivo (administered by stomach tube).[20] Genotoxicity in mouse bone marrow was not observed after intraperitoneal administration of boldine at sublethal doses.[21]

Regulatory Status

See Table 2 for regulatory status in selected countries.

Table 1   **LD_{50} Data Recorded for Boldo Extract and its Constituents**

Substance	Route, Model	LD_{50} Value	Reference
Aqueous ethanolic extract (1:1)	i.p., mice	6 g/kg	15
Boldo essential oil	Oral, rats	130 mg/kg	16
Total alkaloids of boldo	i.p., mice	420 mg/kg	15
Boldine	i.p., mice	250 mg/kg	15

Table **2   Regulatory Status for Boldo
in Selected Countries**

Australia	Boldo is included in Part 4 of Schedule 4 of the Therapeutic Goods Regulations of Australia. However, the recommended daily dose must not exceed 100 mg of volatile oil.
UK & Germany	Boldo is included on the General Sale List, with a maximum single dose of 1.5 g. Boldo leaf is covered by a positive Commission E monograph. Boldo leaf is official in the *European Pharmacopoeia* 4.2.
US	Boldo does not have generally recognised as safe (GRAS) status. However, it is freely available as a "dietary supplement" in the US under DSHEA legislation (Dietary Supplement Health and Education Act of 1994).

REFERENCES

1. British Herbal Medicine Association's Scientific Committee: *British herbal pharmacopoeia*, Bournemouth, 1983, BHMA, pp 155-156.
2. Felter HW, Lloyd JU: *King's American dispensatory*, ed 18, rev 3, vol I; first published 1905, reprinted Portland, 1983, Eclectic Medical Publications, pp 359-360.
3. Bernardes A: *A pocket book of Brazilian herbs: folklore, history, uses*, Brazil, 1983, Shogun Arte, pp 12-13.
4. Gottleland M, Espinoza J, Cassels B, et al: *Rev Med Chil* 123:955-960, 1995.
5. Wagner H, Bladt S: *Plant drug analysis: a thin layer chromatography atlas*, ed 2, Berlin, 1996, Springer-Verlag, p 11.
6. Tisserand R, Balacs T: *Essential oil safety: a guide for health care professionals*, Edinburgh, 1995, Churchill Livingstone, p 123.
7. Vogel H, Razmilic I, Munoz M, et al: *Planta Med* 65:90-91, 1999.
8. Miraldi E, Ferri S: *Riv Ital EPPOS* 20:21-25, 1996.
9. Miraldi E, Ferri S, Franchi GG, et al: *Fitoterapia* 67:227-230, 1996.
10. Bisset NG, ed: *Herbal drugs and phytopharmaceuticals: a handbook for practice on a scientific basis*, Stuttgart, 1994, Medpharm Scientific Publishers, pp 109-111.
11. Almeida ER, Melo AM, Xavier H: *Phytother Res* 14:99-102, 2000.
12. Lambert JP, Cormier A: *Pharmacother* 21:509-512, 2001.
13. Scientific Committee of ESCOP (European Scientific Cooperative on Phytotherapy): *ESCOP monographs: Boldo folium*, UK, March 1996, European Scientific Cooperative on Phytotherapy Secretariat.
14. Osol A, Farrar GE, et al: *The dispensatory of the United States of America*, ed 24, Philadelphia, 1947, Lippincott, p 1370.
15. Levy-Appert-Collin MC, Levy J: *J Pharm Belg* 32:13-22, 1977.
16. Opdyke DL: *Food Cosmet Toxicol* 20:643-644, 1982.
17. Magistretti MJ: *Fitoterapia* 51:67-79, 1980.
18. Kreitmair H: *Pharmazie* 7:507-511, 1952.
19. Moreno PR, Vargas VM, Andreade HH, et al: *Mutat Res* 260:145-152, 1991.
20. Tavares DC, Takahashi CS: *Mutat Res* 321:139-145, 1994.
21. Speisky H, Cassels BK: *Pharmacol Res* 29:1-12, 1994.

BOSWELLIA

Other common names: Indian frankincense, Indian olibanum, Salai guggal
Botanical name: *Boswellia serrata* Roxb. ex Colebr.
Family: Burseraceae
Plant part used: Resin

Safety Summary

Pregnancy category B1: No increase in frequency of malformation or other harmful effects on the foetus from limited use in women. No evidence of increased foetal damage in animal studies.
Lactation category C: Compatible with breastfeeding.
Contraindications: None required on current evidence.
Warnings & precautions: Caution in patients with known allergic tendency.
Adverse reactions: Occasional mild diarrhoea or urticaria.
Interactions: No precautions required on current evidence.

Typical Therapeutic Use

Results from trials conducted in Germany and India indicate that boswellia has benefit over placebo in patients suffering from rheumatoid arthritis,[1] and promising results were obtained in controlled trials for the treatment of chronic colitis, ulcerative colitis and Crohn's disease.[2] Data suggest that the boswellic acids in boswellia are specific nonredox inhibitors of leukotriene synthesis.[3]

Traditional indications for boswellia from Ayurvedic medicine include pulmonary diseases, diarrhoea, menstrual disorders and liver disorders.[4]

Actions

Antiinflammatory, antiarthritic.

Key Constituents

Key constituents of *Boswellia serrata* resin include pentacyclic triterpene acids (mainly β-boswellic acid and the acetylboswellic acids acetyl-β-boswellic acid, acetyl-11-keto-β-boswellic acid (AKBA) and 11-keto-β-boswellic acid).[5] Boswellia resin also contains an essential oil.[6]

Adulteration

No adulterants known.

Typical Dosage Forms & Dosage

Typical adult dosage ranges are:
- 2 to 9 g/day of dried resin or equivalent in tablet or capsule form
- 600 to 1200 mg/day of extract standardised to contain about 60% boswellic acids (corresponding to a resin intake of 2.4 to 4.8 g/day)

Contraindications

None known.

Use in Pregnancy

Category B1: No increase in frequency of malformation or other harmful effects on the foetus from limited use in women. No evidence of increased foetal damage in animal studies.

Treatment of pregnant rats with a boswellic acid fraction (250 to 1000 mg/kg, oral route) revealed no significant effects on gestation period, litter size and weight of offspring at birth. No gross morphological or skeletal abnormalities were recorded. This generation of offspring in turn produced a normal number of normal offspring.[7]

Use in Lactation

Category C: Compatible with breastfeeding.

Warnings & Precautions

Caution in patients with known allergic tendency.

Effect on Ability to Drive or Operate Machinery

No adverse effects expected.

Adverse Reactions

Contact dermatitis has been caused by *Boswellia* spp.[8] Boswellia was well tolerated in clinical trials of treatment of rheumatoid arthritis. Very mild side effects such as diarrhoea and urticaria were reported.[1]

Interactions

None known.

Safety in Children

No information available but adverse effects are not expected.

Overdosage

No incidents found in published literature.

Toxicology

Toxicity studies have shown that the boswellic acid fraction of boswellia resin possesses very low acute toxicity and causes no adverse effects after chronic administration. The oral and intraperitoneal LD_{50} was greater than 2 g/kg in mice and rats. No significant changes were observed in general behaviour, or in clinical, haematological, biochemical, and pathological parameters after chronic oral administration to rats (250 to 1000 mg/kg/day, 180 days) and monkeys (125 to 500 mg/kg/day, 180 days).[7,9]

Regulatory Status

See Table 1 for regulatory status in selected countries.

Table 1   **Regulatory Status for Boswellia in Selected Countries**

Australia	Boswellia is not included in Part 4 of Schedule 4 of the Therapeutic Goods Regulations.
UK & Germany	Boswellia is not included on the General Sale List. It was not included in the Commission E assessment.
US	Boswellia does not have generally recognised as safe (GRAS) status. However, it is freely available as a "dietary supplement" in the US under DSHEA legislation (Dietary Supplement Health and Education Act of 1994).

REFERENCES

1. Etzel R: *Phytomedicine* 3:91-94, 1996
2. Ammon HP: *Wien Med Wochenschr* 152:373-378, 2002.
3. Ammon HPT, Safayhi H, Mack T, et al: *J Ethnopharmacol* 38:113-119, 1993.
4. Kapoor LD: *CRC handbook of Ayurvedic medicinal plants*, Boca Raton, 1990, CRC Press, p 83.
5. Pardhy RS, Bhattacharyya SC: *Indian J Chem Sect B* 16:176-178, 1978.
6. Lawrence BM: *Essential oils 1992-1994*, Carol Stream, IL, 1995, Allured Publishing Corporation, pp 20-23.
7. Singh GB, Bani S, Singh S: *Phytomedicine* 3:87-90, 1996.
8. Mitchell J, Rook A: *Botanical dermatology: plants and plant products injurious to the skin*, Vancouver, 1979, Greengrass, pp 144-145.
9. Singh GB, Singh S, Bani S: *Phytomedicine* 3:81-85, 1996.

BUCHU

Other common name: Bucco
Botanical names: *Agathosma betulina* (Bergius) Pill. (*Barosma betulina* (Bergius) Bartling & Wendl)
Family: Rutaceae
Plant part used: Leaf

Safety Summary

Pregnancy category B2: No increase in frequency of malformation or other harmful effects on the foetus from limited use in women. Animal studies are lacking. This rating only applies for authentic buchu.
Lactation category CC: Compatible with breast-feeding but use caution.
Contraindications: None required on current evidence. Do not use during lactation without professional advice.
Warnings & precautions: None required on current evidence.
Adverse reactions: None found in published literature.
Interactions: No precautions required on current evidence.

Typical Therapeutic Use

Traditional uses of buchu in Western herbal medicine include dysuria, cystitis, urethritis and prostatitis.[1] It is mainly considered to act as a urinary tract antiseptic via its essential oil content. There is concern about the sustainability of wild buchu due to diminished habitat, increased commercial demand, destructive wild harvesting practices and growing genetic vulnerability.[2]

Actions

Urinary antiseptic, mild diuretic.

Key Constituents

Key constituents of *Agathosma betulina* include an essential oil (2%),[3] containing diosphenol and its isomer (ψ-diosphenol) as major constituents. The essential oil also contains pulegone.[4] (Table 1 provides quantitative information for the essential oil components.[4,9-11]) Flavonoids are also present.[3]

Adulteration

The Hottentot (native South African tribe) name "buchu" is applied by them to any aromatic herb or shrub that they find suitable for use as a dusting powder. Hence many species, including those outside the Agathosma genus, are recorded as buchu. The genus Diosma is often referred to as wild buchu, but is used only in cases where true buchu (Barosma) is unprocurable.[5]

Adulterants include: *Agathosma crenulata*, *A. serratifolia*, *A. ericifolia*, *Adenandra fragrans*,[6] *Empleurum serrulatum*, *Psoralea olbiqua* and *Myrtus communis*.[7] Other species also traded as medicinal buchu have included *Diosma oppositifolia* (*Diosma succulentum*), *Agathosma pulchella*, *Empleurum unicapsulare* (*Empleurum ensatum*) and the so-called anise buchu (possibly *A. variabilis*).[8]

Although *A. crenulata* has been used traditionally as true buchu, it is not suitable for therapeutic use due to the lower diosphenol and higher pulegone and isopulegone contents in the essential oil.[4,9] (Pulegone is a potentially toxic constituent. Refer to the pennyroyal (*Mentha pulegium*) monograph for more details.)

The preferred medicinal buchu (*Agathosma betulina*) may be distinguished from *A. crenulata* and *A. serratifolia* by the ratio of leaf length to leaf width.[6] This distinction does not hold for buchu hybrids (considerable hybridisation has taken place between *A. betulina* and *A. crenulata*). Chemical analysis of the essential oil is required.[10] Use of buchu hybrids is not acceptable since the level of pulegone in the essential oil varies enormously (see Table 1).

From chemotaxonomic studies two chemotypes of *A. betulina* have been identified:[9]
- diosphenol chemotype: high concentration of diosphenol (total diosphenol isomers ≥22%), low isomenthone content (<29%)
- isomenthone chemotype: high concentration of isomenthone (>31%), low diosphenol content (total diosphenol isomers ≤0.3%).

No chemotypes of *A. crenulata* were found. The diosphenol chemotype is probably preferable for therapeutic use.

Table **1**   **Comparison of Diosphenol and Pulegone Contents in the Essential Oil Distilled from Various *Agathosma* Species**

	AMOUNT (%)			
Essential Oil Component	***A. betulina***	***A. crenulata***	**Hybrid**	**Reference**
Diosphenol (total of both isomers)	40.9%*	Not detectable*	1.0%*	11
	2.7% to 28% (av 9.5%)[†‡]	0.0[†‡]	3.7% (av)[‡§]	10
	Trace to 49.5%[‖]	Trace[‖]	Trace to 39%[‖]	9
	17%	2%	Not tested	4
Pulegone	0.6% to 4.5%	31.6% to 73.2%	7.6% to 27.8%	9
	0.9%*	53.8%*	15.8%*	11
	31.7%[†‡¶#]	47.0%[†‡]	45.6%[‡§]	10
	3%	50%	Not tested	4

*Sample sourced from 1 plant of each species.
†Average of 6 plants.
‡The buchu leaf samples obtained from South African commercial growers were classified as A. betulina, A. crenulata, or hybrid, on the basis of leaf shape.
§Average of 12 plants.
‖A total of 64 individual plants were harvested from various localities in the Western Cape region of South Africa. All the A. betulina plants with low diosphenol isomer content were obtained from the Piketberg mountain range, although not all plants from this area had a low content.
¶With a lot of variability between samples.
#The high pulegone content found in this sample of A. betulina may have been an aberration, as other studies have not replicated these results.

Typical Dosage Forms & Dosage

Typical adult dosage ranges are:
- 3 to 6 g/day of the dried leaf or by infusion
- 2 to 4.5 mL/day of a 1:2 liquid extract or equivalent in tablet or capsule form

Contraindications

None required on current evidence. Do not use during lactation without professional advice.

Use in Pregnancy

Category B2: No increase in frequency of malformation or other harmful effects on the foetus from limited use in women. Animal studies are lacking.

The *British Herbal Compendium* 1992 suggests that buchu is contraindicated in pregnancy.[1] However, this would only be the case for buchu substitutions (such as *A. crenulata*) that contain much higher levels of pulegone in their essential oil (see above).

Use in Lactation

Category CC: Compatible with breastfeeding but use caution.

Buchu contains an essential oil that may pass into breast milk. As the therapeutic effects provided by buchu are rarely required in infants, its effects in this patient group are unknown, but probably benign.

Warnings & Precautions

None required.

Effect on Ability to Drive or Operate Machinery

No adverse effects expected.

Adverse Reactions

The *British Herbal Compendium* indicates that occasional gastrointestinal intolerance or irritation may occur if buchu is taken on an empty stomach.[1]

Interactions

None required on current evidence.

Safety in Children

No information available but adverse effects are not expected.

Overdosage

No reports of poisoning occur in published literature.[8]

Toxicology

No toxicology data are available for buchu.

Regulatory Status

See Table 2 for regulatory status in selected countries.

Table **2**   **Regulatory Status for Buchu in Selected Countries**

Australia	Buchu is not included in Part 4 of Schedule 4 of the Therapeutic Goods Regulations.
UK & Germany	Buchu is listed on the General Sale List. It is covered by a negative Commission E monograph.
US	Buchu does not have generally recognised as safe (GRAS) status. However, it is freely available as a "dietary supplement" in the US under DSHEA legislation (Dietary Supplement Health and Education Act of 1994).

REFERENCES

1. British Herbal Medicine Association: *British herbal compendium*, vol 1, Bournemouth, 1992, BHMA, pp 43-45.
2. Hoegler N: *HerbalGram* 50:16, 2000.
3. Bisset NG, ed: *Herbal drugs and phytopharmaceuticals: a handbook for practice on a scientific basis*, Stuttgart, 1994, Medpharm Scientific Publishers, pp 102-103.
4. Kaiser R, Lamparsky D, Schudel P: *J Agric Food Chem* 23:943-950, 1975.
5. Watt JM, Breyer-Brandwijk MG: *The medicinal and poisonous plants of Southern and Eastern Africa: being an account of their medicinal and other uses, chemical composition, pharmacological effects and toxicology in man and animal*, ed 2, Edinburgh, 1962, Livingstone, pp 909-910.
6. Spreeth AD: *J S Afr Bot* 42:109-119, 1976.
7. Anonymous: *Flavour Industry* 1:379-382, 1970.
8. Blaschek W, Ebel S, Hackenthal E, et al: *HagerROM 2002: Hagers Handbuch der Drogen und Arzneistoffe*, Heidelberg, 2002, Springer.
9. Collins NF, Graven EH, van Beek, TA et al: *J Essent Oil Res* 8:229-235, 1996.
10. Blommaert KLJ, Bartel E: *J S Afr Bot* 42:121-126, 1976.
11. Posthumus MA, van Beek TA, Collins NF, et al: *J Essent Oil Res* 8:223-228, 1996.

BUGLEWEED & GYPSYWORT

Botanical names: *Lycopus virginicus* L. (common name: bugleweed), *Lycopus europaeus* L. (common name: gypsywort)
Family: Labiatae
Plant part used: Aerial parts

Safety Summary

Pregnancy category C: Has caused or is associated with a substantial risk of causing harmful effects on the foetus or neonate without causing malformations (on the basis of the antithyroid activity).
Lactation category X: Contraindicated in breastfeeding (on the basis of the antiprolactin and antithyroid activities).
Contraindications: Thyroid hypofunction, enlargement of the thyroid without functional disorder, pregnancy and lactation. Do not use during pregnancy or lactation without professional advice.
Warnings & precautions: Caution is advised in women wishing to conceive. Bugleweed should not be suddenly discontinued.
Adverse reactions: Enlarged thyroid; an increase in hyperthyroid symptoms and headache may occur.
Interactions: Do not administer concurrently with preparations containing thyroid hormone or during administration of diagnostic procedures using radioactive isotopes.

Typical Therapeutic Use

Uncontrolled trials indicate benefit for the treatment of overactive thyroid.[1-4] Traditional indications for bugleweed in Western herbal medicine include hyperthyroidism especially with cardiac involvement.[5]

Actions

Thyroid stimulating hormone (TSH) antagonist, antithyroid, mild sedative.

Key Constituents

Lycopus virginicus and *L. europaeus* aerial parts contain flavonoids and phenolic acids, such as derivatives of cinnamic acid (such as caffeic acid), although the pattern varies in each plant.[6-8]

Adulteration

Leonurus marrubiastrum L. may be mistaken for *Lycopus europaeus*, especially when wildcrafted.[9]

Typical Dosage Forms & Dosage

Typical adult dosage ranges are:
- 3 to 9 g/day of dried aerial parts or by infusion
- 3 to 9 mL/day of a 1:1 liquid extract
- 2 to 6 mL/day of a 1:2 liquid extract or equivalent in tablet or capsule form
- 6 to 18 mL/day of a 1:5 tincture

Contraindications

Thyroid hypofunction, enlargement of the thyroid without functional disorder,[10] pregnancy and lactation.[11] Do not use during pregnancy or lactation without professional advice.

Use in Pregnancy

Category C: Has caused or is associated with a substantial risk of causing harmful effects on the foetus or neonate without causing malformations.

Reduction in serum thyroid hormones in vivo suggests that these *Lycopus* spp. should not be taken during pregnancy (see Toxicology section below). Treatment with these *Lycopus* spp. in mice and rats has reduced the number of offspring.[11]

Use in Lactation

Category X: Contraindicated in breastfeeding.

Decreased milk supply has been observed from administration of bugleweed in suckling rats.[11] Although the effect of these *Lycopus* spp. on serum prolactin in experimental models is not clear, these herbs should not be taken while breastfeeding because of the possibility of antithyroid constituents passing into breast milk.

Warnings & Precautions

Caution is advised in women wishing to conceive.

Effect on Ability to Drive or Operate Machinery

No adverse effects expected.

Adverse Reactions

In rare cases, extended therapy and high (undefined) dosages of bugleweed preparations have resulted in an enlargement of the thyroid. Sudden discontinuation of bugleweed preparations can cause increased symptoms of the disease (hyperthyroid function).[10] The following side effects have been reported in the literature between 1941 and 1968 from clinical usage of bugleweed alone or combined with motherwort (*Leonurus cardiaca*): headache, increase in size of thyroid, and occasionally, an increase in hyperthyroid symptoms including nervousness, tachycardia and loss of weight. Increase in thyroid size was observed in patients with goitre not due to thyroid malfunction. The incidence of headache could be avoided by reducing the dosage.[11] Not all trials resulted in such side effects.

Interactions

Interference with uptake of radioactive isotopes has been observed in humans.[11] Bugleweed should not be administered concurrently with preparations containing thyroid hormone.[10]

Safety in Children

No information available, but because of the antithyroid activity caution is advised.

Overdosage

No incidents found in published literature.

Toxicology

Injection of bugleweed freeze dried or aqueous extract exhibited the following activities in rats: suppression of TSH, suppression of pituitary prolactin (but not serum prolactin) and antigonadotropic activity.[12,13]

Pressed juice of *L. europaeus* was lethal to male mice (0.75 mL corresponding to 7.5 g fresh plant, route unknown). Intravenous injection of 1 mL of *L. virginicus* pressed juice was lethal, but 3 mL given orally caused no toxic symptoms.[11]

The main results obtained after oral administration of *L. europaeus* aqueous ethanol extract (1 g/kg) to rats included: a long lasting decrease of T_3 levels (unrelated to TSH levels and due to peripheral T_4 deiodination), decreased serum luteinising hormone (LH), decreased testosterone, and unchanged prolactin levels. These results were different to those obtained from intraperitoneal administration. Previous studies indicating a lack of activity after oral administration of aqueous extracts may have been due to a low concentration of unoxidised phenolic constituents (such as caffeic acid) which are thought to contribute significantly to pharmacological activity.[14]

Caffeic acid has been listed as a possible carcinogen on the basis of in vivo studies in mice and rats using two oral dosage regimes: 2.1 g/kg (males), 3.1 g/kg (females) for 96 weeks; 0.7 g/kg, and 0.8 g/kg over 104 weeks.[15] Given the small amount present in the herb, this research is unlikely to be significant for therapeutic application of bugleweed.[9] Moreover caffeic acid is a common constituent of many plant foods, including fruit, vegetables and coffee, principally in conjugated forms such as chlorogenic acid.

Regulatory Status

See Table 1 for regulatory status in selected countries.

Table 1   **Regulatory Status for Bugleweed in Selected Countries**

Australia	Bugleweed is not included in Part 4 of Schedule 4 of the Therapeutic Goods Regulations.
UK & Germany	Bugleweed is included on the General Sale List. It is covered by a positive Commission E monograph.
US	Bugleweed does not have generally recognised as safe (GRAS) status. However, it is freely available as a "dietary supplement" in the US under DSHEA legislation (Dietary Supplement Health and Education Act of 1994).

REFERENCES

1. Mattausch F: *Hippokrates* 14:168-171, 1943.
2. Leppert H: *Therapiewoche*; 2:571-572, 1951/1952.
3. Frank J: *Munch Med Wschr* 101:203-204, 1959.
4. Fiegel G: *Med Klin* 49:1221-1222, 1954.
5. British Herbal Medicine Association's Scientific Committee: *British herbal pharmacopoeia*, Bournemouth, 1983, BHMA, p 136.

6. Kartnig T, Bucar F: *Planta Med* 61:392, 1995.

7. Bucar F, Kartnig T, Paschek G, et al: *Planta Med* 61:489, 1995.

8. Kartnig T, Bucar F, Neuhold S: *Planta Med* 59:563-564, 1993.

9. Blaschek W, Ebel S, Hackenthal E, et al: *HagerROM 2002: Hagers Handbuch der Drogen und Arzneistoffe*, Heidelberg, 2002, Springer.

10. Blumenthal M, et al, eds: *The complete German Commission E monographs: therapeutic guide to herbal medicines*, Austin, 1998, American Botanical Council, pp 98-99.

11. De Smet PAGM, Keller K, Hansel R, et al, eds: *Adverse effects of herbal drugs*, vol 2, Berlin, 1993, Springer-Verlag, pp 245-251.

12. Sourgens H, Winterhoff H, Gumbinger HG, et al: *Planta Med* 45:78-86, 1982.

13. Kemper F, Loeser A: *Acta Endocrinol* 38:200-206, 1961.

14. Winterhoff H, Gumbinger HG, Vahlensieck U, et al: *Arzneim Forsch* 44: 41-45, 1994.

15. WHO, International Agency for Research on Cancer: *IARC working group on the evaluation of carcinogenic risks to humans*, vol 56, Lyon, 1993, IARC, p 115.

BUPLEURUM

Other common names: Chai Hu, Saiko
Botanical names: Bupleurum falcatum L., Bupleurum scorzonerifolium Willd., Bupleurum chinense DC.
Family: Umbelliferae
Plant part used: Root

Safety Summary

Pregnancy category B1: No increase in frequency of malformation or other harmful effects on the foetus from limited use in women. No evidence of increased foetal damage in animal studies.
Lactation category C: Compatible with breastfeeding.
Contraindications: None required on current evidence.
Warnings & precautions: The use of herbs rich in saponins is possibly inappropriate in coeliac disease, fat malabsorption, and vitamins A, D, E, and K deficiency, some upper digestive irritations, and topically to open wounds. Caution in patients with preexisting cholestasis.
Adverse reactions: Bupleurum has a sedative effect in some patients. Large doses may cause sedation, increased bowel movements and flatulence. Herbs rich in saponins may cause irritation of the gastric mucous membranes and reflux.
Interactions: No precautions required on current evidence.

Typical Therapeutic Use

Therapeutic uses of bupleurum in traditional Chinese medicine (TCM) include alternating chills and fever, the common cold, liver enlargement, prolapse of the uterus and rectum, epigastric pain, nausea and irregular menstruation.[1-3] Bupleurum has demonstrated therapeutic benefit in the treatment of infectious hepatitis (by intravenous injection), influenza, the common cold, and feverish conditions in uncontrolled trials.[1]

Actions

Antiinflammatory, hepatoprotective, diaphoretic, antitussive.

Key Constituents

Constituents of bupleurum root include triterpenoid saponins (saikosaponins), sapogenins, phytosterols,[4] and pectin-like polysaccharides (bupleurans).[5] Since the highest levels of saikosaponins are found in B. falcatum (2.8%) and B. chinense (1.7%), these species are preferred.[1,6]

Adulteration

Although other species of Bupleurum may be used, the toxic plant B. longiradiatum should not be used medicinally.[1,3] Occasionally, adulteration with the roots of Aconitum spp. occurs.[7]

Typical Dosage Forms & Dosage

Typical adult dosage ranges are:
- 3 to 9 g of the dried root per day by decoction
- 3.5 to 8.5 mL/day of a 1:2 liquid extract or equivalent in tablet or capsule form

Contraindications

According to TCM, bupleurum is contraindicated in *deficient yin* cough (i.e., cough in debility) or *liver fire* ascending to the head (i.e., some cases of headache and hypertension). It can occasionally cause nausea or vomiting; if this happens use the smallest dose possible.[2]

Use in Pregnancy

Category B1: No increase in frequency of malformation or other harmful effects on the foetus from limited use in women. No evidence of increased foetal damage in animal studies.

Subcutaneous administration of bupleurum aqueous extract (0.1 to 0.4 mL/day) for 5 days did not affect fertility or exhibit teratogenic effects in mice.[8] Oral administration to female rats, from 2 weeks before mating until day 21 after delivery, of a TCM herbal formula (2 g/kg/day) containing bupleurum did not have teratogenic effects in the F1 generation or F2 foetuses.[9] This formula, also known as Sho-saiko-to, contains bupleurum as the main ingredient (26% to 29% by weight) as well as six other herbs. Another Japanese herbal formula containing bupleurum abolished the teratogenicity of sodium valproate in rats. Oral administration of this formula (up to 3 g/kg/day) to rat foetuses during organogenesis also resulted in no abnormalities.[10]

Use in Lactation

Category C: Compatible with breastfeeding.

Oral administration of Sho-saiko- to to female rats from 2 weeks prior to mating until day 21 after delivery (which includes the lactation period) did not result in any abnormalities in growth, development, behaviour or reproductive ability in the F1 generation or F2 foetuses.[9]

Warnings & Precautions

The use of herbs rich in saponins is possibly inappropriate in coeliac disease, fat malabsorption, and vitamins A, D, E, and K deficiency, some upper digestive irritations, and topically to open wounds. Saponin-containing herbs are best kept to a minimum in patients with preexisting cholestasis.

Effect on Ability to Drive or Operate Machinery

Bupleurum has a sedative effect in some patients, especially in larger doses,[1] therefore these patients should exhibit caution when driving or operating machinery.

Adverse Reactions

Large doses of bupleurum may have a sedative effect, increase bowel movements and flatulence, or decrease appetite in some patients.[1] As with all herbs rich in saponins, oral use may cause irritation of the gastric mucous membranes and reflux.

Three cases of allergic reaction have been reported in patients given intramuscular injections of bupleurum.[1]

The formula Sho-saiko-to has been associated with eosinophilic pneumonia,[11] pulmonary oedema,[12] liver damage,[13] and multiple cases of pneumonitis.[14-16] In Japan, Sho-saiko-to is mainly used to treat liver disease and is the most frequently used herbal remedy for this condition, which may explain the high number of reactions. Pneumonitis induced by herbs is suspected to be caused by an allergic mechanism rather than a toxic mechanism.[14] A review of the literature has found that in addition to reports of hepatotoxicity, Sho-saiko-to is hepatoprotective in humans and animals and has beneficial effects on the liver.[17] Cases of liver toxicity[18] and adult respiratory distress syndrome[19] have also been reported after the use of other TCM herbal preparations containing bupleurum. However, Sho-saiko-to and these preparations contain seven or more different herbs and the particular herb or herbs responsible for these adverse reactions are currently unknown. A provocation test with Baical skullcap (*Scutellaria baicalensis*) suggested that it was this herb that was responsible in another case of drug-induced pneumonitis by a TCM formula which also contained bupleurum.[20] Baical skullcap is also present in Sho-saiko-to.

Interactions

None reported.

Safety in Children

No information available.

Overdosage

No incidents found in published literature.

Toxicology

LD_{50} values in Table 1 indicate that oral and subcutaneous administrations of saikosaponins have low toxicity. However, toxicity is substantially higher after i.p. or i.v. administration. This is a typical finding for saponins and is due to their haemolytic activity.[21,22]

Table 1 **LD_{50} Data Recorded for Bupleurum Extract and Its Constituents**

Substance	Route, Model	LD_{50} Value	Reference
Bupleurum whole plant 50% alcohol extract	i.p., rats	500 mg/kg	21
Bupleurum aerial parts 50% alcohol extract	i.p., rats	50 mg/kg	21
Crude saikosaponins	Oral, mice	4.7 g/kg	22
Crude saikosaponins	s.c., mice	1.9 g/kg	22
Crude saikosaponins	i.p., mice	112 mg/kg	22
Crude saikosaponins	i.p., guinea pigs	58.3 mg/kg	22
Crude saikosaponins	i.v., mice	70.0 mg/kg	22

An aqueous extract of bupleurum root did not show toxic effects in rats or mice at an oral dose of 6 g/kg, but demonstrated potent toxic effects when administered by intraperitoneal injection at the same dose.[23] Repeated oral administration to rats of doses of 1.5 and 3.0 g/kg/day over 21 days decreased liver weight and red blood cell counts and increased serum gamma-glutamyl transpeptidase.[23]

Bupleurum methanolic extract did not demonstrate mutagenic activity in vitro in the Ames test.[24] Bupleurum extract decreased the mutagenicity of the mutagens benzo(α)pyrene and aflatoxin B in the Ames test in one study,[25] but hot water extracts enhanced the mutagenic activity of benzo(α)pyrene in other studies.[26,27] Hot water extracts of bupleurum also demonstrated antimutagenic activity in vivo.[28]

Chronic oral administration of Sho-saiko-to (2 g/kg/day) to male and female rats did not affect their general condition, body weight, food consumption, reproductive ability or gross anatomy. Nor did it cause any abnormalities in the F1 generation or F2 foetuses.[9]

Regulatory Status

See Table 2 for regulatory status in selected countries.

Table **2** **Regulatory Status for Bupleurum in Selected Countries**

Australia	Bupleurum is not included in Part 4 of Schedule 4 of the Therapeutic Goods Regulations.
China	Bupleurum is official in the Pharmacopoeia of the People's Republic of China 1997. The usual adult dosage, usually administered in the form of a decoction, is listed as 3 to 9 g.
UK & Germany	Bupleurum is not included on the General Sale List. It was not included in the Commission E assessment.
US	Bupleurum does not have generally recognised as safe (GRAS) status. However, it is freely available as a "dietary supplement" in the US under DSHEA legislation (Dietary Supplement Health and Education Act of 1994).

REFERENCES

1. Chang HM, But PP: *Pharmacology and applications of Chinese materia medica*, vol 2, Singapore, 1987, World Scientific, pp 967-974.
2. Bensky D, Gamble A: *Chinese herbal medicine materia medica*, Seattle, 1986, Eastland Press, pp 68-69.
3. Pharmacopoeia Commission of the People's Republic of China: *Pharmacopoeia of the People's Republic of China*, English ed, vol 1, Beijing, 1997, Chemical Industry Press, pp 143-144.
4. Tang W, Eisenbrand G: *Chinese drugs of plant origin*, Berlin, 1992, Springer Verlag, pp 223-232.
5. Yamada H, Sun XB, Matsumoto T, et al: *Planta Med* 57:555-559, 1991.
6. Dong YY, Luo SQ: *Zhongguo Zhong Yao Za Zh* 14:678-681, 703-704, 1989.
7. Hansel R, Keller K, Rimpler H, et al: *Hagers Handbuch der Pharmazeutischen Praxis*, 5, Auflage, Bd. 4, Berlin, Springer-Verlag, pp 579-588, 1992.
8. Matsui AS, Rogers J, Woo YK, et al: *Med Pharmacol Exp* 16:414-424, 1967.
9. Shimazu H, Katsumata Y, Takamatsu T, et al: *Yakuri To Chiryo* 25:29-42, 1997.
10. Minematsu S, Taki M, Watanabe M, et al: *Nippon Yakurigaku Zasshi* 96:265-273, 1990.
11. Kobashi Y, Nakajima M, Niki Y, et al: *Nihon Kyobu Shikkan Gakkai Zasshi* 35:1372-1377, 1997.
12. Miyazaki E, Ando M, Ih K, et al: *Nihon Kokyuki Gakkai Zasshi* 36:776-780, 1998.
13. Itoh S, Marutani K, Nishimina T, et al: *Dig Dis Sci* 40:1845-1848, 1995.
14. Mizushima Y, Oosake R, Kobayashi M: *Phytother Res* 11:295-298, 1997.
15. Sato A, Toyoshima M, Kondo A, et al: *Nihon Kyobu Shikkan Gakkai Zasshi* 35:391-395, 1997.
16. Hatakeyama S, Tachibana A, Morita M, et al: *Nihon Kyobu Shikkan Gakkai Zasshi* 35:505-510, 1997.
17. Stickel F, Egerer G, Seitz HK: *Public Health Nutr* 3:113-124, 2000.
18. Kane JA, Kane SP, Jain S: *Gut* 36:146-147, 1995.
19. Shiota T, Wilson JG, Matsumoto H, et al: *Intern Med* 35:494-496, 1996.
20. Takeshita K, Saisho Y, Kitamura K, et al: *Intern Med* 40:764-768, 2001.
21. Sharma ML, Chandokhe N, Ghatak BJR, et al: *Indian J Exp Biol* 16:228-240, 1978.
22. Takagi K, Shibata M: *Yakugaku Zasshi* 89:712-720, 1969.
23. Tanaka S, Takahashi A, Onoda K, et al: *Yakugaku Zasshi* 106:671-686, 1986.
24. Yamamoto H, Mizutani T, Nomura H: *J Pharm Soc Jap* 102:596-601, 1982.
25. Kim JM, Ji HW, Jung YM: *Korean J Vet Public Health* 18:261-268, 1994.
26. Sakai Y, Nagase H, Ose Y, et al: *Mutat Res* 206:327-334, 1988.
27. Niikawa M, Sakai Y, Ose Y, et al: *Chem Pharm Bull (Tokyo)* 38:2035-2039, 1990.
28. Liu DX: *Chung Kuo Tung Yao Tsa Chih* 15:640-642, 1990.

BURDOCK

Botanical names: *Arctium lappa* L. (*Arctium majus* Bernh.), *Arctium minus* Bernh.
Family: Compositae
Plant part used: Root

Safety Summary

Pregnancy category B1: No increase in frequency of malformation or other harmful effects on the foetus from limited use in women. No evidence of increased foetal damage in animal studies.
Lactation category C: Compatible with breastfeeding.
Contraindications: None required on current evidence.
Warnings & precautions: Avoid in patients with known hypersensitivity to plants in the Compositae family. Depuratives can be provocative to skin disease.
Adverse reactions: Contact dermatitis.
Interactions: No precautions required on current evidence.

Typical Therapeutic Use

Traditional indications for burdock in Western herbal medicine include skin eruptions, especially eczema and psoriasis, and rheumatism, cystitis, and gout.[1]

Actions

Depurative, mild diuretic, mild laxative.

Key Constituents

Constituents of burdock root include an essential oil (0.1%, containing sesquiterpenes and sesquiterpene lactones), acetylenic compounds, phenolic acids and inulin (up to 45%).[2]

Adulteration

Confusion is possible with the roots of *Atropa belladonna* (deadly nightshade), *Symphytum officinale* (comfrey), and *Rumex obtusifolius* (bitter dock).[3,4] (See Adverse reactions.)

Typical Dosage Forms & Dosage

Typical adult dosage ranges are:
- 6 to 18 g/day of dried root or by infusion or decoction
- 6 to 24 mL/day of a 1:1 liquid extract
- 1.5 to 3.5 mL/day of a 1:2 liquid extract or equivalent in tablet or capsule form
- 24 to 48 mL/day of a 1:10 tincture
- 500 mL/day of a 1:20 decoction

Contraindications

None known.

Use in Pregnancy

Category B1: No increase in frequency of malformation or other harmful effects on the foetus from limited use in women. No evidence of increased foetal damage in animal studies.

Subcutaneous administration of burdock aqueous extract (0.1 to 0.4 mL/day; plant part unspecified) for 5 days did not affect fertility or demonstrate teratogenic effects in mice.[5]

Burdock (part unspecified) demonstrated uterine stimulant activity.[6] It was unclear whether this research was conducted in vitro or in vivo.

Use in Lactation

Category C: Compatible with breastfeeding.

Warnings & Precautions

Avoid in patients with known hypersensitivity to plants in the Compositae family.

Depuratives can be provocative to skin disease. Care needs to be taken to reduce the prospect of major exacerbations.

Effect on Ability to Drive or Operate Machinery

No adverse effects expected.

Adverse Reactions

Three cases of contact dermatitis from external application of burdock root plasters for antiinflammatory purposes have been confirmed by closed patch testing.[7]

Ingestion of commercial preparations of burdock root tea has been associated with two cases of anticholinergic poisoning. Toxic amounts of atropine were detected in both cases.[8,9] Atropine is not a known constituent of burdock, and its presence was most likely due to adulteration or contamination, possibly with *Atropa belladonna*.[10,11]

Cases of burdock stomatitis in animals, particularly dogs,[12,13] and burdock ophthalmia in humans[14,15] have been reported and are caused by exposure to the burr (the remnant of the fruit).[11]

There is a possible link between the development of chronic active hepatitis and ingestion of a herbal tablet containing burdock. The person was taking a range of herbal tablets containing, respectively: mistletoe; celery seed + guaiacum + burdock root + sarsaparilla; valerian + skullcap + passionflower; and the following conventional medications: verapamil, chlordiazepoxide, thyroxine.[16]

Interactions

None known.

Safety in Children

No information available but adverse effects are not expected.

Overdosage

No incidents found in published literature.

Toxicology

The LD_{50} of burdock root 50% alcohol extract by i.p. administration in rats was assessed at 700 mg/kg.[17]

Burdock root did not demonstrate carcinogenic activity when fed to rats (4% to 33% of the diet) for periods of at least 120 days.[18]

Regulatory Status

See Table 1 for regulatory status in selected countries.

Table 1 **Regulatory Status for Burdock in Selected Countries**

Australia	Burdock is not included in Part 4 of Schedule 4 of the Therapeutic Goods Regulations.
UK & Germany	Burdock is included on the General Sale List. It is covered by a negative Commission E monograph.
US	Burdock does not have generally recognised as safe (GRAS) status. However, it is freely available as a "dietary supplement" in the US under DSHEA legislation (Dietary Supplement Health and Education Act of 1994).

REFERENCES

1. British Herbal Medicine Association's Scientific Committee: *British herbal pharmacopoeia*, Bournemouth, 1983, BHMA, p 128.
2. British Herbal Medicine Association: *British herbal compendium*, vol 1, Bournemouth, 1992, BHMA, pp 48-49.
3. Bisset NG, ed: *Herbal drugs and phytopharmaceuticals: a handbook for practice on a scientific basis*, Stuttgart, 1994, Medpharm Scientific Publishers, pp 99-101.
4. Blaschek W, Ebel S, Hackenthal E, et al: *HagerROM 2002: Hagers Handbuch der Drogen und Arzneistoffe*, Heidelberg, 2002, Springer.
5. Matsui AS, Rogers J, Woo YK, et al: *Med Pharmacol Exp* 16:414-424, 1967.
6. Goto M, Noguchi T, Watanabe T, et al: *Takeda Kenkyusho Nempo* 16:21, 1957. Cited in Farnsworth NR, Bingel AS, Cordell GA, et al: *J Pharm Sci* 64:535-598, 1975.
7. Rodriguez P, Blanco J, Juste S, et al: *Contact Dermatitis* 33:134-135, 1995.
8. Rhoads PM, Tong TG, Banner W Jr, et al: *J Toxicol Clin Toxicol* 22:581-584, 1984-85.
9. Bryson PD, Watanabe AS, Rumack BH, et al: *JAMA* 239:2157, 1978.
10. Bryson PD: *JAMA* 240:1586, 1978.
11. De Smet PAGM. In De Smet PAGM, Keller K, Hansel R, et al, eds: *Adverse effects of herbal drugs*, vol 2, Berlin, 1993, Springer-Verlag, pp 141-146.
12. Thiverge G: *Can Vet J* 14:96-97, 1973.
13. Georgi ME, Harper P, Hyypio PA, et al: *Cornell Vet* 72:43-48, 1982.
14. Breed FB, Kuwabara T: *Arch Ophthalmol* 75:16-20, 1966.
15. Goodwin RA Jr: *J Maine Med Assoc* 59:53-54, 1968.
16. Weeks GR, Proper JS: *Aust J Hosp Pharm* 19:155-157, 1989.
17. Sharma ML, Chandokhe N, Ghatak BJR, et al: *Indian J Exp Biol* 16:228-240, 1978.
18. Hirono I, Mori H, Kato K, et al: *J Environ Pathol Toxicol* 1:71-74, 1978.

BUTCHER'S BROOM

Other common name: Ruscus
Botanical names: *Ruscus aculeatus* L. (*R. ponticus* Woron., *R. hyrcanus* Stankov & Taliev)
Family: Liliaceae
Plant part used: Rootstock (rhizome and roots)

Safety Summary

Pregnancy category BI: No increase in frequency of malformation or other harmful effects on the foetus from limited use in women. No evidence of increased foetal damage in animal studies.
Lactation category C: Compatible with breast-feeding.
Contraindications: Do not apply to broken or ulcerated skin.
Warnings & precautions: The use of herbs rich in saponins is possibly inappropriate in coeliac disease, fat malabsorption, and vitamins A, D, E, and K deficiency, and some upper digestive irritations. Caution in patients with preexisting cholestasis.
Adverse reactions: Chronic diarrhoea (lymphocytic colitis) may occur from long-term use of butcher's broom combined with hesperidin methylchalcone and ascorbic acid. Herbs rich in saponins may cause irritation of the gastric mucous membranes and reflux.
Interactions: No precautions required on current evidence.

Typical Therapeutic Use

Butcher's broom in combination with flavonoids and ascorbic acid has been extensively studied in clinical trials for the treatment of chronic venous insufficiency (CVI).[1,2] A randomised, double-blind, placebo-controlled trial published in 2002 using only butcher's broom extract found it was effective in patients suffering from CVI.[2] Several uncontrolled studies demonstrated efficacy for the isolated sapogenins in the (topical) treatment of haemorrhoids.[1]

Traditional indications for butcher's broom in Western herbal medicine include dropsy, bladder stones, dysuria, ascites, oedema and chronic haemorrhoids. In the case of haemorrhoids, butcher's broom was used both orally and topically.[3,4]

Actions

Antiinflammatory, venotonic.

Key Constituents

Key constituents of the rhizome are steroidal saponins (0.5% to 1.5%) containing the aglycones ruscogenin and neoruscogenin and their glycosides (which are of the spirostanol and furostanol types).[5]

Adulteration

No adulterants known.

Typical Dosage Forms & Dosage

Typical adult dosage ranges are:
- 3.5 to 7 mL/day of a 1:2 liquid extract or equivalent in tablet or capsule form

Contraindications

Because of the irritant effect of the saponins, butcher's broom should not be applied to broken or ulcerated skin.

Use in Pregnancy

Category BI: No increase in frequency of malformation or other harmful effects on the foetus from limited use in women. No evidence of increased foetal damage in animal studies.

Animal studies have not produced any evidence of embryotoxic activity for butcher's broom extract. Butcher's broom combined with sweet clover (*Melilotus officinalis*) or hesperidin methylchalcone has been used topically to treat varicose veins in pregnant women.[6] An uncontrolled trial observed that oral administration of butcher's broom combined with hesperidin methylchalcone and vitamin C to pregnant women (21 to 24 weeks gestation) had no adverse effect on their infants. The assessment included both clinical and ultrasonographic criteria of pregnancy surveillance. The 20 women involved in the study received the herbal treatment for at least 6 weeks and not more than 13 weeks. Postprandial digestive heaviness was noted by 8 patients and was ascribed to the herbal treatment.[7]

Use in Lactation

Category C: Compatible with breastfeeding.

Warnings & Precautions

The use of herbs rich in saponins is possibly inappropriate in coeliac disease, fat malabsorption, and vitamins A, D, E, and K deficiency, and some upper digestive irritations. Saponin-containing herbs are best kept to a minimum in patients with preexisting cholestasis.

Effect on Ability to Drive or Operate Machinery

No adverse effects expected.

Adverse Reactions

As with all herbs rich in saponins, oral use may cause irritation of the gastric mucous membranes and reflux.

Contact allergy to ruscogenins occurs rarely, but may be underestimated. In the 10 years to 1998, 8 cases were reported to the French medical authorities.[8] Contact allergy to butcher's broom extract has also been reported.[9,10] In one of these cases, the cream contained butcher's broom extract and the vehicle thimerosal, and positive patch test results were obtained for both ingredients.[10]

Adverse reactions in association with the oral intake of the butcher's broom extract, combined with hesperidin methylchalcone and ascorbic acid have been reported; in particular, lymphocytic colitis, one case associated with ileal villous atrophy, and most with chronic diarrhoea, many after long term use of the product.[11-14] Other cases of chronic diarrhoea[14-18] including diarrhoea without faeces, mucus or blood,[19] and watery diarrhoea mimicking coeliac disease have been reported (possibly lymphocytic colitis).[20] Faecal fluid measurements were not consistent with an osmotic mechanism.[14] Lymphocytic colitis may be induced secondary to a chronic activation of the mucosal immune system by one or several components of the combination.[21] The results of another six clinical trials found this combination to be very well tolerated and the adverse effects reported were comparable to placebo.[2]

A case of cytolytic hepatitis associated with ingestion of a preparation containing ruscogenins, hesperidin, ascorbic acid, and aesculetol has been reported.[22]

Interactions

No benzodiazepine receptor binding activity was demonstrated in vitro from testing the blood of volunteers pretreated with butcher's broom extract for 3 weeks.[23] Hence any speculated interaction with benzodiazepine drugs is unlikely.

Safety in Children

No information available.

Overdosage

No incidents found in published literature.

Toxicology

Table I lists LD_{50} data recorded for butcher's broom extract and its constituents.[24,25]

Table I **LD_{50} Data Recorded for Butcher's Broom Extract and Its Constituents**

Substance	Route, Model	LD_{50} Value (g/kg)	Reference
Butcher's broom rhizome, fluid extract	Oral, mice	4.6*	24
Butcher's broom rhizome, fluid extract	Oral, rat	>4.6*	24
Ruscogenins (ruscogenin, neoruscogenin)	Oral, mice	>3.0	25
Ruscogenins (ruscogenin, neoruscogenin)	Oral, rats	>3.0	25

*Value expressed as dried herb equivalent.

Intravenous administration of dried butcher's broom extract to dogs resulted in slowing of the heart rate, a marked drop in arterial pressure, and at high doses increased respiration and blood glucose levels. Intraperitoneal doses of 1.5 to 2.0 g/kg of dried ethanolic extract of butcher's broom were lethal in guinea pigs. The authors estimated that the upper level of a safe dose for a human would be about 10 g.[26]

Prolonged oral administration of high doses (300 mg/kg) of saponosides, prosapogenins, and ruscogenins isolated from butcher's broom were well tolerated by rats.[25]

Regulatory Status

See Table 2 for regulatory status in selected countries.

Table **2** **Regulatory Status for Butcher's Broom in Selected Countries**

Australia	Butcher's broom is not included in Part 4 of Schedule 4 of the Therapeutic Goods Regulations.
UK & Germany	Butcher's broom is not included on the General Sale List. It is covered by a positive Commission E monograph.
	Butcher's broom is official in the *British Pharmacopoeia* 2002 and the *European Pharmacopoeia* 4.3.
US	Butcher's broom does not have generally recognised as safe (GRAS) status. However, it is freely available as a "dietary supplement" in the US under DSHEA legislation (Dietary Supplement Health and Education Act of 1994).

REFERENCES

1. Rensen I: *Z Phytother* 21:271-286, 2000.
2. Vanscheidt W, Jost V, Wolna P, et al: *Arzneim Forsch* 52;243-250, 2002.
3. Grieve M: *A modern herbal*, New York, 1971, Dover Publications, pp 128-129.
4. Leclerc H: *Précis de phytothérapie*, ed 5, Paris, 1983, Masson, pp 46-47.
5. Wagner H, Bladt S: *Plant drug analysis: a thin layer chromatography atlas*, ed 2, Berlin, 1996, Springer-Verlag, p 309.
6. Berg D: In Vanhoutte PM, ed: *Return circulation and norepinephrine: an update*, proceedings of the 3rd international symposium held in Cairo (Egypt) March 12-17th, 1990, John Libbey, pp 55-61.
7. Baudet JH, Collet D, Aubard Y et al: In Vanhoutte PM, ed: *Return circulation and norepinephrine: an update*, proceedings of the 3rd international symposium held in Cairo (Egypt) March 12-17th, 1990, John Libbey, pp 63-71.
8. Elbadir S, El-Sayed R, Renaud F, et al: *Rev Fr Allergol* 38: 37-40, 1998.
9. Breuil K, Patte F, Meurice JC, et al: *Rev Fr Allergol Immunol Clin* 29:215, 1989.
10. Landa N, Aguirre A, Goday J, et al: *Contact Dermatitis* 22:290-291, 1990.
11. Dharancy S, Dapvril V, Dupont-Evrard F, et al: *Gastroenterol Clin Biol* 24:134-135, 2000.
12. Pierrugues R, Saingra B: *Gastroenterol Clin Biol* 20:916-917, 1996.
13. Bouaniche M, Chassagne P, Landrin I, et al: *Rev Med Interne* 17:776-778, 1996.
14. Ouyahya F, Codjovi P, Machet MC, et al: *Gastroenterol Clin Biol* 17:65-66, 1993.
15. Mornet M, Boiserie P, Jonville AP, et al: *Therapie* 46:254, 1991.
16. Anon: *Presc Intl* 2:123, 1993.
17. Gendreau-Tranquart C, Barbieux JP, Furet Y, et al: *Presse Med* 18: 1439, 1989.
18. Oliver JM, Bacq Y, Dorval ED, et al: *Gastroenterol Clin Biol* 15:160-162, 1991.
19. Thomas-Anterion C, Guy C, Vial F, et al: *Rev Med Intern* 14:215-217, 1993.
20. Widgren S, De Peyer R, Geissbuhler P, et al: *Schweiz Med Wochenschr* 124:313-318, 1994.
21. Beaugerie L, Luboinski J, Brousse N, et al: *Gut* 35:426-428, 1994.
22. Sgro C, Taque R, Zoll A, et al: *J Hepatol* 22:251, 1995.
23. Blattler W, Schoch P: *Phlebology* 9:32-36, 1994.
24. Seidenberger AV, Muller I, Heindl HJH: *Therapiewoche* 24:866-881, 1974.
25. Capra C: *Fitoterapia* 43:99-113, 1972.
26. Caujolle F, Meriel P, Stanislas E: *Ann Pharm Franc* 11:109-120, 1953.

CALENDULA

Other common names: Marigold, pot marigold
Botanical names: Calendula officinalis L. (Calendula officinalis L. var. prolifera hort.)
Family: Compositae
Plant part used: Flower

Safety Summary

Pregnancy category B2: No increase in frequency of malformation or other harmful effects on the foetus from limited use in women. Animal studies are lacking.
Lactation category C: Compatible with breast-feeding.
Contraindications: Known allergy to calendula.
Warnings & precautions: Avoid in those with known sensitivity to other members of the Compositae family.
Adverse reactions: Occasional allergic contact dermatitis.
Interactions: No precautions required on current evidence.

Typical Therapeutic Use

A randomised, controlled trial found that calendula was efficacious for the topical treatment of burns.[1] Traditional indications for calendula in Western herbal medicine include enlarged or inflamed lymphatic nodes, sebaceous cysts, gastrointestinal ulcers and topical use for leg ulcers, varicose veins, haemorrhoids and skin lesions.[2]

Actions

Vulnerary, antiinflammatory, lymphatic, styptic (haemostatic), antimicrobial.

Key Constituents

Calendula flowers contain an essential oil, sesquiterpenes, flavonoids, saponins (2% to 10%), triterpene alcohols, carotenoids, and sterols.[3]

Adulteration

Adulteration is not common as C. officinalis is usually cultivated, but other species of calendula and of the Compositae family may be mistaken for it.[4] Calendula arvensis (field marigold), although used therapeutically in some traditional systems, is not regarded as therapeutically interchangeable for C. officinalis.

Adulteration may occur for the essential oil, in which case the phototoxic Tagetes spp. are often substituted for absolute of Calendula officinalis.[5] Tagetes tincture (which also has the common name marigold) has also been used to prepare "calendula ointment".[6]

Typical Dosage Forms & Dosage

Typical adult dosage ranges are:
- 3 to 12 g/day of dried flower or by infusion
- 1.5 to 3 mL/day of a 1:1 liquid extract
- 1.5 to 4.5 mL/day of a 1:2 liquid extract or equivalent in tablet or capsule form
- 0.9 to 3.6 mL/day of a 1:5 tincture

Contraindications

Contraindicated in those with known sensitivity to calendula.

Use in Pregnancy

Category B2: No increase in frequency of malformation or other harmful effects on the foetus from limited use in women. Animal studies are lacking.

There is an old, nonspecific reference indicating that calendula has been used as an emmenagogue and abortifacient.[7] It has also been so mentioned in two Ayurvedic texts, although the definition of abortifacient was very broad and included herbs with emmenagogue and ecbolic (uterine contractor) properties.[8] Infusion of calendula demonstrated a uterotonic action on isolated rabbit and guinea pig uterus.[9] This information has led to concerns about use of calendula in pregnancy from some sources,[10,11] but such concerns are obviously highly speculative.

Use in Lactation

Category C: Compatible with breastfeeding.

Warnings & Precautions

The likelihood of calendula preparations causing a contact allergy is low. However, persons with known sensitivity to other members of the Compositae family (such as ragweed, daisies, chrysanthemums) should avoid topical application of calendula or calendula products.[12]

Effect on Ability to Drive or Operate Machinery

No adverse effects expected.

Adverse Reactions

Allergic contact dermatitis has been reported from the use of calendula, but is a low risk. Reports of sensitisation to calendula are extremely rare.[13]

Table 1 shows the frequency of reaction to calendula as indicated by the results of patch testing.[13-17]

Sensitisation to calendula is often accompanied by reactions to other substances such as nickel, fragrance mix and propolis. Sensitisation to calendula cannot be assessed by testing with Compositae mix or sesquiterpene mix alone.[13]

Anaphylactic shock after gargling with an infusion of calendula has been reported.[18]

Interactions

None known.

Safety in Children

No information available but adverse effects are not expected.

Overdosage

No incidents found in published literature.

Toxicology

Table 2 lists LD_{50} data recorded for calendula extracts.[19-23]

Table 1   **Results from Patch Testing with Calendula Preparations**

Reaction Frequency	Patient/Subject Condition	Preparation	Reference
2/1032 (0.2%)	Patients from patch test clinics	Ointment containing 10% calendula tincture	14
9/443 (2%)	Patients	Ether extract of calendula	13
1/119 (0.8%)	Contact allergic dermatitis	10% ethanol extract	15
1/15 (6.7%)	Summer-exacerbated dermatitis	10% calendula in petrolatum	16
0/9 (0%)	"Contact-sensitive" and eczema	Commercial-grade absolute of calendula, 1% in petrolatum	17

Table 2   **LD_{50} Data Recorded for Calendula Extracts**

Substance	Route, Model	LD_{50} Value	Reference
Calendula extract	Oral, rats	>4.6 g/kg	19
Calendula extract	i.p., mice	300 mg/kg	20
Calendula extract (30% ethanol)	i.v., rats	5.3 g/kg	21
Calendula extract (aqueous)	i.v., mice	375 mg/kg	22
Calendula, entire plant, ethanol extract	i.p., mice	300 mg/kg	23

Subcutaneous administration of 10 mL/kg of ethylene glycol extract of calendula (1:2) to albino mice did not result in symptoms of acute toxicity.[24] No symptoms of toxicity were demonstrated after chronic, oral administration of calendula extract (0.15 g/kg, solvent unspecified, in hamsters and rats)[25] or calenduloside B (a minor saponin, up to 200 mg/kg, in rats).[26]

Animal tests showed at most minimal skin irritation and no sensitisation or phototoxicity.[19]

Water extract of calendula was negative in the Drosophila wing somatic mutation and recombination test.[27] Aqueous ethanol extract of calendula was negative in the Ames assay for point mutation in *Salmonella* and only slightly cytotoxic to one of the four strains used in the experimental protocol (50 to 5000 μg/plate). The extract demonstrated mitotic crossing over and chromosome malsegregation in an *Aspergillus nidulans* strain (0.1 to 1 mg solids/mL). The activity was due to the lactone loliolide. The mouse bone marrow micronucleus test, where the extract was dosed orally up to 1 g/kg for 2 days, was negative.[28]

Genotoxic and antigenotoxic activity was demonstrated for calendula extracts in vitro. The concentrations producing genotoxic damage were three orders of magnitude above those that produced protection against the tested carcinogen.[29] Isolated saponins of calendula (400 μg) did not demonstrate mutagenic activity in the Salmonella/microsome assay with strain TA98.[30]

In extensive studies for more than 18 months with groups of rats and hamsters, oral doses of calendula extract (unspecified solvent; 0.15 g/kg) produced no evidence of carcinogenicity.[26]

Regulatory Status

See Table 3 for regulatory status in selected countries.

Table **3**   **Regulatory Status for Calendula in Selected Countries**

Australia	Calendula is not included in Part 4 of Schedule 4 of the Therapeutic Goods Regulations.
UK & Germany	Calendula for external use is included on the General Sale List. It is covered by a positive Commission E monograph. Calendula is official in the *British Pharmacopoeia* 2002 and the *European Pharmacopoeia* 4.3.
US	Calendula does have generally recognised as safe (GRAS) status. It is freely available as a "dietary supplement" in the US under DSHEA legislation (Dietary Supplement Health and Education Act of 1994).

REFERENCES

1. Lievre M, Marichy J, Baux S, et al: *Clin Trials Meta-Analys* 28:9-12, 1992.
2. British Herbal Medicine Association's Scientific Committee: *British herbal pharmacopoeia*, Bournemouth, 1983, BHMA, pp 44-45.
3. Bisset NG, ed: *Herbal drugs and phytopharmaceuticals: a handbook for practice on a scientific basis*, Stuttgart, 1994, Medpharm Scientific Publishers, pp 118-120.
4. Blaschek W, Ebel S, Hackenthal E, et al: *HagerROM 2002: Hagers Handbuch der Drogen und Arzneistoffe*, Heidelberg, 2002, Springer.
5. Tisserand R, Balacs T: *Essential oil safety: a guide for health care professionals*, Edinburgh, 1995, Churchill Livingstone, pp 8, 172.
6. Kartikeyan S, Chaturvedi RM, Narkar SV: *Leprosy Rev* 61:339, 1990.
7. Gessner O: *Gift-und Arzneipflanzen von Mitteleuropa*, ed 3, Heidelberg, 1974, Carl Winter Universitats verlag, pp 275-276.
8. Casey RCD: *Indian J Med Sci* 14:590-600, 1960.
9. Shipochliev T: *Vet Med Nauki* 18:94-98, 1981.
10. Brinker F: *Herb contraindications and drug interactions*, ed 2, Sandy, 1998, Eclectic Medical Publications, p 46.
11. Newall CA, Anderson LA, Phillipson JD: *Herbal medicines, a guide for health-care professionals*, London, 1996, The Pharmaceutical Press, pp 58-59.
12. Scientific Committee of ESCOP (European Scientific Cooperative on Phytotherapy): *ESCOP monographs: Calendulae flos*, UK, March 1996, European Scientific Cooperative on Phytotherapy Secretariat.
13. Reider N, Komericki P, Hausen BM, et al: *Contact Dermatitis* 45:269-272, 2001.
14. Bruynzeel DP, van Ketel WG, Young E, et al: *Contact Dermatitis* 27:278-279, 1992.
15. de Groot AC, Bruynzeel DP, Bos JD, et al: *Arch Dermatol* 124:1525-1529, 1988.
16. Wrangsjo K, Ros AM, Wahlberg JE: *Contact Dermatitis* 22:148-154, 1990.
17. Rodriquez E, Mitchell JC: *Contact Dermatitis* 3:168-169, 1977.

18. Goldman II: *Klin Med* 52:142-143, 1974.
19. No authors listed: *Int J Toxicol* 20(Suppl 2):13-20, 2001.
20. Dhar ML, Dhar MM, Dhawan BN, et al: *Indian J Exp Biol* 6:232-247, 1968.
21. Boyadzhiev TSV: *Nauchni Tr Vissh Med Inst Sofia* 43:15-20, 1964.
22. Manolov P, Boyadzhiev TSV, Nikolov P: *Eksperim Med Morfol* 3:41-45, 1964.
23. Sharma ML, Chandokhe N, Ghatak BJ, et al: *Indian J Exp Biol* 16:228-240, 1978.
24. Russo M: *Riv Ital EPPOS* 54:730-743, 1972.
25. Avramova S, Portarska F, Apostolova B, et al: *MBI Med Biol Inf* 4:28-33, 1988.
26. Iatsyno AI, Belova LF, Lipkina GS, et al: *Farmakol Toksikol* 41:556-560, 1978.
27. Graf U, Alonso Moraga A, Castro R, et al: *Food Chem Toxicol* 32:423-430, 1994.
28. Ramos A, Edreira A, Vizoso A, et al: *J Ethnopharmacol* 61:49-55, 1998.
29. Perez-Carreon JI, Cruz-Jimenez G, Licea-Vega JA, et al: *Toxicol In Vitro* 16:253-258, 2002.
30. Elias R, De Meo M, Vidal-Ollivier E, et al: *Mutagenesis* 5:327-331, 1990.

CALIFORNIA POPPY

Other common name: Californian poppy
Botanical names: *Eschscholzia californica* Cham.
(*Eschscholtzia californica* Cham.)
Family: Papaveraceae
Plant part used: Aerial parts

Safety Summary

Pregnancy category B2: No increase in frequency of malformation or other harmful effects on the foetus from limited use in women. Animal studies are lacking.
Lactation category CC: Compatible with breastfeeding but use caution.
Contraindications: None required on current evidence. Do not use during lactation without professional advice.
Warnings & precautions: Prescribe with caution for pain in children. Other precautions are neurological disease, depression and psychosis, liver and kidney disease, history of allergic or anaphylactic reactions. Long-term therapy with analgesics is not advisable.
Adverse reactions: None found in published literature.
Interactions: Do not prescribe concomitantly with powerful analgesics (theoretical concern).

Typical Therapeutic Use

Traditional uses of California poppy in Western herbal medicine include reducing pain and assisting sleep.[1] Indications include insomnia, neuralgia, anxiety, stress migraine and nervous bowel.[2]

Actions

Anxiolytic, mild sedative, analgesic.

Key Constituents

Key constituents of California poppy are isoquinoline alkaloids including californidine, eschscholtzine, allocryptopine, protopine, sanguinarine, chelerythrine and, in a lesser amount, some protopine derivatives.[3,4] The main alkaloids present are californidine (approx. 0.2%), followed by eschscholtzine, allocryptopine, and protopine (present in approximately the same amounts i.e., each about

0.02% to 0.03%). The other alkaloids are present in lower quantities.[4]

Adulteration

No adulterants known.

Typical Dosage Forms & Dosage

Typical adult dosage ranges are:
- 3 to 6 mL/day of a 1:2 liquid extract or equivalent in tablet or capsule form

Contraindications

None known. Do not use during lactation without professional advice.

Use in Pregnancy

Category B2: No increase in frequency of malformation or other harmful effects on the foetus from limited use in women. Animal studies are lacking.

Despite a Commission E caution for the use of California poppy in pregnancy, the pharmacological activity of California poppy is mild. The reported uterostimulant activity of one of its minor constituents (cryptopine) has been demonstrated in isolated organ and in situ.[5] Uterostimulant activity is not known for California poppy.

Field notes recorded during the 1920s and 1930s indicate that Native American women of the central California region avoided the California poppy plant during pregnancy and lactation because the smell was believed to be poisonous (no further explanation given).[6] However, a toxic effect is not expected.[7]

Use in Lactation

Category CC: Compatible with breastfeeding but use caution.

Warnings & Precautions

The following conditions should be approached with caution when using herbal analgesics: concurrent prescription of powerful analgesics; pain in children; neurological disease; depression and psychosis; liver and kidney disease; history of allergic or anaphylactic reactions. Long-term therapy with analgesics is not advisable.

Effect on Ability to Drive or Operate Machinery

No adverse effects expected.

Adverse Reactions

None known. However some alkaloids in California poppy are closely related to greater celandine (*Chelidonium majus*), so there is the possibility of drug-induced liver damage occurring rarely (see the monograph on greater celandine).

Interactions

Dopamine beta-hydroxylase and monoamine oxidase (MAO-B) have been inhibited in vitro by California poppy aqueous alcohol extracts.[8] The relevance of this in vitro research to humans is currently unknown. As a precaution, do not prescribe concomitantly with powerful analgesics.

Safety in Children

No information available but adverse effects are not expected. California poppy has been used traditionally as a sedative and analgesic for children.[9]

Overdosage

No incidents found in published literature.

Toxicology

Aqueous alcohol extract of California poppy (orally and i.p.) and an aqueous extract (i.p.) did not induce any acute toxic effects in mice. The LD_{50} was over 5 g/kg, indicating low toxicity.[10] The LD_{50} of sanguinarine by i.p. route in the mouse was 0.18 g/kg.[11]

Regulatory Status

See Table 1 for regulatory status in selected countries.

Table **1**   **Regulatory Status for California Poppy in Selected Countries**

Australia	California poppy is not included in Part 4 of Schedule 4 of the Therapeutic Goods Regulations.
UK & Germany	California poppy is not included on the General Sale List. It is covered by a negative Commission E monograph.
US	California poppy does not have generally recognised as safe (GRAS) status. It is not freely available as a "dietary supplement" in the US under DSHEA legislation (Dietary Supplement Health and Education Act of 1994).

REFERENCES

1. Felter HW, Lloyd JU: *King's American dispensatory*, ed 18, rev 3, vol 2; first published 1905, reprinted Portland, 1983, Eclectic Medical Publications, p 1420.
2. Bartram T: *Encyclopedia of herbal medicine*, ed 1, Dorset, 1995, Grace Publishers, p 82.
3. Tome F, Colombo ML, Caldiroli L: *Phytochem Anal* 10:264-267, 1999.
4. Slavic J, Slavikova L: *Coll Czech Chem Commun* 51:1743-1751, 1986.
5. Luduena FP: *Rev Soc Argentina Biol* 14:339-352, 1938.
6. Bocek BR: *Econ Bot* 38:240-255, 1984.
7. Blaschek W, Ebel S, Hackenthal E, et al: *HagerROM 2002: Hagers Handbuch der Drogen und Arzneistoffe*, Heidelberg, 2002, Springer.
8. Kleber E, Schneider W, Schafer HL, et al: *Arzneim Forsch* 45:127-131, 1995.
9. Brinker FJ: *Eclectic dispensatory of botanical therapeutics*, vol 2, sect 1, Sandy, 1995, Eclectic Medical Publications, pp 43-46.
10. Rolland A, Fleurentin J, Lanhers MC, et al: *Phytother Res* 15:377-381, 2001.
11. Watt JM, Breyer-Brandwijk MG: *The medicinal and poisonous plants of Southern and Eastern Africa: being an account of their medicinal and other uses, chemical composition, pharmacological effects and toxicology in man and animal*, ed 2, Edinburgh, 1962, Livingstone, p 822.

CASCARA

Other common name: Cascara sagrada
Botanical names: *Rhamnus purshiana* DC. (*Rhamnus purshianus* DC., *Frangula purshiana* (DC.) Cooper)
Family: Rhamnaceae
Plant part used: Dried whole or fragmented bark

Safety Summary

Pregnancy category B2: No increase in frequency of malformation or other harmful effects on the foetus from limited use in women. Animal studies are lacking. Theoretical questions suggest avoidance unless necessary and particularly in the first trimester.
Lactation category CC: Compatible with breast-feeding with caution.
Contraindications: Inflammation or irritation of the bowel and digoxin prescription. Do not use during lactation without professional advice.
Warnings & precautions: For short-term use only; causes of chronic constipation and any other abdominal symptoms need to be investigated.
Adverse reactions: Griping colic, diarrhoea, potassium and fluid loss, possible hepatic reactions.
Interactions: Digoxin, thiazide diuretics, theoretically others exacerbated by or causing potassium loss.

Typical Therapeutic Use

For short-term use in cases of occasional constipation. Cascara was found to be effective as a laxative in the elderly population in a systematic review.[1] It has an efficacy (along with oral salt solution) comparable even to enemas in hospitalised patients.[2] Cascara has always been a popular and traditional treatment for constipation.[3]

Actions

Laxative.

Key Constituents

The prominent constituents are a complex of anthracenes, of which up to 70% are the anthrones, cascarosides A, B, C, D, E, and F. Aloins, chrysaloins, aloe-emodin, chrysophanol, emodin, and physcion make up the remainder.

The *European Pharmacopoeia* 4.2 recommends that cascara bark contains not less than 8% of hydroxyanthracene glycosides, of which not less than 60% consist of cascarosides, both expressed as cascaroside A.

Adulteration

Cascara bark has been adulterated with the barks of other *Rhamnus* spp. such as *R. frangula* L., *R. catharticus* L. and *R. fallax* (*R. alpinus* L. ssp. *fallax* [Boiss.]).[4,5]

Typical Dosage Forms & Dosage

Adults and children over 10 years.
Bark: 0.3 to 1 g/day in one dose (or up to 2 g by infusion).
Other preparations: equivalent to 20 to 30 mg daily of hydroxyanthracene derivatives, calculated as cascaroside A.
Typical adult dosage ranges are:
- 0.3 to 1 g/day of dried bark
- 3 to 6 mL/day of a 1:2 liquid extract or equivalent in tablet or capsule form
- Other preparations: equivalent to 20 to 30 mg daily of hydroxyanthracene derivatives, calculated as cascaroside A

The dosage should be as low as necessary to be effective.

Contraindications

Cascara should not be used in the case of diarrhoea, or inflammatory or other disease of the colon, lower small intestine or appendix. It should be avoided with the prescription of digoxin, or antiarrhythmic drugs, or in any case where heart disturbances are combined with the prescription of diuretics. It is not advisable to use cascara or other stimulating laxatives where constipation is associated with an irritable or spastic bowel and in any child under the age of 10 years. Do not use during lactation without professional advice.

Use in Pregnancy

Category B2: No increase in frequency of malformation or other harmful effects on the foetus from limited use in women. Animal studies are lacking.

In a prospective study, 53 mother–child pairs were exposed to cascara during the first trimester. There was no evidence for an increased risk of malformations. For use any time during pregnancy, 188 exposures were recorded. The relative risk for benign tumours in the children was higher than expected, but the statistical significance of this is unknown and independent confirmation of this finding is required.[6]

Theoretical questions suggest avoidance unless necessary and particularly in the first trimester. In traditional Chinese medicine, anthraquinone-containing herbs such as rhubarb are contraindicated in pregnancy.

Use in Lactation

Category CC: Compatible with breastfeeding with caution.

The American Academy of Pediatrics has judged cascara as compatible with breastfeeding.[7,8] However, there is insufficient information to rule out the appearance of active levels of the anthracenes in breast milk, in the case of cascara. In the case of senna, significant quantities were not detected (refer to the senna (*Cassia* spp.) monograph).

Warnings & Precautions

Cascara is a stimulating laxative and should not be used for long periods and not beyond 2 weeks without expert supervision. Persistent constipation should be investigated and other appropriate treatment schedules initiated, in which occasional use of cascara may be justified, but which should emphasise dietary changes, bulk laxatives and exercise.

Cascara should not be given when there are any undiagnosed abdominal symptoms.

Effect on Ability to Drive or Operate Machinery

No adverse effects expected.

Adverse Reactions

Diarrhoea: 4% of new cases of diarrhoea at gastroenterology clinics in the west and central belt of Scotland were found to be laxative induced.[9]

Stimulating laxatives may induce griping pains and may best be given with carminative treatments.

Chronic use may cause transient pigmentation of the wall of the colon (pseudomelanosis coli). Associations have been made between pseudomelanosis coli and colorectal cancer, but this has been challenged and is far from conclusive (refer to the senna monograph).

Extended use is likely to lead to tolerance, with diminishing efficacy and the need for increased doses. However, the state of laxative-induced atony of the bowel ("cathartic colon") has been disputed (refer to the senna monograph).

Cascara has been associated in one case with the development of cholestatic hepatitis, complicated by portal hypertension.[10]

There is a confirmed report of cascara provoking IgE-mediated occupational asthma and rhinitis in pharmaceutical employees.[11]

Interactions

Stimulating laxatives may decrease the gastrointestinal transit time and absorption of co-administered agents. Potassium deficiency (resulting from long-term laxative abuse) can potentiate the action of cardiac glycosides and may affect the action of antiarrhythmic agents. Potassium deficiency can be increased by concomitant use of thiazide diuretics, corticosteroids and licorice root.[12,13] There is potential (but not established) interaction for the same reason with quinidine and licorice.

Safety in Children

For children under 10 years, constipation is most often due to excessive activity of the bowel musculation and rarely to the relative atony that marks some later-onset constipation. It is therefore usually inappropriate to provide stimulating laxatives in this age group.

Overdosage

Griping and diarrhoea are most likely symptoms of excessive doses of cascara. Consequent fluid and electrolyte losses (especially of potassium) could result in cardiac and neuromuscular dysfunction. Treatment should include rehydration and electrolyte replacement.

Table 1 **Regulatory Status for Cascara in Selected Countries**

Australia	Cascara is not included in Part 4 of Schedule 4 of the Therapeutic Goods Regulations.
UK & Germany	Cascara bark is included on the General Sale List. It is covered by a positive Commission E monograph.
	Cascara bark is official in the *British Pharmacopoeia* 2002 and the *European Pharmacopoeia* 4.3.
US	Cascara bark is official in the *United States Pharmacopeia-National Formulary* (USP 26-NF 21, 2003).
	Cascara does not have generally recognised as safe (GRAS) status. It is freely available as a "dietary supplement" in the US under DSHEA legislation (Dietary Supplement Health and Education Act of 1994), but must carry the following warning label: "This product contains *Rhamnus purshiana* (cascara). Read and follow directions carefully. Do not use if you have or develop diarrhea, loose stools, or abdominal pain. Consult your physician if you have frequent diarrhea. If you are pregnant, nursing, taking medication, or have a medical condition, consult your physician before using this product".*

*The California Department of Health Services Food and Drug Branch issued an emergency regulation on November 1, 1996, requiring that all herb teas and dietary supplements containing herbs with stimulant laxative activity carry a warning label. The herbs included in this regulation include aloe (Aloe ferox and other related species), buckthorn bark and berry (Rhamnus catharticus), cascara sagrada bark (Rhamnus purshiana), rhubarb root (Rheum palmatum), and senna leaf and pod (Cassia acutifolia, C. angustifolia, C. senna). The ruling exempts herb products made from aloe leaf gel, which normally does not contain significant natural levels of anthraquinones. The new ruling went into effect January 1, 1997.[14]

Toxicology

There are no specific data available for cascara or the cascarosides on mutagenicity, carcinogenicity, or repeated dose toxicity.

Refer to the aloe (*Aloe* spp.) monograph for toxicological information regarding aloe-emodin and to the senna monograph for general toxicological information on anthraquinone glycosides.

Regulatory Status

See Table 1 for regulatory status in selected countries.

REFERENCES

1. Petticrew M, Watt I, Sheldon T: *Health Technol Assess* 1:i-iv, 1-52, 1997.
2. Rosengren JE, Aberg T: *Radiologe* 15:421-426, 1975.
3. British Herbal Medicine Association's Scientific Committee: *British Herbal Pharmacopoeia*, Bournemouth, BHMA, 1983, p 177.
4. Blaschek W, Ebel S, Hackenthal E, et al: *HagerROM 2002: Hagers Handbuch der Drogen und Arzneistoffe*, Heidelberg, 2002, Springer.
5. Bisset NG, ed: *Herbal drugs and phytopharmaceuticals: a handbook for practice on a scientific basis*, Stuttgart, 1994, Medpharm Scientific Publishers, pp 208-210, 412-414.
6. Briggs GG: *Drugs in pregnancy and lactation: a reference guide to fetal and neonatal risk*, ed 6, Philadelphia, 2002, Lippincott Williams & Wilkins, pp 197-198.
7. Hagemann TM: *J Hum Lact* 14:259-262, 1998.
8. American Academy of Pediatrics: *Pediatrics* 108:776-789, 2001.
9. Duncan A, Morris AJ, Cameron A, et al: *J R Soc Med* 85:203-205, 1992.
10. Nadir A, Reddy D, Van Thiel DH: *Am J Gastroenterol* 95:3634-3637, 2000.
11. Giavina-Bianchi PF Jr, Castro FF, Machado ML, et al: *Ann Allergy Asthma Immunol* 79: 449-454, 1997.
12. Blumenthal M, et al, eds: *The complete German Commission E monographs: therapeutic guide to herbal medicines*, Austin, 1998, American Botanical Council, pp 80-81.
13. Scientific Committee of ESCOP (European Scientific Cooperative on Phytotherapy): *ESCOP monographs: Aloe capensis – cape aloes*. UK, June 1997, European Scientific Cooperative on Phytotherapy Secretariat.
14. Blumenthal M: *HerbalGram* 39:26-27, 1997.

CAT'S CLAW

Other common name: Uña de gato
Botanical names: *Uncaria tomentosa* (Willd. ex Schult.) DC (*Nauclea tomentosa* Willd. ex Schult., *N. aculeata* Kunth)
Family: Rubiaceae
Plant part used: Stem bark or root bark

Safety Summary

Pregnancy category D: Has caused or is associated with a substantial risk of causing foetal malformation or irreversible damage.
Lactation category CC: Compatible with breast-feeding but use caution.
Contraindications: Contraindicated in pregnancy and in women wishing to conceive. Do not use during lactation without professional advice.
Warnings & precautions: Manufacturers of standardised pentacyclic oxindole alkaloids (POA) preparations recommend that cat's claw should not be taken by anyone who has recently received or is planning on receiving bone marrow or organ transplantation.
Adverse reactions: Temporary diarrhoea, constipation, indigestion, lymphocytosis, erythrocytosis and aggravation of acne.
Interactions: Manufacturers of standardised POA preparations warn against concurrent administration with immunosuppressive agents, passive vaccines composed of animal sera, intravenous hyperimmunoglobulin therapy, intravenous thymic extracts, hormone therapies with protein-based animal hormones, or cryoprecipitates or fresh blood plasma (in haemophiliacs).

Typical Therapeutic Use

Cat's claw has demonstrated therapeutic benefit in the treatment of rheumatoid arthritis in a randomised, double-blind, placebo-controlled trial[1] and HIV infection and AIDS in uncontrolled trials.[2,3] Traditional indications for cat's claw in Peruvian medicine include cancer, tumours, arthritis, gastric ulcers, diabetes and as a contraceptive.[4]

Actions

Immune enhancing, antiinflammatory, antioxidant.

Key Constituents

Oxindole alkaloids are the key constituents of cat's claw bark. There are two different chemotypes of *U. tomentosa*.[5] The chemotype which predominantly contains pentacyclic oxindole alkaloids (POA) (0.5% to 3%),[6,7] as opposed to tetracyclic oxindole alkaloids (TOA), has been recommended for therapeutic use.[8]

Adulteration

Many thorny plants in the tropical Americas share the common name uña de gato (cat's claw), such as *Uncaria guianensis*.[8] There are no ethnomedical statistical surveys in Peru on the differentiated use of *U. tomentosa* and *U. guianensis*; however, indifferent use of one or the other is quite common.[9] Preparations containing cat's claw often do not distinguish between the *U. tomentosa* TOA-rich chemotype and the POA-rich chemotype.[2] *U. guianensis* bark contains predominantly TOA.[10]

Typical Dosage Forms & Dosage

Typical adult dosage ranges are:
- 2 to 30 g/day of dried bark by decoction
- 4.5 to 11 mL/day of a 1:2 liquid extract or equivalent in tablet or capsule form

Contraindications

Contraindicated in pregnancy and in women wishing to conceive. Do not use during lactation without professional advice.

Use in Pregnancy

Category D: Has caused or is associated with a substantial risk of causing foetal malformation or irreversible damage.

Contraindicated in pregnancy and in women wishing to conceive.

In Peruvian traditional medicine, high doses of cat's claw root decoction are administered as a contraceptive.[11-13] The bark decoction is also traditionally prescribed as a contraceptive in Peru[14] and for irregular menstruation in Bolivia.[15]

Pregnancy was prevented in mice fed *U. tomentosa* aqueous extract (6.25 and 25 mg/kg).[16] A high number of abnormal embryos were observed after pregnant mice were administered *U. tomentosa* (0.125 to 0.5 mg/mL in their drinking water) for 72 hours postcopulation, suggesting an embryotoxic effect.[17]

A tannin-free extract of *U. tomentosa* roots prevented pregnancy in mice when given orally at 6.25 and 25 mg/kg.[18]

Use in Lactation

Category CC: Compatible with breastfeeding but use caution.

Manufacturers of standardised POA preparations recommend that cat's claw is contraindicated in lactating women, due to lack of clinical data of the effect of cat's claw on the immature immune system.[8,19] However, cat's claw is used in traditional Peruvian medicine for recovery after childbirth[20] and use during early lactation can be inferred from this.

Warnings & Precautions

Manufacturers of standardised POA preparations recommend that cat's claw should not be taken by anyone who has recently received or is planning on receiving bone marrow or organ transplantation, due to cat's claw immune enhancing activity and the chance of rejection. They also warn against concurrent administration with immunosuppressive agents, passive vaccines composed of animal sera, intravenous hyperimmunoglobulin therapy, intravenous thymic extracts, hormone therapies with protein-based animal hormones, such as animal insulin, or cryoprecipitates or fresh blood plasma (in haemophiliacs).[19]

Effect on Ability to Drive or Operate Machinery

No adverse effects expected.

Adverse Reactions

Temporary diarrhoea, constipation or indigestion have occurred initially in several patients consuming cat's claw.[8,21] In one of these cases a high (undefined) dosage was consumed over a long period.[21] Sedative effects and circulatory com-

plaints are possible side effects of preparations containing predominantly TOA. Mild lymphocytosis can develop after intake of the POA chemotype. Cases of erythrocytosis in patients with AIDS and aggravation of preexisting acne in patients with HIV have also been reported after use of this chemotype.[8]

U. tomentosa (POA chemotype) had no significant side effects compared to placebo in a randomised, double-blind clinical trial.[1]

Acute renal failure caused by "cat's claw" was reported in a 35-year-old Peruvian female with systemic lupus erythematosus. The ingredients and dosage of the herbal preparation and the duration of treatment were not listed. The contents of the capsules were not analysed. The patient's condition improved one month after discontinuing the preparation. The authors concluded that it was likely that the patient had experienced an idiosyncratic adverse reaction to the herbal preparation.[22]

Interactions

Manufacturers of standardised POA preparations warn against concurrent administration of cat's claw with a number of medicinal products (see Warnings & precautions).

Cat's claw extract and tincture inhibited cytochrome P450 3A4 activity in vitro.[23] However, whether this in vitro effect will result in decreased metabolism of certain drugs is unclear at this stage.

Safety in Children

Use of cat's claw root extracts in children under 3 years of age is said to be contraindicated in Europe due to lack of clinical data rather than any adverse effects.[19,24]

Overdosage

High doses of cat's claw bark decoction are warned against in traditional Peruvian medicine because they can cause diarrhoea.[11]

Toxicology

Table 1 lists LD_{50} data recorded for cat's claw extract and indicate low oral toxicity.[25,26]

Table **1** LD$_{50}$ **Data Recorded for Cat's Claw Extract**

Substance	Route, Model	LD$_{50}$ Value (g/kg)	Reference
Cat's claw root aqueous extract (containing 35 mg/g total POA)	Oral, mice	>16	25
Cat's claw bark aqueous extract	Oral, rats	126.8	26

No toxic effects were observed after oral administration of 1 g/kg/day of an aqueous-acidic root extract (containing 7.5 mg/g total oxindole alkaloids) for 28 days to rats. Kidney weights increased but their histology was normal.[27] Slight histopathological alterations occurred in the kidney, liver, intestines and stomach of rats orally administered cat's claw bark aqueous extract at doses of 800 mg/kg for 24 weeks, or 3 and 6 times this dose for 12 weeks.[26]

Aqueous extract of cat's claw bark (10 to 100 mg/mL) did not exhibit significant cytotoxicity against Chinese hamster ovary cells in three bioassays or against *Photobacterium phosphoreum* cells in the Microtox assay.[28] Cat's claw bark extracts and fractions did not induce mutagenesis in different strains of *Salmonella typhimurium* with and without metabolic activation.[29]

Table **2** **Regulatory Status for Cat's Claw in Selected Countries**

Australia	Cat's claw is not included in Part 4 of Schedule 4 of the Therapeutic Goods Regulations.
UK & Germany	Cat's claw is not included on the General Sale List. It was not included in the Commission E assessment.
US	Cat's claw does not have generally recognised as safe (GRAS) status. However, it is freely available as a "dietary supplement" in the US under DSHEA legislation (Dietary Supplement Health and Education Act of 1994).

Regulatory Status

See Table 2 for regulatory status in selected countries.

REFERENCES

1. Mur E, Hartig F, Eibl G, et al: *J Rheumatol* 29:678-681, 2002.
2. Keplinger K, Laus G, Wurm M, et al: *J Ethnopharmacol* 64:23-34, 1999.
3. Jones K: *Cat's claw: healing vine of Peru*, Seattle, 1995, Sylvan Press, pp 88-89.
4. Jones K: *Cat's claw: healing vine of Peru*, Seattle, 1995, Sylvan Press, pp 21-24.
5. Laus G, Brossner D, Keplinger K: *Phytochemistry* 45:855-860, 1997.
6. Keplinger K, Wurm M, Laus G: 2nd International Congress on Phytomedicine and 7th Congress of the German Society of Phytotherapy in cooperation with ESCOP (European Scientific Cooperative for Phytotherapy). September 11-14, 1996. Munich, Germany.
7. Laus G, Keplinger K: *Z Phytother* 18:122-126, 1997.
8. Reinhard KH: *J Altern Complement Med* 5:143-151, 1999.
9. Obregón Vilches LE: *Cat's claw: Uncaria genus. Botanical, chemical, and pharmacological studies of Uncaria tomentosa and Uncaria guianensis*, English ed, Lima, 1995, Instituto de Fitoterapia Americano, p 48.
10. Lauvault M, Moretti B, Bruneton J: *Planta Med* 47:244-245, 1983.
11. Jones K: *Cat's claw: healing vine of Peru*, Seattle, 1995, Sylvan Press, p 29.
12. De Feo V: *Fitoterapia* 63:417-440, 1992.
13. Obregón Vilches LE: *Cat's claw: Uncaria genus. Botanical, chemical, and pharmacological studies of Uncaria tomentosa and Uncaria guianensis*, English ed, Lima, 1995, Instituto de Fitoterapia Americano, p 51.
14. Jones K: *Cat's claw: healing vine of Peru*, Seattle, 1995, Sylvan Press, p 64.
15. Bourdy G, DeWalt SJ, Chavez de Michell LR, et al: *J Ethnopharmacol* 70:87-109, 2000.
16. Keplinger K: *Composition allowing for modifying the growth of living cells, preparation and utilization of such a composition* [in German], International Patent WO8201130, April 1982.
17. Iziga R, Gutierrez-Pajares J, Pino J: *Boletin de la Sociedad de Biologia de Concepcion* 69:141-145, 1998.
18. Keplinger K: *Cytostat, contraceptive, and antiinflammatory agent from Uncaria tomentosa roots*, PCT Int. Appl. WO 821130 A1, April 1982.
19. Immodal Pharmaka: *Krallendorn®. Uncaria tomentosa (Willd.) DC. mod. pent. root extract. Report on experiences with probands*, Volders/Tirol, Austria, 1996, Immodal Pharmaka GmbH, pp 1-20.

20. Jones K: *Cat's claw: healing vine of Peru*, Seattle, 1995, Sylvan Press, p 25.
21. Obregón Vilches LE: *Cat's claw: Uncaria genus. Botanical, chemical, and pharmacological studies of Uncaria tomentosa and Uncaria guianensis*, English ed, Lima, 1995, Instituto de Fitoterapia Americano, p 124.
22. Hilepo JN, Bellucci AG, Mossey RT: *Nephron* 77:361, 1997.
23. Budzinski JW, Foster BC, Vandenhoek S, et al: *Phytomedicine* 7:273-282, 2000.
24. Jones K: *Cat's claw: healing vine of Peru*, Seattle, 1995, Sylvan Press, p 46.
25. Kynock SR, Lloyd GK: *Acute oral toxicity to mice of substance E-2919*, Huntingdon, 1975, Huntington Research Centre, cited in Reinhard KH: *J Altern Complement Med* 5:143-151, 1999.

26. Pino A, Salazar M, Vargas K, et al: 2nd International Congress on Phytomedicine and 7th Congress of the German Society of Phytotherapy in cooperation with ESCOP (European Scientific Cooperative for Phytotherapy). September 11-14, 1996. Munich, Germany, abstr SL-18.
27. Svendson O, Skydsgaard K: *Test report: extractum radicis Uncariae tomentosae*, Denmark, 1986, Scantox Biological Laboratory, cited in Keplinger K, Laus G, Wurm M, et al: *J Ethnopharmacol* 64:23-34, 1999.
28. Santa Maria A, Lopez A, Diaz MM, et al: *J Ethnopharmacol* 57:183-187, 1997.
29. Rizzi R, Re F, Bianchi A, et al: *J Ethnopharmacol* 38:63-77, 1993.

CELERY SEED

Botanical name: *Apium graveolens* L.
Family: Apiaceae
Plant part used: Ripe fruit (often referred to as seed)

Safety Summary

Pregnancy category B2: No increase in frequency of malformation or other harmful effects on the foetus from limited use in women. Animal studies are lacking.
Lactation category CC: Compatible with breast-feeding but use caution.
Contraindications: Known sensitivity to the birch or mugwort families. Do not use during lactation without professional advice.
Warnings & precautions: Caution is advised in kidney disorders.
Adverse reactions: Allergic reactions are known.
Interactions: May decrease the efficacy of thyroxine replacement therapy.

Typical Therapeutic Use

Traditional indications for celery seed in Western herbal medicine include arthritic disease, gout and urinary tract inflammation.[1]

Actions

Antirheumatic, mild diuretic, mild spasmolytic, antiinflammatory.

Key Constituents

An essential oil containing phthalides (source of the characteristic odour),[2] especially sedanolide and 3-n-butyl phthalide, together with beta-selinene, methoxyphenol, with chemoprotective,[3] insecticidal, nematicidal and fungicidal properties.[4]

Furanocoumarins[5] including methoxsalen (8-methoxypsoralen) and 5-methoxypsoralen, bergapten, and xanthotoxin that can cause photosensitisation in celery field workers and handlers.[6]

Adulteration

Celery seed is potentially susceptible to mould growth and aflatoxin production during storage.[7]

Typical Dosage Forms & Dosage

Typical adult dosage ranges are:
- 1.5 to 3 g/day of dried fruit or by infusion or decoction
- 1.5 to 6 mL/day of a 1:1 liquid extract
- 4.5 to 8.5 mL/day of a 1:2 liquid extract or equivalent in tablet or capsule form

Contraindications

Patients with known sensitivity to the birch or mugwort families. Do not use during lactation without professional advice.

Use in Pregnancy

Category B2: No increase in frequency of malformation or other harmful effects on the foetus from limited use in women. Animal studies are lacking.

Several types of celery seed extract, including aqueous and ethanolic, were inactive when administered orally to rats (100 to 150 mg/kg, days 1 to 7 postcoitum) in several antiimplantation studies.[8]

Use in Lactation

Category CC: Compatible with breastfeeding but use caution.

Warnings & Precautions

Avoid large doses before exposure to UV radiation or sun beds.

Caution is advised in kidney disorders, in particular inflammation of the kidneys, as the essential oil may increase the inflammation by causing epithelial irritation.[9,10]

Effect on Ability to Drive or Operate Machinery

No adverse effects expected.

Adverse Reactions

Individuals sensitised to birch pollen and/or mugwort pollen frequently display allergic symptoms after ingestion of celery.[11-13] An allergenic protein (Api g 1) has been described.[14] Although one case of phototoxicity has been reported in an individual consuming 450 g celery root (celeriac) before the use of a sun bed,[15] no significant psoralens or phototoxic reactions were found even after the ingestion of large amounts of celery root in healthy volunteers.[16] However, there remains a theoretical caution against large doses of celery seed in the case of PUVA treatment or excessive sunbathing.

Interactions

Reduced serums level of thyroxine have been reported in two cases in which patients were taking celery seed tablets in conjunction with thyroxine.[17]

Celery has been claimed to have theoretical effects in increasing bleeding time or to potentiate the effects of warfarin.[18] No confirmatory evidence is available and this appears to be based on a mistaken interpretation of the effects of plant coumarins that it contains.

Pronounced hepatoprotective activity comparable to silymarin has been demonstrated in rats,[19] notably against single high doses of paracetamol.[20] However, a nonspecific decrease in CYP450 in animals has been observed, seen as a prolonged action of aminopyrine and paracetamol.[21] The clinical relevance of these findings is not known.

Safety in Children

No information available.

Overdosage

No incidents found in published literature.

Toxicology

Table 1 lists LD$_{50}$ data recorded for celery seed and its constituents.[22-24]

The phototoxic threshold dose is not reached by the consumption of celery root and other conventional vegetables under normal dietary habits. However, the safety factor between the possible intake of furanocoumarins and the phototoxic threshold dose is about 2 to 10, which is relatively small.[25]

Regulatory Status

See Table 2 for regulatory status in selected countries.

Celery seed is commonly consumed as a spice, and celery root and stalk as foods.

Table **1** **LD$_{50}$ Data Recorded for Celery Seed and Its Constituents**

Substance	Route, Model	LD$_{50}$ Value (g/kg)	Reference
Celery seed 90% methanol extract	i.p., rats	1	22
Celery seed oil	Oral, rats	>5	23
3-n-butylidene phthalide	Oral, rats	2.45	24

Table **2** **Regulatory Status for Celery Seed in Selected Countries**

Australia	Celery seed is not included in Part 4 of Schedule 4 of the Therapeutic Goods Regulations.
UK & Germany	Celery seed is included on the General Sale List. It is covered by a negative Commission E monograph.
US	Celery seed does have generally recognised as safe (GRAS) status. It is freely available as a "dietary supplement" in the US under DSHEA legislation (Dietary Supplement Health and Education Act of 1994).

REFERENCES

1. British Herbal Medicine Association's Scientific Committee: *British herbal pharmacopoeia*, Bournemouth, 1983, BHMA, pp 28-29.
2. Momin RA, Ramsewak RS, Nair MG: *J Agric Food Chem* 48:3785-3788, 2000.
3. Zheng GQ, Kenney PM, Zhang J, et al: *Nutr Cancer* 19:77-86, 1993.
4. Momin RA, Nair MG: *J Agric Food Chem* 49:142-145, 2001.
5. Innocenti G, Dall'Acqua F, Caporale G: *Planta Med* 29:165-170, 1976.
6. Beier RC: *Rev Environ Contam Toxicol* 113:47-137, 1990.
7. Llewellyn GC, Burkett ML, Eadie T: *J Assoc Off Anal Chem* 64:955-960, 1981.
8. Kamboj VP, Dhawan BN: *J Ethnopharmacol* 6:191-226, 1982.
9. British Herbal Medicine Association: *British herbal compendium*, Bournemouth, 1992, BHMA, pp 56-57.

10. Bisset NG, ed: *Herbal drugs and phytopharmaceuticals*, Stuttgart, 1994, Medpharm Scientific Publishers, pp 81-82.

11. Ballmer-Weber BK, Vieths S, Luttkopf D, et al: *J Allergy Clin Immunol* 106:373-378, 2000.

12. Luttkopf D, Ballmer-Weber BK, Wuthrich B, et al: *J Allergy Clin Immunol* 106:390-399, 2000.

13. Vallier P, Dechamp C, Vial O, et al: *Clin Allergy* 18: 491-500, 1988.

14. Breiteneder H, Hoffmann-Sommergruber K, O'Riordain G, et al: *Eur J Biochem* 233:484-489, 1995.

15. Ljunggren B: *Arch Dermatol* 126:1334-1336, 1990.

16. Gral N, Beani JC, Bonnot D, et al: *Ann Dermatol Venereol* 120:599-603, 1993.

17. Moses G: *Australian Prescriber* 24:6, 2001.

18. Heck AM, DeWitt BA, Lukes AL: *Am J Health Syst Pharm* 57:1221-1227, 2000.

19. Ahmed B, Alam T, Varshney M, et al: *J Ethnopharmacol* 79:313-316, 2002.

20. Singh A, Handa SS: *J Ethnopharmacol* 49:119-126, 1995.

21. Jakovljevic V, Raskovic A, Popovic M, et al: *Eur J Drug Metab Pharmacokinet* 27:153-156, 2002.

22. Sharma ML, Chandokhe N, Ghatak BJR, et al: *Indian J Exp Biol* 16:228-240, 1978.

23. Opdyke DLJ: *Food Cosmet Toxicol* 12:849-850, 1974.

24. Opdyke DL: *Food Cosmet Toxicol* 17:251, 1979.

25. Schlatter J, Zimmerli B, Dick R, et al: *Food Chem Toxicol* 29:523-530, 1991.

CHAMOMILE, GERMAN

Other common name: Wild chamomile
Botanical names: *Matricaria recutita* (L) Rauchert (*Matricaria chamomilla* L., *Chamomilla recutita* (L) Rauchert)
Family: Compositae
Plant part used: Flower head

Safety Summary

Pregnancy category A: No proven increase in the frequency of malformation or other harmful effects on the foetus despite consumption by a large number of women.
Lactation category C: Compatible with breastfeeding.
Contraindications: Known allergy.
Warnings & precautions: Known sensitivity to members of the Compositae family.
Adverse reactions: Occasional allergic reactions.
Interactions: No precautions required on current evidence.

Typical Therapeutic Use

Clinical trial data demonstrate topical antiinflammatory effects on the skin.[1,2]

Traditional indications for German chamomile in Western herbal medicine include flatulent nervous dyspepsia, nervous diarrhoea, and restlessness.[3] There is a popular reputation for its use in dysmenorrhoea and amenorrhoea.[4]

Actions

Antiinflammatory, spasmolytic, vulnerary, antimicrobial, mild sedative, diaphoretic.

Key Constituents

Essential oil (0.5% to 1.5%), containing (−)-alpha-bisabolol, chamazulene, bisabolol oxides A, B, C; cis- and trans-en-yn-dicycloethers.[5] The chamazulene is formed from matricine during steam distillation[6]; it has demonstrated antioxidant properties, inhibiting lipid peroxidation in vitro.[7] (−)-Alpha-bisabolol has been shown to protect the gastric mucosa of rats against the toxic effects of acetylsalicylic acid.[8] The herb also contains flavonoids, especially apigenin.[9]

Polysaccharides found in chamomile have demonstrated immunostimulating activity in vitro: these may contribute to topical sensitising properties but are unlikely to survive oral digestion.[10]

Adulteration

There has been much botanical contention over the classification of chamomile. There are various genotypes and it is also easily confused with related species with similar appearance or odour, especially from the genera Anthemis, Matricaria, Chamomilla, Chrysanthemum and Tanacetum. In an authoritative review of the literature it has been suggested that most cases of allergic contact dermatitis involving chamomile may actually concern related species, particularly *Anthemis cotula*, stinking dog fennel, which contains much higher levels of a particularly potent potential allergen, anthecotulide.[11,12]

Typical Dosage Forms & Dosage

Typical adult dosage ranges are:
- 6 to 12 g/day of dried flower heads or by infusion
- 3 to 12 mL/day of a 1:2 liquid extract
- 3 to 6 mL/day of a 1:2 liquid extract or equivalent in tablet or capsule form
- 9 to 30 mL/day of a 1:5 tincture

Infusions or semisolid preparations containing 3% to 10% w/w of the flowers or equivalent for external use as wash or gargle.

Contraindications

Despite reports of skin reactions and dermatitis from topical use of chamomile, the likelihood of chamomile preparations causing a contact sensitivity or an IgE-mediated allergic skin response (from the pollen) is low. However, persons with known sensitivity to the herb should avoid topical application of chamomile products.

Since ingestion of chamomile has been linked to anaphylaxis, its intake should be avoided in cases of known allergy.

Use in Pregnancy

Category A: No proven increase in the frequency of malformation or other harmful effects on the foetus despite consumption by a large number of women.

Chamomile is widely consumed as a tea in many countries and no adverse effects during pregnancy have been documented.

Long-term oral administration of chamomile extracts to rats produced no teratogenicity or signs of changes in prenatal development.[13] A herbal formula containing chamomile, sage and yeast plasmolysate did not produce teratogenic effects in rats. The administered dosage of chamomile extract was 0.4 mL/day.[14,15]

Prenatal development was not affected in rats and rabbits orally administered up to 1 mL/kg of alpha-bisabolol. Teratogenic effects were not observed at this dosage. A dose of 3 mL/kg increased the number of resorptions.[16] Alpha-bisabolol administered orally (250 to 500 mg/kg) to pregnant rats had no effect on the foetus.

There is reference to chamomile infusion causing a stimulating effect on the uterus,[17] but the relevance of this to normal human use is uncertain.

Use in Lactation

Category C: Compatible with breastfeeding.

Warnings & Precautions

Avoid in patients with known hypersensitivity to plants in the Compositae family.

Effect on Ability to Drive or Operate Machinery

No adverse effects expected.

Adverse Reactions

Hypersensitivity reactions as a basis for contact dermatitis to chamomile have been confirmed.[18,19] Chamomile tea allergy,[20] and contact dermatitis,[21-24] including urticaria,[25] including from cosmetics, have been reported.[26] Occasional hypersensitivity reactions to chamomile dust have been reported among tea packers.[27]

Allergic conjunctivitis was observed in seven hay fever sufferers who had used chamomile tea as an eyewash; all cases had positive skin tests to chamomile but there were no reactions after oral consumption. The pollens were judged to be the sensitising components.[28]

A chamomile-containing enema in labour was associated with a fatal anaphylactic attack.[29] One case of severe anaphylactic reaction was observed in an atopic child after taking chamomile tea for the first time. Mugwort was identified as one of the predisposing allergens.[30] Severe anaphylaxis as a result of application of a chamomile tea enema has been reported. The patient had consumed chamomile tea on two occasions in the past without any adverse reaction.[31]

Chamomile allergies are most likely to follow previous sensitising to mugwort (Artemisia vulgaris): cross-reactivity with mugwort sensitivity has been confirmed by skin patch tests to chamomile in 21 out of 24 affected individuals, positive inhalation reactions to chamomile pollen in 16 individuals, and positive reactions to oral consumption of chamomile in 13 out of the 24.[32]

Epidemiological data suggest that chamomile is a significant but not common cause of contact sensitivity.[33] A mixture of Compositae plants used for testing allergic responses has been shown to yield positive results in 3.1% of a sample of 3851 individuals: chamomile was shown to account for 56.5% of this effect; sesquiterpene lactones, polyacetylenes and a thiophene are considered the main contributors to this effect.[34] However, it may be that chamomile is in part a victim of misidentification, as suggested in the Adulteration section above.

Interactions

Speculative interactions with NSAIDs and analgesics,[35] antiepileptics,[36] and warfarin[37] are based on faulty information.

A clinical study has indicated a potential interaction between Matricaria recutita ingestion and reduced iron absorption. An infusion of German chamomile reduced the absorption of iron by 47% from a bread meal (compared to a water control) in adult volunteers. The inhibition was dose dependent and related to its polyphenol content (phenolic acids, monomeric flavonoids, polymerised polyphenols). Inhibition by black tea was 79% to 94%.[38] In anaemia and cases where iron supplementation is required, chamomile should not be taken simultaneously with meals or iron supplements.

Safety in Children

Chamomile is judged as generally benign when taken by children.[39] A chamomile and pectin combination was beneficial for the treatment of diarrhoea in children aged between 6 months and 5.5 years in a placebo-controlled clinical trial.[40]

Overdosage

No incidents found in published literature.

Toxicology

Table 1 lists LD_{50} data recorded for chamomile essential oil.[16,41]

Table 1   **LD_{50} Data Recorded for Chamomile Essential Oil**

Substance	Route, Model	LD_{50} Value	Reference
Chamomile essential oil	Oral, rats	>5 g/kg	41
Chamomile essential oil	Dermal, rabbits	>5 g/kg	41
Alpha-bisabolol	Oral, mice	15.1 mL/kg	16

One study demonstrated no toxicological effects in mice administered up to 1440 mg/kg of a dried preparation of chamomile infusion by intraperitoneal injection. (Reversible depressive effects on the CNS occurred after long-term use at doses beyond 90 mg/kg.) There were no gastrointestinal effects observed in rats for doses up to 5 g/kg.[42]

Regulatory Status

See Table 2 for regulatory status in selected countries. Chamomile is widely consumed as a herbal tea.

Table 2   **Regulatory Status for German Chamomile in Selected Countries**

Australia	German chamomile is not included in Part 4 of Schedule 4 of the Therapeutic Goods Regulations.
UK & Germany	German chamomile is included on the General Sale List. It is covered by a positive Commission E monograph.
	Chamomile flower is official in the *European Pharmacopoeia* 4.3.
US	German chamomile does have generally recognised as safe (GRAS) status. It is also freely available as a "dietary supplement" in the US under DSHEA legislation (Dietary Supplement Health and Education Act of 1994).

REFERENCES

1. Glowania HJ, Raulin Chr, Swoboda M: *Z Hautkr* 62:1262-1271, 1987.
2. Aertgeerts P, Albring M, Klaschka F, et al: *Z Hautkr* 60:270-277, 1985.
3. British Herbal Medicine Association's Scientific Committee: *British herbal pharmacopoeia*, Bournemouth, 1983, BHMA, pp 139-140.
4. Mills S, Bone K: *Principles and practice of phytotherapy: modern herbal medicine*, Edinburgh, 2000, Churchill Livingstone, pp 319-327.
5. Wagner H, Bladt S: *Plant drug analysis: a thin layer chromatography atlas*, ed 2, Berlin, 1996, Springer-Verlag, pp 159-199.
6. Schmidt PC, Weibler K, Soyke B: *Dtsch Apoth Ztg* 131:175-181, 1991.
7. Rekka EA, Kourounakis AP, Kourounakis PN: *Res Commun Mol Pathol Pharmacol* 92:361-364, 1996.
8. Torrado S, Torrado S, Agis A, et al: *Pharmazie* 50: 141-143, 1995.
9. Schreiber A, Carle R, Reinhard E: *Planta Med* 56:179-181, 1990.
10. Uteshev BS, Laskova IL, Afanas'ev VA: *Eksp Klin Farmakol* 62:52-55, 1999
11. De Smet PAGM, Keller K, Hansel R, et al, eds: *Adverse effects of herbal drugs*, vol 1, Berlin, 1993, Springer-Verlag, pp 243-248.
12. Hausen BM, Busker E, Carle R: *Planta Med* 50:229-234, 1984.
13. Mann C, Staba EJ: The chemistry, pharmacology, and commercial formulations of chamomile. In *Herbs, spices, and medicinal plants*, vol 1, Phoenix, 1986, Oryx Press, p 265.

14. Leslie GB, Salmon G: *Swiss Med* 1:43-45, 1979.
15. Bio-Strath AG: Personal communication, September 2003.
16. Habersang S, Leuschner F, Isaac C, et al: *Planta Med* 37:115-123, 1979.
17. Shipochliev T: *Vet Med Nauki* 18:94-98, 1981.
18. Anliker MD, Borelli S, Wuthrich B: *Contact Dermatitis* 46:72-74, 2002.
19. Bossuyt L, Dooms-Goossens A: *Contact Dermatitis* 31:131-132, 1994.
20. Casterline CL: *JAMA* 244:330-331, 1980.
21. Giordano-Labadie F, Schwarze HP, Bazex J: *Contact Dermatitis* 42:247, 2000.
22. Pereira F, Santos R, Pereira A: *Contact Dermatitis* 36:307, 1997.
23. Rodriguez-Serna M, Sanchez-Motilla JM, Ramon R, et al: *Contact Dermatitis* 39:192-193, 1998.
24. Rudzki E, Rebandel P: *Contact Dermatitis* 38:164, 1998.
25. Foti C, Nettis E, Cassano N, et al: *Contact Dermatitis* 42:360-361, 2000.
26. Schempp CM, Schopf E, Simon JC: *Hautarzt* 53:93-97, 2002.
27. Abramson MJ, Sim MR, Fritschi L, et al: *Occup Med (Lond)* 51:259-265, 2001.
28. Subiza J, Subiza JL, Alonso M, et al: *Ann Allergy* 65: 127-132, 1990.
29. Jensen-Jarolim E, Reider N, Fritsch R, et al: *J Allergy Clin Immunol* 102:1041-1042, 1998.
30. Subiza J, Subiza JL, Hinojosa M, et al: *J Allergy Clin Immunol* 84:353-358, 1989.
31. Thien FC: *Med J Aust* 175:54, 2001.
32. de la Torre Morin F, Sanchez Machin I, Garcia Robaina JC, et al: *J Investig Allergol Clin Immunol* 11:118-122, 2001
33. Paulsen E: *Contact Dermatitis* 47:189-198, 2002.
34. Hausen BM: *Am J Contact Dermatitis* 7:94-99, 1996.
35. Abebe W: *J Clin Pharm Ther* 27:391-401, 2002.
36. Spinella M: *Epilepsy Behav* 2:524-532, 2001.
37. Heck AM, DeWitt BA, Lukes AL: *Am J Health Syst Pharm* 57:1221-1227, 2000;
38. Hurrell RF, Reddy M, Cook JD. *Br J Nutr* 81:289-295, 1999.
39. Fugh-Berman A: *Nutr Today* 37:122-124, 2002.
40. de la Motte S, Bose-O'Reilly S, Heinisch M, et al: *Arzneim Forsch* 47:1247-1249, 1997.
41. Opdyke DLJ: *Food Cosmet Toxicol* 12:851-852, 1974.
42. Della Loggia R, Traversa U, Scarcia V, et al: *Pharmacol Res Comm* 14:153-162, 1982.

CHAPARRAL

Other common name: Creosote bush
Botanical names: *Larrea tridentata* (Sessé & Moc. ex DC.) Coville (*Larrea mexicana* Moric.)
Family: Zygophyllaceae
Plant part used: Leaf

Safety Summary

Pregnancy category C: Has caused or is associated with a substantial risk of causing harmful effects on the foetus or neonate without causing malformations.
Lactation category X: Contraindicated in breast-feeding.
Contraindications: Past history of liver disease or damage, pregnancy and lactation.
Warnings & precautions: During chaparral use, decrease exposure to toxins and free radicals; increase intake of antioxidants and inducers of phase II detoxification. Caution is advised for women wishing to conceive. Watch for signs and symptoms of hepatotoxicity.
Adverse reactions: Occasional hepatotoxicity. Autoimmune haemolytic anaemia, stimulation of tumour growth, and contact dermatitis have also been reported.
Interactions: No precautions required on current evidence regarding interactions with drugs.

Typical Therapeutic Use

Chaparral has been used by Native Americans for stomach trouble, diarrhoea and sore throat.[1,2] It was considered a "cure-all" by northern Mexicans and people in the southern United States.[3] A report of regression of malignant melanoma in a man self-medicating with chaparral tea in 1969 led to an interest in its potential as an anticancer remedy.[4] Chaparral contains nordihydroguaiaretic acid (NDGA) which has potent antioxidant activity.[5]

Actions

Depurative, antioxidant, antitumour, antimicrobial.

Key Constituents

L. tridentata mature leaves contain up to 10% dry weight of a thick external resin. Over 80% of the resin is composed of phenolic aglycones, with the major component being the lignan nordihydroguaiaretic acid (5% to 10% of the dry weight). The balance of the resin is a complex mixture of partially o-methylated flavones and flavonols, together with small amounts of acid and basic components.[5,6]

Adulteration

Larrea divaricata is indigenous to South America, and *L. tridentata* to North America.[7] The botanical name *L. divaricata* has been applied to *L. tridentata* (*L. mexicana*) as it was once identified as being the same as the species from Argentina, but in the 1940s they were determined to be distinguishable.[8] There is confusion as to whether *L. divaricata* is medicinally interchangeable with *L. tridentata*. Chaparral is also known by the Hispanic common names jarilla or jarillo. It is possible that *Larrea* spp. indigenous to South America with these common names, such as *Larrea cuneifolia* Cav. and *Larrea nitida* Cav., are sometimes present as adulterants.[9]

Typical Dosage Forms & Dosage

Typical adult dosage ranges are:
- a decoction from 2.25 teaspoons of dried leaf per day
- 1.5 to 3.5 mL/day of a 1:2 liquid extract or equivalent in tablet or capsule form

Contraindications

Past history of liver disease or damage. Pregnancy and lactation.

Use in Pregnancy

Category C: Has caused or is associated with a substantial risk of causing harmful effects on the foetus or neonate without causing malformations.

Qollahuaya Andeans (natives of midwestern Bolivia) use infusion of *Larrea divaricata* as an abortifacient.[10] Infusions of chaparral have been used as a contraceptive agent in Mexico.[11]

Oral administration of extracts of chaparral leaf and twig to female rats during days 1 to 10 of gestation exhibited antiimplantation activity.[12] NDGA (300 mg/kg, s.c.) administered to rats inhibited ovulation.[13] In contrast, oral administration of NDGA

(0.5 g/day) to female rats led to a lower resorption rate (8.1%) than controls (10.6%), which was regarded as beneficial.[14] A lignan isolated from chaparral has demonstrated antiimplantation activity in rats (15 to 60 mg/kg, oral).[15]

Use in Lactation

Category X: Contraindicated in breastfeeding.

Warnings & Precautions

To protect against the reported occasional hepatotoxicity from chaparral ingestion, patients would be well advised to reduce exposure to toxins and free radicals, consume an antioxidant diet (e.g., rich in fruit and vegetables) together with inducers of phase II hepatic detoxification such as the Brassicas. Watch for signs and symptoms of hepatotoxicity.

Effect on Ability to Drive or Operate Machinery

No adverse effects expected.

Adverse Reactions

A review of 18 reports of adverse events associated with the ingestion of chaparral reported to the Food and Drug Administration between 1992 and 1994 found evidence of hepatotoxicity in 13 cases (causal, 10; not followed up, 1; probable, 2; insufficient data, 5). Of the 13 cases, 10 had ingested chaparral only, with the remainder taking products containing chaparral and other herbs and/or ingredients. The total amount of chaparral ingested (where known) was 24.8 to 113.3 g. Adverse events occurred 3 to 52 weeks after the ingestion of chaparral and resolved 1 to 17 weeks after ceasing intake. The predominant pattern of liver injury was characterised as toxic or drug-induced cholestatic hepatitis. In 4 individuals there was progression to cirrhosis and in 2 individuals there was acute fulminant liver failure that required a liver transplant. Of the patients requiring a liver transplant, chaparral was probably not the only cause in one case.[16] Of the 13 cases, information about 4 had been published elsewhere.[17-19]

However, in one study adverse effects were observed in the liver function parameters of 4 patients who consumed low doses of chaparral (34 to 240 mL of 1:2.5 tincture over 1 to 5 months).[20]

Table 1 provides a summary of an additional 7 case reports of adverse reactions associated with ingestion of chaparral.[21-25]

Table 1   **Additional Case Reports of Adverse Reactions Attributed to Chaparral Ingestion**

Case Reports	Adverse Reaction	Ref
1 case, 1999; preparation containing chaparral	Acute hepatitis	21
2 cases, 1995; • chaparral tablets (3 months prior to symptoms) • chaparral tablets (more than 3 tablets/ day for 6 weeks)	Hepatic injury	22
1 case, 1993; chaparral capsules (8 weeks prior to first symptoms)	Severe acute hepatitis; patient had past history of hepatitis A	23
1 case, 1990; chaparral tablets (15 tablets/day, 3 months)	Subacute hepatic necrosis	24
1 case, 1980; chaparral tablets (4 tablets/day)	Autoimmune haemolytic anaemia	25

A case of cystic renal disease and cystic adenocarcinoma of the kidney was reported in 1994 for a 56-year-old woman who admitted drinking chaparral tea (3 to 4 cups/day for 3 months, 1.5 years prior to presentation). The patient had experienced an episode of pyelonephritis earlier in her life (in 1965) and several years later consumed "pau d'arco" tea for a 6-month period.[26] The association between ingestion of chaparral or "pau d'arco" tea and the renal disease is not strong.

In a significant number of patients with advanced incurable malignancy who were participating in an uncontrolled trial with chaparral tea, there appeared to be stimulation of tumour growth.[27,28]

An hypothesis was proposed to explain the possible occasional hepatotoxicity from chaparral ingestion.[5] Under certain conditions, antioxidant compounds such as NDGA can become oxidant and generate free radicals. If hepatic detoxification mechanisms are compromised, these compounds can also have toxic effects. (Every antioxidant compound exists in a reduced and an oxidised form and if the oxidised form predominates, that compound will then act as a pro-oxidant.) Chemical studies of chaparral extracts indicate the presence of a number of reactive free radical species and also the potentially toxic pro-oxidant compound guaiaretic acid diquinone.

Up until the early 1990s sixteen cases of contact dermatitis have been attributed to *Larrea* spp. (sometimes defined as creosote bush or jarilla; 13 cases) or NDGA (3 cases).[29]

Ingestion of chaparral may produce a serological picture resembling that of an autoimmune syndrome. Ingestion of chaparral caused a positive direct antiglobulin test (due to the presence of IgG_1 antibodies) in a male blood donor who was consuming chaparral (4 tablets/day). The association between the chaparral consumption and the abnormal antibody test was confirmed with rechallenge.[25]

Interactions

No drug interactions known.

Safety in Children

No information available.

Overdosage

No incidents found in published literature.

Toxicology

Table 2 lists LD_{50} data recorded for chaparral extract and its constituents, which indicate low acute toxicity.[30,31]

Feeding an aqueous ethanol extract of chaparral (4% for 70 days) to male hamsters resulted in serious signs of toxicity and pathological changes, including a marked hypoplasia of the testes and accessory sex glands.[32]

Table **2** **LD_{50} Data Recorded for Chaparral**

Substance	Route, Model	LD_{50} Value	Reference
Chaparral extract*	i.p., mice (male)	10 g/kg	30
Chaparral extract*	i.p., mice (female)	4 g/kg	30
NDGA	Oral, mice	2-4 g/kg	31
NDGA	Oral, rat	2-5.5 g/kg	31
NDGA	Oral, guinea pig	830 mg/kg	31

Extract prepared by extraction of dried L. divaricata leaves with water and concentrated to a final ratio of 3.75:1.

Preliminary studies with the brine shrimp bioassay and cultured rat hepatocytes indicate that most of the toxic potential of chaparral is accounted for in the methanol-soluble group of components.[5]

NDGA has very strong antioxidant activity and was used as an antioxidant in animal fat, vegetable oil and milk products in U.S. food industries until concern regarding its safety (see below) led to the removal of its GRAS status.[9,33]

Oral administration of NDGA caused kidney cysts and mesenteric lymphadenopathy (0.5% to 1% in diet for 74 weeks) and caecal haemorrhage and enlargement of lymph nodes near the caecum (0.5% in diet for 2 years).[31,34] NDGA (2% in diet) combined with endotoxin acted synergistically in provoking renal damage in germ-free rats.[35] Oral administration of NDGA attenuated ferric–nitrilotriacetate (Fe–NTA)-mediated nephrotoxicity, hepatotoxicity and tumour promotion in mice (Fe–NTA is a known carcinogen).[33] NDGA induced sister-chromatid exchanges in human lymphocytes (in vitro) and in mouse bone marrow cells in vivo.[36]

In vitro studies suggest that the tumour antiproliferative activity of chaparral cannot be attributed to NDGA alone, but this component could add to the activity of other constituents.[37]

Regulatory Status

See Table 3 for regulatory status in selected countries.

Table **3**   **Regulatory Status for Chaparral in Selected Countries**

Australia	Chaparral is not included in Part 4 of Schedule 4 of the Therapeutic Goods Regulations. However, the following warning is required on the labels of products containing chaparral: "Chaparral may harm the liver in some people. Only use under the supervision of a health care professional."
UK & Germany	Chaparral is not included on the General Sale List. It was not included in the Commission E assessment.
US	Chaparral does not have generally recognised as safe (GRAS) status. However, it is freely available as a "dietary supplement" in the US under DSHEA legislation (Dietary Supplement Health and Education Act of 1994).

REFERENCES

1. Vogel VJ: *American Indian medicine*, Norman, 1970, University of Oklahoma Press, pp 296-297.
2. Felger RS, Moser MB: *Econ Bot* 28:414-436, 1974.
3. Sandoval A. *Homegrown healing: traditional home remedies from Mexico*, New York, 1998, Berkley Books, pp 106-107.
4. Smart CR, Hogle HH, Robins RK, et al: *Cancer Chemother Rep* 53:147-151, 1969.
5. Obermeyer WR, Musser SM, Betz JM, et al: *Proc Soc Exp Biol Med* 208:6-12, 1995.
6. Gonzalez-Coloma A, Wisdom CS, Rundel RW: *Biochem Syst Ecol* 16:59-64, 1988.
7. Hunter KL. Betancourt JL, Riddle BR, et al: *Global Ecol Biogeogr* 10:521-533, 2001.
8. Brinker FJ: Section 1: Native healing gifts: *Larrea tridentata*. In *Eclectic dispensatory of botanical therapeutics*, vol 2, Sandy, 1995, Eclectic Medical Publications, pp 69-74.
9. Blaschek W, Ebel S, Hackenthal E, et al: *HagerROM 2002: Hagers Handbuch der Drogen und Arzneistoffe*, Heidelberg, 2002, Springer.
10. Bastien JW: *J Ethnopharmacol* 8:97-111, 1983.
11. Moser MB: *Kiva* 35:201-210, 1970.
12. Konno C, Martin A, Ma BX, et al: *Proceedings of the first Princess Chulabhorn Science Congress, International Congress on Natural Products*, Bangkok, Thailand, 2: 328-337, 10-13 December, 1987.
13. Mikuni M, Yoshida M, Hellberg P, et al: *Biol Reprod* 58:1211-1216, 1998.
14. Telford IR, Woodruff CS, Linford RH: *Am J Anat* 110:29-36, 1962.
15. Konno C, Lu ZZ, Xue HZ, et al: *J Nat Prod* 53:396-406, 1990.
16. Sheikh NM, Philen RM, Love LA: *Arch Intern Med* 157:913-919, 1997.
17. Gordon DW, Rosenthal G, Hart J, et al: *JAMA* 273: 489-490, 1995.
18. Alderman S, Kailas S, Goldfarb S, et al: *J Clin Gastroenterol* 19:242-247, 1994.
19. No authors listed: *MMWR Morb Mortal Wkly Rep* 41:812-814, 1992.
20. Heron S, Yarnell E: *J Altern Complement Med* 7: 175-185, 2001.
21. Shad JA, Chinn CG, Brann OS: *South Med J* 92:1095-1097, 1999
22. Batchelor WB, Heathcote J, Wanless IR: *Am J Gastroenterol* 90:831-833, 1995.
23. Smith BC, Desmond PV: *Aust NZ J Med* 23:526, 1993.
24. Katz M, Saibil F: *J Clin Gastroenterol* 12:203-206, 1990.
25. Tregellas WM, South SF: *Transfusion* 20:647-648, 1980.
26. Smith AY, Feddersen RM, Gardner KD Jr, et al: *J Urol* 152:2089-2091, 1994.
27. Smart CR, Hogle HH, Vogel H, et al: *Rocky Mt Med J* 67:39-43, 1970.
28. The National Academies: *Safety review: draft prototype monograph on chaparral*, Table A, page 1, available via http://wwwsearch.nationalacademies.org/ (downloaded January 2003).
29. De Smet PAGM, Keller K, Hansel R, et al, eds: *Adverse effects of herbal drugs*, vol 2, Berlin, 1993, Springer-Verlag, pp 231-240.
30. Anesini C, Boccio J, Cremaschi G, et al: *Phytother Res* 11:521-523, 1997.
31. Lehman AJ, Fitzhugh OG, Nelson AA, et al: *Adv Food Res* 3:197-208, 1951.
32. Granados H, Cardenas R: *Rev Gastroenterol Mex* 59:31-35, 1994.
33. Ansar S, Iqbal M, Athar M: *Carcinogenesis* 20:599-606, 1999.
34. Grice HC, Becking G, Goodman T: *Food Cosmet Toxicol* 6:155-161, 1968.
35. Gardner KD Jr, Reed WP, Evan AP, et al: *Kidney Int* 32:329-334, 1987.
36. Madrigal-Bujaidar E, Diaz Barriga S, Cassani M, et al: *Mutat Res* 412:139-144, 1998.
37. Anesini C, Ferraro G, Lopez P, et al: *Phytomedicine* 8: 1-7, 2001.

CHASTE TREE

Other common names: Chaste berry, monk's pepper, agnus castus
Botanical name: *Vitex agnus-castus* L.
Family: Labiatae
Plant part used: Fruit

Safety Summary

Pregnancy category BI: No increase in frequency of malformation or other harmful effects on the foetus from limited use in women. No evidence of increased foetal damage in animal studies. (Use cautiously in pregnancy, and only in the early stages, for insufficient corpus luteal function.)
Lactation category C: Compatible with breastfeeding.
Contraindications: None required on current evidence.
Warnings & precautions: Best not taken in conjunction with progesterone drugs, the contraceptive pill or hormone replacement therapy. May aggravate pure spasmodic dysmenorrhoea not associated with premenstrual syndrome.
Adverse reactions: Mainly gastrointestinal disturbances (particularly nausea), skin conditions (acne, pruritus and rashes), and headache.
Interactions: May interact antagonistically with dopamine receptor antagonists (theoretical concern).

Typical Therapeutic Use

Chaste tree has demonstrated therapeutic benefit in randomised, double-blind, placebo-controlled trials for menstrual cycle irregularities due to latent hyperprolactinaemia,[1] some forms of infertility[2] and premenstrual syndrome (PMS),[3-5] including mastalgia.[6-8] Traditional uses of chaste tree in Western herbal medicine include gynaecological problems, insufficient lactation and to decrease libido.[9-11]

Actions

Prolactin inhibitor, dopaminergic agonist, indirectly progesterogenic, galactagogue.

Key Constituents

Constituents of chaste tree berries include an essential oil (0.7%),[12] diterpenes,[13,14] flavonoids, such as casticin[15] and iridoid glycosides including aucubin and agnuside.[16]

Adulteration

Common adulterants of *V. agnus-castus* are *V. negundo, V. rotundifolia* and *V. trifolia*, which are Asiatic species used in Chinese or Ayurvedic medicine.[17]

Typical Dosage Forms & Dosage

Typical adult dosage range is:
- 1.5 to 3 g/day of dried fruit or by decoction
- 1 to 2.5 mL/day of a 1:2 liquid extract or equivalent in tablet or capsule form

Contraindications

None known.

Use in Pregnancy

Category BI: No increase in frequency of malformation or other harmful effects on the foetus from limited use in women. No evidence of increased foetal damage in animal studies. Use cautiously in pregnancy, and only in the early stages, for insufficient corpus luteal function.

There were no significant differences in maternal toxicity, reproductive outcome or foetal developmental parameters compared to placebo in rats and rabbits orally administered a homoeopathic preparation containing chaste tree tincture during the organogenesis period of gestation. The dosages administered corresponded to 6.3 to 51.1 mg/kg chaste tree in rats and 3.7 to 37 mg/kg chaste tree in rabbits. A non-significant increase in foetal body weight, placental weight and number of resorptions was observed in the high dose group for rabbits. For rabbits, three external deformities occurred in the low dose group and one skull deformity (hydrocephalus) in each of the medium dose and high dose groups. It was not determined whether these results were due to chaste tree, the homeopathic preparation, the alcohol content, or spontaneous occurrences.[18]

Oral administration of the same homeopathic preparation to female rats from 2 weeks before mating until up to 28 days postpartum at doses corresponding to 4 to 40 mg/kg chaste tree had no effects on body weight or development, mating behaviour, fertility, reproductive outcome, or lactation. No teratogenic effects were observed in F_1 or F_2 foetuses, and F_1 and F_2 offspring did not differ from controls.[18] Oral administration of chaste tree seeds (1 or 2 g/kg/day) to pregnant rats from day 1 to day 10 of pregnancy did not reduce the number of foetuses compared to controls.[19] Chaste tree (part unspecified) tested negative for antizygotic, antiimplantation and early abortifacient activity.[20]

Use in Lactation

Category C: Compatible with breastfeeding.

Although the dopaminergic activity of chaste tree might suggest that it is best avoided during lactation,[21,22] clinical trials have demonstrated its positive activity on milk production, albeit at low doses of the berry.[23,24]

As described above, a homeopathic preparation containing chaste tree tincture which was orally administered to female rats, at doses corresponding to 4 to 40 mg/kg chaste tree, during their lactation period did not have toxic effects on either the dams or their F_1 and F_2 offspring[18] (see Use in pregnancy section).

Warnings & Precautions

In general, chaste tree is best not taken in conjunction with progesterone drugs, the contraceptive pill or hormone replacement therapy. Chaste tree may aggravate pure spasmodic dysmenorrhoea not associated with PMS. This may be due to the priming effect of progesterone on the endometrial prostaglandin release during the initial stages of menstruation. However, chaste tree is usually beneficial for spasmodic dysmenorrhoea associated with PMS and for congestive dysmenorrhoea.[25]

Effect on Ability to Drive or Operate Machinery

No adverse effects expected.

Adverse Reactions

A review of the literature found that chaste tree was well tolerated in the majority of studies to the mid-1990s. Side effects were reported in only 1% to 2% of participants in most studies and severe side effects were rarely reported. Gastrointestinal disturbances (particularly nausea) and skin conditions (acne, pruritus and rashes) were the most common effects reported. Side effects occasionally reported included headache, fatigue, and hormone-related symptoms, such as menstrual cycle changes, mastalgia, and weight gain.[17] Chaste tree extract (120 to 480 mg/day) was administered to healthy males for 14 days in a placebo-controlled trial. There were no undesired effects on blood pressure, heart rate, blood count, clinical laboratory parameters or testosterone, FSH, and LH values.[26]

A 32-year-old woman with tubal infertility undergoing unstimulated IVF treatment had signs and symptoms suggestive of mild ovarian hyperstimulation syndrome after commencing a herbal preparation containing chaste tree, *Mitchella repens* and *Viburnum opulus* for 13 days (dose not specified). The preparation was discontinued and her next two menstrual cycles were endocrinologically normal. The authors stated that there was no conclusive evidence that the patient's unusual response was due to the herbal preparation.[27,28]

A 45-year-old woman who had been taking separate bottled products of chaste tree, black cohosh and evening primrose oil for 4 months had three nocturnal seizures within a 3-month period. The patient had also consumed one to two beers 24 to 48 hours prior to each incident.[29] It was not established whether the herbal preparations caused the seizures.

A case was reported in 2001 of a woman diagnosed with grade 1 endometrioid adenocarcinoma of the endometrium "whose history was notable for extensive use of supplemental phytoestrogens". Herbs included chaste tree, dong quai, black cohosh, and licorice.[30] No causality was demonstrated.

Interactions

Chaste tree may interact antagonistically with dopamine receptor antagonists.[31] However, this has not been observed clinically.

A survey of U.K. herbalists found that 93.8% of 145 respondents reported that they had not found any orthodox medications to interact with chaste tree, whilst 70.5% of 149 respondents answered that they did not prescribe chaste tree in conjunction with orthodox oestrogenic/progesterogenic medications.[32]

Safety in Children

No information available.

Overdosage

No incidents found in published literature.

Toxicology

The oral and intraperitoneal LD_{50} of chaste tree extract exceeded 2 g/kg in rats and mice, indicating low toxicity. No animals died at this dose. The no-observed-effect-level of chaste tree extract was 50 mg/kg in a subacute oral toxicity study lasting 28 days, and 40 mg/kg in a chronic oral toxicity study lasting 26 weeks.[17]

As described above, oral administration of a homeopathic preparation containing chaste tree tincture to male rats had no effect on mating behaviour, fertility or reproductive outcome. Male rats received the preparation from 10 weeks before mating until the end of the mating period[18] (see Use in pregnancy).

Genotoxic-mutagenic activity was not observed for the same homeopathic preparation in the Ames test in vitro or in the micronucleus test in vivo after oral administration of a dose corresponding to 370 mg/kg chaste tree.[18]

Regulatory Status

See Table 1 for regulatory status in selected countries.

Table 1   **Regulatory Status for Chaste Tree in Selected Countries**

Australia	Chaste tree is not included in Part 4 of Schedule 4 of the Therapeutic Goods Regulations.
UK & Germany	Chaste tree is included on the General Sale List. It is covered by a positive Commission E monograph.
US	Chaste tree does not have generally recognised as safe (GRAS) status. However, it is freely available as a "dietary supplement" in the US under DSHEA legislation (Dietary Supplement Health and Education Act of 1994).

REFERENCES

1. Milewicz A, Gejdel E, Sworen H, et al: *Arzneim-Forsch* 43:752-756, 1993.
2. Gerhard I, Patek A, Monga B, et al: *Forsch Komplementarmed* 5:272-278, 1998.
3. Schellenberg R: *BMJ* 322:134-137, 2001.
4. Mills SY: *Women's medicine: Vitex agnus castus, the herb*, Christchurch, 1992, Amberwood, p 32.
5. Turner S, Mills S: *Complement Ther Med* 1:73-77, 1993.
6. Wuttke W, Solitt G, Gorkow C, et al: *Geb Fra* 57: 569-574, 1997.
7. Kubista E, Muller G, Spona J: *Rev Fr Gynecol Obstet* 82:221-227, 1987.
8. Kubista E, Muller G, Spona J: *Zentralbl Gynakol* 105:1153-1162, 1983.
9. Felter HW, Lloyd JU: *King's American dispensatory*, ed 18, rev 3, vol 2; first published 1905, reprinted Portland, 1983, Eclectic Medical Publications, p 2056.
10. Mills SY: *The essential book of herbal medicine*, London, 1991, Viking Arkana (Penguin), pp 522-524.
11. Mills SY: *Women's medicine: Vitex agnus castus, the herb*, Christchurch, 1992, Amberwood, pp 10-15.
12. Zwaving JH, Bos R: *Planta Med* 62:83-84, 1996.
13. Hoberg E, Orjala J, Meier B, et al: *Phytochemistry* 52:1555-1558, 1999.
14. Hoberg E, Orjala J, Meier B, et al: *Phytochemistry* 63:375, 2003.
15. Wollenweber E, Mann K: *Planta Med* 48:126-127, 1983.
16. Gorler K, Oehlke D, Soicke H: *Planta Med* 50:530-531, 1985.
17. Upton R, Petrone C, Graff A, eds: Chaste tree fruit: *Vitex agnus-castus*. In *American herbal pharmacopoeia and therapeutic compendium*, Santa Cruz CA, 2001, American Herbal Pharmacopoeia.
18. Blaschek W, Ebel S, Hackenthal E, et al: *HagerROM 2002: Hagers Handbuch der Drogen und Arzneistoffe*, Heidelberg, 2002, Springer.
19. Lal R, Sankaranarayanan A, Mathur VS, et al: *Bull Postgrad Inst Med Educ Res Chandigarh* 19:44-47, 1985.
20. Chaudhury RR: *Plants with possible antifertility activity*, New Delhi, 1966, Indian Council of Medical Research, Special report series no. 55, pp 3-19.
21. Sliutz G, Speiser P, Schultz AM, et al: *Horm Metab Res* 25:253-255, 1993.
22. Winterhoff H: *Abstracts of Papers American Chemical Society* 212:AGFD 105, 1996.
23. Mohr W: *Dtsch Med Wschr* 79:1513-1516, 1954.
24. Noack M: *Dtsch Med Wschr* 9:204-206, 1943.
25. Mills S, Bone K: *Principles and practice of phytotherapy: modern herbal medicine*, Edinburgh, 2000, Churchill Livingstone, pp 328-334.
26. Loew D, Gorkow C, Schrodter A, et al: *Z Phytother* 17: 237-240, 243, 1996.
27. Cahill DJ, Fox R, Wardle PG, et al: *Hum Reprod* 9: 1469-1470, 1994.

28. Cahill DJ: *Hum Reprod* 10:2175-2176, 1995.

29. Shuster J: *Hosp Pharm* 31:1553-1554, 1996.

30. Johnson EB, Muto MC, Yanushpolsky EH, et al: *Obstet Gynecol* 98:947-950, 2001.

31. Blumenthal M et al, eds: *The complete German Commission E monographs: therapeutic guide to herbal medicines,* Austin, 1998, American Botanical Council, p 108.

32. Christie S, Walker AF: *Eur J Herbal Med* 3:29-45, 1997.

CHICKWEED

Other common name: Stellaria
Botanical name: *Stellaria media* (L.) Vill.
Family: Caryophyllaceae
Plant part used: Aerial parts

Safety Summary

Pregnancy category B2: No increase in frequency of malformation or other harmful effects on the foetus from limited use in women. Animal studies are lacking.
Lactation category C: Compatible with breast-feeding.
Contraindications: Contraindicated in those with known allergy or sensitivity.
Warnings & precautions: None required on current evidence.
Adverse reactions: None found in published literature.
Interactions: No precautions required on current evidence.

Typical Therapeutic Use

In Western herbal medicine chickweed is used topically as a cooling demulcent and to treat eczema, psoriasis, indolent ulcer, and abscesses. Internal indications include rheumatism.[1,2]

Actions

Demulcent, astringent, refrigerant, antiulcer (peptic), gastrointestinal inflammation.

Key Constituents

The aerial parts of chickweed contain flavonoids, phenolic acids, triterpenoid saponins, phytosterols, carotenoids,[3] and lipids.[4]

Adulteration

No adulterants known.

Typical Dosage Forms & Dosage

Typical adult dosage ranges are:
- 3 to 15 g/day of dried aerial parts or by infusion
- 3 to 15 mL/day of a 1:1 liquid extract
- 3 to 6 mL/day of a fresh plant succus or equivalent in tablet or capsule form
- 6 to 30 mL/day of a 1:5 tincture

Contraindications

Contraindicated in those with known allergy or sensitivity.

Use in Pregnancy

Category B2: No increase in frequency of malformation or other harmful effects on the foetus from limited use in women. Animal studies are lacking.

Use in Lactation

Category C: Compatible with breastfeeding.

Warnings & Precautions

Avoid in patients with known allergy.

Effect on Ability to Drive or Operate Machinery

No adverse effects expected.

Adverse Reactions

Allergic rashes may occasionally result from topical use.

Interactions

None reported.

Safety in Children

No information available but adverse effects are not expected, other than allergy.

Overdosage

There is one case of alleged nitrate toxicity leading to paralysis, but the chickweed implicated in this case may have been contaminated by artificial fertilisers.[5] A typical analysis indicates the nitrate content of chickweed to be 103 mg/100 g of fresh leaf.[6]

Both sheep and lambs are negatively affected by the formation of lumps of chickweed in the stomach, which is followed by fermentation. The seed of chickweed produces gastrointestinal upset when eaten in large amounts by lambs.[7]

Toxicology

The LD_{50} value of 1 g/kg was obtained from i.p. administration of an ethanol extract of aerial parts of chickweed in rats.[8]

The water fraction of a methanol extract of the (nonreproductive) aerial parts of chickweed demonstrated some toxicity in a fruit fly toxicity assay (67% lethality) and zero toxicity in the brine shrimp assay. The cyclohexane extract and the ethyl acetate fraction of the methanol extract produced greater than 80% lethality in the fruit fly assay.[9] The fruit fly and brine shrimp assays are rapid and inexpensive and provide information upon which to base decisions for toxicity evaluation using larger animal assays.

Table **1**   **Regulatory Status for Chickweed in Selected Countries**

Australia	Chickweed is not included in Part 4 of Schedule 4 of the Therapeutic Goods Regulations.
UK & Germany	Chickweed is included on the General Sale List. It was not included in the Commission E assessment.
US	Chickweed does not have generally recognised as safe (GRAS) status. However, it is freely available as a "dietary supplement" in the US under DSHEA legislation (Dietary Supplement Health and Education Act of 1994).

Regulatory Status

See Table 1 for regulatory status in selected countries.

REFERENCES

1. British Herbal Medicine Association's Scientific Committee: *British herbal pharmacopoeia*, Bournemouth, 1983, BHMA, pp 198-199.
2. Felter HW, Lloyd JU: *King's American dispensatory*, ed 18, rev 3, vol 2; first published 1905, reprinted Portland, 1983, Eclectic Medical Publications, pp 1834-1835.
3. Kitanov GM: *Pharmazie* 47:470-471, 1992.
4. Pande A, Shukla YN, Tripathi AK: *Phytochem* 39: 709-711, 1995.
5. McGuffin M, Hobbs C, Upton R, Goldberg A, eds: *American Herbal Products Association's botanical safety handbook*, Boca Raton, 1997, CRC Press, p 110.
6. Guil JL, Rodriguez-Garcia I, Torija E: *Plant Foods Hum Nutr* 51:99-107, 1997.
7. Watt JM, Breyer-Brandwijk MG: *The medicinal and poisonous plants of southern and eastern Africa: being an account of their medicinal and other uses, chemical composition, pharmacological effects and toxicology in man and animal*, ed 2, Edinburgh, 1962, Livingstone, p 177.
8. Sharma ML, Chandokhe N, Ghatak BJ, et al: *Indian J Exp Biol* 16:228-240, 1978.
9. McChesney JD, Adams RP: *Econ Bot* 39:74-86, 1985.

CLEAVERS

Other common name: Clivers
Botanical name: *Galium aparine* L.
Family: Rubiaceae
Plant part used: Aerial parts

Safety Summary

Pregnancy category B2: No increase in frequency of malformation or other harmful effects on the foetus from limited use in women. Animal studies are lacking.
Lactation category C: Compatible with breast-feeding.
Contraindications: None required on current evidence.
Warnings & precautions: None required on current evidence.
Adverse reactions: None found in published literature.
Interactions: No precautions required on current evidence.

Typical Therapeutic Use

Traditional uses of cleavers in Western herbal medicine include psoriasis and other skin diseases, lymphadenopathy, lymphadenitis, enlarged lymph nodes, dysuria.[1,2]

Actions

Diuretic, depurative.

Key Constituents

Key constituents of cleavers include iridoid glycosides (especially monotropein), phenolic acids, and flavonoids.[2] Scopoletin has been isolated from the methanolic extract of cleavers.[3]

Adulteration

No adulterants known.

Typical Dosage Forms & Dosage

Typical adult dosage ranges are:

- 6 to 12 g/day of dried aerial parts or by infusion
- 15 to 45 mL/day of expressed juice
- 6 to 12 mL/day of a 1:1 liquid extract
- 3.5 to 7 mL/day of a 1:2 liquid extract or equivalent in tablet or capsule form
- 12 to 30 mL/day of a 1:5 tincture

Contraindications

None known.

Use in Pregnancy

Category B2: No increase in frequency of malformation or other harmful effects on the foetus from limited use in women. Animal studies are lacking.

Use in Lactation

Category C: Compatible with breastfeeding.

Warnings & Precautions

Depuratives can, in many cases, be provocative to skin disease. Care needs to be taken to reduce the prospect of major exacerbations.

Effect on Ability to Drive or Operate Machinery

No adverse effects expected.

Adverse Reactions

None recorded.

Interactions

None expected.

Safety in Children

No information available but adverse effects are not expected.

Overdosage

No incidents found in published literature.

Toxicology

The LD$_{50}$ value of 1 g/kg was obtained from i.p. administration of an ethanol extract of whole plant of cleavers in rats.[4]

The water fraction of a methanol extract of the (nonreproductive) aerial parts of cleavers demonstrated no toxicity in a brine shrimp and fruit fly toxicity assay. The ethyl acetate fraction produced greater than 80% lethality in both assays.[5] The fruit fly and brine shrimp assays are rapid and inexpensive, and provide information upon which to base decisions for toxicity evaluation using larger animal assays.

Intravenous administration of cleavers extract lowered arterial pressure up to 50% in dogs, without slowing the pulse and without demonstrating toxicity.[6]

Contamination of feed with cleavers seed has caused poisoning in chickens, particularly of the young. The seed surface is covered with small hooks[7] and at least part of the toxicity is mechanical, with gastric obstruction and intestinal atony

occurring.[8] Changes in haematological parameters have also been observed.[9]

Regulatory Status

See Table 1 for regulatory status in selected countries.

Table **1: Regulatory Status for Cleavers in Selected Countries**

Australia	Cleavers is not included in Part 4 of Schedule 4 of the Therapeutic Goods Regulations.
UK & Germany	Cleavers is included on the General Sale List. It was not included in the Commission E assessment.
US	Cleavers does not have generally recognised as safe (GRAS) status. However, it is freely available as a "dietary supplement" in the US under DSHEA legislation (Dietary Supplement Health and Education Act of 1994).

REFERENCES

1. British Herbal Medicine Association's Scientific Committee: *British herbal pharmacopoeia,* Bournemouth, 1983, BHMA, pp 96-97.
2. British Herbal Medicine Association: *British herbal compendium,* vol 1, Bournemouth, 1992, BHMA, pp 61-62.
3. Seabra RM, Silveira JA, Vasconcelos MH: *Plant Med Phytother* 26:49-51, 1993.
4. Sharma ML, Chandokhe N, Ghatak BJ, et al: *Indian J Exp Biol* 16:228-240, 1978.
5. McChesney JD, Adams RP: *Econ Bot* 39:74–86, 1985.
6. Delas R, Dulucq-Mathou Th, Stanislas E, et al: *Toulouse Med* 49:57-64, 1948.
7. Cermakova J: *Veterinarstvi* 38:361-362, 1988.
8. Januszewski J, Lewandowski L, Mazurkiewicz M: *Med Weter* 44:365-367, 1988.
9. Mazurkiewicz M, Gawel A, Kozlik D, et al: *Zest Nauk Akad Roln Wrocl Weter* 49:205-216, 1991.

CODONOPSIS

Other common name: Dang shen
Botanical names: *Codonopsis pilosula* (Franch.) Nannf., *Codonopsis pilosula* Nannf. var *modesta* (Nannf.) L.T. Shen, *Codonopsis tangshen* Oliv., *Codonopsis nervosa* (Chipp.) Nannf., *Codonopsis clematidea* (Schrenk) C.B.Clarke in Hook.f.
Family: Campanulaceae
Plant part used: Root

Safety Summary

Pregnancy category B1: No increase in frequency of malformation or other harmful effects on the foetus from limited use in women. No evidence of increased foetal damage in animal studies.
Lactation category C: Compatible with breast-feeding.
Contraindications: None required on current evidence.
Warnings & precautions: None required on current evidence.
Adverse reactions: None found in published literature.
Interactions: No precautions required on current evidence.

Typical Therapeutic Use

Therapeutic indications for codonopsis in traditional Chinese medicine (TCM) include shortness of breath with chronic cough or palpitations, fatigue, loss of appetite, and diarrhoea.[1-3] It is sometimes used as a cheaper substitute for *Panax ginseng*. Codonopsis has demonstrated therapeutic benefit in patients with coronary heart disease in an uncontrolled trial[4] and as an adjuvant to radiotherapy in the treatment of cancer in a controlled trial.[5]

Actions

Tonic.

Key Constituents

Constituents of codonopsis root include sterols, triterpenes, an essential oil, and phenylpropanoid glucosides named tangshenosides. The alkaloids, codonopsine and codonopsinine, have been isolated from *C. clematidea*.[6] Triterpenoid saponins, including ginseng saponins, have not been found in codonopsis.[7]

Adulteration

Campanumoea javania and *Platysodon grandiflorus* are listed as adulterants of codonopsis.[8]

Typical Dosage Forms & Dosage

Typical adult dosage ranges are:
- 9 to 30 g of dried root per day by decoction
- 4.5 to 8.5 mL/day of a 1:2 liquid extract or equivalent in tablet or capsule form

Contraindications

None known.

Use in Pregnancy

Category B1: No increase in frequency of malformation or other harmful effects on the foetus from limited use in women. No evidence of increased foetal damage in animal studies.

Subcutaneous administration of codonopsis aqueous extract (0.1 to 0.4 mL/day) for 5 days did not affect fertility or exhibit teratogenic effects in mice.[9]

Use in Lactation

Category C: Compatible with breastfeeding.

Warnings & Precautions

According to TCM,[1] codonopsis is incompatible with Rhizoma et Radix Veratri (*Veratrum nigrum*, li lu).

Effect on Ability to Drive or Operate Machinery

No adverse effects expected.

Adverse Reactions

No adverse reactions documented.

Interactions

None reported.

Safety in Children

No information available but adverse effects are not expected.

Overdosage

Doses of codonopsis exceeding 60 g may cause precordial discomfort (chest pain) and arrhythmia.[2]

Toxicology

Table 1 lists LD$_{50}$ data recorded for codonopsis.[2]

Table 1   **LD$_{50}$ Data Recorded for Codonopsis**

Substance	Route, Model	LD$_{50}$ Value	Reference
Codonopsis	i.p., mice	79.2 g/kg	2
Codonopsine	i.p., mice	66 to 79 mg/kg	2

Codonopsis did not produce toxic reactions when administered to rats by subcutaneous injection (0.5 g) for 13 days or to rabbits by intraperitoneal injection (1 g) for 15 days.[2]

Regulatory Status

See Table 2 for regulatory status in selected countries.

Table 2   **Regulatory Status for Codonopsis in Selected Countries**

Australia	Codonopsis is not included in Part 4 of Schedule 4 of the Therapeutic Goods Regulations.
China	Codonopsis is official in the *Pharmacopoeia of the People's Republic of China* 1997. The usual adult dosage, usually administered in the form of a decoction, is listed as 9 to 30 g.
UK & Germany	Codonopsis is not included on the General Sale List. It was not included in the Commission E assessment.
US	Codonopsis does not have generally recognised as safe (GRAS) status. However, it is freely available as a "dietary supplement" in the US under DSHEA legislation (Dietary Supplement Health and Education Act of 1994).

REFERENCES

1. Pharmacopoeia Commission of the People's Republic of China: *Pharmacopoeia of the People's Republic of China*, vol 1, English ed, Beijing, 1997, Chemical Industry Press, p 145.
2. Chang HM, But PP: *Pharmacology and applications of Chinese materia medica*, vol 2, Singapore, 1987, World Scientific, pp 975-978.
3. Bensky D, Gamble A: *Chinese herbal medicine materia medica*, Seattle, 1986, Eastland Press, pp 454-455.
4. Xu X, Wang SR, Lin Q: *Chung Kuo Chung Hsi I Chieh Ho Tsa Chih* 15:398-400, 1995.
5. Zneg XL, Li XA, Zhang BY: *Chung Kuo Chung Hsi I Chieh Ho Tsa Chih* 12:607-608, 581, 1992.
6. Tang W, Eisenbrand G: *Chinese drugs of plant origin*, Berlin, 1992, Springer-Verlag, pp 357-359.
7. Wong MP, Chiang TC, Chang HM: *Planta Med* 49:60, 1983.
8. Fu RZ, Wang J, Zhang YB, et al: *Planta Med* 65:648-650, 1999.
9. Matsui AS, Rogers J, Woo YK, et al: *Med Pharmacol Exp* 16:414-424, 1967.

CORN SILK

Other common name: Zea
Botanical name: *Zea mays* L.
Family: Gramineae
Plant part used: Style and stigma

Safety Summary

Pregnancy category B2: No increase in frequency of malformation or other harmful effects on the foetus from limited use in women. Animal studies are lacking.
Lactation category C: Compatible with breastfeeding.
Contraindications: None required on current evidence.
Warnings & precautions: None required on current evidence.
Adverse reactions: None found in published literature.
Interactions: No precautions required on current evidence.

Typical Therapeutic Use

Traditional indications for corn silk in Western herbal medicine include inflammatory conditions and infections of the prostate and urinary system.[1] In addition to its use as a diuretic, corn silk is used to reduce blood pressure in traditional Chinese medicine. Diuretic activity has been demonstrated in uncontrolled trials.[2]

Actions

Diuretic, antilithic, urinary demulcent.

Key Constituents

Key constituents of corn silk are flavonoids, especially 6-C-glycosylflavones, the major one of which is maysin. Like many diuretic herbs, corn silk contains potassium.[3]

Adulteration

No adulterants known.

Typical Dosage Forms & Dosage

Typical adult dosage ranges are:

- 12 to 24 g/day of dried style and stigma or by infusion
- 2 to 6 mL/day of a 1:1 liquid extract or equivalent in tablet or capsule form
- 15 to 45 mL/day of a 1:5 tincture

Contraindications

None known.

Use in Pregnancy

Category B2: No increase in frequency of malformation or other harmful effects on the foetus from limited use in women. Animal studies are lacking.

Use in Lactation

Category C: Compatible with breastfeeding.

Warnings & Precautions

None required.

Effect on Ability to Drive or Operate Machinery

No adverse effects expected.

Adverse Reactions

No adverse reactions documented for corn silk. Dermatitis has occurred from contact with leaf and cob.[4]

Interactions

None reported.

Safety in Children

No information available, but adverse effects are not expected. Eclectic physicians recommended corn silk to be of value in bladder disorders of children.[5]

Overdosage

No incidents found in published literature for poisoning associated with corn silk. Corn used as grain, forage, or silage has been responsible for a variety of diseases in livestock. This may result from an abnormally high nitrate content or from ingestion of mouldy or unripe corn.[6,7]

Toxicology

The methanol-insoluble fraction of corn silk aqueous extract has an LD_{50} of 250 mg/kg in rabbits when administered by intravenous injection. (The effective diuretic dose was 1.5 mg/kg by i.v. injection and 6 mg/kg by oral administration.) Oral preparations are described as "almost nontoxic".[2]

The constituents of corn silk were investigated in the early 20th century and were found to have no significant toxicity.[8]

The results of a toxicology study published in 1992 indicate that the aqueous extract of corn silk was not significantly toxic at the low and medium oral doses tested (50 and 100 mg/kg, in rats).[9]

Regulatory Status

See Table 1 for regulatory status in selected countries.

Table 1 **Regulatory Status for Corn Silk in Selected Countries**

Australia	Corn silk is not included in Part 4 of Schedule 4 of the Therapeutic Goods Regulations.
UK & Germany	Corn silk is not included on the General Sale List. It was not included in the Commission E assessment.
US	Corn silk does have generally recognised as safe (GRAS) status. It is freely available as a "dietary supplement" in the US under DSHEA legislation (Dietary Supplement Health and Education Act of 1994).

REFERENCES

1. British Herbal Medicine Association's Scientific Committee: *British herbal pharmacopoeia*, Bournemouth, 1983, BHMA, pp 238-239.
2. Chang HM, But PP: *Pharmacology and applications of Chinese materia medica*, vol 1, Singapore, 1987, World Scientific, pp 293-297.
3. British Herbal Medicine Association: *British herbal compendium*, vol 1, Bournemouth, 1992, BHMA, pp 69-70.
4. Mitchell J, Rook A: Botanical dermatology: *Plants and plant products injurious to the skin*, Vancouver, 1979, Greengrass, pp 344-345.
5. Felter HW, Lloyd JU: *King's American dispensatory*, ed 18, rev 3, vol 2, first published 1905, reprinted Portland, 1983, Eclectic Medical Publications, pp 2092-2093.
6. Kingsbury JM: *Poisonous plants for the United States and Canada*, Englewood Cliffs, 1964, Prentice Hall, pp 495-500.
7. Chopra RN, Badhwar RL, Ghosh S: *Poisonous plants of India*, vol II, New Delhi, 1965, Indian Council of Agricultural Research, pp 943-945.
8. Watt JM, Breyer-Brandwijk MG: *The medicinal and poisonous plants of Southern and Eastern Africa: Being an account of their medicinal and other uses, chemical composition, pharmacological effects and toxicology in man and animal*, ed 2, Edinburgh, 1962, Livingstone, pp 489-494.
9. Garg DK, Goyal RN: *J Appl Toxicol* 12:359-363, 1992.

COUCH GRASS

Botanical names: *Agropyron repens* (L.) Beauv (*Elymus repens* (L.) Gould, *Elytrigia repens* (L.) Desv. ex B.D. Jackson, *Triticum repens* L.)
Family: Gramineae
Plant part used: Rhizome

Safety Summary

Pregnancy category B2: No increase in frequency of malformation or other harmful effects on the foetus from limited use in women. Animal studies are lacking.
Lactation category C: Compatible with breastfeeding.
Contraindications: None required on current evidence.
Warnings & precautions: Copious fluid intake should not be undertaken if oedema due to impaired cardiac or renal function exists (Commission E warning).
Adverse reactions: None found in published literature.
Interactions: No precautions required on current evidence.

Typical Therapeutic Use

Couch grass extract demonstrated therapeutic benefit in patients with urinary tract infection or irritable bladder in a postmarketing surveillance study.[1] Traditional indications for couch grass in Western herbal medicine include cystitis, urethritis, prostatitis, benign prostatic hyperplasia, and urinary calculi.[2]

Actions

Soothing diuretic, urinary demulcent.

Key Constituents

Constituents of couch grass include polysaccharides (triticin), sugar alcohols, and possibly saponins.[3]

Adulteration

The principal adulterant is the rhizome of *Cynodon dactylon*. *Imperata cylindrica* and *Carex* spp. have also been noted as adulterants.[3,4]

Typical Dosage Forms & Dosage

Typical adult dosage ranges are:

- 12 to 24 g/day of dried rhizome or by decoction
- 3 to 6 mL/day of a 1:1 liquid extract or equivalent in tablet or capsule form
- 15 to 30 mL/day of a 1:5 tincture

Contraindications

None known.

Use in Pregnancy

Category B2: No increase in frequency of malformation or other harmful effects on the foetus from limited use in women. Animal studies are lacking.

Use in Lactation

Category C: Compatible with breastfeeding.

Warnings & Precautions

The Commission E advises that copious fluid intake should not be undertaken if oedema due to impaired cardiac or renal function exists.[5]

Effect on Ability to Drive or Operate Machinery

No adverse effects expected.

Adverse Reactions

In an uncontrolled study, patients allergic to the pollen of a number of taxonomically diverse species were shown to have IgE antibodies to couch grass pollen.[6] Intradermal skin tests with couch grass pollen demonstrated a positive reaction in 15% of 1000 dogs with a history of atopic dermatitis in south-eastern Australia.[7] However, pollen should not be present in preparations of couch grass rhizome.

Interactions

None known.

Safety in Children

No information available, but adverse effects are not expected.

Overdosage

No incidents found in published literature.

Toxicology

Couch grass extract tested negative for in vitro mutagenic activity in the Ames test.[8]

Regulatory Status

See Table 1 for regulatory status in selected countries.

Table 1   **Regulatory Status for Couch Grass in Selected Countries**

Australia	Couch grass is not included in Part 4 of Schedule 4 of the Therapeutic Goods Regulations.
UK & Germany	*Agropyron* (*Triticum*) is included on the General Sale List, although the species is not defined. It is covered by a positive Commission E monograph.
	Couch grass is official in the *British Pharmacopoeia* 2002 and the *European Pharmacopoeia* 4.3.
US	Couch grass does have generally recognised as safe (GRAS) status. It is freely available as a "dietary supplement" in the US under DSHEA legislation (Dietary Supplement Health and Education Act of 1994).

REFERENCES

1. Hautmann C, Scheithe K: *Z Phytother* 21:252-255, 2000.
2. British Herbal Medicine Association's Scientific Committee: *British herbal pharmacopoeia*, Bournemouth, 1983, BHMA, pp 17-18.
3. Bisset NG (ed): *Herbal drugs and phytopharmaceuticals: A handbook for practice on a scientific basis.* Stuttgart, 1994, Medpharm Scientific Publishers, pp 241-242.
4. Blaschek W, Ebel S, Hackenthal E, et al: *HagerROM 2002: Hagers Handbuch der Drogen und Arzneistoffe*, Heidelberg, 2002, Springer.
5. Blumenthal M, et al (eds): *The complete German Commission E monographs: Therapeutic guide to herbal medicines*, Austin, 1998, American Botanical Council, p 118.
6. Pham NH, Baldo BA: *Clin Exp Allergy* 25:599-606, 1995.
7. Mueller RS, Bettenay SV, Tideman L: *Aust Vet J* 78:392-399, 2000.
8. Schimmer O, Kruger A, Paulini H, et al: *Pharmazie* 49:448-451, 1994.

CRAMP BARK

Botanical names: *Viburnum opulus* L., *V. opulus* L. var. *americanum* Ait.
Family: Caprifoliaceae
Plant part used: Bark

Safety Summary

Pregnancy category B2: No increase in frequency of malformation or other harmful effects on the foetus from limited use in women. Animal studies are lacking.
Lactation category C: Compatible with breastfeeding.
Contraindications: None required on current evidence.
Warnings & precautions: None required on current evidence.
Adverse reactions: None found in published literature.
Interactions: No precautions required on current evidence.

Typical Therapeutic Use

Traditional indications for cramp bark in Western herbal medicine include spasmodic muscular cramps, hypertension, ovarian and uterine pains, threatened miscarriage, and as a partus praeparator.[1,2]

Actions

Spasmolytic, mild sedative, astringent, hypotensive, peripheral vasodilator.

Key Constituents

The constituents of cramp bark are not well defined, but the presence of catechin and epicatechin and the absence of amentoflavone are considered characteristic (for differentiation from *Viburnum prunifolium* [black haw]). The coumarins scopoletin and scopolin are also present, although apparently only in trace amounts.[2]

Adulteration

Historically, adulterants of cramp bark have included mountain maple or false cramp bark (*Acer spicatum*) and other *Viburnum* spp., such as black haw (*V. prunifolium*) and the toxic southern cramp bark (*V. alnifolium*). Black haw is the main adulterant presently, and *V. trilobum* is used interchangeably in some

areas. Pharmacological studies conducted prior to 1940 cannot be relied upon for correct identification of plant material.[2-4]

Typical Dosage Forms & Dosage

Typical adult dosage ranges are:
- 6 to 12 g/day of dried bark or by decoction
- 6 to 12 mL/day of a 1:1 liquid extract
- 2 to 4.5 mL/day of a 1:2 liquid extract or equivalent in tablet or capsule form
- 15 to 30 mL/day of a 1:5 tincture

Contraindications

None known.

Use in Pregnancy

Category B2: No increase in frequency of malformation or other harmful effects on the foetus from limited use in women. Animal studies are lacking.

Cramp bark has long been used in Western herbal medicine for threatened miscarriage and as a partus praeparator to facilitate childbirth.[1,2,5]

Scopoletin did not demonstrate teratogenic activity in rats after oral intubation during the organogenesis period.[6]

Use in Lactation

Category C: Compatible with breastfeeding.

Warnings & Precautions

None required.

Effect on Ability to Drive or Operate Machinery

No adverse effects expected.

Adverse Reactions

Investigating physicians in the late 1900s reported that "high" (undefined) doses caused some nervous system depression.[2]

Interactions

None known.

Safety in Children

No information available for cramp bark, but adverse effects are not expected.

Mild cases of poisoning in children due to the ingestion of berries have been reported (see Overdosage section).

Overdosage

An early source reports that large doses or prolonged use of cramp bark extract can cause vertigo, vomiting, disturbances of speech, movement and consciousness, dyspnoea, and dry mouth.[7]

The berries, but not the bark, of cramp bark have been associated with serious poisoning in 19th-century literature. However, only mild cases of poisoning in children have been reported recently, due to the ingestion of unripe berries or large quantities of berries.[8] Nineteen cases have been reported in the database DIMDI Intox. Only mild symptoms were observed, such as diarrhoea, vomiting, nausea, and mild burning in the mouth. In an evaluation of 400 cases (1965 to 1991), where the children ate 10 to 20 berries or an unknown quantity, symptoms of nausea, vomiting, flank pain, and diarrhoea developed in only 10% of cases.[7]

Toxicology

Rats fed rations containing 70 mg scopoletin per 100 g for up to 12 months showed brain histology suggestive of neuropathic pathogenesis.[9] However, the relevance of this research to the safe use of cramp bark would be very low.

Regulatory Status

See Table 1 for regulatory status in selected countries.

Table **1**   **Regulatory Status for Cramp Bark in Selected Countries**

Australia	Cramp bark is not included in Part 4 of Schedule 4 of the Therapeutic Goods Regulations.
UK & Germany	Cramp bark is not included on the General Sale List. It was not included in the Commission E assessment.
US	Cramp bark does not have generally recognised as safe (GRAS) status. However, it is freely available as a "dietary supplement" in the US under DSHEA legislation (Dietary Supplement Health and Education Act of 1994).

REFERENCES

1. British Herbal Medicine Association's Scientific Committee: *British herbal pharmacopoeia*, Bournemouth, 1983, BHMA, p 230.
2. American Herbal Pharmacopoeia: *Cramp bark – Viburnum opulus: Analytical, quality control, and therapeutic monograph*, Santa Cruz, February 2000, American Herbal Pharmacopoeia.
3. Lloyd JU: *Druggist Circ* 59:87-90, 1915.
4. Costello CH, Lynn EV: *J Am Pharm Assoc* 32:20-22, 1943.
5. Felter HW, Lloyd JU: *King's American dispensatory*, ed 18, rev 3, vol 2, first published 1905, reprinted Portland, 1983, Eclectic Medical Publications, pp 2058-2059.
6. Ruddick JA, Harwig J, Scott PM: *Teratology* 9:165-168, 1974.
7. Blaschek W, Ebel S, Hackenthal E, et al: *HagerROM 2002: Hagers Handbuch der Drogen und Arzneistoffe*, Heidelberg, 2002, Springer.
8. Frohne D, Pfander HJ: *A colour atlas of poisonous plants: A handbook for pharmacists, doctors, toxicologists, and biologists*, translated from the 2nd German ed by NG Bisset, London, 1984, Wolfe Publishing, p 85.
9. Ezeanyika LU, Obidoa O, Shoyinka VO: *Plant Foods Hum Nutr* 53:351-358, 1999.

CRANBERRY

Botanical name: *Vaccinium macrocarpon* Ait.
Family: Ericaceae
Plant part used: Fruit

Safety Summary

Pregnancy category A: No proven increase in the frequency of malformation or other harmful effects on the foetus despite consumption by a large number of women.
Lactation category C: Compatible with breastfeeding.
Contraindications: None required on current evidence.
Warnings & precautions: Use with caution if there is a history of oxalate urinary stones. The commercial juice may be unsuitable for diabetics.
Adverse reactions: None of significance found in published literature.
Interactions: Caution in patients taking warfarin.

Typical Therapeutic Use

Cranberry juice was shown to reduce bacteriuria in older women in a randomised double-blind placebo-controlled trial,[1] and the tablet form was shown to be even more cost effective.[2] There may be a direct reduction in adhesion of Gram-negative bacteria (such as *Escherichia coli*, *Proteus*, *Klebsiella*, *Enterobacter*, and *Pseudomonas*) on the walls of the urinary tract,[3,4] which may, in turn, be mediated by nonspecific competitive binding of bacterial lectins by elements in the cranberry juice, a property which may have application to bacterial infections in the mouth and even to *Helicobacter pylori* infection.[5] A high-molecular-weight, low-sugar extract of cranberry has been shown to reduce aggregation of plaque-forming bacteria in vitro.[6]

Actions

Bacteriostatic, especially in the urinary tract; astringent.

Key Constituents

Key constituents of cranberry include: procyanidins (also known as proanthocyanidins and polyphenols), including catechin and epicatechin[7,8]; anthocyanins (glycosides of cyanidin and peonidin)[9]; flavonoids,[10] including quercetin and myricetin[11]; organic acids (quinic, malic, citric and benzoic acids)[12,13]; vitamin C; sugars (glucose to fructose ratio of 3.55, which is unusual for a fruit juice)[14]; amino acids, and peptides.[15]

Adulteration

Due to widespread cultivation, adulteration of cranberry with other species of *Vaccinium* is unlikely. *Vaccinium corymbosum* has occasionally been found as an adulterant in the United States, and *V. uliginosum* has been found historically as an adulterant in Europe, although not in recent years. Cranberry juice products have been adulterated with colouring agents.[9]

Typical Dosage Forms & Dosage

Typical adult dosage ranges are:
- 10 to 20 g/day of fresh fruit or equivalent in tablet or capsule form
- 400 to 800 mg/day of dry concentrate (25:1)
- 75 to 300 mL/day of a commercial juice

Contraindications

None required on current evidence.

Use in Pregnancy

Category A: No proven increase in the frequency of malformation or other harmful effects on the foetus, despite consumption by a large number of women. Subject to urinary oxalate increases, cranberry is safe and widely used prophylactically as a beverage against urinary infections in pregnancy.

Use in Lactation

Category C: Compatible with breastfeeding.

Warnings & Precautions

Cranberries contain moderate levels of oxalates. A 47-year-old man with a history of calcium oxalate kidney stones developed recurrent stones. He had been taking cranberry concentrate tablets twice daily for the previous 6 months. Intake of cranberry concentrate tablets at recommended dosage for 7 days in five healthy volunteers on a normal diet increased urinary oxalate levels by an average of 43.4%, with rises also in urinary calcium, phosphate, and sodium. Inhibitors of stone formation, specifically magnesium and potassium, also increased.[16] (This study has been criticised for not measuring intakes of calcium and vitamin C, both contributors to urinary oxalates, and for failing to measure the content of oxalate in the tablets.[17]) A review of the effect of dietary oxalate and calcium on urinary oxalate, and risk of formation of kidney stones, found that cranberry juice had no effect on urinary oxalate excretion. Only eight foods (spinach, rhubarb, beets, nuts, chocolate, tea, wheat bran, and strawberries) caused a significant increase in urinary oxalate excretion.[18] The use of cranberry juice should be limited in those with a history of urinary stones.

Earlier studies involving healthy volunteers have not found cranberry to have a large effect on urinary oxalates.[19,20] The value for urinary oxalate excretion was high for spinach (1.2 g), moderate for chocolate (126 mg) and tea (66 mg), and low for cranberry juice, vegetable juice, pecans, and orange juice (2 to 26 mg).[19]

The high sugar content of commercial juices may make regular use unsuitable; they should be avoided in diabetes.

Effect on Ability to Drive or Operate Machinery

No adverse effects expected.

Adverse Reactions

A Cochrane review that analysed five controlled trials for the prevention of urinary tract infections found a high dropout rate, which suggests that drinking considerable amounts of cranberry juice over a long period may not be acceptable to patients.[21] Details are provided in Table 1, which indicates a low incidence of reported side effects.

In a study group of normal and uraemic men, cranberry consumption increased the renal excretion of hippuric acid and increased acid secretory

Table 1   **Adverse Event Information for Well-Designed, Randomised or Quasi-Randomised, Controlled, Double-Blind Trials Evaluating Cranberry**

Study, Dosage, Duration	No. of Patients (Total)	No. of Patients Withdrawn or Lost to Follow-up	Adverse Events
Walker (1997)*; cranberry capsules containing 400 mg of cranberry solids (number per day not stated) for 6 months total	19	9	No participants reported side effects; withdrawals were due to pregnancy, unrelated infections requiring antibiotics, or moving from the area
Avorn (1994); elderly women, 300 mL/day cranberry juice cocktail containing 30% cranberry concentrate for 6 months	192	39	No data were provided for side effects or for the reasons for withdrawal
Haverkorn (1994)*; elderly men and women; 30 mL/day cranberry juice (concentration not specified) for 8 weeks total	38	22	No data were provided for side effects or for the reasons for withdrawal
Foda (1995)*; children with neuropathic bladder, managed by intermittent catheterisation; 15 mL/kg/day cranberry juice cocktail containing 30% cranberry concentrate for 12 months total	40	19	17 dropouts from cranberry group: 12 specified cranberry as the reason – taste (9), caloric load (2), cost (1); other 5 – too busy (2), no reason (2), nonurologic death (1) 2 dropouts in placebo (water) group, no reason given

Table I   **Adverse Event Information for Well-Designed, Randomised or Quasi-Randomised, Controlled, Double-Blind Trials Evaluating Cranberry—Cont'd**

Study, Dosage, Duration	No. of Patients (Total)	No. of Patients Withdrawn or Lost to Follow-up	Adverse Events
Schlager (1999)*; children with neuropathic bladder and managed by intermittent catheterisation; 300 mL/day cranberry juice cocktail containing 30% cranberry concentrate for 6 months total	15	None	No side effects were reported

Duration: total = active + placebo for crossover trials.

activity in the nephron. This effect is inadvisable in patients with renal insufficiency.[22]

Interactions

The U.K. Committee on Safety and Medicines has received five reports since 1999 suggesting that cranberry juice had an effect on increasing the potency of warfarin. One death was attributed to this interaction[23]; however, the robustness of the association is not known. It is also not known if supplements prepared from cranberry might also have the same effect, and whether the interaction was due to an excessive intake of cranberry juice. Until further information is available, patients taking warfarin should limit or avoid intake of cranberry juice.

Omeprazole causes protein-bound vitamin B_{12} malabsorption, and ingestion of an acidic drink improves protein-bound vitamin B_{12} absorption. A clinical study involving healthy, elderly volunteers verified that, with cranberry juice ingestion, the omeprazole-treated group showed increased absorption of protein-bound vitamin B_{12}.[24]

Twenty-seven patients with indwelling urinary catheters and chronic bacteriuria were studied for methenamine (hexamine hippurate) efficacy. Supplementation with ascorbic acid alone or ascorbic acid plus cranberry cocktail had no significant effect on mean urine pH or methenamine efficacy.[25,26] (For patients with an alkaline urine, acidification is recommended to assist the action of the drug.[27])

In 1981, a Russian study indicated that an increase in the acidity of the urine of patients with urinary infections caused by *Pseudomonas aeruginosa* occurred after administration of the antibiotic novobiocin and cranberry juice. Ex vivo, an increase in activity of novobiocin against Gram-negative bacteria, particularly *P. aeruginosa* and *Proteus* spp., in urine was shown.[28]

Urinary acidification is widely used to increase the excretion rate of the hallucinogen phencyclidine (PCP, angel dust) in abusers. Cranberry juice alone, or with lysine, ammonium chloride, or ascorbic acid, is recommended as an acidification procedure.[29]

Interference with dipstick tests for glucose and haemoglobin in urine has been reported in patients who drank up to 150 mL/day of cranberry juice for 7 weeks.[30]

Safety in Children

Adverse effects are not expected if taken at the recommended dosage.

Intoxication characterized by diarrhoea, hyperglycaemia, and metabolic acidosis has been observed in a 4-month-old baby after the administration of 180 mL of cranberry juice.[31]

Overdosage

A 37-year-old man with a history of traumatic incomplete paraplegia, head injury, and urinary problems presented with hyperkalaemia. He had been drinking more than 2 L of cranberry juice daily for a few days and was taking other medications. No treatment for the hyperkalaemia was required, and it subsequently resolved within 10 days.[32]

Toxicology

No information available on cranberry.

Furfural has an LD_{50} value of 127 mg/kg after oral administration to rats[33]; however, cranberry contains only trace amounts of this constituent (0.1 to 0.3 ppm). (Traces of furfural occur naturally in several foods, including fruit, bread, tea [2 to 7 ppm, black tea], coffee, and cocoa [55 to 255 ppm].[34])

Regulatory Status

See Table 2 for regulatory status in selected countries. Cranberry is widely available as a food and beverage.

Table **2   Regulatory Status for Cranberry in Selected Countries**

Australia	Cranberry is not included in Part 4 of Schedule 4 of the Therapeutic Goods Regulations.
UK & Germany	Cranberry is not included on the General Sale List. It was not included in the Commission E assessment.
US	Cranberry is official in the *United States Pharmacopeia-National Formulary* (USP 26-NF 21, 2003). Cranberry does not have generally recognised as safe (GRAS) status. However, it is freely available as a "dietary supplement" in the US under DSHEA legislation (Dietary Supplement Health and Education Act of 1994).

REFERENCES

1. Avorn J, Monane M, Gurwitz JH, et al: *JAMA* 271:751-754, 1994

2. Stothers L: *Can J Urol* 9:1558-1562, 2002.

3. Schmidt DR, Sobota AE: *Microbios* 55:173-181, 1988.

4. Sobota AE: *J Urol* 131:1013-1016, 1984.

5. Sharon N, Ofek I: *Crit Rev Food Sci Nutr* 42:267-272, 2002.

6. Weiss EL, Lev-Dor R, Sharon N, et al: *Crit Rev Food Sci Nutr* 42:285–292, 2002.

7. Howell AB, Vorsa N, Der Marderosian A, et al: *N Engl J Med* 339:1085–1086, 1998.

8. Wang PL, Du CT, Francis FJ: *J Food Sci* 43:1402–1404, 1978.

9. American Herbal Pharmacopoeia: *Cranberry fruit – Vaccinium macrocarpon: Standards of analysis, quality control, and therapeutics*, Santa Cruz, 2002, American Herbal Pharmacopoeia.

10. Torronen R, Hakkinen S, Karenlampi S, et al: *Cancer Lett* 114:191-192, 1997.

11. Haekkinen SH, Kaerenlampi SO, Heinonen I, et al: *J Agric Food Chem* 47:2274-2279, 1999.

12. Coppola ED, Conrad EC, Cotter R: *J Assoc Off Anal Chem* 61:1490-1492, 1978.

13. United States Patent 5646178: Cranberry extract and biologically active compounds derived therefrom, Utah, July 1997, JLB Inc.

14. Kuzminski LN: *Nutr Rev* 54:S87-S90, 1996.

15. United States Patent 4775477: Cranberry color extraction, New York, October 1988, General Foods Corporation.

16. Terris MK, Issa MM, Tacker JR: *Urology* 57:26-29, 2001.

17. Leachy M, Roderick R, Brilliant K: *Nutr Today* 36:254-265, 2001.

18. Massey LK, Roman-Smith H, Sutton RA: *J Am Diet Assoc* 93:901-906, 1993.

19. Brinkley L, McGuire J, Gregory J, et al: *Urology* 17:534-538, 1981.

20. Finch AM, Kasidas GP, Rose GA: *Clin Sci* 60: 411-418, 1981.

21. Jepson RG, Mihaljevic L, Craig J: *Cochrane Database Syst Rev* (3):CD001321, 2001.

22. Cathcart-Rake W, Porter R, Whittier F, et al: *Am J Clin Nutr* 28:1110-1115, 1975.

23. Committee on Safety of Medicines: *Current Problems in Pharmacovigilance* 29:8, 2003.

24. Saltzman JR, Kemp JA, Golner BB, et al: *J Am Coll Nutr* 13:584-591, 1994.

25. Nahata MC, Cummins BA, McLeod DC, et al: *Eur J Clin Pharmacol* 22:281-284, 1982.

26. Nahata MC, Cummins BA, McLeod DC, et al: *J Am Geriatr Soc* 29:236-239, 1981.

27. E-MIMS, Version 4.00.0457, St Leonards NSW Australia, 2000, MIMS Australia Pty Ltd.

28. Chernomordik AB, Vasilenko EG: *Antibiotiki* 26:456-460, 1981.

29. Simpson GM, Khajawall AM: *Hillside J Clin Psychiatry* 5:161-168, 1983.

30. Kilbourn JP: *Clin Chem* 33:1297, 1987.

31. Garcia-Calatayud S, Larreina Cordoba JJ, Lozano De La Torre MJ: *An Esp Pediatr* 56:72-73, 2002.

32. Thomson F: *Farm Portug* 11:215-216, 2001.

33. Jenner PM, Hagan EC, Taylor JM, et al: *Food Cosmet Toxicol* 2:327-343, 1964.

34. Fifty-first meeting of the Joint FAO/WHO Expert Committee on Food Additives (JECFA): *Safety evaluation of certain food additives*, WHO Food Additives Series 42, Geneva, 1999, World Health Organization.

CRANESBILL

Other common name: American cranesbill
Botanical name: *Geranium maculatum* L.
Family: Geraniaceae
Plant part used: Root

Safety Summary

Pregnancy category B2: No increase in frequency of malformation or other harmful effects on the foetus from limited use in women. Animal studies are lacking.
Lactation category C: Compatible with breastfeeding.
Contraindications: In principle, the use of herbs containing high levels of tannins is contraindicated, or at least inappropriate, in constipation, iron deficiency anaemia, and malnutrition.
Warnings & precautions: Because of the tannin content of this herb, long-term use should be avoided. Use cautiously in highly inflamed or ulcerated conditions of the gastrointestinal tract.
Adverse reactions: None found in published literature for cranesbill root. A potential adverse reaction due to the high tannin content is irritation of the mouth and gastrointestinal tract.
Interactions: Take separately from oral thiamin, metal ion supplements, or alkaloid-containing medications.

Typical Therapeutic Use

Traditional indications for cranesbill in Western herbal medicine include diarrhoea, dysentery, haemorrhoids, duodenal or peptic ulcer, haematemesis, melaena, and menorrhagia.[1]

Actions

Astringent, antidiarrhoeal, antihaemorrhagic.

Key Constituents

Tannins are key constituents of cranesbill root (up to 30%).[2] The main hydrolysable tannin is geraniin.[3]

Adulteration

No adulterants known.

Typical Dosage Forms & Dosage

Typical adult dosage ranges are:

- 3 to 6 g/day of dried root or by infusion
- 3 to 6 mL/day of a 1:1 liquid extract
- 2 to 5 mL/day of a 1:2 liquid extract or equivalent in tablet or capsule form
- 6 to 12 mL/day of a 1:5 tincture

Contraindications

In principle, the use of tannins is contraindicated, or at least inappropriate, in constipation, iron deficiency anaemia, and malnutrition.

Use in Pregnancy

Category B2: No increase in frequency of malformation or other harmful effects on the foetus from limited use in women. Animal studies are lacking.

Use in Lactation

Category C: Compatible with breastfeeding.

Warnings & Precautions

Because of the tannin content of this herb, long-term use should be avoided (for both internal and topical use). Use cautiously in highly inflamed or ulcerated conditions of the gastrointestinal tract.

Effect on Ability to Drive or Operate Machinery

No adverse effects expected.

Adverse Reactions

None known for cranesbill root. High doses of tannins lead to excessive astringency on mucous membranes, which has an irritating effect.

Interactions

None known for cranesbill root.

Tannins complex metal ions and inhibit their absorption. A study with rats found that as long as tea (which is rich in tannins) and iron are consumed separately, iron absorption was not affected.[4] Cases of iron deficiency due to tannin intake have been documented for heavy tea drinkers.[5,6] A marked reduction in iron absorption was observed in human volunteers who consumed sorghum containing 0.15% tannins.[7]

Animal studies also indicate that tannins can react with thiamin and decrease its absorption.[8] A thiamin deficiency status has been shown among people who have the habit of chewing fermented tea leaves.[9]

A study involving healthy volunteers indicated that tea consumption showed a small, but not statistically significant, adverse effect on zinc bioavailability.[10]

Tannins are able to bind to and precipitate alkaloids at an acidic pH. An in vitro study confirmed this well-known chemical phenomenon. Tannic acid or geraniin in solution (up to 1.5%) precipitated solutions containing 0.01% alkaloids, such as berberine, papaverine, or quinine, at pH 5.4. No precipitation occurred when tannin levels reached 3%.[11]

Cranesbill root should be taken separately from oral thiamin, metal ion supplements, or alkaloid-containing medications.

Safety in Children

No information available, but adverse effects are not expected if taken within the recommended dosage.

Overdosage

No incidents found in published literature. However, long-term use with high doses of tannins is to be avoided.

Toxicology

Hydrolysable tannins are polymers of gallic or ellagic acid esterified to a core molecule, commonly glucose or a polyphenol such as catechin. Condensed tannins are flavonoid polymers such as proanthocyanidins. Tannins are also referred to as polyphenols.

Chronic intake of tannins (predominantly hydrolysable gallotannins) at levels of 13.5 to 50 g/kg by broiler cockerels resulted in inhibition of digestive enzymes, especially the membrane-bound enzymes of the small intestinal mucosa. Pancreas weight showed a significant increase with increasing levels of dietary tannin, while liver weight remained unaffected. Growth of the birds was also adversely affected by the tannin-containing diets.[12]

Tannins have been reported to be responsible for decreases in feed intake, growth rate, feed efficiency, net metabolisable energy, and protein digestibility in experimental animals. However, it is now thought that the major effect of tannins was not due to their inhibition on food consumption or digestion, but rather the decreased efficiency in converting the absorbed nutrients to new body substances. Incidences of certain cancers, such as oesophageal cancer, have been reported to be related to consumption of tannin-rich foods such as betel nuts and herbal teas, suggesting that tannins might be carcinogenic on repeated contact. However, other reports indicated that the carcinogenic activity of tannins might be related to components associated with tannins, rather than tannins themselves, and other social factors such as social class and smoking may also be involved.[7] (Toxicity studies relating to betel nut polyphenols are not conclusive, with both carcinogenic and anticarcinogenic effects being reported. There is also inconclusive evidence regarding the contribution of the alkaloids in betel nut. It appears that betel nut toxicity is not completely due to its polyphenol and alkaloid contents.[13]) Several studies have also shown that the increased risk of oesophageal cancer from ingestion of very hot tea may be due to the hot temperature rather than the tea itself.[7]

Reports have also indicated a negative association between tea consumption and the incidence of certain cancers. Tea polyphenols and many tannin components were suggested to be anticarcinogenic. Many tannin molecules have also been shown to reduce the mutagenic activity of a number of mutagens. The anticarcinogenic and antimutagenic potentials of tannins may be related to their antioxidant property. There is an extensive amount of literature supporting the antioxidant activity of tannins.[7]

Hydrolysable tannins are potentially toxic to ruminants. Pyrogallol, a hepatotoxin and nephrotoxin, is a product of hydrolysable tannin degradation by ruminal microbes.[14] Tannic acid administered by feeding tube to rats, in a single dose of 2 g/kg, induced acute hepatocellular changes. Neither orally nor parenterally administered tannic acid induced noticeable DNA damage, detectable as single-strand breaks on alkaline-sucrose gradients.[15] Although tannic acid is hepatotoxic when given orally to mice (2 to 4.6 g/kg) or intraperitoneally to sheep (0.1 g/kg), it does not produce renal or significant hepatic injury in sheep when given orally (8 g/kg), but rather causes metabolic acidosis and methaemoglobinaemia.[16]

For information regarding the toxicity in humans from topical use of tannic acid, refer to *Principles and practice of phytotherapy*.[17]

Regulatory Status

See Table I for regulatory status in selected countries.

Table I   **Regulatory Status for Cranesbill in Selected Countries**

Australia	Cranesbill is not included in Part 4 of Schedule 4 of the Therapeutic Goods Regulations.
UK & Germany	Cranesbill is included on the General Sale List. It was not included in the Commission E assessment.
US	Cranesbill does not have generally recognised as safe (GRAS) status. However, it is freely available as a "dietary supplement" in the US under DSHEA legislation (Dietary Supplement Health and Education Act of 1994).

REFERENCES

1. British Herbal Medicine Association's Scientific Committee: *British herbal pharmacopoeia*, Bournemouth, 1983, BHMA, pp 101-102.
2. Wren RC: *Potter's new cyclopaedia of botanical drugs and preparations*, Essex, 1989, The C.W. Daniel Company Limited, p 95.
3. Haslam E, Lilley TH, Cai Y, et al: *Planta Med* 55:1-8, 1989.
4. South PK, House A, Miller DD: *Nutr Res* 17:1303-1310, 1997.
5. Zijp IM, Korver O, Tijburg LB: *Crit Rev Food Sci Nutr* 40:371-398, 2000.
6. Gabrielli GB, De Sandre G: *Haematologica* 80:518-520, 1995.
7. Chung KT, Wong TY, Wei CI, et al: *Crit Rev Food Sci Nutr* 38:421-464, 1998.
8. Ruenwongsa P, Pattanavibag S: *Experientia* 38:787-788, 1982.
9. Vimokesant SL, Nakornchai S, Dhanamitta S, et al: *Nutr Rep Int* 9:371-376, 1974.
10. Ganji V, Kies CV: *Plant Foods Hum Nutr* 46:267-276, 1994.
11. Okuda T, Mori K, Shiota M: *Yakugaku Zasshi* 102:854-858, 1982.
12. Ahmed AE, Smithard R, Ellis M: *Br J Nutr* 65:189-197, 1991.
13. Jeng JH, Chang MC, Hahn LJ: *Oral Oncol* 37:477-492, 2001.
14. Reed JD: *J Anim Sci* 73:1516-1528, 1995.
15. Oler A, Neal MW, Mitchell EK: *Food Cosmet Toxicol* 14:565-570, 1976.
16. Zhu J, Filippich LJ, Alsalami MT: *Res Vet Sci* 53:280-292, 1992.
17. Mills S, Bone K: *Principles and practice of phytotherapy: Modern herbal medicine*, Edinburgh, 2000, Churchill Livingstone, p 37.

CRATAEVA

Botanical names: *Crataeva nurvala* Buch.-Ham., *Crataeva religiosa* G. Forst.
Note: Crataeva is also spelt as Crateva.
Family: Capparidaceae (= Capparaceae)
Plant part used: Bark

Safety Summary

Pregnancy category B3: No increase in frequency of malformation or other harmful effects on the foetus from limited use in women. Evidence of increased foetal damage in animal studies exists, although the relevance to humans is unknown.
Lactation category CC: Compatible with breastfeeding but use caution.
Contraindications: None required on current evidence. Do not use during pregnancy or lactation without professional advice.
Warnings & precautions: None required on current evidence.
Adverse reactions: None found in published literature.
Interactions: No precautions required on current evidence.

Typical Therapeutic Use

Crataeva demonstrated therapeutic benefit in uncontrolled trials involving patients with urinary tract disorders including urinary tract infection, hypotonic, atonic or neurogenic bladder, kidney, ureter or bladder stones and incontinence.[1] Traditional uses of crataeva in Ayurvedic medicine include disorders of the urinary system, especially kidney and bladder stones.[2]

Actions

Antilithic, bladder tonic, antiinflammatory.

Key Constituents

Constituents of crataeva bark include sterols (especially lupeol, a pentacyclic triterpene) and flavonoids. The Capparidaceae family is characterised by the presence of glucosinolates,[3] and glucocapparin has been isolated from *C. nurvala* stem bark.[4]

Adulteration

No adulterants known.

Typical Dosage Forms & Dosage

Typical adult dosage ranges are:
- 5.5 to 8.5 g/day of dried bark as a decoction
- 6 to 14 mL/day of a 1:2 liquid extract or equivalent in tablet or capsule form

Contraindications

None known. Do not use during pregnancy or lactation without professional advice.

Use in Pregnancy

Category B3: No increase in frequency of malformation or other harmful effects on the foetus from limited use in women. Evidence of increased foetal damage in animal studies exists, although the relevance to humans is unknown.

Ethanolic extract of crataeva bark demonstrated antifertility activity in rats after oral administration from day 1 to day 7 postcoitum at a dose of 250 mg/kg/day.[5,6]

Use in Lactation

Category CC: Compatible with breastfeeding but use caution.

Warnings & Precautions

Due to potential mutagenicity and goitrogenicity, herbs containing glucosinolates should not be taken in doses exceeding the maximum therapeutic range in the long term. However, the relevance of this caution to crataeva is unknown.

Effect on Ability to Drive or Operate Machinery

No adverse effects expected.

Adverse Reactions

Topical application of freshly ground leaves of crataeva are known to have a blistering effect. However, the decoction of the root and stem bark is well tolerated.[7]

Interactions

None known.

Safety in Children

No information available but adverse effects are not expected.

Overdosage

No incidents found in published literature.

Toxicology

The LD_{50} value of crataeva bark 50% ethanol extract administered by intraperitoneal injection to rats was assessed at greater than 1 g/kg.[8]

Regulatory Status

See Table 1 for regulatory status in selected countries.

Table 1   **Regulatory Status for Crataeva in Selected Countries**

Australia	Crataeva is not included in Part 4 of Schedule 4 of the Therapeutic Goods Regulations.
UK & Germany	Crataeva is not included on the General Sale List. It was not included in the Commission E assessment.
US	Crataeva does not have generally recognised as safe (GRAS) status. However, it is freely available as a "dietary supplement" in the US under DSHEA legislation (Dietary Supplement Health and Education Act of 1994).

REFERENCES

1. Deshpande PJ, Sahu M, Kamur P: *Indian J Med Res* 76(Suppl):46-53, 1982.
2. Chopra RN, Chopra IC, Handa KL, et al: *Chopra's indigenous drugs of India*, ed 2, 1958; reprinted Calcutta, 1982, Academic Publishers, pp 502, 671.
3. Prabhakar YS, Suresh Kumar D: *Fitoterapia* 61:99-111, 1990.
4. Regional Research Laboratory and Indian Drug Manufacturers' Association: *Indian herbal pharmacopoeia*, Jammu-Tawi, 1998, Indian Drug Manufacturers' Association, Mumbai and Regional Research Laboratory, pp 56-63.
5. Sharma BB, Varshney MD, Gupta DN, et al: *Int J Crude Drug Res* 21:183-187, 1983.
6. Prakash AO: *Contracept Deliv Syst* 5:9-10, 1984.
7. Bharatiya Vidya Bhavan's Swami Prakashananda Ayurveda Research Centre: *Selected medicinal plants of India*, Bombay, 1992, Chemexcil, pp 108-111.
8. Sharma ML, Chandokhe N, Ghatak BJR, et al: *Indian J Exp Biol* 16:228-240, 1978.

DAMIANA

Botanical names: *Turnera diffusa* Willd. ex J.A. Schultes (*Turnera aphrodisiaca* Ward, *Turnera microphylla* Desv.), *Turnera diffusa* Willd. ex J.A. Schultes var. *aphrodisiaca* (G.H. Ward) Urban
Family: Turneraceae
Plant part used: Leaf

Safety Summary

Pregnancy category B2: No increase in frequency of malformation or other harmful effects on the foetus from limited use in women. Animal studies are lacking.
Lactation category ND: No data available.
Contraindications: None required on current evidence.
Warnings & precautions: None required on current evidence.
Adverse reactions: None found in published literature.
Interactions: No precautions required on current evidence.

Typical Therapeutic Use

Traditional uses of damiana in Western herbal medicine include depression, anxiety (particularly due to sexual factors), sexual inadequacy, nervous dyspepsia and constipation.[1] Therapeutic uses of damiana in traditional Mexican medicine include nervous debility, impotence, frigidity and stomach pains and as an aphrodisiac and invigorator.[2]

Actions

Nervine tonic, tonic, mild laxative.

Key Constituents

Constituents of damiana include an essential oil (0.5%), resins (14%) and tannins (3.5%). A small amount of a cyanogenic glycoside (tetraphyllin B, 0.26%) is present.[3,4]

Adulteration

The leaves of other Mexican shrubs which are also called damiana but are unrelated to Turnera, such as *Aplopappus venetus*, *A. discoideus* and *Chrysactinia mexicana*, have been substituted in the past.[2,5]

Typical Dosage Forms & Dosage

- Typical adult dosage ranges are:
- 6 to 12 g/day of dried leaf or by infusion
- 6 to 12 mL/day of a 1:1 liquid extract
- 3 to 6 mL/day of a 1:2 liquid extract or equivalent in tablet or capsule form

Contraindications

None known.

Use in Pregnancy

Category B2: No increase in frequency of malformation or other harmful effects on the foetus from limited use in women. Animal studies are lacking.

Damiana has been used as an emmenagogue and as an aid to childbirth in traditional Mexican medicine.[2,6]

Use in Lactation

Category ND: No data available.

Warnings & Precautions

None required.

Effect on Ability to Drive or Operate Machinery

No adverse effects expected.

Adverse Reactions

No adverse reactions documented.

Interactions

None reported.

Safety in Children

No information available (on safety). However, there is documented use of damiana in Mexico as a stimulating tea which was also served to children.[7]

Overdosage

A case of overdose has been reported where an alcoholic consumed 8 ounces (227 mL) of an extract of damiana, which resulted in tetanus-like convulsions and paroxysms.[2]

Toxicology

An extract of damiana tested negative for in vitro mutagenic activity in the Ames test.[8]

Regulatory Status

See Table 1 for regulatory status in selected countries.

Table **1**   **Regulatory Status for Damiana in Selected Countries**

Australia	Damiana is not included in Part 4 of Schedule 4 of the Therapeutic Goods Regulations.
UK & Germany	Damiana is included on the General Sale List. It is covered by a negative Commission E monograph.
US	Damiana does not have generally recognised as safe (GRAS) status. However, it is freely available as a "dietary supplement" in the US under DSHEA legislation (Dietary Supplement Health and Education Act of 1994).

REFERENCES

1. British Herbal Medicine Association's Scientific Committee: *British herbal pharmacopoeia*, Bournemouth, 1983, BHMA, pp 219-220.
2. Brinker FJ: *Eclectic dispensatory of botanical therapeutics: history*, vol 2, Sandy OR, 1995, Eclectic Medical Publications, pp 101-103.
3. British Herbal Medicine Association: *British herbal compendium*, vol 1, Bournemouth, 1992, BHMA, pp 71-72.
4. Spencer KC, Seigler DS: *Planta Med* 43:175-178, 1981.
5. Felter HW, Lloyd JU: *King's American dispensatory*, ed 18, rev 3, vol 1. First published 1905; reprinted Portland, 1983, Eclectic Medical Publications, pp 645-647.
6. Ellingwood F, Lloyd JU: *American materia medica, therapeutics and pharmacognosy*, ed 11, *Naturopathic Medical Series: Botanical* vol 2, Portland, 1983, Eclectic Medical Publications, pp 459-460.
7. Lloyd JU: *Damiana*, Mexico, 1904, La Paz, p 6.
8. Schimmer O, Kruger A, Paulini H, et al: *Pharmazie* 49:448-451, 1994.

DANDELION

Botanical name: *Taraxacum officinale* Weber
Family: Compositae
Plant part used: Leaf or root

Safety Summary

Pregnancy category B2: No increase in frequency of malformation or other harmful effects on the foetus from limited use in women. Animal studies are lacking.
Lactation category C: Compatible with breastfeeding.
Contraindications: Known allergy.
Warnings & precautions: None required on current evidence.
Adverse reactions: None found in published literature.
Interactions: No precautions required on current evidence.

Typical Therapeutic Use

Traditional indications of dandelion leaf and root in Western herbal medicine include gallbladder conditions, oedema and oliguria, dyspeptic conditions and skin and arthritic diseases associated with these symptoms.[1]

Actions

Diuretic (especially leaf), choleretic, mild laxative, antirheumatic.

Key Constituents

Germacranolide sesquiterpene lactones[2]; triterpenes; phytosterols; flavonoids[3]; potassium (up to 4.5% in dried leaf)[4]; taraxalisin—a serine proteinase in the fresh latex (particularly in spring).[5]

Adulteration

Rarely with leaves of *Leontodon autumnalis* L. and roots of *Cichorium intybus* L.

Typical Dosage Forms & Dosage

Typical adult dosage ranges are:
- 12 to 30 g/day of dried leaf or by infusion
- 6 to 24 g/day of dried root or by infusion or decoction

- 6 to 11.5 mL/day of a 1:1 liquid extract of dandelion leaf or equivalent in tablet or capsule form
- 3 to 6 mL/day of a 1:2 liquid extract of dandelion root or equivalent in tablet or capsule form
- 6 to 15 mL/day of a 1:5 tincture of dandelion leaf
- 15 to 30 mL/day of a 1:5 tincture of dandelion root

Contraindications

Known allergy.

Official monographs have listed occlusion of the bile ducts, gallbladder empyema, obstructive ileus. There are few data to support these warnings, however, and it may arise out of a theoretical view of a choleretic action.

Use in Pregnancy

Category B2: No increase in frequency of malformation or other harmful effects on the foetus from limited use in women. Animal studies are lacking.

Use in Lactation

Category C: compatible with breastfeeding.

Warnings & Precautions

Dandelion Leaf

Despite reports of skin reactions and dermatitis from topical use of dandelion aerial parts, the likelihood of dandelion leaf preparations causing a contact allergy is low. However, persons with known sensitivity to other members of the Compositae family (such as ragweed, daisies, chrysanthemums) should avoid topical application of dandelion leaf or dandelion leaf products.

Dandelion Root

Caution is required if gallstones are present.[6]

Effect on Ability to Drive or Operate Machinery

No adverse effects expected.

Adverse Reactions

Dandelion pollen has been implicated, as a Compositae and relative of ragweed, in allergic reactions to a bee pollen supplement.[7] Around 75% of those suffering allergic reactions to honey are also sensitive to dandelion pollen within honey.[8] Contact reactions to other Compositae, including dandelion, have also been reported, notably among gardeners, florists and those with outside hobbies.[9-13] A contact sensitivity to dandelion leaves provoked eczematous reactions in one case of erythema multiforme.[14] A cross reaction in some patients with photoallergies has also been established.[15] However, unlike other Compositae allergies, reaction to a standard mixture of sesquiterpene lactones is not predictive of dandelion sensitivity.[16,17] Another constituent, taraxinic acid 1'-O-beta-D-glucopyranoside, has been implicated as a major allergen.[18]

Interactions

Dandelion tea added to the drinking water of rats decreased CYP2E and CYP1A2 activity by 48% and 15% respectively, together with a dramatic increase in activity of the phase II detoxifying enzyme UDP-glucuronosyl transferase: the net effect of these changes may reduce the prospect of harmful hepatic effects, but might theoretically increase the half-life of some other medication.[19]

Safety in Children

No information available, but adverse effects are not expected.

Overdosage

There is an early report of poisoning in children making daisy chains with fresh plant (after sucking the latex from the flower stems).[20]

Toxicology

Table 1 lists LD_{50} data recorded for dandelion.[21]

Rabbits treated orally with dandelion whole plant (3 to 6 g/kg) showed no visible signs of acute toxicity.[22] Dandelion root ethanol extract showed a very low toxicity when administered to rats and mice in doses of 10 g/kg (orally) and 4 g/kg (i.p.) (doses refer to dried herb equivalent).[23]

Regulatory Status

See Table 2 for regulatory status in selected countries. Roasted dandelion root is commonly consumed as a coffee substitute.

Table **1**   **LD_{50} Data Recorded for Dandelion**

Substance	Route, Model	LD_{50} Value (g/kg)	Reference
Dandelion leaf 1:1 fluid extract*	i.p., mice	28.8	21
Dandelion root 1:1 fluid extract*	i.p., mice	36.6	21

Doses refer to dried herb equivalent.

Table **2**   **Regulatory Status for Dandelion in Selected Countries**

Australia	Dandelion is not included in Part 4 of Schedule 4 of the Therapeutic Goods Regulations.
UK & Germany	Dandelion is included on the General Sale List. The whole dandelion plant is covered by two positive Commission E monographs (dandelion herb; dandelion root with herb).
US	Dandelion has generally recognised as safe (GRAS) status and is freely available as a "dietary supplement" in the US under DSHEA legislation (Dietary Supplement Health and Education Act of 1994).

REFERENCES

1. British Herbal Medicine Association's Scientific Committee: *British herbal pharmacopoeia*, Bournemouth, 1983, BHMA, pp 207-208.
2. Michalska K, Kisiel W: *Planta Med* 69:181-183, 2003.
3. Williams CA, Goldstone F, Greenham J: *Phytochemistry* 42:121-127, 1996.
4. Rácz G, Bodon J, Tölgyesi G: *Herba Hung* 17:43-54, 1978.
5. Rudenskaya GN, Bogacheva AM, Preusser A, et al: *FEBS Lett* 437:237-240, 1998.
6. Blumenthal M et al, eds: *The complete German Commission E monographs: therapeutic guide to herbal medicines*, Austin, 1998, American Botanical Council, pp 118-119.
7. Cohen SH, Yunginger JW, Rosenberg N, et al: *J Allergy Clin Immunol* 64:270-274, 1979.
8. Helbling A, Peter C, Berchtold E, et al: *Allergy* 47:41-49, 1992.
9. Davies MG, Kersey PJ: *Contact Dermatitis* 14:256-257, 1986.
10. Dawe RS, Green CM, MacLeod TM, et al: *Contact Dermatitis* 35:109-110, 1996.
11. Fernandez C, Martin-Esteban M, Fiandor A, et al: *J Allergy Clin Immunol* 92:660-667, 1993.
12. Guin JD, Skidmore G: *Arch Dermatol* 123:500-502, 1987.
13. Ingber A: *Contact Dermatitis* 43:49, 2000.
14. Jovanovic M, Mimica-Dukic N, Poljacki M, et al: *Contact Dermatitis* 48:17-25, 2003.
15. Mark KA, Brancaccio RR, Soter NA, et al: *Arch Dermatol* 135:67-70, 1999.
16. Goulden V, Wilkinson SM: *Br J Dermatol* 138:1018-1021, 1998.
17. Lovell CR, Rowan M: *Contact Dermatitis* 25:185-188, 1991.
18. Hausen BM: *Dermatosen Beruf Umwelt* 30:51-53, 1982.
19. Maliakal PP, Wanwimolruk S: *J Pharm Pharmacol* 53:1323-1329, 2001.
20. Gessner O: *Gift- und Arzneipflanzen von Mitteleuropa*, ed 3, Heidelberg, 1974, Carl Winter Universitatsverlag, pp 382-383.
21. Racz-Kotilla E, Racz G, Solomon A: *Planta Med* 26:212-217, 1974.
22. Akhtar MS, Khan QM, Khaliq T: *J Pak Med Assoc* 35:207-210, 1985.
23. Tita B, Bello U, Faccendini P, et al: *Pharmacol Res* 27(Suppl 1):23-24, 1993.

DEVIL'S CLAW

Other common names: Harpagophytum, grapple plant

Botanical name: *Harpagophytum procumbens* (Burch.) DC. ex Meisn.

Family: Pedaliaceae

Plant part used: Secondary root tubers

Safety Summary

Pregnancy category B2: No increase in frequency of malformation or other harmful effects on the foetus from limited use in women. Animal studies are lacking.

Lactation category C: Compatible with breastfeeding (in low doses).

Contraindications: None required on current evidence.

Warnings & precautions: Gastric or duodenal ulcers. Bitters should be used with caution in oesophageal reflux and in states of hyperacidity. Prescribe with caution for pain in children. Other precautions are neurological disease, depression and psychosis, liver and kidney disease, history of allergic or anaphylactic reactions. Long-term therapy with analgesics is not advisable.

Adverse reactions: Mild gastrointestinal complaints, allergic reactions of the skin, eyes, and respiratory passages.

Interactions: May potentiate the effect of warfarin (one case report of possible interaction). Do not prescribe concomitantly with powerful analgesics (theoretical concern).

Typical Therapeutic Use

Devil's claw has demonstrated therapeutic benefit in the treatment of patients with arthrosis, articular pain, osteoarthritis, and chronic back pain in randomised, double-blind, controlled trials.[1-5] Traditional indications for devil's claw in Western herbal medicine include rheumatism, arthritis, gout, and lumbago.[6] Traditional uses in South Africa include lack of appetite and as an analgesic.[7]

Actions

Antiinflammatory, antirheumatic, analgesic, bitter tonic.

Key Constituents

Constituents of devil's claw root include iridoid glycosides (0.5% to 3.0%), primarily harpagoside.[8]

Adulteration

Occasionally the harpagoside-poor primary roots of devil's claw are found as an adulterant, as are the roots of other intensely bitter tasting African plants, such as *Elephantorrhiza* spp. and *Acanthosicyos naudinianus* and *Harpagophytum zeyheri*.[9] Even though *Harpagophytum procumbens* and *H. zeyheri* can easily be distinguished in the field, it is impossible to tell them apart visually when in the form of dried and sliced tubers. Both species are harvested and traded as devil's claw in Namibia. Between 1985 and 1986 it was estimated that about 50% of the harvested wild material was mixed *H. procumbens* and *H. zeyheri*.[10] Devil's claw was proposed for inclusion in Appendix II of the Convention on International Trade in Endangered Species (CITES) in April 2000, but the proposal was not accepted,[11] and it remains off the list as of May 2003.

Typical Dosage Forms & Dosage

Typical adult dosage ranges are:
- 1.5 to 6 g/day of dried root or by decoction
- 3 to 11.5 mL/day of a 1:2 liquid extract or equivalent in tablet or capsule form
- standardised extract containing 36 to 87 mg/day iridoid glycosides or 50 to 100 mg/day harpagoside

Contraindications

None known.

Use in Pregnancy

Category B2: No increase in frequency of malformation or other harmful effects on the foetus from limited use in women. Animal studies are lacking.

In South African traditional medicine, low doses of the dried tuber (such as 0.25 g three times daily) are administered to pregnant women to relieve pain, and this is continued postpartum at a reduced dose. The fresh tuber is made into an ointment and applied to the abdomen of women who anticipate a difficult birth.[12]

Use in Lactation

Category C: Compatible with breastfeeding (in very low doses).

Devil's claw has been used in low doses in the postpartum period in traditional South African medicine.[12]

Warnings & Precautions

The Commission E advises that use of devil's claw is contraindicated in patients with gastric or duodenal ulcers and should only be used with professional supervision in patients with gallstones.[13] However, any health risks are theoretical in nature and have been projected from the bitter tonic activity of the herb. Bitters should be used with caution in oesophageal reflux and in states of hyperacidity.

The following conditions should be approached with caution when using herbal analgesics: concurrent prescription of powerful analgesics; pain in children; neurological disease; depression and psychosis; liver and kidney disease; history of allergic or anaphylactic reactions. Long-term therapy with analgesics is not advisable.

Effect on Ability to Drive or Operate Machinery

No adverse effects expected.

Adverse Reactions

Mild gastrointestinal complaints are the most frequently reported adverse reaction.[14] Devil's claw–specific allergic skin reactions have also been reported in a clinical trial.[15] One case of conjunctivitis, rhinitis and asthma has been reported after occupational exposure to devil's claw. Allergy was confirmed by a provocation test.[16]

Interactions

Devil's claw may potentiate the effect of warfarin. A case of purpurea was reported in a patient taking warfarin and devil's claw.[17] The patient's medical condition, other medications, and the doses and duration of the warfarin and devil's claw ingestion were not reported.

Devil's claw has demonstrated a protective effect against arrhythmia in vitro and in vivo[18,19] and it has been proposed that it may interact with antiarrhythmic drugs.[1] However, this is a theoretical concern of unknown clinical relevance.

As a precaution, do not prescribe concomitantly with powerful analgesics.

Safety in Children

No information available but adverse effects are not expected.

Overdosage

No incidents found in published literature.

Toxicology

Table 1 lists LD_{50} data recorded for devil's claw extract and its constituents.[20-22]

Table 1   **LD_{50} Data Recorded for Devil's Claw Extract and Its Constituents**

Substance	Route, Model	LD_{50} Value	Reference
Devil's claw	Oral, mice	>13.5 g/kg	20
Devil's claw purified extract (85% harpagoside)	i.v., mice	511 mg/kg	21
Harpagoside	i.p., mice	1 g/kg	22

Devil's claw has demonstrated low toxicity in acute and subacute toxicity studies.[20,21] No significant haematological or gross pathological findings were evident in rats after oral administration of 7.5 g/kg devil's claw for 21 days. Hepatotoxic effects could not be demonstrated with respect to liver weight, levels of microsomal protein and liver enzymes after 7 days of oral treatment with 2 g/kg.[20]

Regulatory Status

See Table 2 for regulatory status in selected countries.

Table **2** **Regulatory Status for Devil's Claw in Selected Countries**

Australia	Devil's claw is not included in Part 4 of Schedule 4 of the Therapeutic Goods Regulations.
UK & Germany	Devil's claw is not included on the General Sale List. It is covered by a positive Commission E monograph.
	Devil's claw is official in the *British Pharmacopoeia* 2002 and the *European Pharmacopoeia* 4.3.
US	Devil's claw does not have generally recognised as safe (GRAS) status. However, it is freely available as a "dietary supplement" in the US under DSHEA legislation (Dietary Supplement Health and Education Act of 1994).

REFERENCES

1. Scientific Committee of ESCOP (European Scientific Cooperative on Phytotherapy): *ESCOP monographs: Harpagophytum radix*, UK, March 1996, European Scientific Cooperative on Phytotherapy Secretariat.
2. Chantre P, Cappelaere A, Leblan D, et al: *Phytomed* 7:177-183, 2000.
3. Leblan D, Chantre P, Fournie B: *Joint Bone Spine* 67:462-467, 2000.
4. Chrubasik S, Zimpfer CH, Schutt U, et al: *Phytomed* 3:1-10, 1996.
5. Chrubasik S, Junck H, Breitschwerdt H, et al: *Eur J Anaesthesiol* 16:118-129, 1999.
6. British Herbal Medicine Association's Scientific Committee: *British herbal pharmacopoeia*, Bournemouth, 1983, BHMA, p 111.
7. van Wyk B-E, van Oudtshoorn B, Gericke N: *Medicinal plants of South Africa*, Arcadia, 1997, Briza Publications, p 144.
8. Wagner H, Bladt S: *Plant drug analysis: a thin layer chromatography atlas*, ed 2, Berlin 1996, Springer-Verlag, p 76.
9. Bisset NG, ed: *Herbal drugs and phytopharmaceuticals: a handbook for practice on a scientific basis*, Stuttgart, 1994, Medpharm Scientific Publishers, p 250.
10. Hachfeld B, Schippmann U: *Medicinal plant conservation*, vol 6, Bonn, 2000, Bundesamt fur Naturschutz, pp 3-9.
11. Convention of International Trade in Endangered Species of Wild Fauna and Flora, Eleventh meeting of the Conference of the Parties, Gigiri (Kenya), 10-20 April, 2000.
12. Watt JM, Breyer-Brandwijk MG: *The medicinal and poisonous plants of southern and eastern Africa: being an account of their medicinal and other uses, chemical composition, pharmacological effects and toxicology in man and animal*, ed 2, Edinburgh, 1962, Livingstone, p 830.
13. Blumenthal M et al, eds: *The complete German Commission E monographs: therapeutic guide to herbal medicines*, Austin, 1998, American Botanical Council, p 120.
14. Chrubasik S: *Phytomedicine* 7(Suppl 2):41, 2000.
15. Chrubasik S, Thanner J, Kunzel O, et al: *Phytomedicine* 9:181-194, 2002.
16. Altmeyer N, Garnier R, Rosenberg N, et al: *Arch Mal Prof* 53:289-291, 1992.
17. Shaw D, Leon C, Kolev S, et al: *Drug Saf* 17:342-356, 1997.
18. Costa De Pasquale R, Busa G, Circosta C, et al: *J Ethnopharmacol* 13:193-199, 1985.
19. Circosta C, Occhiuto F, Ragusa S, et al: *J Ethnopharmacol* 11:259-274, 1984.
20. Whitehouse LW, Znamirowska M, Paul CJ: *Can Med Assoc J* 129:249-251, 1983.
21. Erdos A, Fontaine R, Friehe H et al: *Planta Med* 34:97-108, 1978.
22. Van Haelen M, Van Haelen-Fastre R, Samaey-Fontaine J, et al: *Phytotherapy* 5:7-13, 1983.

DONG QUAI

Other common name: Dang gui
Botanical names: *Angelica sinensis* (Oliv.) Diels
(*Angelica polymorpha* Maxim. var. *sinensis* Oliv.)
Family: Umbelliferae
Plant part used: Root

Safety Summary

Pregnancy category C: On the basis of traditional writing, has caused or is associated with a substantial risk of causing harmful effects on the foetus or neonate without causing malformations. Contraindicated in the first trimester of pregnancy and in women with a tendency to spontaneous abortion.
Lactation category C: Compatible with breastfeeding.
Contraindications: Traditional contraindications include diarrhoea caused by weak digestion, haemorrhagic disease, acute viral infections such as the common cold and influenza, tendency to spontaneous abortion and the first trimester of pregnancy. Do not use during pregnancy without professional advice.
Warnings & precautions: Do not prescribe concomitantly with warfarin.
Adverse reactions: Gynaecomastia (one case report of uncertain validity).
Interactions: May potentiate the effects of warfarin.

Typical Therapeutic Use

Dong quai demonstrated therapeutic benefit in the treatment of dysmenorrhoea (in combination with other Chinese herbs),[1] chronic hepatitis and hepatic cirrhosis[2] and as a douche for infertility due to tubal occlusion[3] in uncontrolled trials. Therapeutic use of dong quai in traditional Chinese medicine (TCM) includes anaemia with dizziness and palpitations, irregular menstruation, dysmenorrhoea, amenorrhoea, constipation and rheumatism.[4-6]

Actions

Antiinflammatory, antianaemic, antiplatelet, female tonic, mild laxative, antiarrhythmic.

Key Constituents

A main constituent of *Angelica sinensis* root is ligustilide (Z-ligustilide). Other key constituents include 3-n-butylidene phthalide and ferulic acid.[7-9] Other constituents which have been detected in dong quai root include the coumarin scopoletin[10] and, in the essential oil, safrole.[8]

Adulteration

Ligusticum glaucescens and *Levisticum officinale* are regarded as substitutes of lower quality for dong quai.[8] *Angelica acutiloba* is a therapeutically interchangeable species for *A. sinensis* in Japan (but in China would be regarded as a substitute of lower quality).[8,9] *A. dahurica*, *A. pubescens* and *Ligusticum chuanxiong* are also used in TCM, while *Ligusticum porteri* is traditionally used in Mexico and is sold in the United States. These plants are morphologically similar to *Angelica sinensis* and may occur as substitutes.[9]

A. acutiloba contains phthalides as main constituents and can be difficult to distinguish from *A. sinensis* by thin layer chromatography,[7] although ferulic acid was detected in *A. sinensis* and not in *A. acutiloba*.[11]

Typical Dosage Forms & Dosage

Typical adult dosage ranges are:
- 4.5 to 9 g of dried root per day by decoction
- 4.5 to 8.5 mL/day of a 1:2 liquid extract or equivalent in tablet or capsule form.

Contraindications

In TCM dong quai is contraindicated in diarrhoea caused by weak digestion, haemorrhagic disease, acute viral infections such as the common cold and influenza, tendency to spontaneous abortion, and the first trimester of pregnancy.[7] Do not use during pregnancy without professional advice.

Use in Pregnancy

Category C: Has caused or is associated with a substantial risk of causing harmful effects on the foetus or neonate without causing malformations. (Apparently, based on traditional considerations, dong quai is contraindicated in the first trimester of pregnancy and in women with a tendency to spontaneous abortion.[8])

The essential oil relaxed the isolated uterus, but other components of dong quai increased uterine contraction. Some experiments on the whole root have shown a stimulant effect in vivo, while others have shown that it can relax or coordinate (make more rhythmic) uterine contractions, depending on uterine tone.[4,12] Subcutaneous administration of dong quai aqueous extract (0.1 to 0.4 mL/day) for 5 days did not affect fertility or exhibit teratogenic effects in mice.[13]

Use in Lactation

Category C: Compatible with breastfeeding.

Warnings & Precautions

Do not prescribe concomitantly with warfarin (see below).

Effect on Ability to Drive or Operate Machinery

No adverse effects expected.

Adverse Reactions

A 35-year-old man developed gynaecomastia (mammary glandular hyperplasia) after ingestion of dong quai capsules for one month. The label indicated "100% dong quai (*Angelica sinensis*) root powder. No fillers or additives." The patient discontinued the pills and the gynaecomastia had regressed completely when he was reviewed 3 months later.[14]

"Angelica-Paeonia Powder" has been reported to cause mild lassitude, drowsiness and urticaria after oral administration.[4] The species of *Angelica* and the formula was not defined.

A case of liver toxicity in a female patient was reported after the ingestion of a Chinese herbal preparation for six months. *A. sinensis* was one of nine herbs in the formula. The patient's liver function normalised within several months of ceasing the herbal mixture.[15] It is not known if the dong quai was implicated.

A case was reported in 2001 of a woman diagnosed with grade 1 endometrioid adenocarcinoma of the endometrium, "whose history was notable for extensive use of supplemental phytoestrogens". Herbs included chaste tree, dong quai, black cohosh and licorice.[16] No causality was demonstrated.

Interactions

Caution is advised for patients receiving chronic treatment with warfarin, as dong quai may potentiate its effects. One female patient stabilised on warfarin presented with widespread bruising and an increased international normalised ratio (INR),[17] and another developed an increased INR and prothrombin time after taking dong quai concurrently for 4 weeks.[18]

Oral administration of dong quai extract (4 g of dried herb/kg/day) for 3 days significantly lowered prothrombin time in rabbits when it was coadministered with a single dose of warfarin (2 mg/kg, s.c.), but not when it was administered alone. However, when dong quai was administered at the same dose after a steady state of warfarin (0.6 mg/kg/day, s.c.) had been reached, mean prothrombin times significantly increased. This was not due to alteration of plasma warfarin concentration, as the steady state concentration did not change significantly.[19]

Safety in Children

No information available, but no adverse effects expected.

Overdosage

No incidents found in published literature.

Toxicology

Table 1 lists LD$_{50}$ data recorded for dong quai and its constituents.[7,20]

The minimum lethal dose of dong quai root was 30 to 90 g/kg in mice (route unknown).[4] Respiration

Table 1 **LD$_{50}$ Data Recorded for Dong Quai and Its Constituents**

Substance	Route, Model	LD$_{50}$ Value (g/kg)	Reference
Concentrated dong quai extract*	Oral, rats	100	7
3-n-butylidene phthalide	Oral, rats	2.45	20

*According to information supplied by the author, this concentrated extract was 8 to 16:1.[7]

was inhibited and blood pressure fell in anaesthetised rabbits, cats and dogs intravenously administered the essential oil (1 mg/kg).[4]

Dong quai significantly induced the proliferation of MCF-7 human breast cancer cells in vitro, but failed to demonstrate oestrogenic activity in vitro or in vivo after oral administration.[21]

Ferulic acid, which also occurs naturally in many fruits and vegetables, demonstrated chromosome-damaging activity in vitro at a concentration of 25 mg/mL.[22,23] However, it has also demonstrated antigenotoxic and anticarcinogenic activity in vivo after oral and intraperitoneal administration and topical application.[23] In any case, it occurs at quite low levels in dong quai.

Safrole, a carcinogenic compound, has been detected in dong quai root,[8] although not confirmed. If present it is likely to occur at very low levels.

Regulatory Status

See Table 2 for regulatory status in selected countries.

Table 2   Regulatory Status for Dong Quai in Selected Countries

Australia	Dong quai is not included in Part 4 of Schedule 4 of the Therapeutic Goods Regulations.
China	Dong quai is official in the *Pharmacopoeia of the People's Republic of China* 1997. The usual adult dosage, usually administered in the form of a decoction, is listed as 4.5 to 9 g.
UK & Germany	Angelica is included on the General Sale List. However, the species is undefined. Dong quai was not included in the Commission E assessment.
US	Dong quai does not have generally recognised as safe (GRAS) status. However, it is freely available as a "dietary supplement" in the US under DSHEA legislation (Dietary Supplement Health and Education Act of 1994).

REFERENCES

1. Liu MA, Qi CH, Yang JC: *Beijing J Trad Chin Med* 5:30-31, 1988.
2. Zhou QJ. In: Chang HM, Yeung HW, Tso WW, et al, eds: *Advances in Chinese medicinal materials research*, Singapore, 1985, World Scientific, p 217.
3. Fu YF, Xia Y, Shi YP, et al: *Jiangsu J Trad Chin Med* 9:15-16, 1988.
4. Chang HM, But PP: *Pharmacology and applications of Chinese materia medica*, vol 1. Singapore, 1987, World Scientific, pp 489-505.
5. Pharmacopoeia Commission of the People's Republic of China: *Pharmacopoeia of the People's Republic of China*, vol 1, English ed, Beijing, 1997, Chemical Industry Press, pp 138-139.
6. Bensky D, Gamble A: *Chinese herbal medicine materia medica*, Seattle, 1986, Eastland Press, pp 474-476.
7. Wagner H, Bauer R, Peigen X, et al, eds: *Chinese drug monographs and analysis: radix Angelicae sinensis – danggui*, Kotzting/Bayer, 2001, Verlag fur Ganzheitliche Medizin.
8. Zhu DP: *Am J Chin Med* 15:117-125, 1987.
9. Zschocke S, Liu JH, Stuppner H, et al: *Phytochem Anal* 9:283-290, 1998.
10. Tang W, Eisenbrand G: *Chinese drugs of plant origin*, Berlin, 1992, Springer-Verlag, pp 111-125.
11. Sheu SJ, Ho YS, Chen YP, et al: *Planta Med* 53:377-378, 1986.
12. Mei QB, Tao JY, Cui B: *Chin Med J* 104:776-781, 1991.
13. Matsui AS, Rogers J, Woo YK, et al: *Med Pharmacol Exp* 16:414-424, 1967.
14. Goh SY, Loh KC: *Singapore Med J* 42:115-116, 2001.
15. Kane JA, Kane SP, Jain S: *Gut* 36:146-147, 1995.
16. Johnson EB, Muto MC, Yanushpolsky EH, et al: *Obstet Gynecol* 98:947-950, 2001.
17. Ellis GR, Stephens MR: *BMJ* 319:650, 1999.
18. Page RL, Lawrence JD: *Pharmacotherapy* 19:870-876, 1999.
19. Lo AC, Chan K, Yeung JH, et al: *Eur J Drug Metab Pharmacokinet* 20:55-60, 1995.
20. Opdyke DL: *Food Cosmet Toxicol* 17:251, 1979.
21. Amato P, Christophe S, Mellon PL: *Menopause* 9:145-150, 2002.
22. Stich HF, Rosin MP, Wu CH, et al: *Cancer Lett* 14:251-260, 1981.
23. Stich HF: *Mutat Res* 259:307-324, 1991.

ECHINACEA

Other common name: Purple coneflower
Botanical names: *Echinacea angustifolia* DC, *Echinacea purpurea* (L.) Moench, *Echinacea pallida* (Nutt.) Nutt.
Family: Compositae
Plant part used: Root; Aerial parts

Safety Summary

Pregnancy category A: No proven increase in the frequency of malformation or other harmful effects on the foetus despite consumption by a large number of women.
Lactation category C: Compatible with breastfeeding.
Contraindications: Transplant patients taking immunosuppressant medication – use echinacea for short-term therapy only.
Warnings & precautions: Allergic reactions may occur in susceptible patients, particularly if the aerial parts are administered.
Adverse reactions: Unpleasant taste, digestive upset, allergic skin reactions (mainly when using aerial parts). Leucopenia and erythema nodosum attributed to echinacea have been documented in case reports.
Interactions: Immunosuppressant medication (theoretical concern).

Typical Therapeutic Use

A review of clinical trials concluded that some echinacea preparations may be better than placebo for preventing and treating the common cold.[1]

Traditional indications for the root of *Echinacea angustifolia* and *Echinacea pallida* in Western herbal medicine include septicaemia, upper respiratory tract catarrh, tonsillitis, boils and abscesses.[2] Although used less extensively than *E. angustifolia* (and *E. pallida*), *Echinacea purpurea* root was used by Native Americans, particularly for cough.[3] There is a record of the use of *E. purpurea* root by Eclectic physicians for the treatment of syphilis,[4] although it is more likely to have been *E. angustifolia*.[3] Native Americans also used *E. angustifolia* leaf, although usually in combination with root and often for only topical application.[2] *Echinacea angustifolia* flowering plant and root were used in homoeopathy in Europe in the mid-1930s. The subsequent use of *E. purpurea* in European herbal medicine occurred

from the cultivation of imported seed from America.[5] *Echinacea pallida* is considered by some authors to be the least effective of the three species.[6]

Actions

Immune modulating, immune enhancing, depurative, antiinflammatory, vulnerary, lymphatic, sialagogue.

Key Constituents

Notable constituents occurring in echinacea are the caffeic acid derivatives, polysaccharides and the lipophilic components (mainly alkylamides and polyacetylenes). The alkylamides, which cause a characteristic tingling in the mouth, include the subgroup of isobutylamides. The level of certain key constituents can vary markedly (even being reduced to zero) depending upon the time of harvest, the quality of postharvest handling (especially drying), geographical location, hybridisation and the subsequent manufacture of the raw material into a herbal product.

Table 1 illustrates the differences between the species and plant parts for two groups of these chemical constituents. The root is often considered to be the most active part.[7,8]

In the past *E. angustifolia* and *E. pallida* have been regarded as varieties of the same species or even identical plants. A revision of the genus Echinacea in 1968 saw them classified as two distinct species. In 1987 it became apparent that a considerable amount of commercial *E. angustifolia* cultivated in Europe was in fact *E. pallida*. Data on *E. angustifolia* published prior to 1987 which was based on European commercial material should be reviewed with caution.[9]

More recently, the designation *E. angustifolia* has been reclassified as a variety of *E. pallida*, namely *E. pallida* var. *angustifolia*.[10]

Adulteration

Echinacea has been readily adulterated, particularly in the United States by species of *Parthenium* such as *P. integrifolium*.[11] The roots of *E. angustifolia* and *E. pallida* are very similar, both macroscopically and microscopically,[12] and are often confused. They can, however, be chemically differentiated.[13]

Table I   **Chemical Profile by Echinacea Species and Plant Part**

ROOT

Alkylamides

Highest quantity in *E. angustifolia*, less in *E. purpurea* and largely absent from *E. pallida*

Caffeic Acid Esters

Echinacoside: present in *E. angustifolia* and *E. pallida* in similar quantities (0.3% to 1.7%); absent from *E. purpurea*

Cichoric acid: present in significant quantities in *E. purpurea* only (0.6% to 2.1%)

Cynarin: characteristic constituent of *E. angustifolia*; not present in *E. purpurea* or *E. pallida*

AERIAL PARTS

Alkylamides

Present in substantially lower quantities than in the roots

Caffeic Acid Esters

Cichoric acid: abundant in the flower of *E. purpurea* (1.2% to 3.1%); smaller amounts present in *E. pallida* (1.2%) and *E. angustifolia* (<0.2%)

In the Unites States, native species of echinacea are dwindling in the wild from loss of habitat and over-harvesting. *E. purpurea* is not as threatened as *E. angustifolia,* since *E. purpurea* is the most widely used species for cultivation.[14]

Typical Dosage Forms & Dosage

Table 2 illustrates the typical adult dosage ranges. Higher doses are often recommended by herbalists during acute infections.

Contraindications

Echinacea is contraindicated in patients taking immunosuppressant medication (such as transplant patients). Short-term therapy only is suggested in this instance.

The German Commission E monograph states that, in principle, echinacea should not be used in "progressive conditions" such as tuberculosis, leukaemia, collagen disorders, multiple sclerosis, AIDS, HIV infection, and other autoimmune disease.[15] However, the key words here are "in principle". There are no clinical studies or case reports which document any adverse effect resulting from echinacea use in any of these conditions. Other authoritative sources do not support these restrictions.[2,9]

A 1999 publication suggested that echinacea is not beneficial for the immune systems of people living with HIV.[16] The basis for this recommendation appears to be extrapolated from the results of an

Table **2**   **Typical Adult Dosage Ranges for Echinacea**

	Dried Herb*	Liquid Extract	Tincture, Juice
E. angustifolia root	3 g/day	0.75 to 3 mL/day of 1:1 3 to 6 mL/day of 1:2†	3 to 15 mL/day of 1:5
E. purpurea root	—	3 to 6 mL/day of 1:2†	4.5 to 8.5 mL/day of 1:3
E. purpurea aerial parts	—	—	6 to 9 mL/day of expressed juice
E. pallida root	3 g/day	0.75 to 3 mL/day of 1:1	3 to 6 mL/day of 1:5

*Or by infusion or decoction.
†Or equivalent in tablet or capsule form.

in vitro study, for which incubation with fresh expressed juice of *E. purpurea* stimulated the production of cytokines from human peripheral blood macrophages.[17] Seven other in vitro and two in vivo studies also reported stimulation of cytokines after application of echinacea. However, six of the seven in vitro studies used either purified polysaccharides or extracts containing glycoproteins and polysaccharides; these same extracts were administered by intravenous injection to mice in the in vivo studies.[17-19] How the results of such studies relate to oral use of echinacea is not known, particularly since the polysaccharides and glycoproteins may not be bioavailable. Oral administration of *E. purpurea* leaf to mice with experimentally-induced leukaemia resulted in increased survival time and decreased size of lymphoma. Production of endogenous IFN-gamma was increased, but the change in production of other cytokines such as TNF-α and IL-12 was minimal.[20] On the other hand, a clinical study found no significant alteration in the production of cytokines in patients orally administered a preparation containing *E. angustifolia*, *Eupatorium perfoliatum* and *Thuja occidentalis* when compared to controls.[21] The above in vitro research may have triggered the concern expressed in a 1997 article published in the *Australian Medical Observer*, which cautioned that echinacea is a danger to asthmatic patients.[22] There is currently no sound evidence to suggest that echinacea cannot be used for the treatment of HIV, or that it should be used with caution in asthma.

The suggestion that echinacea is contraindicated in autoimmune disease assumes that any enhancement of any aspect of immune function is detrimental. There is growing evidence that an inappropriate response to infectious microorganisms, through phenomena such as molecular mimicry, may be a factor in the pathogenesis of autoimmune disorders. If so, echinacea may be beneficial in these disorders because it may decrease the chronic presence of microorganisms. There are several herbalists who routinely prescribe echinacea in autoimmune disease without apparent adverse effects in their patients.

Use In Pregnancy

Category A: No proven increase in the frequency of malformation or other harmful effects on the foetus despite consumption by a large number of women.

A prospective, controlled study published in 2000 concluded that gestational use of echinacea (typically for 5 to 7 days) during organogenesis was not associated with an increased risk of major malformations. There were no significant differences in pregnancy outcome between the study group consisting of 206 women who had used echinacea during pregnancy (112 during the first trimester, 17 for all three trimesters) and 206 matched controls. In the echinacea group there was a total of 195 live births, 14 abortions, and 6 major malformations (note there were multiple births for some women). Four of these malformations occurred with echinacea exposure in the first trimester. In the matched controls there was a total of 198 live births, 8 abortions, and 7 major malformations.[23]

Expressed juice of *E. purpurea* (up to 2.7 g/kg, oral) did not cause any embryotoxic effects in rats and rabbits. Postnatal development was not affected in rats.[24] Injection of *E. purpurea* solution did not affect early development in chick embryos.[25]

Use In Lactation

Category C: Compatible with breastfeeding.

Warnings & Precautions

Allergic reactions, mainly contact dermatitis, may occur rarely in susceptible patients sensitised to echinacea aerial parts and to plants from the Compositae family. The likelihood of echinacea root preparations causing allergy is very low.

There is no sound evidence that it is detrimental to use echinacea for long periods. Indications listed in traditional sources (such as prophylaxis and treatment of chronic infections) suggest long-term usage is warranted.[2,9] A risk–benefit assessment of expressed juice of *E. purpurea* found it was well tolerated on long-term oral administration (up to 12 weeks).[26] A randomised, double-blind, placebo-controlled trial investigating the efficacy of two herbal formulas in preventing the common cold in highly stressed medical students over a period of 15 weeks also found *E. angustifolia* root and *E. purpurea* root blend to be effective and well tolerated.[27]

There is no evidence to suggest that echinacea causes immune system tachyphylaxis. In a clinical study, the oral administration of *E. purpurea* tincture over a 5-day period increased phagocytic activity compared to controls.[28] Only when the echinacea was stopped did phagocytic activity decline to normal (pretest) values, demonstrating a typical washout effect. This demonstrated that there was in fact a residual stimulating effect, which lasted for about two days after echinacea was ceased.[29]

Effect on Ability to Drive or Operate Machinery

No adverse effects expected.

Adverse Reactions

Adverse reactions to echinacea are relatively infrequent and typically consist of digestive upset.[26] The unpleasant taste and increased salivation with liquid preparations may cause inexperienced patients to panic.

Contact dermatitis may occur rarely in susceptible patients. In Europe, echinacea is one of many species of the Compositae family, which is known to cause sensitisation or dermatitis. For exposure to echinacea, the occurrence is rare.[30] Allergenicity is likely to be due to the presence of protein in the pollen (see Chapter 10).

A review of clinical trials to 1997 indicated that echinacea appeared to be a safe treatment.[31] Table 3 provides details of case reports of adverse reactions associated with ingestion of echinacea.[26,32-38,40]

A critical review of ADRAC reports received between April 1990 and November 2001, which involved echinacea (54 in total), found that the limited information presented made it difficult to find a causal association with echinacea. Not a single report stated the species or plant part taken, and in

Table **3   Case Reports of Adverse Reactions Associated with Ingestion of Echinacea**

Case Reports	Adverse Reaction	Additional Details	Ref
1 case, 2002; echinacea (1500 mg/day, 2 months), also taking buproprion, vitamins and minerals	Leucopenia	White blood cell count fluctuated in direct association with echinacea intake over 11 months.	32
5 cases, 2002; echinacea (undefined)*	Anaphylaxis (2) Acute asthma attack (1) Recurrent mild asthma (1) Maculopapular rash (1)	Three patients had positive results on SPT[†]	33
1 case, 2001; echinacea (undefined)	Recurrent erythema nodosum		34
51 case reports, received by ADRAC[‡] Jan 1979 to Mar 2000; echinacea products	Allergic response (26)[§] Nonurticarial rash (12) Hepatitis (7) Fatigue, arthralgia, myalgia, headache, increased blood pressure, dizziness, atrial fibrillation, vasculitis, acute renal failure, nausea, epistaxis (remainder)[‖]	In 41 cases, echinacea was implicated as the sole suspected trigger (See also critical review, below)	33
1 case, 1999; echinacea	Hyperglycaemia	Patient had insulin-dependent diabetes	35
1 case, 1998; preparation containing *E. angustifolia* whole plant and *E. purpurea* root; other dietary supplements	Anaphylaxis		36

Table **3** **Case Reports of Adverse Reactions Associated with Ingestion of Echinacea—Cont'd**

Case Reports	Adverse Reaction	Additional Details	Ref
3 cases, over a 6-year period, reported in German media in 1996	Death (unsubstantiated)	No action taken by the authorities, as no causal link between the deaths and the taking of echinacea could be established	37
13 adverse reactions, 1989 to 1995, received by German authorities; expressed juice of *E. purpurea*	Allergic skin reactions	In only 4 cases were the adverse events considered causally related to echinacea treatment[¶]	26

Patch Testing	Result	Additional Details	Ref
100 atopic patients, 2002	20 patients had positive results on SPT[†] Only 3 of these had taken echinacea previously	Previous echinacea use unknown, but none experienced a reaction when taking it[#]	33
1032 patients from 6 patch test clinics, July 1988 to early 1989	2 had positive reaction to echinacea	Ointment containing *E. angustifolia* (part undefined) and components of the ointment bases tested. Not certain that the reaction was to the plant material	38

*Correspondence with the authors indicated that in one of the 5 cases, a tablet consisting of E. angustifolia root powder (250 mg) and extract equivalent to dry E. purpurea flowering herb (1.5 g) had been taken.[39]
[†]The aqueous and glycerinated extracts used in the skin prick test (SPT) were made from a combination of E. purpurea whole plant and E. angustifolia root.
[‡]Adverse Drug Reactions Advisory Committee, Australia.
[§]Of the 24 cases for which information was available, causality was indicated in ADRAC data as certain (2 cases), probable (10) and possible (12).
[||]Listed as incidence of side effect.
[¶]Compared to several million patient courses the reported adverse reaction rate, and hence the estimated risk, is quite small.[40]
[#]It is possible that crossreactivity between echinacea and other environmental allergens may trigger allergic reactions in those who have not taken echinacea.*

the majority of cases even the dosage taken by the patient was not included. In many cases there was concomitant use of drugs that had the potential to cause the observed adverse reactions. Considering the extensive use of echinacea and echinacea-containing products in Australia, there have been relatively very few reported cases of allergy. Allergic reactions to echinacea are likely to occur in a few susceptible individuals. These reactions are most likely to occur in preparations containing the whole plant and unlikely to occur with products made from root.[39]

Misinformation exists that echinacea is potentially hepatotoxic due to the presence of pyrrolizidine alkaloids (PAs). However the PAs found in echinacea do not contain the 1,2-unsaturated necrine ring system essential for such reactions.

Interactions

Do not prescribe echinacea long term with immunosuppressant medication, as it may decrease the effectiveness of the drug. This is a theoretical concern based on the immune-enhancing activity of echinacea. No case reports of this interaction have been published.

Safety in Children

No information available, but adverse effects are not expected. Echinacea is being investigated for the prevention of recurrent otitis media in children,[41] and for the treatment of upper respiratory tract infections in children 2 to 11 years old.[42]

Overdosage

No incidents found in published literature.

Toxicology

Table 4 lists LD_{50} data recorded for echinacea expressed juice.[43]

The acute oral toxicity of an *E. purpurea* root extract has been determined to be greater than 3 g/kg in mice.[44] No significant toxicity was found in rats orally administered the expressed juice of *E. purpurea* over 4 weeks in doses up to 8 g/kg/day. In vitro and in vivo tests for mutagenicity gave negative results and carcinogenicity was not evident in vitro. There was no evidence of mutagenicity either in bacterial and mammalian cells or in vivo (oral, 25 g/kg, mice) or of carcinogenicity (in vitro test).[43]

Regulatory Status

See Table 5 for regulatory status in selected countries.

Table **4** **LD_{50} Data Recorded for Echinacea Expressed Juice**

Substance	Route, Model	LD_{50} Value	Reference
Expressed juice of *E. purpurea*	Oral, rats	>15 g/mg	43
Expressed juice of *E. purpurea*	Oral, mice	>30 g/kg	43

Table **5** **Regulatory Status for Echinacea in Selected Countries**

Australia	Echinacea is not included in Part 4 of Schedule 4 of the Therapeutic Goods Regulations.
UK & Germany	Echinacea is included on the General Sale List. *E. purpurea* aerial parts and *E. pallida* root are covered by a positive Commission E monograph. *E. angustifolia* aerial parts, *E. angustifolia* root, *E. purpurea* root and *E. pallida* aerial parts are covered by a negative Commission E monograph.
US	Rhizome with roots of *E. angustifolia*, *E. purpurea* and *E. pallida* are official in the *United States Pharmacopeia-National Formulary* (USP 26-NF 21, 2003).
	Echinacea does not have generally recognised as safe (GRAS) status. However, *E. angustifolia*, *E. purpurea* and *E. pallida* are freely available as a "dietary supplement" in the US under DSHEA legislation (Dietary Supplement Health and Education Act of 1994).

REFERENCES

1. Melchart D, Linde K, Fischer P, et al: *Cochrane Database Syst Rev* 2:CD000530, 2000.
2. British Herbal Medicine Association's Scientific Committee: *British herbal pharmacopoeia*, Bournemouth, 1983, BHMA, pp 80-81.
3. Bergner P: *The healing power of echinacea & goldenseal and other immune system herbs*, Rocklin, 1997, Prima Publishing, pp 10-17.
4. Felter HW, Lloyd JU: *King's American dispensatory*, ed 18, rev 3, vol 1; first published 1905, reprinted Portland, 1983, Eclectic Medical Publications, p 677.
5. Corrigan D: *Indian medicine for the immune system*, Surrey, 1994, Amberwood Publishing Ltd, pp 11-12.
6. Hobbs C: *Echinacea: the immune herb*, Santa Cruz, 1990, Botanica Press, pp 25-28.
7. Wagner H, Farnsworth NR, eds: *Economic and medicinal plant research*, vol 5, London, 1991, Academic Press, pp 258-285.
8. Bauer R: Chemistry, analysis and immunological investigations of echinacea phytopharmaceuticals. In Wagner H, ed: *Immunomodulatory agents from plants*, Basel, 1999, Birkauser Verlag, pp 42-73.

9. British Herbal Medicine Association: *British herbal compendium*, vol 1, Bournemouth, 1992, BHMA, pp 81-83.

10. Binns SE, Baum BR, Arnason JT: *Syst Bot* 27:610-632, 2002.

11. Hobbs C: *Echinacea: the immune herb*, Santa Cruz, 1990, Botanica Press, p 70.

12. Bisset NG, ed: *Herbal drugs and phytopharmaceuticals: a handbook for practice on a scientific basis*, Stuttgart, 1994, Medpharm Scientific Publishers, pp 182-184.

13. Blaschek W, Ebel S, Hackenthal E, et al: *HagerROM 2002: Hagers Handbuch der Drogen und Arzneistoffe*, Heidelberg, 2002, Springer.

14. Natural Resources Conservation Service: *Plant guide: eastern purple coneflower Echinacea purpurea (L.) Moench*, United States Department of Agriculture. Available via http://plants.usda.gov (accessed May 2003).

15. Blumenthal M, et al, eds: *The complete German Commission E monographs: therapeutic guide to herbal medicines*, Austin, 1998, American Botanical Council, pp 121-123, 327-328, 391-393.

16. No authors listed: *Treatmentupdate* 11:3, 1999.

17. Burger RA, Torres AR, Warren RP, et al: *Int J Immunopharmacol* 19:371-379, 1997.

18. Bauer R: Chemistry, analysis and immunological investigations of echinacea phytopharmaceuticals. In Wagner H, ed: *Immunomodulatory agents from plants*, Basel, 1999, Birkauser Verlag, pp 49-53, 56-57, 62-65, 73-77.

19. Rininger JA, Kickner S, Chigurupati P, et al: *J Leukoc Biol* 68:503-510, 2000.

20. Hayashi I, Ohotsuki M, Suzuki I, et al: *Nihon Rinsho Meneki Gakkai Kaishi* 24:10-20, 2001.

21. Elsasser-Beile U, Willenbacher W, Bartsch HH, et al: *J Clin Lab Anal* 10:441-445, 1996.

22. Sharp R: Echinacea a danger to asthmatics, *Medical Observer* 8 August 1997, p 1.

23. Gallo M, Sarkar M, Au W, et al: *Arch Intern Med* 160:3141-3143, 2000.

24. Mengs U, Leuschner J, Marshall RR: *Phytomedicine* 7(Suppl 2):32, 2000.

25. Nuckols JT, Chopin SF: *J Investig Med* 48:113A, 2000.

26. Parnham MJ: *Phytomedicine* 3:95-102, 1996.

27. MacIntosh A, D'Huyvetter K, Goldberg B, et al: *Prevention of colds by two herbal formulas in a high stress population*, unpublished data on file, Warwick, Australia, 2001, MediHerb Pty Ltd.

28. Jurcic K, Melchart D, Holzmann M, et al: *Z Phytother* 10:67-70, 1989.

29. Mills S, Bone K: *Principles and practice of phytotherapy: modern herbal medicine*, Edinburgh, 2000, Churchill Livingstone, pp 354-362.

30. Paulsen E: *Contact Dermatitis* 47:189-198, 2002.

31. Giles JT, Palat CT 3rd, Chien SH, et al: *Pharmacotherapy* 20:690-697, 2000.

32. Kemp DE, Franco KN: *J Am Board Fam Pract* 15:417-419, 2002.

33. Mullins RJ, Heddle R: *Ann Allergy Asthma Immunol* 88:42-51, 2002.

34. Soon SL, Crawford RI: *J Am Acad Dermatol* 44:298-299, 2001.

35. Finlay P: *Diabetes Forecast* 52:15-16, 1999.

36. Mullins RJ: *Med J Aust* 168:170-171, 1998.

37. Bauer R, Wagner H: *Z Phytother* 17:251-252, 1996.

38. Bruynzeel DP, Van Ketel WG, Young E, et al: *Contact Dermatitis* 27:278-279, 1992.

39. Burgoyne B: Information on file, Warwick, Australia, March 2002, MediHerb Pty Ltd.

40. Barrett B, Vohmann M, Calabrese C: *J Fam Pract* 48:628-635, 1999.

41. Mark JD, Grant KL, Barton LL: *Clin Pediatr* 40:265-269, 2001.

42. Taylor JA: Crisp data base, National Institutes of Health, 2000.

43. Mengs U, Clare CB, Poiley JA: *Arzneim-Forsch* 41:1076-1081, 1991.

44. Blumenthal M, et al, eds: *The complete German Commission E monographs: therapeutic guide to herbal medicines*, Austin, 1998, American Botanical Council, pp 391-393.

ELDER FLOWER

Other common name: Sambucus
Botanical name: *Sambucus nigra* L.
Family: Caprifoliaceae
Plant part used: Flower

Safety Summary

Pregnancy category B2: No increase in frequency of malformation or other harmful effects on the foetus from limited use in women. Animal studies are lacking.
Lactation category C: Compatible with breast-feeding.
Contraindications: None required on current evidence.
Warnings & precautions: None required on current evidence.
Adverse reactions: None found in published literature.
Interactions: No precautions required on current evidence.

Typical Therapeutic Use

Traditional indications for elder flower in Western herbal medicine include influenza, the common cold, and sinusitis.[1]

Actions

Diaphoretic, anticatarrhal.

Key Constituents

Constituents of elder flower include flavonoids, phenolic acids, triterpenes and an essential oil.[2]

Adulteration

Sambucus nigra flowers may occasionally be adulterated with *S. ebulus* (leaf, fruit and root of *S. ebulus* are used therapeutically, but are not medicinally interchangeable with *S. nigra*).[3]

Typical Dosage Forms & Dosage

Typical adult dosage ranges are:
- 6 to 12 g/day of dried flower or by infusion
- 6 to 12 mL/day of a 1:1 liquid extract
- 2 to 6 mL/day of a 1:2 liquid extract or equivalent in tablet or capsule form
- 30 to 75 mL/day of a 1:5 tincture

Contraindications

None known.

Use in Pregnancy

Category B2: No increase in frequency of malformation or other harmful effects on the foetus from limited use in women. Animal studies are lacking.

Use in Lactation

Category C: Compatible with breastfeeding.

Warnings & Precautions

None required.

Effect on Ability to Drive or Operate Machinery

No adverse effects expected.

Adverse Reactions

In large doses, elder flower may produce nausea, diarrhoea,[4] and polyuria.[5] Elder berries eaten raw can cause nausea and vomiting in humans.[6]

Interactions

None reported in humans. Elder flower decoction (2 mL/kg of 1:10) caused a significant decrease of the sleep induction time of pentobarbitone and increased sleeping time when compared with rats administered pentobarbitone only. Elder flower had no significant effect on the analgesic activity of morphine at this dosage.[7]

Safety in Children

No information available.

Overdosage

No incidents were found in the published literature for poisoning in humans with flower of *Sambucus nigra.* There have been reports of poisoning in children with European red elder berry (species undefined).[8] Livestock do not spontaneously eat the elder plant and in the very rare cases of poisoning that have been recorded, the symptoms and lesions are those of superpurgation.[4]

Toxicology

No significant toxicity was observed in rabbits administered an ethanol extract of elder flowers intragastrically (39 mg/kg/day of dried herb) over a period of 3 days. Parameters measured included rate of breathing, pulse rate, red blood count, Quick value (prothrombin time), and serum calcium, potassium, and sodium.[9]

Regulatory Status

See Table 1 for regulatory status in selected countries.

Table 1   **Regulatory Status for Elder Flower in Selected Countries**

Australia	Elder is not included in Part 4 of Schedule 4 of the Therapeutic Goods Regulations.
UK & Germany	Elder is included on the General Sale List. Elder flower is covered by a positive Commission E monograph.
	It is official in the *British Pharmacopoeia* 2002 and the *European Pharmacopoeia* 4.3.
US	Elder flower does have generally recognised as safe (GRAS) status. It is freely available as a "dietary supplement" in the US under DSHEA legislation (Dietary Supplement Health and Education Act of 1994).

REFERENCES

1. British Herbal Medicine Association's Scientific Committee: *British herbal pharmacopoeia,* Bournemouth, 1983, BHMA, pp 186-187.
2. British Herbal Medicine Association. *British herbal compendium,* vol 1. Bournemouth, 1992, BHMA, pp 84-85.
3. Blaschek W, Ebel S, Hackenthal E, et al: *HagerROM 2002: Hagers Handbuch der Drogen und Arzneistoffe,* Heidelberg, 2002, Springer.
4. Chopra RN, Badhwar RL, Ghosh S: *Poisonous plants of India,* vol 1, New Delhi, 1965, Indian Council of Agricultural Research, pp 447-448.
5. Gessner O: *Gift- und Arzneipflanzen von Mitteleuropa,* ed 3, Heidelberg, 1974, Carl Winter Universitatsverlag, pp 317-319.
6. Munro DB: Canadian Poisonous Plants Information System. Ottawa, 1993, Centre for Land and Biological Resources Research. Electronic file, also available via http://sis.agr.gc.ca/pls/pp/poison?p_x=px within the Agriculture and Agri-Food Canada webpage.
7. Jakovljevic V, Popovic M, Mimica-Dukic N, et al: *Pharm Biol* 39:142-145, 2001.
8. Lamminpaa A, Kinos M: *Hum Exp Toxicol* 15:245-249, 1996.
9. Chibanguza G, Marz R, Sterner W: *Arzneim Forsch* 34:32-36, 1984.

ELECAMPANE

Botanical name: *Inula helenium* L.
Family: Compositae
Plant part used: Root

Safety Summary

Pregnancy category B2: No increase in frequency of malformation or other harmful effects on the foetus from limited use in women. Animal studies are lacking.

Lactation category SD: Strongly discouraged in breastfeeding (on the basis of the presence of the sesquiterpene lactone alantolactone, which can act as a contact allergen).

Contraindications: Known sensitivity. Do not use during lactation without professional advice.

Warnings & precautions: Avoid in patients with known hypersensitivity to plants in the Compositae family and other plants containing sesquiterpene lactones.

Adverse reactions: Allergic contact dermatitis.

Interactions: No precautions required on current evidence.

Typical Therapeutic Use

Traditional indications for elecampane in Western herbal medicine include bronchial or tracheal catarrh and irritating cough, especially bronchitis or pulmonary tuberculosis.[1] Therapeutic indications for elecampane in traditional Chinese medicine (TCM) include distending pain in the chest, hypochondrium and epigastrium, vomiting and diarrhoea.[2] Constituents of elecampane have demonstrated therapeutic benefit in patients with peptic ulcer disease[3] and in children with *Ascaris*·infestation.[4]

Actions

Expectorant, diaphoretic, antibacterial, spasmolytic, bronchospasmolytic.

Key Constituents

Constituents of elecampane root include sesquiterpene lactones of the eudesmanolide type (such as alantolactone, isoalantolactone and their derivatives), and essential oil.[5]

Adulteration

Adulteration is very rare, but Belladonna roots are sometimes encountered.[6,7]

Typical Dosage Forms & Dosage

Typical adult dosage ranges are:
- 4.5 to 12 g/day of dried root or by decoction
- 4.5 to 12 mL/day of a 1:1 liquid extract
- 3 to 6 mL/day of a 1:2 liquid extract or equivalent in tablet or capsule form
- 9 to 15 mL/day of a 1:5 tincture

Contraindications

Contraindicated in those with known sensitivity. Do not use during lactation without professional advice.

Use in Pregnancy

Category B2: No increase in frequency of malformation or other harmful effects on the foetus from limited use in women. Animal studies are lacking.

Elecampane is listed as contraindicated in pregnancy in the *British Herbal Compendium*.[5] However, it is indicated for threatened abortion in TCM.[2]

Use in Lactation

Category SD: Strongly discouraged in breastfeeding.

The *British Herbal Compendium* lists elecampane as contraindicated in lactation,[5] perhaps on the basis of the presence of the sesquiterpene lactone alantolactone, which is a contact allergen.

Warnings & Precautions

Avoid in patients with known hypersensitivity to plants in the Compositae family and other plants containing sesquiterpene lactones.

Effect on Ability to Drive or Operate Machinery

No adverse effects expected.

Adverse Reactions

Occasional allergic contact dermatitis reactions may occur, due to sensitivity caused by the sesquiterpene lactones present in elecampane.[8-11]

Interactions

None reported.

Safety in Children

No information available.

Overdosage

Large doses of alantolactone or overdose with elecampane can lead to nausea, vomiting, diarrhoea, stomach cramps, rash and symptoms of paralysis.[7,12]

Toxicology

Parenteral administration of helenin to animals led to vomiting, convulsions, paralysis and breathing difficulty. The oral lethal dose of helenin in rabbits was 1.2 g/kg.[7] (The crystalline portion of steam distilled elecampane root, which is primarily a mixture of sesquiterpene lactones, has been referred to as helenin [or alant camphor], particularly in older literature. These names have also been applied to alantolactone itself.[5,7]) Alantolactone (1 μg/mL) exhibited toxic effects in vitro in leukocyte cultures.[13]

Regulatory Status

See Table 1 for regulatory status in selected countries.

Table 1   **Regulatory Status for Elecampane in Selected Countries**

Australia	Elecampane is not included in Part 4 of Schedule 4 of the Therapeutic Goods Regulations.
China	Elecampane is official in the *Pharmacopoeia of the People's Republic of China*, 1997. The usual adult dosage, used mostly in making pills or powder, is listed as 3 to 9 g.
UK & Germany	Elecampane is included on the General Sale List. It is covered by a negative Commission E monograph.
US	Elecampane does not have generally recognised as safe (GRAS) status. However, it is freely available as a "dietary supplement" in the US under DSHEA legislation (Dietary Supplement Health and Education Act of 1994).

REFERENCES

1. British Herbal Medicine Association's Scientific Committee: *British herbal pharmacopoeia*, Bournemouth, 1983, BHMA, p 118.
2. Pharmacopoeia Commission of the People's Republic of China: *Pharmacopoeia of the People's Republic of China*, English ed, vol I, Beijing, 1997, Chemical Industry Press, p 155.
3. Luchkova MM: *Vrachebnoe Delo* 6:69-71, 1978.
4. Ozeki S, Kotake M, Hayashi K: *Proc Imp Acad* 12:233-234, 1936.
5. British Herbal Medicine Association: *British herbal compendium*, Bournemouth, 1992, BHMA, pp 87-88.
6. Bisset NG, ed: *Herbal drugs and phytopharmaceuticals: a handbook for practice on a scientific basis*, Stuttgart, 1994, Medpharm Scientific Publishers, pp 254-256.
7. Blaschek W, Ebel S, Hackenthal E, et al: *HagerROM 2002: Hagers Handbuch der Drogen und Arzneistoffe*, Heidelberg, 2002, Springer.
8. Lamminpaa A, Estlander T, Jolanki R, et al: *Contact Dermatitis* 34:330-335, 1996.
9. Alonso Blasi N, Fraginalis R, Lepoittevin JP, et al: *Arch Dermatol Res* 284:297-302, 1992.
10. P'iankova ZP, Nugmanova ML: *Vestn Dermatol Venerol* 12:52-54, 1975.
11. Pazzaglia M, Venturo N, Borda G, et al: *Contact Dermatitis* 33:267, 1995.
12. Blumenthal M, et al, eds: *The complete German Commission E monographs: therapeutic guide to herbal medicines*, Austin, 1998, American Botanical Council, pp 328-329.
13. Dupuis G, Brisson J: *Chem Biol Interact* 15:205-217, 1976.

EPHEDRA

Other common name: Ma Huang
Botanical names: *Ephedra sinica* Stapf, *E. intermedia* Schrenk et C.A. Mey, *E. equisetina* Bge (*E. shennungiana* Tang), *E. gerardiana* Wall, *E. nebrodensis* Tineo
Family: Ephedraceae
Plant part used: Stem and branch

Safety Summary

Pregnancy category B3: No increase in frequency of malformation or other harmful effects on the foetus from limited use in women. Evidence of increased foetal damage in animal studies exists, although the relevance to humans is unknown.
Lactation category SD: Strongly discouraged in breastfeeding.
Contraindications: Contraindications for use of ephedra include anxiety, hypertension, glaucoma, impaired cerebral circulation, heart disease, benign prostatic hyperplasia associated with urine retention, phaeochromocytoma, thyrotoxicosis and concurrent use with monoamine oxidase (MAO) inhibitor drugs (see also the Interactions section below). Do not use during pregnancy or lactation without professional advice.
Warnings & precautions: Caution during pregnancy, especially in the first trimester. Ephedra should not be taken long term since tolerance and dependency are associated with ephedrine use. Concurrent use of ephedra with sympathomimetic drugs is best avoided. Ephedra should be discontinued at least one week prior to surgery.
Adverse reactions: Typical adverse effects include insomnia, restlessness, irritability, headache, nausea, vomiting, disturbance of urination, hypertension and cardiac arrhythmias. Rare and serious adverse events could include seizures, psychiatric disturbances, hepatotoxicity, stroke and myocardial infarction. Deaths have been attributed to the use of ephedra.
Interactions: Ephedra is best avoided in conjunction with cardiac glycosides, halothane, guanethidine, ergot alkaloid derivatives, and oxytocin. Caution should also be exercised for concurrent use of ephedra with CNS stimulants, antihypertensive drugs, α and β adrenergic agonists and selective serotonin reuptake inhibitor drugs. Use of ephedra in conjunction with MAO inhibitor drugs is contraindicated.

Typical Therapeutic Use

Two patterns of use have developed for ephedra in recent times. On the one hand, there are the ongoing traditional uses for fever, asthma, upper respiratory tract congestion and oedema in traditional Chinese medicine (TCM)[1] and for asthma, allergies and enuresis in Western herbal medicine.[2] On the other hand, ephedra and its main alkaloid ephedrine have become popular, particularly in the United States, for assisting weight loss and boosting athletic performance.[3] There are controlled clinical trials with positive outcomes to support these recent uses[3] and the RAND report concluded that, despite methodological weaknesses in the studies, there is evidence that ephedrine-containing dietary supplements (with or without other stimulants such as caffeine) do provide a statistically significant increase in short-term weight loss (compared to placebo).[4]

Actions

Antiallergic, decongestant, central nervous system stimulant, sympathomimetic, diaphoretic (TCM), diuretic (TCM).

Key Constituents

Ephedra typically contains 2.5% to 3% total alkaloids including L-ephedrine (0.75% to 1%), norephedrine, (+)-pseudoephedrine and norpseudoephedrine.[5] The Chinese pharmacopoeia specifies that ephedra should contain not less than 0.8% total alkaloids (as determined by the method provided in that text) calculated as ephedrine.[6]

Adulteration

Sida cordifolia has been mentioned as a possible adulterant.[7]

Typical Dosage Forms & Dosage

Typical traditional adult dosage ranges are:
- 3 to 12 g/day of dried stem or by decoction
- 3 to 9 mL/day of a 1:1 liquid extract
- 1.5 to 4.5 mL/day of a 1:2 liquid extract or equivalent in tablet or capsule form

For assisting weight loss and boosting athletic performance, tablet or capsule products typically recommend doses equivalent to 60 to 90 mg/day of ephedrine (either as the herb, herb extract or pure ephedrine).

Contraindications

Contraindications listed by the Commission E are anxiety and restlessness, high blood pressure, glaucoma, impaired cerebral circulation, benign prostatic hyperplasia associated with urine retention, phaeochromocytoma, and thyrotoxicosis.[8]

The WHO monograph adds coronary thrombosis, heart disease, and diabetes, and additionally contraindicates coadministration with MAO inhibitors, which can lead to severe, possibly fatal, hypertension.[9] (See also the Interactions section below.)

The proposed U.S. herbal industry label warning for products containing ephedra is as follows:

> *"WARNING: Not intended for use by anyone under the age of 18. Do not use this product if you are pregnant or nursing. Consult a health care professional before using this product if you have heart disease, thyroid disease, diabetes, high blood pressure, depression or other psychiatric condition, glaucoma, difficulty in urinating, prostate enlargement, or seizure disorder, if you are using a MAO inhibitor, or any other prescription drug, or you are using an over-the-counter drug containing ephedrine, pseudoephedrine or phenylpropanolamine (PPA) (ingredients found in certain allergy, asthma, cough/cold and weight control products). Exceeding recommended serving will not improve results and may cause serious adverse health effects. Discontinue use and call a health care professional immediately if you experience rapid heartbeat, dizziness, severe headache, shortness of breath, or other similar symptoms."*

As noted on the label warning, some writers feel that ephedra is contraindicated during pregnancy,[3] although this concern is not reiterated in TCM,[1] nor by the Commission E.[8] (See also Use in pregnancy below.) Do not use during pregnancy or lactation without professional advice.

Use in Pregnancy

Category B3: No increase in frequency of malformation or other harmful effects on the foetus from limited use in women. Evidence of increased foetal damage in animal studies exists, although the relevance to humans is unknown.

Maternal consumption of a herbal mixture containing ephedra was implicated in the premature birth and death of an infant.[10] However, the relevance of this finding to ephedra is not known. Intake of ephedrine in the first trimester was not associated with an increased incidence of congenital malformations,[11] but foetal irritability and tachycardia have been observed following maternal ingestion of ephedrine during labour.[12]

Ephedra was not abortifacient in rats and did not exhibit teratogenic effects.[13] An antifertility effect was noted for ephedra in one animal study.[14]

Administration of ephedrine caused cardiovascular malformations in the embryonic chick[15] and in rats.[16] Ephedrine administered to pregnant rabbits resulted in cardiovascular abnormalities in the offspring and incidences of foetal loss.[17]

Use in Lactation

Category SD: Strongly discouraged in breastfeeding.

Warnings & Precautions

Caution during pregnancy, especially in the first trimester. Ephedra should not be taken long term since tolerance and dependency are associated with ephedrine use. Concurrent use of ephedra with sympathomimetic drugs is best avoided.

Intake of ephedra could result in a positive drug test for ephedrine.[18] The ephedrine content of most commercially available cold remedies is well in excess of the amount necessary to cause users to exceed current International Olympic Committee cutoffs. Healthy volunteers given realistic doses of an ephedrine-containing nasal spray (roughly 14 mg) were found to have urine levels ranging from 0.09 to 1.65 µg/mL.[19] It has also been speculated that intake of ephedrine or ephedra may result in a positive drug test to amphetamines, due to the poor specificity of some test methodologies.[20]

Ephedra should be discontinued at least one week prior to surgery.[21]

Effect on Ability to Drive or Operate Machinery

Excessive and prolonged doses may cause impairment of judgement. A major road accident in Australia was attributed to the use of ephedrine by a truck driver.[22]

Adverse Reactions

Adverse effects from typical doses of ephedra are listed by the Commission E as insomnia, restlessness, irritability, headache, nausea, vomiting, disturbance of urination, and tachycardia.[8] In higher doses ephedra is said to cause hypertension, cardiac arrhythmia, and possible development of dependency.[8] The WHO monograph also notes that prolonged use (>3 days) of topical nasal preparations containing ephedra may cause rebound congestion and chronic rhinitis.[9]

The distinct possibility exists that ephedra or ephedrine may rarely cause serious adverse reactions including hepatotoxicity, stroke, and myocardial infarction.[3] Deaths, including sudden death, have been linked to the use of ephedra and ephedrine.[3]

Since its widespread promotion and use in the United States, numerous adverse reactions to ephedra have been recorded. However, it is difficult to assess meaningfully the majority of these, due to insufficient information, the failure to distinguish between ephedrine and ephedra as treatments, and the tendency to combine ephedra with other stimulants in weight loss products (which may potentiate its ability to cause serious side effects).

Nonetheless, the RAND report undertook a comprehensive analysis of adverse consequences from both clinical trials and case reports submitted to the FDA.[4] In terms of clinical trials, the report concluded that there is sufficient evidence that the use of ephedrine and/or ephedra, or ephedrine plus caffeine, is associated with two to three times the risk of nausea, vomiting, psychiatric symptoms such as anxiety and change in mood, autonomic hyperactivity, and palpitations. It was not possible to determine the contribution of caffeine to these events. There were no reports of serious adverse events in the controlled trials.[4]

From the adverse events reported to one manufacturer of ephedra-containing dietary supplements and to the U.S. FDA, the RAND report identified what it termed to be "sentinel events" (classification of a sentinel event does not mean to imply a proven cause and effect relationship). These included two deaths, three myocardial infarctions, nine strokes, three seizures and five psychiatric cases, with prior ephedra consumption. The report also identified 43 additional cases as possible sentinel events and noted that about half of all the sentinel events occurred in those aged 30 years or younger.[4]

Hepatotoxicity has been linked to the use of ephedra both in traditional Chinese formulations and in weight loss supplements.[23-25]

One unlikely hypothesis put forth in the literature was that the use of ephedra and ephedrine is associated with kidney stones.[26] It was claimed that these alkaloids could be detected in patients' stones.

Interactions

According to the Commission E, interactions are possible with cardiac glycosides and halothane (heart rhythm disturbances), guanethidine (may negate the antihypertensive effect), MAO inhibitors, ergot alkaloid derivatives and oxytocin (may increase risk of hypertension).[8] Caution should be exercised in these instances (use of ephedra with MAO inhibitors is contraindicated).

Interactions are theoretically possible with central nervous system stimulants (such as caffeine and amphetamines), antihypertensive drugs (negation of effect) and α and β adrenergic agonists (reinforcement of effect). As stated above, intake of ephedra should be discontinued prior to surgery.

Serotonin syndrome was reported in a patient taking the selective serotonin reuptake inhibitor paroxetine and a cold medicine containing ephedrine.[27]

Ephedra (oral administration) decreased the plasma concentration of aminophylline in rabbits.[28]

Safety in Children

Only to be used in children older than six and the corresponding herb dose should not deliver in excess of 0.5 mg/kg total alkaloids for a single dose, or more than 2.0 mg/kg per daily dose.[8]

Overdosage

Overdose of ephedra has caused the expected symptoms of excessive intake of sympathomimetic agents, such as severe hypertension and cerebral vasospasm with vomiting, sweating, headache, palpitations, and peripheral weakness and numbness.[29]

Toxicology

The toxicological data for ephedrine and ephedra were extensively reviewed in the CANTOX review and will not be repeated here.[30] In summary, the vast majority of studies were on ephedrine, but those on ephedra indicated low acute oral toxicity (for example, LD_{50} of 24.0 g/kg in mice). The toxicity of ephedrine in subacute and subchronic studies was expressed as the typical sympathomimetic effects (hyperactivity, reduced weight gain). Carcinogenicity studies in rats and mice found that the no observable effect level was greater than 250 ppm (or around 10 mg/kg/day respectively) of ephedrine in the feed.[30] No treatment-related tumours were observed.

All in vitro and in vivo genotoxicity or mutagenicity studies on ephedrine or ephedra extract produced negative responses.[30]

Ephedrine is a secondary amine which can be N-nitrosated. N-nitrosoephedrine was found to be mutagenic in vitro and carcinogenic.[31] However, the relevance of this reaction to the normal human use of ephedra is unknown.

Regulatory Status

See Table 1 for regulatory status in selected countries.

At the time of writing this monograph (May 2003), the regulatory status of ephedra-based dietary supplements was the subject of considerable debate. In May 1995 the Texas Medical Association adopted a policy that ephedrine and ephedra should be prohibited from dietary supplements and over-the-counter drugs. Laws regulating ephedra, which include the herbal industry standards and recommendations, have been passed in several U.S. states.[3]

In June 1997 the FDA issued proposed regulations on ephedra-containing dietary supplements that would see the maximum daily dose limited to 24 mg ephedrine. This proposal was subsequently withdrawn.[3]

In February 2003, U.S. federal officials announced a proposal for new label warnings on ephedra-based supplements and ordered 24 companies to stop advertising ephedra as a way to enhance athletic performance.

Fear of litigation and substantial increases in product liability insurance premiums have resulted in several companies withdrawing their ephedra products from the U.S. market.

In a submission to the FDA, the American Herbalists Guild (AHG) stressed that the traditional use of the herb ephedra was different to both the uses of ephedrine, and those products promoted for weight loss and athletic performance.[32] The AHG urged the FDA to take this difference into account in future legislation, and not to unnecessarily restrict the traditional use of ephedra (as has happened in other countries such as Australia).

Table **1**   **Regulatory Status for Ephedra in Selected Countries**

Australia	Ephedra is included in Schedule 4 of the Standard for the Uniform Scheduling of Drugs and Poisons (SUSDP), except in preparations containing <0.001% of ephedrine. It is only available by a doctor's prescription.
China	Ephedra is official in the *Pharmacopoeia of the People's Republic of China* 1997. The usual adult dosage, usually administered in the form of a decoction, is listed as 2 to 9 g.
UK & Germany	Ephedra is not included on the General Sale List. It is listed in Part II and III of the Statutory Instrument SI 2130 (Retail Sale or Supply of Herbal Remedies) Order 1977 and may be prescribed at a maximum single dose of 600 mg and a maximum daily dose of 1800 mg.
	Ephedra stem is covered by a positive Commission E monograph.
US	Ephedra does not have generally recognised as safe (GRAS) status. However, it is freely available as a "dietary supplement" in the US under DSHEA legislation (Dietary Supplement Health and Education Act of 1994).

REFERENCES

1. Bensky D, Gamble A: *Chinese herbal medicine materia medica*, Seattle, 1986, Eastland Press, pp 32-34.
2. British Herbal Medicine Association's Scientific Committee: *British herbal pharmacopoeia*, Bournemouth, 1983, BHMA, pp 82-83.
3. Blumenthal M, Brinckmann J, Wollschlaeger B: *The ABC clinical guide to herbs*, Austin, Texas, 2003, American Botanical Council, pp 110-121.
4. Shekelle P, Morton S, Maglione M, et al: *Ephedra and ephedrine for weight loss and athletic performance enhancement: clinical efficacy and side effects*. Evidence report/technology assessment no. 76 (prepared by Southern California Evidence-Based Practice Center, RAND, under contract no 290-97-0001, task order no 9), AHRQ publication no. 03-E022, Rockville, MD, February 2003, Agency for Healthcare Research and Quality.
5. Wagner H, Bladt S: *Plant drug analysis: a thin layer chromatography atlas*, ed 2, Berlin, 1996, Springer-Verlag, p 11.
6. Pharmacopoeia Commission of the People's Republic of China: *Pharmacopoeia of the People's Republic of China*, English ed, vol I, Beijing, 1997, Chemical Industry Press, pp 92-93.
7. Means C: *Vet Clin Small Anim* 32:367-382, 2002.
8. Blumenthal M et al, eds: *The complete German Commission E monographs: therapeutic guide to herbal medicines*, Austin, 1998, American Botanical Council, pp 125-126.
9. World Health Organization: *WHO monographs on selected medicinal plants*, vol I, Geneva, 1999, WHO, pp 145-153.
10. The Special Nutritional Adverse Event Monitoring System. Accessed 17/10/01. vm.cfsan.fda.gov/~dms/aems.html
11. Heinonen OP, Slone D, Shapiro S: *Birth defects and drugs in pregnancy*, Littleton, 1977, Publishing Sciences Group, pp 395, 438, 442, 497.
12. Berkowitz RL, Coustan DR, Nochizuki TK: *Handbook for prescribing medications during pregnancy*, Boston, 1981, Little, Brown & Company.
13. Lee EB: *Korean J Pharmacogn* 13:116-121, 1982.
14. Prakash AO: *Int J Crude Drug Res* 24:19-24, 1986.
15. Nishikawa THJ, Bruyere HJ Jr, Takagi Y, et al: *Toxicol Lett* 29:59-63, 1985.
16. Kanai T, Nishikawa T, Satoh A, et al: *Teratology* 34:469, 1986.
17. Gilbert-Barnes E, Drut RM: *Vet Human Toxicol* 42:168-171, 2000.
18. Ros JJW, Pelders M, De Smet AGM: *Pharm World Sci* 21:44-46, 1999.
19. Lefebvre RA, Surmont F, Bouckaert J, et al: *J Pharm Pharmacol* 44:672-675, 1992.
20. Cupp MJ, ed: *Toxicology and clinical pharmacology of herbal products*, Totowa, NJ, 2000, Humana Press, pp 16-30.
21. Ang-Lee MK, Moss J, Yuan C-S: *JAMA* 286:208-216, 2001.
22. State of New South Wales: Glebe Coroners' Court Reports on Grafton and Kempsey bus crashes, 7 February 1990 and 1 June 1990.
23. Borum ML: *AJG* 96:1654-1655, 2001.
24. Nadir A, Agrawal S, King PD, et al: *Am J Gastroenterol* 91:1436-1438, 1996.
25. Stolpman DR, Petty J, Ham J, et al: *Hepatology* 36:168A, 2002.
26. Powell T, Hsu FF, Turk J, et al: *Am J Kidney Dis* 32:153-159, 1998.
27. Skop BP, Finkelstein JA, Mareth TR, et al: *Am J Emerg Med* 12:642-644, 1994.
28. Zhang SF, Zhang M: *Chin J Hosp Pharm* 6:97-102, 1986.
29. Pace S: *J Toxicol Clin Toxicol* 34:598, 1996.
30. CANTOX Health Sciences International: *Safety assessment and determination of a tolerable upper limit for ephedra*, Washington, DC, December 19, 2000, prepared for Council for Responsible Nutrition.
31. Tang W, Eisenbrand G: *Chinese drugs of plant origin*, Berlin, 1992, Springer Verlag, pp 223-232.
32. American Herbalists Guild: Docket no 095N-0304 before the United States of America Department of Health and Human Services, Food and Drug Administration. Submitted April 7, 2003.

EUPHORBIA

Other common name: Pill-bearing spurge
Botanical names: *Euphorbia hirta* L. (*E. pilulifera* L., *Chamaesyce hirta* (L.) Millsp., *E. capitata* Lam.)
Family: Euphorbiaceae
Plant part used: Aerial parts

Safety Summary

Pregnancy category B2: No increase in frequency of malformation or other harmful effects on the foetus from limited use in women. Animal studies are lacking.
Lactation category C: Compatible with breastfeeding.
Contraindications: None required on current evidence.
Warnings & precautions: None required on current evidence.
Adverse reactions: Gastrointestinal upset and nausea occur occasionally.
Interactions: No precautions required on current evidence.

Typical Therapeutic Use

Traditional indications for euphorbia in Western herbal medicine include asthma, bronchitis, upper respiratory catarrh and intestinal amoebiasis.[1] Uncontrolled trials in the mid-1960s indicate that euphorbia can remove intestinal protozoal parasites.[2,3]

Actions

Expectorant, antiasthmatic, spasmolytic, antiprotozoal.

Key Constituents

Constituents of euphorbia include triterpenes, flavonoids, phenolic acids, shikimic acid and choline,[4] and polyphenols (about 2%, and including hydrolysable tannins such as the euphorbins).[5,6] Diterpene esters of the tigliane and ingenol type have been isolated from aerial parts and roots of *E. hirta* of Indian origin, but were absent from plant material of American origin.[6] These compounds are potentially toxic (see Toxicology section below).

Adulteration

Eclectic texts indicate that euphorbia may be adulterated with *E. parviflora*.[7] Also *Euphorbia indica* may be confused for *E. hirta*.[8] Succulent species of *Euphorbia*, excluding artificially propagated specimens of cultivars of *Euphorbia trigona*, are listed on Appendix II of the Convention on International Trade in Endangered Species (CITES) as of May 2003. In addition, ten species (not medicinal *Euphorbia*) are listed in Appendix I. (Succulent plants are those that have tissues specialised for storage of water, such as cacti. Euphorbias of the African deserts are succulent, but *Euphorbia hirta* is not.)

Typical Dosage Forms & Dosage

Typical adult dosage ranges are:
- 0.4 to 0.9 g/day of dried aerial parts or by infusion
- 0.4 to 0.9 mL/day of a 1:1 liquid extract
- 0.7 to 2 mL/day of a 1:2 liquid extract* or equivalent in tablet or capsule form
- 1.8 to 6 mL/day of a 1:5 tincture

Contraindications

None known.

Use in Pregnancy

Category B2: No increase in frequency of malformation or other harmful effects on the foetus from limited use in women. Animal studies are lacking.

Use in Lactation

Category C: Compatible with breastfeeding.
In Ayurvedic medicine, euphorbia is administered to nursing mothers as a galactagogue. The herb is most probably given after boiling, as it is irritant to the stomach without boiling.[9]

Warnings & Precautions

None required.

---

*In chronic cases of intestinal protozoal infestation, daily dosage can be increased to 15 to 20 mL of 1:2 extract for up to 7 days' continuous treatment.

Effect on Ability to Drive or Operate Machinery

No adverse effects expected.

Adverse Reactions

Euphorbia is an irritant to the gastrointestinal tract and may occasionally cause epigastric upset with nausea.[7] Early animal studies confirm this irritant effect.[9]

Euphorbia spp. produce a latex which has often been used in Africa as an ingredient in arrow poison. The constituents responsible for the irritant property are diterpene esters.[10]

The latex of the fresh plant (*E. hirta*) has caused dermatitis.[11] Gardeners who pull the weed out of their lawns can develop dermatitis, particularly along the sides of the fingers.[12] Contact dermatitis and positive follow-up patch testing using *Euphorbia hirta* extract has been recorded.[13]

Interactions

None reported.

Safety in Children

No information available, but adverse effects are not expected if taken within the recommended dosage range.

Euphorbia has been used to treat children with diarrhoea and dysentery[14] and in Ayurvedic medicine is used for a variety of childhood disorders.[9]

Overdosage

There is mention of euphorbia causing death in an Eclectic text, but with no details provided.[15]

Euphorbia hirta has been suspected of causing sickness in cattle,[11] but this has been disputed.[16]

Toxicology

Ethanol extract of *E. hirta* plant of Indian origin had a maximum tolerated dose of 1 g/kg after oral administration to mice.[17] Early experimental studies indicate that euphorbia extract had a depressant action on the cardiovascular system and produced a fall in blood pressure.[9]

Freeze-dried aqueous extract of euphorbia did not induce any toxic effect when administered intraperitoneally and orally (up to the dose of 6 g dried plant/kg).[18] Whole plant fed to rats (5% of their diet) for 97 days caused no symptoms and no gross pathology was found on autopsy.[19]

Ether extract of *E. hirta* whole plant of Malaysian origin demonstrated activity in an in vitro tumour-promotion assay at concentrations of 10 to 30 µg/mL. Diterpene esters from Euphorbiaceae had previously been found to exert this activity, hence only ether extracts were tested in this study.[20] Tigliane and ingenane diterpene esters of the Euphorbiaceae are contact irritants and considered to be active tumour promoters (conditional [non-genotoxic] carcinogens).[21] An earlier study, using the same in vitro assay (human lymphoblastoid cells latently infected with Epstein-Barr virus) found ether extract of *E. hirta* "branches" to be inactive. Other species from *Euphorbia* and other genera within the Euphorbiaceae exhibited strong activity.[22]

Regulatory Status

See Table 1 for regulatory status in selected countries.

Table 1   **Regulatory Status for Euphorbia in Selected Countries**

Australia	Euphorbia is not included in Part 4 of Schedule 4 of the Therapeutic Goods Regulations.
UK & Germany	Euphorbia is included on the General Sale List. It was not included in the Commission E assessment.
US	Euphorbia does not have generally recognised as safe (GRAS) status. However, it is freely available as a "dietary supplement" in the US under DSHEA legislation (Dietary Supplement Health and Education Act of 1994).

REFERENCES

1. British Herbal Medicine Association's Scientific Committee: *British herbal pharmacopoeia*, Bournemouth, 1983, BHMA, pp 88-89.
2. Ridet J, Chartol A: *Med Trop* 24:119-143, 1964.
3. Martin M, Chartol A, Porte L, et al: *Med Trop* 24:250-261, 1964.
4. Leung AY, Foster S: *Encyclopedia of common natural ingredients used in food, drugs and cosmetics*, ed 2, New York–Chichester, 1996, John Wiley, pp 234-235.
5. Yoshida T, Chen L, Shingu T, et al: *Chem Pharm Bull* 36:2940-2949, 1988.
6. Blaschek W, Ebel S, Hackenthal E, et al: *HagerROM 2002: Hagers Handbuch der Drogen und Arzneistoffe*, Heidelberg, 2002, Springer.
7. Felter HW, Lloyd JU: *King's American dispensatory*, ed 18, rev 3, vol 1. First published 1905; reprinted Portland, 1983, Eclectic Medical Publications, pp 750-751.
8. Chu X, Cao L, Yuan C: *Zhong Yao Cai* 24:28-29, 2001.
9. Chopra RN, Badhwar RL, Ghosh S: *Poisonous plants of India*, vol II, New Delhi, 1965, Indian Council of Agricultural Research, pp 784-785.
10. Vlietinck AJ: Biologically active substances from traditional drugs. In Hostettmann K, Lea PJ, eds: *Annual Proceedings of the Phytochemical Society of Europe* vol 27: *Biologically active natural products*, Oxford, 1987, Clarendon Press, pp 40-42.
11. Watt JM, Breyer-Brandwijk MG: *The medicinal and poisonous plants of southern and eastern Africa: being an account of their medicinal and other uses, chemical composition, pharmacological effects and toxicology in man and animal*, ed 2, Edinburgh, 1962, Livingstone, pp 408-411.
12. Mitchell J, Rook A: *Botanical dermatology: plants and plant products injurious to the skin*, Vancouver, 1979, Greengrass, p 275.
13. Rajai AK, Govil DC, Bhargava SN: *Indian J Dermatol Venereol* 48:268-270, 1982.
14. Noumi E, Dibakto TW: *Fitoterapia* 71:406-412, 2000.
15. Culbreth DMR: *A manual of materia medica and pharmacology*, Naturopathic Medical Series: Botanical vol 3. First published 1922; reprinted Portland, 1983, Eclectic Medical Publications, pp 382-383.
16. Everist SL: *Poisonous plants of Australia*, revised ed, London, 1981, Angus & Robertson, pp 269-270.
17. Dhar ML, Dhar MM, Dhawan BN, et al: *Indian J Exp Biol* 6:232-247, 1968.
18. Lanhers MC, Fleurentin J, Cabalion P, et al: *J Ethnopharmacol* 29:189-198, 1990.
19. Hazleton LW, Hallerman RC: *J Am Pharm Assoc* 37:491-497, 1948.
20. Norhanom AW, Yadav M: *Br J Cancer* 71:776-779, 1995.
21. Zayed SM, Farghaly M, Soliman SM, et al: *J Cancer Res Clin Oncol* 127:40-47, 2001.
22. Ito Y, Yanase S, Fujita J, et al: *Cancer Lett* 13:29-37, 1981.

EVENING PRIMROSE OIL

Botanical name: *Oenothera biennis* L.
Family: Onagraceae
Plant part used: Fixed oil from the seed

Safety Summary

Pregnancy category B1: No increase in frequency of malformation or other harmful effects on the foetus from limited use in women. No evidence of increased foetal damage in animal studies.
Lactation category C: Compatible with breastfeeding.
Contraindications: None required on current evidence.
Warnings & precautions: None required on current evidence.
Adverse reactions: Most commonly headache and mild nausea; rarely, epilepsy in schizophrenic patients.
Interactions: No precautions required on current evidence.

Typical Therapeutic Use

Evening primrose oil (EPO) is used for a variety of disorders, primarily as an antiinflammatory agent. The key constituent, γ-linolenic acid (GLA), is converted in the body to dihomo-γ-linolenic acid which is a precursor of monoenoic prostaglandins such as PGE_1. Clinical trials began investigating the use of EPO for the treatment of atopic eczema in the 1980s. A recent systematic review found insufficient evidence to recommend EPO for the treatment of atopic eczema.[1] A more recent clinical trial concluded that EPO could be highly effective in the treatment of a grossly noninflammatory type of atopic dermatitis, perhaps by modulation of the immunological mechanism involving interferon-γ.[2] Reviews of EPO treatment have found some credible evidence for benefits in rheumatoid arthritis[3]; inconsistent or inconclusive results for premenstrual syndrome,[4] Raynaud's phenomenon, Sjogren syndrome, discomfort of fibrocystic breast conditions[5]; no greater efficacy than placebo for cyclical mastalgia[6]; and no clear benefit for schizophrenia.[7]

Actions

Antiinflammatory, antiallergic, corrects omega-6 essential fatty acid deficiency, hypotensive.

Key Constituents

The key constituent of evening primrose (fixed) oil is GLA (8% to 14%). EPO also contains linoleic acid (65% to 80%). EPO is unique among vegetable oils because of its high content of GLA.[8] GLA (also known as gamolenic acid) and linoleic acid are essential fatty acids of the omega-6 series. (Omega-3 series essential fatty acids are present in fish oils.)

Adulteration

No adulterants known.

Typical Dosage Forms & Dosage

Typical adult dosage ranges are:
- EPO equivalent to 250 to 500 mg/day GLA for atopic dermatitis and mastalgia
- EPO equivalent to 500 to 2000 mg/day GLA for diabetes, inflammatory and cardiovascular disorders

Contraindications

None required.

Use in Pregnancy

Category B1: No increase in frequency of malformation or other harmful effects on the foetus from limited use in women. No evidence of increased foetal damage in animal studies.

A retrospective study involving 108 nulliparous women found that oral administration of evening primrose oil from the 37th gestational week until birth did not shorten gestation or decrease the overall length of labour. There was a trend for the EPO group to have a more protracted active phase, prolonged rupture of membranes, oxytocin augmentation and arrest of descent. The prescribed dosage of EPO was 1500 mg/day for the first week, then 500 mg/day until labour began. The babies were slightly larger in the EPO group, but this is unlikely to account for the differences observed.[9] EPO has been trialled in pre-eclampsia with mixed results.[10,11] Diastolic pressor response to angiotensin II was significantly reduced in midtrimester pregnant women who received EPO (320 mg/day GLA) and vitamins, compared to controls.[12]

In a 1999 survey of certified nurse–midwives in the United States, EPO was reported as used by 60% of the 90 respondents who used herbal medicine to stimulate labour. It was often applied topically for this purpose. There were no reported complications from the use of EPO.[13]

The diet of male and female blue foxes was supplemented with EPO (4.5 g/day), zinc sulphate (2.5 mg/day) and vitamin E (90 mg/day) to observe the effect on reproduction. Compared to the control group, there was an increased rate of abortion in the EPO group, but simultaneously a nonsignificant decrease in the frequency of barren females. A tendency for increased litter size in the EPO group was found mainly as an effect of male treatment (suggesting an effect on semen quality).[14] EPO supplementation had a beneficial effect in pregnant zinc-deficient rats and subsequently in their newborn pups.[15] EPO had no effect on parturition or postnatal growth when fed to rats prior to mating.[16]

Use in Lactation

Category C: Compatible with breastfeeding.

GLA and linoleic acid are normally found in human milk.[17-19] A comparative study noted that the breast milk of allergic mothers contained less GLA than that of healthy mothers. The serum lipid fatty acid levels in atopic infants did not correlate with those in maternal breast milk.[20]

A placebo-controlled trial observed that maternal supplementation with EPO during breast-feeding raised the essential fatty acid and total fat content of breast milk.[21]

Warnings & Precautions

EPO may have potential to instigate previously undiagnosed temporal lobe epilepsy, especially in those receiving phenothiazines. This is unlikely on current evidence, but caution should apply (see Adverse reactions below).

Effect on Ability to Drive or Operate Machinery

No adverse effects expected.

Adverse Reactions

The most common adverse effects recorded in clinical trials to the early 1990s were headache, mild nausea and abdominal discomfort.[22,23]

GLA administration has been shown to increase arachidonate levels. GLA (2 g/day) given to previously obese women increased the arachidonate content of their serum phospholipids. Prolonged administration of GLA over more than a year may result in accumulation of arachidonate in tissue, thus possibly counteracting the early therapeutic effects of GLA, since tissue build-up of arachidonate might promote subsequent inflammation, thrombosis and immunosuppression. Symptoms may rebound in patients after discontinuation of GLA.[24]

In recent years, concerns have been expressed over the use of EPO in patients with a history of epilepsy. The concerns arose originally from case reports (three schizophrenics, reported in 1981)[25] and from a 1983 trial involving a small group of patients with chronic schizophrenia.[26]

Three hospitalised schizophrenics who had failed to respond to conventional antipsychotic medication were treated with EPO (8 g/day in one case, dosage undisclosed in others). In each case their schizophrenia became worse and EEG features of temporal lobe epilepsy became apparent. They improved when the EPO was stopped and anticonvulsant medication begun. GLA was administered in an attempt to correct abnormal prostaglandin E1 levels. The patients were at the time or previously taking phenothiazine and other antipsychotic drugs.[25]

In a double-blind, crossover trial that enrolled 23 chronic schizophrenics, three patients experienced grand mal seizures. EPO (4 g/day) and vitamins were administered in the experimental part of the trial (4 months). Two of the three patients who had seizures were receiving EPO and vitamins. The seizure/s occurred at 3 months into the treatment and both patients were taking phenothiazines. One patient had no history of epilepsy. No definite link to the EPO treatment was established.[26]

Phenothiazines can lower the seizure threshold and in some cases induce a discharge pattern in the EEG that is associated with epileptic seizure disorders. Dosage adjustment of anticonvulsant medications can be necessary when taking phenothiazines.[27] In two clinical trials conducted since this time, psychiatric patients (predominantly schizophrenics) who received EPO (540 to 600 mg/day GLA) did not experience such adverse effects.[28,29] There have been no other reports of an epileptic attack being associated with EPO monotherapy in humans (however, see next paragraph).[30]

A 45-year-old woman who had been taking herbal preparations containing black cohosh, chaste tree and evening primrose oil for 4 months had three seizures within a 3-month period. The herbal preparations were stopped and the patient was treated with anticonvulsants.[31] No causal link between the seizures and the herbal treatment was established.

Blood tests of patients with Raynaud's phenomenon who received EPO (6 g/day EPO, containing 8% GLA) indicated an antiplatelet effect. This was significant during the first 2 to 6 weeks of treatment, and there was a "fall off" in effect by week 8.[32] In multiple sclerosis patients treated with EPO for 6 weeks (20 g/day EPO, containing 8% GLA), only platelet aggregation to thrombin was significantly reduced compared to controls. Overall EPO did not show a significant effect on platelets of MS patients.[33] In hypertriglyceridaemic patients, GLA supplementation did not affect platelet function.[34]

Interactions

There is insufficient evidence to suggest avoiding concomitant use of EPO with phenothiazines (see Adverse reactions section above).

There are no reports of an interaction between EPO and anticoagulants or antiplatelet drugs.

Safety in Children

Adverse effects are not expected. EPO and GLA have been administered to children in clinical trials.

Of the randomised clinical trials for the treatment of atopic eczema examined to the year 2000, seven trials involved children, with ages ranging from 0.8 to 16 years and treatment from 4 to 16 weeks. In most cases 0.5 to 4 g/day of EPO was administered.[1] In one of these trials 48 atopic children aged 2.2 to 8.5 years received placebo, low dose EPO or high dose EPO for 8 weeks. The high dose amounted to 500 mg/kg/day of EPO. No adverse effects were observed.[35]

In other trials EPO was administered to children with atopic eczema,[36] hyperactivity,[37-40] insulin-dependent diabetes (90 mg/day GLA for 4 months increasing to 180 mg/day for 4 months)[41] and cystic fibrosis (20 g/day EPO for 12 months).[42]

Overdosage

No incidents found in published literature. It is known that an excess of omega-6 essential fatty acids can reduce the metabolism of α-linolenic acid, possibly leading to a deficit of eicosapentaenoic acid and other metabolites.[3]

Toxicology

Being an intermediate of normal human metabolism, GLA is unlikely to be harmful or toxic if it is consumed in quantities which are comparable to those formed within the human body; 20 mg/kg/day of GLA is likely to be formed from linolenic acid in a normal adult woman and 23 to 65 mg/kg/day of GLA may be consumed by a breastfed baby.[19]

In two sets of toxicity studies, effects of oral administration of EPO (containing 8.5% to 9% GLA, and 70% to 73% linoleic acid) were compared with corn oil (60% linoleic acid) and controls, which received no oil.[43,44] In rats (fed up to 2.5 mL/kg/day over 53 weeks) and dogs (fed up to 5 mL/kg/day over 52 weeks) there were no significant differences between tested groups in terms of clinical signs, food consumption or body weight changes. No consistent differences were seen in haematology or urinalysis results for rats or dogs, or in clinical chemistry for male rats. Serum potassium was marginally increased in female rats on the highest EPO dose. Male EPO-treated rats showed modestly reduced liver weights and a greater proportion showed testicular shrinkage or softening than in the control group. The authors concluded that no important adverse effects were produced by EPO administration and it is as safe a nutritional supplement as corn oil.[43] No significant effect on tumour incidence was observed in the rats fed EPO compared to the other groups.[44]

Regulatory Status

See Table 1 for regulatory status in selected countries.

Table 1   **Regulatory Status for Evening Primrose in Selected Countries**

Australia	Evening primrose oil is not included in Part 4 of Schedule 4 of the Therapeutic Goods Regulations.
UK & Germany	Evening primrose oil is not included on the General Sale List. It was not included in the Commission E assessment.
US	Evening primrose oil does not have generally recognised as safe (GRAS) status. However, it is freely available as a "dietary supplement" in the US under DSHEA legislation (Dietary Supplement Health and Education Act of 1994).

REFERENCES

1. Hoare C, Li Wan Po A, Williams H: *Health Technol Assess* 4:1-191, 2000.
2. Yoon S, Lee J, Lee S: *Skin Pharmacol Appl Skin Physiol* 15:20-25, 2002.
3. Belch JJF, Hill A: *Am J Clin Nutr* 71(Suppl 1):352S-356S, 2000.
4. Carter J, Verhoef MJ: *Womens Health Issues* 4:130-137, 1994.
5. Horner NK, Lampe JW: *J Am Diet Assoc* 100:1368-1380, 2000.
6. Mellanby A, Best L, Stevens A: DEC Report No. 65, Southampton, 1996, Wessex Institute for Health Research and Development.
7. Joy CB, Mumby-Croft R, Joy LA: *Cochrane Database Syst Rev* 2:CD001257, 2000.
8. Blaschek W, Ebel S, Hackenthal E, et al: *HagerROM 2002: Hagers Handbuch der Drogen und Arzneistoffe*, Heidelberg, 2002, Springer.
9. Dove D, Johnson P: *J Nurse Midwifery* 44:320-324, 1999.
10. Laivuori H, Hovatta O, Viinikka L, et al: *Prostaglandins Leukot Essent Fatty Acids* 49:691-694, 1993.
11. D'Almeida A, Carter JP, Anatol A, et al: *Women Health* 19:117-131, 1992.
12. O'Brien PMS, Morrison R, Pipkin FB: *Br J Clin Pharmacol* 19:335-342, 1985.
13. McFarlin BL, Gibson MH, O'Rear J, et al: *J Nurse Midwifery* 44:205-216, 1999.
14. Tauson AH, Forsberg M: *Acta Vet Scand* 32:345-351, 1991.
15. Dib A, Carreau JP: *Ann Nutr Metab* 31:312-319, 1987.
16. Leaver HA, Lytton FD, Dyson H, et al: *Prog Lipid Res* 25:143-146, 1986.
17. Gibson RA, Kneebone GM: *Am J Clin Nutr* 34:252-257, 1981.
18. Harzer G, Haug M, Dieterich I, et al: *Am J Clin Nutr* 37:612-621, 1983.
19. Carter JP: *Food Technol* 42:72-82, 1988.
20. Kankaanpaa P, Nurmela K, Erkkila A, et al: *Allergy* 56:633-638, 2001.
21. Cant A, Shay J, Horrobin DF: *J Nutr Sci Vitaminol* 37:573-579, 1991.
22. Joe LA, Hart LL: *Ann Pharmacother* 27:1475-1477, 1993.
23. LiWan Po A: *Pharmaceutical J* June 1:676-678, 1991.
24. Phinney S: *Ann Intern Med* 120:692, 1994.
25. Vaddadi KS: *Prostaglandins Med* 6:375-379, 1981.
26. Holman CP, Bell AFJ: *J Orthomolec Psychiatry* 12: 302-304, 1983.
27. E-MIMS version 4.00.0457, Havas, 2000, MediMedia International.
28. Vaddadi KS, Courtney P, Gilleard CJ, et al: *Psychiatry Res* 27:313-323, 1989.
29. Wolkin A, Jordan B, Peselow E, et al: *Am J Psychiatry* 143:912-914, 1986.
30. Dobbin SN: *Vet Rec* 131:591, 1992.
31. Shuster J: *Hosp Pharm* 31:1553-1554, 1996.
32. Belch JJ, Shaw B, O'Dowd A, et al: *Thromb Haemost* 54:490-494, 1985.
33. McGregor L, Smith AD, Sidey M, et al: *Acta Neurol Scand* 80:23-27, 1989.
34. Boberg M, Vessby B, Selinus I: *Acta Med Scand* 220:153-160, 1986.
35. Biagi PL, Bordoni A, Hrelia S, et al: *Drugs Exp Clin Res* 20:77-84, 1994.
36. Biagi PL, Bordoni A, Masi M, et al: *Drugs Exp Clin Res* 14:285-290, 1988.
37. Aman MG, Mitchell EA, Turbott SH: *J Abnorm Child Psychol* 15:75-90, 1987.
38. Arnold LE, Kleykamp D, Votolato NA, et al: *Biol Psychiatry* 25:222-228, 1989.
39. Colquhoun I, Bunday S: *Med Hypotheses* 7:673-679, 1981.
40. Gibson RA: *Proc Nutr Soc Aust* 10:196, 1985.
41. Arisaka M, Arisaka O, Yamashiro Y: *Prostaglandins Leukot Essent Fatty Acids* 43:197-201, 1991.
42. Horrobin DF: *Prog Lipid Res* 31:163-194, 1992.
43. Everett DJ, Greenough RJ, Perry CJ, et al: *Med Sci Res* 16:863-864, 1988.
44. Everett DJ, Perry CJ, Bayliss P: *Med Sci Res* 16:865-866, 1988.

EYEBRIGHT

Botanical name: *Euphrasia* spp.
Family: Scrophulariaceae
Plant part used: Aerial parts (harvested during the flowering season)

Safety Summary

Pregnancy category B2: No increase in frequency of malformation or other harmful effects on the foetus from limited use in women. Animal studies are lacking.
Lactation category C: Compatible with breastfeeding.
Contraindications: None required on current evidence.
Warnings & precautions: Topical eye preparations need to be sterile. Do not apply herbal tinctures or extracts directly to the eyes.
Adverse reactions: None found in published literature.
Interactions: No precautions required on current evidence.

Typical Therapeutic Use

Traditional uses of eyebright in Western herbal medicine include nasal catarrh, sinusitis and as a topical treatment for conjunctivitis.[1] The efficacy and tolerability of treatment with eyebright eye drops was assessed to be good to very good in more than 85% of 65 patients with inflammatory or catarrhal conjunctivitis in a prospective, open, multicentre trial.[2]

Actions

Astringent, anticatarrhal, mucous membrane tonic, antiinflammatory.

Key Constituents

Constituents of eyebright include iridoid glycosides (such as aucubin, catalpol, euphroside and ixoroside), lignans, and flavonoids (such as quercetin and apigenin glycosides).[3]

Adulteration

The nomenclature for this species is under debate. Medicinal eyebright includes various *Euphrasia* species, but especially the taxa grouped around *E. rostkoviana* Hayne (which includes *E. officinalis* L. –

an ambiguous name) and *E. stricta* D. Wolff ex J.F. Lehm, as well as their hybrids. The classification of the genus *Euphrasia* differs greatly in the literature.[4] The U.S. Department of Agriculture lists *E. rostkoviana* Hayne as preferred to the previous *E. officinalis* L., nom. ambig.[5] The *Flora Europaea* continues to list *Euphrasia officinalis* L., nom. ambig., albeit with a provisional name status.

A nomenclature study published in 1991 suggests *Euphrasia officinalis* L. may be divided into several subspecies including *E. officinalis* spp. *rostkoviana* (Hayne) Townsend (synonym *Euphrasia rostkoviana* Hayne).[6] In addition to the species listed here, many other species of *Euphrasia* are regarded as medicinal. Due to the different systematic organisations of the genus *Euphrasia* and/or the ambiguity of some species or varieties within the species, adulteration is probable.[7]

Typical Dosage Forms & Dosage

Typical adult dosage ranges are:
- 6 to 12 g/day of dried aerial parts or by infusion
- 6 to 12 mL/day of a 1:1 liquid extract
- 2 to 4.5 mL/day of a 1:2 liquid extract or equivalent in tablet or capsule form
- 6 to 18 mL/day of a 1:5 tincture

For use in eyebaths, a decoction with greater than 10 minutes at boiling point, followed by transfer to a sterile container, is recommended. Allow to cool before applying to the eyes.

Contraindications

None known.

Use in Pregnancy

Category B2: No increase in frequency of malformation or other harmful effects on the foetus from limited use in women. Animal studies are lacking.

Use in Lactation

Category C: Compatible with breastfeeding.

Warnings & Precautions

Topical eye preparations need to be sterile. Normal herbal tinctures or extracts should never be applied directly to the eyes because of their ethanol content.

Effect on Ability to Drive or Operate Machinery

No adverse effects expected.

Adverse Reactions

No adverse reactions documented.

Interactions

None reported.

Safety in Children

No information available but adverse effects are not expected.

Overdosage

No incidents found in published literature.

Toxicology

No symptoms indicating toxicity were observed over a 72-hour period in rats which were orally administered an aqueous extract of *E. officinalis* leaf (0.1 to 6 g/kg).[8] Respiratory depression and hypothermia were observed after intraperitoneal administration of aucubin (100 mg/kg) to rats.[9]

Eyebright tincture demonstrated in vitro mutagenic activity in the Ames test.[10]

Regulatory Status

See Table 1 for regulatory status in selected countries.

Table **1**   **Regulatory Status for Eyebright in Selected Countries**

Australia	Eyebright is not included in Part 4 of Schedule 4 of the Therapeutic Goods Regulations.
UK & Germany	Eyebright is not included on the General Sale List. It is covered by a negative Commission E monograph.
US	Eyebright does not have generally recognised as safe (GRAS) status. However, it is freely available as a "dietary supplement" in the US under DSHEA legislation (Dietary Supplement Health and Education Act of 1994).

REFERENCES

1. British Herbal Medicine Association's Scientific Committee: *British herbal pharmacopoeia*, Bournemouth, 1983, BHMA, pp 89-90.
2. Stoss M, Michels C, Peter E, et al: *J Altern Complement Med* 6:499-508, 2000.
3. Wagner H, Bladt S: *Plant drug analysis: a thin layer chromatography atlas*, ed 2, Berlin, 1996, Springer-Verlag, p 75.
4. Bisset NG, ed: *Herbal drugs and phytopharmaceuticals: a handbook for practice on a scientific basis*, Stuttgart, 1994, Medpharm Scientific Publishers, pp 195-196.
5. Wiersema JH, Leon B: *World economic plants: a standard reference*, Boca Raton, Florida, 1999, CRC Press, p 221.
6. Silverside AJ: *Watsonia* 18:343-350, 1991.
7. Blaschek W, Ebel S, Hackenthal E, et al: *HagerROM 2002: Hagers Handbuch der Drogen und Arzneistoffe*, Heidelberg, 2002, Springer.
8. Porchezhian E, Ansari SH, Shreedharan NKK: *Fitoterapia* 71:522-526, 2000.
9. Ortiz de Urbina AV, Martin ML, Fernandez B, et al: *Planta Med* 60:512-515, 1994.
10. Schimmer O, Kruger A, Paulini H, et al: *Pharmazie* 49:448-451, 1994.

FALSE UNICORN

Other common name: Helonias root
Botanical name: *Chamaelirium luteum* (L.) A. Gray
Family: Liliaceae
Plant part used: Root and rhizome

Safety Summary

Pregnancy category B2: No increase in frequency of malformation or other harmful effects on the foetus from limited use in women. Animal studies are lacking.
Lactation category C: Compatible with breastfeeding.
Contraindications: None required on current evidence.
Warnings & precautions: The use of herbs rich in saponins is possibly inappropriate in coeliac disease, fat malabsorption and vitamins A, D, E, and K deficiency, some upper digestive irritations, and topically to open wounds. Caution in patients with preexisting cholestasis.
Adverse reactions: Herbs rich in saponins may cause irritation of the gastric mucous membranes and reflux.
Interactions: No precautions required on current evidence.

Typical Therapeutic Use

Traditional indications for false unicorn root in Western herbal medicine include amenorrhoea, dysmenorrhoea, threatened miscarriage,[1] menopausal symptoms, and to promote fertility.[2]

Actions

Uterine tonic, ovarian tonic, oestrogen modulating.

Key Constituents

Saponins, including chamaelirin (approximately 9.5%).[3,4]

Adulteration

No adulterants known.

Typical Dosage Forms & Dosage

Typical adult dosage ranges are:

- 3 to 6 g/day of dried root and rhizome or by infusion or decoction
- 3 to 6 mL/day of a 1:1 liquid extract
- 2 to 6 mL/day of a 1:2 liquid extract or equivalent in tablet or capsule form
- 6 to 15 mL/day of 1:5 tincture

Contraindications

None known.

Use in Pregnancy

Category B2: No increase in frequency of malformation or other harmful effects on the foetus from limited use in women. Animal studies are lacking.

Use in Lactation

Category C: Compatible with breastfeeding.

Warnings & Precautions

The use of herbs rich in saponins is possibly inappropriate in coeliac disease, fat malabsorption and vitamins A, D, E, and K deficiency, some upper digestive irritations, and topically to open wounds. Saponin-containing herbs are best kept to a minimum in patients with preexisting cholestasis.

Effect on Ability to Drive or Operate Machinery

No adverse effects expected.

Adverse Reactions

Excessive doses may produce nausea and vomiting.[3] As with all herbs rich in saponins, oral use may cause irritation of the gastric mucous membranes and reflux.

Interactions

None known.

Safety in Children

No information available.

Overdosage

No incidents found in published literature. Excessive doses may produce nausea and vomiting.

Toxicology

No information available.

Regulatory Status

See Table 1 for regulatory status in selected countries.

Table 1   Regulatory Status for False Unicorn Root in Selected Countries

Australia	False unicorn root is not included in Part 4 of Schedule 4 of the Therapeutic Goods Regulations.
UK & Germany	False unicorn root is included on the General Sale List. It was not included in the Commission E assessment.
US	False unicorn root does not have generally recognised as safe (GRAS) status. However, it is freely available as a "dietary supplement" in the US under DSHEA legislation (Dietary Supplement Health and Education Act of 1994).

REFERENCES

1. British Herbal Medicine Association's Scientific Committee: *British herbal pharmacopoeia*, Bournemouth, 1983, BHMA, pp 59-60.
2. Mills SY: *The essential book of herbal medicine*, London, 1991, Penguin Arkana (Penguin), pp 520-522.
3. British Herbal Medicine Association: *British herbal compendium*, Bournemouth, 1992, BHMA, p 125.
4. Blaschek W, Ebel S, Hackenthal E, et al: *HagerROM 2002: Hagers Handbuch der Drogen und Arzneistoffe*, Heidelberg, 2002, Springer.

FENNEL

Other common names: Bitter fennel, sweet fennel
Botanical names: *Foeniculum vulgare* Mill., *Foeniculum vulgare* Mill. subsp. *vulgare* var. *vulgare* (bitter fennel), *Foeniculum vulgare* Mill. subsp. *vulgare* var. *dulce* (Mill.) Thellung (sweet fennel)
Family: Umbelliferae
Plant part used: Cremocarps and mericarps (fruit, sometimes referred to as seed)

Safety Summary

Pregnancy category B3: No increase in frequency of malformation or other harmful effects on the foetus from limited use in women. Evidence of increased foetal damage in animal studies exists, although the relevance to humans is unknown.
Lactation category C: Compatible with breastfeeding. Traditionally used to enhance lactation.
Contraindications: Known sensitivity to Umbelliferae species. Do not use during pregnancy without professional advice.
Warnings & precautions: None required on current evidence.
Adverse reactions: Occasional allergic or hypersensitivity reactions.
Interactions: No precautions required on current evidence.

Typical Therapeutic Use

From clinical trials an inhalation of fennel essential oil resulted in a 1.5- to 2.5-fold increase in relative sympathetic activity compared with inhalation of an odourless solvent (p <0.05).[1]

Traditional indications of fennel in Western herbal medicine include flatulent dyspepsia and colic, and loss of appetite.[2] There is a European tradition of use for upper respiratory conditions, especially in children, and to encourage lactation.

Actions

Carminative, spasmolytic, galactagogue, possible oestrogenic, antimicrobial, expectorant.

Key Constituents

The essential oil of bitter fennel contains predominantly anethole and fenchone (up to 7.5%) and at most 5% estragole[3]; also α-pinene, limonene, cam-

phene, p-cymene, β-pinene, β-myrcene, α-phellandrene, sabinene, γ-terpinene, and terpinolene.[4] The essential oil of sweet fennel contains more anethole and estragole and less fenchone.

Adulteration

Contamination with aflatoxin-producing fungi has been reported.[5] Other mycoflora, including *Aspergillus* and *Penicillium*, have also been detected.[6]

Typical Dosage Forms & Dosage

Typical adult dosage ranges are:
- 0.9 to 1.8 g/day of dried fruit (cremocarps and mericarps) or by infusion
- 3 to 6 mL/day of a 1:2 liquid extract or equivalent in tablet or capsule form
- 7 to 14 mL/day of a 1:5 tincture

Contraindications

Known sensitivity to Umbelliferae species. Do not use during pregnancy without professional advice.

Use in Pregnancy

Category B3: No increase in frequency of malformation or other harmful effects on the foetus from limited use in women. Evidence of increased foetal damage in animal studies exists, although the relevance to humans is unknown.

Intragastric administration of water extract of fennel (0.05 g/day of dried herb) reduced the fertility of female mice. Of the six treated females only three became pregnant.[7]

Oestrogenic effects have been demonstrated as possibly due to polymers of anethole, such as dianethole and photoanethole.[8] The acetone extract of the whole seed over 15 days decreased the protein concentration in testes and vas deferens, and increased protein in the prostate and seminal vesicles, in male rats. In females, oestrogenic effects (increased weight of mammary glands at moderate doses, increased weight of oviduct, endometrium, myometrium, cervix, and vagina with higher doses) were also seen.[9]

Use in Lactation

Category C: Compatible with breastfeeding. Traditionally used to enhance lactation.

Warnings & Precautions

None required.

Effect on Ability to Drive or Operate Machinery

No adverse effects expected.

Adverse Reactions

Occasional immediate hypersensitivity reactions to the ingestion of fennel have been reported.[10] Cross-sensitivity to fennel and other members of the Apiaceae (Umbelliferae) has been found in a high proportion of patients with positive skin tests to birch, mugwort, and celery[11] and in one study fennel sensitivity was found in one case among 200 children with food allergies that were investigated for their causes.[12]

Skin prick tests showed a positive immediate response to a range of other spices in one subject allergic to aniseed: asparagus, caraway, coriander, cumin, dill, and fennel extracts.[13] A positive skin test to fresh fennel seed was found in one case of occupational asthma,[14] and in one case as a partial allergen in atopic dermatitis in children.[15]

However some diagnosed "spice allergies" to Apiaceae such as fennel, anise, coriander, and cumin may not have an immunological component and may be best characterised as food intolerances.[16]

No adverse effects were reported in one cohort study of 30 females with primary dysmenorrhoea treated with fennel essential oil.[17]

Interactions

Concomitant oral dosing of the aqueous fennel extract (2 g dried herb/kg) reduced the bioavailabil-ity of the antibiotic ciprofloxacin in rats. None of the phytochemical components of fennel seemed to cause this interaction, which may have been due to the presence of relatively large amounts of metal cations in the extract.[18]

trans-Anethole injected intraperitoneally into mice prolonged the sleeping time of pentobarbital. Fennel oil (also by injection) was marginally effective in prolonging sleeping times.[19]

Safety in Children

Apart from the rare case of allergic reaction, no adverse effects are expected in children.[20]

Overdosage

No incidents found in published literature.

Toxicology

Table 1 lists LD_{50} data recorded for fennel oil.[21-24]

No toxic effects were observed in mice administered single oral doses of 0.5, 1.0 and 3.0 g/kg of fennel ethanolic extract (equivalent to 5, 10, and 30 g of fennel seed). In the chronic toxicity study, 100 mg/kg of fennel extract orally administered per day over 90 days caused no significant differences in mortality, external morphology, haematology, or spermatogenesis compared to controls. After 40 days, alopecia in the snout area developed in some male animals. The average body weight of the male animals increased, while that of the female mice decreased or remained the same.[25] In another study using the same dosages, only the 3 g/kg dose showed signs of reduced locomotor activity and piloerection in mice. All other parameters were negative.[26]

Table 1   **LD_{50} Data Recorded for Fennel Oil**

Substance	Route, Model	LD_{50} Value	Reference
Essential oil of fennel	Oral, rats	1326 mg/kg	21
Essential oil of fennel (sweet?)	Oral, rats	4.5 mL/kg	22,23
Essential oil of fennel (bitter)	Oral, rats	4.5 mL/kg	23,24

It is desirable to have low estragole-containing fennel. High-dosage estragole studies in rats indicate potential hepatocarcinogenicity. However, since estragole is metabolised differently in humans, and with only limited absorption,[25,27] any suggested carcinogenic risk in humans is tenuous.

Methanolic and water extracts of bitter and sweet fennel were not mutagenic in the Ames test and had no DNA-damaging activity in the *Bacillus subtilis* rec-assay.[25] A fennel fruit extract prepared by percolation with 95% ethanol, and concentrated by vacuum, demonstrated intermediate mutagenic results in the Ames test and significant toxic activity in the brine shrimp bioassay.[28]

The mutagenic potential of fennel oil is not conclusive, as indicated by the conflicting results obtained in the following in vitro tests. Fennel oil, sweet fennel oil, and estragole were negative, but anethole was positive in Ames tests.[29,30] In another study, fennel oil and anethole showed weakly positive results.[19] Sweet fennel oil and anethole were negative in the *Escherichia coli* reversion test. Sweet fennel oil, but not anethole, demonstrated DNA-damaging activity in the *Bacillus subtilis* rec-assay; however, the authors indicated problems with this test with respect to the testing of oils.[30] Fennel oil demonstrated negative results in the chromosomal aberration test on hamster fibroblasts.[29]

Regulatory Status

See Table 2 for regulatory status in selected countries.

Table **2**   **Regulatory Status for Fennel in Selected Countries**

Australia	Fennel is not included in Part 4 of Schedule 4 of the Therapeutic Goods Regulations.
China	Fennel is official in the *Pharmacopoeia of the People's Republic of China* 1997. The usual adult dosage, usually administered in the form of a decoction, is listed as 3 to 6 g.
UK & Germany	Fennel is included on the General Sale List. It is covered by a positive Commission E monograph. Fennel is official in the *European Pharmacopoeia* 4.3.
US	Fennel does have generally recognised as safe (GRAS) status. It is freely available as a "dietary supplement" in the US under DSHEA legislation (Dietary Supplement Health and Education Act of 1994).

REFERENCES

1. Haze S, Sakai K, Gozu Y: *Jpn J Pharmacol* 90:247-253, 2002.
2. British Herbal Medicine Association's Scientific Committee: *British herbal pharmacopoeia,* Bournemouth, 1983, BHMA, pp 92-93.
3. De Vincenzi M, Silano M, Mialetti F, et al: *Fitoterapia* 71:725-729, 2000.
4. Piccaglia R, Marotti M: *J Agric Food Chem* 49:239-244, 2001.
5. El-Kady IA, El-Maraghy SS, Eman Mostafa M: *Folia Microbiol (Praha)* 40:297-300, 1995.
6. Moharram AM, Abdel-Mallek AY, Abdel-Hafez AI: *J Basic Microbiol* 29:427-435, 1989.
7. Alkofahi A, Al-Hamood MH, Elbetieha AM: *Arch STD/HIV Res* 10:189-196, 1996.
8. Albert-Puleo M: *J Ethnopharmacol* 2:337-344, 1980.
9. Malini T, Vanithakumari G, Megala N, et al: *Indian J Physiol Pharmacol* 29:21-26, 1985.
10. Asero R: *Ann Allergy Asthma Immunol* 84:460-462, 2000.
11. Stager J, Wuthrich B, Johansson SG: *Allergy* 46:475-478, 1991.
12. Rance F, Dutau G: *Pediatr Allergy Immunol* 8:41-44, 1997.
13. Garcia-Gonzalez JJ, Bartolome-Zavala B, Fernandez-Melendez S, et al: *Ann Allergy Asthma Immunol* 88:518-522, 2002.
14. Schwartz HJ, Jones RT, Rojas AR, et al: *Ann Allergy Asthma Immunol* 78:37-40, 1997.
15. Ottolenghi A, De Chiara A, Arrigoni S, et al: *Pediatr Med Chir* 17:525-530, 1995.
16. Jensen-Jarolim E, Leitner A, Hirshwerh R, et al: *Clin Exp Allergy* 27:1299-1306, 1997.
17. Namavar Jahromi B, Tartifizadeh A, Khabnadideh S: *Int J Gynaecol Obstet* 80:153-157, 2003.
18. Zhu M, Wong PY, Li RC: *J Pharm Pharmacol* 51:1391-1396, 1999.
19. Marcus C, Lichtenstein EP: *J Agric Food Chem* 30:563-568, 1982.
20. Fugh-Berman A: *Nutr Today* 37:122-124, 2002.
21. Ostad SN, Soodi M, Shariffzadeh M, et al: *J Ethnopharmacol* 76:299-304, 2001.

22. Opdyke DL: *Food Cosmet Toxicol* 12:309, 1974.
23. De Smet PAGM, Keller K, Hansel R, et al (eds): *Adverse effects of herbal drugs*, vol 1, Berlin, 1993, Springer-Verlag, pp 135-142.
24. Opdyke DL: *Food Cosmet Toxicol* 14:309, 1976.
25. Caldwell J, Sutton JD: *Food Chem Toxicol* 26:87-91, 1988.
26. Tanira MOM, Shah AH, Mohsin A, et al: *Phytother Res* 10:33-36, 1996.
27. Sangster SA, Caldwell J, Smith RL: *Food Chem Toxicol* 22:707-713, 1984.
28. Mahmoud I, Alkofahi A, Abdelaziz A: *Int J Pharmacognosy* 30:81-85, 1992.
29. Ishidate M Jr, Sofuni T, Yoshikawa K, et al: *Food Chem Toxicol* 22:623-636, 1984.
30. Sekizawa J, Shibamoto T: *Mutat Res* 101:127-140, 1982.

FENUGREEK

Botanical name: *Trigonella foenum-graecum* L.
Family: Leguminosae (Papilionoideae)
Plant part used: Ripe seeds

Safety Summary

Pregnancy category B3: No increase in frequency of malformation or other harmful effects on the foetus from limited use in women. Evidence of increased foetal damage in animal studies exists, although the relevance to humans is unknown.
Lactation category C: Compatible with breastfeeding. Widely used to enhance lactation.
Contraindications: None required on current evidence. Do not use during pregnancy without professional advice.
Warnings & precautions: The use of herbs rich in saponins is possibly inappropriate in coeliac disease, fat malabsorption and vitamins A, D, E, and K deficiency, some upper digestive irritations, and topically to open wounds. Caution in patients with preexisting cholestasis. Avoid where known spice allergies exist. Caution with high doses (>20 g/day) in patients with low thyroid activity.
Adverse reactions: Occasional allergic reactions. Herbs rich in saponins may cause irritation of the gastric mucous membranes and reflux.
Interactions: May inhibit iron absorption.

Typical Therapeutic Use

Preliminary human and animal trials suggest possible hypolipidaemic,[1-3] hypoglycaemic,[4-7] gastroprotective,[8] antioxidant[9-11] (especially in diabetic disease[12]) and immunomodulatory[13] properties of orally administered fenugreek seed powder.

Traditional indications of fenugreek in Western herbal medicine include loss of appetite, dyspepsia, gastritis, and as a remedy to aid convalescence. It has been used topically for wounds, and skin and subdermal inflammations.[14] Fenugreek has a long history of medical uses in Ayurvedic and Chinese medicine, and has been used for numerous indications, including labour induction, aiding digestion, and as a general tonic to improve metabolism and health.[15] It has traditionally been used in the Middle East for diabetes,[16] (with modern recommendation as an adjunct in type 2 diabetes[1]) and widely to stimulate lactation,[17] and as a treatment for inflammatory bowel disease.[18]

Actions

Hypoglycaemic, hypocholesterolaemic, demulcent, nutritive, galactagogue.

Key Constituents

Flavonoids: vitexin, tricin, naringenin, quercetin, and tricin-7-O-β-D-glucopyranoside[19]; diosgenin (0.70% to 0.87%)[20]; furostanol-type steroid saponins (5% to 6%).[21] The steroid saponin fraction added with the diet has been shown to have appetite enhancing and hypocholesterolaemic effects in rats.[22,23] An amino acid, 4-hydroxyisoleucine, potentiates insulin secretion from pancreatic β-cells in a glucose-dependent manner in vivo.[24] Fenugreek galactomannan (a soluble fibre containing a relatively high level of galactose) reduced postprandial cholesterolaemia, not by affecting cholesterol absorption, but apparently by decreasing the rate of hepatic cholesterol synthesis.[25] The unique dietary fibre composition and high saponin content, together, appear to be responsible for its hypoglycaemic and hypocholesterolaemic properties.[26]

Adulteration

No adulterants known.

Typical Dosage Forms & Dosage

Typical adult dosage ranges are:
- 2 g/day of dried seed (although much higher doses have been used, up to 25 g/day, for hypoglycaemic and hypolipidaemic activities)
- 2 mL/day of a 1:1 liquid extract
- 2 to 4.5 mL/day of a 1:2 liquid extract or equivalent in tablet or capsule form
- 10 mL/day of a 1:5 tincture

Contraindications

None known. Do not use during pregnancy without professional advice.

Use in Pregnancy

Category B3: No increase in frequency of malformation or other harmful effects on the foetus from limited use in women. Evidence of increased foetal damage in animal studies exists, although the relevance to humans is unknown.

Some theoretical concern has been expressed,[27] but there is no evidence to justify caution, given the widespread use of fenugreek as a foodstuff in pregnancy. Some surveys below suggest a reputation for abortifacient activity. However, even if this is the case, the doses likely to be involved would be well in excess of normal therapeutic doses.

A review of traditional Ayurvedic literature notes that fenugreek is listed as an abortifacient in two of the five sources checked. However, the definition of abortifacient was very broad and included emmenagogue, ecbolic (uterine contractor), and "antimetabolite".[28] A survey of herbal remedies used for abortion was conducted in the northern area of Morocco in the late 1990s. Barley and fenugreek seed soaked overnight in water containing squill bulb (*Urginea maritima*) was ingested by pregnant women to provoke abortion.[29]

A survey of indigenous medicinal plants used for abortion in some districts of Uttar Pradesh, India in 1987 found that 60% of pregnant women used fenugreek seed. Of the 100 fertile women that were interviewed, 50 were pregnant at the time. The survey plants were used singly at a time, but in many cases women used more than one plant during the entire period of pregnancy.[30]

Fenugreek seeds (known as methi) form an important constituent of a special maternal food consumed during pregnancy and lactation in western India (methipak, see below). Its use in pregnancy is less common because of the belief that it has abortifacient activity. Dietary fenugreek seed (5% and 20% of diet) had no adverse effect on fertility or birth outcome in rats. Fenugreek seed powder was administered in raw form and incorporated into biscuits with or without casein.[31] This is in contrast to earlier research published in 1969 indicating that aqueous and alcoholic fenugreek extracts had a stimulating effect on isolated uterus (and highlights the issue that herbal research on isolated organs often has little relevance to effects after oral intake).[32]

The addition of fenugreek to the mother's diet during pregnancy and lactation, or only during lactation, did not increase the weight gain of young rat pups compared with controls.[33]

Petroleum extract of fenugreek demonstrated antifertility activity (approximately 60%) when administered orally to rats (0.5 to 1.25 g/kg/day)

from days 1 to 10 of pregnancy.[34] Crude fenugreek extracts have been reported to be abortifacient and cause embryo resorption in female rats.[35]

Use in Lactation

Category C: Compatible with breastfeeding.

Fenugreek seed (10 g/day) significantly increased milk yield in goats compared to controls.[36] See also the Pregnancy section above for further experimental information.

Fenugreek is traditionally used to enhance lactation in Western herbal medicine[37] and Ayurveda.[38] Fenugreek is recommended to assist lactating women in the Sudan.[39] Methipak (a bittersweet confection made from wheat, fat, sugar, and generous amounts of fenugreek powder) is a well-accepted food throughout western India. It is considered to be a galactagogue that strengthens the bond between mother and child. Fenugreek is rich in iron (6.5 mg/100 g) and, since 1994, an Indian government health programme has been encouraging lactating mothers to use methipak to enhance nutritional status in infants.[40] (Note the study below which suggests that fenugreek may inhibit iron absorption.) A survey of 662 women in western India in 1985 found that 85% of women consumed methipak during lactation. Major benefits were minimising body aches, galactogogue, and strengthening qualities. It was consumed in the last trimester (for 1 to 2 months) and from 10 days postpartum (for 1 to 2 months), at the level of 50 g/day in the morning.[41]

Warnings & Precautions

The use of herbs rich in saponins is possibly inappropriate in coeliac disease, fat malabsorption, and vitamins A, D, E, and K deficiency, some upper digestive irritations, and topically to open wounds. Caution in patients with preexisting cholestasis. Avoid in patients with known allergy to spices.

Intragastric administration of a dried, aqueous ethanol extract of fenugreek seed (0.1 g/kg) to both mice and rats significantly decreased serum triiodothyronine (T_3) concentration and T_3/T_4 ratio, but increased thyroxine (T_4) levels. The inhibition in T_4 to T_3 conversion was not peroxidation-mediated.[42] Caution with high doses (>20 g/day) in patients with low thyroid activity.

Effect on Ability to Drive or Operate Machinery

No adverse effects expected.

Adverse Reactions

None expected for internal use if fenugreek is taken within the recommended dosage range. Mild gastrointestinal upset has been recorded in a small percentage of patients during a clinical trial using high doses of fenugreek seed (25 g/day).[2]

Asthmatic symptoms have been reported in workers exposed to fenugreek powder.[43] Anaphylactic symptoms to curry powder as a whole have also been reported that may or may not be linked to the presence of fenugreek.[44] In one survey carried out on patients with food allergy, two cases of severe allergy to fenugreek were identified. In the first case, inhalation of fenugreek seed powder resulted in rhinorrhoea, wheezing, and fainting. In the second, a patient with chronic asthma developed numbness of head, facial angioedema, and wheezing after application of fenugreek paste to her scalp as a treatment for dandruff. Skin scratch tests for the patients revealed strong sensitivity to fenugreek and chickpeas (another legume).[45]

A 2-year follow-up of a controlled clinical trial demonstrating improved glucose tolerance and reduced low-density lipoprotein (LDL) cholesterol levels in non–insulin-dependent diabetics showed no long-term adverse effects of a herbal powder containing fenugreek.[46] In a separate placebo-controlled study, this effect of fenugreek (at 2.5 g twice daily) on diabetic patients was confirmed, but there were no changes in postprandial glucose and lipid levels in healthy subjects. Fenugreek administration did not affect platelet aggregation, fibrinolytic activity, or fibrinogen.[3]

Frequent consumption of (dietary) fenugreek has been associated with anaemia in Ethiopian children due to inhibition of iron absorption. The plant part and quantity ingested were undefined.[47]

Maple syrup urine disease is an autosomal recessive inherited disorder of branched-chain amino acid metabolism. Fenugreek, maple syrup, and the urine of maple syrup urine disease patients all share a characteristic odour, originating from a common component, sotolone (4,5-dimethyl-3-hydroxy-2[5H]-furanone).[48] Ingestion of fenugreek by mothers during labour resulted in a maple syrup-like odour in their newborn infants, leading to a false suspicion of the inherited disease.[49,50]

As with all herbs rich in saponins, oral use may cause irritation of the gastric mucous membranes and reflux.

Interactions

A herbal product combining fenugreek with boldo (Peumus boldus) was identified as leading to an increase in international normalised ratio (INR), and therefore a potential increase in bleeding time, when warfarin was being prescribed.[51] Although it is not known which was the responsible factor in the mix, fenugreek has been listed as having a theoretical risk of interaction with warfarin.[52] Nevertheless, the observation in the above clinical trial[3] should be taken into account.

Large or frequent doses of fenugreek may inhibit iron absorption.[47] Fenugreek should be prescribed cautiously with hypoglycaemic drugs and insulin due to its potential blood glucose lowering activity.

Safety in Children

No information available but adverse effects are not expected.

Overdosage

No incidents found in published literature.

Toxicology

The LD_{50} of fenugreek 50% ethanol extract administered by intraperitoneal injection in rats was measured at 0.5 g/kg.[53] At doses of 1 to 2 g/kg no mortality was observed during the bi-weekly oral administration of an aqueous extract of fenugreek seed (1:2). Animals received the extract for 4 weeks. Gross examination of the organs did not reveal any pathological changes, although histopathological evaluation revealed necrosis of kidney and liver tissue.[54] In acute toxicology studies, debitterised fenugreek powder intragastrically administered to albino mice and albino rats of both sexes failed to induce any signs of toxicity or mortality up to a maximum practical dosage of 2 and 5 g/kg body weight, respectively. No significant alterations were discernible either in relative organ weights or their histology. In a 90-day subchronic study, the same powder fed to weanling rats of both sexes at dietary doses of 0%, 1%, 5%, and 10% in a pure diet had no effect either on the daily food intake or growth. There were no alterations in relative organ weights of various vital organs, or their histoarchitecture. Levels of glutamic-pyruvic transaminase (GPT), glutamic-oxaloacetic transaminase (GOT), and alkaline phosphatase (ALP), as well as many serum constituents such as proteins, cholesterol, urea, and creatinine, were not significantly changed at any of the dietary levels.[55]

Fenugreek herb has been known to cause myopathy in grazing animals.[56] Toxic effects were observed in chicken fed fenugreek seed saponins (0.5 g/kg/day for 21 days.)[57]

Regulatory Status

See Table 1 for regulatory status in selected countries. Fenugreek is widely consumed as a spice.

Table **1**   **Regulatory Status for Fenugreek in Selected Countries**

Australia	Fenugreek is not included in Part 4 of Schedule 4 of the Therapeutic Goods Regulations.
China	Fenugreek is official in the *Pharmacopoeia of the People's Republic of China* 1997. The usual adult dosage, usually administered in the form of a decoction, is listed as 4.5 to 9 g.
UK & Germany	Fenugreek is included on the General Sale List. It is covered by a positive Commission E monograph. Fenugreek is official in the *European Pharmacopoeia* 4.3.
US	Fenugreek does have generally recognised as safe (GRAS) status. It is freely available as a "dietary supplement" in the US under DSHEA legislation (Dietary Supplement Health and Education Act of 1994).

REFERENCES

1. Gupta A, Gupta R, Lal B: *J Assoc Physicians India* 49:1057-1061, 2001.
2. Sharma RD, Sarkar A, Hazra DK, et al: *Phytother Res* 10:332-334, 1996.
3. Bordia A, Verma SK, Srivastava KC: *Prostaglandins Leukot Essent Fatty Acids* 56:379-384, 1997.
4. Sharma RD, Raghuram TC, Rao NS: *Eur J Clin Nutr* 44:301-306, 1990.
5. Madar Z, Abel R, Samish S, et al: *Eur J Clin Nutr* 42:51-54, 1988.
6. Vats V, Grover JK, Rathi SS: *J Ethnopharmacol* 79:95-100, 2002.
7. Zia T, Hasnain SN, Hasan SK: *J Ethnopharmacol* 75:191-195, 2001.
8. Pandian RS, Anuradha CV, Viswanathan P: *J Ethnopharmacol* 81:393-397, 2002.
9. Anuradha CV, Ravikumar P: *Indian J Physiol Pharmacol* 45:408-420, 2001.
10. Choudhary D, Chandra D, Choudhary S, et al: *Food Chem Toxicol* 39:989-997, 2001.
11. Genet S, Kale RK, Baquer NZ: *Mol Cell Biochem* 236:7-12, 2002.
12. Ravikumar P, Anuradha CV: *Phytother Res* 13:197-201, 1999.
13. Bin-Hafeez B, Haque R, Parvez S, et al: *Int Immunopharmacol* 3:257-265, 2003.
14. British Herbal Medicine Association's Scientific Committee: *British herbal pharmacopoeia,* Bournemouth, 1983, BHMA, pp 216-217.
15. Brasch E, Ulbricht C, Kuo G, et al: *Altern Med Rev* 8:20-27, 2003.
16. Al-Rowais NA: *Saudi Med J* 23:1327-1331, 2002.
17. Gabay MP: *J Hum Lact* 18:274-279, 2002.
18. Langmead L, Dawson C, Hawkins C, et al: *Aliment Pharmacol Ther* 16: 197-205, 2002.
19. Shang M, Cai S, Han J, et al: *Zhongguo Zhong Yao Za Zhi* 23:614-616, 639, 1998.
20. Taylor WG, Zulyniak HJ, Richards KW, et al: *J Agric Food Chem* 50:5994-5997, 2002.
21. Waller GR, Yamasaki K (eds): *Saponins used in food and agriculture: advances in experimental medicine and biology,* vol 405, New York, 1996, Plenum Press, pp 37-46.
22. Petit PR, Sauvaire YD, Hillaire-Buys DM, et al: *Steroids* 60:674-680, 1995.
23. Sauvaire Y, Baissac Y, Leconte O, et al: *Adv Exp Med Biol* 405:37-46, 1996.
24. Broca C, Gross R, Petit P, et al: *Am J Physiol* 277:617-623, 1999.
25. Evans AJ, Hood RL, Oakenfull DG, et al: *Br J Nutr* 68:217-229, 1992.

26. Madar Z, Stark AH: *Br J Nutr* 88(suppl 3):287-292, 2002.
27. McGuffin M, Hobbs C, Upton R, Goldberg A (eds): *Botanical safety handbook*, Boca Raton, Florida, 1997, CRC Press, p 117.
28. Casey RCD: *Indian J Med Sci* 14:590-600, 1960.
29. Merzouki A, Ed-derfoufi F, Molero Mesa J: *J Ethnopharmacol* 73:501-503, 2000.
30. Nath D, Sethi N, Srivastav S, et al: *Fitoterapia* 68:223-225, 1997.
31. Mital N, Gopaldas T: *Nutr Rep Int* 33:363-369, 1986.
32. Abdo MS, Al-Kafawi AA: *Planta Med* 17:14-18, 1969.
33. Mital N, Gopaldas T: *Nutr Rep Int* 33:477-484, 1986.
34. Adhikary P, Banerji J, Choudhury D, et al: *Indian J Pharmacol* 22:24-25, 1990.
35. Al-Habori M, Raman A: *Med Arom Plants Indust Profile* 11:162-182, 2002.
36. Kholif AM, Abd El-Gawad MAM: *Egypt J Dairy Sci* 29:139-150, 2001.
37. Bartram T: *Encyclopedia of herbal medicine*, ed 1, Dorset, 1995, Grace Publishers, pp 181-182.
38. Kapoor LD: *CRC handbook of Ayurvedic medicinal plants*, Boca Raton, 1990, CRC Press, p 327.
39. Bedri NM: *Ahfad J* 12:74-86, 1995.
40. Gopaldas T: India's control programs for iron deficiency anemia in preschool children: past, present, and future. In Nestel P (ed.): *Proceedings: Interventions for child survival, London, 17-18 May 1995,* available online: www.jsi.com/intl/omni/ironmain.htm (accessed August 2003).
41. Mital N: *Ecol Food Nutr* 16:243-252, 1985.
42. Panda S, Tahiliani P, Kar A: *Pharmacol Res* 40:405-409, 1999.
43. Dugue P, Bel J, Figueredo M: *Presse Med* 22:922, 1993.
44. Ohnuma N, Yamaguchi E, Kawakami Y: *Allergy* 53:452-454, 1998.
45. Patil SP, Niphadkar PV, Bapat MM: *Ann Allergy Asthma Immunol* 78:297-300, 1997.
46. Bhardwaj PK, Dasgupta DJ, Prashar BS, et al: *J Assoc Physicians India* 42:33-35, 1994.
47. Adish AA, Esrey SA, Gyorkos TW, et al: *Public Health Nutr* 2:243-252, 1999.
48. Podebrad F, Heil M, Reichert S, et al: *J Inherit Metab Dis* 22:107-114, 1999.
49. Korman SH, Cohen E, Preminger A: *J Paediatr Child Health* 37:403-404, 2001.
50. Sewell AC, Mosandl A, Bohles H: *N Engl J Med* 341:769, 1999.
51. Lambert JP, Cormier A: *Pharmacotherapy* 21:509-512, 2001.
52. Heck AM, DeWitt BA, Lukes AL: *Am J Health Syst Pharm* 57:1221-1227, 2000.
53. Sharma ML, Chandokhe N, Ghatak BJR, et al: *Indian J Exp Biol* 16:228-240, 1978.
54. Effraim KD, Jaxks TW, Nwafor PA: *Pakistan Vet J* 19:13-16, 1999.
55. Muralidhara K, Narasimhamurthy K, Viswanatha S, et al: *Food Chem Toxicol* 37:831-838, 1999.
56. Shlosberg A, Egyed MN: *Arch Toxicol Suppl* 6:194-196, 1983.
57. Nakhla HB, Mohamed OS, Abu IM, et al: *Vet Hum Toxicol* 33:561-564, 1991.

FEVERFEW

Botanical names: *Tanacetum parthenium* (L.) Sch. Bip. (*Chrysanthemum parthenium* (L.) Bernh., *Leucanthemum parthenium* (L.) Gren. & Godr., *Matricaria parthenium* L., *Pyrethrum parthenium* (L.) Sm.)
Family: Compositae
Plant part used: Leaf

Safety Summary

Pregnancy category B3: No increase in frequency of malformation or other harmful effects on the foetus from limited use in women. Evidence of increased foetal damage in animal studies exists (at very high doses), but the relevance to humans is unknown.
Lactation category ND: No data available.
Contraindications: Patients with known sensitivity to feverfew, parthenolide, or other members of the Compositae family should not take feverfew internally. Do not use during pregnancy without professional advice.
Warnings & precautions: It is advisable to reduce the dosage gradually over a month if treatment is to be ceased.
Adverse reactions: Mild gastrointestinal symptoms, mouth ulceration, sore tongue, swollen lips/mouth, heavier periods, palpitations, dizziness, weight gain, skin rash (after oral use), contact dermatitis, urinary problems, and headache. Side effects appear to be more common after consuming the fresh leaves.
Interactions: No precautions required on current evidence.

Typical Therapeutic Use

Reviews of randomised, double-blind, placebo-controlled trials found that feverfew demonstrated therapeutic benefit for the prophylaxis of migraine headaches in the majority of trials.[1,2] Traditional indications for feverfew in Western herbal medicine include fever, prophylaxis of migraines, and arthritic conditions.[3,4]

Actions

Antiinflammatory, antiallergic, bitter tonic, emmenagogue (in high doses), anthelmintic.

Key Constituents

Key constituents of feverfew leaf include sesquiterpene lactones containing an α-methylene-γ-lactone group, including parthenolide (up to 1.68%).[5]

Adulteration

No adulterants known.

Typical Dosage Forms & Dosage

Typical adult dosage ranges are:
- 50 to 200 mg/day of dried leaf (usually as tablets/capsules)
- 0.7 to 2 mL/day of a 1:1 fresh plant tincture
- 1 to 3 mL/day of a 1:5 dried plant tincture or equivalent in tablet or capsule form
- standardised preparations corresponding to 0.2 to 0.6 mg/day of parthenolide

Contraindications

Patients with known sensitivity to feverfew, parthenolide, or other members of the Compositae family should not take feverfew internally.[6] Do not use during pregnancy without professional advice.

Use in Pregnancy

Category B3: No increase in frequency of malformation or other harmful effects on the foetus from limited use in women. Evidence of increased foetal damage in animal studies exists (at very high doses), but the relevance to humans is unknown.

Doses during pregnancy should be kept to a minimum (no more than 500 mg/day or equivalent). A decoction of the flowers in wine was combined with nutmeg or mace in traditional Western herbal medicine to bring on menstruation and to expel the afterbirth and stillborn children.[7]

Very high oral doses of feverfew (0.86 g/kg/day) reduced foetal weights when administered to rats from day 8 to 15 of gestation, and caused enlarged placentae when administered from day 1 to 8, or day 8 to 15, of gestation. The percentages of implantation loss and litter size were not significantly different from controls, and major malformations were relatively rare. The herb was administered as an ethanol extract and the dose administered was the highest possible for which the ethanol remained below the teratogenic threshold.[8]

According to one source, feverfew is reputed to cause abortion in grazing cows (presumably after intake of large amounts), but no specific information was provided.[9]

Use in Lactation

Category ND: No data available.

Warnings & Precautions

It is advisable to reduce the dosage gradually over a month if treatment is to be ceased.

Effect on Ability to Drive or Operate Machinery

No adverse effects expected.

Adverse Reactions

A review in 2000 of six randomised, double-blind, placebo-controlled trials found that feverfew use was associated with only mild and transient adverse effects.[2] Adverse reactions were reported in four of the trials and included mild gastrointestinal symptoms, mouth ulceration, heavier periods, palpitations, dizziness, weight gain, and skin rash. Feverfew was administered in capsule form or as an extract in these trials.[10-13] Reactions were reported more frequently in the placebo group than in the feverfew group in two of the trials,[10,11] including the incidence of mouth ulceration.[11]

A survey conducted in the early 1980s, of 270 migraine patients who had eaten fresh feverfew leaves every day for prolonged periods, found that side effects occurred in 17.9%. They included mouth ulcers/sore tongue (6.4%), abdominal pain/indigestion (3.9%), unpleasant taste (3.0%), tingling sensation (0.9%), urinary problems (0.9%), headache (0.9%), swollen lips/mouth (0.4%), and diarrhoea (0.4%). Symptoms were reported in the first week of treatment in some users, whereas in others they appeared gradually over the first 2 months. Of an additional 164 users who had stopped taking fresh feverfew, 21% did so because of side effects, which mainly affected the gastrointestinal tract.[14,15]

Migraine patients who had used feverfew long-term to control their symptoms found that the frequency and severity of headache, nausea, and vomiting increased when they ceased using feverfew. Other symptoms reported by these patients after ceasing feverfew included increased nervousness, tension headache, insomnia/disturbed sleep, and joint stiffness. These symptoms have been described as "postfeverfew syndrome".[10]

A 27-year-old woman who had been taking feverfew for 6 months had an abnormally high prothrombin time reading and was refused surgery.[16]

Cases of allergic contact dermatitis due to feverfew, particularly from occupational exposure, have been reported. The sesquiterpene lactones are responsible. Cross-reactivity with other members of the Compositae family is very common.[6,17,18]

Interactions

None known.

Safety in Children

No information available.

Overdosage

No incidents found in published literature.

Toxicology

No toxic effects were observed in rats and guinea pigs fed 100 to 150 times the human daily dose of feverfew each day for 5 to 7 weeks.[14] In a subacute study, the highest nontoxic oral dose of feverfew in rats was 0.86 g/kg/day as an alcohol extract.[19]

Detailed haematological analysis found no significant differences between 60 migraine patients who were feverfew users, nonuser migraine patients, and nonuser healthy volunteers. Some feverfew-users had used feverfew daily for more than 1 year.[14]

No significant differences in the frequency of chromosomal aberrations or sister chromatid exchanges were found in the circulating peripheral lymphocytes of chronic feverfew users (over 11 consecutive months) and nonuser migraine patients. The mutagenicity of urine from feverfew users was not different from that of urine from nonusers.[20,21] Parthenolide at concentrations up to 800 μM was found to be nonmutagenic in a forward mutation assay using Salmonella typhimurium.[22]

Regulatory Status

See Table 1 for regulatory status in selected countries.

Table **I**   **Regulatory Status for Feverfew in Selected Countries**

Australia	Feverfew is not included in Part 4 of Schedule 4 of the Therapeutic Goods Regulations.
UK & Germany	Feverfew is not included on the General Sale List. It was not included in the Commission E assessment. Feverfew is official in the *British Pharmacopoeia* 2002 and the *European Pharmacopoeia* 4.3.
US	Feverfew is official in the *United States Pharmacopeia-National Formulary* (USP 26-NF 21, 2003). Feverfew does not have generally recognised as safe (GRAS) status. However, it is freely available as a "dietary supplement" in the US under DSHEA legislation (Dietary Supplement Health and Education Act of 1994).

REFERENCES

1. Vogler BK, Pittler MH, Ernst E, et al: *Cephalalgia* 18:704-708, 1998.
2. Ernst E, Pittler MH: *Public Health Nutr* 3:509-514, 2000.
3. British Herbal Medicine Association: *British herbal compendium*, vol 1, Bournemouth, 1992, BHMA, pp 96-98.
4. le Strange R: *A history of herbal plants*, London, 1977, Angus & Robertson, p 74.
5. Cutlan AR, Bonilla LE, Simon JE, et al: *Planta Med* 66:612-617, 2000.
6. Hausen BM: Sesquiterpene lactones—*Tanacetum parthenium*. In De Smet PAGM, Keller K, Hansel R, et al (eds): *Adverse effects of herbal drugs*, vol 1, Berlin, 1992, Springer-Verlag, p 257.
7. Culpeper N: *Culpeper's complete herbal and english physician*, first published 1826, reprinted Bath, 1981, Harvey Sales, p 58.
8. Yao M, Brown-Woodman PDC, Ritchie H: *Birth Defects Res (Part A)* 67:141-147, Abstract 9, 2003.
9. Johnson S: *Feverfew: a traditional herbal remedy for migraine and arthritis*, London, 1984, Sheldon Press, p 89.
10. Johnson ES, Kadam NP, Hylands DM, et al: *BMJ (Clin Res Ed)* 291:569-573, 1985.
11. Murphy JJ, Heptinstall S, Mitchell JR: *Lancet* 2:189-192, 1988.
12. De Weerdt CJ, Bootsma HP, Hendriks H: *Phytomedicine* 3:225-230, 1996.
13. Pfaffenrath V, Fischer M, Friede M, et al: Clinical dose-response study for the investigation of efficacy and tolerability of *Tanacetum parthenium* in migraine prophylaxis. *Proceedings of Deutscher Schmerzkongress*, 1999.
14. Johnson ES: *MIMS Mag* 15:32-35, 1983.
15. Johnson S: *Feverfew: a traditional herbal remedy for migraine and arthritis*, London, 1984, Sheldon Press, pp 78-83.
16. Murphy LM: *Assoc Operat Room Nurses J* 69:173-183, 1999.
17. Baldwin CA, Anderson LA, Phillipson JD: *Pharm J* 239:237-238, 1987.
18. Paulsen E, Andersen KE, Hausen BM: *Contact Dermatitis* 45:197-204, 2001.
19. Yao M, Brown-Woodman PD, Ritchie H: *Teratology* 64:323-324, 2001.
20. Anderson D, Jenkinson PC, Dewdney RS, et al: *Hum Toxicol* 7:145-152, 1988.
21. Johnson ES, Kadam NP, Anderson D, et al: *Hum Toxicol* 6:533-534, 1987.
22. Marles RJ, Pazos-Sanou L, Compadre CM, et al: Sesquiterpene lactones revisited. In Arnason JT, et al (eds): *Recent advances in phytochemistry*, vol 29, *Phytochemistry of medicinal plants*, New York, 1995, Plenum Press, pp 333-356.

FRINGE TREE

Other common name: Chionanthus
Botanical name: *Chionanthus virginicus* L.
Family: Oleaceae
Plant part used: Root bark

Safety Summary

Pregnancy category B2: No increase in frequency of malformation or other harmful effects on the foetus from limited use in women. Animal studies are lacking.
Lactation category C: Compatible with breastfeeding.
Contraindications: None required on current evidence.
Warnings & precautions: None required.
Adverse reactions: None found in published literature.
Interactions: No precautions required on current evidence.

Typical Therapeutic Use

Traditional indications for fringe tree in Western herbal medicine include liver disease, cholecystitis, duodenitis, enlarged spleen, portal congestion, glycosuria, skin, and bowel disorders.[1,2]

Actions

Cholagogue, choleretic, mild laxative, antiemetic, depurative.

Key Constituents

The constituents of fringe tree are not well researched. The occurrence of a saponin, which was first reported in 1875, was confirmed in 1942.[3] A lignan glycoside known as phillyrin or chionanthin was isolated from the root (2.2%) in 1959.[4]

Adulteration

John Uri Lloyd wrote in 1915 "up to 1904, this much employed drug [Chionanthus] had never, under my observation, been contaminated . . . At the present time, this statement is erroneous." He goes on to describe adulteration of commercial fringe tree by an unidentified bark.[5] Commercial samples were also known to be adulterated with stem bark.[3]

Typical Dosage Forms & Dosage

Typical adult dosage ranges are:
- 6 to 12 g/day of dried root bark or by infusion
- 3 to 9 mL/day of a 1:1 liquid extract
- 3 to 6 mL/day of a 1:2 liquid extract or equivalent in tablet or capsule form
- 6 to 9 mL/day of a 1:5 tincture

Contraindications

None required on current evidence.

Use in Pregnancy

Category B2: No increase in frequency of malformation or other harmful effects on the foetus from limited use in women. Animal studies are lacking.

Eclectic physicians recommended fringe tree as a fast-acting treatment for jaundice during pregnancy.[6]

Use in Lactation

Category C: Compatible with breastfeeding.

Warnings & Precautions

None required.

Effect on Ability to Drive or Operate Machinery

No adverse effects expected.

Adverse Reactions

No adverse reactions documented. Some herbal texts refer to fringe tree being "narcotic", although this has been disputed.[2,6]

Interactions

None reported.

Safety in Children

No adverse effects are expected. Eclectic physicians recommended fringe tree as a gentle and effective treatment for infantile jaundice.[6]

Overdosage

No incidents found in published literature.

Toxicology

No information available.

Regulatory Status

See Table 1 for regulatory status in selected countries

Table 1   Regulatory Status for Fringe Tree in Selected Countries

Australia	Fringe tree is not included in Part 4 of Schedule 4 of the Therapeutic Goods Regulations.
UK & Germany	Fringe tree is included on the General Sale List. It was not included in the Commission E assessment.
US	Fringe tree does not have generally recognised as safe (GRAS) status. However, it is freely available as a "dietary supplement" in the US under DSHEA legislation (Dietary Supplement Health and Education Act of 1994).

REFERENCES

1. British Herbal Medicine Association's Scientific Committee: *British herbal pharmacopoeia*, Bournemouth, 1983, BHMA, pp 63-64.
2. Felter HW, Lloyd JU: *King's American dispensatory*, ed 18, rev 3, vol 1, first published 1905, reprinted Portland, 1983, Eclectic Medical Publications, pp 500-502.
3. Youngken HW, Feldman HS: *J Am Pharm Assoc* 31:129-135, 1942.
4. Blaschek W, Ebel S, Hackenthal E, et al: *HagerROM 2002: Hagers Handbuch der Drogen und Arzneistoffe*, Heidelberg, 2002, Springer.
5. Lloyd JU: *Druggist Circ* 59:87-90, 1915.
6. Lloyd JU: *Treatise no. V: Chionanthus virginica*. Cincinnati, 1904, Lloyd Brothers.

GARLIC

Botanical name: *Allium sativum* L.
Family: Alliaceae (broadly Liliaceae)
Plant part used: Clove

Safety Summary

Pregnancy category A: No proven increase in the frequency of malformation or other harmful effects on the foetus despite consumption by a large number of women.
Lactation category C: Compatible with breast-feeding.
Contraindications: Contraindicated in those with known sensitivity. Doses greater than the equivalent of 5 g/day of fresh garlic are contraindicated with concurrent use of warfarin.
Warnings & precautions: Due to its antiplatelet activity, discontinue intake of garlic 10 days before undergoing surgery. Prolonged and high doses of fresh raw garlic and allicin-releasing garlic products should not be taken during pregnancy or in conjunction with antiplatelet or anticoagulant drugs. On current information, caution should also be observed for concurrent use of garlic and protease inhibitor drugs.
Adverse reactions: Typical adverse reactions include allergy, contact dermatitis and other skin reactions, increased body odour, and minor gastrointestinal symptoms. Increased bleeding tendency has been reported for prolonged and high intake of garlic. Occupational allergy to garlic (contact dermatitis, asthma) has also been observed.
Interactions: See above in Contraindications and Warnings & precautions.

Typical Therapeutic Use

A meta-analysis of 39 trials (which analysed the data of 13 trials meeting the inclusion criteria) concluded that garlic is superior to placebo in reducing total cholesterol levels in hypercholesterolaemia, although the effect is modest. Products included in the analysis were garlic powder (11 trials, 10 of which used one standardised product) and steam-distilled oil (two trials). It was noted that there was possibly incomplete formation of active constituents in batches of the standardised garlic-powder product manufactured from 1995 to 1997, which may have adversely affected the results.[1] Another meta-analysis noted that, compared to placebo, standardised garlic powder reduced blood pressure in mild hypertension (with 8 of 11 trials eligible for inclusion).[2] Generally many trials had methodological shortcomings and more rigorous trials were suggested.[2-4] A meta-analysis of the epidemiological literature indicated that a high intake of raw or cooked garlic may be associated with a protective effect against stomach and colorectal cancers.[5] There are also clinical trials supporting the use of aged garlic products for lowering cholesterol and for antiplatelet activity.[6]

Traditional indications for garlic in Western herbal medicine include chronic bronchitis, respiratory catarrh, whooping cough, bronchitic asthma, and worm infestation.[7,8] In addition to these indications, garlic has been used in traditional Chinese medicine for indigestion and diarrhoea, and in Ayurveda for fevers, including those of an intermittent nature, dyspepsia, and debilitated conditions.[9,10]

As can be seen from the above, several types of garlic products are consumed:

- fresh raw garlic
- garlic oil products (macerated or distilled)
- aged garlic products (produced by fermentation)
- garlic-powder products (which aim to mimic the chemistry of fresh crushed garlic).

The safety issues for the various products will obviously vary and data are provided below for fresh raw garlic, garlic powder (similar in effects to fresh garlic), and aged garlic.

Actions

Diaphoretic, stimulant, diuretic, expectorant, antiseptic, hypolipidaemic, mild hypotensive.

Key Constituents

The chemistry of garlic is complex. Key constituents are the sulphur compounds, of which S-allyl-cysteine sulphoxide (also known as alliin) is the most important. Allicin (an odorous compound) is generated in garlic when an enzyme (allinase) initiates its formation from the odourless precursor alliin. The allinase is released when the garlic bulb is cut or crushed. Allicin is rather unstable and decomposes further, producing a range of compounds, including diallyl sulphides (diallyl disulphide as the major product), ajoenes, and vinyldithiins. The total sulphur content of garlic is about 1% of its dry weight.[11]

Garlic products contain the following key constituents[11]:

- Garlic powder: preserves alliin and the enzyme allinase, and the objective is that when the alliin comes into contact with allinase in the digestive tract, conversion to allicin occurs.
- Aged garlic products: contain modified sulphur compounds such as S-allylcysteine.
- Garlic oils: when obtained by steam-distillation these are rich in diallyl and dimethyl sulphides.

Adulteration

No adulterants known; however, garlic-powder products may not produce biologically active levels of key constituents (such as allicin) when ingested. A 2001 survey of 24 brands of enteric-coated garlic-powder tablets found that nearly all brands met their claims for allicin potential when crushed and suspended in water, but all except one gave substandard dissolution release of allicin under simulated gastrointestinal conditions.[12]

Typical Dosage Forms & Dosage

Typical adult dosage ranges are:
- 6 to 11.5 mL/day of a 1:1 liquid extract
- 6 to 12 mL/day of a 1:5 tincture
- doses in tablet or capsule form corresponding to 5 to 12 mg/day of allicin or total thio-sulphinates
- 0.5 to 1 g/day of dried garlic powder
- 0.9 to 4.8 g/day of aged garlic extract (powder)

Contraindications

Contraindicated in those with known sensitivity. Doses greater than the equivalent of 5 g/day of fresh garlic are contraindicated with concurrent use of warfarin.

Use in Pregnancy

Category A: No proven increase in the frequency of malformation or other harmful effects on the foetus despite consumption by a large number of women. However, large doses of fresh raw garlic or allicin-releasing products should not be consumed during pregnancy.

A small clinical trial observed that garlic ingestion by pregnant women significantly alters the odour of their amniotic fluid.[13] Garlic has been noted on more than one occasion on the breath of the newborn infant delivered from mothers of Pakistani origin.[14]

A randomised, single blind trial investigated the effect of garlic on nulliparous pregnant women at high risk of preeclampsia. One hundred women, 28 to 32 weeks pregnant, received tablets of dried garlic powder (providing 2 mg/day allicin) or placebo for 8 weeks. There was no significant difference between the two groups with regard to outcome of pregnancy and perinatal characteristics. Garlic also significantly decreased total cholesterol and the risk of hypertension alone, but had no effect on the levels of other lipids, platelet aggregation, and the incidence of preeclampsia. Reported side effects for the treatment and placebo group, respectively, were odour (34% versus 4%) and slight nausea (16% versus 4%).[15] (This trial was not included in the above meta-analysis.)

Use in Lactation

Category C: Compatible with breastfeeding.

A small placebo-controlled study investigated the effects of garlic ingestion by the mother on the odour of her breast milk and the suckling behaviour of her infant. Garlic ingestion significantly and consistently increased the perceived intensity of the milk odour, which peaked in strength 2 hours after ingestion. The babies detected these changes, as indicated by an increased time of attachment to the breast and more suckling when the milk smelled like garlic. There was also a tendency for infants to ingest more milk.[16]

Warnings & Precautions

Due to its antiplatelet activity, discontinue intake of garlic 10 days before undergoing surgery. Prolonged and high doses of fresh raw garlic and allicin-releasing garlic products should not be taken during pregnancy or in conjunction with antiplatelet or antico-agulant drugs. On current information, caution should also be observed for concurrent use of garlic and protease inhibitor drugs.

Effect on Ability to Drive or Operate Machinery

No adverse effects expected.

Adverse Reactions

Ten of the 13 trials assessed in the first meta-analysis referred to above (see Typical therapeutic use) provided information regarding adverse events. This information is listed in Table 1. Gastrointestinal symptoms and garlic breath were most frequently reported.

For the meta-analysis investigating the effect of garlic on blood pressure, 7 of the 8 included trials mentioned that adverse effects were not significantly increased as a result of garlic treatment. (Four of the trials were also analysed in the hypercholesterolaemia meta-analysis and are listed in Table 1: Auer 1990, Vorberg and Schneider 1990, de Santos and Grunwald 1993, and Jain 1993.[2]) A review of 45 randomised trials and 73 additional studies (mostly case reports or small case series) noted that reported adverse effects of garlic ingestion (in addition to those already listed here and those listed in the Interactions section) were rhinitis, asthma, and Menière's disease. The frequency of adverse effects and variation according to each particular preparation were not studied. In most case reports and case series, adverse effects could not be attributed directly to garlic because chance, coincidence, or confounding factors could have been responsible for the adverse effect. Alternative causes of reported adverse effects were possible in 22% of the reviewed studies and could not be definitively excluded in 69%. The review also noted that a modest but significant decrease in platelet aggregation was demonstrated for garlic compared with placebo treatment in the four trials for which participants were prohibited from taking antiplatelet medication.[17,18]

Table 2 lists additional case reports of adverse reactions to garlic. Of concern are a few reports of an increased bleeding tendency.[19-24]

Quite high doses of garlic can be consumed by many people without apparent adverse effects. Participants have consumed 3 to 15 g/day fresh garlic in clinical trials assessing the reduction of serum lipids. In China during the mid-1980s the average consumption of fresh garlic was recorded at 20 g/day.[25] No adverse effects were observed in an uncontrolled clinical trial during which patients received essential oil of garlic in capsules. The daily dose was equivalent to 50 g of raw garlic.[26] In a clinical study investigating fibrinolytic activity, volunteers and patients received, in capsule form, a daily dose of essential oil equivalent to 1 g/kg of raw garlic for a period of 3 months. No side effects were observed.[27] However, high doses of garlic have been noted to cause vomiting and diarrhoea, due to a strong irritant activity on the gastrointestinal mucosa.[28]

Garlic can cause allergic reactions. Such garlic-related adverse reactions include irritant contact dermatitis (with the rare variant of zosteriform dermatitis), induction of pemphigus, allergic asthma and rhinitis, contact urticaria, protein contact dermatitis, allergic contact dermatitis (including the haematogenic variant), and combinations thereof.[29] Fresh garlic applied to skin is corrosive and will burn, as is evidenced by case reports. Many reports of contact dermatitis and respiratory symptoms caused by inhalation of garlic dust occur as a result of occupational exposure.[30]

A case of contact dermatitis occurred from oral ingestion of garlic tablets. Allergy to garlic was confirmed by patch test and rechallenge.[31] Garlic has been observed to be an allergen in a double-blind, placebo-controlled food challenge involving 163 asthmatic children with food allergy. Of the foods tested, it recorded the lowest frequency of allergic response, at 1.2%.[32] In a telephone survey investigating food allergies in 132 children, garlic was identified as a food allergen in 3% of those reactions for which the cause was able to be identified.[33] There are other reports of allergic reactions following garlic ingestion in people without occupational exposure.[30]

Sensitisation to garlic has been confirmed in skin-prick tests.[34] Garlic-sensitive patients have shown positive tests to diallyldisulphide, allylpropyldisulphide, allylmercaptan, and allicin. Despite the positive patch-test results, an irritative type of reaction could not be excluded. Cross-sensitisation between onion and garlic has also been observed.[35]

Interactions

See Table 3 for information on the interactions between garlic and orthodox drugs.[36-42]

Table I   **Adverse Event Information for Well-Designed, Randomised, Placebo-Controlled, Double-Blind Trials Evaluating Garlic for the Treatment of Hypercholesterolaemia**

Study and Dosage	Number of Patients[†]	Adverse Events in Garlic Treatment Group	Adverse Events in Placebo Group
Bordia (1981)*; steam-distilled garlic oil[‡] (0.25 mg/kg/day, 20 weeks)	62	Diarrhoea (1); epigastric distress (3)[§]	
Auer (1990)*; standardised garlic powder[∥] (600 mg/day, 12 weeks)	47	Odour (3)[§]	
Mader (1990)*; standardised garlic powder (800 mg/day, 16 weeks)	221	Odour (30); gastrointestinal symptoms (1)	Odour (12); gastrointestinal symptoms (2); allergy (1)
de Santos and Grunwald (1993); standardised garlic powder (900 mg/day, 24 weeks)	52	Flatulence and aftertaste (1)	
Jain (1993); standardised garlic powder (900 mg/day, 12 weeks)	42	Odour and belching (1)	Abdominal symptoms (2); minor rash (1); increased bleeding (1)
Neil (1996)*; standardised garlic powder (900 mg/day, 24 weeks)	115	Odour (19); abdominal symptoms (4)	Odour# (5); abdominal symptoms (2); myocardial infarction (1)
Alder and Holub (1997); standardised garlic powder (900 mg/day, 12 weeks)	23	Odour (20% of participants)	
McCrindle (1998); standardised garlic powder (900 mg/day, 8 weeks)	30	Headache and upset stomach (31% of participants)	Headache and upset stomach (36% of participants)
Isaacsohn (1998); standardised garlic powder (900 mg/day, 12 weeks)	42	Odour (5); abdominal symptoms (2); intestinal obstruction (1)	Epigastric burning (1); myocardial infarction (1); chest pain (1)
Berthold (1998)*; steam-distilled garlic oil (10 mg/day,[¶] 12 weeks)	25	Odour and abdominal symptoms (a few participants)	Odour# and abdominal symptoms (a few participants)

The information in this table was obtained from the Stevinson review,[1] and, where asterisked, supplemented with information from the individual research papers. Trials not providing adverse event details were Plengvidhya (1988), Vorberg and Schneider (1990), and Saradeth (1994).

[†]Number of patients who completed the trial and were included in the data analysis.

[‡]1 mg of oil corresponded to approximately 2 g of raw garlic.

[§]Trial did not specify the group in which the symptoms occurred.

[∥]600 to 900 mg of this standardised garlic powder corresponded approximately to 1.8 to 2.7 g of fresh garlic.[2]

[¶]Daily dose corresponded to approximately 4 to 5 fresh cloves, 4000 units of allicin-equivalents.

[#]The placebo used had a coating that tasted like garlic.

Table **2**   **Adverse Reactions Possibly Associated with Garlic Intake**

Clinical Study and Case Reports	Adverse Reaction	Ref.
One case, 2002; odourless garlic tablet taken regularly, 5 tablets (= 5 g fresh bulb) taken the day prior to surgery	Bilateral retrobulbar haemorrhage with elevated intraocular pressure during strabismus surgery	19
One case, 1995; "heavy garlic intake" prior to cosmetic surgery (preparation and dosage undefined)	Bleeding complications and prolonged clotting time	20
One case, 1995; garlic tablets taken for many years (preparation and dosage undefined)	Haemorrhage during surgery; anticoagulant effect confirmed 3 months after resuming garlic	21
One case, 1990; garlic ingestion (4 cloves/day, approx. 2 g)	Spontaneous spinal epidural haematoma associated with prolonged bleeding time despite adequate platelet count	22
Pharmacological study, 1983; 5 volunteers: ingestion of fresh garlic extract (10 to 25 mL, single dose on an empty stomach)	Burning sensation in mouth, oesophagus, and stomach lasting 15 minutes (10 mL dose); nausea, diaphoresis, light-headedness lasting 30 minutes (25 mL dose)	23
One case, 1982; ingestion of a whole garlic bulb	Mechanical bowel obstruction (no previous history of obstruction)	24

Table **3**   **Possible Interactions Between Garlic and Orthodox Drugs**

Clinical Studies and Case Reports of Possible Interaction	Adverse Reaction	Ref.
HIV PROTEASE INHIBITORS		
Pharmacokinetic study, 2000/2002; healthy volunteers: garlic caplets, twice daily (equivalent to 8 g/day cloves, standardised for allicin and alliin) from days 5 to 24, saquinavir administered to overlap on days 22 to 24	Decreased plasma concentration of saquinavir	36, 37
Pharmacokinetic study, 2000; 10 healthy volunteers: single-dose ritonavir, garlic capsule for 4 days	Insignificant decrease of ritonavir*	38
WARFARIN		
Two cases; 1991; taking garlic products (garlic oil, garlic tablet; no more information), previously stabilised on warfarin	Increased international normalised ratio (INR), increase in clotting time (about doubled)	39
Pilot study, 2000; eight patients stabilised on warfarin: garlic (aged extract 1200 mg/day) or placebo for 4 weeks	No significant effect of aged garlic extract on INR	40
OTHER		
Clinical study (experimental, chemopreventative model), 16 volunteers: aged garlic extract (equivalent to 6 to 7 cloves/day) for 3 months	Increase in peak plasma paracetamol concentration, decreased paracetamol renal clearance, increased plasma levels of paracetamol metabolites	41
One case, 1979; woman with non–insulin-dependent diabetes mellitus taking chlorpropamide, consumed curry containing garlic and karela (*Momordica charantia*)	Hypoglycaemia	42

*The lack of effect may be due to short duration of garlic intake and non-steady state concentration of ritonavir.[37,38]

On the basis of case reports and a clinical study summarised in Table 3, caution is advised when patients are taking warfarin and HIV protease inhibitors such as saquinavir. Since heavy garlic use has been associated with an increased bleeding tendency (see Table 2), it is contraindicated in patients taking warfarin when prescribed in doses equivalent to greater than 5 g/day of fresh garlic.

On the basis of the antiplatelet activity and documented increased bleeding tendency from garlic intake (see Table 2), caution is advised in those also taking aspirin and other antiplatelet drugs.

A clinical study demonstrated that garlic consumption is a potential confounder when monitoring human exposure to allylhalides and other chemicals. Consumption of garlic leads to acetyl-S-allyl-L-cysteine excretion, which is also a biomarker of such exposure.[43]

Safety in Children

No information available, but adverse effects are not expected other than possible mild gastrointestinal discomfort. Garlic should not be administered to children younger than 3 years.

Overdosage

Large doses of garlic oil can cause violent vomiting, diarrhoea, kidney inflammation, and possibly kidney damage.[28]

Toxicology

Table 4 lists LD$_{50}$ data recorded for garlic products and garlic constituents.[44,45]

The effect of the administration of garlic products on gastric mucosa was investigated using endoscopy in dogs. Raw garlic powder caused severe mucosal damage, including erosion. Dehydrated boiled garlic powder caused reddening of the mucosa, but aged garlic extract did not cause any undesirable effects.[46]

Serious stomach injury and death occurred in female rats fed raw garlic juice (5 mL/kg) for 21 days. Swelling of the liver, hypertrophy of the spleen and adrenal glands, and alterations in red blood count and morphology were observed after 3 and 8 days. These effects were not observed in animals fed aged garlic juice.[47] No toxic symptoms were demonstrated in rats orally administered aged garlic extract, even at a dose level of 2 g/kg five times a week for a period of 6 months.[48]

Garlic tincture (prepared according to the German pharmacopoeia, 6th Edition, Supplement) was negative in the Ames assay utilising tester strains TA98 and TA100 with and without the addition of S9 mix.[49] The juice of fresh garlic (10% v/v of the test medium) in the absence of S9 induced significant levels of chromosomal damage in vitro relative to control treatments, predominantly in the form of chromatid breaks and exchanges.[50] Two garlic constituents (diallyl sulphide and diallyl disulphide) also induced chromosomal aberrations and sister chromatid exchanges. The addition of S9 to the assays modified the effects of the two compounds in a nonconsistent manner.[51] Oral administration of freshly prepared garlic extract alone did not significantly induce chromosomal aberrations in vivo (mice, bone marrow tissue). Using the same model, this extract also demonstrated chemopreventative potential

Table **4   LD$_{50}$ Data Recorded for Garlic Products and Garlic Constituents**

Substance	Route, Model	LD$_{50}$ Value	Reference
Aqueous extract of crushed fresh garlic	Undefined*, rats	173.8 mL/kg	44
Allicin (as an oil)	Undefined*, mice	0.2 mL/kg	44
Allicin	i.p., mice	60 mg/kg	45
Allicin	s.c., mice	120 mg/kg	45

*Route undefined, but very likely oral.

Table **5**   **Regulatory Status for Garlic in Selected Countries**

Australia	Garlic is not included in Part 4 of Schedule 4 of the Therapeutic Goods Regulations.
UK & Germany	Garlic and garlic oil are included on the General Sale List. It is covered by a positive Commission E monograph. Garlic is official in the *British Pharmacopoeia* 2002 and the *European Pharmacopoeia* 4.3.
US	Garlic is official in the *United States Pharmacopeia-National Formulary* (USP 26-NF 21, 2003). Garlic does have generally recognised as safe (GRAS) status. It is freely available as a "dietary supplement" in the US under DSHEA legislation (Dietary Supplement Health and Education Act of 1994).

against cyclophosphamide-induced chromosomal mutations.[52]

Regulatory Status

See Table 5 for regulatory status in selected countries. Garlic is widely consumed as a food throughout the world.

REFERENCES

1. Stevinson C, Pittler MH, Ernst E: *Ann Intern Med* 133:420-429, 2000.
2. Silagy CA, Neil HA: *J Hypertens* 12:463-468, 1994.
3. Silagy C, Neil A: *J R Coll Physicians Lond* 28:39-45, 1994.
4. Ackermann RT, Mulrow CD, Ramirez G, et al: *Arch Intern Med* 161:813-824, 2001.
5. Fleischauer AT, Poole C, Arab L: *Am J Clin Nutr* 72:1047-1052, 2000.
6. Blumenthal M, Brinckmann J, Wollschlaeger B: *The ABC clinical guide to herbs*, Austin, 2003, American Botanical Council, pp 155-170.
7. British Herbal Medicine Association's Scientific Committee: *British herbal pharmacopoeia*, Bournemouth, 1983, BHMA, pp 20-21.
8. Felter HW, Lloyd JU: *King's American dispensatory*, ed 18, rev 3, vol 1, first published 1905, reprinted Portland, 1983, Eclectic Medical Publications, pp 145-146.
9. Chopra RN, Chopra IC, Handa KL, et al: *Chopra's indigenous drugs of India*, ed 2, first published 1958, reprinted Calcutta, 1982, Academic Publishers, pp 271-274.
10. Chang HM, But PP: *Pharmacology and applications of Chinese materia medica*, vol 1, Singapore, 1987, World Scientific, pp 84-93.
11. Sendl A: *Phytomedicine* 4:323-339, 1995.
12. Lawson LD, Wang ZJ: *J Agric Food Chem* 49:2592-2599, 2001.
13. Mennella JA, Johnson A, Beauchamp GK: *Chem Senses* 20:207-209, 1995.
14. Snell SB: *Lancet* 2:43, 1973.
15. Ziaei S, Hantoshzadeh S, Rezasoltani P, et al: *Eur J Obstet Gynecol Reprod Biol* 99:201-206, 2001.
16. Mennella JA, Beauchamp GK: *Pediatrics* 88:737-744, 1991.
17. Ackermann RT, Mulrow CD, Ramirez G, et al: *Arch Intern Med* 161:813-824, 2001.
18. US Department of Health and Human Services, Agency for Healthcare Research and Quality: *Garlic: effects on cardiovascular risks and disease, protective effects against cancer, and clinical adverse effects*, Evidence Report No. 20, October 2000, AHRQ Pub. No. 01-E022, available online: http://hstat.nlm.nih.gov/hq/Hquest/db/local.epc.er.garl/screen/DLTocDisplay/s/56051/action/DLToc (accessed May 2003).
19. Carden SM, Good WV, Carden PA, et al: *Clin Experiment Ophthalmol* 30:303-304, 2002.
20. Burnham BE: *Plast Reconstr Surg* 95:213, 1995.
21. German K, Kumar U, Blackford HN: *Br J Urol* 76:518, 1995.
22. Rose KD, Croissant PD, Parliament CF, et al: *Neurosurgery* 26:880-882, 1990.
23. Caporaso N, Smith SM, Eng RH: *Antimicrob Agents Chemother* 23:700-702, 1983.
24. Szybejko J, Zukowski A, Herbec R: *Wiad Lek* 35:163-164, 1982.
25. Koch HP: Toxicity, side effects, and unwanted effects of garlic. In Koch HP, Lawson LD (eds): *Garlic: the science and therapeutic application of Allium sativum L. and related species*, ed 2, Baltimore, 1996, Williams & Wilkins, p 221.
26. Anon: *J Trad Chin Med* 6:117-120, 1986.
27. Bordia AK, Joshi HK, Sanadhya YK, et al: *Atherosclerosis* 28:55-159, 1977.
28. Gessner O: *Gift- und Arzneipflanzen von Mitteleuropa*, ed 3, Carl Winter Universitatsverlag, 1974, Heidelberg, pp 324-328.
29. Jappe U, Bonnekoh B, Hausen BM, et al: *Am J Contact Dermat* 10:37-39, 1999.
30. Morbidoni L, Arterburn JM, Young V, et al: *J Herbal Pharmacother* 1:63-83, 2001.
31. Burden AD, Wilkinson SM, Beck MH, et al: *Contact Dermatitis* 30:299-300, 1994.
32. Rance F, Dutau G: *Arch Pediatr* 9(suppl 3):402s-407s, 2002.

33. Nowak-Wegrzyn A, Conover-Walker MK, Wood RA: *Arch Pediatr Adolesc Med* 155:790-795, 2001.

34. Moneret-Vautrin DA, Morisset M, Lemerdy P, et al: *Allerg Immunol (Paris)* 34:135-140, 2002.

35. Papageorgiou C, Corbet JP, Menezes-Brandao F, et al: *Arch Dermatol Res* 275:229-234, 1983.

36. Piscitelli SC, Burstein AH, Welden N, et al: *8th Conference on retroviruses and opportunistic infections, Chicago, 4-7 February 2000,* Abstract No. 734.

37. Piscitelli SC, Burstein AH, Welden N, et al: *Clin Infect Dis* 34:234-238, 2002.

38. Gallicano K, Foster B, Choudhri S: *Br J Clin Pharmacol* 55:199-202, 2003.

39. Sunter W: *Pharm J* 246:722, 1991.

40. Rozenfeld V, Sisca TS, Callahan AK, et al: *35th Annual ASHP (American Society of Health-System Pharmacists) Midyear Clinical Meeting, Las Vegas, 3-7 December 2000.*

41. Gwilt PR, Lear CL, Tempero MA, et al: *Cancer Epidemiol Biomarkers Prev* 3:155-160, 1994.

42. Aslam M, Stockley IH: *Lancet* 1:607, 1979.

43. de Rooij BM, Boogaard PJ, Rijksen DA, et al: *Arch Toxicol* 70:635-639, 1996.

44. Chowdhury AK, Ahsan M, Islam SN, et al: *Indian J Med Res* 93:33-36, 1991.

45. Calallito CJ, Bailey JH: *J Am Chem Soc* 66:1950-1951, 1944.

46. Hoshino T, Kashimoto N, Kasuga S: *J Nutr* 131:1109S-1113S, 2001.

47. Nakagawa S, Masamoto K, Sumiyoshi H, et al: *J Toxicol Sci* 5:91-112, 1980.

48. Sumiyoshi H, Kanezawa A, Masamoto K, et al: *J Toxicol Sci* 9:61-75, 1984.

49. Schimmer O, Kruger A, Paulini H, et al: *Pharmazie* 49:448-451, 1994.

50. Charles GD, Linscombe VA, Tornesi B, et al: *Food Chem Toxicol* 40:1391-1402, 2002.

51. Musk SR, Clapham P, Johnson IT: *Food Chem Toxicol* 35:379-385, 1997.

52. Shukla Y, Taneja P: *Cancer Lett* 176:31-36, 2002.

GENTIAN

Botanical name: *Gentiana lutea* L.
Family: Gentianaceae
Plant part used: Root and rhizome

Safety Summary

Pregnancy category B2: No increase in frequency of malformation or other harmful effects on the foetus from limited use in women. Animal studies are lacking.
Lactation category C: Compatible with breastfeeding.
Contraindications: Possible care with peptic ulceration and hyperacidity conditions.
Warnings & precautions: See Contraindications.
Adverse reactions: None found in published literature.
Interactions: No precautions required on current evidence.

Typical Therapeutic Use

Traditional indications for gentian in Western herbal medicine include anorexia and atonic dyspepsia.[1] It is thought to increase gastric acid and other digestive secretions.[2]

Actions

Bitter tonic, digestive stimulant.

Key Constituents

Secoiridoids: gentiopicroside (1% to 4%; metabolised to erythrocentaurin, gentiopicral, and others by human intestinal bacteria[3]), amarogentin, swertiamarine, and sweroside. Triterpenes: 2,3-seco-3-oxours-12-en-2-oic acid, 2,3-seco-3-oxoolean-12-en-2-oic acid, and betulin 3-*O*-palmitate.[4] Oligosaccharides, including bitter-tasting gentianose and gentiobiose; xanthones (approximately 0.1%), mainly gentisin, isogentisin, and gentioside; traces of essential oil.

Adulteration

Inexperienced collection of the plant in the wild can lead to substitution with a plant in the same locality and of similar appearance: *Veratrum album*. This contains toxic alkaloids. The roots of *Rumex* species and

other species of *Gentiana* are also possible adulterants.[5] *Gentiana lutea* is protected, and/or has restrictions for wildcrafting, in several areas of Europe.[6] Human poisoning has been documented for the ingestion of *Veratrum album* mistaken for gentian.[5]

Typical Dosage Forms & Dosage

Typical adult dosage ranges are:
- 1.8 to 6 g/day dried rhizome and root or by infusion or decoction
- 0.7 to 2 mL/day of a 1:2 extract or equivalent in tablet or capsule form
- 3 to 12 mL/day of a 1:5 tincture

Contraindications

Established monographs state that gentian is contraindicated in gastric or duodenal ulcers and gastric conditions associated with hyperacidity. These are not corroborated in modern times, although some care is necessary in using gentian in these conditions.

Use in Pregnancy

Category B2: No increase in frequency of malformation or other harmful effects on the foetus from limited use in women. Animal studies are lacking. Some clinicians state that gentian is poorly tolerated by pregnant women.

Use in Lactation

Category C: Compatible with breastfeeding.

Warnings & Precautions

See Contraindications above.

Effect on Ability to Drive or Operate Machinery

No adverse effects expected.

Adverse Reactions

Occasional headaches may occur.[7]

Interactions

None known.

Safety in Children

No information available, but adverse effects are not expected apart from a reaction to the strong, bitter taste.

Overdosage

Overdose may lead to nausea or even vomiting. Given at very high doses in animals (250 and 500 mg/kg by intraperitoneal injection), the methanol extract of *Gentiana lutea* roots caused a significant increase in stamina and a slight analgesic activity without sedation, fatigue, or toxicity. The secoiridoid fraction was shown to be the most active.[8]

Toxicology

No significant toxicity was observed in rabbits administered an ethanol extract of gentian root intragastrically (6.5 mL/kg/day of 0.6 g dried herb/100 mL extract) over a period of 3 days. Parameters measured included rate of breathing, pulse rate, red blood count, Quick value (prothrombin time) and serum calcium, potassium, and sodium. Only the red blood count was slightly, but significantly, reduced compared to control groups.[9]

Regulatory Status

See Table 1 for regulatory status in selected countries.

Table 1   **Regulatory Status for Gentian in Selected Countries**

Australia	Gentian is not included in Part 4 of Schedule 4 of the Therapeutic Goods Regulations.
UK & Germany	Gentian is included on the General Sale List. It is covered by a positive Commission E monograph. Gentian root is official in the *European Pharmacopoeia* 4.3.
US	Gentian does not have generally recognised as safe (GRAS) status. However, it is freely available as a "dietary supplement" in the US under DSHEA legislation (Dietary Supplement Health and Education Act of 1994).

REFERENCES

1. British Herbal Medicine Association's Scientific Committee: *British herbal pharmacopoeia*, Bournemouth, 1983, BHMA, pp 99-100.
2. Mills S, Bone K: *Principles and practice of phytotherapy: modern herbal medicine*; Edinburgh, 2000, Churchill Livingstone, pp 38-41.
3. el-Sedawy Al, Hattori M, Kobashi K, et al: *Chem Pharm Bull (Tokyo)* 37:2435-2437, 1989.
4. Toriumi Y, Kakuda R, Kikuchi M, et al: *Chem Pharm Bull (Tokyo)* 51:89-91, 2003.
5. Blaschek W, Ebel S, Hackenthal E, et al: *HagerROM 2002: Hagers Handbuch der Drogen und Arzneistoffe*, Heidelberg, 2002, Springer.
6. Lange D: *Europe's medicinal and aromatic plants: their use, trade and conservation*, Cambridge, 1998, TRAFFIC International, p III.
7. Blumenthal M, et al (eds): *The complete German Commission E monographs: therapeutic guide to herbal medicines*, Austin, 1998, American Botanical Council, p 135.
8. Ozturk N, Husnu Can Baser K, Ozturk Y, et al: *Phytother Res* 16:627-631, 2002.
9. Chibanguza G, Marz R, Sterner W: *Arzneim Forsch* 34:32-36, 1984.p

GINGER

Botanical name: *Zingiber officinale* Roscoe
Family: Zingiberaceae
Plant part used: Rhizome

Safety Summary

Pregnancy category A: No proven increase in the frequency of malformation or other harmful effects on the foetus despite consumption by a large number of women.
Lactation category C: Compatible with breastfeeding.
Contraindications: None required on current evidence.
Warnings & precautions: Avoid high doses with anticoagulant prescription; proceed only with expert advice in peptic ulceration, gallstones, and pregnancy.
Adverse reactions: Mild gastrointestinal reactions are known and there are occasional cases of spice allergies to ginger.
Interactions: Possible interaction at high doses with warfarin and other anticoagulants. There is a possible increase in bioavailability for a wide range of other medication.

Typical Therapeutic Use

A systematic review of randomised controlled trials has evaluated the efficacy of ginger for nausea and vomiting. Six trials conducted prior to the year 2000 were evaluated. The pooled absolute risk reduction for the incidence of postoperative nausea calculated from three trials indicated a nonsignificant difference between the ginger and placebo groups. The dose was 1 g powdered ginger given preoperatively. Two of these trials suggested that ginger was superior to placebo and equally efficacious as metoclopramide. Three studies (investigating seasickness, morning sickness, and chemotherapy-induced nausea) collectively favoured ginger over placebo.[1] The Cochrane Review of treatments for vomiting of pregnancy suggests that ginger may be of benefit (based on two clinical trials) but that the evidence was weak to date (year 2000).[2]

Traditional indications for ginger in Western herbal medicine include dysmenorrhoea, flatulent dyspepsia, and colic.[3] In folk use, ginger has been used as a prophylactic against nausea and vomiting of motion sickness.

It was one of the most popular herbal remedies in one survey of patients presenting at an emergency department in an urban teaching hospital.[4]

Actions

Carminative, antiemetic, spasmolytic, peripheral circulatory stimulant, antiinflammatory, digestive stimulant.

Key Constituents

Essential oil (1% to 3%)[5] including monoterpenes (mainly geranial and neral) and sesquiterpenes (30% to 70%), mainly β-sesquiphellandrene, β-bisabolene, *ar*-curcumene and α-zingiberene[6]; pungent principles (4% to 7.5% w/w),[7] including the gingerols, shogaols, and related phenolic ketone derivatives.[8]

The components β-sesquiphellandrene and zingiberene are highest in fresh ginger, and decompose on drying and storage. The gingerols gradually decompose into shogaols on storage. Two of the pungent constituents of ginger, (6)-shogaol and (6)-gingerol, have been investigated separately. Both inhibited spontaneous motor activity, had analgesic and antipyretic effects, and suppressed gastric contraction in vivo. (6)-Shogaol was generally the strongest of the two and also had pronounced antitussive effects. Both also produced depressor responses on blood pressure regulation.[9]

Adulteration

There is a history of adulterations in the commercial spice trade, with substitutions such as turmeric and cayenne to bolster flavour, ferric oxide to add colour, and there is also a tradition of washing with lime. Sourcing whole roots is advisable. Substitution by other species of *Zingiber* and *Alpinia* is occasionally reported.

"Jamaican ginger paralysis" has entered the literature as an apparent toxic event associated with ginger. However, it has little to do with the spice. In 1930, thousands were poisoned by an illicit extract of Jamaica ginger ("jake") used to circumvent the Prohibition laws in America. A neurotoxic organophosphate compound, triorthocresyl phosphate, had been used as an adulterant.[10]

Typical Dosage Forms & Dosage

Typical adult dosage ranges are:
- 1 to 2 g of dried rhizome in single dose as an antiemetic

- 0.75 to 3 g/day of dried rhizome or by infusion or decoction
- 1.5 to 3 g/day of fresh rhizome
- 0.7 to 2 mL/day of a 1:2 liquid extract or equivalent in tablet or capsule form
- 1.7 to 5 mL/day of a 1:5 tincture

For antiemetic activity the dose is usually taken 30 minutes before travel.

Contraindications

In the Commission E monograph, ginger is contraindicated in patients with gallstones, except under close supervision, and should not be administered for morning sickness during pregnancy (however, see below).[11]

Use in Pregnancy

Category A: No proven increase in the frequency of malformation or other harmful effects on the foetus despite consumption by a large number of women. Widely used in pregnancy with some proven benefits; however, expert views on its safety are not consistent. In accordance with good practice, the herb should not be used during pregnancy and lactation without expert advice.

There is no consensus in the literature about whether ginger is safe to take in pregnancy.[12] The Commission E monograph proscription differs from that in Chinese medical texts.[13] Advice to use ginger in pregnancy is often given,[14] sometimes based on good clinical evidence[15]: in one double-blind crossover clinical study on 27 women with hyperemesis gravidarum which showed efficacy for ginger, no significant effects on the subsequent births were observed.[16] Ginger is also the most popular remedy for self-medication among pregnant women.[17-19] The evidence of an effect on nausea and vomiting in early pregnancy includes two studies that have not conclusively demonstrated the benefit.[2,20]

Given this uncertainty, the herb should not be used during pregnancy or lactation without expert advice. In any case, a daily dose of 2 g of dried ginger should not be exceeded in pregnancy.

Ginger included in the drinking water of pregnant rats (at levels of 20 and 50 g/L) led to increased embryo loss compared with controls, but increased weight and development of foetuses, and no other adverse effects on developed foetuses or mothers.[21] However, another study, with a ginger-alpinia standardised extract, showed no effect on organogenesis or other adverse effects on pregnancy in rats.[22]

Use in Lactation

Category C: Compatible with breastfeeding.

Warnings & Precautions

Daily doses of ginger in excess of 4 g should particularly be prescribed with caution in patients who are already taking blood-thinning drugs such as warfarin or aspirin, or who have increased risk of haemorrhage (see Interactions section below).[23]

Proceed with caution in cases of peptic ulceration or other gastric diseases. Any exacerbation in such cases should be immediately apparent and transient. However, do not proceed if symptoms such as heartburn occur.

Effect on Ability to Drive or Operate Machinery

No adverse effects expected.

Adverse Reactions

Occupational allergic contact dermatitis from spices is relatively rare, but needs to be taken into consideration in patients who have hand dermatitis and work with spices and foods. Acute spice reactions may also be linked to respiratory symptoms (although the possibility is that these are due to direct irritation of the lungs).[24] Ginger is known to be a significant contributor to such allergies.[25,26] Patients at risk of spice allergy are young adults sensitised to mugwort and birch allergens, sharing cross-sensitisation with various food plant allergens: this group makes up 6.4% of all food allergies in adults.[27] However, there are doubts about the consistency of a link with celery-birch allergy patterns.[28]

Gastrointestinal symptoms, including heartburn, are relatively common, especially at higher doses.[29]

A standardised extract of *Zingiber* and *Alpinia galanga* moderately reduced symptoms of osteoarthritis of the knee in a randomised double-blind placebo-controlled clinical trial ($n = 247$) over 6 weeks. In this study almost half those taking ginger experienced mild gastrointestinal symptoms (compared to 17% with similar symptoms in the placebo group).[30] The main symptom was heartburn.

Interactions

Ginger is claimed to have antiplatelet activity and potential interactions with anticoagulant medication.[31-35] This is thought to involve the effect of ginger on thromboxane synthetase activity.[36] However, such concerns have been specifically refuted in a randomised double-blind placebo-controlled trial in healthy volunteers. There was no difference between 2 g of dried ginger or placebo on platelet function, bleeding time, platelet count, and aggregation up to 24 hours after consumption. It was concluded that any effect on thromboxane synthetase would require higher doses or the use of the fresh plant.[37] Nor were there any changes in coagulation parameters or on warfarin-induced effects of a ginger-alpinia standardised extract in rats.[38]

Powdered ginger given at a dose of 4 g daily to 30 patients with coronary artery disease (CAD) did not affect platelet aggregation measured after 1.5 and 3 months of administration. In addition, no change in fibrinolytic activity and fibrinogen level was observed. No information was provided for controls. However, a single dose of 10 g ginger to each of 10 CAD patients produced a significant reduction in platelet aggregation after 4 hours ($P < 0.05$). There was a small, nonsignificant rise in platelet aggregation for the placebo group.[23]

There is one report of a reduction in platelet count from 1.8 million to 240,000 in a patient with Kawasaki disease the day after consuming a beverage comprising a half-teaspoon of ground ginger plus sugar steeped in boiling water, which had soda water added to it after cooling. The effect was believed to be due to ginger and carbon dioxide, both regarded as thromboxane synthetase inhibitors.[39]

Theoretical concerns about taking ginger preoperatively have been expressed,[40] and there are also doubts about the efficacy of ginger so taken in reducing postoperative nausea. In a double-blind, randomised, placebo-controlled trial, 0.5 g or 1 g of ginger or placebo was given to patients ($n = 108$) an hour before gynaecological laparoscopic surgery and the degree of nausea monitored 3 hours postoperatively. The ginger had no significant effect on symptoms of nausea and vomiting.[41] A separate study with two doses of ginger in a randomised, double-blind trial ($n = 180$) of patients also undergoing gynaecological laparoscopy also showed no effect in postoperative nausea and vomiting.[42] However, there are studies indicating efficacy in controlling the emetic effects of some cytotoxic drugs.[43] Ginger demonstrated highly significant protection against gastric irritation by nonsteroidal antiinflammatory drugs (NSAIDs) in rats.[44] This may support the view that the interaction of ginger with other treatments (and its effect on emesis generally) is primarily at the gastric mucosa rather than systemically.[45]

There is a suggestion that ginger is one of a number of hot spices that increase bioavailability of other drugs, either by increasing their absorption rate from the gastrointestinal tract or by protecting the drug from being metabolised/oxidised in its first passage through the liver after being absorbed.[46] This means that concurrent administration of ginger, and other hot spices, could increase the activity of other medication.

Safety in Children

Ginger is generally considered a safe remedy for children.[47]

Overdosage

No incidents found in published literature.

Toxicology

Table 1 lists LD_{50} data recorded for ginger and its constituents.[48,49]

Ginger extract caused no mortality at doses of up to 2.5 g/kg in mice (equivalent to about 75 g/kg of fresh rhizome).[50] This low acute toxicity was confirmed in a separate study, which also found that ginger extract at 100 mg/kg/day for 3 months caused no signs of chronic toxicity.[51]

Some cytotoxicity has been reported for ginger in vitro,[52] but in another study showed no signs of mutagenicity, unlike other spices,[53] and other investigations have demonstrated some antimutagenicity.[54,55]

Ginger failed to show any mutagenicity in one trial,[56] and has demonstrated anticarcinogenic effects in others.[57]

Regulatory Status

See Table 2 for regulatory status in selected countries.

Table **1** **LD$_{50}$ Data Recorded for Ginger and Its Constituents**

Substance	Route, Model	LD$_{50}$ Value (g/kg)	Reference
Dried ginger	Oral, rats	250	48
Ginger oil	Oral, rats	>5	49

Table **2** **Regulatory Status for Ginger in Selected Countries**

Australia	Ginger is not included in Part 4 of Schedule 4 of the Therapeutic Goods Act Regulations of Australia. However, products containing ginger with an equivalent dry weight per dosage unit of 2 g and above are required to carry warnings regarding concomitant use with anticoagulants and advising that those with bleeding problems seek medical advice.
China	Ginger is official in the *Pharmacopoeia of the People's Republic of China* 1997. The usual adult dosage, usually administered in the form of a decoction, is listed as 3 to 9 g.
UK & Germany	Ginger is included on the General Sale List. It is covered by a positive Commission E monograph. Ginger is official in the *British Pharmacopoeia* 1988.
US	Ginger is official in the *United States Pharmacopeia-National Formulary* (USP 26-NF 21, 2003). Ginger does have generally recognised as safe (GRAS) status. It is also freely available as a "dietary supplement" in the US under DSHEA legislation (Dietary Supplement Health and Education Act of 1994).

REFERENCES

1. Ernst E, Pittler MH: *Br J Anaesth* 84:367-371, 2000.
2. Jewell D, Young G: *Cochrane Database Syst Rev* CD000145, 2000.
3. British Herbal Medicine Association's Scientific Committee: *British herbal pharmacopoeia*, Bournemouth, 1983, BHMA, p 239-240.
4. Hung OL, Shih RD, Chiang WK, et al: *Acad Emerg Med* 4:209-213, 1997.
5. Wagner H, Bladt S: *Plant drug analysis: a thin layer chromatography atlas*, ed 2, Berlin, 1996, Springer-Verlag, p 293.
6. MacLeod AJ, Pieris NM: *Phytochemistry* 23:353-359, 1984.
7. Steinegger E, Stucki K: *Pharm Acta Helv* 57:66-71, 1982.
8. Yoshikawa M, Hatakeyama S, Chatani N, et al: J. *Yakugaku Zasshi* 113:307-315, 1993.
9. Suekawa M, Ishige A, Yuasa K, et al: *J Pharmacobiodyn* 7:836-848, 1984.
10. Morgan JP, Penovich P: *Arch Neurol* 35:530-532, 1978.
11. Blumenthal M, et al (eds): *The complete German Commission E monographs: therapeutic guide to herbal medicines*, Austin, 1998, American Botanical Council, pp 135-136.
12. Wilkinson JM: *Midwifery* 16:224-228, 2000.
13. Bensky D, Gamble A: *Chinese herbal medicine materia medica*, Seattle, 1986, Eastland Press, pp 431-432.
14. Ernst E, Schmidt K: *Wien Med Wochenschr* 152:190-192, 2002.
15. Niebyl JR: *Curr Opin Obstet Gynecol* 4:43-47, 1992.
16. Fischer-Rasmussen W, Kjaer SK, Dahl C, et al: *Eur J Obstet Gynecol Reprod Biol* 38:19-24, 1991.
17. Hollyer T, Boon H, Georgousis A, et al: *Complement Altern Med* 2:5, 2002.
18. Tiran D: *Complement Ther Nurs Midwifery* 8:191-196, 2002.
19. Tsui B, Dennehy CE, Tsourounis C: *Am J Obstet Gynecol* 185:433-437, 2001.
20. Niebyl JR, Goodwin TM: *Am J Obstet Gynecol* 185:S253-255, 2002.
21. Wilkinson JM: *Reprod Toxicol* 14:507-512, 2000.
22. Weidner MS, Sigwart K: *Reprod Toxicol* 15:75-80, 2001.
23. Bordia A, Verma SK, Srivastava KC: *Prostaglandins Leukot Essent Fatty Acids* 56:379-384, 1997.
24. Zuskin E, Kanceljak B, Skuric Z, et al: *Environ Res* 47:95-108, 1988.
25. Futrell JM, Rietschel R: *Cutis* 52:288-290, 1993.
26. Kanerva L, Estlander T, Jolanki R: *Contact Dermatitis* 35:157-162, 1996.
27. Moneret-Vautrin DA, Morisset M, Lemerdy P, et al: *Allerg Immunol (Paris)* 34:135-140, 2002.
28. Stager J, Wuthrich B, Johansson SG: *Allergy* 46:475-478, 1991.
29. De Smet PAGM, Keller K, Hansel R, et al (eds): *Adverse effects of herbal drugs*, vol 3, Berlin, 1992, Springer-Verlag, p 221.

30. Altman RD, Marcussen KC: *Arthritis Rheum* 44:2531-2538, 2001.
31. Abebe W: *J Clin Pharm Ther* 27:391-401, 2002.
32. Heck AM, DeWitt BA, Lukes AL: *Am J Health Syst Pharm* 57:1221-1227, 2000.
33. Pribitkin ED, Boger G: *Arch Facial Plast Surg* 3:127-132, 2001.
34. Argento A, Tiraferri E, Marzaloni M: *Ann Ital Med Int* 15:139-143, 2000.
35. Barrett B, Kiefer D, Rabago D: *Altern Ther Health Med* 5:40-49, 1999.
36. Backon J: *Anaesthesia* 46:705-706, 1991.
37. Lumb AB: *Thromb Haemost* 71:110-111, 1994.
38. Weidner MS, Sigwart K: *J Ethnopharmacol* 73:513-520, 2000.
39. Backon J: *Med Hypotheses* 34:230-231, 1991.
40. Hodges PJ, Kam PC: *Anaesthesia* 57:889-899, 2002.
41. Arfeen Z, Owen H, Plummer JL, et al: *Anaesth Intensive Care* 23:449-452, 1995.
42. Eberhart LH, Mayer R, Betz O, et al: *Anesth Analg* 96:995-998, 2003.
43. Yamahara J, Rong HQ, Naitoh Y, et al: *J Ethnopharmacol* 27:353-355, 1989.
44. al Yahya MA, Rafatullah S, Mossa JS, et al: *Am J Chin Med* 17:51-56, 1989.
45. Holtmann S, Clarke AH, Scherer H, et al: *Acta Oto Laryngologica* 108:168-174, 1989.
46. Atal CK, Zutshi U, Rao PG: *J Ethnopharmacol* 4:229-232, 1981.
47. Fugh-Berman A: *Nutr Today* 37:122-124, 2002.
48. Wu H, Ye D, Bai Y, et al: *Zhongguo Zhong Yao Za Zhi* 15:278-280, 317-318, 1990.
49. Opdyke DLJ: *Food Cosmet Toxicol* 12:901-902, 1974.
50. Mascolo N, Jain R, Jain SC, et al: *J Ethnopharmacol* 27:129-140, 1989.
51. Qureshi S, Shah AH, Tariq M, et al: *Am J Chin Med* 17:57-63, 1989.
52. Unnikrishnan MC, Kuttan R: *Nutr Cancer* 11:251-257, 1988.
53. Sivaswamy SN, Balachandran B, Balanehru S, et al: *Indian J Exp Biol* 29:730-737, 1991.
54. Soudamini KK, Unnikrishnan MC, Sukumaran K, et al: *Indian J Physiol Pharmacol* 39:347-353, 1995.
55. Surh YJ, Lee E, Lee JM: *Mutat Res* 402:259-267, 1998.
56. Sivaswamy SN, Balachandran B, Balanehru S, et al: *Indian J Exp Biol* 29:730-737, 1991.
57. Tarjan V, Csukas I: *Mutat Res* 216:297, 1989.

GINKGO

Other common name: Maidenhair tree
Botanical name: *Ginkgo biloba* L.
Family: Ginkgoaceae
Plant part used: Leaf

Safety Summary

Pregnancy category B1: No increase in frequency of malformation or other harmful effects on the foetus from limited use in women. No evidence of increased foetal damage in animal studies.
Lactation category ND: No data available.
Contraindications: Known sensitivity to ginkgo preparations.
Warnings & precautions: Caution should be exercised when prescribing ginkgo to patients with coagulation disorders, or concomitantly with anticoagulant or antiplatelet medication. Patients about to undergo surgery are advised to stop taking ginkgo 3 days beforehand. Ginkgo preparations high in alkylphenols may pose a risk of allergic reaction.
Adverse reactions: Mild gastrointestinal complaints, headache, dizziness, allergic skin reactions, and palpitations. Cases of spontaneous cerebral or extracerebral bleeding, seizure, manic psychosis, and Stevens-Johnson syndrome have been attributed to ginkgo use.
Interactions: No cases of definite drug interactions have been reported but caution should be exercised when prescribing ginkgo concomitantly with anticoagulant or antiplatelet medication. Ginkgo may potentiate the efficacy of haloperidol and decrease the efficacy of sodium valproate.

Typical Therapeutic Use

Meta-analyses of randomised, double-blind, placebo-controlled trials concluded that standardised ginkgo extract is of therapeutic benefit for the early stages of primary degenerative dementia (Alzheimer-type),[1] peripheral arterial occlusive disease,[2] and cerebral insufficiency (restricted cerebral blood flow) and its related symptoms.[3]

Actions

Antioxidant, anti-PAF (anti-platelet activating factor), tissue perfusion enhancing, circulatory stimulant, cognition enhancing, neuroprotective.

Key Constituents

Constituents of ginkgo leaf include flavonol glycosides, terpene lactones (including bilobalide and ginkgolides), biflavonoids, and traces of alkylphenols (around 100 ppm; including ginkgolic acids).[4-6] Pharmacological and clinical studies have used a special concentrated extract of ginkgo leaves standardised to contain 22.5% to 25% flavonol glycosides (ginkgo flavone glycosides) and 6% to 8% terpenoids (ginkgolides and bilobalide). Ginkgolic acids and biflavonoids are generally absent, or present in only minute quantities in these extracts.[7] The German Commission E and the World Health Organization (WHO) stipulate that extracts should contain less than 5 ppm ginkgolic acids.[8,9]

Adulteration

Considerable variability has been found in total terpene content and in individual terpene levels in commercial ginkgo leaf extracts.[10] A study by the Hong Kong Consumer Council found that 13 of 14 commercial products contained levels of ginkgolic acids exceeding WHO recommendations by 16 to 733 times.[11]

Typical Dosage Forms & Dosage

Typical adult dosage ranges are:
- 3 to 4 mL/day of a standardised 2:1 liquid extract containing 9.6 mg/mL of ginkgo flavone glycosides or equivalent in tablet or capsule form
- 120 to 240 mg/day of a standardised 50:1 dry extract containing 24% ginkgo flavone glycosides and 6% terpene lactones (corresponding to 6 to 12 g/day of dried leaf)

Contraindications

Contraindicated in those with known sensitivity to ginkgo preparations.

Use in Pregnancy

Category B1: No increase in frequency of malformation or other harmful effects on the foetus from limited use in women. No evidence of increased foetal damage in animal studies.

One review hypothesised that ginkgo may be a risk factor for excessive blood loss during delivery, but there are no reports of this in the literature.[10]

Oral administration of standardised ginkgo extract to rats (up to 1600 mg/kg/day) and rabbits (up to 900 mg/kg/day) did not cause teratogenicity or embryotoxicity, or affect reproduction.[12,13]

A commercial ginkgo extract, and fractions of ginkgo extract containing high concentrations of ginkgolic acids, demonstrated embryotoxic effects in the hen's egg test when injected into freshly fertilised chick eggs[14,15] (see Toxicology). The dose of commercial ginkgo extract injected was not specified.[14]

A recent study claimed to have identified the highly toxic alkaloid colchicine in a commercial ginkgo preparation, and linked this to their discovery of the presence of colchicine in the placental blood of women who had used herbal supplements. The herbal supplements taken by the women were not identified, and it was not clear whether ginkgo was one of them.[16] Colchicine has never been detected in ginkgo previously and studies conducted since the findings were released have failed to detect colchicine in commercial preparations.[17-19] The validity of the findings and the conclusions drawn from them have been vigorously criticised.[17,20]

Pretreatment of hamster oocytes in vitro with ginkgo (1 mg/mL) significantly reduced penetration by human sperm compared to control. However, significant reduction of sperm penetration was not observed at a concentration of 0.1 mg/mL, which represents typical human exposure for in vitro research.[21]

Use in Lactation

Category ND: No data available.

Only small amounts of flavonol glycosides and terpene lactones accumulate in the serum, and the serum half-life of terpene lactones is relatively short. This would reduce the amount available to enter the breast milk and the possibility of accumulation in the infant.[10]

Warnings & Precautions

Standardised ginkgo extract should be given to patients for at least 6 to 8 weeks before any clinical benefit is assessed. The German Commission E advises that treatment with ginkgo extract should be reviewed after 3 months.[8]

Caution should be exercised when prescribing ginkgo to patients with coagulation disorders or concomitantly with anticoagulant or antiplatelet medication (see Adverse reactions and Interactions).

Patients about to undergo surgery are advised to stop taking ginkgo 3 days beforehand, due to possible risk of increased bleeding tendency.[22,23]

Ginkgo preparations which contain appreciable quantities of ginkgolic acids may pose a risk of allergic reaction.

Effect on Ability to Drive or Operate Machinery

Possible improvement of these functions, especially in older subjects.

Adverse Reactions

Reviews and meta-analyses of clinical trials have shown that standardised ginkgo extract has a remarkably low incidence of side effects,[2,12,24,25] and there were no differences between ginkgo and placebo in the adverse event profile.[12,26,27] Two adverse events were reported in 314,000 patient years of use in 1988. Only 0.5% of 9772 patients reported adverse events over 44 clinical trials. Adverse events reported have included mild gastrointestinal complaints, headache, dizziness, allergic skin reactions, and palpitations.[12] Palpitations and ventricular arrhythmia have been associated with ginkgo use in a case report.[28]

More than 5 million units of ginkgo preparations were sold in Germany in 1998 alone.[29] German authorities have recorded 117 reports of adverse effects in connection with preparations containing ginkgo from 1990 to 2000, including nonstandardised extracts, homoeopathics, and multi-ingredient preparations. Ginkgo was indicated as the only medication in 65 cases.[30] By 2002 the number of adverse reactions was 185 (see Interactions).

A number of cases of seizure[31,32] or spontaneous cerebral or extracerebral bleeding[33-38] attributed to the intake of ginkgo preparations have been reported. It was not possible to establish ginkgo as the cause in any of these cases. Prolonged bleeding times were noted in two of the bleeding cases,[33,35] although the bleeding time quoted in one is widely considered to be within the normal range.[35] In another case involving spontaneous hyphema, the authors state that, after extensive ophthalmological and haematological investigations, no putative causes were recorded other than ginkgo intake.[39] Use of ginkgo has also been attributed to one case of postoperative bleeding following laparoscopic cholecystectomy.[23] Other isolated cases of spontaneous bleeding and seizure have been attributed to drug interactions with ginkgo (see Interactions).

It has been established conclusively that the antiplatelet activity of ginkgo extract is due to platelet activating factor (PAF)-antagonism.[40,41] Since PAF is mainly involved in pathological thrombus formation, the use of ginkgo extract may have no effect whatsoever on normal physiological mechanisms of platelet aggregation and therefore on bleeding time, as is supported by the studies below.

In studies with healthy volunteers, acute oral administration of standardised ginkgo extract (15 mL) and ginkgolide mixture (80 mg and 120 mg) inhibited PAF-induced platelet aggregation.[42,43] The effect with ginkgo extract was only transient and there were no concomitant changes in coagulation, skin bleeding time, haematological, and biochemical laboratory tests, blood pressure, or pulse.[42] Longer-term oral administration with standardised extract (120 mg/day for 3 months) inhibited collagen-induced platelet aggregation but failed to inhibit three other inducers, including PAF (1 μmol/L), ex vivo.[44] Oral administration of standardised extract (112.5 mg) to healthy volunteers has been shown to reduce erythrocyte aggregation, but had no effect on plasma viscosity, platelet aggregation, or blood pressure.[45] Another study reported a significant decrease in both diastolic and systolic blood pressure in healthy volunteers ingesting standardised extract (120 mg/day at bedtime) for 3 months. Bleeding times and fibrinogen levels showed no change.[46]

Cases of Stevens-Johnson syndrome associated with the use of preparations containing ginkgo have also been reported.[30,47] Stevens-Johnson syndrome is an acute inflammatory skin disease which affects the skin and mucous membranes of the face and mouth.

Severe circulatory disturbances, local phlebitis, allergic skin reactions, and anaphylactic shock may occur with parenteral use of standardised ginkgo extracts.[24] Injectable preparations have been disallowed in some European countries.[48]

Hypersensitivity reactions to standardised extracts of the leaf are extremely rare, indicating that it has a very low potential for sensitisation.[12,49] However, cases of allergic contact dermatitis due to ginkgo fruit pulp have been reported repeatedly.[50] Gastrointestinal disturbances (tenesmus, stomatitis, proctitis) have also been reported after consumption of the fruit.[24,51] Provocation tests in patients, and animal experiments, have identified alkylphenols such as ginkgolic acids as causative constituents.[52] Tests in guinea pigs have shown that although sensitisation developed with purified ginkgolic acids, it failed to occur to leaf extract containing approximately 1000 ppm ginkgolic acids,[50] which is 200 times higher than the level deemed acceptable in standardised extracts. Nonetheless, consumption of ginkgo extracts containing ginkgolic acids above acceptable levels may constitute a risk to those who are allergic to plants from the Anacardiaceae family, such as poison ivy and cashew, because of cross-reactivity between the alkylphenols of the two families.[53]

A diffuse morbilliform eruption occurred in a 66-year-old woman about 1 week after the ingestion of a ginkgo preparation, which was suspected to be due to alkylphenols.[54] The alkylphenol level of the preparation was not measured.

Manic psychosis has been questionably associated with the use of ginkgo in two sisters, who had been consuming the herb for approximately 2 years at a dosage twice that recommended. A few months before the onset of symptoms the dosage had been further increased. The family psychiatric history was significant for paranoid schizophrenia on the paternal side. They were stabilised on medication and 6 months later were free of all medications and were not manifesting psychiatric symptoms. Almost 1 year after the first episode one sister had a relapse; she was not taking ginkgo.[55]

Interactions

No cases of definite drug interactions have been reported, even though patients taking standardised ginkgo extracts are often taking many other drugs simultaneously.[10]

Caution should be exercised when prescribing ginkgo with anticoagulant or antiplatelet medication, as an increased bleeding tendency has been observed in isolated case reports with warfarin[56] and aspirin,[57] suggesting possible interaction.

A 2002 publication lists 185 reports of adverse effects in connection with ginkgo, with 20 reports related to coagulation disorders. It was concluded that patients using ginkgo extracts are in danger of suffering complications during surgery or spontaneous bleeding, and there is an increased danger of bleeding with concomitant use of anticoagulant agents.[58] However, there is still no strong evidence for this. Concomitant treatment with a standardised ginkgo extract (100 mg/day) for 4 weeks in patients who were stabilised on long-term warfarin treatment had no significant influence on their response to warfarin in a randomised, double-blind, placebo-controlled, crossover trial (average age of patients was 64.5 years). The stability of international normalised ratio (INR) values was confirmed and major bleedings or thromboembolic events were not observed.[59] A substudy within the National Institutes of Health-funded Dementia Prevention Study investigated whether ginkgo standardised extract would affect platelet function. Fifty-one patients had platelet function analysis performed at baseline and at 6-month follow-up. Patients were randomised to receive ginkgo (240 mg/day) or placebo. There was no significant difference between the placebo and ginkgo groups. Fifteen patients were taking aspirin, but there was no difference in closure time at either time point, and aspirin did not show any interaction with ginkgo.[60]

Ginkgo (253 mg/day; not specified whether this was extract) was suspected of interacting with rofecoxib (a nonsteroidal antiinflammatory drug [NSAID]) in another case of spontaneous bleeding. The patient had an abnormal bleeding time, which returned to normal upon discontinuation of all vitamin supplements and rofecoxib, and remained normal upon resuming low-dose rofecoxib. Apart from ginkgo, the patient had also been taking "Siberian ginseng" (162 mg/day), fish oil tablets (1000 mg/day) and vitamin E (30 IU/day), and multivitamins "for years".[61] Rofecoxib is a cyclooxygenase (COX-2) inhibitor and should not cause bleeding. Fish oil has been shown to prolong bleeding time and inhibit platelet aggregation in many studies.[62]

Two patients with well-controlled epilepsy presented with recurrent seizures within 2 weeks of commencing ginkgo extract. Ginkgo was discontinued and both patients were seizure-free several months later. Both patients were taking the anticonvulsant sodium valproate in combination with other medications.[32] Ginkgo could not be identified as the causative agent; however, intraperitoneal injection of ginkgo (50 mg/kg) has been shown to reduce the effectiveness of sodium valproate and carbamazepine in mice.[63]

An elderly patient with Alzheimer's disease developed a coma a few days after starting the selective serotonin reuptake inhibitor (SSRI) antidepressant trazodone (40 mg/day), which has hypnotic and sedative effects, in conjunction with ginkgo extract (160 mg/day). Previously she had been taking bromazepam (3.5 mg/day), donazepil (5 mg/day), and vitamin E (1200 mg/day). It was postulated that sedation was caused by increased GABAergic activity via ginkgo flavonoids acting directly at the benzodiazepine receptor, and indirectly by inducing the cytochrome P450 enzyme CYP34A to increase the metabolism of trazodone to an active compound which also has GABAergic activity.[64] However, standardised ginkgo extract has been shown to have no effect on the hepatic drug microsomal drug oxidation system, including CYP34A activity,[65,66] or an effect suggestive of CYP34A inhibition,[67] in clinical trials of healthy volunteers. In vitro studies have demonstrated that ginkgolides have no effect on cytochrome P450 enzymes, including CYP34A.[68] Ginkgolic acids, which are absent or present in minute quantities in standardised extracts, were shown to have an inhibitory effect.

Ginkgo leaf extract may potentiate the efficiency of haloperidol in patients with schizophrenia.[69,70]

An elderly patient started treatment with a thiazide diuretic for elevated blood pressure. She then started taking ginkgo, and after a week her blood pressure was found to have increased further. Her blood pressure decreased gradually when both medications were ceased.[71] It was unclear how soon the ginkgo was started after the thiazide diuretic, and the interpretation of this case as a herb-drug interaction is highly questionable.

Concerns have been raised that ginkgo extract may increase the hepatic metabolic clearance rate of insulin and hypoglycaemic agents in non–insulin-dependent diabetes mellitus patients, resulting in reduced insulin-mediated glucose metabolism and elevated blood glucose.[72] However, no adverse effects of any significance have been reported regarding blood glucose levels and laboratory results of glucose control in ten trials conducted from 1980 to 1998, where ginkgo extract was administered to diabetics and nondiabetics.[10,73]

In a crossover trial involving eight healthy volunteers, the concomitant use of standardised ginkgo extract and digoxin did not have any significant effect on the pharmacokinetics of orally administered digoxin.[74]

Safety in Children

No side effects were observed in infants (2 to 7 months old) with hypoxic-ischaemic encephalopathy treated with standardised ginkgo extract (0.5 mL/day p.o.) for 2 months.[75] Standardised ginkgo extract has also been used to treat asthma in children.[76]

Cases of poisoning have been reported in young children after ingestion of a large number of ginkgo seeds, 50 or more in some cases[77-80] (see Overdosage). Japanese authorities advise that children should not eat more than five seeds (nuts) per day, and that they should not eat seeds every day.[81]

Overdosage

Intoxication generally occurs after ingestion of large numbers of seeds, and so young children are often more vulnerable to poisoning. Those under age six comprise about 74% of cases.[81] Symptoms include vomiting, diarrhoea, irritability, seizure and, in some cases, death.[77-80] The number of seeds consumed in reported fatalities ranged from 15 to 574.[77] The neurotoxin 4′-O-methylpyroxidine, which can cause vitamin B_6 deficiency symptoms, is thought to be responsible.[79,80] Intravenous vitamin B_6 (2 mg/kg) has been used to treat ginkgo seed poisoning.[77]

The stems and leaves of ginkgo also contain 4′-O-methylpyroxidine.[82,83] This toxin has been measured at levels of 42 µg/g fresh weight of stem[83] and up to 80 µg per raw seed.[82] The highest concentration of 4′-O-methylpyroxidine in the medicinal preparations tested conferred a daily dose of 60 µg.[83] In contrast, the acute oral toxic dose was measured at 11 mg/kg in guinea pigs.[79,80] The ingestion of ginkgo extracts and of boiled ginkgo seeds (eaten in Japan) is not expected to cause detrimental effects,[82,83] although ingestion of seeds should be limited, particularly in children.

Toxicology

Table 1 lists LD_{50} data recorded for ginkgo extract and its constituents.[12,13,15]

Standardised ginkgo extract has very low toxicity. No deaths occurred in rats orally administered up to 10 g/kg of standardised extract. Chronic oral toxicity studies showed no evidence of biochemical, haematological, or histological damage, or impairment of hepatic or renal function, in rats and dogs administered standardised ginkgo extract orally for 6 months. Doses began at 20 and 100 mg/kg/day and gradually increased to 500 mg/kg/day in rats and 400 mg/kg/day in dogs. Light and transient vasodilatory effects were observed in dogs at the 100 mg/kg dose, and became more pronounced with increasing dose. These effects were noticed in the head area.[12,13]

No carcinogenic effects were observed in rats orally administered standardised leaf extract for 104 weeks at doses of 4, 20, and 100 mg/kg,[13] or in rats fed ginkgo seed for almost a year.[84] Standardised

Table 1 **LD$_{50}$ Data Recorded for Gingko Extract and Its Constituents**

Substance	Route, Model	LD$_{50}$ Value	Reference
Standardised ginkgo extract	Oral, mice	7.7 g/kg	12,13
Standardised ginkgo extract	i.p., mice	1.9 g/kg	13
Standardised ginkgo extract	i.v., mice	1.1 g/kg	13
Standardised ginkgo extract	i.p., rats	2.1 g/kg	13
Standardised ginkgo extract	i.v., rats	1.1 g/kg	13
Ginkgo leaf extract fraction (ginkgolic acids 16%; biflavones 6.7%)	Injection, hen's eggs	1.8 mg/egg (33 ppm)	15
Ginkgo leaf extract fraction (ginkgolic acids 58%; biflavones 0.02%)	Injection, hen's eggs	3.5 mg/egg (64 ppm)	15
Ginkgo leaf extract fraction (ginkgolic acids 1%; biflavones 16%)	Injection, hen's eggs	250 mg/egg (4540 ppm)	15

leaf extract did not demonstrate mutagenic activity in in vitro tests with and without metabolic activation, or in vivo tests in mice after oral administration of doses up to 20 g/kg.[12,13]

No adverse effects were observed in human volunteers administered pure ginkgolides at doses of 720 mg (acute) or 360 mg/day for 1 week.[85]

Fractions of ginkgo leaf extract containing high concentrations of ginkgolic acids have been shown to be cytotoxic against human and animal cell lines in vitro[86] and immunotoxic in vivo after subplantar injection.[52,53] They were embryotoxic in the hen's egg test. The authors of the latter study did not exclude the possibility that other constituents, such as the biflavones, may amplify the adverse effects of ginkgolic acids.[15] Ginkgolic acids demonstrated neurotoxic,[87] genotoxic, and tumour-promoting[88] activities in vitro.

Regulatory Status

See Table 2 for regulatory status in selected countries.

Table **2**   **Regulatory Status for Gingko in Selected Countries**

Australia	Ginkgo is not included in Part 4 of Schedule 4 of the Therapeutic Goods Regulations.
UK & Germany	Ginkgo is not included on the General Sale List. Standardised ginkgo leaf extract is covered by a positive Commission E monograph, but ginkgo leaf is covered by a negative Commission E monograph. Ginkgo is official in the *British Pharmacopoeia* 2002 and the *European Pharmacopoeia* 4.3.
US	Ginkgo is official in the *United States Pharmacopeia-National Formulary* (USP 26-NF 21, 2003). Ginkgo does not have generally recognised as safe (GRAS) status. However, it is freely available as a "dietary supplement" in the US under DSHEA legislation (Dietary Supplement Health and Education Act of 1994).

REFERENCES

1. Oken BS, Storzbach DM, Kaye JA: *Arch Neurol* 55:1409-1415, 1998.
2. Pittler MH, Ernst E: *Am J Med* 108:276-281, 2000.
3. Hopfenmuller W: *Arzneim Forsch* 44:1005-1013, 1994.
4. Wagner H, Bladt S: *Plant drug analysis: a thin layer chromatography atlas*, ed 2, Berlin, 1996, Springer-Verlag, p 237.
5. DeFeudis FV: Ginkgo biloba *extract (EGb 761): pharmacological activities and clinical applications*. Amsterdam, 1991, Elsevier, pp 10-13.
6. Schotz K: *Pharmazie* 57:508-510, 2002.
7. Siegers CP: *Phytomedicine* 6:281-283, 1999.
8. Blumenthal M, et al (eds): *The complete German Commission E monographs: therapeutic guide to herbal medicines*, Austin, 1998, American Botanical Council, p 137.
9. World Health Organization: *WHO monographs on selected medicinal plants*, vol 1, Geneva, 1999, WHO, p 158.
10. McKenna DJ, Jones K, Hughes K, et al: *Botanical medicines: the desk reference for major herbal supplements*, ed 2, New York, 2002, The Haworth Herbal Press, pp 480-488.
11. Hong Kong Consumer Council: Test casts doubt on clinical benefits of Ginkgo leaf products with non-standardized extract. *Choice*, No. 289, 15 November 2002.
12. DeFeudis F: Gingko biloba *extract (EGb 761): pharmacological activities and clinical applications*, Amsterdam, 1991, Elsevier, pp 143-146.
13. Blaschek W, Ebel S, Hackenthal E, et al: *HagerROM 2002: Hagers Handbuch der Drogen und Arzneistoffe*, Heidelberg, 2002, Springer.
14. Flossiac M, Chopin S: *FASEB J* 13:A1031, 1999.
15. Baron-Ruppert G, Luepke NP: *Phytomedicine* 8:133-138, 2001.
16. Petty HR, Fernando M, Kindzelskii AL, et al: *Chem Res Toxicol* 14:1254-1258, 2001.
17. American Botanical Council: Herbal science group debunks research suggesting presence of toxin colchicine in Ginkgo, News release to national media, 30 August 2001.
18. Li W, Fitzloff JF, Farnsworth NR, et al: *Phytomedicine* 9:442-446, 2002.
19. Li W, Sun Y, Fitzloff JF, et al: *Chem Res Toxicol* 15:1174-1178, 2002.
20. Bone K: *Townsend Letter for Doctors and Patients* 225:143-144, 2002.
21. Ondriek RR, Chan PJ, Patton WC, et al: *Fertil Steril* 71:517-522, 1999.
22. Ang-Lee MK, Moss J, Yuan CS: *JAMA* 286:208-216, 2001.

23. Fessenden JM, Wittenborn W, Clarke L: *Am Surg* 67:33-35, 2001.
24. Woerdenbag HJ, Van Beek TA: In De Smet PAGM, Keller K, Hansel R, et al (eds): *Adverse effects of herbal drugs*, vol 3, Berlin, 1997, Springer-Verlag, pp 57-60.
25. Ernst E, Pittler MH: *Clin Drug Invest* 17:301-308, 1999.
26. Le Bars PL, Kastelan J: *Public Health Nutr* 3:495-499, 2000.
27. Birks J, Grimley EV, Van Dongen M: *Cochrane Database Syst Rev* CD003120, 2002.
28. Cianfrocca C, Pelliccia F, Auriti A, et al: *Ital Heart J* 3:689-691, 2002.
29. Schwabe U, Paffrath D: *Arzneiverordnungs-Report 1999*, Berlin, 2000, Springer Verlag.
30. Arzneimittelkommission der deutschen Ärzteschaft: *Dtsch Ärztebl* 97:A474, 2000.
31. Gregory PJ: *Ann Intern Med* 134:344, 2001.
32. Granger AS: *Age Ageing* 30:523-525, 2001.
33. Rowin J, Lewis SL: *Neurology* 46:1775-1776, 1996.
34. Gilbert GJ: *Neurology* 48:1137, 1997.
35. Vale S: *Lancet* 352:36, 1998.
36. Benjamin J, Muir T, Briggs K, et al: *Postgrad Med J* 77:112-113, 2001.
37. Purroy Garcia F, Molina C, Alvarez Sabin J: *Med Clin (Barc)* 119:596-597, 2002.
38. Miller LG, Freeman B: *J Herbal Pharmacother* 2:57-63, 2002.
39. Schneider C, Bord C, Misse P, et al: *J Fr Ophtalmol* 25:731-732, 2002.
40. Braquet P, Touqui L, Shen TY, et al: *Pharmacol Revs* 39:97-145, 1987.
41. Braquet P: *Adv Prostaglandin Thromboxane Leukot Res* 16:179-198, 1986.
42. Guinot P, Caffrey E, Lambe R, et al: *Haemostasis* 19:219-223, 1989.
43. Chung KF, Dent G, McCusker M, et al: *Lancet* 1:248-251, 1987.
44. Kudolo G: *Altern Ther Health Med* 7:105, 2001.
45. Jung C, Mrowietz H, Kiesewetter H, et al: *Arzneim Forsch* 40:589-593, 1990.
46. Kudolo GB: *J Clin Pharmacol* 40:647-654, 2000.
47. Davydov L, Stirling AL: *J Herbal Pharmacother* 1:65-69, 2001.
48. Sticher O, Hasler A, Meier B: *Dtsch Apoth Ztg* 131:1827-1835, 1991.
49. Mossabeb R, Kraft D, Valenta R: *Wien Klin Wochenschr* 113:580-587, 2001.
50. Hausen BM: *Am J Contact Dermat* 9:146-148, 1998.
51. Becker LE, Skipworth GB: *JAMA* 231:1162-1163, 1975.
52. Koch E, Jaggy H, Chatterjee SS: *Int J Immunopharmacol* 22:229-236, 2000.
53. Jaggy H, Koch E: *Pharmazie* 52:735-738, 1997.
54. Chiu AE, Lane AT, Kimball AB: *J Am Acad Dermatol* 46:145-146, 2002.
55. La Monaca G, Klesmer J, Kata JL: *Prim Psychiat* 8:63-64, 2001.
56. Matthews MK Jr: *Neurology* 50:1933-1934, 1998.
57. Rosenblatt M, Mindel J: *New Engl J Med* 336:1108, 1997.
58. Arzneimittelkommission der deutschen Ärzteschaft: *Dtsch Ärztebl* 99:A2214, 2002.
59. Engelsen J, Nielsen JD, Winther K: *Thromb Haemost* 87:1075-1076, 2002.
60. DeLoughery TG, Kaye JA, Morris CD, et al: *Blood* 11:Abstract #3809, 2002.
61. Hoffman T: *Hawaii Med J* 60:290, 2001.
62. Pizzorno JE, Murray MT (eds): *A textbook of natural medicine*, ed 2, vol 1, Edinburgh, 1999, Churchill Livingstone, p 740.
63. Manocha A, Pillai KK, Husain SZ: *Indian J Pharmacol* 28:84-87, 1996.
64. Galluzzi S, Zanetti O, Binetti G, et al: *J Neurol Neurosurg Psychiatry* 68:679-680, 2000.
65. Duche JC, Barre J, Guinot P, et al: *Int J Clin Pharmacol Res* 9:165-168, 1989.
66. Gurley BJ, Gardner SF, Hubbard MA, et al: *Clin Pharmacol Ther* 72:276-287, 2002.
67. Smith M, Lin KM, Zheng YP: *Clin Pharmacol Ther* 69:P86, 2001.
68. Zou L, Harkey MR, Henderson GL: *Life Sci* 71:1579-1589, 2002.
69. Zhang XY, Zhou DF, Su JM, et al: *J Clin Psychopharmacol* 21:85-88, 2001.
70. Zhang XY, Zhou DF, Zhang PY, et al: *J Clin Psychiatry* 62:878-883, 2001.
71. Shaw D, Leon C, Kolev S, et al: *Drug Saf* 17:342-356, 1997.
72. Kudolo GB: *J Clin Pharmacol* 41:600-611, 2001.
73. Appleton G: *Health Notes Rev Complement Integr Med* 7:298-300, 2000.
74. Mauro VF, Mauro LS, Kleshinski JF, et al: *Am J Ther* 10:247-251, 2003.
75. Shprakh VV, Saiutina SB, Revezova TV, et al: *Zh Nevrol Psikhiatr Im S S Korsakova* 100:33-35, 2000.
76. Borgain-Reuse M: 6th International conference on prostaglandins and related compounds, Florence, June 1986. Cited in Braquet P: *Adv Prostaglandin Thromboxane Leukot Res* 16:179-198, 1986.
77. Kajiyama Y, Fujii K, Takeuchi H, et al: *Pediatrics* 109:325-327, 2002.
78. Yagi M, Wada K, Sakata M, et al: *Yakugaku Zasshi* 113:596-599, 1993.
79. Wada K, Ishigaki S, Ueda K, et al: *Chem Pharm Bull (Tokyo)* 33:3555-3557, 1985.
80. Wada K, Ishiaki S, Ueda K, et al: *Chem Pharm Bull* 36:1779-1782, 1988.
81. Wada K: Food poisoning by Ginkgo seeds: The role of 4-O-methylpyroxidine. In van Beek TA (ed.): *Ginkgo Biloba*, Amsterdam, 2000, Harwood Academic, pp 453-465.
82. Arenz A, Klein M, Fiehe K, et al: *Planta Med* 62:548-551, 1996.
83. Leistner E, Arenz A: *Z Phytother* 18:230-231, 1997.

84. Hirono I, Shibuya C, Shinizu M, et al: *Gann* 63:383-386, 1972.

85. Bonvoison B, Guinot P: Clinical studies of BN 52063 a specific PAF antagonist. In Braquet P (ed.): *Ginkgolides – chemistry, biology, pharmacology and clinical perspectives*, vol 2, Barcelona, 1989, JR Prous Science Publishers, pp 845-854.

86. Siegers CP: *Phytomedicine* 6:281-283, 1999.

87. Ahlemeyer B, Selke D, Schaper C, et al: *Eur J Pharmacol* 430:1-7, 2001.

88. Westendorf J, Regan J: *Phytomedicine* 7(suppl 2):104, 2000.

GINSENG

Other common names: Korean ginseng, Asian ginseng

Botanical names: *Panax ginseng* C. Meyer (*Panax schinseng* Nees)

Family: Araliaceae

Plant part used: Root (main and lateral roots)

Safety Summary

Pregnancy category A: No proven increase in the frequency of malformation or other harmful effects on the foetus despite consumption by a large number of women.

Lactation category C: Compatible with breastfeeding.

Contraindications: Traditionally contraindicated in acute asthma, signs of heat, excessive menstruation, or nose bleeds. It is best not used during acute infections. Avoid in patients with hypertension.

Warnings & precautions: Concurrent use with stimulants such as caffeine and amphetamines is best avoided. Overstimulation may occur in susceptible patients, especially at higher doses.

Adverse reactions: Ginseng is generally safe and well tolerated but high doses may cause overstimulation. Rare side effects associated with the use of ginseng include mania, cerebral arteritis, oestrogenic effects, and Stevens-Johnson syndrome.

Interactions: The use of ginseng in conjunction with monoamine oxidase inhibitors should be avoided. Caution should be exercised for concurrent use of ginseng and warfarin.

Typical Therapeutic Use

Results from clinical trials on ginseng are often contradictory. However, significant benefits have been demonstrated for athletic and psychomotor performance, general well being, and sexual dysfunction.[1]

Traditional indications for ginseng in Western herbal medicine include neurasthenia and depressive states associated with sexual inadequacy.[2] Uses from traditional Chinese medicine include: prostration with impending collapse marked by cold limbs, faint pulse, and sweating; heart failure, shock; palpitation with anxiety, forgetfulness, and restlessness[3,4]; general weakness with irritability and insomnia in chronic diseases[3]; impotence or frigidity[3]; and organ prolapse.[4]

Actions

Adaptogenic, tonic, immune modulating, cardiotonic, male tonic, cancer preventative, cognition enhancing.

Key Constituents

Ginseng root contains:
- A complex mixture of dammarane saponins (3%), called ginsenosides, and an oleanolic saponin.[5]
- Polysaccharides and essential oil.[6]
- Polyacetylenes, peptides, and trilinolein and other lipids.[7-9]

Adulteration

The main and lateral roots of ginseng can be adulterated with the inferior root hairs and aerial parts. Despite the rarity of wild ginseng, only the population of *Panax ginseng* from the Russian Federation is listed on Appendix II of the Convention on International Trade in Endangered Species (CITES) as of May 2003.

Typical Dosage Forms & Dosage

Typical adult dosage ranges are:
- 1.8 to 9 g/day of dried root or by decoction
- 1.5 to 6 mL/day of a 1:2 liquid extract or equivalent in tablet or capsule form
- 100 to 200 mg/day of a 5:1 concentrated extract in tablet or capsule form

The Commission E advises that *Panax ginseng* can be used for up to 3 months, with a repeat course if necessary.[10] Continuous use in the unwell and elderly is appropriate. Doses in excess of 1 g/day may cause overstimulation.

Contraindications

Ginseng is traditionally contraindicated in acute asthma, signs of heat, excessive menstruation, or nose bleeds. It is best not used during acute infections.[11]

As the clinical implications of the effect of ginseng on blood pressure are not clear, it should be avoided in patients with hypertension.[11]

Use in Pregnancy

Category A: No proven increase in the frequency of malformation or other harmful effects on the foetus despite consumption by a large number of women.

Ginseng consumption during pregnancy is popular in Hong Kong. Eighty-eight patients taking ginseng during their pregnancy were matched with control patients with similar characteristics who delivered within the same period but were not taking ginseng. Eight patients in the control group had preeclampsia, but only one patient in the ginseng group suffered this condition ($P < 0.02$). The control group also had higher mean blood pressures in the second and third trimesters, but the differences were not statistically significant. The authors suggested that further studies are necessary to clarify this possible benefit of ginseng during pregnancy.[12]

The effect of a 5:1 extract of ginseng root on reproductive performance was studied in male and female rats at oral doses of 1.5, 5, and 15 mg/kg/day. No adverse effects were seen in two generations of offspring.[13]

The isolated ginsenoside Rb$_1$ caused significant morphological changes in vitro using a whole rat embryo culture model at a concentration of 30 μg/mL.[14] Despite the considerable publicity given to this finding at the time of its release, due to the high levels of exposure and the uncertain bioavailability of the ginsenosides as such, this is likely to have little relevance to the oral use of normal doses of ginseng, and stands in stark contrast to the human and in vivo studies which have shown no adverse effects on pregnancy.

Use in Lactation

Category C: Compatible with breastfeeding.

Ginseng is traditionally prescribed for lactating mothers (often in combination) as a tonic.

Warnings & Precautions

Concurrent use with stimulants such as caffeine and amphetamines is best avoided. Overstimulation may occur in susceptible patients, especially at higher doses.[11]

Effect on Ability to Drive or Operate Machinery

No adverse effects expected.

Adverse Reactions

Results from controlled clinical trials using a daily dose of 1 g indicate that ginseng is generally safe and well-tolerated. However, higher doses may cause side effects, and ginseng abuse syndrome (GAS) has been described.[15] GAS is defined as hypertension, together with nervousness, euphoria, insomnia, skin eruptions, and morning diarrhoea, and is thought to be related to ginseng's interaction with glucocorticoid production in the body. However, since this particular study did not differentiate the species of ginseng used, its reliability can be questioned. Moreover, a follow-up study found that many subjects with reported GAS were actually taking *Eleutherococcus senticosus* (Siberian ginseng).[16] Nonetheless, it is likely that high doses of ginseng can cause overstimulation, and symptoms of GAS have been reported in independent studies.[17,18]

Ginseng may cause side effects related to an oestrogen-like activity in women.[19] Cases of mastalgia[20] and vaginal bleeding in a 72-year-old woman[21] have been reported. A case of postmenopausal bleeding attributed to the use of a ginseng face cream has also been published.[22] The potential adulteration of these products with hormonal agents needs to be considered.

Ginseng is widely used, and several other adverse reactions have been reported which are at best possibly related to ginseng or may otherwise reflect on contamination, adulteration, or coincidence. These include Stevens-Johnson syndrome,[23,24] diuretic resistance,[25] cerebral arteritis (possibly due to overdose),[26] and mydriasis.[27,28]

Following an earlier case report of mania,[29] two other reports have emerged.[30,31] One case involved a female patient with major depression who was also taking clomipramine and haloperidol.[30] The other was in a healthy male with no history of psychiatric illness.[31]

A systematic review of adverse effects involving ginseng observed that the most commonly experienced events were mild and similar to those with placebo.[32]

Interactions

Two independent reports of a possible interaction of the monoamine oxidase inhibitor phenelzine with ginseng have been reported.[33,34] A case of a possible interaction between warfarin and ginseng has been described. Ginseng intake appeared to reduce the anticoagulant activity of the warfarin, but the mode of action was unclear.[35]

Interactions with sildenafil, hypoglycaemic drugs, and central nervous system (CNS) stimulants are also theoretically possible, but no cases have been reported. For more information see the herb-drug interaction table in Chapter 6.

Safety in Children

No information available but adverse effects are not expected.

Overdosage

Cerebral arteritis with severe headaches and chest tightness, nausea, and vomiting developed in two women who consumed an extract from around 25 g of ginseng root.[26]

Toxicology

Ginseng root has very low toxicity. A 5:1 extract of ginseng root was found to be safe (no effect at up to 6 g/kg in mice when administered i.p. and at 30 g/kg given orally in a single dose).[36] Subacute toxicity studies at 1.5 to 15 mg/kg/day of the same extract revealed no treatment-related effects on body weight, food consumption, haematology, biochemical parameters, and histopathological findings.[37]

A 5:1 extract of ginseng root administered to male rabbits and rats as part of their feed at 100 mg/kg/day for 30 to 60 days caused a reduction in testicular germ cell counts, size and number of Leydig cells, and other features of reduced fertility.[38]

Regulatory Status

See Table 1 for regulatory status in selected countries.

Table 1   **Regulatory Status for Ginseng in Selected Countries**

Australia	Ginseng is not included in Part 4 of Schedule 4 of the Therapeutic Goods Regulations.
China	Ginseng is official in the *Pharmacopoeia of the People's Republic of China* 1997. The usual adult dosage, usually administered in the form of a decoction, is listed as 3 to 9 g.
UK & Germany	Ginseng is included on the General Sale List. It is covered by a positive Commission E monograph. Ginseng is official in the *British Pharmacopoeia* 2002 and the *European Pharmacopoeia* 4.3.
US	Ginseng is official in the *United States Pharmacopeia-National Formulary* (USP 26-NF 21, 2003). Ginseng does not have generally recognised as safe (GRAS) status. However, it is freely available as a "dietary supplement" in the US under DSHEA legislation (Dietary Supplement Health and Education Act of 1994).

REFERENCES

1. Mills S, Bone K: *Principles and practice of phytotherapy: modern herbal medicine*, Edinburgh, 2000, Churchill Livingstone, pp 418-432.
2. British Herbal Medicine Association's Scientific Committee: *British herbal pharmacopoeia*, Bournemouth, 1983, BHMA, p 152.
3. Pharmacopoeia Commission of the People's Republic of China: *Pharmacopoeia of the People's Republic of China*, English ed, Beijing, 1997, Chemical Industry Press.
4. Bensky D, Gamble A: *Chinese herbal medicine materia medica*, Seattle, 1986, Eastland Press.
5. Wagner H, Bladt S: *Plant drug analysis: a thin layer chromatography atlas*, ed 2, Berlin, 1996, Springer-Verlag, p 307.
6. Chang HM, But PP: *Pharmacology and applications of chinese materia medica*, vol 1, World Scientific, 1986, Singapore, pp 17-31.
7. Kwon BM, Nam JY, Lee SH, et al: *Chem Pharm Bull* 44:444-445, 1996.
8. Yagi A, Ishizu T, Okamura N, et al: *Planta Med* 62: 115-118, 1996.
9. Wang YH, Hong CY, Chen CF, et al: *J Liq Chromatograph Relat Tech* 20:899-905, 1997.
10. Blumenthal M, et al (eds): *The complete German Commission E monographs: therapeutic guide to herbal medicines*, Austin, 1998, American Botanical Council.
11. British Herbal Medicine Association: *British herbal compendium*, vol 1, Bournemouth, 1992, BHMA.
12. Chin RK: *Asia Oceania J Obstet Gynaecol* 17:379-380, 1991.

13. Hess FG Jr, Parent RA, Cox GE, et al: *Food Chem Toxicol* 20:189-192, 1982.
14. Chan LY, Chiu PY, Lau TK: *Hum Reprod* 18:2166-2168, 2003.
15. Siegel RK: *JAMA* 241:1614-1615, 1979.
16. Siegel RK: *JAMA* 243:32, 1980.
17. Chen KJ: *J Trad Chin Med* 1:69-72, 1981.
18. Hammond TG, Whitworth JA: *Med J Aust* 1:492, 1981.
19. Punnonen R, Lukola A: *BMJ* 281:1110, 1980.
20. Palmer BV, Montgomery ACV, Monteiro JCMP: *BMJ* 1:1284, 1978.
21. Greenspan EM: *JAMA* 249:2018, 1983.
22. Hopkins MP, Androff L, Benninghoff AS: *Am J Obstet Gynecol* 159:1121-1122, 1988.
23. Faleni R, Soldati F: *Lancet* 348:267, 1996.
24. Dega H, Laporte JL, Frances C, et al: *Lancet* 347:1344, 1996.
25. Becker BN, Greene J, Evanson J, et al: *JAMA* 276:606-607, 1996.
26. Ryu SJ, Chien YY: *Neurology* 45:829-830, 1995.
27. Chan TY: *Vet Hum Toxicol* 37:156-157, 1995.
28. Lou BY, Li CF, Li PY, et al: *Yen Ko Hsueh Pao* 5:96-97, 1989.
29. Gonzalez-Seijo JC, Ramos YM, Lastra I: *J Clin Psychopharmacol* 15:447-448, 1995.
30. Vazquez I, Aguera-Ortiz LF: *Acta Psychiatr Scand* 105:76-78, 2002.
31. Engelberg D, McCutcheon A, Wiseman S: *J Clin Psychopharmacol* 21:535-537, 2001.
32. Coon JT, Ernst E: *Drug Saf* 25:323-344, 2002.
33. Jones BD, Runikis AM: *J Clin Psychopharmacol* 7:201-202, 1987.
34. Shader RI, Greenblatt DJ: *J Clin Psychopharmacol* 8:235, 1988.
35. Janetzky K, Morreale AP: *Am J Health-Syst Pharm* 54:692-693, 1997.
36. Singh VK, George CX, Singh N, et al: *Planta Med* 47:234-236, 1983.
37. Hess FG Jr, Parent RA, Stevens KR, et al: *Food Chem Toxicol* 21:95-97, 1983.
38. Sharma KK, Sharma A, Chaturvedi M, et al: *International Ginseng Conference '99 programme and abstracts, 8-11 July 1999, Hong Kong.* Hong Kong, China, 1999, BDG Communications Management Ltd.

GLOBE ARTICHOKE

Botanical name: *Cynara scolymus* L.
Family: Compositae
Plant part used: Leaf

Safety Summary

Pregnancy category B2: No increase in frequency of malformation or other harmful effects on the foetus from limited use in women. Animal studies are lacking.
Lactation category C: Compatible with breastfeeding.
Contraindications: Obstructed bile ducts.
Warnings & precautions: Known allergy to globe artichoke or to other plants of the Compositae family. Use cautiously in unconjugated hyperbilirubinaemia, acute or severe hepatocellular disease, septic cholecystitis, intestinal spasm or ileus, liver cancer.
Adverse reactions: Flatulence, feeling of weakness and hunger, contact dermatitis (fresh plant), urticaria-angioedema (fresh or boiled plant).
Interactions: No precautions required on current evidence.

Typical Therapeutic Use

A review of the clinical data from mostly uncontrolled trials indicated that globe artichoke leaf extract was able to lower lipid levels (cholesterol and/or triglycerides).[1] The choleretic activity of the herb has been confirmed in a randomised, double-blind, placebo-controlled trial.[2] Traditional indications for globe artichoke leaf in Western herbal medicine include jaundice and gout.[3]

Actions

Hepatoprotective, hepatic trophorestorative, choleretic, cholagogue, bitter tonic, hypocholesterolaemic, antiemetic, diuretic, depurative.

Key Constituents

Key constituents of globe artichoke leaf include caffeic acid derivatives (especially cynarin), sesquiterpene lactones (0.5% to 6%; including cynaropicrin) and flavonoids (0.1% to 1%).[4]

Adulteration

Occasionally globe artichoke is confused with Jerusalem artichoke (*Helianthus tuberosus*).[3]

Typical Dosage Forms & Dosage

Typical adult dosage ranges are:
- 3 to 8 mL/day of a 1:2 liquid extract or equivalent in tablet or capsule form.
- Clinical studies indicate that doses need to be relatively high, especially to achieve a clinically relevant reduction in cholesterol levels (in the range of the equivalent of 4 to 9 g/day of dried leaves)

Contraindications

Obstructed bile ducts.[5]

Use in Pregnancy

Category B2: No increase in frequency of malformation or other harmful effects on the foetus from limited use in women. Animal studies are lacking.

Use in Lactation

Category C: Compatible with breastfeeding.

Warnings & Precautions

Use only with professional supervision in cholelithiasis (gallstones). The Commission E advises caution for patients with known allergy to globe artichoke and to other plants of the Compositae family.[5] The likelihood of globe artichoke preparations causing an allergy is very low.

Choleretics and cholagogues should be used cautiously and may be inappropriate in the following:
- Unconjugated hyperbilirubinaemia (jaundice following haemolytic diseases, hereditary disease like Gilbert's and Crigler-Najjar syndromes)
- Acute or severe hepatocellular disease (e.g., following viral hepatitis, cirrhosis, adverse reactions to drugs such as anaesthetics, steroids, oestrogen, chlorpromazine)
- Septic cholecystitis (where there is a risk of peritonitis)
- Intestinal spasm or ileus
- Liver cancer.

Effect on Ability to Drive or Operate Machinery

No adverse effects expected.

Adverse Reactions

A 1997 review stated that globe artichoke leaf extract has good tolerability with a very low rate of side effects.[1] Mild side effects such as flatulence and a feeling of weakness and hunger have been reported in 1.3% of 553 dyspeptic patients in post-marketing surveillance studies.[6,7] However, as with other members of the Compositae family, contact with the fresh plant can cause contact dermatitis.[8,9] This is presumably due to the content of potentially allergenic sesquiterpene lactones.[10] One case of urticaria-angioedema from ingestion of both raw and boiled globe artichoke has been described. Allergy was confirmed by skin prick testing.[11]

Interactions

None known.

Safety in Children

No information available, but adverse effects are not expected.

Overdosage

No incidents found in published literature.

Toxicology

Table 1 lists LD_{50} data recorded for globe artichoke extract.[12]

Globe artichoke has low toxicity. No toxic effects were observed in rats after oral administration of globe artichoke extract (10 to 200 mg/kg) for four months[13] or dermal application (1 g/kg and 3 g/kg) for 21 days.[14] The dermal LD_0 was 6 g/kg in rats (LD_0 is the highest dose at which none of the test organisms die). Globe artichoke extract did not demonstrate skin-irritant or eye-irritant activity in rabbits, nor skin-sensitising potential in guinea pigs.[14]

Aqueous extract of globe artichoke (35.7 and 150 mg/kg) administered to sexually mature male rats five times per week for 75 days did not lead to any significant change in the structure of the semen.[15]

Globe artichoke leaf extract was cytotoxic to rat hepatocytes in culture at concentrations greater than 1 mg/mL.[16]

Regulatory Status

See Table 2 for regulatory status in selected countries.

Table 1   **LD_{50} Data Recorded for Globe Artichoke Extract**

Substance	Route, Model	LD_{50} Value	Reference
Purified globe artichoke extract	Oral, rats	>2 g/kg	12
Purified globe artichoke extract (containing 46% caffeoylquinic acids)	i.p., rats	265 mg/kg	12
Total extract of globe artichoke (containing 19% caffeoylquinic acids)	i.p., rats	1 g/kg	12

Table 2   **Regulatory Status for Globe Artichoke in Selected Countries**

Australia	Globe artichoke is not included in Part 4 of Schedule 4 of the Therapeutic Goods Regulations.
UK & Germany	Artichoke is included on the General Sale List; however, the botanical name is undefined. Globe artichoke is covered by a positive Commission E monograph.
US	Globe artichoke does not have generally recognised as safe (GRAS) status. However, it is freely available as a "dietary supplement" in the US under DSHEA legislation (Dietary Supplement Health and Education Act of 1994).

REFERENCES

1. Kraft K: *Phytomedicine* 4:369-378, 1997.
2. Kirchhoff R, Beckers Ch, Kirchhoff GM, et al: *Phytomedicine* 1:107-115, 1994.
3. Felter HW, Lloyd JU: *King's American dispensatory*, ed 18, 3rd revision, vol 1. First published 1905, reprinted Portland, 1983, Eclectic Medical Publications, p 641.
4. Wagner H, Bladt S: *Plant drug analysis: a thin layer chromatography atlas*, ed 2, Berlin, 1996, Springer-Verlag, p 77.
5. Blumenthal M, et al, eds: *The complete German Commission E monographs: therapeutic guide to herbal medicines*, Austin, 1998, American Botanical Council, pp 84-85.
6. Fintelmann V: *Z Allg Med* 72:3-19, 1996.
7. Fintelmann V, Menaen HG: *Dtsch Apoth Ztg* 136:63-74, 1996.
8. Meding B: *Contact Dermatitis* 9:314, 1983.
9. Quirce S, Tabar AI, Olaguibel JM, et al: *J Allergy Clin Immunol* 97:710-711, 1996.
10. Mitchell JC, Dupuis G: *Brit J Dermatol* 84: 139-150, 1971.
11. Romano C, Ferrara A, Falagiani P: *J Investig Allergol Clin Immunol* 10:102-104, 2000.
12. Lietti A: *Fitoterapia* 48:153-158, 1977.
13. Halkova Z, Zaikov C, Shumkov N, et al: *Khig Zdraveopazvane* 40:9-12, 1997.
14. Halkova Z: *Probl Khig* 21:74-80, 1996.
15. Ilieva P, Khalkova Zh, Zaikov Kh, et al: *Probl Khig* 19:105-111, 1994.
16. Gebhardt R: *Toxicol Appl Pharmacol* 144:279-286, 1997.

GOAT'S RUE

Botanical name: *Galega officinalis* L.
Family: Leguminosae (Papilionoideae)
Plant part used: Aerial parts

Safety Summary

Pregnancy category B1: No increase in frequency of malformation or other harmful effects on the foetus from limited use in women. No evidence of increased foetal damage in animal studies.
Lactation category C: Compatible with breastfeeding.
Contraindications: None required on current evidence.
Warnings & precautions: Prescribe with caution in patients stabilised on hypoglycaemic drugs or insulin.
Adverse reactions: Adverse reactions are not expected at the recommended dosage.
Interactions: Enhanced reduction of blood glucose is theoretically possible in combination with hypoglycaemic drugs or insulin.

Typical Therapeutic Use

Traditional indications for goat's rue in Western herbal medicine include diabetes mellitus.[1] A recent patent has suggested the use of a goat's rue constituent (galegine) for weight loss.[2] However, an agent that causes weight loss in an animal experiment may be exhibiting a toxic effect.

Actions

Hypoglycaemic, antidiabetic, galactagogue.

Key Constituents

Key constituents of goat's rue aerial parts include the guanidine derivative galegine. Also present are flavonoids and small amounts of saponins and chromium (3.7 ppm).[3]

Adulteration

No adulterants known.

Typical Dosage Forms & Dosage

Typical adult dosage ranges are:
- 3 to 6 g/day of dried aerial parts or by infusion
- 3 to 6 mL/day of a 1:1 liquid extract
- 4.5 to 8 mL/day of a 1:2 liquid extract or equivalent in tablet or capsule form
- 6 to 12 mL/day of a 1:10 tincture

Contraindications

None known.

Use in Pregnancy

Category B1: No increase in frequency of malformation or other harmful effects on the foetus from limited use in women. No evidence of increased foetal damage in animal studies.

Oral administration of goat's rue (above-ground parts) to pregnant ewes at various stages of gestation produced no recognisable damage in the newborn lambs. The dosage regime is listed in Table 1.[4]

Use in Lactation

Category C: Compatible with breastfeeding.

Goat's rue in combination with mineral salts increased milk volume in lactating women in a controlled trial published in 1968.[5]

Warnings & Precautions

Prescribe with caution in patients stabilised on hypoglycaemic drugs or insulin.

Effect on Ability to Drive or Operate Machinery

No adverse effects expected.

Adverse Reactions

Side effects were not observed in a small group of diabetic patients who took goat's rue extract within the recommended dosage, with the exception of increased perspiration, which occurred at the high end of the dosage range. A patient who by error consumed 20 times the therapeutic dose had some nausea and vomiting, but showed no other signs of toxicity.[6]

Interactions

There are no documented case histories, but the combination of goat's rue with hypoglycaemic drugs

Table 1 Doses of Goat's Rue Administered to Pregnant Ewes

Dosage	Plant Material
2 to 3.5 g/kg/day on days 20 to 35 of gestation	Semimature seed stage
1.6 to 2.3 g/kg on day 60 of gestation followed by 1.1 to 2.3 g/kg/day on days 60 to 90	Early seed stage
1.1 to 2.3 g/kg/day on days 100 to 130 of gestation	Mature seed stage

and insulin may result in enhanced reduction of blood glucose. In these circumstances prescribe cautiously, monitor blood sugar regularly, and warn the patient about possible hypoglycaemia.

Safety in Children

No information available.

Overdosage

No incidents were found in published literature for poisoning by goat's rue in humans. The plant has caused poisoning and death in sheep. The dosage causing toxicity varied (0.8 to 24 g/kg) and was likely to be a result of a variation in the individual animal's susceptibility.[4,7] Other galegine-containing plants have caused toxicosis with similar effects and galegine has been shown to be responsible.[8,9]

Toxicology

Table 2 lists LD_{50} data recorded for goat's rue extract and its constituents.[10,11]

Toxicological studies conducted in 1969 suggested that substances other than galegine contributed to the acute toxicity of goat's rue leaf extract in mice.[11]

Regulatory Status

See Table 3 for regulatory status in selected countries.

Table 2 LD_{50} Data Recorded for Goat's Rue Extract and Its Constituents

Substance	Route, Model	LD_{50} Value	Reference
Goat's rue dry methanol extract	i.g., mice	4.4 g/kg (= 30 g/kg of dried herb)	10
Galegine sulphate	i.g., mice	122 mg/kg	10
Galegine sulphate	s.c., mice	77.5 mg/kg	11

Table 3 Regulatory Status for Goat's Rue in Selected Countries

Australia	Goat's rue is not included in Part 4 of Schedule 4 of the Therapeutic Goods Regulations.
UK & Germany	Goat's rue is not included on the General Sale List. It is covered by a negative Commission E monograph.
US	Goat's rue does not have generally recognised as safe (GRAS) status. However, it is freely available as a "dietary supplement" in the US under DSHEA legislation (Dietary Supplement Health and Education Act of 1994).

REFERENCES

1. British Herbal Medicine Association's Scientific Committee: *British herbal pharmacopoeia*, Bournemouth, 1983, BHMA, p 96.
2. Palit et al: *Amine and amidine containing compounds as weight reducing agents*, United States Patent 5945455, August 1999.
3. Bisset NG, ed: *Herbal drugs and phytopharmaceuticals: a handbook for practice on a scientific basis*, Stuttgart, 1994, Medpharm Scientific Publishers, pp 220-221.
4. Keeler RF, Johnson AE, Stuart LD, et al: *Vet Hum Toxicol* 28:309-315, 1986.
5. Heiss H: *Wien Med Wochenschr* 24:546-548, 1968.
6. Parturier G, Hugonot G: *Presse Med* 43:258-260, 1935.
7. Keeler RF, Baker DC, Evans JO: *Vet Hum Toxicol* 30:420-423, 1988.
8. Keeler RF, Baker DC, Panter KE: *J Environ Pathol Toxicol Oncol* 11:11-17, 1992.
9. Huxtable CR, Dorling PR, Colegate SM: *Aust Vet J* 70:169-171, 1993.
10. Petricic J, Kalodera Z: *Acta Pharm Jugosl* 32:219-223, 1982.
11. Koehler H: *Biol Zentralbl* 88:165-167, 1969.

GOLDEN ROD

Other common name: Goldenrod
Botanical names: Solidago virgaurea L. (Solidago virga-aurea L.)
Family: Compositae
Plant part used: Aerial parts

Safety Summary

Pregnancy category B2: No increase in frequency of malformation or other harmful effects on the foetus from limited use in women. Animal studies are lacking.
Lactation category C: Compatible with breastfeeding.
Contraindications: Contraindicated in those with known allergy to golden rod.
Warnings & precautions: Allergic reactions may occur in susceptible patients sensitised to plants from the Compositae family. Copious fluid intake should not be undertaken if oedema due to impaired cardiac or renal function exists (Commission E warning).
Adverse reactions: Allergic reaction is possible.
Interactions: No precautions required on current evidence.

Typical Therapeutic Use

Golden rod has been successfully used for treating urological complaints in uncontrolled trials.[1,2] Traditional indications for golden rod in Western herbal medicine include inflammation of the nasopharynx with persistent catarrh, flatulent dyspepsia, cystitis and topically in nose and throat infection.[3]

Actions

Antiinflammatory, diaphoretic, diuretic, anticatarrhal.

Key Constituents

Constituents of golden rod include flavonoids, anthocyanidins, saponins (2.4%, including virgaureasaponins), diterpenes, phenolic acids, catechol tannins (10% to 15%) and a small amount of essential oil (<0.5%).[4]

Adulteration

Solidago virgaurea is often adulterated with another therapeutic herb with the common name, namely early golden rod (Solidago giganteae) and Canadian golden rod (S. canadensis). As S. virgaurea has been difficult to source, these other species are often offered commercially.[4,5] The phenolic glycosides leiocarposide and virgaureoside A, which are present in S. virgaurea, have not been detected in S. giganteae or S. canadensis.[5,6] Although these species may have medicinal properties, they are not regarded interchangeable for S. virgaurea.

Typical Dosage Forms & Dosage

Typical adult dosage ranges are:
- 1.5 to 6 g/day of dried aerial parts or by infusion
- 1.5 to 6 mL/day of a 1:1 liquid extract
- 3 to 6 mL/day of a 1:2 liquid extract or equivalent in tablet or capsule form
- 1.5 to 3 mL/day of a 1:5, 1:8, 1:10 tincture

Contraindications

Contraindicated in those with known allergy to golden rod. Golden rod is a medium level sensitiser[7] and has caused allergic contact dermatitis after oral administration.[8] Contact dermatitis has been reported in field workers exposed to the plant.[9]

Use in Pregnancy

Category B2: No increase in frequency of malformation or other harmful effects on the foetus from limited use in women. Animal studies are lacking.

Use in Lactation

Category C: Compatible with breastfeeding.

Warnings & Precautions

Allergic reactions may occur in susceptible patients sensitised to plants from the Compositae family.

The Commission E advises that copious fluid intake is recommended to assist in the reduction of microorganisms in the urinary tract without loss of electrolytes, but should not be undertaken if oedema due to impaired cardiac or renal function exists.[10] This caution relates to the use of golden rod during urinary tract infections.

Effect on Ability to Drive or Operate Machinery

No adverse effects expected.

Adverse Reactions

Allergic reaction is possible, but rare.

Interactions

None known.

Safety in Children

No information available, but adverse effects are not expected.

Overdosage

No incidents found in published literature of poisoning in humans. An early mention is made of *Solidago virgaurea* in North America causing intoxication in livestock, particularly horses.[6]

Toxicology

Table 1 lists LD_{50} data recorded for golden rod extract and one of its constituents.[11,12]

Regulatory Status

See Table 2 for regulatory status in selected countries.

Table 1   **LD_{50} Data Recorded for Golden Rod and Leiocarposide**

Substance	Route, Model	LD_{50} Value	Reference
Golden rod, entire plant, ethanol extract	i.p., mice	600 mg/kg	11
Leiocarposide	Oral, rats	1.55 g/kg	12

Table **2**   **Regulatory Status for Golden Rod in Selected Countries**

Australia	Golden rod is not included in Part 4 of Schedule 4 of the Therapeutic Goods Regulations.
UK & Germany	Golden rod is not included on the General Sale List. It is covered by a positive Commission E monograph.
	The related species *Solidago giganteae* and *S. canadensis* are official in the *British Pharmacopoeia* 2002 and the *European Pharmacopoeia* 4.3.
US	Golden rod does not have generally recognised as safe (GRAS) status. However, it is freely available as a "dietary supplement" in the US under DSHEA legislation (Dietary Supplement Health and Education Act of 1994).

REFERENCES

1. Pfannkuch A, Stammwitz U: *Z Phytother* 23:20-25, 2002.
2. Bruhwiler K, Frater-Schroder M, Kalbermatten R, et al: 4th and International Congress on Phytotherapy, Munich, September 10-13, 1992, Abstract SL 20.
3. British Herbal Medicine Association's Scientific Committee: *British herbal pharmacopoeia*, Bournemouth, 1983, BHMA, pp 234-235.
4. Bisset NG, ed: *Herbal drugs and phytopharmaceuticals: a handbook for practice on a scientific basis*, Stuttgart, 1994, Medpharm Scientific Publishers, pp 530-533.
5. Bisset NG, ed: *Herbal drugs and phytopharmaceuticals: a handbook for practice on a scientific basis*, Stuttgart, 1994, Medpharm Scientific Publishers, pp 476-479.
6. Blaschek W, Ebel S, Hackenthal E, et al: *HagerROM 2002: Hagers Handbuch der Drogen und Arzneistoffe*, Heidelberg, 2002, Springer.
7. Zeller W, de Gols M, Hausen BM: *Arch Dermatol Res* 277:28-35, 1985.
8. Schatzle M, Agathos M, Breit R: *Contact Dermatitis* 39:271-272, 1998.
9. Mitchell J, Rook A: *Botanical dermatology: plants and plant products injurious to the skin*, Vancouver, 1979, Greengrass, pp 216-217.

10. Blumenthal M, et al, eds: *The complete German Commission E monographs: therapeutic guide to herbal medicines,* Austin, 1998, American Botanical Council.

11. Sharma ML, Chandokhe N, Ghatak BJ, et al: *Indian J Exp Biol* 16:228-240, 1978.

12. Chodera A, Dabrowska K, Senczuk M, et al: *Acta Pol Pharm* 42:199-204, 1985.

GOLDEN SEAL

Other common names: Hydrastis, goldenseal
Botanical name: *Hydrastis canadensis* L.
Family: Ranunculaceae
Plant part used: Root and rhizome

Safety Summary

Pregnancy category C: Has caused or is associated with a substantial risk of causing harmful effects on the foetus or neonate without causing malformations (on the basis of the presence of berberine and related alkaloids and the implications for neonatal jaundice).
Lactation category SD: Strongly discouraged in breastfeeding (on the basis of the presence of berberine and related alkaloids).
Contraindications: Jaundiced neonates. Do not use during pregnancy or lactation without professional advice.
Warnings & precautions: None required on current evidence.
Adverse reactions: None found in published literature worthy of note.
Interactions: Drugs which displace the protein binding of bilirubin, such as phenylbutazone.

Typical Therapeutic Use

Traditional indications for golden seal in Western herbal medicine include skin disorders, dyspepsia, gastritis, peptic ulcer, colitis, anorexia, menorrhagia, dysmenorrhoea, sinusitis, and mucosal inflammations.[1,2]

Actions

Antihaemorrhagic, anticatarrhal, mucous membrane trophorestorative, antimicrobial, antibacterial, bitter tonic, antiinflammatory, depurative, vulnerary, choleretic, reputed oxytocic.

Key Constituents

Key constituents include isoquinoline alkaloids (especially β-hydrastine [1.5% to 4%], berberine [2.5%], canadine [0.5%]) and other alkaloids.[2]

Adulteration

Due to the price of genuine golden seal, commercial products have been found not to contain the authentic plant material.[3]

Golden seal was listed on Appendix II of the Convention on International Trade in Endangered Species (CITES) as of 18 September 1997,[4] and is currently listed. It is preferable to use cultivated sources (rather than wildcrafted sources) of golden seal because of its endangered status.

Typical Dosage Forms & Dosage

Typical adult dosage ranges are:
- 1.5 to 3 g/day of dried root and rhizome or by decoction
- 0.9 to 3 mL/day of a 1:1 liquid extract or equivalent in tablet or capsule form
- 2 to 4.5 mL/day of a 1:3 tincture
- 6 to 12 mL/day of a 1:10 tincture

Contraindications

The *British Herbal Pharmacopoeia* 1983 advises that golden seal is contraindicated in pregnancy and hypertensive conditions.[1] The contraindication for hypertension may be based on the cardiovascular activity of berberine. The *British Herbal Compendium* 1992 does not list hypertension as a contraindication.[2] An Eclectic text notes that "the whole drug... arterial tension is augmented, and blood pressure in the capillaries increased, rendering it valuable, like belladonna and ergot, in overcoming blood stasis".[5]

Although berberine-containing plants have been used in traditional Chinese medicine for the treatment of jaundiced neonates, berberine is thought to cause severe acute haemolysis and neonatal jaundice in babies with glucose-6-phosphate dehydrogenase (G6PD) deficiency.[6] However, a review published in 2001 questioned the causal relationship between the berberine-containing herb *Coptis chinensis* and haemolysis in G6PD deficient infants (see Pregnancy section below).[7]

Do not use during pregnancy or lactation without professional advice.

Use in Pregnancy

Category C: Has caused or is associated with a substantial risk of causing harmful effects on the foetus or neonate without causing malformations (on the basis of the presence of berberine and related alkaloids and the implications for neonatal jaundice).

Golden seal is best avoided during pregnancy except for short-term use to assist labour (see above and below).

Hydrastine (0.5 g) induced labour when taken orally by pregnant women.[8]

At a very high oral dosage of 1.86 g/kg administered from days 1 to 15 of gestation, golden seal did not have an adverse effect on reproductive outcome in rats. Foetal weights were slightly increased when the herb was administered from days 1 to 8 and days 8 to 15 of gestation. There was no difference in placental weight, number of resorptions, or litter size. There were no externally visible malformations. The herb was administered as an ethanol extract and the dose administered was the highest possible in which ethanol remained below the teratogenic threshold.[9]

Reduction in average foetal body weight per litter was observed in the offspring of mated mice fed golden seal root powder (7.7 g/kg/day) from days 6 to 17. No significant developmental toxicity was observed below this dosage. Maternal liver weights were increased at greater than 2 g/kg/day, but histopathological lesions were absent.[10]

Golden seal demonstrated antispasmodic activity in experimentally-induced uterine contractions (isolated uterus).[11,12]

Refer to the barberry (*Berberis vulgaris*) monograph for information on the developmental toxicology of berberine.

Use in Lactation

Category SD: Strongly discouraged in breastfeeding. Infants have been exposed to berberine via breast milk following maternal ingestion of berberine-containing plants.[13]

Warnings & Precautions

None required.

Effect on Ability to Drive or Operate Machinery

No adverse effects expected.

Adverse Reactions

In popular literature, golden seal is often described as toxic in large doses and/or that it should be restricted to short term use. It is possible that this information comes from a misinterpretation of the writings of the homoeopath Dr Edwin Hale, who

noted side effects (such as exhaustion of the mucous membranes) after many homoeopathic provings in the mid-nineteenth century.[14] The results of homoeopathic provings do not necessarily translate to herbal practice.

Native Americans and Eclectic physicians have used golden seal topically, particularly for ophthalmias (eye inflammation). One objection to this use was its ability to stain the conjunctiva.[5]

Interactions

Berberine demonstrated potent displacement of bilirubin in vitro and in vivo after chronic administration to rats (10 to 20 mg/kg i.p.). Berberine at this dosage range caused elevation in serum levels of bilirubin (since the binding of bilirubin to albumin decreased). However, at a dose of 2 mg/kg, the displacement was not signficant.[13] Hence berberine may reinforce the effects of other drugs that displace the protein binding of bilirubin.

The notion that ingestion of golden seal could mask illicit drugs in urinalysis has appeared in the popular literature since the late 1970s. A number of scientific studies have verified that this is a fallacy.[14,15] This notion is likely to have come from a novel written in 1900 by the well-known American herbalist John Uri Lloyd.[15]

Chronic use of golden seal is said to decrease absorption of vitamin B.[16] There is no further information available to support this claim.

Safety in Children

Berberine has been used to treat diarrhoea and giardiasis in children, which suggests that berberine-containing plants such as golden seal may also be used in this way. Treatment of newborns with neonatal jaundice is contraindicated.

Overdosage

Golden seal has been said to cause irritation of the mouth, throat and stomach as well as convulsions when taken in toxic (undefined) doses.[16]

The Commission E notes that death from berberine poisoning has occurred. At doses higher than 0.5 g, berberine may cause dizziness, nose bleeds, dyspnoea, skin and eye irritation, gastrointestinal irritation, nausea, diarrhoea, nephritis and urinary tract disorders.[17] Such doses of berberine will not be reached from berberine-containing herbs used at the recommended therapeutic doses. In two clinical trials for acute diarrhoea due to enterotoxigenic *E. coli* and *Vibrio cholerae*, berberine was well tolerated in dosages of 0.8 to 1.2 g/day.[18,19]

Refer also to the barberry (*Berberis vulgaris*) monograph for toxicology information and LD_{50} values for berberine.

Hydrastine tested negative in the *Salmonella* mutagenicity test.[21]

Toxicology

Table 1 lists LD_{50} data recorded for golden seal extract and hydrastine, one of its key constituents.[11,20]

Regulatory Status

See Table 2 for regulatory status in selected countries.

Table 1   **LD_{50} Data Recorded for Golden Seal Extract and Hydrastine**

Substance	Route, Model	LD_{50} Value	Reference
Golden seal extract	Oral, mice	1.62 g/kg	11
Hydrastine	i.p., rats	104 mg/kg	20

Table 2   **Regulatory Status for Golden Seal in Selected Countries**

Australia	Golden seal is not included in Part 4 of Schedule 4 of the Therapeutic Goods Regulations.
UK & Germany	Golden seal is included on the General Sale List. It was not included in the Commission E assessment.
US	Golden seal is official in the *United States Pharmacopeia-National Formulary* (USP 26-NF 21, 2003).
	Golden seal does not have generally recognised as safe (GRAS) status. However, it is freely available as a "dietary supplement" in the US under DSHEA legislation (Dietary Supplement Health and Education Act of 1994).

REFERENCES

1. British Herbal Medicine Association's Scientific Committee: *British herbal pharmacopoeia*, Bournemouth, 1983, BHMA, pp 113-115.
2. British Herbal Medicine Association: *British herbal compendium*, vol 1, Bournemouth, 1992, BHMA, pp 119-120.
3. Govindan M, Govindan G: *Fitoterapia* 71:232-235, 2000.
4. Bannerman J: *HerbalGram* 41:51-52, 1997.
5. Felter HW, Lloyd JU: *King's American dispensatory*, ed 18, rev 3, vol 2. First published 1905; reprinted Portland, 1983, Eclectic Medical Publications, pp 1020-1030.
6. Ho NK: *Singapore Med J* 37: 645-651, 1996.
7. Fok TF: *J Perinatol* 21(Suppl 1):S98-S100, 2001.
8. Grismondi GL, Scivoli L, Cetera C: *Min Ginecol* 31:19-32, 1979.
9. Yao M, Brown-Woodman PDC, Ritchie H: *Teratology* 64:320-325, 2001.
10. NTP Study TER99004: *Final study report developmental toxicity evaluation for goldenseal (Hydrastis canadensis) root powder administered in the feed to Swiss (CD1®) mice on gestational days 6-17*, available from the National Toxicology Program website: ntp-server.niehs.nih.gov/
11. Haginiwa J, Harada M: *Yakugaku Zasshi* 82:726-731, 1962.
12. Cometa MF, Abdel-Haq H, Palmery M: *Phytother Res* 12(Suppl 1):S83-S85, 1998.
13. Chan E: *Biol Neonate* 63:201-208, 1993.
14. Bergner P: *Medical Herbalism* 8:1, 4-6, 1996-1997.
15. Foster S: *HerbalGram* 21:7, 35, 1989.
16. Hamon NW: *Can Pharm J* 123:508-510, 1990.
17. Blumenthal M, et al, eds: *The complete German Commission E monographs: therapeutic guide to herbal medicines*, Austin, 1998, American Botanical Council, pp 309-310.
18. Rabbani GH, Butler T, Knight J, et al: *J Infect Dis* 155:979-984, 1987.

19. Khin-Maung U, Myo-Khin, Nyunt-Nyunt-Wai et al: *J Diarrhoeal Dis Res* 5:184-187, 1987.

20. Poe CF, Johnson CC: *Acta Pharmacol Toxicol* 10:338-346, 1954.

21. National Toxicology Program website: ntp-server.niehs.nih.gov

GOTU KOLA

Other common names: Indian pennywort, man-dukaparni

Botanical names: *Centella asiatica* (L.) Urban (*Hydrocotyle asiatica* L., *H. erecta* L. f., *Centella coriacea* Nannf.)

Family: Umbelliferae

Plant part used: Aerial parts

Safety Summary

Pregnancy category B1: No increase in frequency of malformation or other harmful effects on the foetus from limited use in women. No evidence of increased foetal damage in animal studies.

Lactation category C: Compatible with breast-feeding.

Contraindications: Known allergy to gotu kola.

Warnings & precautions: The use of herbs rich in saponins is possibly inappropriate in coeliac disease, fat malabsorption, and vitamins A, D, E, and K deficiency, some upper digestive irritations, and topically to open wounds. Caution in patients with preexisting cholestasis.

Adverse reactions: Allergic contact dermatitis occurs rarely. Herbs rich in saponins may cause irritation of the gastric mucous membranes and reflux.

Interactions: No precautions required on current evidence.

Typical Therapeutic Use

The triterpene fraction of gotu kola has demonstrated benefit in well designed clinical trials assessing the treatment of venous diseases, including venous insufficiency, and for wound healing.[1]

Traditional indications for gotu kola in Western herbal medicine include rheumatic and skin conditions and topically for indolent wounds, leprosy and to assist healing in surgical wounds.[2] It has a long history of use in traditional Ayurvedic medicine for the treatment of leprosy and as a brain tonic.[3] This herb has also been used in many other traditional systems.

Actions

Vulnerary, antiinflammatory, depurative, adaptogenic, nervine tonic.

Key Constituents

The main constituents of gotu kola aerial parts are the triterpene saponins asiaticoside and madecassoside and their aglycones asiatic acid and madecassic acid. The quantity of triterpenes in gotu kola varies, but good quality herb should contain 2.5% to 3% total triterpenes (the four constituents listed above). The occurrence of an alkaloid designated as hydrocotyline was noted in 1947 but could not be verified by later investigations.[4]

A number of preparations consisting of various proportions of the triterpenoid saponins have been tested in pharmacological and clinical studies. For simplicity, they are referred to in this monograph as the triterpene fraction of gotu kola (TFGK).

Adulteration

Unintentional adulteration may occur due to confusion over the common name of gotu kola. In Ayurveda both *Centella asiatica* and *Bacopa monnieri* are known by the local name "brahmi".[5]

Typical Dosage Forms & Dosage

Typical adult dosage ranges are:
- 1.8 g/day of dried aerial parts or by infusion
- 3 to 6 mL/day of a 1:2 liquid extract or equivalent in tablet or capsule form
- 60 to 180 mg/day of TFGK (approximately 2.5 to 7.0 g/day of dried herb equivalent)

Contraindications

Gotu kola is contraindicated in patients with known allergy.

Use in Pregnancy

Category B1: No increase in frequency of malformation or other harmful effects on the foetus from limited use in women. No evidence of increased foetal damage in animal studies.

Gotu kola has been traditionally used in Bengal as a contraceptive agent. However, compared to controls, a reduction in conception rate was observed in female mice fed gotu kola (juice of whole plant, equivalent to 20 to 80 g fresh whole plant/kg) by gavage. Two sets of animals received the herb for 14 days (7 days before and 7 days during cohabitation) and 21 days (7 days before and 14 days during cohabitation). In the first set, sterile mating occurred for 50% to 60% of animals vs. 15% in the controls, and for the second set 50% to 55% vs. 20%. An isolated triterpenoid glycoside (40 to 120 mg/kg) and a compound derived from it also demonstrated antifertility activity. In all treatment groups, there was no significant decrease in the number of young per litter, and birth weights of the young were normal. The authors noted that the isolated glycoside and the compound derived from it caused consistent reduction of fertility.[6] These were very high doses, well above those normally used in clinical practice. Moreover, an antifertility effect does not imply harm during pregnancy.

Antifertility activity was demonstrated in vivo in an early study for *Centella asiatica* (part undefined). Gotu kola was tested for antizygotic, antiimplantation and early abortifacient activity. There is no more information regarding these studies.[7] The teratological effects have been studied in the rabbit and found to be negative for that animal.[8]

Use in Lactation

Category C: Compatible with breastfeeding.

Warnings & Precautions

The use of herbs rich in saponins is possibly inappropriate in coeliac disease, fat malabsorption, and vitamins A, D, E, and K deficiency, some upper digestive irritations, and topically to open wounds. Saponin-containing herbs are best kept to a minimum in patients with preexisting cholestasis.

Effect on Ability to Drive or Operate Machinery

No adverse effects expected.

Adverse Reactions

As with all herbs rich in saponins, oral use may cause irritation of the gastric mucous membranes and reflux.

Cases of allergic contact dermatitis have been reported from the use of gotu kola, TFGK and asiaticoside, but they are considered to be low risk treatments.[9-16] Both the extract and the triterpene constituents are weak sensitisers,[9] although asiaticoside has been classified as a contact allergen.[17] Patch

tests in many cases confirmed that gotu kola or its constituents were responsible,[10,11,14,15] although in some cases other constituents in the preparations were also responsible (e.g., propylene glycol,[13] geraniol, lavender essence, and neomycin[12]).

Traditional sources indicate that gotu kola may produce photosensitisation when used in tropical areas, although whether from use by oral or topical application is not indicated.[2,3] Occasional gastric intolerance has been observed.[8] A review of the use of TFGK for the treatment of chronic venous insufficiency indicated that it was safe and well tolerated. Most trials used dosage of TFGK in the range 60 to 120 mg/day.[18]

Interactions

In an in vivo study investigating wound healing with drugs, the antiinflammatory drugs dexamethasone and phenylbutazone individually combined with asiaticoside caused a reduction in the tensile strength (and hence therapeutic effect) produced by asiaticoside alone.[19] In this study the test substances were administered by intramuscular injection (asiaticoside is a saponin and has surfactant activity), so it is not known if the observed results extrapolate to the topical use of asiaticoside or oral use of gotu kola in humans.

In open trials asiaticoside has been used topically in combination with an antibiotic and corticosteroid,[20] and was well tolerated.[21]

Safety in Children

Adverse effects are not expected. Gotu kola dried herb has been assessed in a clinical trial in India as a mental tonic for mentally disabled children.[22] Gotu kola is used in leaf concentrate meals, which are prepared as a porridge for preschool children in Sri Lanka to combat nutritional deficiencies.[23] (Although leaf composition varies with location, fresh gotu kola leaves typically contain 2% protein, 7 mg/100 g vitamin C, 0.09 mg/100 g vitamin B_1 and 5.6 mg/100 g iron.[24])

Overdosage

There are no reliable reports of overdose with gotu kola.

An early case (prior to 1896) is recorded concerning a "Dr Boiteau who, in treating himself, progressively increased the dose and found that after two months the drug had produced all the effects of a violent, cumulative poison. ... the plant, properly prepared and administered, is a powerful stimulant of the circulatory system, its action chiefly affecting the vessels of the skin and mucous membrane."[25] Traditional sources writing in the early to mid 20th century indicate that the plant is a stupefying narcotic in large doses, and in some cases produces headache or vertigo with a tendency to coma.[3]

Toxicology

Gotu kola has been consumed as a leafy vegetable, particularly in Bangladesh, Thailand, Indonesia (West Java), Sri Lanka, and South Africa,[26-28] and appears to have no harmful effect when used as a food.[29] The leaf and stolon is eaten raw and cooked.[30]

Acute toxicity testing indicated a low toxicity following oral administration to rats (LD_{50} >675 mg/kg of gotu kola extract, equivalent to >4 g/kg dried leaf). Chronic administration of 150 mg/kg/day of extract (equivalent to 0.9 g/kg dried leaf) for a period of 30 days did not produce any adverse effects.[31] Mice receiving up to 1 g/kg of gotu kola extract (2.5 g/kg dried plant) by mouth did not exhibit adverse effects.[32] Aqueous ethanol extract of gotu kola entire plant demonstrated an MTD value of 250 mg/kg after i.p. injection in mice.[33]

Subcutaneous injection of 40 to 50 mg/kg of asiaticoside was toxic to mice and rabbits while 20 to 250 mg/kg resulted in increased bleeding time. An oral dose of 1 g/kg was well tolerated.[34]

The local toxicity of asiaticoside was investigated by the measurement of skin respiration and histological analysis (the death of a cell is accompanied by loss of respiratory activity). Compared with other therapeutic agents, the toxicity of asiaticoside was not excessive and was comparable to that of many common antibiotics. Histological effects on guinea pig skin indicated moderate concentrations of asiaticoside produced swollen and abnormally staining cells. Higher concentrations resulted in necrotic cultures, showing signs of "thickening" of the epidermis even though the cells had mostly disintegrated. This may have been due to the cells becoming rapidly keratinised. Although fairly high concentrations of asiaticoside were required to produce this effect, it occurred in vivo (5 mg, s.c.) as well as in vitro.[35]

An ethanol extract of gotu kola exhibited mutagenic activity to strain TA98 (Salmonella/microsome test) only in the presence of S9 mix.[36] A water extract of gotu kola was not toxic towards TA98 and TA100 with or without addition of S9 mix at the tested concentration (5 mg/plate). Gotu kola weakly inhibited the mutagenicity of the indirect mutagen IQ (2-amino-3-methylimidazo[4,5-f]quinoline).[37] In another experiment, gotu kola water extract (1 mL of a 1:5 decoction) showed mutagenic activity in strain TA98 with metabolic activation only.[38] Gotu kola methanol extract induced abnormal metaphases and an increase in chromosome aberrations in the *Vicia faba* root meristem assay.[39]

Asiaticoside was found to be a weak tumour promoter in the hairless mouse epidermis model and was very weakly carcinogenic to the dermis after topical application.[40]

Regulatory Status

See Table 1 for regulatory status in selected countries.

Table 1   **Regulatory Status of Gotu Kola in Selected Countries**

Australia	Gotu kola is not included in Part 4 of Schedule 4 of the Therapeutic Goods Regulations.
China	Gotu kola is official in the *Pharmacopoeia of the People's Republic of China* 1997. The usual adult dosage, usually administered in the form of a decoction, is listed as 15 to 30 g, or 30 to 60 g of the fresh herb.
UK & Germany	Gotu kola for external use is included on the General Sale List. It was not included in the Commission E assessment.
	Gotu kola is official in the *British Pharmacopoeia* 2002 and the *European Pharmacopoeia* 4.3.
US	Gotu kola does not have generally recognised as safe (GRAS) status. However, it is freely available as a "dietary supplement" in the US under DSHEA legislation (Dietary Supplement Health and Education Act of 1994).

REFERENCES

1. Brinkhaus B, Lindner M, Schuppan D, et al: *Phytomedicine* 7: 427-448, 2000.
2. British Herbal Medicine Association's Scientific Committee: *British herbal pharmacopoeia*, Bournemouth, 1983, BHMA, pp 56-57.
3. Chopra RN, Chopra IC, Handa KL, et al: *Chopra's indigenous drugs of India*, ed 2, 1958; reprinted Calcutta, 1982, Academic Publishers, pp 351-353.
4. Gunther B, Wagner H: *Phytomedicine* 3:59-65, 1996.
5. Chopra RN, Chopra IC, Handa KL, et al: *Chopra's indigenous drugs of India*, ed 2, 1958; reprinted Calcutta, 1982, Academic Publishers, p 341.
6. Dutta T, Basu UP: *Indian J Exp Biol* 6:181-182, 1968.
7. Chaudhury RR: *Spec Rep Ser Indian Counc Med Res* 55:3-19, 1966.
8. Bosse JP, Papillon J, Frenette G, et al: *Ann Plast Surg* 3:13-21, 1979.
9. Hausen BM: *Contact Dermatitis* 29:175-179, 1993.
10. Danese P, Carnevali C, Bertazzoni MG: *Contact Dermatitis* 31:201, 1994.
11. Santucci B, Picardo M, Cristaudo A: *Contact Dermatitis* 13:39, 1985.
12. Izu R, Aguirre A, Gil N, et al: *Contact Dermatitis* 26:192-193, 1992.
13. Eun HC, Lee AY: *Contact Dermatitis* 13:310-313, 1985.
14. Huriez C, Martin P: *G Ital Dermatol Minerva Dermatol* 44:463-464, 1969.
15. Gonzalo Garijo MA, Revenga Arranz F, Bobadilla Gonzalez P: *Allergol Immunopathol* 24:132-134, 1996.
16. Vena GA, Angelini GA: *Contact Dermatitis* 15:108-109, 1986.
17. Goossens A, Beck MH, Haneke E, et al: *Contact Dermatitis* 40:112-113, 1999.
18. Incandela L, Cesarone MR, Cacchio M, et al: *Angiology* 52(Suppl 2):S9-S13, 2001.
19. Velasco M, Romero E: *Curr Ther Res Clin Exp* 19:121-125, 1976.
20. Kartnig T: *Herb Spice Med Plant* 3:145-173, 1988.
21. Hadida E, Sayag J, Bonerandi JJ, et al: *Bull Soc Fr Dermatol Syphiligr* 77:522-525, 1970.
22. Appa Rao MVR, Srinivasan K, Koteswara Rao T: *J Res Indian Med* 8:9-15, 1973.
23. Cox DN, Rajasuriya S, Soysa PE, et al: *Int J Food Sci Nutr* 44:123-132, 1993.
24. Peiris KHS, Kays SJ: *Hort Tech* 6:13-18, 1996.
25. Chopra RN, Badhwar RL, Ghosh S: *Poisonous plants of India*, vol 1, New Delhi, 1965, Indian Council of Agricultural Research, pp 433-434.
26. Bagchi CD, Puri HS: *Herba Hung* 27:137-140, 1988.
27. Dharma AP: *Indonesian medicinal plants*, Jakarta, 1987, Balai Pustaka, pp 24-25.
28. van Wyk B-E, Gericke N: *People's plants: a guide to useful plants of Southern Africa*, Arcadia, 2000, Briza Publications, pp 68, 142.
29. Rattanapanone V, Sanpitak N, Phornphibul B: *Chiang Mai Med Bull* 10:17-23, 1971.
30. Kays SJ, Silva Dias JC: *Econ Bot* 49:115-152, 1995.
31. de Lucia R, Sertie JAA: *Fitoterapia* 68:413-416, 1997.
32. Sakina MR, Dandiya PC: *Fitoterapia* 61:291-296, 1990.
33. Dhar ML, Dhar MM, Dhawan BN, et al: *Indian J Exp Biol* 6:232-247, 1968.
34. Boiteau P, Ratsimamanga AR: *Therapie* 11:125-149, 1956.
35. Lawrence JC: *Eur J Pharmacol* 1:414-424, 1967.
36. Ieamworapong C, Kangsadalumpai K, Rojanapo W: *Environ Mol Mutagen* 14(Suppl 15): 93, 1989.
37. Yen GC, Chen HY, Peng HH: *Food Chem Toxicol* 39:1045-1053, 2001.
38. Rivera IG, Martins MT, Sanchez PS, et al: *Environ Toxicol Water Qual* 9:87-93, 1996.
39. Gopalan HNB, Wairimu AN: *Environ Mol Mutagen* 14(Suppl 15):73, 1989.
40. Laerum OD, Iversen OH: *Cancer Res* 32:1463-1468, 1972.

GREATER CELANDINE

Botanical name: *Chelidonium majus* L.
Family: Papaveraceae
Plant part used: Aerial parts

Safety Summary

Pregnancy category C: Has caused or is associated with a substantial risk of causing harmful effects on the foetus or neonate without causing malformations.
Lactation category SD: Strongly discouraged in breastfeeding.
Contraindications: Preexisting liver disease, pregnancy and lactation.
Warnings & precautions: Do not use for extended periods and discontinue use if evidence of liver damage arises. Use cautiously in unconjugated hyperbilirubinaemia, acute or severe hepatocellular disease, septic cholecystitis, intestinal spasm or ileus, liver cancer.
Adverse reactions: Cases of hepatotoxicity and one case of haemolytic anaemia.
Interactions: No precautions required on current evidence.

Typical Therapeutic Use

In an uncontrolled study involving 60 Berlin practices, a high-dose standardised preparation of greater celandine demonstrated good or very good therapeutic effect on symptoms of cramp-like abdominal pains. The dose was initially 5 tablets/day (containing 2.85 mg/tablet of total alkaloids) and this was reduced to 3 tablets/day in patients who responded to treatment.[1]

Traditional indications for greater celandine in Western herbal medicine include gallstones, gallbladder inflammation and topically for warts and other skin tumours.[2] A traditional use in middle Europe is the treatment of tumours—a high alkaloid extract, marketed as Ukrain, is used as an agent in the treatment of carcinoma.

Actions

Choleretic, cholagogue, mild laxative, spasmolytic, antiinflammatory.

Key Constituents

Isoquinoline alkaloids, such as sanguinarine, chelidonine, chelerythrine, berberine and coptisine; the total content of alkaloids reaches 1.3%.[3] These have antiviral, antitumour and antimicrobial properties both in vitro and in vivo.[4]

Adulteration

No adulterants known.

Typical Dosage Forms & Dosage

Typical adult dosage ranges are:
- 6 to 12 g/day of dried aerial parts or by infusion
- 3 to 6 mL/day of a 1:1 liquid extract
- 1 to 2 mL/day of a 1:2 liquid extract or equivalent in tablet or capsule form
- 6 to 12 mL/day of a 1:10 tincture

Note: Doses at the high end of the dosage range are for short-term use only.

Contraindications

Preexisting liver disease. Do not use during pregnancy or lactation without professional advice.

Use in Pregnancy

Category C: Has caused or is associated with a substantial risk of causing harmful effects on the foetus or neonate without causing malformations.

Intramuscular injection of Ukrain (thiophosphoric acid alkaloid derivatives from greater celandine) on days 6 to 11 of gestation to hamsters and on days 6 to 15 of gestation to rats (0.1 to 28 mg/kg/day) did not produce teratogenic effects in either species compared to controls. Slight embryotoxic effects (increased postimplantation losses) and, in consequence, decreased number of average litter size were noted in hamsters exposed to Ukrain at doses which were otherwise not embryotoxic to rats.[5]

Use in Lactation

Category SD: Strongly discouraged in breastfeeding.

Warnings & Precautions

Do not use for extended periods and discontinue use if evidence of liver damage arises. Do not combine with heavy alcohol consumption.

Choleretics and cholagogues should be used cautiously and may be inappropriate in the following:

- Unconjugated hyperbilirubinaemia (jaundice following haemolytic diseases, hereditary disease like Gilbert's and Crigler-Najjar syndromes)
- Acute or severe hepatocellular disease (e.g., following viral hepatitis, cirrhosis, adverse reactions to drugs such as anaesthetics, steroids, oestrogen, chlorpromazine)
- Septic cholecystitis (where there is a risk of peritonitis)
- Intestinal spasm or ileus
- Liver cancer.

Effect on Ability to Drive or Operate Machinery

No adverse effects expected.

Adverse Reactions

The potential association of greater celandine with hepatotoxicity was first reported in 1996. A 69-year-old woman developed symptoms of acute hepatitis after taking tablets containing several herbs, including greater celandine, over a period of 6 weeks. Symptoms returned with rechallenge.[6] Three additional cases were then reported (1997, 1998).[7-9] In one series of observations over 2 years (1997 to 1999) in an area of approximately 1 million inhabitants in Germany, preparations of greater celandine apparently induced 10 cases of acute hepatitis. Investigations and tests excluded viral causes and alcohol intake and hereditary causes were also eliminated. Although immunological factors cannot safely be excluded, the evidence, including liver biopsy, suggested a drug-related pathology. In half the cases cholestasis was observed, but there were no cases of liver failure. In all cases the condition improved quickly when greater celandine was stopped. In one case a rechallenge led to a second attack of hepatitis.[10] Three cases of acute hepatitis associated with greater celandine were reported in

the literature in 2002 to May 2003.[11,12] Generally, hepatotoxicity has been observed after using high dose German products.

A case of haemolytic anaemia has also been observed, with kidney failure and thrombocytopenia.[13] The general safety of greater celandine has been called into question,[14] which prompted a review by the Australian regulatory authorities. The Complementary Medicines Evaluation Committee examined the evidence on 30 May 2003 and deferred making a recommendation on the need for any stronger controls over the herb's availability until a full review is completed.[15]

A case of contact dermatitis has been linked to exposure to the plant.[16]

Interactions

None known.

Safety in Children

No information available, but prolonged use is probably unsuitable in children.

Overdosage

Critical consideration of the often-cited fatal case of poisoning in a 4-year-old boy, observed in 1936, suggests that it is by no means certain that greater celandine should be ascribed to the case. More than 500 g of greater celandine is said to be required to cause toxic effects in horses and cattle.[17]

Toxicology

Table 1 lists LD_{50} data recorded for greater celandine and its constituents.[18,19]

Regulatory Status

See Table 2 for regulatory status in selected countries.

Table 1　**LD_{50} Data Recorded for Greater Celandine and Its Constituents**

Substance	Route, Model	LD_{50} Value	Reference
Decoction of greater celandine	i.p., mice	9.5 g/kg	18
Alkaloids of greater celandine	s.c., mice	300 mg/kg	19

Table **I** **Regulatory Status for Greater Celandine in Selected Countries**

Australia	Greater celandine is not included in Part 4 of Schedule 4 of the Therapeutic Goods Regulations.
UK & Germany	Greater celandine is listed in Part III of the Statutory Instrument SI 2130 (Retail Sale or Supply of Herbal Remedies) Order 1977 and may be prescribed at a maximum single dose of 2 g and a maximum daily dose of 6 g. It is covered by a positive Commission E monograph.
US	Greater celandine does not have generally recognised as safe (GRAS) status. However, it is freely available as a "dietary supplement" in the US under DSHEA legislation (Dietary Supplement Health and Education Act of 1994).

REFERENCES

1. Kniebel R, Urlacher W: *Zeit Allg Med* 69:680-684, 1993.
2. British Herbal Medicine Association's Scientific Committee: *British herbal pharmacopoeia*, Bournemouth, 1983, BHMA, pp 61-62.
3. Wagner H, Bladt S: *Plant drug analysis: a thin layer chromatography atlas*, ed 2, Berlin, 1996, Springer-Verlag, p 10.
4. Colombo ML, Bosisio E: *Pharmacol Res* 33:127-134, 1996.
5. Juszkiewicz T, Minta M, Wlodarczyk B, et al: *Drugs Exp Clin Res* 18(Suppl):23-29, 1992.
6. De Smet PA, Van den Eertwegh AJ, Lesterhuis W, et al: *BMJ* 313:92, 1996.
7. Greving I, Niedereichholz U, Meister V, et al: Poster no. PO19, Europäischer Pharmakovigilanz Kongress, Berlin, February 1997.
8. Greving I, Meister V, Monnerjahn C, et al: *Pharmacoepidemiol Drug Saf* 7:S66-S69, 1998.
9. Strahl S, Ehret V, Dahm HH, et al: *Dtsch Med Wschr* 123:1410-1414, 1998.
10. Benninger J, Schneider HT, Schuppan D, et al: *Gastroenterology* 117:1234-1237, 1999.
11. Crijns AP, de Smet PA, van den Heuvel M, et al: *Ned Tijdschr Geneeskd* 146:124-128, 2002.
12. Stickel F, Poschl G, Seitz HK, et al: *Scand J Gastroenterol* 38:565-568, 2003.
13. Pinto Garcia V, Vicente PR, Barez A, et al: *Sangre (Barc)* 35:401-403, 1990.
14. De Smet P: *Lancet* 360:1336, 2002.
15. Therapeutic Goods Administration: *Concerns about the herb greater celandine (Chelidonium majus)*, available from http://www.health.gov.au/tga/docs/html/celandine.htm, accessed 27 June 2003.
16. Etxenagusia MA, Anda M, Gonzales-Mahave I, et al: *Contact Dermatitis* 43:47, 2000.
17. Frohne D, Pfander HJ: *A colour atlas of poisonous plants: a handbook for pharmacists, doctors, toxicologists, and biologists*, translated from the German ed 2 by Bisset NG, London, 1984, Wolfe Publishing, pp 160-162.
18. Chang HM, But PP: *Pharmacology and applications of Chinese materia medica*, vol 1, Singapore, 1987, World Scientific, pp 390-394.
19. Huang KC: *The pharmacology of Chinese herbs*, Boca Raton, 1993, CRC Press, pp 144-145.

GRINDELIA

Botanical names: *Grindelia camporum* Greene, *G. robusta* Nutt., *G. squarrosa* (Pursh) Dunal, *G. humilis* Hook. et Arn
Family: Compositae
Plant part used: Aerial parts

Safety Summary

Pregnancy category B2: No increase in frequency of malformation or other harmful effects on the foetus from limited use in women. Animal studies are lacking.
Lactation category C: Compatible with breastfeeding.
Contraindications: None required on current evidence.
Warnings & precautions: None required on current evidence.
Adverse reactions: Possible contact dermatitis.
Interactions: No precautions required on current evidence.

Typical Therapeutic Use

Traditional indications for grindelia in Western herbal medicine include asthma, bronchitis and whooping cough.[1]

Actions

Expectorant, spasmolytic, bronchospasmolytic.

Key Constituents

Constituents of the medicinal *Grindelia* spp. include a resin containing diterpenoid acids; phenolic acids, flavonoids, an essential oil, and small amounts of saponins.[2-4]

Adulteration

No adulterants known.

Typical Dosage Forms & Dosage

Typical adult dosage ranges are:
- 6 to 9 g/day of dried aerial parts or by infusion
- 1.8 to 3.6 mL/day of a 1:1 liquid extract
- 1.5 to 3 mL/day of a 1:2 liquid extract or equivalent in tablet or capsule form
- 1.5 to 3 mL/day of a 1:5, 1:8, 1:10 tincture

Contraindications

None known.

Use in Pregnancy

Category B2: No increase in frequency of malformation or other harmful effects on the foetus from limited use in women. Animal studies are lacking.

Use in Lactation

Category C: Compatible with breastfeeding.

Warnings & Precautions

None required.

Effect on Ability to Drive or Operate Machinery

No adverse effects expected.

Adverse Reactions

An unidentified species of *Grindelia*, which was a constituent of a proprietary remedy, produced positive patch test reactions in four patients who had previously suffered from dermatitis caused by contact with plants.[5]

Interactions

None reported.

Safety in Children

No information available, but adverse effects are not expected.

Overdosage

Large doses are reported to cause renal irritation.[1] This warning may be due to the presence of saponins.

No incidents found in the published literature attributable to grindelia. Abuse of asthma powders (burnt and inhaled) attributed to stramonium and belladonna, but containing grindelia, is recorded.[6]

An Eclectic text indicated that overdose with grindelia is toxic, causing paralysis of the muscles of respiration.[7]

Toxicology

No information available.

Regulatory Status

See Table 1 for regulatory status in selected countries.

Table 1   **Regulatory Status for Grindelia in Selected Countries**

Australia	Grindelia is not included in Part 4 of Schedule 4 of the Therapeutic Goods Regulations.
UK & Germany	Grindelia is included on the General Sale List. It is covered by a positive Commission E monograph.
US	Grindelia does not have generally recognised as safe (GRAS) status. However, it is freely available as a "dietary supplement" in the US under DSHEA legislation (Dietary Supplement Health and Education Act of 1994).

REFERENCES

1. British Herbal Medicine Association's Scientific Committee: *British herbal pharmacopoeia*, Bournemouth, 1983, BHMA, p 106.
2. Bruneton J: *Pharmacognosy, phytochemistry, medicinal plants*, Paris, 1995, Lavoisier Publishing, pp 518-519.
3. Kreutzer S, Schimmer O, Waibel R: *Planta Med* 56:392-394, 1990.
4. El-Shamy AM, El-Hawary SS, El-Shabrawy AO, et al: *J Essent Oil Res* 12:631-634, 2000.
5. Mitchell J, Rook A: *Botanical dermatology: plants and plant products injurious to the skin*, Greengrass, 1979, Vancouver, pp 205-206.
6. Gowdy JM: *JAMA* 221:585-587, 1972.
7. Ellingwood F, Lloyd JU: *American materia medica, therapeutics and pharmacognosy*, ed 11, *Naturopathic Medical* series, Botanical vol 2, Portland, 1983, Eclectic Medical Publications, p 247.

GUGGUL

Botanical names: *Commiphora mukul* (Hook. ex Stocks) (*Balsamodendron mukul* Hook. ex Stocks), *Commiphora wightii* (Arn.) Bhand.
Family: Burseraceae
Plant part used: Resinous exudate from the stem

Safety Summary

Pregnancy category C: Has caused or is associated with a substantial risk of causing harmful effects on the foetus or neonate without causing malformations.
Lactation category SD: Strongly discouraged in breastfeeding (on the basis of allergenic potential).
Contraindications: None required on current evidence. Do not use during pregnancy or lactation without professional advice.
Warnings & precautions: Hyperthyroidism. Caution should be exercised when prescribing guggul to patients with coagulation disorders or concomitantly with anticoagulant or antiplatelet medication. Caution is also advised for pregnant women or those wishing to conceive.
Adverse reactions: Mainly mild gastrointestinal upset and headache for guggul fractions and purified gum guggul; a skin rash may also occur with the use of guggul fractions and the crude herb.
Interactions: Propranolol, diltiazem and medications that reduce thyroid activity.

Typical Therapeutic Use

Traditional Ayurvedic uses of guggul include rheumatism, asthma, tuberculosis, debility, indigestion, diarrhoea, amenorrhoea, and menorrhagia. It is also used topically for gum disease and chronic tonsillitis.[1,2]

Guggul gum has been used successfully to lower serum cholesterol in patients with hyperlipidaemia, but mixed results have been obtained for obesity.[3] A semi-refined and standardised extract of guggul resin has shown benefit for the treatment of acne[4] and hyperlipidaemia[5] in clinical trials, although a trial conducted in the United States found this extract did not reduce serum cholesterol.[6]

Actions

Hypocholesterolaemic, antiplatelet, antiinflammatory.

Key Constituents

Key constituents include steroidal compounds such as the guggulsterones (E- and Z-guggulsterone [cis- and trans-4,17(20)-pregnadiene-3,16-dione]) and guggulsterols.[3,7,8] The crude resin contains approximately 2% guggulsterone.[9] The essential oil (within the resin) contains monoterpenes.[10]

Adulteration

The main adulterants of guggul available on the Indian market in the early 1980s were the gums of plants such as *Albizia lebbeck*, *Acacia senegal*, *Acacia arabica*, *Boswellia serrata* and *Moringa oleifera*.[11] Most adulteration is effected by mixing guggul with the cheaper gums.[12] The plant has been overexploited in recent decades and is currently considered an endangered species in the arid regions of India.[13] Both *Commiphora mukul* and *C. wightii* are listed as endangered in these regions.[12,13]

Typical Dosage Forms & Dosage

Typical adult dosage ranges are:
- 6 g/day of guggul gum
- 1 to 1.5 g/day of the petroleum ether fraction of gum guggul
- 1.2 to 6 g/day of the ethyl acetate fraction of gum guggul standardised to contain 40% guggulsterones

Contraindications

None known. Do not use during pregnancy or lactation without professional advice.

Use in Pregnancy

Category C: Has caused or is associated with a substantial risk of causing harmful effects on the foetus or neonate without causing malformations.

Guggul and its acid fraction demonstrated an antifertility effect in vivo (200 and 20 mg/kg/day respectively) for 7 days after oral doses. A reduction in the weights of the uterus, ovaries and cervix of rats was observed with a concomitant increase in the glycogen and sialic acid levels in uterus and ovaries.[14] On the basis of this finding, caution is advised for women wishing to conceive.

In teratogenic studies in rats, monkeys and dogs, the ethyl acetate fraction of gum guggul showed no adverse effects.[15]

Use in Lactation

Category SD: Strongly discouraged in breastfeeding (on the basis of allergenic potential; see below).

Warnings & Precautions

Guggul extract (0.2 g/kg/day, orally for 15 days) induced an increase in serum triiodothyronine (T_3) concentrations in mice.[16] Although the relevance of this research to humans is unknown, caution is advised in patients with hyperthyroidism.

Caution should be exercised when prescribing guggul to patients with coagulation disorders or concomitantly with anticoagulant or antiplatelet medication (see Adverse reactions below).

Effect on Ability to Drive or Operate Machinery

No adverse effects expected.

Adverse Reactions

Crude Guggul: Unpurified and Purified

A traditional Ayurvedic text notes that guggul sometimes produces an erythematous rash and, rarely, symptoms of kidney irritation may appear, but these rapidly disappear when the herb is discontinued.[1] Guggul gum is purified in Ayurveda by several means. One method is to boil guggul gum in a solution in which neem and fresh turmeric paste are dissolved. Undissolved sediments are sifted out when guggul has completely dissolved. The solution is boiled repeatedly until the water has evaporated. The semi-solid guggul is fried in ghee or castor oil and then used. Guggul gum may also be decocted with *Terminalia bellerica*, *Terminalia chebula* and *Phyllanthus emblica* for purification. The unpurified gum causes itching and inflammation when applied locally,[17] and in an early clinical study produced side effects such as skin rashes, diarrhoea, and irregular menstruation. Skin rashes were controlled by reducing the dose.[3]

The incidence of side effects reported in clinical trials of crude guggul gum and purified guggul gum varies and is not dose dependent.[18-20] The most common side effect reported was mild gastrointestinal upset. In one trial this was minimised by taking the herb after food.[19]

Guggul gum and its alcohol-soluble fraction were found to increase coagulation time, prothrombin time and fibrinolytic activity in clinical trials, although there was no change in fibrinogen levels and no observed effect on bleeding time or platelet count.[3]

Guggul: Fractions and Isolated Constituents

Clinical trials on guggul in the late 1970s to mid-1980s investigated a "fraction A" which in some cases was not defined,[21] but was most frequently the petroleum ether fraction of crude gum guggul.[22-25] The most frequent side effect reported was mild diarrhoea, which occurred in 12% to 15% of patients,[22,23] although in other trials no side effects were observed.[3,21,24,25] Other reported side effects from use of this preparation included hiccup and anxiety.[23]

Serum fibrinolytic activity increased and the platelet adhesive index was reduced after administration of a petrol-soluble fraction to both healthy individuals and patients with coronary artery disease.[26]

Later clinical trials investigated the ethyl acetate fraction of gum guggul (EAGG) and its isolated steroidal ketones (guggulsterones). Some trials reported no side effects[1,27-29] and another two trials each reported a single patient with mild gastrointestinal upset.[1,27] Reports of headache and mild gastrointestinal upset occurred 22 and 25 times respectively among 31 patients who received EAGG in a placebo-controlled trial.[30] In another trial there was no difference in the rate of gastrointestinal side effects among EAGG-treated patients and a placebo. However, 11.7% of patients in a high dose group developed a skin rash within 3 days of starting EAGG, compared to 3% in the low dose group and 2.7% in the placebo group.[6]

No adverse effect was recorded for haematological parameters and liver function tests in two trials where such tests were undertaken.[27,30]

Interactions

Coadministration of EAGG (1 g) reduced the peak plasma concentration and area under the curve of single doses of propranolol (40 mg) and diltiazem (60 mg) in healthy volunteers.[31] The bioavailability of digoxin was not significantly reduced by concomitant administration of EAGG in healthy volunteers.[32]

Coadministration of guggulsterones with carbimazole counteracted the decrease in radiolabelled iodine uptake and hypertrophy of the thyroid gland induced by carbimazole in chickens.[33]

Safety in Children

No information available.

Overdosage

No incidents found in published literature.

Toxicology

Table 1 lists LD_{50} data recorded for guggul.[34,35]

No mortality was observed in acute toxicity studies for up to 72 hours after administration of 5 mg/kg dose of petroleum ether fraction of guggul to rats, mice, and dogs. In chronic toxicity studies no mortality occurred in dogs with a dose of 1 g/day over a period of 3 months. However, a 50% mortality rate occurred in rats with a dose of 250 mg/kg per day over 3 months compared to 20% mortality in control groups.[23] The ethyl acetate insoluble portion, which contains carbohydrate constituents, was found to be toxic to animals.[36,37]

EAGG demonstrated no adverse effects in toxicity and mutagenic studies in rats, monkeys, and dogs.[15]

Regulatory Status

See Table 2 for regulatory status in selected countries.

Table 1 **LD_{50} Data Recorded for Guggul**

Substance	Route, Model	LD_{50} Value	Reference
Ethyl acetate fraction of gum guggul	Oral and i.p., mice	>2 g/kg	34
Essential oil	i.p., mice	705 mg/kg	35
Essential oil	Oral, mice	1.7 g/kg	35

Table 2 **Regulatory Status for Guggul in Selected Countries**

Australia	Guggul is not included in Part 4 of Schedule 4 of the Therapeutic Goods Regulations. However, it is also not included on the Herbal Substances Australian Approved Name (AAN) list. Without an AAN, a herb cannot be included in products for supply in or export from Australia without prior evaluation by an expert committee.
UK & Germany	Guggul is not included on the General Sale List. It was not included in the Commission E assessment.
US	Guggul does not have generally recognised as safe (GRAS) status. However, it is freely available as a "dietary supplement" in the US under DSHEA legislation (Dietary Supplement Health and Education Act of 1994).

REFERENCES

1. Chopra RN, Chopra IC, Handa KL, et al: *Chopra's indigenous drugs of India*, ed 2, 1958; reprinted Calcutta, 1982, Academic Publishers, pp 285-287.
2. Thakur RS, Puri HS, Husain A: *Major medicinal plants of India*, Lucknow, 1989, Central Institute of Medicinal and Aromatic Plants, pp 208-211.
3. Satyavati GV: Guggulipid: a promising hypolipidaemic agent from gum guggul (*Commiphora wightii*). In Wagner H, Farnsworth NR, eds: *Economic and medicinal plant research*, vol 5, London, 1991, Academic Press, pp 47-82.
4. Thappa DM, Dogra J: *J Dermatol* 21:729-731, 1994.
5. Nityanand S, Srivastava JS, Asthana OP: *J Assoc Physicians India* 37:323-328, 1989.

6. Szapary PO, Wolfe ML, Bloedon LT, et al: Abstract presented at the Third Annual Conference of Alternative and Complementary Medicine, Chicago, December 2001.

7. Kapoor LD: *CRC handbook of Ayurvedic medicinal plants*, Boca Raton, 1990, CRC Press, pp 131-132.

8. Patil VD, Nayak UR, Sukh Dev: *Tetrahedron* 28:2341-2352, 1972.

9. Mesrob B, Nesbitt C, Misra R, et al: *J Chromatogr B Biomed Sci Appl* 720:189-196, 1998.

10. Saxena VK, Sharma RN: *J Med Arom Plant Sci* 20:55-56, 1998.

11. Central Council for Research in Ayurveda and Siddha: *CCRAS New Lett* 4:1-7, 1982.

12. Indrayan AK, Shukla RK, Dwivedi S, et al: *J Med Arom Plant Sci* 22/23:686-689, 2001.

13. Dixit AM, Rao SVS: *Trop Ecol* 41:81-88, 2000.

14. Amma MK, Malhotra N, Suri RK, et al: *Indian J Exp Biol* 16:1021-1023, 1978.

15. Gugulipid studies, Lucknow, India, 1986, Central Drug Research Institute.

16. Panda S, Kar A: *Life Sci* 65:PL137-PL141, 1999.

17. Shanavaskhan AE, Binu S, Unnithan CM, et al: *Fitoterapia* 68:69-74, 1997.

18. Sharma KP, Sharma R, Prakash S: *J Res Indian Med Yoga Homoeo* 11:132-134, 1976.

19. Kuppurajan K, Rajagopalan SS, Koteswara Rao T, et al: *J Res Indian Med* 8:1-8, 1973.

20. Verma SK, Bordia A: *Indian J Med Res* 87:356-360, 1988.

21. Sharma JN, Sharma JN, Shastri HD, et al: *Rheumatism* 8:21-53, 1972.

22. Malhotra SC, Ahuja MMS, Sundaram KR: *Indian J Med Res* 65:390-395, 1977.

23. Malhotra SC, Ahuja MMS: *Indian J Med Res* 59:1621-1632, 1971.

24. Kuppurajan K, Rajagopalan SS, Koteswara Rao T, et al: *J Assoc Physicians India* 26:367-373, 1978.

25. Kotiyal JP, Bisht DB, Singh DS: *J Res Indian Med Yoga Homoeo* 14:11-15, 1979.

26. Bordia A, Chuttani SK: *Indian J Med Res* 70:992-996, 1979.

27. Agarwal RC, Singh SP, Saran RK et al: *Indian J Med Res* 84:626-634, 1986.

28. Gopal K, Saran RK, Nityanand S et al: *J Assoc Physicians India* 34:249-251, 1986.

29. Beg M, Singhal KC, Afzaal S: *Indian J Physiol Pharmacol* 40:237-240, 1996.

30. Singh RB, Niaz MA, Ghosh S: *Cardiovasc Drugs Ther* 8:659-664, 1994.

31. Dalvi SS, Nayak VK, Pohujani SM et al: *J Assoc Physicians India* 42:454-455, 1994.

32. Moghe VV, Dalvi SS, Joshi MV et al: *Indian J Hosp Pharm* 31:172-174, 1994.

33. Tripathi SN, Gupta M, Sen SP et al: *Indian J Exp Biol* 13:15-18, 1975.

34. Shanker G, Singh HK: *Indian J Pharmacol* 33:296-308, abstract no. 220, 2001.

35. Bagi MK, Kakrani HK, Kalyani GA, et al: *Fitoterapia* 56:245-248, 1985.

36. Nityanand S, Kapoor NK: *Indian J Exp Biol* 11:395-396, 1973.

37. Sukh Dev: *Proc Indian Natl Sci Acad* 49A:359-385, 1983.

GYMNEMA

Botanical name: *Gymnema sylvestre* (Retz.) Schultes
Family: Asclepiadaceae
Plant part used: Leaf

Safety Summary

Pregnancy category B2: No increase in frequency of malformation or other harmful effects on the foetus from limited use in women. Animal studies are lacking.
Lactation category ND: No data available.
Contraindications: None required on current evidence.
Warnings & precautions: Prescribe cautiously with hypoglycaemic drugs and insulin. The use of herbs rich in saponins is possibly inappropriate in coeliac disease, fat malabsorption, and vitamins A, D, E, and K deficiency, some upper digestive irritations, and topically to open wounds. Caution in patients with preexisting cholestasis.
Adverse reactions: Herbs rich in saponins may cause irritation of the gastric mucous membranes and reflux.
Interactions: Prescribe cautiously with hypoglycaemic drugs and insulin.

Typical Therapeutic Use

Gymnema reduced appetite, calorie intake and sense of taste for sweet foods[1] and demonstrated therapeutic benefit in the treatment of diabetes mellitus (both insulin-dependent and non–insulin-dependent)[2,3] in controlled clinical trials. Traditional indications for gymnema in Ayurveda include diabetes, glycosuria and urinary disorders.[4,5]

Actions

Antidiabetic, hypoglycaemic, hypocholesterolaemic, weight reducing.

Key Constituents

Constituents of gymnema leaves include saponins which are present as both nonacylated glycosides, known as gymnemasaponins, and the acylated gymnemic acids.[6] The total gymnemic acid content in leaf samples was 3.9% to 4.6%.[7]

Adulteration

No adulterants known.

Typical Dosage Forms & Dosage

Typical adult dosage ranges are:
- 6 to 60 g/day of dried leaf by infusion
- 3.5 to 11 mL/day of a 1:1 liquid extract or equivalent in tablet or capsule form

Contraindications

None known.

Use in Pregnancy

Category B2: No increase in frequency of malformation or other harmful effects on the foetus from limited use in women. Animal studies are lacking.

Folk use of the root of gymnema to promote abortion has been reported.[8]

Use in Lactation

Category ND: No data available.

Warnings & Precautions

Gymnema should be prescribed cautiously with hypoglycaemic drugs and insulin due to its potential blood glucose lowering activity. The patient should be warned about possible hypoglycaemia and have their blood sugar monitored regularly. If the dose of their drug medication needs to be reduced, this should be done in conjunction with the prescribing physician.

The use of herbs rich in saponins is possibly inappropriate in coeliac disease, fat malabsorption, and vitamins A, D, E, and K deficiency, some upper digestive irritations and topically to open wounds. Saponin-containing herbs are best kept to a minimum in patients with preexisting cholestasis.

Effect on Ability to Drive or Operate Machinery

No adverse effects expected.

Adverse Reactions

As with all herbs rich in saponins, oral use may cause irritation of the gastric mucous membranes and reflux.

Interactions

Although no cases of interaction have been described in the literature, gymnema should be prescribed cautiously with hypoglycaemic drugs and insulin, due to its potential blood glucose lowering activity.

Safety in Children

No information available, but adverse effects are not expected.

Overdosage

No incidents found in published literature.

Toxicology

In acute toxicity studies no gross behavioural, neurological, or autonomic effects were observed in mice orally administered graded doses (0.25 to 8 g/kg) of an aqueous–alcoholic concentrate of gymnema (19.5:1). The oral LD_{50} for this concentrate was 3.99 g/kg (equivalent to 78 g/kg of dried gymnema leaf).[9] Daily oral administration of 33 mg/kg of an aqueous–alcoholic extract of gymnema leaf (containing 2.4% gymnemic acids) for 10 weeks to rats did not affect food intake, body weight, haematological and biochemical parameters, organ weights, or renal and hepatic histology compared to controls.[10]

Regulatory Status

See Table 1 for regulatory status in selected countries.

Table 1   **Regulatory Status for Gymnema in Selected Countries**

Australia	Gymnema is not included in Part 4 of Schedule 4 of the Therapeutic Goods Regulations.
UK & Germany	Gymnema is not included on the General Sale List. It was not included in the Commission E assessment.
US	Gymnema does not have generally recognised as safe (GRAS) status. However, it is freely available as a "dietary supplement" in the US under DSHEA legislation (Dietary Supplement Health and Education Act of 1994).

REFERENCES

1. Brala PM, Hagen RL: *Physiol Behav* 30:1-9, 1983.
2. Shanmugasundaram ER, Rajeswari G, Baskaran K, et al: *J Ethnopharmacol* 30:281-294, 1990.
3. Baskaran K, Kizar Ahamath B, Radha Shanmugasundaram K, et al: *J Ethnopharmacol* 30:295-300, 1990.
4. Thakur RS, Puri HS, Husain A: *Major medicinal plants of India*, Lucknow, 1989, Central Institute of Medicinal and Aromatic Plants, pp 299-302.
5. Chopra RN, Chopra IC, Handa KL, et al: *Chopra's indigenous drugs of India*, ed 2, 1958; reprinted Calcutta, 1982, Academic Publishers, pp 336-339.
6. Hostettmann K, Marston A: *Chemistry & pharmacology of natural products: saponins*, Cambridge, 1995, Cambridge University Press, p 281.
7. Yokota T, Mizutani K, Kenzo O, et al: *Nippon Shokuhin Kogyo Gakkaishi* 41:202-205, 1994.
8. Tarafder CR: *J Econ Taxon Bot* 4:507-516, 1983.
9. Chattopadhyay RR: *J Ethnopharmacol* 67:367-372, 1999.
10. Shigematsu N, Asano R, Shimosaka M, et al: *Biol Pharm Bull* 24:643-649, 2001.

HAWTHORN LEAF & FLOWER

Botanical names: *Crataegus monogyna* Jacq. (Lindm.), *Crataegus laevigata* (Poir.) DC (*C. oxyacantha* auct., *C. oxyacanthoides* Thuill.)
Family: Rosaceae
Plant part used: Leaf and flower

Safety Summary

Pregnancy category B1: No increase in frequency of malformation or other harmful effects on the foetus from limited use in women. No evidence of increased foetal damage in animal studies.
Lactation category C: Compatible with breastfeeding.
Contraindications: None required on current evidence.
Warnings & precautions: Not to be used concomitantly with heart and blood pressure medication unless supervised by a qualified herbal practitioner or physician.
Adverse reactions: Very rare various minor adverse effects.
Interactions: Hawthorn may act in synergy with digitalis glycosides, beta-blockers and other hypotensive drugs. Modification of drug dosage may be required.

Typical Therapeutic Use

Hawthorn has been thoroughly researched. In vitro and in vivo studies have suggested the following pharmacological actions[1]:
(1) cAMP-independent positive inotropy;
(2) peripheral and coronary vasodilation;
(3) protection against ischaemia-induced ventricular arrhythmias;
(4) antioxidative properties; and
(5) antiinflammatory effects.

It has also been the subject of a number of positive clinical trials, including a major long-term multicentre study on the survival and prognosis of congestive heart failure.[2]

Traditional indications for hawthorn in Western herbal medicine include cardiac failure, angina, hypertension, and symptoms of arteriosclerosis.[3]

Actions

Cardiotonic (mild), cardioprotective, antioxidant, collagen stabilising, astringent, hypotensive, antiarrhythmic.

Key Constituents

Oligomeric procyanidins (1% to 3%), mainly procyanidin B-2, based on the condensation of catechin and/or epicatechin.[4]

Flavonoids (1% to 2%), including quercetin glycosides (hyperoside, rutin) and flavone-C-glycosides (vitexin).[5] The flowers contain the highest levels of flavonoids and the leaves contain the highest levels of oligomeric procyanidins.

Adulteration

No adulterants known.

Typical Dosage Forms & Dosage

Typical adult dosage ranges:
- 0.75 to 6 g/day of dried flower, leaf or by infusion
- 3 to 6 mL/day of a 1:2 liquid extract of hawthorn leaf or equivalent in tablet or capsule form
- 3.5 to 17.5 mL/day of a 1:5 tincture of hawthorn leaf
- concentrated extracts and powders (3:1 to 5:1), standardised to various levels of flavonoid and/or oligomeric procyanidin content

Contraindications

None known.

Use in Pregnancy

Category B1: No increase in frequency of malformation or other harmful effects on the foetus from limited use in women. No evidence of increased foetal damage in animal studies.

At a very high oral dosage of 2.8 g/kg administered from days 1 to 15 of gestation, hawthorn (part undefined) did not have an adverse effect on reproductive outcome in rats. Foetal weights were slightly increased when the herb was administered from days 8 to 15 of gestation. There was no difference in placental weight, the number of resorptions, or litter size. There were no externally visible malformations. The herb was administered as an ethanol extract and the dose administered was the highest possible for which ethanol remained below the teratogenic threshold.[6]

Use in Lactation

Category C: Compatible with breastfeeding.

Warnings & Precautions

Not to be used concomitantly with heart and blood pressure medication unless supervised by a qualified herbal practitioner or physician.

Effect on Ability to Drive or Operate Machinery

No adverse effects expected.

Adverse Reactions

There was very low reporting of adverse effects in a placebo-controlled clinical trial of two doses of standardised extract taken by patients with heart failure over 16 weeks.[7] This was also observed in a larger placebo-controlled study over 24 weeks[8] and further studies over 12 weeks[9,10] and 8 weeks.[11,12] In all cases, efficacy of the product compared to placebo was demonstrated. The general lack of adverse reports in clinical research studies on hawthorn was confirmed in another study.[13]

At therapeutic dosages, hawthorn has been reported to cause a mild rash, headache, sweating, dizziness, palpitations, sleepiness, agitation, and gastrointestinal symptoms.[14] However, these are, in the experience of most clinicians, rare and mild events.

One case of a type I hypersensitivity reaction to hawthorn has been reported.[15]

Interactions

Speculation on a harmful interaction with digoxin[16] has not been borne out in any study. A large number of patients, previously treated unsuccessfully with digoxin alone, were compensated for rest and slight stress with relatively low oral doses of the glycoside in combination with hawthorn and without evidence of adverse effects.[17,18] A randomised, crossover trial published in June 2003, involving eight healthy volunteers, confirmed that standardised hawthorn extract (leaf and flower extract, 900 mg/day) and digoxin may be coadministered safely.[19] However, an in vivo effect, blocking repolarising potassium currents in ventricular cells (thus reducing contractility), is suggested as showing a similarity in action to some antiarrhythmic drugs.[20]

Hawthorn may act in synergy with digitalis glycosides, beta-blockers, and other hypotensive drugs. Modification of drug dosage may be required.

Safety in Children

No information available, but adverse effects are not expected.

Overdosage

No incidents found in published literature.

Toxicology

Studies involving excessive dosing of hawthorn flower extract (600 mg/kg/day; undefined extract strength, 4.4% flavonoids) over 30 days in rats showed unremarkable adverse effects.[21]

The acute oral toxicity in undefined animals of hawthorn was 6 g/kg. No target-organ toxicity was defined at 100 times the human dose (2.7 mg/kg) of concentrated hawthorn extract. Standard mutagenic and clastogenic tests were also negative.[22]

Schimmer and co-workers found that an ethanolic extract of Crataegus was weakly mutagenic in the *Salmonella* test, a finding which they attributed to the quercitin content of the extract.[23] Popp and coworkers found a DNA-damaging potency of commercial *Crataegus* preparations in human lymphocyte cultures.[24] The active principles were not identified, but were probably flavonoids. Several procyanidins with different degrees of polymerisation (dimers, a trimer, and a polymer) were found to be nonmutagenic in the *Salmonella* mutagenesis assay system.[25]

Regulatory Status

See Table 1 for regulatory status in selected countries.

Table **I**   **Regulatory Status for Hawthorn in Selected Countries**

Australia	Hawthorn is not included in Part 4 of Schedule 4 of the Therapeutic Goods Regulations.
UK & Germany	Hawthorn is not included on the General Sale List. Hawthorn leaf and flower combined are covered by a positive Commission E monograph. Hawthorn berry, flower and leaf are each individually covered by negative assessments. Hawthorn berries and hawthorn leaf and flower are both official in the *European Pharmacopoeia* 4.3.
US	Hawthorn does not have generally recognised as safe (GRAS) status. However, it is freely available as a "dietary supplement" in the US under DSHEA legislation (Dietary Supplement Health and Education Act of 1994). Hawthorn flower and leaf is official in the *United States Pharmacopeia-National Formulary* (USP 26-NF 21, 2003).

REFERENCES

1. Loew D: *Wien Med Wochenschr* 149:226-228, 1999.
2. Holubarsch CJ, Colucci WS, Meinertz T, et al: *Eur J Heart Fail* 2:431-437, 2000.
3. British Herbal Medicine Association's Scientific Committee: *British herbal pharmacopoeia*, Bournemouth, 1983, BHMA, pp 74-75.
4. British Herbal Medicine Association's Scientific Committee: *British herbal pharmacopoeia*, Bournemouth, 1983, BHMA, pp 198.
5. Rehwald A, Meier B, Sticher O: *J Chromatogr A* 677:25-33, 1994.
6. Yao M, Brown-Woodman PDC, Ritchie H: *Teratology* 64:320-325, 2001.
7. Tauchert M: *Am Heart J* 143:910-915, 2002.
8. Tauchert M, Gildor A, Lipinski J: *Herz* 24:465-474, 1999.
9. Zapfe G Jr: *Phytomedicine* 8:262-266, 2001.
10. Rietbrock N, Hamel M, Hempel B, et al: *Arzneim Forsch* 51:793-798, 2001.
11. Weikl A, Assmus KD, Neukum-Schmidt A, et al: *Fortschr Med* 114:291-296, 1996.
12. Leuchtgens H: *Fortschr Med* 111:352-354, 1993.
13. Weihmayr T, Ernst E: *Fortschr Med* 114:27-29, 1996.
14. Rigelsky JM, Sweet BV: *Am J Health Syst Pharm* 59:417-422, 2002.
15. Steinman HK, Lovell CR, Cronin E: *Contact Dermatitis* 11:321, 1984.
16. Miller LG: *Arch Intern Med* 158:2200-2211, 1998.
17. Wolkerstorfer H: *MMW* 108:438-441, 1966.
18. Jaursch U, Landers E, Schmidt R, et al: *Med Welt* 27:1547-1552, 1969.
19. Tankanow R, Tamer HR, Streetman DS, et al: *J Clin Pharmacol* 43:637-642, 2003.
20. Muller A, Linke W, Klaus W: *Planta Med* 65:335-339, 1999.
21. Fehri B, Aiache JM, Boukef K, et al: *J Pharm Belg* 46:165-176, 1991.
22. Schlegelmilch R, Heywood R: *J Am Coll Toxicol* 13:103-111, 1994.
23. Schimmer O, Hafele F, Kruger A: *Mutat Res* 206:201-208, 1988.
24. Popp R, Paulini H, Volkl S, et al: *Planta Med* 55:644-645, 1989.
25. Yu CL, Swaminathan B: *Food Chem Toxicol* 25:135-140, 1987.

HOPS

Botanical name: *Humulus lupulus* L.
Family: Cannabinaceae
Plant part used: Female inflorescence or strobile

Safety Summary

Pregnancy category B2: No increase in frequency of malformation or other harmful effects on the foetus from limited use in women. Animal studies are lacking.
Lactation category CC: Compatible with breastfeeding but use caution.
Contraindications: Possibly depressive illness. Do not use during lactation without professional advice.
Warnings & precautions: In principle, herbal sedatives are best avoided in depression and insomnia marked by increasing restlessness during the early hours of the morning. Use of herbal sedatives should ideally be limited in duration.
Adverse reactions: Rare contact allergies.
Interactions: No precautions required on current evidence.

Typical Therapeutic Use

Traditional use of hops in Western herbal medicine include nervous tension, anxiety, restlessness, and difficulty in falling asleep.[1]

Actions

Mild sedative,[2] hypnotic, spasmolytic,[3] aromatic bitter.

Key Constituents

Key constituents of hops are the bitter resinoid principles (15% to 25%).[4] The essential oil contains mainly myrcene, humulene, and caryophyllene, with a trace of 2-methyl-3-buten-2-ol, increasing to a maximum (approximately 0.15%) after storage.[5] Other constituents include the chalcone xanthohumol,[6] phyto-oestrogenic constituents, especially 8-prenylnaringenin,[7] and other flavonoids and tannins (2% to 4%).[8]

Adulteration

Medicinal hops is rarely adulterated with wild hops, which has a lower content of bitter acids.[9]

Typical Dosage Forms & Dosage

Typical adult dosage ranges are:
- 1.5 to 3 g/day of dried strobile or by infusion
- 1.5 to 3 mL/day of a 1:1 liquid extract
- 1.5 to 3 mL/day of a 1:2 liquid extract or equivalent in tablet or capsule form
- 3 to 6 mL/day of a 1:5 tincture

Contraindications

In one tradition depressive illness,[10] but this is not universally accepted. Do not use during lactation without professional advice.

Use in Pregnancy

Category B2: No increase in frequency of malformation or other harmful effects on the foetus from limited use in women. Animal studies are lacking.

There is postulated oestrogenic action[11,12] (linked to the competitive binding of hops extract to oestrogenic receptors,[13] and in vitro and in vivo activity of 8-prenylnaringenin[14]) that might raise theoretical safety concerns. However, very high doses of hops would be required and, for example, the consumption of beer required for these effects would be considerable.[15,16] (Oestrogenic stimulation of the vaginal epithelium in an experimental model required concentrations of 100 μg/mL, about 500-fold greater than is found in beer.[15]) The polyphenol xanthohumol has oestrogenic activity and, although present in freshly harvested hops, it disappears rapidly through oxidation, even on cold storage.[17]

Use in Lactation

Category CC: Compatible with breastfeeding but use caution due to possible sedating effects in the infant.

Warnings & Precautions

In principle, herbal sedatives are best avoided in depression and insomnia marked by increasing restlessness during the early hours of the morning. Use of herbal sedatives should ideally be limited in duration.

Effect on Ability to Drive or Operate Machinery

No adverse effects expected, since the sedative effects are mild.

Adverse Reactions

Contact reactions including urticaria have been reported to hops, especially fresh strobiles and hop dust.[18,19] In one case there was previous urticaria-angioedema from peanut, chestnut, and banana.[20] However, these are very rare events, they do not cause respiratory problems,[21] and do not transfer to a sensitivity to ingested hops products such as beer.[22]

Interactions

None known.

Safety in Children

No information available, but adverse effects are not expected.

Overdosage

No incidents found in published literature.

Toxicology

Table 1 lists LD_{50} data recorded for hops extracts and its constituents.[23]

Large daily intragastric doses of lupulone may be given to common laboratory animals without appreciable effect. Mice fed 2% to 4% lupulone in food for 40 days showed a leucocytic infiltration into the lungs and sometimes bronchopneumonia.[24]

Regulatory Status

See Table 2 for regulatory status in selected countries.

Hops are widely consumed as the alcoholic beverage beer.

Table 1 **LD_{50} Data Recorded for Hops Extracts and Its Constituents**

Substance	Route, Model	LD_{50} Value	Reference
Ethanol extract of hops	Oral, mice	3.5 g/kg	23
Ethanol extract of hops	Oral, rats	2.7 g/kg	23
Ethanol dry extract of hops	Oral, mice	2.7 g/kg	23
Ethanol dry extract of hops	Oral, rats	415 mg/kg	23
Lupulone	Oral, mice	525 mg/kg	23

Table 2 **Regulatory Status for Hops in Selected Countries**

Australia	Hops is not included in Part 4 of Schedule 4 of the Therapeutic Goods Regulations.
UK & Germany	Hops is included on the General Sale List. It is covered by a positive Commission E monograph.
US	Hops does have generally recognised as safe (GRAS) status. It is freely available as a "dietary supplement" in the US under DSHEA legislation (Dietary Supplement Health and Education Act of 1994).

REFERENCES

1. British Herbal Medicine Association's Scientific Committee: *British herbal pharmacopoeia*, Bournemouth, 1983, BHMA, pp 111-112.
2. Wohlfart R, Hansel R, Schmidt H: *Planta Med* 48:120-123, 1983.
3. Caujolle F, Chanh PH, Duch-Kan P, et al: *Agressologie* 10:405-410, 1969.
4. Hölzl J: *Z Phytotherapie* 13:155-161, 1992.
5. Hänsel R, Wohlfart R, Schmidt H: *Planta Med* 45:224-228, 1982.
6. Gerhauser C, Alt A, Heiss E, et al: *Mol Cancer Ther* 1:959-969, 2002.
7. Coldham NG, Sauer MJ: *Food Chem Toxicol* 39:1211-1224, 2001.
8. Bisset NG (ed.): *Herbal drugs and phytopharmaceuticals: a handbook for practice on a scientific basis.*

Stuttgart, 1994, Medpharm Scientific Publishers, pp 305-308.

9. Blaschek W, Ebel S, Hackenthal E, et al: *HagerROM 2002: Hagers Handbuch der Drogen und Arzneistoffe.* Heidelberg, 2002, Springer.

10. British Herbal Medicine Association: *British herbal compendium*, vol 1, Bournemouth, 1992, BHMA, pp 128-130.

11. Hesse R, Hoffmann B, Karg H, et al: *Zbl Vet Med* 28:442-454, 1981.

12. Kumai A, Okamoto R: *Toxicol Lett* 21:203-207, 1984.

13. Liu J, Burdette JE, Xu H, et al: *J Agric Food Chem* 49:2472-2479, 2001.

14. Coldham NG, Sauer MJ: *Food Chem Toxicol* 39:1211-1224, 2001.

15. Milligan S, Kalita J, Pocock V, et al: *Reproduction* 123:235-242, 2002.

16. Rong H, Boterberg T, Maubach J, et al: *Eur J Cell Biol* 80:580-585, 2001.

17. Verzele M: *J Inst Brew* 92:32-48, 1986.

18. Pradalier A, Campinos C, Trinh C: *Allerg Immunol (Paris)* 34:330-332, 2002.

19. Hogan DJ, Lane P: *Occup Med State Art Rev* 1:285-300, 1986.

20. Estrada JL, Gozalo F, Cecchini C, et al: *Contact Dermatitis* 46:127, 2002.

21. Meznar B, Kajba S: *Plucne Bolesti* 42:27-29, 1990.

22. Raith L, Jager K: *Contact Dermatitis* 11:53, 1984.

23. Hänsel R, Wagener HH: *Arzneim Forsch* 17:79–81, 1967.

24. Chin YC, Anderson HH: *Arch Int Pharmacodyn Ther* 82:1-15, 1950.

HORSECHESTNUT

Other common name: Horse chestnut
Botanical name: *Aesculus hippocastanum* L.
Family: Hippocastanaceae
Plant part used: Seed

Safety Summary

Pregnancy category B3: No increase in frequency of malformation or other harmful effects on the foetus from limited use in women. Evidence of increased foetal damage in animal studies exists, although the relevance to humans is unknown.
Lactation category CC: Compatible with breast-feeding but use caution.
Contraindications: Do not apply to broken or ulcerated skin. Do not use during pregnancy or lactation without professional advice.
Warnings & precautions: The use of herbs rich in saponins is possibly inappropriate in coeliac disease, fat malabsorption, and vitamins A, D, E and K deficiency and some upper digestive irritations. Caution in patients with preexisting cholestasis.
Adverse reactions: Gastrointestinal complaints, dizziness, nausea, headache, and pruritus. Herbs rich in saponins may also cause reflux.
Interactions: No precautions required on current evidence.

Typical Therapeutic Use

Meta-analysis and review of randomised, double-blind, controlled trials and observational studies have concluded that horsechestnut seed extract is an effective treatment for chronic venous insufficiency.[1,2] Traditional indications for horsechestnut in Western herbal medicine include conditions involving venous congestion or throbbing pain and fullness, such as varicose veins, haemorrhoids, rectal neuralgia, and proctitis.[3]

Actions

Venotonic, antioedematous, antiinflammatory, antiecchymotic (against bruises).

Key Constituents

Constituents of horsechestnut seed include saponins (3% to 6%), collectively referred to as aescin, and flavonoids. Aescin is a complex mixture of over 30 individual pentacyclic triterpene diester glycosides.[4,5] The toxic coumarin esculin (aesculin) has been found in the bark, bud, and pericarp of the fruit of horsechestnut, but not in the seed.[6,7] Aescin (also known as escin) is registered as a therapeutic drug in parts of Europe, and is often administered by injection.

Adulteration

No adulterants known.

Typical Dosage Forms & Dosage

Typical adult dosage ranges are:
- 1 to 2 g/day of dried seed or by decoction
- 2 to 5 mL/day of a 1:2 liquid extract or equivalent in tablet or capsule form
- 5 to 15 mL/day of a 1:5 tincture
- standardised extract corresponding to 100 mg/day of aescin

Contraindications

Because of the irritant effect of the saponins, horsechestnut should not be applied to broken or ulcerated skin. Do not use during pregnancy or lactation without professional advice.

Use in Pregnancy

Category B3: No increase in frequency of malformation or other harmful effects on the foetus from limited use in women. Evidence of increased foetal damage in animal studies exists, although the relevance to humans is unknown.

Standardised horsechestnut seed extracts have been used successfully in clinical studies[8-11] to treat venous conditions in pregnant women at dosages of 600 mg/day (containing 100 mg aescin) for 2 to 4 weeks. Some studies excluded women in the third trimester of pregnancy.[9,10]

Intravenous administration of standardised horsechestnut seed extract (9 and 30 mg/kg/day) to rats (days 6 to 15 gestation) and rabbits (days 6 to 18 gestation) did not result in teratogenicity or embryotoxicity. The same results were demonstrated in rats (100 and 300 mg/kg/day) and rabbits (100 mg/kg/day) after oral administration. Although no teratogenic effects were observed in rabbits orally administered very high doses of extract (300 mg/kg/day), foetal body weights were significantly reduced compared to controls.[12]

Use in Lactation

Category CC: Compatible with breastfeeding but use caution.

Warnings & Precautions

The use of herbs rich in saponins is possibly inappropriate in coeliac disease, fat malabsorption, and vitamins A, D, E and K deficiency, and some upper digestive irritations. Saponin-containing herbs are best kept to a minimum in patients with preexisting cholestasis.

Effect on Ability to Drive or Operate Machinery

No adverse effects expected.

Adverse Reactions

A 2002 review of 14 randomised, double-blind, controlled trials concluded that oral horsechestnut seed extract (standardised to 50 to 150 mg/day aescin) for 20 days to 12 weeks is a safe and effective treatment for chronic venous insufficiency. Eight trials reported on adverse reactions, with four of these trials reporting that there were no treatment-related reactions. Over all eight trials, 2.6% of 575 patients reported mild adverse reactions, which included mild gastrointestinal complaints, dizziness, nausea, headache, and pruritus.[2] A 2002 meta-analysis of adverse reactions found no significant difference between horsechestnut seed extract and placebo.[1] Meta-analysis of three postmarketing surveillance studies, which included 10,725 patients, found that an average of 1.51% of patients treated with horsechestnut seed extract reported mild adverse reactions.[1] From 1968 until 1989 nearly 900 million individual doses of one brand of standardised horsechestnut seed extract were prescribed. In that time, only 15 patients reported significant side effects.[13]

A case has been reported in Japan where pruritus, jaundice, elevated liver enzymes, liver cholestasis, centrilobular necrosis, and mild eosinophilia developed 60 days after intramuscular injection of a product containing horsechestnut extract for pathological bone fracture. Drug-induced hepatic injury was suspected.[14] The product has been in use in Japan since 1967 and only mild side effects, such as nausea, vomiting, urticaria and, rarely, spasm and shock, have been reported.[14,15]

Cases of pseudolupus (an autoimmune syndrome) after use of a product containing phenopyrazone, horsechestnut extract and cardiac glycosides have been reported.[16] The ingredient or ingredients responsible for this reaction were not established. Urticaria and dyspnoea have been reported after topical application of aescin.[17,18]

As with all herbs rich in saponins, oral use may cause irritation of the gastric mucous membranes and reflux. This can be minimised by the use of enteric-coated tablets. Saponins and sapogenins are generally recognised as having haemolytic properties, but this effect is negligible at the oral doses used.

Interactions

A case of acute renal insufficiency after therapy with aescin and the antibiotic gentamycin has been reported.[19] (It is likely that aescin was administered by injection.) High doses of intravenous aescin have been implicated in acute renal failure[20] (see the Overdosage section below.) Aescin is a saponin which can cause haemolysis after injection. The liberated haemoglobin can deposit in the kidneys and cause renal failure. The risk of haemolysis after oral intake of horsechestnut is minimal.

Safety in Children

Poisonings in children due to the ingestion of horsechestnut seeds or infusions made from the leaves and twigs have been reported, including fatalities.[21] However, in an analysis of human exposures to *Aesculus* spp., which included 1527 children aged 0 to 5 years, serious toxicity was not reported and no effect or a nontoxic effect occurred in the majority of cases.[22] Cases of toxicity in children attributed to horsechestnut seed might have actually resulted from ingestion of the seed capsule (pericarp).

Overdosage

Very high doses will result in gastrointestinal irritation. If sufficient quantities of aescin are absorbed through damaged or irritated gastrointestinal mucous membranes, haemolysis with associated kidney damage could result.[23]

Cases of acute renal failure have been reported which were suspected to have been caused by high doses of aescin (510 to 540 µg/kg) administered intravenously for postoperative oedema.[20,24] However, in trials designed to assess the effects of intravenous aescin on renal function, no signs of impaired renal function developed in patients with normal renal function, and renal function did not worsen in patients with preexisting renal impairment. Adults received (10 to 25 mg/day) intravenous aescin for 3 to 10 days, and two children with normal renal function were prescribed 0.2 mg/day for 6 days.[17,25-27]

In the United States, an analysis of 3099 cases of human exposure to plant parts from eight different *Aesculus* spp. from 1985 to 1994 found that no effect or a nontoxic effect was recorded in 76.6% of cases. Most exposures (49.2%) occurred in children aged 0 to 5 years. Analysis of the 1993 to 1994 subset (571 cases) found that no cases of serious toxicity were reported and gastrointestinal symptoms occurred in only 5% of cases.[22]

Toxicology

Table 1 lists LD_{50} data recorded for horsechestnut extract and its constituents.[12,28,29]

Horsechestnut seed extract has low oral toxicity. The substantially higher toxicity after i.p. or i.v. administration is probably a reflection of the haemolytic activity of aescin.

No toxic effects were observed in the behaviour, growth, food consumption, haematological and biochemical tests, or organ histology of rats fed horsechestnut seed extract at dosages of 100 to 400 mg/kg/day for 34 weeks. The only toxic effect observed in dogs orally administered the extract (20 to 80 mg/kg/day 5 days per week) for the same time period was vomiting in the highest dosage

Table 1   **LD_{50} Data Recorded for Horsechestnut Extract and Its Constituents**

Substance	Route, Model	LD_{50} Value	Reference
Horsechestnut seed extract	Oral, mice	99 mg/kg	12
Horsechestnut seed extract	Oral, rats	2.15 g/kg	12
Horsechestnut seed extract	Oral, guinea pigs	1.12 g/kg	12
Horsechestnut seed extract	Oral, rabbits	1.53 g/kg	12
Horsechestnut seed extract (water-soluble portion)	Oral, chicks	10.6 g/kg	28
Horsechestnut seed extract (water-soluble portion)	Oral, hamsters	10.7 g/kg	28
Horsechestnut dried seed	Oral, chicks	6.5 g/kg	28
Horsechestnut seed extract	i.p., mice	342 mg/kg	12
Horsechestnut seed extract	i.v., mice	138 mg/kg	12
Horsechestnut seed extract	i.v., rats	165 mg/kg	12
Horsechestnut seed extract	i.v., guinea pigs	465 mg/kg	12
Horsechestnut seed extract	i.v., rabbits	18 mg/kg	12
Aescin	i.v., mice	9.3 mg/kg	29
Aescin	i.v., rats	16.8 mg/kg	29
Aescin	i.v., guinea pigs	9.1 mg/kg	29
Aescin	i.v., rabbits	5 mg/kg	29
Aescin	i.v., dogs	Approximately 3 mg/kg	29
Aescin	i.v., pigs	Approximately 4 mg/kg	29

group at 8 weeks. This was eliminated by the use of enteric-coated tablets. No toxic effects were observed in rats after daily intravenous injection of 9 mg/kg of extract for 8 weeks. Lesions were observed primarily in the kidneys after administration of acutely toxic oral and intravenous doses.[12]

Oral administration of the sodium salt of aescin (10 mg/kg, 70 mg/kg) to rats did not induce fatty degeneration of the liver.[30] Intraperitoneal administration of aescin (10 mg/kg) to juvenile male rats did not affect fertility or cause renal toxicity.[31] Toxic effects in rodents following intravenous injection of high doses of aescin were due to massive haemolysis. Continuous administration of aescin (1.1 mg/kg/day) for 1 month was associated with minimal haemolysis in rabbits,

which was only detectable by increased erythropoiesis.[17,32] The route of administration was not clearly specified. However, as the dose was one-fifth of the LD_{50}, aescin was probably administered by injection.

Horsechestnut seed extract has demonstrated weak mutagenic activity in the Ames test in vitro. It was suggested that this effect might be due to the flavonoid quercetin.[33] The potential genotoxicity of quercetin has been studied extensively and the results have been interpreted as being not relevant to human intake.[34]

Regulatory Status

See Table 2 for regulatory status in selected countries.

Table **2   Regulatory Status for Horsechestnut in Selected Countries**

Australia	Horsechestnut is not included in Part 4 of Schedule 4 of the Therapeutic Goods Regulations.
UK & Germany	Horsechestnut for external use is included on the General Sale List. It is covered by a positive Commission E monograph.
US	Horsechestnut does not have generally recognised as safe (GRAS) status. However, it is freely available as a "dietary supplement" in the US under DSHEA legislation (Dietary Supplement Health and Education Act of 1994).

REFERENCES

1. Siebert U, Brach M, Sroczynski G, et al: *Int Angiol* 21:305-315, 2002.
2. Pittler MH, Ernst E: *Cochrane Database Syst Rev* CD003230, 2002.
3. Felter HW: *The eclectic materia medica, pharmacology and therapeutics*, first published 1922, reprinted Portland, 1983, Eclectic Medical Publications, pp 990-992.
4. Hostettmann K, Marston A: *Chemistry & pharmacology of natural products: saponins*, Cambridge, 1995, Cambridge University Press, p 318.
5. Wagner H, Bladt S: *Plant drug analysis: a thin layer chromatography atlas*, ed 2, Berlin, 1996, Springer-Verlag, p 308.
6. Krueger M: *Dtsch Hailpfl* 9:82, 1943.
7. Bombardelli E, Morazzoni P, Griffini A: *Fitoterapia* 68:483-511, 1996.
8. Alter H: *Z Allgemeinmed* 49:1301-1304, 1973.
9. Steiner M, Hillemanns HG: *Munch Med Wochenschr* 128:551-552, 1986.
10. Steiner M, Hillemanns HG: *Phlebology* 5:41-44, 1990.
11. Steiner M: *Phebol Proktol* 19:239-242, 1990.
12. Liehn HD, Franco PA, Hampel H, et al: *Panminerva Med* 14:84-91, 1972.
13. Hitzenberger G: *Wien Med Wochenschr* 139:385-389, 1989.
14. Takegoshi K, Tohyama T, Okuda K, et al: *Gastroenterol Jpn* 21:62-65, 1986.
15. McKenna DJ, Jones K, Hughes K, et al: *Botanical medicines: the desk reference for major herbal supplements*, ed 2, New York, 2002, The Haworth Herbal Press, p 688.
16. Grob PJ, Muller-Schoop JW, Hacki MA, et al: *Lancet* 2:144-148, 1975.
17. Sirtori CR: *Pharmacol Res* 44:183-193, 2001.
18. Escribano MM, Munoz-Bellido FJ, Velazquez E, et al: *Contact Dermatitis* 37:233, 1997.
19. Voigt E, Junger H: *Anaesthesist* 27:81-83, 1978.
20. Hellberg K, Ruschewski W, de Vivie R: *Thoraxchir Vask Chir* 23:396-399, 1975.
21. Hardin JW, Arena JM: *Human poisoning from native and cultivated plants*, Durham, NC, 1965, Duke University Press, p 80.
22. Maytunas N, Krenzelok E, Jacobsen T, et al: *J Toxicol Clin Toxicol* 35:527-528, 1997.
23. Mills S, Bone K: *Principles and practice of phytotherapy: modern herbal medicine*, Edinburgh, 2000, Churchill Livingstone, pp 448-455.
24. Grasso A, Corvaglia E: *Gazz Med Ital* 135:581-584, 1976.

25. Wilhelm R, Feldmeier C: *Med Klin* 70:2079-2083, 1975.
26. Bastian HP, Vahlensieck W: *Med Klin* 71:1295-1299, 1976.
27. Ascher PW: *Therapiewoche* 52:3-10, 1977.
28. Williams M, Olsen JD: *Am J Vet Res* 45:539-542, 1984.
29. Blaschek W, Ebel S, Hackenthal E, et al: *HagerROM 2002: Hagers Handbuch der Drogen und Arzneistoffe,* Heidelberg, 2002, Springer.
30. Ulicna O, Volmut J, Kupcova V, et al: *Bratisl Lek Listy* 94:158-161, 1993.
31. von Kreybig T, Prechtel K: *Arzneim-Forsch* 27:1465, 1977.
32. Pangiati D: *Boll Chim Farm* 131:320-321, 1992.
33. Schimmer O, Kruger A, Paulini H, et al: *Pharmazie* 49:448-451, 1994.
34. Ito N: *Jpn J Cancer Res* 83:312-313, 1992.

HORSETAIL

Other common names: Equisetum, scouring rush
Botanical name: *Equisetum arvense* L.
Family: Equisetaceae
Plant part used: Aerial part

Safety Summary

Pregnancy category B2: No increase in frequency of malformation or other harmful effects on the foetus from limited use in women. Animal studies are lacking.
Lactation category C: Compatible with breastfeeding.
Contraindications: None required on current evidence.
Warnings & precautions: Copious fluid intake should not be undertaken if oedema due to impaired cardiac or renal function exists (Commission E warning).
Adverse reactions: A rare allergic reaction is possible in patients susceptible to nicotine as a hapten.
Interactions: No precautions required on current evidence.

Typical Therapeutic Use

Traditional indications for horsetail in Western herbal medicine include inflammation or mild infections of the genitourinary tract.[1]

Actions

Diuretic, astringent, styptic (haemostatic).

Key Constituents

Key constituents of the aerial parts of *Equisetum arvense* include phenolic compounds: flavonoids (such as quercetin and kaempferol glycosides) and hydroxycinnamic acid derivatives (such as caffeic acid esters).[2] The flavonoid composition reveals the existence of two chemotypes of *E. arvense* (one from Asia and North America and the other from Europe).[3] A hydroxycinnamic acid (di-E-caffeoyl-meso-tartaric acid) provides a marker for both chemotypes to distinguish them from other *Equisetum* spp.[4] Traces of alkaloids, including nicotine, are reported.[3] The amount of nicotine obtained from 5 kg of dried horsetail (including *E. arvense*) was estimated by ultraviolet spectrophotometry as not more than 2 mg.[5]

Horsetail also contains appreciable amounts of silica (1.2% to 6.9%).

Adulteration

Medicinal horsetail is frequently adulterated, usually with other *Equisetum* species including the potentially toxic *E. palustre* (which contains the alkaloid palustrine). In addition to genuine *E. arvense*, there are also hydrids which are difficult to characterise and with unknown alkaloidal contents.[3,6]

Typical Dosage Forms & Dosage

Typical adult dosage ranges are:
- 3 to 12 g/day of dried aerial parts or by infusion or decoction
- 3 to 12 mL/day of a 1:1 liquid extract
- 2 to 6 mL/day of a 1:2 liquid extract or equivalent in tablet or capsule form
- 6 to 18 mL/day of a 1:5 tincture

Contraindications

None known.

Use in Pregnancy

Category B2: No increase in frequency of malformation or other harmful effects on the foetus from limited use in women. Animal studies are lacking.

Use in Lactation

Category C: Compatible with breastfeeding.

Warnings & Precautions

The Commission E advises that copious fluid intake should not be undertaken if oedema due to impaired cardiac or renal function exists.[7]

Effect on Ability to Drive or Operate Machinery

No adverse effects expected.

Adverse Reactions

Allergic reaction is possible in patients susceptible to nicotine as a hapten (an antigen capable of causing an immune response only when coupled to a carrier). After passive inhalation of tobacco smoke, a patient regularly in contact with horsetail in the proximity of his house developed dermatitis on his hand and face which resembled seborrhoeic dermatitis. A fresh exposure to horsetail induced a more rapid reaction which necessitated local application of adrenaline and oral antihistamines. His history of atopic reactions to nicotine as a hapten (in tobacco smoke) correlated with the possible presence of nicotine in horsetail.[8]

Interactions

None known.

Safety in Children

No information available.

Overdosage

Toxicity is possible from eating large amounts of *E. arvense*. This has occurred in children who used the stems as blowguns and whistles.[9]

Toxicology

A diet with increasing quantities of horsetail (0.1 to 0.8 mg/kg/day) was not found to be toxic to voles (rodents) in terms of liver and kidney function.[10] This study investigated the effect of forage grasses on the animal's physiology (hence the low dosage) and was not a toxicology model.

Much information has been collated about the poisoning of livestock by ingestion of horsetail (equisetosis). Due to the uncertainty in defining the species, it is not clear whether the reports from the early to mid 20th century relate to *E. arvense*. Feeding experiments reported in 1904 investigating the toxicity of several *Equisetum* species with several animal species found *E. arvense* to be harmless and *E. palustre*, in particular, to be toxic. These and other studies conducted at the time concluded that the silica and aconitic acid (present in both *E. arvense* and *E. palustre*) were not to blame. An alkaloid isolated from *E. palustre* was considered responsible,[11] but subsequently ruled out. The focus then shifted to a thiamine-destroying substance, such as thiaminase, as at least partially responsible. Mechanical injury to the mouth and intestinal tract may also be involved.[12] However, it is not known if this activity exists in extracts of dried horsetail.

The occurrence of horsetail poisoning was observed in three horses. Horsetail-contaminated hay was found to be responsible. Two of the horses were treated successfully with subcutaneous injections of thiamine hydrochloride (100 mg/day for 4 days). In vitro tests demonstrated that horsetail destroyed thiamine via enzymatic activity.[13] Cattle fed the horsetail-contaminated hay over the same period showed no ill effects.

Regulatory Status

See Table 1 for regulatory status in selected countries.

Table 1 **Regulatory Status for Horsetail in Selected Countries**

Australia	Horsetail is not included in Part 4 of Schedule 4 of the Therapeutic Goods Regulations.
UK & Germany	*Equisetum* (species undefined) is included on the General Sale List. Horsetail is covered by a positive Commission E monograph. Horsetail is official in the *British Pharmacopoeia* 2002 and the *European Pharmacopoeia* 4.3.
US	Horsetail does not have generally recognised as safe (GRAS) status. However, it is freely available as a "dietary supplement" in the US under DSHEA legislation (Dietary Supplement Health and Education Act of 1994).

REFERENCES

1. British Herbal Medicine Association: *British herbal compendium*, vol 1, Bournemouth, 1992, BHMA, pp 92-94.
2. Veit M, Becket C, Hohne C, et al: *Phytochem* 38: 881-891, 1995.
3. Bisset NG (ed.): *Herbal drugs and phytopharmaceuticals: A handbook for practice on a scientific basis*, Stuttgart, 1994, Medpharm Scientific Publishers, pp 188-191.
4. Veit M, Strack D, Czygan FC, et al: *Phytochem* 30:527-529, 1991.
5. Phillipson JD, Melville C: *J Pharm Pharmacol* 12:506-508, 1960.
6. Veit M: *Dtsch Apoth Ztg* 127:2049-2056, 1987.
7. Blumenthal M, et al (eds): *The complete German Commission E monographs: therapeutic guide to herbal medicines*, Austin, 1998, American Botanical Council, pp 150-151.
8. Sudan BJ: *Contact Dermatitis* 13:201-202, 1985.
9. Hamon NW, Awang DV: *Can Pharm J* 125:399-401, 1992.
10. Jean Y, Bergeron JM: *Can J Zool* 64:158-162, 1986.
11. Long HC: *Plants poisonous to live stock*, ed 2, revised, Cambridge, 1924, Cambridge University Press, pp 85-89.
12. Kingsbury JM: *Poisonous plants for the United States and Canada*, Englewood Cliffs, 1964, Prentice Hall, pp 114-118.
13. Henderson JA, Evans EV, McIntosh RA: *J Am Vet Med Assoc* 120:375-378, 1952.

HYDRANGEA

Other common name: Seven barks
Botanical name: *Hydrangea arborescens* L.
Family: Hydrangeaceae
Plant part used: Root

Safety Summary

Pregnancy category B2: No increase in frequency of malformation or other harmful effects on the foetus from limited use in women. Animal studies are lacking.
Lactation category C: Compatible with breastfeeding.
Contraindications: None required on current evidence.
Warnings & precautions: None required on current evidence.
Adverse reactions: None found in published literature associated with hydrangea.
Interactions: No precautions required on current evidence.

Typical Therapeutic Use

Traditional indications for hydrangea in Western herbal medicine include inflammation of the bladder, urethra and prostate; kidney stones, and enlarged prostate.[1,2]

Actions

Diuretic, antilithic.

Key Constituents

The constituents of hydrangea are not well researched. In 1887 hydrangea was reported as containing a characteristic glycoside which was named hydrangin. Other constituents included resin and saponin.[3] Hydrangin is now listed as a synonym for the coumarin umbelliferone (7-hydroxycoumarin).[4]

Adulteration

No adulterants known.

Typical Dosage Forms & Dosage

Typical adult dosage ranges are:
- 6 to 12 g/day of dried root or by decoction
- 6 to 12 g/day of a 1:1 liquid extract
- 2 to 7 mL/day of a 1:2 liquid extract or equivalent in tablet or capsule form
- 6 to 30 mL/day of a 1:5 tincture

Contraindications

None known.

Use in Pregnancy

Category B2: No increase in frequency of malformation or other harmful effects on the foetus from limited use in women. Animal studies are lacking. Hydrangea is a herb used predominantly by men.

Use in Lactation

Category C: Compatible with breastfeeding.

Warnings & Precautions

None required.

Effect on Ability to Drive or Operate Machinery

No adverse effects expected.

Adverse Reactions

A case of protracted cholestatic hepatitis after the use of a herbal and nutritional preparation has been reported. The herbal preparation contained hydrangea, saw palmetto (*Serenoa repens*), *Pygeum africanum*, *Panax ginseng*, zinc picolinate, pyridoxine, alanine, glutamic acid, *Apis mellifica* pollen, and silica.[5] The ingredient causing the adverse reaction was not identified.

Interactions

None reported.

Safety in Children

No information available but adverse effects are not expected.

Overdosage

Poisoning has occurred in animals and humans after consumption of hydrangea leaf or bud, respectively.[6] No incidents were found in the published literature for hydrangea root. Eclectic texts indicate that if hydrangea is taken in overdose it produces some unpleasant side effects, such as dizziness and oppression of the chest.[2]

Toxicology

No information available.

Regulatory Status

See Table 1 for regulatory status in selected countries.

Table 1 **Regulatory Status for Hydrangea in Selected Countries**

Australia	Hydrangea is not included in Part 4 of Schedule 4 of the Therapeutic Goods Regulations.
UK & Germany	Hydrangea is included on the General Sale List. It was not included in the Commission E assessment.
US	Hydrangea does not have generally recognised as safe (GRAS) status. However, it is freely available as a "dietary supplement" in the US under DSHEA legislation (Dietary Supplement Health and Education Act of 1994).

REFERENCES

1. British Herbal Medicine Association's Scientific Committee: *British herbal pharmacopoeia*, Bournemouth, 1983, BHMA, p 112.
2. Felter HW, Lloyd JU: *King's American dispensatory*, ed 18, rev 3, vol 2, first published 1905, reprinted Portland, 1983, Eclectic Medical Publications, pp 1000-1001.
3. Bondurant CS: *Am J Pharm* 59:123, 1887.
4. Budavari S, et al (eds): *The Merck index: an encyclopedia of chemicals, drugs and biologicals*, ed 12, Whitehouse Station, 1996, Merck & Co, p 1680.
5. Hamid S, Bojter S, Vierling J: *Ann Intern Med* 127:169-170, 1997.
6. Kingsbury JM: *Poisonous plants for the United States and Canada*, Englewood Cliffs, 1964, Prentice Hall, pp 370-371.

JAMAICA DOGWOOD

Other common names: Jamaican dogwood, piscidia
Botanical names Piscidia erythrina L. (*Piscidia piscipula* L. Sarg., *Erythrina piscipula* L.)
Family: Leguminosae (Papilionoideae)
Plant part used: Root bark

Safety Summary

Pregnancy category D: Has caused or is associated with a substantial risk of causing foetal malformation or irreversible damage (on the basis of its rotenone content).
Lactation category SD: Strongly discouraged in breastfeeding.
Contraindications: Contraindicated in pregnancy, bradycardia, and cardiac insufficiency. Do not use during lactation without professional advice.
Warnings & precautions: In principle, herbal sedatives are best avoided in depression and insomnia marked by increasing restlessness during the early hours of the morning. Prescription of herbal sedatives should ideally be limited in duration. Prescribe with caution for pain in children. Other precautions are neurological disease, depression and psychosis, liver and kidney disease, history of allergic or anaphylactic reactions. Long-term therapy with analgesics is not advisable. Caution is advised for women wishing to conceive.
Adverse reactions: May cause nausea and headache in susceptible patients.
Interactions: Do not prescribe concomitantly with powerful analgesics (theoretical concern).

Typical Therapeutic Use

Traditional indications for Jamaica dogwood in Western herbal medicine include neuralgia, migraine, insomnia, and dysmenorrhoea.[1]

Actions

Analgesic, spasmolytic, mild sedative.

Key Constituents

Key constituents of Jamaica dogwood root bark include complex isoflavones, including erythbigenin, piscidone, piscerythrone, ichthynone, and jamaicin and the rotenoids (including rotenone). The isoflavone profile varies depending upon the source.[2]

Adulteration

No adulterants known.

Typical Dosage Forms & Dosage

Typical adult dosage ranges are:
- 3 to 6 g/day of dried root bark or by decoction
- 3 to 6 mL/day of a 1:1 liquid extract*
- 3 to 6 mL/day of a 1:2 liquid extract or equivalent in tablet or capsule form
- 15 to 45 mL/day of a 1:5 tincture

Contraindications

Contraindicated in pregnancy, bradycardia, and cardiac insufficiency.[2] Do not use during lactation without professional advice.

Use in Pregnancy

Category D: Has caused or is associated with a substantial risk of causing foetal malformation or irreversible damage (on the basis of its rotenone content).

Oral administration of rotenone (10 mg/kg) to rats on days 6 to 15 of pregnancy was associated with an increased number of nonpregnant rats and resorptions. Reductions in maternal body weight gain, foetal weight, and skeletal ossification, as well as an increased incidence of an extra rib, were observed at a dosage of 5 and 10 mg/kg. No significant effects were observed at 2.5 mg/kg.[3] Rotentone inhibited experimentally induced ovulation in rats, with nearly complete inhibition at the dosage of 0.5 mg/kg (route unknown).[4]

Use in Lactation

Category SD: Strongly discouraged in breastfeeding.

Warnings & Precautions

In principle, herbal sedatives are best avoided in depression and insomnia marked by increasing

---

*The British Pharmaceutical Codex 1934 also lists a higher dosage of 2 to 8 mL, 3 to 4 times per day.

restlessness during the early hours of the morning. Prescription of herbal sedatives should ideally be limited in duration.

The following conditions should be approached with caution when using herbal analgesics: concurrent prescription of powerful analgesics; pain in children; neurological disease; depression and psychosis; liver and kidney disease; history of allergic or anaphylactic reactions. Long-term therapy with analgesics is not advisable.

Caution is advised for women wishing to conceive.

Effect on Ability to Drive or Operate Machinery

No adverse effects expected.

Adverse Reactions

Traditional texts record that Jamaica dogwood may cause nausea, vomiting, and headache in patients prescribed even small, therapeutic doses. Convulsions were provoked in a woman given a 0.5-drachm dose for hemicrania. (This dosage is probably referring to use of the fluid extract: 0.5 fluid drachm is approximately 1.7 mL.) In overdose, Jamaica dogwood is said to be toxic (no further detail given).[5,6] Another traditional text notes that it does not produce toxic or adverse effects in therapeutic doses.[7]

Interactions

None known for Jamaica dogwood. As a precaution do not prescribe concomitantly with powerful analgesics.

Safety in Children

No information available.

Overdosage

No incidents found in published literature.

Toxicology

Table 1 lists LD_{50} data recorded for Jamaica dogwood extract and one of its key constituents.[8,9]

Jamaica dogwood has been used as a fish and insect poison (due to its rotenone content) but has negligible toxicity in warm-blooded animals. Jamaica dogwood extract (1.5 g/kg, i.v.) induced a death rate of 30% in mice after 24 hours. Chronic administration over 5 weeks (20 to 500 mg/kg, rats, i.p.; 100 mg/kg, rabbits, i.p.) did not produce substantial differences in haematological parameters or weight when compared to controls.[8] Earlier acute toxicity studies indicated that Jamaica dogwood had a low relative toxicity when fed orally to rats. The fluid extract was nontoxic at a dosage of 20 g/kg. In another series of tests, two rats out of a group of seven died after receiving an isopropyl alcohol dried extract (10 g/kg, equivalent to 106 g of the dried bark).[10]

In vivo studies indicate that rotenone induces impairment of the myocardial contractile force and rate, a hypotensive effect, and stimulation of respiration.[11] The oral lethal dose of rotenone in humans is approximately 200 g.[9]

Regulatory Status

See Table 2 for regulatory status in selected countries.

Table 1   **LD_{50} Data Recorded for Jamaica Dogwood and Rotenone**

Substance	Route, Model	LD_{50} Value	Reference
Jamaica dogwood extract	Oral, mice	3.75 g/kg	8
Rotenone	Oral, rats	60 mg/kg	9

Table **2**   **Regulatory Status for Jamaica Dogwood in Selected Countries**

Australia	Jamaica dogwood is not included in Part 4 of Schedule 4 of the Therapeutic Goods Regulations.
UK & Germany	Jamaica dogwood is included on the General Sale List. It was not included in the Commission E assessment.
US	Jamaica dogwood does not have generally recognised as safe (GRAS) status. However, it is freely available as a "dietary supplement" in the US under DSHEA legislation (Dietary Supplement Health and Education Act of 1994).

REFERENCES

1. British Herbal Medicine Association's Scientific Committee: *British herbal pharmacopoeia*, Bournemouth, 1983, BHMA, p 163.
2. British Herbal Medicine Association: *British herbal compendium*, vol 1, Bournemouth, 1992, BHMA, pp 139-141.
3. Khera KS, Whalen C, Angers G: *J Toxicol Environ Health* 10:111-120, 1982.
4. Koshida M, Takenaka A, Okamura H, et al: *Acta Obstet Gynaecol Jpn* 36:2474-2475, 1984.
5. Grieve M: *A modern herbal*, New York, 1971, Dover Publications, pp 261-262.
6. Felter HW, Lloyd JU: *King's American dispensatory*, ed 18, rev 3, vol 2, first published 1905, reprinted Portland, 1983, Eclectic Medical Publications, pp 1509-1511.
7. Ellingwood F, Lloyd JU: *American materia medica, therapeutics and pharmacognosy*, ed 11, Naturopathic Medical Series, Botanical vol 2, Portland, 1983, Eclectic Medical Publications, pp 110-112.
8. Aurousseau M, Berny C, Albert O: *Ann Pharm Franc* 23:251-257, 1965.
9. Anonymous: *Food Cosmet Toxicol* 4:108, 1966.
10. Costello CH, Butler CL: *J Am Pharm Assoc* 37:89-97, 1948.
11. Santi FM, Toth ER: *Farmaco* 21:689-703, 1966.

KAVA

Other common name: Kava kava
Botanical name *Piper methysticum* G. Forst.
Family: Piperaceae
Plant part used: Root (rootstock)

Safety Summary

Pregnancy category B1: No increase in frequency of malformation or other harmful effects on the foetus from limited use in women. No evidence of increased foetal damage in animal studies.

Lactation category CC: Compatible with breastfeeding but use caution (on the basis of the presence of kava lactones).

Contraindications: None required on current evidence. Do not use during lactation without professional advice.

Warnings & precautions: Kava has been implicated in rare cases of liver damage; it should be taken under professional supervision and continuous use should best not exceed 4 weeks. Caution is advised in disorders related to dopamine deficiency, elderly patients, and those with Parkinson's disease, pregnancy, lactation, endogenous depression, and in children under 12 years of age. In principle, herbal sedatives are best avoided in insomnia marked by increasing restlessness during the early hours of the morning. Prescription of herbal sedatives should ideally be limited in duration.

Adverse reactions: Skin reactions, gastrointestinal complaints, headache, dizziness, dopamine antagonism, rare cases of hepatotoxicity.

Interactions: Excessive alcohol consumption, benzodiazepines, L-dopa and other disease medications for Parkinson's disease.

Typical Therapeutic Use

Kava is mainly used in Western countries for the treatment of anxiety. The results of a systematic review of clinical trials which was updated in August 2002 is as follows. Eleven randomised, double-blind, placebo-controlled trials involving a total of 645 participants met the inclusion criteria. A meta-analysis of six studies using the total score on the Hamilton Anxiety scale as a common outcome measure suggested a significant reduction in anxiety for patients receiving kava extract compared with those receiving placebo. The dosage of standardised kava extract prescribed varied from the equivalent of 105 to 210 mg/day of kava lactones. The duration of treatment ranged from 4 to 24 weeks.[1] One of the trials included in this meta-analysis found that kava treatment reduced depression and menopausal symptoms in addition to menopausal anxiety.[2]

Traditional indications for kava in Western herbal medicine include infection and inflammation of the genitourinary tract.[3] Therapeutic uses in the Pacific Islands, where kava is extensively cultivated and consumed as a social and ceremonial beverage, include treatment of inflammation and infection of the urogenital system (including gonorrhoea), pain relief, and as a tonic.[4]

Actions

Anxiolytic, hypnotic, anticonvulsant, mild sedative, skeletal muscle relaxant, local anaesthetic, mild analgesic, antipruritic (topically).

Key Constituents

Key constituents of kava rhizome are the kava pyrones (5% to 9%, depending upon geographical location), including kavain (or kawain), dihydrokavain, methysticin, dihydromethysticin (DHM), yangonin, and desmethoxyyangonin.[5]

Adulteration

Instead of a rhizome with the periderm and roots removed, kava may be presented for commerce as an unpeeled rhizome covered with the cork or with the roots attached.[6] Peelings from the root and stump are also used in commerce.[7]

Typical Dosage Forms & Dosage

Typical adult dosage ranges are:
- 6 to 12 g/day of dried root or by decoction
- 6 to 12 mL/day of a 1:1 liquid extract
- 3 to 8.5 mL/day of a 1:2 liquid extract
- doses in tablet or capsule form corresponding to 105 to 210 mg/day of kava lactones

Contraindications

The German Commission E lists the following contraindications: pregnancy, lactation, and endogenous depression. However, these have resulted from a lack of positive safety data rather than any reported safety concerns. Do not use during lactation without professional advice.

Use in Pregnancy

Category B1: No increase in frequency of malformation or other harmful effects on the foetus from limited use in women. No evidence of increased foetal damage in animal studies.

The Australian Therapeutic Goods Administration recommends that kava-containing medicines should not be taken by pregnant women.

In traditional societies in the Pacific Islands, women have less access to, and use of, kava than men. Hence the interpretation of information from the traditional literature regarding use in pregnancy needs to take this lower usage into account. In addition, these societies held a number of cultural myths relating to kava which affected women.[8,9]

Kava has been used as an abortifacient on Pohnpei (although this has been said to be denied by another source),[10] and in south-east coastal Irian Jaya, although combined with other herbs such as various "pepper-roots", chillies, and *Citrus* spp.[11] In Hawaii, women avoided any kava use immediately upon becoming pregnant.[12] There are several references to kava leaf used topically to induce miscarriage (Hawaii and Polynesia).[13] Both the rhizome and leaf are used orally as a contraceptive.[14,15] Folk theory suggests that kava use renders women infertile.[13,16] Yet therapeutic use during pregnancy is also noted: to induce an easy labour and to correct displacement of the womb.[17,18]

Synthetic kavain orally administered on days 6 to 17 of gestation (100 and 500 mg/kg, rats; 20 and 200 mg/kg, rabbits) did not produce teratogenic effects in terms of the foetal parameters measured. No teratogenic effects were seen in the F_1 and F_2 generations of rats given dihydromethysticin (50 mg/kg, i.p.) three times weekly over a period of 3 months.[19]

Use in Lactation

Category CC: Compatible with breastfeeding but use caution (on the basis of the presence of kava lactones).

Traditionally, women in some areas of New Guinea drank kava beverage (prepared by grating and maceration) during their pregnancy, to promote the flow of milk.[17]

The Australian Therapeutic Goods Administration (TGA) recommends that kava-containing medicines should not be taken by nursing women.

Warnings & Precautions

Due to possible dopamine antagonism, kava should be used cautiously in elderly patients, especially those with Parkinson's disease (see Adverse reactions below).

In August 2002, the Australian TGA advised that the kava-containing medicines carry a label warning that kava has been implicated in serious liver damage; it be taken only under the supervision of a health care practitioner; and it be used only for short periods of time, not exceeding 6 weeks. An expert committee of the TGA that reviewed the safety of kava decided in August 2003 that only certain forms of kava were suitable for use in listed medicines. Products must be made from water extract/dispersion or whole rhizome and the daily dosage of kava lactones must be capped (at 250 mg).

In principle, herbal sedatives are best avoided in depression and insomnia marked by increasing restlessness during the early hours of the morning. Prescription of herbal sedatives should ideally be limited in duration.

Consideration of pharmacokinetic data and the possibility for a potentiation of the sedative effects of anaesthetics has led to the recommendation that patients taking kava should discontinue use at least 24 hours prior to surgery.[20]

Effect on Ability to Drive or Operate Machinery

No negative influence is expected at normal therapeutic doses. In a randomised, double-blind study, 40 healthy volunteers received either standardised kava extract (equivalent to 210 mg/day kava lactones) or placebo for 15 days. Kava extract did not significantly affect performance capability relevant to operating machines and driving.[21] Administration of kava extract (equivalent to 240 mg/day of kava lactones) to volunteers did not affect performance parameters (stress tolerance, vigilance, and motor coordination) compared to baseline values.[22]

Adverse Reactions

Refer to Chapter 12 for a discussion of the cases of hepatotoxicity attributed to kava.

In Germany to the year 2000, about 60 adverse reactions to kava-containing preparations had been reported since their introduction.[23] This is a very small rate considering that the annual use of kava products was estimated at the time at over 70 million daily doses in Germany.[24]

The meta-analysis referred to above (see Typical therapeutic use) reported that the adverse events noted in the reviewed clinical trials were mild, transient, and infrequent. The 68 documented cases of suspected hepatotoxicity were not included in this analysis, but were noted together with a brief critique. From the information available in early 2002 (which included four postmarketing surveillance studies [Table 1[25-28]]), the authors questioned whether the frequency of liver damage in kava users differed significantly from that of nonkava users.[1] Table 2[1,29] lists adverse reactions observed from well-controlled clinical trials for both kava and placebo treatments.

A controlled study found that acute administration of kava (500 mL of a 1:5 decoction) did not significantly affect cognition compared to placebo, although there was a trend to poorer performance. Those receiving kava reported subjective feelings of intoxication (apparent from increased body sway)

which peaked approximately 1 hour after ingestion, but there was a high degree of individual variation. Three of the 12 volunteers who received kava reported feeling nauseous.[30]

An early clinical trial investigating the anticonvulsant activity of kava found that a dose of up to 6 g/day of root and an alcohol extract of 1 g/day helped control seizures but caused skin yellowing after several weeks. Daily doses of dihydromethysticin (800 mg/day) also produced side effects (reddening of the conjunctiva, vomiting, and diarrhoea) after 1 month of treatment.[31,32]

An early clinical pharmacological evaluation of dihydromethysticin found that doses of 300 to 800 mg/day produced a scaly skin rash in a high percentage of subjects.[33] Other reported adverse reactions are provided in Table 3.[23,34-41]

Five cases of adverse reactions, ranging from minor to major, occurred from ingestion of "herbal ecstasy" tablets in New Zealand. The composition of these tablets varied and may have included ephedrine, caffeine, and kava.[42]

Kava was falsely implicated in health complications in a group of people believed to have consumed a product containing kava at a "rave" (dance party) in Los Angeles on New Year's Eve, 1996. Samples tested

Table 1   **Postmarketing Studies of Kava Extract and Kavain**

Treatment	Number of Patients	Tolerability and Adverse Events (AEs)	Ref.
Standardised kava extract (equivalent to 105 mg/day kava lactones, 7 weeks)	4049	• Tolerability good to very good in 96% of patients • 61 AEs (1.5%), mainly gastrointestinal complaints or allergic reactions which were mild and reversible • 50% of these cases were rated as probably due to kava	25
Standardised kava extract (equivalent to 120 to 240 mg/day kava lactones, minimum of 4 weeks)	3029	• Tolerability good to very good in 93% of patients • 69 patients reported AEs (2.3%), mainly allergic reactions (nine reports), gastrointestinal complaints (31 reports), and CNS symptoms (22 reports, headache, dizziness) which were mild and reversible • 37 patients who reported AEs withdrew from the study (1.2%)	26
Standardised kava extract (equivalent to 120 mg/day kava lactones, 5 weeks)	1673	• Tolerability good to very good in 93% of patients • 29 patients reported mild AEs (1.7%)	27
Kavain (400 mg/day, 4 weeks)	2944	• 3.3% side effects, very rarely with causal connection to the test preparation	28

Table **2**　**Adverse Event Information for Well-designed, Randomised, Placebo-controlled, Double-blind Trials Evaluating Kava**

Study and Dosage	Number of Patients (Total)	Adverse Events in Kava Treatment Group	Adverse Events in Placebo Group
Bhate (1989)*: kava extract (equivalent to 60 mg kava lactones × 2 prior to operation)	59	• Postoperative hangover (2)	• Postoperative hangover (4)
Gastpar (2002): kava extract (equivalent to 105 mg/day kava lactones, 4 weeks)	141	• Tiredness (1) • Unrelated to the kava treatment (undefined, 4) • Symptom aggravation (3)	• Information not available
Geier (2002): kava extract (equivalent to 105 mg/day kava lactones, 4 weeks)	50	• General condition deteriorated due to pneumonia (1) • Deterioration of preexisting fibrosis (1)	• Information not available
Kinzler (1991): kava extract (equivalent to 210 mg/day kava lactones, 4 weeks)	58	• None	• None
Lehmann (1998): kava extract (equivalent to 150 mg/day kava lactones, 1 week)	20	• Undefined (1)	• Undefined (3)
Lehrl (2002): kava extract (equivalent to 140 mg/day kava lactones, 4 weeks)	57	• None	• Information not available
Malsch (2001): kava extract (increase dose equivalent to 35 to 210 mg/day kava lactones over 1 week, then 210 mg/day for 3 weeks)	40	• Unspecific symptoms due to the withdrawal of benzodiazepine (5 patients)	• Unspecific symptoms due to the withdrawal of benzodiazepine (10 patients)
Singh (1998): kava extract (equivalent to 240 mg/day kava lactones, 4 weeks)	60	• None	• None
Volz (1997)*: kava extract (equivalent to 210 mg/day kava lactones, 24 weeks)	100	• Undefined and unrelated to kava (4) • Stomach upset (2)	• Undefined and unrelated to placebo (12) • Vertigo, palpitation (3)
Warnecke (1990): kava extract (equivalent to 60 mg/day kava lactones, 4 weeks)	40	• Headache, tiredness, lack of energy (5) • Stomach complaints, heartburn, and diarrhoea (3)	• Gastrointestinal symptoms (2)
Warnecke (1991): kava extract (equivalent to 210 mg/day kava lactones, 8 weeks)	40	• Restlessness, stomach complaints, drowsiness, tremor (4)	• Restlessness, stomach complaints, drowsiness, tremor (6)

*The information in this table was obtained from the Cochrane review,[1] a safety review,[29] and, where asterisked, supplemented with information from the individual research papers.

Table **3**   **Case Reports of Adverse Reactions Possibly Associated with Kava Intake**

Case Reports	Adverse Reaction	Ref.
SKIN REACTIONS		
I case, 2000: kava extract containing 120 mg/day kava lactones, for 3 weeks	Generalised rash, diagnosed as delayed-type hypersensitivity reaction	23
I case, 1999: kava extract, for 2 weeks	Dermatomyositis	34
2 cases, 1998:		35
• Kava extract (quantity unknown, plus yohimbine and several drugs), for 2 to 3 weeks	• Induced erythema with lymphocytic attack on sebaceous glands not caused by other agents or disease; reaction occurred after sunlight exposure for several hours	
• Kava extract (quantity unknown), for 3 weeks	• Induced erythema with lymphocytic attack on sebaceous glands	
I case, 1996: standardised kava extract (dosage undefined), taken for several weeks	Systemic contact dermatitis (confirmed by rechallenge)	36
I case, 1986: kava tea (> 4 cups) taken on the previous night; 3 months prior he had drunk kava tea and had been hospitalised with generalised erythema	Skin erythema with facial oedema	37
OTHER REACTIONS		
I case (2002): kava extract (65 mg/day for 10 days); family history of essential tremor; reaction occurred 2 to 3 weeks after ingestion; prior to kava ingestion was treated for depression with benzodiazepines and sertraline	Severe and persistent parkinsonism	38
I case, 2000: weight trainer taking herbal product containing guarana (500 mg), ginkgo (200 mg) and kava (100 mg)	Myoglobinuria	39
4 cases, 1995:	Clinical signs suggestive of dopamine antagonism*	40
• 2 cases: kava extract containing 70 mg kava lactones, reaction began 90 minutes and 4 hours after the first dose		
• 2 cases: kava extract (2 to 3 × 150 mg/day, for 4 to 10 days)		

*A central dopaminergic antagonism seems unlikely to be involved in these reported cases. Cholinergic hyperactivity may be involved.[41]

initially by the Los Angeles Police Department and subsequently by the American Botanical Council showed no kava lactones present. The product was found to contain caffeine and 1,4-butanediol (an industrial solvent which is metabolised to gamma-hydroxybutyrate).[43] A Californian chiropractor was sentenced in February 1998 after pleading guilty to misbranding the product.[44]

Interactions

Normal therapeutic doses of kava do not dampen alertness, interact with mild alcohol consumption, or cause physiological tolerance.

A crossover clinical study evaluated whether simultaneous administration of bromazepam (9 mg/day) and kava extract (containing 240 mg/day of kava lactones) would produce an effect on safety-related performance over and above those anticipated by the single treatment. The study found that kava extract plus a benzodiazepine was unlikely to produce greater effects on general well-being and mental performance aspects required for safety than the benzodiazepine alone.[22] According to the German Commission E, a synergistic effect is possible for substances acting on the central nervous system such as alcohol, barbiturates, and psychopharmacological agents.

High doses of ethanol potentiated the sedative and hypnotic activity of kava resin and markedly increased the toxicity in mice.[45] In a placebo-controlled, double-blind study involving 40 healthy volunteers, the effect of a standardised kava extract (equivalent to 210 mg/day kava lactones, for 8 days) combined with ethanol (0.05% blood alcohol concentration) on safety-relevant performance parameters was investigated. No negative effects were caused by the kava extract, in fact it tended to counter the adverse effect of the alcohol on mental concentration.[46] In a more recent randomised, placebo-controlled trial, acute administration of a very high dose of kava (1 g/kg) combined with alcohol (0.75 g/kg) potentiated both the perceived and measured impairment of motor and cognitive function produced by alcohol alone.[47]

Kava may interact with central dopamine agonists or antagonists[40] and should not be administered to patients taking L-dopa and other medications for Parkinson's disease. Table 4 lists case reports of possible interactions.[48,49]

Safety in Children

The Australian Therapeutic Goods Administration recommends that kava-containing medicines should not be taken by children under 12 years of age.

In Polynesia kava has been used traditionally in children for general debility, stomach disorders, and for fretting.[18]

Overdosage

Kava dermopathy is an acquired reversible ichthyosis (scaly skin eruption) that arises after excessive and chronic use of kava. It appears as a generalised, shiny, scaly skin resembling a cracked porcelain glaze. At the time of Western arrival in some Pacific islands this skin disorder was a mark of prestige.[50] The cutaneous effects were reported in the late 18th century by members of Captain James Cook's Pacific expeditions,[51] although other references date back to ancient times.[52] The cause is unknown, but the phenomenon is not due to a deficiency of one of the B vitamins, since a clinical trial of nicotinamide (100 mg/day) in kava drinkers with prominent skin changes failed to have a significant effect. Kava may interfere with the cholesterol metabolism necessary for proper keratinocyte formation.[52] This skin condition is unlikely to occur after normal therapeutic use. The rash quickly regresses if kava intake is ceased.

Excessive kava drinking may cause pupil dilation, reduced light reflexes, photophobia, bloodshot eyes, and poor attention to diet.[53]

Kava was introduced from Fiji in late 1981[54] to Aboriginal communities of northern Australia and rapidly became a drug of abuse, probably because of a lack of ceremonial or traditional restraints controlling its use. Estimates for individual consumption have been as high as 100 times the amount of kava habitually consumed in the Pacific Islands.[55] A survey of three Aboriginal communities in the mid-1980s found that the average consumption per drinker was 14 to 53 g/day of kava powder, although a

Table **4   Case Reports of Possible Interactions Associated with Kava Intake**

Case Reports of Possible Interactions	Adverse Reaction	Ref.
1 case 2001: long-term intake of benzodiazepines (recently flunitrazepam); reaction within 36 hours of beginning kava tablets	Confusion, auditory, and visual hallucinations	48
1 case, 1996: kava extract + a benzodiazepine drug (alprazolam); other medications: cimetidine, terazosin; no alcohol consumed; reaction within 3 days of beginning kava tablets	Lethargy, disorientation (inaccurately described in the paper as coma)	49

review in the early 1990s suggested consumption may have been as high as 88.3 g/day.[56]

Subsequently, a large amount of information regarding the adverse effects observed from excessive intake of kava in Australian Aboriginal[55,57-59] and Fijian communities[60] was documented. Intake most commonly ranged from 100 to 500 g/week,[58,60] but could be as high as 900 g/week.[58] Common adverse reactions included scaly skin, weight loss, watery eyes, headache, decreased blood lymphocytes, and an increase in liver enzymes (not due to alcohol consumption).[55,57-60] Ischaemic cardiac events (including sudden death), chest pain, and pulmonary hypertension were noted.[55,58-60] There was no impairment in cognitive function and some improvement in psychotic individuals.[55,57] There is also record of three cases of sudden cardiac death in young Aboriginals who drank kava on the evening before an Australian Rules football game.[61] However, there is no electrocardiographic or epidemiological evidence to show that sudden deaths are more frequent in kava-using communities than in other Aboriginal communities.[58]

Some of the findings of a pilot survey[58] and the anecdotal reports from health care workers[59] have been questioned.[62-65] The effect of kava abuse on liver enzymes is not conclusive,[62,65] and the involvement of factors other than kava ingestion in the occurrence of the reported adverse events cannot be ruled out.[63-65]

In addition, three cases arising from abuse of traditionally prepared kava have been documented.[59,66,67] Adverse reactions included visual disturbance,[66] acute neurological syndrome,[59] scaly skin, confusion, hypotonic limbs, and elevated gamma-glutamyl transpeptidase (in a nonalcohol drinker).[67] This last find may have been due to enzyme induction by kava, rather than hepatotoxicity.

Toxicology

Table 5 lists LD_{50} data recorded for kava extracts and its constituents, indicating low acute toxicity.[19,68]

Chronic administration of dihydrokavain (50 mg/kg/day i.p.) three times a week for 3 months to rats produced no evidence of chronic toxicity. Six single doses to cats also did not produce chronic toxicity in terms of the haematological parameters measured, although a reversible dermopathy occurred.[19]

An ether extract of kava administered by stomach tube did not affect the fertility of male rats. The dosage was equivalent to 8 g of dry rhizome twice a week for 2.5 months.[69]

Regulatory Status

The regulatory status of kava (Table 6) has recently changed in many countries due to concerns over hepatotoxicity.

Table **5**   **LD_{50} Data Recorded for Kava Extract and Its Constituents**

Substance	Route, Model	LD_{50} Value	Reference
Standardised kava extract (containing 70% kava lactones)	Oral, mice	1.8 g/kg	19
Standardised kava extract (containing 70% kava lactones)	Oral, rats	16 g/kg	19
Standardised kava extract (containing 70% kava lactones)	i.p., mice	380 mg/kg	19
Standardised kava extract (containing 70% kava lactones)	i.p., rats	370 mg/kg	19
Kava extract (undefined)	i.p., rats	250 mg/kg	68
Dihydrokavain	Oral, mice	980 mg/kg	19
Dihydromethysticin	Oral, mice	1050 mg/kg	19
Kavain	Oral, mice	1130 mg/kg	19
Methysticin	Oral, mice	>800 mg/kg	19
Yangonin	Oral, mice	>1.5 mg/kg	19

Table **6** **Regulatory Status for Kava in Selected Countries**

Australia	Kava is subject to control under the Customs Import/Export Legislation. Those intending to import kava must have the appropriate licence and permit(s) to import. In July 1988 the Western Australian government restricted the sale and supply of kava under the Poisons Act 1964 to cultural uses and medical/scientific research. However, the sale of kava as a therapeutic good was not restricted in the other states of Australia. In May 1998 the Northern Territory government restricted the use and sale of kava in order to control the use of kava as a beverage in Australian Aboriginal communities. This did not affect the use of kava as a therapeutic good. In July 2002 the Therapeutic Goods Administration (TGA) initiated a voluntary withdrawal of all over-the-counter complementary medicines containing kava. The listable (automatic registration) status of kava was reviewed in 2003, with the result that kava is now included in Part 4 of Schedule 4 of the Therapeutic Goods Regulations of Australia. Preparations for oral (nonhomoeopathic) use must be either an aqueous dispersion or an aqueous extract of whole or peeled rhizome or dried whole or peeled rhizome. The following conditions must be adhered to: • the preparation does not contain, for its recommended daily dose, more than 250 mg of kava lactones; and • if the preparation is in the form of a tablet or capsule, the amount of kava lactones does not exceed 125 mg for each tablet or capsule; and if the preparation is in the form of a tea bag, the amount of dried whole or peeled rhizome does not exceed 3 g for each tea bag • if the preparation contains more than 25 mg of kava lactones per dose, the label on the goods includes the following warnings (or words to the same effect): Not for prolonged use. If symptoms persist, seek advice from a health care practitioner. Not recommended for use by pregnant or lactating women. May harm the liver.
UK & Germany	Kava was included on the General Sale List, with a maximum single dose of 625 mg. In December 2002 legislation was enacted to prohibit the sale of food consisting of, or containing, kava (Statutory Instrument No. 3169 The Kava-kava in Food (England) Regulations 2002), and to prohibit the sale of any medicinal product which consists of or contains kava (Statutory Instrument No. 3170 The Medicines for Human Use (Kava-kava) (Prohibition) Order 2002). Kava is covered by a positive Commission E monograph. However, in June 2002 the German Health Authority (BfArM) banned the therapeutic use of kava.
US	Kava does not have generally recognised as safe (GRAS) status. However, it is freely available as a "dietary supplement" in the US under DSHEA legislation (Dietary Supplement Health and Education Act of 1994).

REFERENCES

1. Pittler MH, Ernst E: *Cochrane Database Syst Rev* CD003383, 2003.
2. Warnecke G: *Fortschr Med* 109:119-122, 1991.
3. British Herbal Medicine Association's Scientific Committee: *British herbal pharmacopoeia*, Bournemouth, 1983, BHMA, pp 162-163.
4. Lebot V, Merlin M, Lindstrom L: *Kava - the Pacific elixir: the definitive guide to its ethnobotany, history and chemistry*, New Haven, 1992, Yale University Press, pp 112-118.
5. Wagner H, Bladt S: *Plant drug analysis: a thin layer chromatography atlas*, ed 2, Berlin, 1996, Springer-Verlag, pp 258-259.
6. Pharmaceutical Society of Great Britain: *British pharmaceutical codex 1934*, London, 1941, The Pharmaceutical Press, pp 573-574.
7. Dragull K, Yoshida WY, Tang CS: *Phytochemistry* 63:193-198, 2003.
8. Lebot V, Merlin M, Lindstrom L: *Kava - the Pacific elixir: the definitive guide to its ethnobotany, history and chemistry*, New Haven, 1992, Yale University Press, pp 119-174.
9. Alexander K: *Kava in the North. A study of kava in Arnhem Land Aboriginal Communities*, Casuarina, 1985, Australian National University North Australia Research Unit, p 9.
10. Riesenberg SH: *The native polity of Ponape*, Washington, 1968, Smithsonian Institution Press, p 103.
11. Serpenti LM: *Cultivators in the swamps: social structure and horticulture in a New Guinea society (Frederik-Hendrik Island West New Guinea)*. Assen, 1965, Van Gorcum, p 145.
12. Gutmanis J, 1976, cited in McKenna DJ, Jones K, Hughes K, et al: *Botanical medicines: the desk reference*

for major herbal supplements, ed 2, New York, 2002, Haworth Herbal Press, p 720.

13. Lebot V, Merlin M, Lindstrom L: *Kava - the Pacific elixir: the definitive guide to its ethnobotany, history and chemistry*, New Haven, 1992, Yale University Press, pp 111, 135-136.

14. Cambie RC, Ash J: *Fijian medicinal plants*, 1994, CSIRO Australia, pp 239-240.

15. Lebot V, Merlin M, Lindstrom L: *Kava - the Pacific elixir: the definitive guide to its ethnobotany, history and chemistry*, New Haven, 1992, Yale University Press, p 114.

16. Steinmetz EF: Piper Methysticum *(Kava - Kawa - Yaqona): famous drug plant of the South Sea islands*, Amsterdam, 1960, E.F. Steinmetz, p 43.

17. Steinmetz EF: Piper Methysticum *(Kava - Kawa - Yaqona): famous drug plant of the South Sea islands*. Amsterdam, 1960, E.F. Steinmetz, p 31.

18. Titcomb M: *J Polynes Soc* 57:105-171, 1948.

19. Hansel R, Woelk H: *Spektrum Kava-Kava (Arzneimitteltherapie heute: Phytopharmaka; Band 6)*, Basel, 1994, Aesopus Verlag, pp 40-41.

20. Ang-Lee MK, Moss J, Yuan CS: *JAMA* 286:208-216, 2001.

21. Herberg KW: *Z Allg Med* 67:842-846, 1991.

22. Herberg KW: *Z Allg Med* 72:973-977, 1996.

23. Schmidt P, Boehncke WH: *Contact Dermatitis* 42:363-364, 2000.

24. Gruenwald J, Freder J: Kava – the present European situation. *Nutraceuticals World* Jan/Feb:22-24, 2002.

25. Siegers CP, Honold E, Krall B, et al: *Arztl Forsch* 39:7-11, 1992.

26. Hofmann R, Winter U: *Psycho Zeitschrift Praxis Klin* 22:51-53, 1996.

27. Spree MH, Croy HH: *Der Kassenarzt* 17:44-51, 1992.

28. Unger L: *Therapiewoche* 38:3171-3174, 1988.

29. Stevinson C, Huntley A, Ernst E: *Drug Saf* 25:251-261, 2002.

30. Prescott J, Jamieson D, Emdur N, et al: *Drug Alcohol Rev* 12:49-58, 1993.

31. Pfeiffer CC, Murphree HB, Goldstein L, 1967, cited in Efron DH, Holmstedt B, Kline NS (eds): *Ethnopharmacologic search for psychoactive drugs: Proceedings of a Symposium held in San Francisco, CA, January 28-30*, Public Health Service Publication No. 1645, 1967, pp 155-161.

32. Hansel R: *Z Phytother* 17:180-195, 1996.

33. Keller F, Klohs MW: *Lloydia* 26:1-15, 1963.

34. Guro-Razuman S, Anand P, Hu Q, et al: *J Clin Rheumatol* 5/6:342-345, 1999.

35. Jappe U, Franke I, Reinhold D, et al: *J Am Acad Dermatol* 38:104-106, 1998.

36. Suss R, Lehmann P: *Hautarzt* 47:459-461, 1996.

37. Levine R, Taylor WB: *Arch Dermatol* 122:856, 1986.

38. Meseguer E, Taboada R, Sanchez V, et al: *Mov Disord* 17:195-196, 2002.

39. Donadio V, Bonsi P, Zele I, et al: *Neurol Sci* 21:124, 2000.

40. Schelosky L, Raffauf C, Jendroska K, et al: *J Neurol Neurosurg Psychiatry* 58:639-640, 1995.

41. Nolder M, Chatterjee SS: *Phytomedicine* 6:285-286, 1999.

42. Yates KM, O'Connor A, Horsley CA: *NZ Med J* 113:315-317, 2000.

43. Blumenthal M: *Natural Pharmacy* April 1997; pp 12-15.

44. Nordenberg T: *FDA Consumer. FDA Investigators' Reports - July/August 1998*, vol 43, no. 4, Washington DC, 1998, FDA.

45. Jamieson DD, Duffield PH: *Clin Exp Path Physiol* 17:509-514, 1990.

46. Herberg KW: *Blutalkohol* 30:96-105, 1993.

47. Foo H, Lemon J: *Drug Alcohol Rev* 16:147-155, 1997.

48. Cartledge A, Rutherford J: Rapid response (electronic letter), *BMJ* 12 Feb, 2001, available online: bmj.com/cgi/eletters/322/7279/139#12643 (accessed 21 February 2002).

49. Almeida JC, Grimsley EW: *Ann Intern Med* 125:940-941, 1996.

50. Norton SA: *Hawaii Med J* 57:382-386, 1998.

51. Norton SA, Ruze P: *J Am Acad Dermatol* 31:89-97, 1994.

52. Ruze P: *Lancet* 335:1442-1445, 1990.

53. Lebot V, Merlin M, Lindstrom L: *Kava - the Pacific elixir: the definitive guide to its ethnobotany, history and chemistry*, New Haven, 1992, Yale University Press, pp 59-60.

54. Alexander K: *Kava in the North. A study of kava in Arnhem Land Aboriginal Communities*, Casuarina, 1985, Australian National University North Australia Research Unit, p 10.

55. Cawte J: *Aust NZ J Psychiatry* 20:70-76, 1986.

56. d'Abbs P, Burns C: *Report on inquiry into the issue of kava regulation*, Prepared for the Sessional Committee on the Use and Abuse of Alcohol by the Community, Legislative Assembly of the Northern Territory, Darwin, 1997, Menzies School of Health Research.

57. Cairney S, Clough AR, Maruff P, et al: *Neuropsychopharmacology* 28:389-396, 2003.

58. Mathews JD, Riley MD, Fejo L, et al: *Med J Aust* 148:548-555, 1988.

59. Spillane PK, Fisher DA, Currie BJ: *Med J Aust* 167:172-173, 1997.

60. Kava R: *Pacific Health Dialog* 8:115-118, 2001.

61. Young MC, Fricker PA, Thomson NJ, et al: *Med J Aust* 170: 425-428, 1999.

62. Markey P: *Proceedings of the 28th Annual Conference of the Public Health Association of Australia*, Perth, 1996, p 192.

63. Douglas W: *Med J Aust* 149:341-342, 1988.

64. Lebot V, Merlin M, Lindstrom L: *Kava - the Pacific elixir: the definitive guide to its ethnobotany, history and chemistry*, New Haven, 1992, Yale University Press, p 201.

65. Mathews D, Riley MD: *Med J Aust* 149:342, 1988.

66. Garner LF, Klinger JD: *J Ethnopharmacol* 13:307-311, 1985.

67. Giles Chanwai L: *Emerg Med* 12:142-145, 2000.

68. Edwards J, Wang M, Pecore N, et al: *FASEB J* 12:A464, 1998.

69. van Dam-Bakker AWI, de Groot AP, Luyken R: *Trop Geogr Med* 10:68-70, 1958.

LAVENDER

Botanical names: *Lavandula officinalis* Chaix (*Lavandula angustifolia* Mill., *Lavandula vera* DC., *Lavandula spica* L., *Lavandula angustifolia* Mill. subsp. *angustifolia*)
Family: Labiatae
Plant part used: Flower

Safety Summary

Pregnancy category B2: No increase in frequency of malformation or other harmful effects on the foetus from limited use in women. Animal studies are lacking.
Lactation category C: Compatible with breast-feeding.
Contraindications: None required on current evidence.
Warnings & precautions: Avoid in patients with cross-sensitivity to other members of the Labiatae family.
Adverse reactions: None found in published literature.
Interactions: No precautions required on current evidence.

Typical Therapeutic Use

Traditional indications for lavender in Western herbal medicine include depression, digestive dysfunction, colic, and headache.[1]

Actions

Carminative, spasmolytic, antidepressant, anxiolytic.

Key Constituents

A key component of lavender is the essential oil (1% to 3%) which contains mainly linalyl acetate and linalool.[2]

Adulteration

No adulterants known.

Typical Dosage Forms & Dosage

Typical adult dosage ranges are:
- 3 to 6 g/day of dried flower or by infusion
- 2 to 4.5 mL/day of a 1:2 liquid extract or equivalent in tablet or capsule form
- 6 to 12 mL/day of a 1:5 tincture

Contraindications

None known.

Use in Pregnancy

Category B2: No increase in frequency of malformation or other harmful effects on the foetus from limited use in women. Animal studies are lacking.

Use in Lactation

Category C: Compatible with breastfeeding.

Lavender contains an essential oil which may pass into breast milk, providing a mild carminative effect in the baby.

Warnings & Precautions

Avoid in patients with cross-sensitivity to other members of the Labiatae family (see Adverse reactions below).

Effect on Ability to Drive or Operate Machinery

No adverse effects expected.

Adverse Reactions

Cross-sensitivity with plants belonging to the Labiatae family is possible. A positive result was obtained for lavender extract using the skin prick technique in a patient who demonstrated systemic allergic reactions after ingestion of oregano (*Origanum vulgare*) and thyme (*Thymus vulgaris*). Positive skin tests and specific IgE in serum to the Labiatae plants tested were not detected in control patients.[3] Lavender powder produced a strong positive patch test reaction in a patient with atopic eczema.[4]

Traditional herbal texts indicate that too frequent ingestion of lavender infusion will cause griping and colic.[5,6] Contact allergy to lavender oil is recorded,[7,8] although not common.[7]

Interactions

None known.

Safety in Children

No information available, but adverse effects are not expected.

Overdosage

No incidents found in published literature.

Toxicology

Table 1 lists LD_{50} data recorded for lavender.[9,10]

Regulatory Status

See Table 2 for regulatory status in selected countries.

Table 1   **LD_{50} Data Recorded for Lavender**

Substance	Route, Model	LD_{50} Value (g/kg)	Reference
Lavender oil	Rats, oral	>5	9
Lavender absolute*	Rats, oral	4.25	10

* Lavender absolute is an alcohol extract of lavender concrete (which is obtained from the fresh lavender flowers by an organic solvent extraction). The above results indicate low toxicity.

Table 2   **Regulatory Status for Lavender in Selected Countries**

Australia	Lavender is not included in Part 4 of Schedule 4 of the Therapeutic Goods Regulations.
UK & Germany	Lavender oil is included on the General Sale List. Lavender is covered by a positive Commission E monograph. Lavender is official in the *British Pharmacopoeia* 2002 and the *European Pharmacopoeia* 4.3.
US	Lavender does have generally recognised as safe (GRAS) status. It is freely available as a "dietary supplement" in the US under DSHEA legislation (Dietary Supplement Health and Education Act of 1994).

REFERENCES

1. British Herbal Medicine Association's Scientific Committee: *British herbal pharmacopoeia*, Bournemouth, 1983, BHMA, pp 128-129.
2. Wagner H, Bladt S: *Plant drug analysis: a thin layer chromatography atlas*, ed 2, Berlin, 1996, Springer-Verlag, p 157.
3. Benito M, Jorro G, Morales C, et al: *Ann Allergy Asthma Immunol* 76:416-418, 1996.
4. Mitchell J, Rook A: *Botanical dermatology: plants and plant products injurious to the skin*, Vancouver, 1979, Greengrass, pp 360-361.
5. Grieve M: *A modern herbal*, New York, 1971, Dover Publications, pp 467-473.
6. Felter HW, Lloyd JU: *King's American dispensatory*, ed 18, rev 3, vol 2, first published 1905, reprinted Portland, 1983, Eclectic Medical Publications, pp 1123-1124.
7. Rademaker M: *Contact Dermatitis* 31:58-59, 1994.
8. Sugiura M, Hayakawa R, Kato Y, et al: *Contact Dermatitis* 43:157-160, 2000.
9. Opdyke DL: *Food Cosmet Toxicol* 14:451, 1976.
10. Opdyke DL: *Food Cosmet Toxicol* 14:449, 1976.

LEMON BALM

Other common names: Melissa, balm mint
Botanical name *Melissa officinalis* L.
Family: Labiatae
Plant part used: Aerial parts

Safety Summary

Pregnancy category B2: No increase in frequency of malformation or other harmful effects on the foetus from limited use in women. Animal studies are lacking.
Lactation category C: Compatible with breast-feeding.
Contraindications: None required on current evidence.
Warnings & precautions: None required on current evidence.
Adverse reactions: There is low evidence of allergy from topical use.
Interactions: No precautions required on current evidence.

Typical Therapeutic Use

Lemon balm in combination with valerian (*Valeriana officinalis*) produced higher quality of sleep in volunteers and patients with light insomnia.[1,2] Topical treatment with lemon balm has shown significant benefit over placebo for recurring herpes labialis.[3] Traditional indications for lemon balm in Western herbal medicine include flatulent dyspepsia, depression, fever, and painful menstruation.[4,5]

Actions

Carminative, spasmolytic (antispasmodic), mild sedative, diaphoretic, thyroid stimulating hormone (TSH) antagonist, antiviral (topically).

Key Constituents

The essential oil (0.02% to 0.3%) is a key constituent of lemon balm aerial parts and contains monoterpenes (especially citronellal and citral) and sesquiterpenes. (Citral is a mixture of two geometric isomers: citral a [geranial] and citral b [neral].) Other constituents include phenolic acids and flavonoids.[6]

Adulteration

Adulteration occurs occasionally, especially by *Nepeta cataria* var. *citriodora*. Lemon balm can be distinguished from the leaves of possible adulterant species of *Stachys* and *Ballota* using microscopic techniques.[6] *Melissa officinalis* subsp. *officinalis* is the subspecies of lemon balm in official use. The other two subspecies (*M. officinalis* subsp. *inodora* and *M. officinalis* subsp. *altissima*) are regarded as adulterants.[7]

Typical Dosage Forms & Dosage

Typical adult dosage ranges are:
- 6 to 12 g/day of dried aerial parts or by infusion
- 6 to 12 mL/day of a 1:1 liquid extract
- 3 to 6 mL/day of a 1:2 liquid extract or equivalent in tablet or capsule form
- 6 to 18 mL/day of a 1:5 tincture

Contraindications

None required on current evidence.

Use in Pregnancy

Category B2: No increase in frequency of malformation or other harmful effects on the foetus from limited use in women. Animal studies are lacking.

Use in Lactation

Category C: Compatible with breastfeeding.

Lemon balm contains an essential oil which may pass into breast milk, producing a mild sedative effect in the baby. Adverse effects are not expected.

Warnings & Precautions

None required.

Effect on Ability to Drive or Operate Machinery

No adverse effects expected.

Adverse Reactions

Adverse effects are not expected. In a double-blind clinical trial for treatment of herpes simplex, the incidence of side effects from topical treatment was similar in both the lemon-balm-treated and placebo groups.[8] In an experimental model, lemon balm extract demonstrated very low sensitising power compared to the antiviral drug tromantadine.[9]

Contact urticaria occurred in a woman who applied a cosmetic formulation to her face. Testing of the face mask components on the skin indicated allergy to aloe gel, chamomile extract, lemon balm extract, allantoin, lecithin, and whole egg.[10]

Interactions

None expected.

Safety in Children

No information available, but adverse effects are not expected.

Overdosage

No incidents found in published literature.

Toxicology

A review of the toxicological literature revealed that administration of citral to rats for 13 weeks via the diet (1 to 10 g/kg) caused no macroscopic organ changes. However, in a later study, citral-induced hepatomegaly was observed which was accompanied by an altered distribution of lipid and glycogen in the liver, and peroxisome proliferation was present.[11]

Acute administration of lemon balm extract to normal rats (25 mg/kg by intravenous injection) resulted in reduced TSH concentrations in serum and the pituitary gland. An aqueous ethanol extract was prepared, the ethanol removed, and then the extract was freeze dried. Thyroid hormone concentration remained unchanged after the 3-hour observation period. Lemon balm did not lower TSH concentration in goitrous rats. The authors interpreted the loss of activity observed for lemon balm in hypothyroid rats as a weak thyroxine (T_4) agonism that was insufficient to induce pituitary TSH-repletion. At the administered dose (25 mg/kg) serum prolactin was not significantly altered in normal rats or goitrous rats.[12] The mild antithyrotropic activity of lemon balm may be due to its polyphenolic constituents combining with the protein groups of TSH to form an adduct which has a reduced ability to bind to the TSH receptor.[13]

Lemon balm tincture produced a negative result in the Ames test using *Salmonella typhimurium* strains (TA48, TA100) with or without metabolic activation.[14] Lemon balm tincture did not demonstrate mutagenicity in another in vitro model (*Aspergillus nidulans* for detection of somatic segregation).[15]

Regulatory Status

See Table 1 for regulatory status in selected countries.

Table 1 **Regulatory Status for Lemon Balm in Selected Countries**

Australia	Lemon balm is not included in Part 4 of Schedule 4 of the Therapeutic Goods Regulations.
UK & Germany	Lemon balm is not included on the General Sale List. It is covered by a positive Commission E monograph. Lemon balm is official in the *British Pharmacopoeia* 2002 and the *European Pharmacopoeia* 4.3.
US	Lemon balm does have generally recognised as safe (GRAS) status. It is freely available as a "dietary supplement" in the US under DSHEA legislation (Dietary Supplement Health and Education Act of 1994).

REFERENCES

1. Dressing H, Kohler S, Muller WE: *Psychopharmakother* 3:123-130, 1996.
2. Cerny A, Schmid K: *Fitoterapia* 70:221-228, 1999.
3. Koytchev R, Alken RG, Dundarov S: *Phytomedicine* 6:225-230, 1999.
4. British Herbal Medicine Association's Scientific Committee: *British herbal pharmacopoeia*, Bournemouth, 1983, BHMA, p 141.
5. Felter HW, Lloyd JU: *King's American dispensatory*, ed 18, rev 3, vol 2, first published 1905, reprinted Portland, 1983, Eclectic Medical Publications, pp 1252-1253.

6. Bisset NG (ed): *Herbal drugs and phytopharmaceuticals: a handbook for practice on a scientific basis*, Stuttgart, 1994, Medpharm Scientific Publishers, pp 329-332.

7. van den Berg T, Freundl E, Czygan FC: *Pharmazie* 52:802-808, 1997.

8. Wolbling RH, Leonhardt K: *Phytomedicine* 1:25-31, 1994.

9. Hausen BM, Schulze R: *Derm Beruf Umwelt* 34:163-170, 1986.

10. West I, Maibach HI: *Contact Dermatitis* 32:121, 1995.

11. de Vincenzi M, Maialetti F, Dessi MR: *Fitoterapia* 66:203-210, 1995.

12. Sourgens H, Winterhoff H, Gumbinger HG, et al: *Planta Med* 45:78-86, 1982.

13. Auf'mkolk M, Ingbar JC, Kubota K, et al: *Endocrinology* 116:1687-1693, 1985.

14. Schimmer O, Kruger A, Paulini H, et al: *Pharmazie* 49:448-451, 1994.

15. Ramos Ruiz A, De la Torre RA, Alonso N, et al: *J Ethnopharmacol* 52:123-127, 1996.

LICORICE

Other common name: Liquorice
Botanical name: *Glycyrrhiza glabra* L.
Family: Leguminosae (Papilionoideae)
Plant part used: Root and stolon

Safety Summary

Pregnancy category A: No proven increase in the frequency of malformation or other harmful effects on the foetus despite consumption by a large number of women. However, excessive intake should be avoided.
Lactation category C: Compatible with breastfeeding.
Contraindications: High blood pressure, lowered blood potassium, anorexia nervosa, cholestatic and cirrhotic liver disease, kidney failure, oedema, and congestive heart failure.
Warnings & precautions: High doses should not be taken for prolonged periods without professional advice. Caution in the elderly and those with cardiac, renal, or hepatic disease.
Adverse reactions: Lowered blood potassium levels, raised sodium and blood pressure are frequently recorded, but mainly from use of the confectionery.
Interactions: Do not prescribe concomitantly with digoxin and with diuretics, laxatives, and other potassium-depleting drugs.

Typical Therapeutic Use

Traditional indications for licorice in Western herbal medicine include bronchitis, gastritis, peptic ulceration, and adrenal insufficiency.[1]

Licorice preparations have been shown to be effective in the treatment of gastric and duodenal ulceration in clinical trials.[2,3]

Actions

Antiinflammatory, expectorant, demulcent, adrenal tonic.

Key Constituents

Triterpenoid saponins (at between 2% and 6%), especially glycyrrhizin (glycyrrhizic acid)[4] present in the form of potassium and calcium salts.[5,6] Glycyrrhetinic acid, the aglycone of glycyrrhizin, is also present in the root (0.5% to 0.9%).[7]

Flavonoids (1% to 1.5%) mainly liquiritin, chalcones, and isoflavonoids.[8]

Glycyrrhizin (but not glycyrrhetinic acid) has an intensely sweet taste (between 50 and 170 times sweeter than sugar).

Adulteration

Supplies of licorice from the Far East are likely to contain quantities of *Glycyrrhiza uralensis*, the favoured licorice in Chinese medicine. However, this species is at least comparable in effect.

Typical Dosage Forms & Dosage

Typical adult dosage ranges are:
- 3 to 12 g/day of dried root and stolon or by decoction or infusion
- 2 to 6 mL/day of a 1:1 liquid extract
- 1.5 to 4.5 mL/day of a 1:1 high glycyrrhizin liquid extract or equivalent in tablet or capsule form
- 1.2 to 4.8 mL/day of deglycyrrhizinised licorice extract BP

High-dose treatments should be of limited duration, not more than 4 to 6 weeks.[8] The Commission E indicates that when licorice is used as a flavouring component, a maximum daily dosage of less than 100 mg glycyrrhizin is acceptable.

Contraindications

Contraindications listed by the Commission E include: cholestatic liver disorders, liver cirrhosis, hypertension, hypokalaemia, severe kidney insufficiency, and pregnancy.[9]

The hypokalaemic effects may be particularly serious for patients with anorexia nervosa who have additional causes of lowered potassium levels, and permanent renal damage has been reported in one such case where high levels of licorice were consumed.[10] Licorice is also contraindicated if there is oedema or congestive heart failure.

Use in Pregnancy

Category A: No proven increase in the frequency of malformation or other harmful effects on the foetus despite consumption by a large number of women. However, the following study indicates that heavy licorice consumption (as a confectionery) was associated with the incidence of preterm delivery.

An epidemiological study involving 1049 Finnish women and their healthy babies in 1998 observed that heavy glycyrrhizin exposure (500 mg/week or greater) during pregnancy did not significantly affect birth weight or maternal blood pressure, but was significantly associated with lower gestational age. Consumption of this level of glycyrrhizin shortened the mean duration of gestation by 2.5 days.[11] A follow-up study in 2000 to 2001 with 95 Finnish women who delivered preterm babies noted that heavy glycyrrhizin consumption was associated with a more than twofold increased risk of preterm (<37 weeks) delivery. The association was stronger when only the 40 births classified as early preterm delivery (<34 weeks) were included. The authors suggest that heavy glycyrrhizin exposure may be a novel marker for preterm delivery.[12]

European authorities advise that licorice generally is contraindicated in pregnancy, and there are theoretical concerns about the link between prematurity and the health of the newborn. However, doses up to 3 g/day are likely to be safe.

For other reasons referred to here, women with hypertension in pregnancy (preeclampsia) should avoid licorice.

Ethanol extract of licorice root (250 mg/kg) did not demonstrate any significant antiimplantation activity when administered orally to female rats.[13]

Use in Lactation

Category C: Compatible with breastfeeding.

Warnings & Precautions

Patients who are prescribed licorice preparations high in glycyrrhizin for prolonged periods should be placed on a high potassium and low sodium diet. They should be closely monitored for blood pressure increases and weight gain. Hypokalaemia is the earliest threat and can occur at relatively low doses.

Special precautions should be taken with elderly patients and patients with hypertension or cardiac, renal, or hepatic disease. They should not receive licorice preparations high in glycyrrhizin for prolonged periods.

Do not prescribe concomitantly with digoxin or with diuretics, laxatives, and other potassium-depleting drugs.

The Commission E advises that (at the high doses of 5 to 15 g used in Germany) licorice should not be taken for longer than 6 to 8 weeks without professional supervision.

Avoid high doses in pregnancy and lactation.

Effect on Ability to Drive or Operate Machinery

No adverse effects expected.

Adverse Reactions

Chronic use of licorice can lead to an acquired form of "apparent mineralocorticoid excess" syndrome, with sodium retention, potassium loss, and suppression of the renin-angiotensin-aldosterone system. This is thought to follow inactivation of 11-beta-hydroxysteroid dehydrogenase and the binding of cortisol to mineralocorticoid receptors in the kidneys. In addition to clinical consequences such as raised blood pressure and oedema,[14] there are reversible effects on angiotensin I and the renin-aldosterone axis from chronic use.[15] There are early reports of severe hypertension, heart enlargement, and congestive heart failure in those consuming licorice candy (up to 100 g/day) for extended periods of time. Symptoms disappeared after cessation of licorice ingestion.[16-18]

Long-term high consumption with consequent hypokalaemia has also been associated with embolism.[19] Licorice-induced pseudoaldosteronism has been associated with a hypokalaemic myopathy and ECG findings suggesting dilated cardiomyopathy.[20]

There is an argument that the effect of licorice can be selective on sodium-retention and not necessarily on blood pressure itself: for example, a case is reported of generalised oedema without any increase in blood pressure, with biochemical and hormonal features of apparent mineralocorticoid excess, in a young woman who had been ingesting substantial amounts of licorice for several years.[21]

However, a clinical study observed that licorice significantly raised the blood pressure of volunteers even with doses as low as 50 g of licorice (75 mg glycyrrhizin) consumed daily for 2 weeks. A linear dose-response relationship was observed and the degree of individual response to licorice consumption followed the normal distribution curve.[22] A literature review published in 1993 indicates that there is individual variation in the susceptibility to glycyrrhizin. Regular daily intake of 100 mg glycyrrhizin produced adverse effects. There were no adverse effects documented for consumption below this value. Most individuals who consume 400 mg glycyrrhizin daily experience adverse effects. The authors considered that a regular intake of 100 mg/day of glycyrrhizin is the lowest observed adverse effect level and, using a safety factor of 10, a daily intake of 10 mg glycyrrhizin would represent a safe dose for most healthy adults.[23] A clinical trial published in 2003 concluded that patients with essential hypertension are more sensitive to the inhibition of 11-beta-hydroxysteroid dehydrogenase by licorice than normotensive patients, and that this inhibition causes more clinical symptoms in women than in men. Participants consumed 100 g of licorice daily, for 4 weeks, corresponding to a daily intake of 150 mg glycyrrhizin.[24]

Inhibition of 11-beta-hydroxysteroid dehydrogenase in susceptible individuals has been associated with rare cases of hypertension encephalopathy, following regular daily intake of doses of licorice equating to around 100 mg/day of glycyrrhizin.[25]

There are case reports of rhabdomyolysis, resulting in acute renal failure and deposition of calcium into damaged skeletal and cardiac muscles, associated with licorice ingestion.[26,27]

A study reported in the *New England Journal of Medicine* published in October 1999 that serum testosterone was reduced by 35% after 4 days of licorice consumption in seven men. The administered dose was 7 g/day of a licorice preparation containing 0.5 g of glycyrrhizin (since good-quality licorice contains about 5% glycyrrhizin, this dose corresponds to around 10 g/day of licorice root).[28] Replication of the results of this trial were twice attempted by a research team using the same dosage of glycyrrhizin. A statistically insignificant decrease in testosterone concentration was observed in both studies. The authors disagreed with the recommendation that men with low libido should avoid licorice consumption[29] (see also the Overdosage section below).

A case was reported in 2001 of a woman diagnosed with adenocarcinoma of the endometrium "whose history was notable for extensive use of supplemental phytoestrogens". Herbs included chaste tree, dong quai, black cohosh, and licorice.[30] No causality was demonstrated.

Interactions

Diuretics and laxatives are among a range of important drugs that deplete the body fluids of potassium.

These drugs should therefore not be taken together with licorice. There is one case report of hypokalaemic crises with neuromuscular paralysis in a woman taking excessive doses of the diuretic furosemide along with high licorice consumption.[31] Since the toxicity of digoxin and other cardiac glycosides is enhanced by low serum potassium levels, licorice should be prescribed cautiously in conjunction with this drug.[32] A case of aggravated congestive heart failure caused by digoxin toxicity has been reported in an elderly man who also took a Chinese herbal laxative containing licorice (400 mg) and rhubarb (1600 mg), three times a day for 7 days. The patient, who had mitral regurgitation with atrial fibrillation, was being treated with furosemide (80 mg) and digoxin (25 mg). Blood tests indicated elevated digoxin and lowered potassium levels.[33]

There is a theoretical risk that licorice may counteract the contraceptive pill, and long term use of high levels of licorice is best avoided in this circumstance. The intake of licorice may exaggerate the effects of a high-salt diet.

Safety in Children

As children often like licorice confectionery, care should be taken not to expose them to too much. The use of licorice as a flavouring in herbal tinctures should be moderate.

Overdosage

Six male volunteers took 7 g/day of a commercial preparation of licorice for 7 days, corresponding to an intake of 500 mg/day of glycyrrhizin. Pseudoaldosteronism was evident during the treatment, with an increase of body weight, suppression of plasma renin activity and plasma aldosterone, and reduction of serum potassium.[28]

Graded daily doses of dried, aqueous extract of licorice root, containing 108, 217, 380, and 814 mg of glycyrrhizin, were administered to four groups of six healthy volunteers of both sexes for 4 weeks. No significant effects occurred in groups 1 and 2. After 2 weeks, side effects leading to withdrawal from the protocol occurred in a female in group 3 (headache), a male with a family history of hypertension in group 4 (arterial hypertension), and a female also taking oral contraceptives in group 4 (hypertension, hypokalaemia, and peripheral oedema). In group 4, transient reduction in kalaemia and an increase in body weight were found after

1 and 2 weeks, respectively. A depression of plasma renin activity occurred in groups 3 and 4. In healthy subjects, only the highest doses of licorice led to untoward effects. These were favoured by subclinical disease or oral contraceptives, and were less common and less pronounced than adverse effects reported after the intake of glycyrrhizin taken as such or as a flavouring agent in confectionery products.[34]

Excessive consumption of licorice confectionery (¼ lb to 2 lbs or approximately 113 to 907 g) has been shown to lead to transient visual loss. It is believed that licorice derivatives can cause retinal or occipital vasospasm, giving rise to transient monocular or binocular visual loss/aberrations.[35]

Consumption of 300 to 400 g/day of licorice confectionery has induced reversible growth retardation in one child with Addison's disease.[36]

Toxicology

Doses of 100, 250, and 500 mg/kg in rats showed strong dose-dependent suppression of the adrenal-pituitary axis, with significant decreases in the concentration of cortisol, adrenocorticotrophic hormone, aldosterone, and potassium, as well as stimulation of renin production.[37]

Long-term administration of glycyrrhizin to mice did not induce tumours.[38] Oral consumption of glycyrrhetinic acid by rats (0.1 to 1.0 mg/mL) caused an increase in right atrial pressure and thickening of the pulmonary vessels, suggesting pulmonary hypertension.[39]

At doses of 100 to 1000 mg/kg/day (intragastric route, for a 1-year period) no significant changes were observed in rats. Dogs given the highest dose displayed decreased body weight gain and increased transaminase levels. The maximum tolerated dose is 300 mg/kg/day for dogs.[40]

Glycyrrhizin is mainly absorbed as glycyrrhetinic acid, the more potent agent at causing the aldosterone-like effects. Once absorbed, glycyrrhetinic acid is transported, mainly taken up into the liver by capacity-limited carriers, where it is metabolised into glucuronide and sulphate conjugates. These conjugates are transported efficiently into the bile. After outflow of the bile into the duodenum, the conjugates are hydrolysed to glycyrrhetinic acid by commensal bacteria; glycyrrhetinic acid is subsequently reabsorbed, causing a pronounced delay in the terminal plasma clearance. Physiologically based pharmacokinetic modelling indicated that, in humans, the transit rate of gastrointestinal contents through the small and large intestines predominantly determines to what extent these glycyrrhetinic acid conjugates will be reabsorbed. This parameter, which can be estimated noninvasively, may serve as a useful risk estimator for glycyrrhizin-induced adverse effects, because in subjects with prolonged gastrointestinal transit times, glycyrrhetinic acid might accumulate after repeated intake.[41]

In pharmacokinetic studies, significantly lower glycyrrhizin and glycyrrhetinic acid plasma levels were found in rats and humans treated with aqueous licorice root extract compared to the levels obtained with those in which glycyrrhizin alone was administered. This was attributed to the interaction during intestinal absorption between glycyrrhizin and several components in the whole-root extract.[42] Furthermore, whole-root extract demonstrated a significant choleretic effect and, as the bile was shown to excrete glycyrrhizin, this could be expected to further lower plasma levels.[43]

Regulatory Status

See Table 1 for regulatory status in selected countries.

Licorice is commonly consumed as a confectionery, especially in Europe.

Table 1   Regulatory Status for Licorice in Selected Countries

Australia	Licorice is not included in Part 4 of Schedule 4 of the Therapeutic Goods Regulations.
China	Licorice is official in the *Pharmacopoeia of the People's Republic of China* 1997. The usual adult dosage, usually administered in the form of a decoction, is listed as 1.5 to 9 g.
UK & Germany	Licorice is included on the General Sale List. It is covered by a positive Commission E monograph with the average daily dosage prescribed as 5 to 15 g of root, equivalent to 200 to 600 mg of glycyrrhizin or equivalent preparations. Licorice is official in the *European Pharmacopoeia* 4.3.
US	Licorice does have generally recognised as safe (GRAS) status. It is also freely available as a "dietary supplement" in the US under DSHEA legislation (Dietary Supplement Health and Education Act of 1994). Licorice is official in the *United States Pharmacopeia-National Formulary* (USP 26-NF 21, 2003).

REFERENCES

1. British Herbal Medicine Association's Scientific Committee: *British herbal pharmacopoeia*, Bournemouth, 1983, BHMA, pp 104-105.

2. Gutz HJ, Berndt H, Jackson D, et al: *Practitioner* 222:849-853, 1979.

3. Morgan AG, McAdam WA, Pacsoo C, et al: *Gut* 23:545-551, 1982.

4. Wagner H, Bladt S: *Plant drug analysis: a thin layer chromatography atlas*, ed 2, Berlin, 1996, Springer-Verlag, p 308.

5. Hostettmann K, Marston A: *Chemistry and pharmacology of natural products: saponins*, Cambridge, 1995, Cambridge University Press, pp 312-318.

6. Takino Y, Koshioka M, Shiokawa M, et al: *Planta Med* 36:74-78, 1979.

7. Killacky J, Ross MS, Turner TD, et al: *Planta Med* 30:310-316, 1976.

8. British Herbal Medicine Association: *British herbal compendium*, Bournemouth, 1992, BHMA, pp 145-148.

9. Blumenthal M, et al (eds): *The complete German Commission E monographs: therapeutic guide to herbal medicines*, Austin, 1998, American Botanical Council, pp 161-162.

10. Ishikawa S, Kato M, Tokuda T, et al: *Int J Eat Disord* 26:111-114, 1999.

11. Strandberg TE, Jarvenpaa AL, Vanhanen H, et al: *Am J Epidemiol* 153:1085-1088, 2001.

12. Strandberg TE, Andersson S, Jarvenpaa AL, et al: *Am J Epidemiol* 156:803-805, 2002.

13. Sharma BB, Varshney MD, Gupta DN, et al: *Int J Crude Drug Res* 21:183-187, 1983.

14. Olukoga A, Donaldson D: *J R Soc Health* 120:83-89, 2000.

15. Megia A, Herranz L, Martin-Almendra MA, et al: *Nephron* 65:329-330, 1993.

16. Chamberlain TJ: *JAMA* 213:1343, 1970.

17. Koster M, David GK: *N Engl J Med* 278:1381-1383, 1968.

18. Conn JW, Rovner DR, Cohen EL: *JAMA* 205:492-496, 1968.

19. Lozano P, Flores D, Martinez S, et al: *J Cardiovasc Surg (Torino)* 41:631-632, 2000.

20. Hasegawa J, Suyama Y, Kinugawa T, et al: *Cardiovasc Drugs Ther* 12:599-600, 1998.

21. Negro A, Rossi E, Regolisti G, et al: *Ann Ital Med Int* 15:296-300, 2000.

22. Sigurjonsdottir HA, Franzson L, Manhem K, et al: *J Hum Hypertens* 15:549-552, 2001.

23. Stormer FC, Reistad R, Alexander J: *Food Chem Toxicol* 31:303-312, 1993.

24. Sigurjonsdottir HA, Manhem K, Axelson M, et al: *J Hum Hypertens* 17:125-131, 2003.

25. Russo S, Mastropasqua M, Mosetti MA, et al: *Am J Nephrol* 20:145-148, 2000.

26. Firenzuoli F, Gori L: *Recenti Prog Med* 93:482-483, 2002.

27. Saito T, Tsuboi Y, Fujisawa G, et al: *Nippon Jinzo Gakkai Shi* 36:1308-1314, 1994.

28. Armanini D, Bonanni G, Palermo M: *N Engl J Med* 341:1158, 1999.

29. Josephs RA, Guinn JS, Harper ML, et al: *Lancet* 358:1613-1614, 2001.

30. Johnson EB, Muto MC, Yanushpolsky EH, et al: *Obstet Gynecol* 98:947-950, 2001.

31. Famularo G, Corsi FM, Giacanelli M: *Acad Emerg Med* 6:960-964, 1999.

32. E-MIMS: *Version 4.00.0457*, St Leonards NSW Australia, 2000, MIMS Australia Pty Ltd.

33. Harada T, Ohtaki E, Misu K, et al: *Cardiology* 98:218, 2002.

34. Bernardi M, D'Intino PE, Trevisani F, et al: *Life Sci* 55:863-872, 1994.

35. Dobbins KR, Saul RF: *J Neuroophthalmol* 20:38-41, 2000.

36. Doeker BM, Andler W: *Horm Res* 52:253-255, 1999.

37. Al-Qarawi AA, Abdel-Rahman HA, Ali BH, et al: *Food Chem Toxicol* 40:1525-1527, 2002.

38. Kobuke K, Inai K, Nambu S, et al: *Food Chem Toxicol* 23:979-983, 1985.

39. Ruszymah BH, Nabishah BM, Aminuddin S, et al: *Clin Exp Hypertens* 17:575-591, 1995.

40. Kelloff GJ, Crowell JA, Boone CW, et al: *J Cell Biochem Suppl* 20:166-175, 1994.

41. Ploeger B, Mensinga T, Sips A, et al: *Drug Metab Rev* 33:125-147, 2001.

42. Cantelli-Forti G, Maffei F, Hrelia P, et al: *Environ Health Perspect* 102(Suppl 9):65-68, 1994.

43. Cantelli-Forti G, Raggi MA, Bugamelli F, et al: *Pharmacol Res* 35:463-470, 1997.

LIME FLOWERS

Other common names: Tilia, linden flower, lime blossom
Botanical names: *Tilia cordata* Mill. (*Tilia parvifolia* Ehrh., *Tilia ulmifolia* Scop.), *Tilia platyphyllos* Scop. (*Tilia grandifolia* Ehrh.), *Tilia* × *europaea* L. (*Tilia* × *vulgaris* Hayne)
Family: Tiliaceae
Plant part used: Flower

Safety Summary

Pregnancy category B2: No increase in frequency of malformation or other harmful effects on the foetus from limited use in women. Animal studies are lacking.
Lactation category C: Compatible with breastfeeding.
Contraindications: None required on current evidence.
Warnings & precautions: Avoid in patients with known allergy.
Adverse reactions: Rare allergic reaction.
Interactions: May reduce iron absorption if taken simultaneously with meals or iron supplements.

Typical Therapeutic Use

Traditional indications for lime flowers in Western herbal medicine include upper respiratory catarrh, restlessness, headache, and hypertension.[1]

Actions

Spasmolytic, peripheral vasodilator, mild sedative, diaphoretic.

Key Constituents

Lime flowers contain flavonoids, phenolic acids, procyanidin dimers, and an essential oil.[1]

Adulteration

Lime flower adulterants include *T. tomentosa* (*T. argentea*), *T.* × *euchlora*, *T. americana*, *T. pubescens* and, in Chinese products, *T. chinensis* and *T. mandschurica*. Hybrids of these plants are also considered adulterants.[2,3]

Many other species of *Tilia* are used in herbal medicine, depending upon the locality. The following species were used by the Eclectics: *T. americana* and *T. heterophylla*.[4] *T. tomentosa* (*T. argentea*) and *T. rubra* are used for similar purposes in Turkish folk medicine.[5] These species are regarded as inferior. Lime flower commercial samples from Europe in the mid-1980s were found to contain the species *T. argentea*.[6]

Typical Dosage Forms & Dosage

Typical adult dosage ranges are:
- 6 to 12 g/day of dried flower or by infusion
- 6 to 12 mL/day of a 1:1 liquid extract
- 2 to 4.5 mL/day of a 1:2 liquid extract or equivalent in tablet or capsule form
- 12 to 30 mL/day of a 1:5 tincture

Contraindications

None known.

Use in Pregnancy

Category B2: No increase in frequency of malformation or other harmful effects on the foetus from limited use in women. Animal studies are lacking.

Use in Lactation

Category C: Compatible with breastfeeding.

Warnings & Precautions

Avoid in patients with known allergy.

Effect on Ability to Drive or Operate Machinery

No adverse effects expected.

Adverse Reactions

A case of contact urticaria following the use of a shampoo containing lime flower extract has been reported. Patch testing of this patient indicated a positive reaction to lime flower extract and eugenol (which was also present at a low concentration in the shampoo).[7] Allergic rhinitis following ingestion of lime flower tea has been reported. Patch testing with dilute lime flower extract yielded a positive result.[8] Allergic rhinitis from lime flowers is well described, but allergic asthma is not.[9] Exposure to lime flower pollen can induce IgE-mediated rhinoconjunctivitis and cough.[10]

Interactions

A clinical study has indicated a potential interaction between lime flower ingestion and reduced iron absorption. An infusion of lime flowers reduced the absorption of iron by 52% from a bread meal (compared to a water control) in adult volunteers. The inhibition was dose-dependent and related to its polyphenol content (phenolic acids, monomeric flavonoids, polymerised polyphenols). Inhibition by black tea was 79% to 94%.[11] In anaemia and cases where iron supplementation is required, lime flowers should not be taken simultaneously with meals or iron supplements.

Safety in Children

No information available.

Overdosage

No reliable information found in published literature. A report of a tea prepared from very old flowers causing narcotic intoxication is regarded as unreliable, as is the notion that too frequent use of lime flower tea will cause damage to the heart.[8]

Toxicology

No information available for the flower of the therapeutic *Tilia* spp.

Regulatory Status

See Table 1 for regulatory status in selected countries.

Table 1   **Regulatory Status for Lime Flowers in Selected Countries**

Australia	Lime flowers is not included in Part 4 of Schedule 4 of the Therapeutic Goods Regulations.
UK & Germany	Lime flowers is included on the General Sale List. It is covered by a positive Commission E monograph. Lime flowers is official in the *British Pharmacopoeia* 2002 and the *European Pharmacopoeia* 4.3.
US	Lime flowers does have generally recognised as safe (GRAS) status. It is freely available as a "dietary supplement" in the US under DSHEA legislation (Dietary Supplement Health and Education Act of 1994).

REFERENCES

1. British Herbal Medicine Association: *British herbal compendium*, vol 1, Bournemouth, 1992, BHMA, pp 142-144.
2. Bisset NG (ed.): *Herbal drugs and phytopharmaceuticals: a handbook for practice on a scientific basis*, Stuttgart, 1994, Medpharm Scientific Publishers, pp 496-498.
3. Blaschek W, Ebel S, Hackenthal E, et al: *HagerROM 2002: Hagers Handbuch der Drogen und Arzneistoffe*, Heidelberg, 2002, Springer.
4. Felter HW, Lloyd JU: *King's American dispensatory*, ed 18, rev 3, vol 2, first published 1905, reprinted Portland, 1983, Eclectic Medical Publications, pp 1940-1941.
5. Toker G, Aslan M, Yesilada E, et al: *J Pharm Biomed Anal* 26:111-121, 2001.
6. Ulmann RM: *Pharm Weekbl* 120:482-483, 1985.
7. Picardo M, Rovina R, Cristaudo A, et al: *Contact Dermatitis* 19:72-73, 1988.
8. de Smet PAGM, Keller K, Hansel R, et al (eds): *Adverse effects of herbal drugs*, vol 2, Berlin, 1993, Springer-Verlag, pp 303-306.
9. Weber RW: *Ann Allergy Asthma Immunol* 88:A4, 2002.
10. Mur P, Feo Brio F, Lombardero M, et al: *Allergy* 56: 457-458, 2001.
11. Hurrell RF, Reddy M, Cook JD: *Br J Nutr* 81:289-295, 1999.

MARSHMALLOW

Botanic name: *Althaea officinalis* L.
Family: Malvaceae
Plant part used: Root and leaf

Safety Summary

Pregnancy category B2: No increase in frequency of malformation or other harmful effects on the foetus from limited use in women. Animal studies are lacking.
Lactation category C: Compatible with breast-feeding.
Contraindications: None required on current evidence.
Warnings & precautions: None required on current evidence.
Adverse reactions: None found in published literature.
Interactions: The absorption of other drugs taken simultaneously may be retarded, but this effect is likely to be a minor one.

Typical Therapeutic Use

Traditional indications for marshmallow in Western herbal medicine include gastritis, peptic ulceration, cough, inflammation of the upper respiratory tract, and cystitis.[1] These uses are attributed largely to the local effects of the mucilage content of the herb.[2]

Actions

Demulcent, urinary demulcent.
Topically: emollient, vulnerary.

Key Constituents

Mucilage polysaccharides (5% to 10%) in the root,[3] lower levels in the leaf.

Adulteration

Marshmallow leaf is rarely adulterated by leaves of other Malvaceae and particularly by *Lavatera thuringiaca* L.[4] The roots of *Althaea rosea* L. are occasionally encountered as medicinal marshmallow.[5] *Althaea officinalis* is protected and/or has restrictions for wildcrafting in several areas of Europe.[6]

Typical Dosage Forms & Dosage

Typical adult dosage ranges are:
- 6 to 15 g/day of dried leaf or root (extraction is best by cold infusion in water)
- 3 to 6 mL/day of a 1:2 extract of leaf
- 3 to 6 mL/day of a 1:5 liquid extract of root (best extracted in a glycerol-water mixture)

Contraindications

None known.

Use in Pregnancy

Category B2: No increase in frequency of malformation or other harmful effects on the foetus from limited use in women. Animal studies are lacking.

A weak antioestrogenic and androgenic effect of the extract of a relative of marshmallow (the hollyhock, *Althaea rosea*) has been shown in rats.[7] These effects were considered to be due to stimulation by phyto-oestrogens (possibly anthocyanidins and flavonoids) of aromatase and beta-oestrogen receptors.[8] They are unlikely to have implications for use in pregnancy.

Use in Lactation

Category C: Compatible with breastfeeding.

Warnings & Precautions

None required.

Effect on Ability to Drive or Operate Machinery

No adverse effects expected.

Adverse Reactions

None known.

Interactions

The absorption of drugs taken simultaneously may be retarded, but this effect is likely to be minor.[9]

Safety in Children

No information available but adverse effects are not expected.

Overdosage

No incidents found in published literature.

Toxicology

No information available.

Regulatory Status

See Table 1 for regulatory status in selected countries.

Table **1**   **Regulatory Status for Marshmallow in Selected Countries**

Australia	Marshmallow is not included in Part 4 of Schedule 4 of the Therapeutic Goods Regulations.
UK & Germany	Marshmallow root is included on the General Sale List. Marshmallow leaf and root are each covered by a positive Commission E monograph.
US	Marshmallow does not have generally recognised as safe (GRAS) status. However, it is freely available as a "dietary supplement" in the US under DSHEA legislation (Dietary Supplement Health and Education Act of 1994).

REFERENCES

1. British Herbal Medicine Association's Scientific Committee: *British herbal pharmacopoeia*, Bournemouth, 1983, BHMA, pp 22-23.
2. Mills S, Bone K: *Principles and practice of phytotherapy: modern herbal medicine*, Edinburgh, 2000, Churchill Livingstone, pp 26-27.
3. Rosik J, Kardosova A, Toman R, et al: *Cesk Farm* 33: 68-71, 1984.
4. Blaschek W, Ebel S, Hackenthal E, et al: *HagerROM 2002: Hagers Handbuch der Drogen und Arzneistoffe*, Heidelberg, 2002, Springer.
5. Bisset NG (ed.): *Herbal drugs and phytopharmaceuticals: a handbook for practice on a scientific basis*. Stuttgart, 1994, Medpharm Scientific Publishers, pp 65-66.
6. Lange D: *Europe's medicinal and aromatic plants: their use, trade and conservation*, Cambridge, 1998, TRAFFIC International, p 11.
7. Papiez M: *Folia Histochem Cytobiol* 39:219-220, 2001.
8. Papiez M, Gancarczyk M, Bilinska B: *Folia Histochem Cytobiol* 40:353-359, 2002.
9. Scientific Committee of ESCOP (European Scientific Cooperative on Phytotherapy): *ESCOP Monographs: Althaeae radix*, UK, March 1996, ESCOP Secretariat.

MEADOWSWEET

Botanical names: *Filipendula ulmaria* (L.) Maxim., *Filipendula ulmaria* (L.) Maxim. subsp. *ulmaria* (*Spiraea ulmaria* L.)
Family: Rosaceae
Plant part used: Aerial parts

Safety Summary

Pregnancy category B3: No increase in frequency of malformation or other harmful effects on the foetus from limited use in women. Evidence of increased foetal damage in animal studies exists, although the relevance to humans is unknown. (Recommendation on the basis of the salicylaldehyde content.)
Lactation category CC: Compatible with breastfeeding but use caution.
Contraindications: In principle, the use of herbs containing high levels of tannins is contraindicated, or at least inappropriate, in constipation, iron deficiency anaemia, and malnutrition. Do not use during pregnancy or lactation without professional advice.
Warnings & precautions: Avoid, or use with caution, in patients with salicylate sensitivity, bleeding disorders, or glucose-6-phosphate dehydrogenase deficiency. The use of tannins can be inappropriate in constipation, iron deficiency anaemia, or malnutrition. Long-term therapy with high doses of tannins is best avoided. Use cautiously in highly inflamed or ulcerated conditions of the gastrointestinal tract.
Adverse reactions: None found in published literature for meadowsweet. A potential adverse reaction due to the high tannin content is irritation of the mouth and gastrointestinal tract.
Interactions: Use with caution if patients are taking anticoagulant medication. Take separately from oral thiamine, metal ion supplements, or alkaloid-containing medications.

Typical Therapeutic Use

Traditional uses of meadowsweet in Western herbal medicine include atonic dyspepsia with heartburn and hyperacidity, diarrhoea, acute cystitis, rheumatic pain, and prophylaxis and treatment of gastric ulcer.[1] Therapeutic benefit was demonstrated in an uncontrolled trial of patients with cervical dysplasia treated with an ointment containing meadowsweet.[2]

Actions

Antiulcerogenic, antacid, antiinflammatory, mild urinary antiseptic, astringent.

Key Constituents

Constituents of meadowsweet aerial parts include flavonoids (3% to 5%); phenolic glycosides, such as spiraein (salicylaldehyde primveroside), monotropitin (methyl salicylate primveroside), and isosalicin; an essential oil (0.2%) containing salicylaldehyde (75%), phenylethyl alcohol (3%), benzyl alcohol (2%), and methylsalicylate (1.3%); and tannins (10% to 15%), such as rugosin-D.[3,4] Meadowsweet also contains salicylic acid (0.6% to 0.8%) and its methylester (0.14%).[4]

The salicylate content of high quality 1:2 liquid extracts of meadowsweet is expected to be approximately 400 µg/mL.

Adulteration

Confusion with *Filipendula hexapetala* and *Sambucus nigra* (elder flower) has occurred.[5,6]

Typical Dosage Forms & Dosage

Typical adult dosage ranges are:
- 12 to 18 g/day of dried aerial parts or by infusion
- 4.5 to 18 mL/day of a 1:1 liquid extract
- 3 to 6 mL/day of a 1:2 liquid extract or equivalent in tablet or capsule form
- 6 to 12 mL/day of a 1:5 tincture

Contraindications

In principle, the use of tannins is contraindicated, or at least inappropriate, in constipation, iron deficiency anaemia, and malnutrition. Do not use during pregnancy or lactation without professional advice.

Use in Pregnancy

Category B3: No increase in frequency of malformation or other harmful effects on the foetus from limited use in women. Evidence of increased foetal damage in animal studies exists, although the relevance to humans is unknown.

An aqueous infusion (1:20) of meadowsweet flowers increased the tone and force of contraction of smooth muscle from sections of the uterine horns of rats, guinea pigs, and cats.[7]

Foetal toxicity, measured as the number of resorptions, deaths, and malformations, was 46.1% in pregnant rats subcutaneously administered salicylaldehyde (400 mg/kg) on day 11 of gestation, compared to 2.7% in the control group.[8] This dose of salicylaldehyde is considerably higher than the amount contained in a therapeutic dose of meadowsweet, and the study is unlikely to be relevant to therapeutic use of meadowsweet.

Use in Lactation

Category CC: Compatible with breastfeeding but use caution.

Salicylates excreted in breast milk have been reported to cause macular rashes in breast-fed babies.

Warnings & Precautions

The use of tannins can be inappropriate in constipation, iron deficiency anaemia, and malnutrition. Because of the tannin content of this herb, long-term use should be avoided (for both internal and topical use). Use cautiously in highly inflamed or ulcerated conditions of the gastrointestinal tract.

Meadowsweet contains salicylates and should be avoided, or used with caution, in patients with salicylate sensitivity or glucose-6-phosphate dehydrogenase deficiency (in this condition salicylic acid causes haemolytic anaemia).

Meadowsweet should be used with caution in patients with bleeding disorders, as anticoagulant activity for extracts of the flowers and seeds has been demonstrated in vitro and in vivo after oral administration.[9]

Effect on Ability to Drive or Operate Machinery

No adverse effects expected.

Adverse Reactions

None known for meadowsweet. High doses of tannins lead to excessive astringency on mucous membranes, which has an irritating effect.

Interactions

None known. Due to the experimental anticoagulant activity,[9] meadowsweet should be used with caution in patients taking anticoagulant medication.

Tannins can bind metal ions, thiamine, and alkaloids, reducing their absorption. Refer to the cranesbill root (*Geranium maculatum*) monograph for information regarding the interactions of tannins. Meadowsweet should be consumed at least 2 hours away from oral thiamine, mineral supplements such as iron, and alkaloid-containing drugs.

Safety in Children

Clinicians should be aware of the possibility of Reye's syndrome, an acute sepsis-like illness encountered exclusively in children below 15 years of age. The cause is unknown, although viral agents and drugs, especially salicylate derivatives, have been implicated.[10] However, it is unknown whether the salicylates in meadowsweet are capable of causing this reaction.

Overdosage

No incidents found in published literature. However, long-term use with high doses of tannins is to be avoided.

Toxicology

LD_{50} data for salicylaldehyde, which is a minor component of meadowsweet, is provided in Table 1.[11-14]

Animal studies of the flowers and alcoholic and aqueous extracts have suggested that meadowsweet is without toxic effects.[15]

Refer to the cranesbill root (*Geranium maculatum*) monograph for information regarding interactions of tannins (see Interactions section).

Regulatory Status

See Table 2 for regulatory status in selected countries.

Table 1 **LD$_{50}$ Data Recorded for Meadowsweet**

Substance	Route, Model	LD$_{50}$ Value	Reference
Salicylaldehyde	Oral, rats	520 mg/kg	11
Salicylaldehyde	i.p., mice	2.2 mg/kg	12
Salicylaldehyde	s.c., rats	900 mg/kg	13
Salicylaldehyde	Topical, rats	600 mg/kg	14
Salicylaldehyde	Topical, rabbits	3 g/kg	11

Table 2 **Regulatory Status for Meadowsweet in Selected Countries**

Australia	Meadowsweet is not included in Part 4 of Schedule 4 of the Therapeutic Goods Regulations.
UK & Germany	Meadowsweet is included on the General Sale List. It is covered by a positive Commission E monograph.
US	Meadowsweet does not have generally recognised as safe (GRAS) status. However, it is freely available as a "dietary supplement" in the US under DSHEA legislation (Dietary Supplement Health and Education Act of 1994).

REFERENCES

1. British Herbal Medicine Association's Scientific Committee: *British herbal pharmacopoeia.* Bournemouth, 1983, BHMA, pp 91-92.
2. Peresun'ko AP, Bespalov VG, Limarenko AI, et al: *Vopr Onkol* 39:291-295, 1993.
3. British Herbal Medicine Association: *British herbal compendium,* vol 1, Dorset, 1992, BHMA, pp 158-160.
4. Wagner H, Bladt S: *Plant drug analysis: a thin layer chromatography atlas,* ed 2, Berlin, 1996, Springer-Verlag, p 199.
5. Bisset NG (ed.): *Herbal drugs and phytopharmaceuticals: a handbook for practice on a scientific basis,* Stuttgart, 1994, Medpharm Scientific Publishers, pp 480-482.
6. Blaschek W, Ebel S, Hackenthal E, et al: *HagerROM 2002: Hagers Handbuch der Drogen und Arzneistoffe.* Heidelberg, 2002, Springer.
7. Barnaulov OD, Bukreeva TB, Kokarev AA, et al: *Rastit Resur* 14:573–579, 1978.
8. Saito H, Yokoyama A, Takeno S, et al: *Res Commun Chem Pathol Pharmacol* 38:209-220, 1982.
9. Liapina LA, Koval'chuk GA: *Izv Akad Nauk Ser Biol* 4:625-628, 1993.
10. Isselbacher KJ, Podolsky DK. In Harrison TR, Fauci AS (eds): *Harrison's principles of internal medicine,* ed 14, CD-ROM, New York, 1998, McGraw-Hill.
11. Moreno OM: *Report to RIFM,* 27 January 1977. In Opdyke DLJ: *Food Cosmet Toxicol* 17(Suppl 2):903, 1979.
12. Williams LA, Howell RC, Young R, et al: *Comp Biochem Physiol C Toxicol Pharmacol* 128:119-125, 2001.
13. Fassett DW. In Patty FA (ed.): *Industrial hygiene and toxicology,* ed 2, vol 2, New York, 1963, Interscience Publishers, p 1987.
14. Moeser E, Bien E, Jung F: *Acta Biol Med Germ* 21:693, 1968.
15. Barnaulov OD, Boldina IG, Galushko VV, et al: *Rastitel'Nye Resursy* 15:399-407, 1979.

MOTHERWORT

Botanical names: *Leonurus cardiaca* L. (*L. villosus* Desf. ex Spreng., *L. quinquelobatus* Usteri, *L. tataricus* L., *L. glaucescens* Ledeb.), *Leonurus quinquelobatus* Gilib.
Family: Labiatae
Plant part used: Aerial parts

Safety Summary

Pregnancy category B3: No increase in frequency of malformation or other harmful effects on the foetus from limited use in women. Evidence of increased foetal damage in animal studies exists, although the relevance to humans is unknown (on the basis of leonurine).
Lactation category C: Compatible with breastfeeding.
Contraindications: None required on current evidence. Do not use during pregnancy without professional advice.
Warnings & precautions: None required on current evidence.
Adverse reactions: None found in published literature.
Interactions: No precautions required on current evidence.

Typical Therapeutic Use

Traditional indications for motherwort in Western herbal medicine include cardiac debility, tachycardia and amenorrhoea.[1]

Actions

Nervine tonic, cardiotonic, hypotensive, antiarrhythmic, antithyroid, spasmolytic, emmenagogue.

Key Constituents

Motherwort contains bitter glycosides, diterpenoids, triterpenes, flavonoids, alkaloids (leonurine, stachydrine), tannins (5% to 9%) and an iridoid glycoside (leonuride).[2] The alkaloids leonurine and stachydrine are present in very small amounts: 0.007% and 0.06% respectively.[3,4]

Adulteration

Leonurus glaucescens Bunge (*L. cardiaca* subsp. *glaucescens* (Bunge) Schmalh) is regarded as an adulterant.[4]

Typical Dosage Forms & Dosage

Typical adult dosage ranges are:
- 6 to 12 g/day of dried aerial parts or by infusion
- 6 to 12 mL/day of a 1:1 liquid extract
- 2 to 3.5 mL/day of a 1:2 liquid extract or equivalent in tablet or capsule form
- 6 to 18 mL/day of a 1:5 tincture

Contraindications

None recommended. See Use in pregnancy section below. Do not use during pregnancy without professional advice.

Use in Pregnancy

Category B3: No increase in frequency of malformation or other harmful effects on the foetus from limited use in women. Evidence of increased foetal damage in animal studies exists, although the relevance to humans is unknown (on the basis of leonurine).

The *British Herbal Compendium* recommends that motherwort is contraindicated in pregnancy. This contraindication is probably an extrapolation from studies on the constituent leonurine, which has increased tone and contractions in isolated uterus.[5] A very slight stimulating effect on isolated uterus was observed for *L. cardiaca* ethanol extract in an early study,[6] although it failed to show activity in other studies.[7,8] The Commission E advises there are no known contraindications.

Use in Lactation

Category C: Compatible with breastfeeding.

Warnings & Precautions

None required.

Effect on Ability to Drive or Operate Machinery

No adverse effects expected.

Adverse Reactions

No adverse reactions are known for ingestion of motherwort aerial parts. The plant can cause contact dermatitis in sensitive individuals.[9]

Interactions

None known.

Safety in Children

No information available.

Overdosage

No incidents found in published literature.

Toxicology

Leonurine injected in mice produced irritation, convulsions and respiratory paralysis. Small doses in cats act as a respiratory stimulant; excessive doses produce respiratory paralysis.[5]

Motherwort extract tested negative for in vitro mutagenic activity in the Ames test.[10]

Regulatory Status

See Table 1 for regulatory status in selected countries.

Table 1   **Regulatory Status for Motherwort in Selected Countries**

Australia	Motherwort is not included in Part 4 of Schedule 4 of the Therapeutic Goods Regulations.
UK & Germany	Motherwort is included on the General Sale List. It is covered by a positive Commission E monograph.
US	Motherwort does not have generally recognised as safe (GRAS) status. However, it is freely available as a "dietary supplement" in the US under DSHEA legislation (Dietary Supplement Health and Education Act of 1994).

REFERENCES

1. British Herbal Medicine Association's Scientific Committee: *British herbal pharmacopoeia*, Bournemouth, 1983, BHMA, pp 129-130.
2. British Herbal Medicine Association: *British herbal compendium*, vol 1, Bournemouth, 1992, BHMA, pp 161-162.
3. Gulubov AZ, Chervenkova VB: *Nauch Tr Vissh Pedagog Inst Plovdiv Mat Fiz Khim Biol* 8:129-132, 1970.
4. Blaschek W, Ebel S, Hackenthal E, et al: *HagerROM 2002: Hagers Handbuch der Drogen und Arzneistoffe*, Heidelberg, 2002, Springer.
5. Kubota S, Nakashima S: *Folia Pharmacol Japon* 11:159-167, 1930.
6. Erspamer LV: *Arch Int Pharmacodyn* 76:132-152, 1948.
7. Pilcher JD: *J Pharmacol Exp Therapeut* 8:110-111, 1916.
8. Pilcher JD, Mauer RT: *Surg Gynecol Obstet* 27:97-99, 1918.
9. Munro DB: Canadian Poisonous Plants Information System. Centre for Land and Biological Resources Research, Ottawa, 1993. Electronic file, also available via http://sis.agr.gc.ca/pls/pp/poison?p_x=px within the Agriculture and Agri-Food Canada webpage.
10. Schimmer O, Kruger A, Paulini H, et al: *Pharmazie* 49:448-451, 1994.

MULLEIN

Botanical names: *Verbascum thapsus* L., *V. phlomoides* L., *V. densiflorum* Bertol. (*V. thapsiforme* Schrad.)
Family: Scrophulariaceae
Plant part used: Leaf

Safety Summary

Pregnancy category B2: No increase in frequency of malformation or other harmful effects on the foetus from limited use in women. Animal studies are lacking.
Lactation category C: Compatible with breastfeeding.
Contraindications: None required on current evidence.
Warnings & precautions: None required on current evidence.
Adverse reactions: None found in published literature.
Interactions: No precautions required on current evidence.

Typical Therapeutic Use

Traditional indications for mullein leaf in Western herbal medicine include inflammation and congestion of the respiratory tract and influenza.[1]

Actions

Expectorant, demulcent, anticatarrhal, vulnerary.

Key Constituents

Mullein leaf contains iridoid glycosides (especially aucubin), flavonoids, and an undefined saponin.[2] The leaves of *V. thapsus* were also found to contain a small amount of rotenone, which varies with the time of year.[3]

Adulteration

No adulterants known, although poor quality material evidenced by noncompliance with quality standards has been observed in commercial samples, which appears to be independent of the (medicinally interchangeable) species provided.[4]

The Unani medicinal herb bantamaku is referred to in the literature as both *Atropa acuminata* and

Verbascum thapsus. Pharmacognostic studies conducted on dried stem and leaf plant samples indicate that bantamaku is derived from *Atropa acuminata*.[5] Although no cases have been reported, attention has been drawn to the use of local common names as providing risk of adulteration. *Verbascum thapsus* has been sold in California (1947) and Chicago (1977) under the common name of gordolobo. Other plants with this name sold near the Mexican border include *Gnaphalium macounii* and the toxic *Senecio longilobus*. The latter plant has been responsible for several cases of poisoning in Arizona. Also, at this time, *V. thapsus* was sold under five other common names, one of which was also common to *Nicotiana tabacum*.[6]

Typical Dosage Forms & Dosage

Typical adult dosage ranges are:
- 12 to 24 g/day of dried leaf or by infusion
- 12 to 24 mL/day of a 1:1 liquid extract
- 4.5 to 8.5 mL/day of a 1:2 liquid extract or equivalent in tablet or capsule form

Contraindications

None known.

Use in Pregnancy

Category B2: No increase in frequency of malformation or other harmful effects on the foetus from limited use in women. Animal studies are lacking.

Use in Lactation

Category C: Compatible with breastfeeding.

Warnings & Precautions

None required on current evidence.

Effect on Ability to Drive or Operate Machinery

No adverse effects expected.

Adverse Reactions

Occupational dermatitis from mullein has been reported.[7] Contact with aerial parts must have occurred, but it is not known whether the plant was flowering.

Interactions

None reported.

Safety in Children

No information available, but adverse effects are not expected.

Overdosage

No incidents found in published literature.

Toxicology

Ethanol extract of whole plant of *V. thapsus* produced the LD_{50} value of 1 g/kg when administered to mice by intraperitoneal injection.[8]

Verbascum thapsus extracts demonstrated toxicity in the brine shrimp assay (at concentrations around 1 g/L) and to radish seed germination and growth (>1 g/L). In the brine shrimp assay of aqueous extracts, a decoction was more toxic than an infusion.[9]

Regulatory Status

See Table 1 for regulatory status in selected countries.

Table 1   **Regulatory Status for Mullein in Selected Countries**

Australia	Mullein is not included in Part 4 of Schedule 4 of the Therapeutic Goods Regulations.
UK & Germany	Mullein is not included on the General Sale List. Mullein leaf was not included in the Commission E assessment.
US	Mullein does not have generally recognised as safe (GRAS) status. However, it is freely available as a "dietary supplement" in the US under DSHEA legislation (Dietary Supplement Health and Education Act of 1994).

REFERENCES

1. British Herbal Medicine Association's Scientific Committee: *British herbal pharmacopoeia*, Bournemouth, 1983, BHMA, pp 226-227.
2. Blaschek W, Ebel S, Hackenthal E, et al: *HagerROM 2002: Hagers Handbuch der Drogen und Arzneistoffe*, Heidelberg, 2002, Springer.
3. Obdulio F, Lobete MP: *Farm Nueva* 8:204-206, 1943.
4. Purbrick P: Information on file, Warwick, Queensland 4072, Australia, 2003, MediHerb Pty Ltd.
5. Ghauri EG: *Pak J Sci Ind Res* 32:754-759, 1989.
6. Huxtable RJ: *Perspect Biol Med* 24:1-14, 1980.
7. Romaguera C, Grimalt F, Vilaphana J: *Contact Dermatitis* 12:176, 1985.
8. Bhakuni DS, Dhar ML, Dhar MM, et al: *Indian J Exp Biol* 7:250-262, 1969.
9. Turker A, Camper N: *J Ethnopharmacol* 82:117-125, 2002.

MYRRH

Botanical names: *Commiphora molmol* Engl.[*][1-7] (*Balsamodendron myrrha* Nees, *C. myrrha* (Nees) Engl.)
Family: Burseraceae
Plant part used: Oleo-gum resin

Safety Summary

Pregnancy category B1: No increase in frequency of malformation or other harmful effects on the foetus from limited use in women. No evidence of increased foetal damage in animal studies.
Lactation category CC: Compatible with breast-feeding but use caution.
Contraindications: Known allergy. Do not use during lactation without professional advice.
Warnings & precautions: Long-term use and intake during pregnancy are best avoided.
Adverse reactions: Contact dermatitis and allergy.
Interactions: No precautions required on current evidence.

Typical Therapeutic Use

Traditional indications of myrrh in Western herbal medicine include pharyngitis, aphthous ulceration, respiratory infections and topically for furunculosis.[8] Myrrh is used traditionally in the Middle East as a treatment for diabetes[9] and for gastric inflammation and ulceration.[10]

A clinical study was carried out on 204 patients with schistosomiasis, a widespread worm infestation. At a dose of 10 mg/kg of body weight/day for 3 days, a combination of resin and volatile oil extracted from myrrh permanently cleared the infection in 91.7%.[11] Effective elimination of *Fasciola* eggs were demonstrated in infected human patients

from a resin/volatile oil extract of myrrh (12 mg/kg) administered orally for 6 days.[12]

There are some indications of an effect inhibiting dental plaque regrowth.[13]

Actions

Astringent, antiseptic, antiinflammatory, vulnerary.

Key Constituents

Volatile oil (2% to 10%) including sesquiterpenes[14]; resin (25% to 40%) including commiphoric acids; gum (30% to 60%)[15]; also furanosesquiterpenoids,[16] and triterpenoid resins.[17]

Adulteration

Small stones may be found in the gum. Gum arabic has been found as an adulterant. Products from many other *Commiphora* species are probably occasionally passed off as myrrh. Adulterants of plant origin include *C. mukul* Hook. (Engl.), *C. erythraea* (Ehrenb.) Engl., *C. agallocha* (Roxb.) Engl., *C. ugogensis* Engl.,[3,4,7,18] *C. sphaerocarpa* Chiov., *C. holtziana* Engl., and *C. kataf* (Forssk.) Engl.[19]

Typical Dosage Forms & Dosage

Typical adult dosage range is:
* 1.5 to 4.5 mL/day of a 1:5 liquid extract

Contraindications

Known allergy. Do not use during lactation without professional advice.

Use in Pregnancy

Category B1: No increase in frequency of malformation or other harmful effects on the foetus from limited use in women. No evidence of increased foetal damage in animal studies.

Administration of a combination of resin and volatile oil extracted from myrrh to pregnant rats (50 to 200 mg/kg from days 6 to 15) caused no abnormalities in the foetal skeleton.[20]

According to traditional Chinese medicine, myrrh is contraindicated in pregnancy and in cases of excessive uterine bleeding.[21]

---

[*] Authoritative texts and pharmacopoeias define medicinal myrrh as *Commiphora molmol* and/or other *Commiphora* species.[1-5] The German Commission E regards other Commiphora species as those with comparable chemical composition to *C. molmol*.[6] Other *Commiphora* species may be used if the chemical composition compares favourably with that specified in the German pharmacopoeia (DAB 10).[7] Other possible acceptable species could include *C. abyssinica* (Berg) Engl. (*C. madagascariensis* Jacq.) and *C. schimperi* (Berg) Engl.[1,7] See also the Adulteration section below.

Use in Lactation

Category CC: Compatible with breastfeeding but use caution due to the potential for allergy.

Warnings & Precautions

The alcohol content may cause a transient burning sensation on the skin or mucous membranes. Myrrh should not be ingested for prolonged periods (more than a few weeks) because of the potential of allergic contract dermatitis.

Effect on Ability to Drive or Operate Machinery

No adverse effects expected.

Adverse Reactions

Contact allergy has been reported in the use of myrrh for topical application.[22-25] Continued topical use of essential oils, including those of myrrh, were associated with a deterioration of symptoms in a study on children with atopic eczema, suggesting a possible build up of contact sensitivity.[26]

Cases of allergy due to oral administration of myrrh have been reported in traditional Chinese medicine literature. In both cases the patients received a formulation containing processed myrrh, which was subsequently identified as the allergen.[27]

Interactions

None known.

Safety in Children

No information available, but no adverse effects anticipated.

Overdosage

No incidents found in published literature.

Toxicology

The LD50 for an oil of myrrh was given as 1.65 g/kg in rats.[28] Doses of an ethanolic extract given by mouth at 1000 mg/kg to male Wistar rats for 2 weeks led to depression, jaundice, ruffled hair, hepatonephropathy, haemorrhagic myositis, and death, accompanied by increases in serum ALP and ALT activities, bilirubin, cholesterol, and creatinine concentrations, decreases in total protein and albumin levels, and macrocytic anaemia, and leucopenia.[29] In acute toxicity testing, myrrh oleo-gum resin exhibited no visible signs of toxicity and no mortality was observed up to 3 g/kg in mice. A decrease in locomotor activity was noticed at 3 g/kg. In chronic oral testing (100 mg/kg/day, 90 days) there was no significant difference in mortality compared to controls. At the end of treatment there was a significant increase in weight of testes, caudae epididymides and seminal vesicles and in red blood count and haemoglobin levels in the myrrh-treated group.[30]

Death occurred after consumption of between 5 g and 16 g plant resin/kg/day in goats. Enterohepatonephrotoxicity was accompanied by anaemia, leucopenia, increases in serum ALP activity and concentrations of bilirubin, cholesterol, triglycerides, and creatinine, and decreases in total protein and albumin. The oral dose of 0.25 g plant resin/kg/day was not toxic.[31]

The intravenous administration of 4 mg/kg of the aqueous extract immediately depressed systemic arterial blood pressure by 20% ($P < 0.01$) and reduced the heart rate of anaesthetised rats by 14%, an effect apparently mediated by the stimulation of muscarinic cholinergic receptors (i.e., blocked by atropine sulphate).[32]

Regulatory Status

See Table 1 for regulatory status in selected countries.

Table 1 **Regulatory Status for Myrrh in Selected Countries**

Australia	Myrrh is not included in Part 4 of Schedule 4 of the Therapeutic Goods Regulations.
UK & Germany	Myrrh is included on the General Sale List. It is covered by a positive Commission E monograph.
US	Myrrh does not have generally recognised as safe (GRAS) status. However, it is freely available as a "dietary supplement" in the US under DSHEA legislation (Dietary Supplement Health and Education Act of 1994). Myrrh is official in the *United Pharmacopeia-National Formulary* (USP 26-NF 21, 2003).

REFERENCES

1. British Herbal Medicine Association: *British herbal compendium*, vol 1, Bournemouth, 1992, BHMA, pp 163-165.
2. *British pharmacopoeia*, CD-ROM, 2002.
3. *European pharmacopoeia* 4.2, CD-ROM, 2002.
4. *The United States Pharmacopeia: The national formulary*, USP26-NF21, 2003.
5. Scientific Committee of ESCOP: *ESCOP monographs: myrrha*, UK, October 1999, European Scientific Cooperative on Phytotherapy Secretariat.
6. Blumenthal M, et al, eds: *The complete German Commission E monographs: therapeutic guide to herbal medicines*, Austin, 1998, American Botanical Council, pp 173-174.
7. Blaschek W, Ebel S, Hackenthal E, et al: *HagerROM 2002: Hagers Handbuch der Drogen und Arzneistoffe*, Heidelberg, 2002, Springer.
8. British Herbal Medicine Association's Scientific Committee: *British herbal pharmacopoeia*, Bournemouth, 1983, BHMA, pp 72-73.
9. Al-Rowais NA: *Saudi Med J* 23:1327-1331, 2002.
10. Borrelli F, Izzo AA: *Phytother Res* 14:581-591, 2000.
11. Sheir Z, Nasr AA, Massoud A, et al: *Am J Trop Med Hyg* 65:700-704, 2001.
12. Massoud A, El Sisi S, Salama O, et al: *Am J Trop Med Hyg* 65:96-99, 2001.
13. Moran J, Addy M, Roberts S: *J Clin Periodontol* 19:578-582, 1992.
14. Kreis P, Hener U, Mosandl A: *Dtsch Apoth Ztg* 130:985–988, 1990.
15. Wiendl RM, Franz G: *Dtsch Apoth Ztg* 134:25-30, 1994.
16. Zhu N, Kikuzaki H, Sheng S, et al: *J Nat Prod* 64:1460-1462, 2001.
17. Brody RH, Edwards HG, Pollard AM: *Biopolymers* 67:129-141, 2002.
18. Bisset NG, ed: *Herbal drugs and phytopharmaceuticals: a handbook for practice on a scientific basis*, Stuttgart, 1994, Medpharm Scientific Publishers, pp 345-347.
19. Dekebo A, Dagne E, Sterner O: *Fitoterapia* 73:48-55, 2002;
20. Massoud AM, El-Ashmawy, Ibrahim M, et al: *Alex J Pharm Sci* 14:61-68, 2000.
21. Bensky D, Gamble A: *Chinese herbal medicine materia medica*, Seattle, 1986, Eastland Press, pp 407-408.
22. Lee TY, Lam TH: *Contact Dermatitis* 29:279, 1993.
23. Al-Suwaidan SN, Gad el Rab MO, Al-Fakhiry S, et al: *Contact Dermatitis* 39:137, 1998.
24. Gallo R, Rivara G, Cattarini G, et al: *Contact Dermatitis* 41:230-231, 1999.
25. Lee TY, Lam TH: *Contact Dermatitis* 28:89-90, 1993.
26. Anderson C, Lis-Balchin M, Kirk-Smith M: *Phytother Res* 14:452-456, 2000.
27. Bian HZ, Pan MS: *Bull Chin Materia Med* 12:565, 1987.
28. Opdyke DLJ: *Food Cosmet Toxicol* 14:621, 1976.
29. Omer SA, Adam SE, Khalid HE: *Vet Hum Toxicol* 41:193-196, 1999.
30. Rao RM, Khan ZA, Shah AH: *J Ethnopharmacol* 76:151-154, 2001.
31. Omer SA, Adam SE: *Vet Hum Toxicol* 41:299-301, 1999.
32. Abdul-Ghani AS, Amin R: *J Ethnopharmacol* 57:219-222, 1997.

NETTLE

Botanical names: *Urtica dioica* L., *Urtica urens* L.
Family: Urticaceae
Plant part used: Leaf and root

Safety Summary

Pregnancy category B2: No increase in frequency of malformation or other harmful effects on the foetus from limited use in women. Animal studies are lacking.
Lactation category C: Compatible with breastfeeding.
Contraindications: Known allergy (for topical use of fresh or unprocessed dried leaves).
Warnings & precautions: The use of nettle root for benign prostatic hyperplasia should occur under professional supervision to include monitoring of the state of the prostate.
Adverse reactions: Apart from nettle stings from the fresh plant only, occasional minor gastrointestinal symptoms from use of the root.
Interactions: No precautions required on current evidence.

Typical Therapeutic Use

Nettle root has demonstrated, in controlled clinical trials, an improvement of urological symptoms in benign prostatic hyperplasia.[1,2]

Traditional indications for nettle leaf in Western herbal medicine include uterine haemorrhage, epistaxis and cutaneous eruptions.[3] Both ESCOP and Commission E support the use of nettle leaf in rheumatic conditions.[4,5]

Actions

Nettle leaf: antirheumatic, antiallergic, depurative, styptic (haemostatic), mild diuretic.[6]

Nettle root: reducing benign prostatic hyperplasia.[7]

Key Constituents

Nettle leaf: flavonoids[8]; nettle hairs contain leukotrienes, neutrophil chemotactic activity and histamine. They therefore resemble insect venoms and cutaneous mast cells with regard to their spectrum of mediators.[9] Nettle hairs also contain silicon.

Nettle root: lectin (*Urtica dioica* agglutinin)[10]; lignans: (+)-neoolivil, (−)-secoisolariciresinol, dehy-drodiconiferyl alcohol, isolariciresinol, pinoresinol and 3,4-divanillyltetrahydrofuran.[11]

Adulteration

A woman showing the symptoms of atropine poisoning after drinking nettle tea was found to have consumed a tea mixture containing belladonna (*Atropa belladonna*) among other contaminants.[12]

Typical Dosage Forms & Dosage

Typical adult dosage ranges are:
- 6 to 12 g/day of dried leaf or by infusion
- 4 to 6 g/day of dried root or by decoction or infusion
- 6 to 12 mL/day of 1:1 liquid extract of nettle leaf
- 1.5 to 7.5 mL/day of 1:1 liquid extract of nettle root
- 2 to 6 mL/day of 1:2 liquid extract of nettle leaf or equivalent in tablet or capsule form
- 4.5 to 8.5 mL/day of 1:2 liquid extract of nettle root or equivalent in tablet or capsule form
- 7 to 14 mL/day of 1:5 tincture of nettle leaf

Contraindications

Known allergy (for topical use of fresh or unprocessed dried leaves).

Use in Pregnancy

Category B2: No increase in frequency of malformation or other harmful effects on the foetus from limited use in women. Animal studies are lacking.

The lignans in nettle, as well as their intestinal transformation products (enterodiol and enterolactone), are known to bind to sex hormone binding globulin in vitro.[13] The affinity of (−)-3,4-divanillyltetrahydrofuran was notably high.[11] This may provide a mechanism for the claimed benefit of nettle root in benign prostatic hyperplasia, but is not thought to pose a risk in pregnancy.

Ethanol extract of nettle aerial parts (250 mg/kg) did not demonstrate any significant antiimplantation activity when administered orally to female rats.[14]

Use in Lactation

Category C: Both leaf and root are compatible with breastfeeding.

Warnings & Precautions

The use of nettle root for benign prostatic hyperplasia should occur under professional supervision to include monitoring of the state of the prostate.[5]

Effect on Ability to Drive or Operate Machinery

No adverse effects expected.

Adverse Reactions

Nettle stings are due to histamine and serotonin introduced by the nettle hair (each hair containing 6.1 ng and 33.25 pg, respectively). However, the persistence of the stinging sensation might suggest the presence of substances in nettle fluid directly toxic to nerves or capable of secondary release of other mediators.[15] The results are an urticaria that generally, but not always, passes quickly. No such reaction is expected from ingesting extracted leaf.

Both an immediate and a delayed hypersensitivity reaction were exhibited in a child after falling into a nettle patch.[16] A man who had developed a contact dermatitis after treating his eczema with a poultice of herbs including chamomile also manifested a diffuse oedematous gingivostomatitis. He regularly drank nettle tea. This reaction was believed to be an allergic contact reaction to the chamomile and also the nettle (and not an irritant reaction).[17]

In a multicentre trial of the effect of nettle root on 4051 prostatic patients, mild side effects affecting the gastrointestinal tract were experienced in 0.7% of cases.[18]

Interactions

None known.

Safety in Children

No information available, but adverse effects are not expected.

Overdosage

No incidents found in published literature.

Toxicology

Table 1 lists LD_{50} data recorded for nettle leaf.[19]

Nettle leaf ethanol extract showed low toxicity in both mice and rats, when administered orally and by i.p. injection in doses up to 2 g/kg (dried herb equivalent).[20]

Nettle leaf tea demonstrated weak genotoxic activity comparable to the flavonoids quercetin and rutin.[21]

Regulatory Status

See Table 2 for regulatory status in selected countries.

Table 1 **LD_{50} Data Recorded for Constituents of Nettle Leaf**

Substance	Route, Model	LD_{50} Value (g/kg)	Reference
Nettle leaf infusion	Oral, rats	1.31	19
Nettle leaf infusion	i.v., mice	1.92	19
Nettle leaf decoction	i.v., mice	1.72	19

Table **2** **Regulatory Status for Nettle in Selected Countries**

Australia	Nettle is not included in Part 4 of Schedule 4 of the Therapeutic Goods Regulations.
UK & Germany	Nettle is included on the General Sale List. Nettle leaf and root are each covered by positive Commission E monographs.
US	Nettle does not have generally recognised as safe (GRAS) status. However, it is freely available as a "dietary supplement" in the US under DSHEA legislation (Dietary Supplement Health and Education Act of 1994).

REFERENCES

1. Vontobel HP, Herzog R, Rutishauser G, et al: *Urologe A* 24:49-51, 1985.
2. Fischer M, Wilbert D. In Rutishauser G, ed: *Benigne Prostatahyperplasie III*, München, 1992, Zuckschwerdt, pp 79-84.
3. British Herbal Medicine Association's Scientific Committee: *British herbal pharmacopoeia*, Bournemouth, 1983, BHMA, pp 224-225.
4. Scientific Committee of ESCOP: *ESCOP monographs: urticae folium/herba*, UK, July 1997, European Scientific Cooperative on Phytotherapy Secretariat.
5. Blumenthal M, et al, eds: *The complete German Commission E monographs: therapeutic guide to herbal medicines*, Austin, 1998, American Botanical Council, pp 216-217.
6. Tahri A, Yamani S, Legssyer A, et al: *J Ethnopharmacol* 73:95-100, 2000.
7. Hirano T, Homma M, Oka K: *Planta Med* 60:30-33, 1994.
8. Chaurasia N, Wichtl M: *Planta Med* 53:432-434, 1987.
9. Czarnetzki BM, Thiele T, Rosenbach T: *Int Arch Allergy Appl Immunol* 91:43-46, 1990.
10. Broekaert WF, Van Parijs J, Leyns F, et al: *Science* 245:1100-1102, 1989.
11. Schottner M, Gansser D, Spiteller G: *Planta Med* 63:529-532, 1997.
12. Scholz H, Kascha S, Zingerle H: *Fortschr Med* 98:1525-1526, 1980.
13. Gansser D, Spiteller G: *Z Naturforsch [C]* 50:98-104, 1995.
14. Sharma BB, Varshney MD, Gupta DN, et al: *Int J Crude Drug Res* 21:183-187, 1983.
15. Oliver F, Amon EU, Breathnach A, et al: *Clin Exp Dermatol* 16:1-7, 1991.
16. Edwards EK Jr, Edwards EK Sr: *Contact Dermatitis* 27:264-265, 1992.
17. Bossuyt L, Dooms-Goossens A: *Contact Dermatitis* 31:131-132, 1994.
18. Geiger WN, Haak C, Wagner H: 2nd International Congress on Phytomedicine, Munich, September 11-14, 1996.
19. Baraibar C, Broncano FJ, Lazaro-Carrasco MJ, et al: *An Bromatol* 35:99-103, 1984.
20. Tita B, Bello U, Faccendini P, et al: *Pharmacol Res* 27(Suppl 1):21-22, 1993.
21. Graf U, Moraga AA, Castro R, et al: *Food Chem Toxicol* 32:423-430, 1994.

OREGON GRAPE

Botanical names: *Mahonia aquifolium* (Pursh.) Nutt.
(*Berberis aquifolium* Pursh.)
Family: Berberidaceae
Plant part used: Root and rhizome

Safety Summary

Pregnancy category C: Has caused or is associated with a substantial risk of causing harmful effects on the foetus or neonate without causing malformations (on the basis of the presence of berberine and related alkaloids and the implications for neonatal jaundice).
Lactation category SD: Strongly discouraged in breastfeeding (on the basis of the presence of berberine and related alkaloids).
Contraindications: Pregnancy, jaundiced neonates. Do not use during pregnancy or lactation without professional advice.
Warnings & precautions: Care needs to be taken to reduce the prospect of exacerbating chronic skin conditions.
Adverse reactions: Occasional skin reaction from topical use may occur.
Interactions: Drugs which displace the protein binding of bilirubin, such as phenylbutazone.

Typical Therapeutic Use

Traditional indications for Oregon grape in Western herbal medicine include skin disease, especially psoriasis and eczema; gastritis, and cholecystitis.[1]

Actions

Antipsoriatic, antiinflammatory, depurative, mild cholagogue, antimicrobial.

Key Constituents

The following alkaloids have been isolated from Oregon grape root: magnoflorine, berberine, jatrorrhizine, columbamine, oxyacanthine, oxyberberine, berbamine, aromoline, baluchistine, and aquifoline. The presence of palmatine is not certain as it was absent in one sample and isolated from another.[2-5]

Oregon grape is not a rich source of berberine compared to herbs such as barberry (*Berberis vulgaris*) and golden seal (*Hydrastis canadensis*).

Adulteration

No adulterants known.

Typical Dosage Forms & Dosage

Typical adult dosage ranges are:
- 3 to 6 g/day of dried root and rhizome or by decoction
- 3 to 6 mL/day of a 1:1 liquid extract
- 3.5 to 7 mL/day of a 1:2 liquid extract or equivalent in tablet or capsule form

Contraindications

Although berberine-containing plants have been used in traditional Chinese medicine for the treatment of jaundiced neonates, berberine is thought to cause severe acute haemolysis and neonatal jaundice in babies with glucose-6-phosphate dehydrogenase (G6PD) deficiency.[6] However, a review published in 2001 questioned the causal relationship between the berberine-containing herb *Coptis chinensis* and haemolysis in G6PD deficient infants (see Pregnancy section below).[7] Do not use during pregnancy or lactation without professional advice.

Use in Pregnancy

Category C: Has caused or is associated with a substantial risk of causing harmful effects on the foetus or neonate without causing malformations (on the basis of the presence of berberine and related alkaloids and the implications for neonatal jaundice).

Magnoflorine was not toxic in the rat embryo culture (REC) in vitro assay at concentrations of 0.1 to 500 μg/mL.[8] Magnoflorine induced contractions in isolated pregnant rat uterus.[9]

Refer to the barberry (*Berberis vulgaris*) monograph for the toxicology of berberine.

Use in Lactation

Category SD: Strongly discouraged in breastfeeding.

Infants have been exposed to berberine via breast milk following maternal ingestion of berberine-containing plants.[10]

Warnings & Precautions

Depuratives can in many cases be provocative to skin disease. Care needs to be taken to reduce the prospect of major exacerbations.

Effect on Ability to Drive or Operate Machinery

No adverse effects expected.

Adverse Reactions

Adverse reactions such as itching and burning sensation were reported in 4% of patients treated with a topical preparation of Oregon grape stem bark in an intraindividual study (in which placebo and herb ointments were each applied to one arm).[11]

Interactions

Berberine demonstrated potent displacement of bilirubin in vitro and in vivo after chronic administration to rats (10 to 20 mg/kg; i.p.). Berberine at this dosage range caused elevation in serum levels of bilirubin (since the binding of bilirubin to albumin decreased). However, at a dose of 2 mg/kg the displacement was not signficant.[10] Hence berberine may reinforce the effects of other drugs that displace the protein binding of bilirubin.

Safety in Children

Berberine has been used to treat diarrhoea and giardiasis in children, which suggests that berberine-containing plants may also be used in this way. Treatment of newborns with neonatal jaundice is contraindicated.

Overdosage

An Eclectic text notes that overdose of Oregon grape may produce tremor of the limbs, lack of muscular power, dullness of the mind, drowsiness, and active diuresis; however, it is not regarded as a poisonous agent.[12] Although undefined, it is likely that this refers to extract of root.

Refer to the barberry (*Berberis vulgaris*) monograph for overdosage information of berberine.

Toxicology

Table 1 lists LD_{50} data recorded for constituents of Oregon grape.[13,14]

Oxyacanthine was nonmutagenic towards both *Salmonella typhimurium* strains (TA98, TA100) with or without addition of S9 mix.[15]

Refer to the barberry (*Berberis vulgaris*) monograph for toxicology and LD_{50} values for berberine.

Regulatory Status

See Table 2 for regulatory status in selected countries.

Table 1   **LD_{50} Data Recorded for Constituents of Oregon Grape**

Substance	Route, Model	LD_{50} Value	Reference
Berbamine hydrochloride	i.g., mice	1.5 g/kg	13
Berbamine	i.p., mice	75 mg/kg	14
Oxyacanthine	i.p., mice	50 mg/kg	14

Table 2   **Regulatory Status for Oregon Grape in Selected Countries**

Australia	Oregon grape is not included in Part 4 of Schedule 4 of the Therapeutic Goods Regulations.
UK & Germany	Oregon grape is not listed on the General Sale List (GSL). *Berberis* (species undefined) is included on the GSL, with a maximum single dose equivalent to 0.5 mg berberine. Oregon grape was not included in the Commission E assessment.
US	Oregon grape does not have generally recognised as safe (GRAS) status. However, it is freely available as a "dietary supplement" in the US under DSHEA legislation (Dietary Supplement Health and Education Act of 1994).

REFERENCES

1. British Herbal Medicine Association's Scientific Committee: *British herbal pharmacopoeia*, Bournemouth, 1983, BHMA, pp 40-41.
2. Kostalova D, Brazdovicova B, Tomko J: *Chem Zvesti* 35:279-283, 1981.
3. Schwabe W: *Dtsch Apoth Ztg* 54:326-327, 1939.
4. Kostalova D, Hrochova V, Tomko J: *Chem Pap* 40:389-394, 1986.
5. Kostalova D, Uhrin D, Hrochova V, et al: *Collect Czech Chem Commun* 52: 242-246, 1987.
6. Ho NK: *Singapore Med J* 37:645-651, 1996.
7. Fok TF: *J Perinatol* 21(Suppl 1):S98-S100, 2001.
8. Kennelly EJ, Flynn TJ, Mazzola EP, et al: *J Nat Prod* 62:1385-1389, 1999.
9. El-Tahir KEH: *Int J Pharmacogn* 29:101-110, 1991.
10. Chan E: *Biol Neonate* 63:201-208, 1993.
11. Wiesenauer M, Ludtke R: *Phytomedicine* 3:231-235, 1996.
12. Ellingwood F, Lloyd JU: *American materia medica, therapeutics and pharmacognosy*, ed 11, *Naturopathic Medical Series*: Botanical vol 2, Portland, 1983, Eclectic Medical Publications, p 369.
13. Chang HM, But PP: *Pharmacology and applications of Chinese materia medica*, vol 1, Singapore, 1987, World Scientific, p 68.
14. Kuroda H, Nakazawa S, Katagiri K, et al: *Chem Pharm Bull* 24:2413-2420, 1976.
15. Nozaka T, Watanabe F, Tadaki S, et al: *Mutat Res* 240:267-279, 1990.

PASQUE FLOWER

Other common name: Pulsatilla
Botanical names: *Anemone pulsatilla* L. (*Pulsatilla vulgaris* Mill.), *Anemone pratensis* L., (*Pulsatilla pratensis* (L.) Mill.)
Family: Ranunculaceae
Plant part used: Aerial parts (dried)

Safety Summary

Pregnancy category C: Has caused or is associated with a substantial risk of causing foetal malformation or irreversible damage (on the basis of the possible presence of traces of protoanemonin).
Lactation category SD: Strongly discouraged in breastfeeding.
Contraindications: Pregnancy and lactation.
Warnings & precautions: Administer within the recommended dosage. Prescribe with caution for pain in children. Other precautions are neurological disease, depression and psychosis, liver and kidney disease, history of allergic or anaphylactic reactions. Long-term therapy with analgesics is not advisable.
Adverse reactions: None found in published literature for dried plant preparations consumed within the recommended dosage.
Interactions: Do not prescribe concomitantly with powerful analgesics (theoretical concern).

Typical Therapeutic Use

Traditional indications for dried pasque flower preparations in Western herbal medicine include inflammation or painful conditions of the female or male reproductive tract, headache, hyperactivity, insomnia and skin eruptions.[1] Eclectic physicians used fresh plant preparations and at lower doses[2] than British herbalists, who were mainly using dried plant preparations.[1]

Actions

Spasmolytic, analgesic, sedative.

Key Constituents

Fresh, intact aerial parts of *Anemone pulsatilla* (and other species of the Ranunculaceae) contain a lactonic glucoside called ranunculin.[3,4] Ranunculin degrades to form protoanemonin (not strictly the

aglycone) in the presence of water (e.g., in solution or by steam distillation of the fresh plant), by an enzymatic process upon crushing the plant material,[4] or by freeze drying.[5] Protoanemonin dimerises to form anemonin,[4] although the extent to which and under what conditions it undergoes this reaction during the drying process,[6] or within a liquid extract over time, is not fully known. (Protoanemonin causes side effects including blistering,[7,8] but anemonin is not a blistering agent.[4]) Other constituents in small or unknown quantities include triterpenoid saponins, tannins, and volatile oil.[7,9]

Adulteration

The danger of adulteration arises from other more toxic species of *Pulsatilla*, such as *P. patens*. There is concern for the possible endangered status of *Pulsatilla pratensis* and *P. vulgaris* in some regions of Europe. *Pulsatilla* species are protected in Germany.[9,10]

Typical Dosage Forms & Dosage

Typical adult dosage ranges are:
- 0.4 to 0.9 g/day of dried aerial parts or by infusion or decoction
- 0.4 to 0.9 mL/day of a 1:1 liquid extract (made from dried plant)
- 0.4 to 1.5 mL/day of a 1:2 liquid extract (made from dried plant) or equivalent in tablet or capsule form
- 0.9 to 3 mL/day of a 1:10 tincture (made from dried plant)

Fresh plant preparations of pasque flower need to be used with caution.

Contraindications

Contraindicated in pregnancy and lactation.[7]

Use in Pregnancy

Category C: Has caused or is associated with a substantial risk of causing harmful effects on the foetus or neonate without causing malformations (on the basis of the possible presence of traces of protoanemonin).

Dried plant preparations of pasque flower are said to be contraindicated in pregnancy.[6,7] The ingestion of protoanemonin-containing fresh plants by grazing animals has been observed to lead to abortion and teratogenic effects.[6]

A fresh plant preparation of pasque flower was recommended by Eclectic physicians for nervous manifestations and urinary dysfunction during pregnancy.[2] Doses much lower than those given above were prescribed.

Use in Lactation

Category SD: Strongly discouraged in breastfeeding.

Dried plant preparations of pasque flower are said to be contraindicated in lactation.[7] Despite this suggested contraindication, fresh plant of pasque flower was recommended by Eclectic physicians as a galactagogue in anxious women with painful, swollen breasts (albeit at quite low doses).[11]

Warnings & Precautions

Administer pasque flower within the recommended dosage.

The following conditions should be approached with caution when using herbal analgesics: concurrent prescription of powerful analgesics; pain in children; neurological disease; depression and psychosis; liver and kidney disease; history of allergic or anaphylactic reactions. Long-term therapy with analgesics is not advisable.

Effect on Ability to Drive or Operate Machinery

No adverse effects expected.

Adverse Reactions

Excessive (undefined) doses of pasque flower dried plant extract can cause violent gastritis.[7] Use of high doses of dried plant preparations results in irritation to the kidneys and the urinary tract.[6] These observations suggest that protoanemonin is retained to some extent in dried plant preparations.

Use of fresh plant preparations, or preparations containing (substantial) protoanemonin, produces severe irritations of the skin and mucosa with itch-

ing, rashes, and pustules (ranunculus dermatitis).[6] Fresh pasque flower taken in sufficient amounts produces gastroenteritis with vomiting and purging, often accompanied by evidence of irritation of the kidneys.[12]

Interactions

None reported for pasque flower. As a precaution, do not prescribe concomitantly with powerful analgesics.

Safety in Children

No information available.

Overdosage

Fresh plant of pasque flower taken in overdose acts as a gastric irritant, producing burning and pain in the stomach, attempts to vomit, and marked prostration. A case of poisoning with these symptoms has been recorded.[11] Convulsions have occurred after poisoning with pasque flower dried plant extract.[13]

Toxicology

The LD_{50} value for anemonin administered by i.p. injection in mice is 150 mg/kg.[14] In anaesthetised animals, i.v. injection of anemonin quickly arrests respiration and is soon followed by heart failure.[15]

Haematuria, diarrhoea, and inflammation of the stomach and intestines may occur in livestock fed on the fresh plant.[16] Death occurred within 6 hours in dogs administered 15 g of fresh juice.[9]

In animal experiments, protoanemonin caused stimulation followed by paralysis of the central nervous system. Irritation occurred in the kidney and the urinary tract, which may be due to the alkylating action of protoanemonin.[6]

Regulatory Status

See Table 1 for regulatory status in selected countries.

Table **1** **Regulatory Status for Pasque Flower in Selected Countries**

Australia	Pasque flower is not included in Part 4 of Schedule 4 of the Therapeutic Goods Regulations.
UK & Germany	Pasque flower (pulsatilla) is included on the General Sale List. It is covered by a negative Commission E monograph.
US	Pasque flower does not have generally recognised as safe (GRAS) status. However, it is freely available as a "dietary supplement" in the US under DSHEA legislation (Dietary Supplement Health and Education Act of 1994).

REFERENCES

1. British Herbal Medicine Association's Scientific Committee: *British herbal pharmacopoeia*, Bournemouth, 1983, BHMA, pp 173-174.
2. Ellingwood F, Lloyd JU: *American materia medica, therapeutics and pharmacognosy*, ed 11, *Naturopathic Medical Series*: Botanical vol 2, Portland, 1983, Eclectic Medical Publications, pp 149-152.
3. Budavari S, O'Neil MJ, Smith A, et al, eds: *The Merck index: an encyclopedia of chemicals, drugs and biologicals*, ed 12, Whitehouse Station, 1996, Merck & Co, p 108.
4. Hill R, van Heyningen R: *Biochem J* 49:332-335, 1951.
5. Bai Y, Benn MH, Majak W, et al: *J Agric Food Chem* 44:2235-2238, 1996.
6. Blumenthal M, et al, eds: *The complete German Commission E monographs: therapeutic guide to herbal medicines*, Austin, 1998, American Botanical Council, p 363.
7. British Herbal Medicine Association: *British herbal compendium*, vol 1. Bournemouth, 1992, BHMA, pp 179-180.
8. Turner NJ: *J Ethnopharmacol* 11:181-201, 1984.
9. Blaschek W, Ebel S, Hackenthal E, et al: *HagerROM 2002: Hagers Handbuch der Drogen und Arzneistoffe*, Heidelberg, 2002, Springer.
10. Lange D: *Europe's medicinal and aromatic plants: their use, trade and conservation*, Cambridge, 1998, TRAFFIC International, pp XVII-XVIII.
11. Felter HW, Lloyd JU: *King's American dispensatory*, ed 18, rev 3, vol 2. First published 1905; reprinted Portland, 1983, Eclectic Medical Publications, pp 1588-1592.
12. Osol A, Farrar GE, et al: *The dispensatory of the United States of America*, ed 24, Philadelphia, 1947, Lippincott, pp 1559-1560.
13. Grieve M: *A modern herbal*, New York, 1971, Dover Publications, pp 32-33.
14. Brodersen R, Kjaer A: *Acta Pharmacol* 2:109-120, 1946.
15. Chopra RN, Badhwar RL, Ghosh S: *Poisonous plants of India*, vol 1, New Delhi, 1965, Indian Council of Agricultural Research, p 98.
16. Long HC: *Plants poisonous to live stock*, ed 2, revised, Cambridge, 1924, Cambridge University Press, pp 9-10.

PASSIONFLOWER

Other common names: Passion flower, Passiflora
Botanical name: *Passiflora incarnata* L.
Family: Passifloraceae
Plant part used: Aerial parts

Safety Summary

Pregnancy category B1: No increase in frequency of malformation or other harmful effects on the foetus from limited use in women. No evidence of increased foetal damage in animal studies.
Lactation category C: Compatible with breastfeeding.
Contraindications: None required on current evidence.
Warnings & precautions: None required on current evidence.
Adverse reactions: Side effects occur rarely, and most often are of an allergic nature.
Interactions: No precautions required on current evidence.

Typical Therapeutic Use

In randomised, double-blind, clinical trials passionflower was efficacious for the treatment of generalised anxiety disorder,[1] and in the management of mental symptoms during outpatient detoxification of opiate addicts.[2]

Traditional indications for passionflower in Western herbal medicine include insomnia, neuralgia and nervous tachycardia.[3]

Actions

Anxiolytic, spasmolytic, mild sedative, hypnotic.

Key Constituents

Key constituents of *Passiflora incarnata* aerial parts include flavonoids (up to 1.2%), especially flavone-C-glycosides including isovitexin.[4] Small amounts of maltol (0.05%) and the cyanogenic glycoside gynocardin (0.01%) are present.[5]

The presence of trace amounts of the harmane alkaloids (such as harman) appears to be dependent upon the stage of development of the plant and they are absent in many samples.[5,6] The German Commission E recommends that passionflower contains not more than 0.01% of harman alkaloids.[7]

In Australia, harmala alkaloids are scheduled, except for herbs or preparations that contain less than 0.1% of harmala alkaloids, or in divided preparations containing 2 mg or less of these alkaloids per recommended daily dose.[8] (These β-carboline alkaloids are referred to in the literature as harman, harmane or harmala alkaloids.) One of these alkaloids, harman (3-methyl-4-carboline) is also denoted as harmane and passiflorin.

High performance liquid chromatographic analyses of dried herb and methanol extracts of *P. incarnata* indicate the following levels: harman (0 to 0.1 ppm) and harmine (0 to 0.3 ppm). (Previous methods [paper chromatography, acidic titration] were neither selective nor accurate and resulted in large overestimates of alkaloid concentrations.[9,10])

Adulteration

Passiflora incarnata is often adulterated with material derived from other species of *Passiflora* including *P. edulis* and *P. coerulea*.[11,12] *P. edulis* is mainly cultivated for its edible fruits,[12] although the leaves are used in the traditional medicine of Brazil as a sedative.[13] Authenticated *P. edulis* does not exert the anxiolytic activity in vivo demonstrated by *P. incarnata*.[12] A survey of the botanical literature on the genus *Passiflora* noticed that in many references *P. incarnata* and *P. edulis* are mentioned synonymously. The prevailing confusion may have led to inconclusive and contradictory pharmacological reports on the plants.[14]

Typical Dosage Forms & Dosage

Typical adult dosage ranges are:
- 0.75 to 6 g/day of dried aerial parts or by infusion
- 1.5 to 3 mL/day of a 1:1 liquid extract
- 3 to 6 mL/day of a 1:2 liquid extract or equivalent in tablet or capsule form
- 1.5 to 6 mL/day of a 1:8 tincture

Contraindications

None required on current evidence.

Use in Pregnancy

Category B1: No increase in frequency of malformation or other harmful effects on the foetus from limited use in women. No evidence of increased foetal damage in animal studies.

Teratogenic effects were not observed in rats administered *Passiflora incarnata* extract.[15,16]

Use in Lactation

Category C: Compatible with breastfeeding.

Warnings & Precautions

None required.

Effect on Ability to Drive or Operate Machinery

No adverse effects expected.

Adverse Reactions

Cardiovascular and gastrointestinal side effects were observed in a woman self-medicating with a *Passiflora incarnata* product. She had taken a dosage below the maximum therapeutic level. The tablets were verified by a government agency as containing *Passiflora incarnata* by chromatographic analysis.[17]

A case of cutaneous vasculitis and urticaria caused by an idiosyncratic hypersensitivity reaction has been associated with ingestion of passionflower.[18]

There is a possible link between the development of chronic active hepatitis and ingestion of herbal tablets containing passionflower. The person was taking three different herbal products: mistletoe; celery seed + Guaiacum + burdock root + sarsaparilla; valerian + skullcap + passionflower and the following conventional medications: verapamil, chlordiazepoxide, thyroxine.[19]

Passiflora alata and *Rhamnus purshiana* (cascara) caused IgE-mediated asthma and rhinitis in a person who worked with herbal products in a pharmacy.[20] IgE-mediated anaphylaxis caused by ingestion of a herbal product containing *Passiflora incarnata* has been reported in a latex-allergic patient. Cross-reactivity between latex and passionflower was demonstrated by laboratory tests.[21]

Interactions

None known.

Safety in Children

No information available but adverse effects are not expected.

Overdosage

No incidents were found in published literature for the aerial parts of *Passiflora incarnata*. Altered consciousness has been reported from ingestion of a herbal product containing mainly the fruit of *Passiflora incarnata*.[22]

Harmaline and its derivatives cause visual troubles, loss of coordination, agitation and delirium. At high doses they can produce paralysis.[23] Passionflower does not contain enough of these alkaloids to cause these symptoms.

Toxicology

Intraperitoneal administration of hydrochloric acid soluble fraction of *P. incarnata* dry extract (1 g/kg) in mice caused tremor-like symptoms followed by death. Administration of the dry extract (0.5 g/kg) caused no significant changes in behaviour.[24] Passionflower extract had an acute toxicity value higher than 900 mg/kg in mice. An aqueous ethanol extract had the ethanol removed and was administered by the i.p. route.[25] Subacute oral treatment of male rats with an aqueous ethanol extract of *P. incarnata* (5 g/kg/day, 21 days) produced no change in weight, rectal temperature or motor coordination compared to controls.[26] This indicates very low oral toxicity for the extract.

Maltol has the LD_{50} value 820 mg/kg for subcutaneous administration in mice.[24]

Fluid extract of *Passiflora incarnata* leaf did not demonstrate mutagenicity in an in vitro model (*Aspergillus nidulans* for detection of somatic segregation).[27] Harman is a co-mutagen which interacts directly or indirectly with DNA.[28] Harman, if present in passionflower, is present in very low quantities.[9,10]

Regulatory Status

See Table 1 for regulatory status in selected countries.

Table **I**   **Regulatory Status for Passionflower in Selected Countries**

Australia	Passionflower is not included in Part 4 of Schedule 4 of the Therapeutic Goods Regulations.
UK & Germany	Passionflower (Passiflora) is included on the General Sale List. It is covered by a positive Commission E monograph. Passionflower is official in the *British Pharmacopoeia* 2002 and the *European Pharmacopoeia* 4.3.
US	Passionflower does not have generally recognised as safe (GRAS) status. However, it is freely available as a "dietary supplement" in the US under DSHEA legislation (Dietary Supplement Health and Education Act of 1994).

REFERENCES

1. Akhondzadeh S, Naghavi HR, Vazirian M, et al: *J Clin Pharm Ther* 26:363-367, 2001.
2. Akhondzadeh S, Kashani L, Mobaseri M, et al: *J Clin Pharm Ther* 26:369-373, 2001.
3. British Herbal Medicine Association's Scientific Committee: *British herbal pharmacopoeia*, Bournemouth, 1983, BHMA, pp 153-154.
4. Wagner H, Bladt S: *Plant drug analysis: a thin layer chromatography atlas*, ed 2, Berlin, 1996, Springer-Verlag, p 202.
5. British Herbal Medicine Association: *British herbal compendium*, Bournemouth, 1992, BHMA, pp 171-173.
6. Blaschek W, Ebel S, Hackenthal E, et al: *HagerROM 2002: Hagers Handbuch der Drogen und Arzneistoffe*, Heidelberg, 2002, Springer.
7. Blumenthal M, et al, eds: *The complete German Commission E monographs: therapeutic guide to herbal medicines*, Austin, 1998, American Botanical Council, pp 179-180.
8. *Standard for the Uniform Scheduling of Drugs and Poisons*, no. 17, effective 2nd June 2002, Canberra, 2002, Commonwealth Department of Health and Aged Care, p 220.
9. Rehwald A, Sticher O: *Phytochem Anal* 6:96-100, 1995.
10. Grice ID, Ferreira LA, Griffiths LR: *J Liq Chrom Rel Technol* 24:2513-2523, 2001.
11. Bisset NG, ed: *Herbal drugs and phytopharmaceuticals: a handbook for practice on a scientific basis*, Stuttgart, 1994, Medpharm Scientific Publishers, pp 363-365.
12. Dhawan K, Kumar S, Sharma A: *Fitoterapia* 72:698-702, 2001.
13. Mors WB, Rizzini CT, Pereira NA: *Medicinal plants of Brazil. Medicinal plants of the world*, no. 6, Algonac, 2000, Reference Publications, p 269.
14. Dhawan K, Kumar R, Kumar S, et al: *J Med Food* 4:137-144, 2001.
15. Schardein JL: *Chemically induced birth defects*, ed 2, New York, 1993, Marcel Dekker, pp 800-822.
16. Hirakawa T, Suzuki T, Sano Y, et al: *Kiso To Rinsho* 15:3431-3451, 1981.
17. Fisher AA, Purcell P, Le Couteur DG: *J Toxicol Clin Toxicol* 38:63-66, 2000.
18. Smith GW, Chalmers TM, Nuki G: *Br J Rheumatol* 32:87-88, 1993.
19. Weeks GR, Proper JS: *Aust J Hosp Pharm* 19:155-157, 1989.
20. Giavina-Bianchi PF Jr, Castro FF, Machado ML, et al: *Ann Allergy Asthma Immunol* 79:449-454, 1997.
21. Echechipia S, Garcia BE, Alvarez MJ, et al: *Allergy* 51(Suppl 31): 49, 1996.
22. Solbakken AM, Rorbakken G, Gundersen T: *Tidsskr Nor Laegeforen* 117:1140-1141, 1997.
23. Lamchouri F, Settaf A, Cherrah Y, et al: *Ann Pharm Fr* 60:123-129, 2002.
24. Aoyagi N, Kimura R, Murata T: *Chem Pharm Bull* 22:1008-1013, 1974.
25. Speroni E, Minghetti A: *Planta Med* 54:488-491, 1988.
26. Sopranzi N, de Feo G, Mazzanti G, et al: *Clin Ter* 132:329-333, 1990.
27. Ramos Ruiz A, De la Torre RA, Alonso N, et al: *J Ethnopharmacol* 52:123-127, 1996.
28. de Meester C: *Mutat Res* 339:139-153, 1995.

PAU D'ARCO

Other common names: Lapacho, ipe, taheebo
Botanical names: *Tabebuia avellanedae* Lorentz ex Griseb. (*T. impetiginosa* (Mart. ex DC.) Standl.), *T. ipe* (Mart. ex K. Schum.) Standl. (*T. heptaphylla* (Vell.) Toledo)
Family: Bignoniaceae
Plant part used: Bark, especially inner bark.

Safety Summary

Pregnancy category D: Has caused or is associated with a substantial risk of causing foetal malformation or irreversible damage.
Lactation category CC: Compatible with breast-feeding but use caution.
Contraindications: Pregnancy and patients on anti-coagulant therapy. Do not use during lactation without professional advice.
Warnings & precautions: Pau d'arco should not be relied upon as a sole treatment for cancer or infections. Caution is advised for women wishing to conceive.
Adverse reactions: Allergic contact dermatitis.
Interactions: Anticoagulant drugs.

Typical Therapeutic Use

Pau d'arco became popular in the West after anecdotal report of successful use by physicians for the treatment of terminal cancer and leukaemia in Brazil in the late 1960s.[1]

The main species of "purple" pau d'arco used medicinally in Brazil are: *T. avellanedae* (used most frequently), *T. heptaphylla* (now *T. ipe*), and *T. roseoalba*. (Purple pau d'arco is not always purple and may include pink-, red-, magenta-, and violet-flowered varieties.) South American uses of *T. avellanedae* and *T. impetiginosa* bark include impetigo, cancer, and topical use for scabies and mouth inflammation. Traditional uses for the yellow-flowered *T. serratifolia* bark include cancer and oral inflammation. Other yellow-flowering species (*T. chrysantha*, *T. neochrysantha*, *T. aurea* [*T. argentea*]) are used for chronic anaemia, ulcer, stomach ache, fevers, and malaria. The bark of *T. rosea* (*T. pentaphylla*, the pink variety used in preference to the white) is used in Mexico and Central America for uterine cancer, malaise, headache, and pain.[2-7]

Actions

Immune-enhancing, antitumour, antibacterial, antifungal, antiparasitic, depurative.

Key Constituents

Key constituents of *Tabebuia impetiginosa* heartwood and stem bark include naphthoquinones of the 1,4 type, especially β-lapachol (3.6%) in the heartwood with minor amounts of lapachenol, β-lapachone, xyloidone (dehydro-α-lapachone), α-lapachone and deoxylapachol.[8] Other constituents include naphtho-furandiones (or furanonaphthoquinones), iridoids, and very small quantities of anthraquinones.[8-12] (Naphthofurandiones are naphthoquinones with a furan ring attached to carbons at the 2 and 3 positions.) Levels of lapachol are lower in the inner stem bark compared to the heartwood.

Lapachol is only slightly soluble in hot water,[13] and so may only be present in a minute amount in decoction and aqueous extracts. A survey in 1994 of commercial pau d'arco products obtained in Canada found the levels of naphthoquinones was highly variable.[14]

Adulteration

"Pau d'arco" is a common name in South America referring to trees of the *Tabebuia* and *Tecoma* genera. Throughout the Amazon a number of species of *Tabebuia* are used medicinally. The western preference for *Tabebuia avellanedae* originates from the Brazilian clinical investigations in the late 1960s in which the investigating scientist observed that the "purple" species were superior to the yellow-flowered pau d'arco. However, there is evidence to suggest that the yellow-flowered *T. serratifolia* is used for similar therapeutic purposes by natives in other parts of South America.[15]

Traditional Brazilian sources indicate that side effects may occur from ingestion of the bark of the yellow-flowered pau d'arco plants *T. umbellata* and *T. pedicellata*. Reported side effects from ingestion of *T. umbellata* include swelling, burning and vomiting.[16]

Exploitation of *Tabebuia impetiginosa* has been to such an extent (for timber) that a 1994 article noted significant population declines in Brazil and at a local level in Argentina.[17] In the 1997 review of the application of the 1994 Convention on International

Trade in Endangered Species of Wild Fauna and Flora (CITES) listing criteria to timber species, there was insufficient information available on *Tabebuia impetiginosa* to recommend its inclusion.

Typical Dosage Forms & Dosage

Typical adult dosage ranges are:
* 3 to 6 cups/day of decoction (e.g., 4 teaspoons of bark per pint of water), with larger amounts taken in serious illness
* 3 to 7 mL/day of a 1:2 liquid extract or equivalent in tablet or capsule form

Contraindications

Pau d'arco is contraindicated in pregnancy. Patients on anticoagulant therapy should not be prescribed pau d'arco due to the potential warfarin-like action of naphthoquinones at high doses. (Lapachol has a chemical structure similar to vitamin K, differing only in its side chain.) Do not use during lactation without professional advice.

Use in Pregnancy

Category D: Has caused or is associated with a substantial risk of causing foetal malformation or irreversible damage.

In Argentinian folk medicine, decoction of *Tabebuia heptaphylla* (in formulations) is recommended for inducing abortion, although it is possible that other plants in the formula are the abortifacients.[18] Yellow-flowered *Tabebuia argentea* (*T. aurea*) is part of a formula used by indigenous people of Paraguay to induce abortion. Other plants in the formula include rue (*Ruta graveolens*) and caroa (*Jacaranda mimosifolia*). The part of the *Tabebuia* species used was not defined.[16,19]

The results of animal studies investigating the effect of lapachol on reproduction are summarised in Table 1.[20-27]

Use in Lactation

Category CC: Compatible with breastfeeding but use caution.

Table 1   **Results of Animal Studies Investigating the Effect of Lapachol on Reproduction**

Lapachol Administration, Route and Pregnancy Model	Day Administered	Results	Ref
10 mg (approx. 56 mg/kg), oral, rats	Days 8 to 12	99.2% foetal mortality rate	20
20 mg (approx. 112 mg/kg), oral, rats	Days 8 to 12	100% foetal mortality rate	21
100 mg/kg, oral, rats	Days 17 to 20	No effect on implantation or resorption Foetal growth retardation occurred	22
100 mg/kg, oral, rats	Days 1 to 5	100% foetal resorption	23
100 mg/kg, oral, rats	Days 7 to 12	78.7% foetal resorption Foetal malformation observed at day 21 (5.8% exophthalmia, 11.6% leporine lip)	23
100 mg/kg, oral, rats	Days 14 to 19	No foetal resorption	23
20 mg/kg, i.m., mice	Days 1 to 7	100% inhibition of pregnancy	24
20 mg/kg, i.m., mice	Days 1 to 3	71.2% inhibition of pregnancy	24
20 mg/kg, i.m., mice	Days 4 to 6	84.5% inhibition of pregnancy	24
100 to 200 mg/kg, oral, rats	Days 3 to 5	No effect on implantation or resorption	25, 26
100 mg/kg, oral, rats	Days 1 to 5	No effect on embryonic development	26, 27

Warnings & Precautions

Although pau d'arco contains constituents that can generate free radicals and interfere with mitochondrial respiration and blood coagulation, there is no evidence that the pau d'arco will cause adverse effects if taken within the recommended dosage and guidelines. The therapeutic effects of pau d'arco are likely to be mild and it should not be relied upon as a sole treatment for cancer or infections. Caution is advised for women wishing to conceive.

Effect on Ability to Drive or Operate Machinery

No adverse effects expected.

Adverse Reactions

A case was reported of hepatic failure in a man who was self-treating mild multiple sclerosis with zinc, skullcap tablets and pau d'arco tablets. The authors postulated that the skullcap tablets were adulterated.[28]

Adverse effects were recorded in patients taking high doses of lapachol during an uncontrolled clinical trial. No toxicity was observed at oral doses below 1.5 g. Above this dosage, nausea and vomiting were usual, although the unpalatable nature of the formulation may have contributed. Liver function tests were normal. At doses above 2 g/day, prothrombin time was often markedly prolonged and required correction with parenteral vitamin K. The results of other tests for clotting were normal.[29] This is a high dose of lapachol, and there is no evidence to suggest that pau d'arco would cause similar effects at its recommended dosage.

Allergic contact dermatitis caused by exposure to lapachol and other naphthoquinones has been reported in wood workers.[30,31]

Interactions

Although there is no evidence that pau d'arco has any effect on blood coagulation, it should not be combined with anticoagulant drugs. High doses of lapachol have caused prolonged prothrombin time in patients (see Adverse effects above).

Safety in Children

Information provided to the Brazilian Ministry of Health in 1967 indicated that purple pau d'arco was suitable to administer to children.[18]

Overdosage

No incidents found in published literature. Information provided to the Brazilian Ministry of Health in 1967 indicated that patients taking an extract of purple pau d'arco in a dose, "will feel a slight irritation, a sort of itchiness, although it is of no consequence . . . A person can take 5 g/kg (of extract) daily with no damage"[18] (although not defined, it is possible that these were aqueous extracts).

Toxicology

Table 2 lists LD_{50} data recorded for pau d'arco.[32-34]

No lethal effect was observed in dogs given daily oral doses of 0.25, 0.5, 1, or 2 g/kg of lapachol, 6 days per week for 4 weeks. Monkeys were treated on the same schedule (at doses of 0.0625, 0.125, 0.25, 0.5, or 1 g/kg) and death occurred after 6 doses of 0.5 g/kg and after 5 doses of 1 g/kg. Severe anaemia, elevated alkaline phosphatase activity, and other blood changes also occurred in dogs and monkeys. Haemorrhage was not observed, but clotting times in dogs remained normal even though prothrombin times were elevated.[32]

Information provided to the Brazilian Ministry of Health in 1967 indicated that purple pau d'arco had "no toxicity".[18] Studies conducted 2 years later confirmed a low toxicity for *T. avellanedae* extracts in rats.[35] It was not possible to measure the LD_{50} due to the lack of mice deaths, even at the high concentration of inner bark aqueous extract administered (1 to 5 g/kg, oral).[36] No toxic effect was observed from an ethanol extract of the inner bark of *T. serratifolia* (1 g/kg, oral or 100 mg/kg, i.v.).[16]

A study investigating the mutagenicity of naphthoquinones using the Ames test found lapachol was not mutagenic towards any of the tested strains.[37]

Regulatory Status

See Table 3 for regulatory status in selected countries.

Table **2** **LD$_{50}$ Data Recorded for Pau d'Arco**

Substance	Route, Model	LD$_{50}$ Value	Reference
Lapachol	Oral, mice	621 mg/kg	32
Lapachol	Oral, male mice	487 mg/kg	32
Lapachol	Oral, female mice	792 mg/kg	32
Lapachol	Oral, rats	>2.4 g/kg	32
Lapachol	i.p., mice	400 mg/kg	33
Lapachol	i.p., mice	1.6 g/kg	34
Xyloidone	i.p., mice	600 mg/kg	34
β-Lapachone	i.p., mice	80 mg/kg	34

Table **3** **Regulatory Status for Pau d'Arco in Selected Countries**

Australia	Pau d'arco is not included in Part 4 of Schedule 4 of the Therapeutic Goods Regulations.
UK & Germany	Pau d'arco is not included on the General Sale List. It was not included in the Commission E assessment.
US	Pau d'arco does not have generally recognised as safe (GRAS) status. However, it is freely available as a "dietary supplement" in the US under DSHEA legislation (Dietary Supplement Health and Education Act of 1994).

REFERENCES

1. Jones K: *Pau d'arco: immune power from the rain forest,* Vermont, 1995, Healing Arts Press, pp 1-4, 16.
2. Jones K: *Pau d'arco: immune power from the rain forest,* Vermont, 1995, Healing Arts Press, pp 34, 37, 38, 40, 46, 54, 98.
3. Mors WB, Rizzini CT, Pereira NA: *Medicinal plants of Brazil. Medicinal plants of the world,* no. 6, Algonac, 2000, Reference Publications, pp 82-83.
4. Davis EW: *J Ethnopharmacol* 9:225-236, 1983.
5. Evans Schultes R, Raffauf RF: *The healing forest: medicinal and toxic plants of the northwest Amazonia,* Portland, 1990, Dioscorides Press.
6. Boom BM, Moestl S: *Econ Bot* 44:416-419, 1990.
7. Dominguez XA, Alcorn JB: *J Ethnopharmacol* 13:139-156, 1985.
8. Blaschek W, Ebel S, Hackenthal E, et al: *HagerROM 2002: Hagers Handbuch der Drogen und Arzneistoffe,* Heidelberg, 2002, Springer.
9. Steinert J, Khalaf H, Rimpler M: *J Chromatogr A* 693:281-287, 1995.
10. Fujimoto Y, Eguchi T, Murasaki C, et al: *J Chem Soc Perkin Trans* 10:2323-2327, 1991.
11. Wagner H, Kreher B, Lotter H, et al: *Helv Chim Acta* 72:659-667, 1989.
12. Nakano K, Maruyama K, Murakami K, et al: *Phytochem* 32:371-374, 1993.
13. Budavari S, O'Neil MJ, Smith A, et al, eds: *The Merck index: an encyclopedia of chemicals, drugs and biologicals,* ed 12, Whitehouse Station, 1996, Merck & Co, p 917.
14. Awang DVC, Dauson BA, Ethier JC, et al: *J Herb Spice Med Plant* 2:27-43, 1994.
15. Jones K: *Pau d'arco: immune power from the rain forest,* Vermont, 1995, Healing Arts Press, pp 4, 33, 34, 45, 46.
16. Jones K: *Pau d'arco: immune power from the rain forest,* Vermont, 1995, Healing Arts Press, p 98.
17. Annex 2. Profiles of tree species: the Americas. Available from UNEP-WCMC website: *www.unep-wcmc.org* (accessed June 2003).
18. Jones K. Pau d'Arco: *Immune power from the rain forest,* Vermont, 1995, Healing Arts Press, p 99.
19. Arenas P, Moreno Azorero R: *Econ Bot* 31:298-301, 1977.
20. Guerra Mde O, Mazoni AS, Brandao MA, et al: *Braz J Biol* 61:171-174, 2001.
21. Guerra MO, Mazoni AS, Brandao MA, et al: *Contraception* 60:305-307, 1999.
22. Felicio AC, Chang CV, Brandao MA, et al: *Contraception* 66:289-293, 2002.
23. Rodrigues de Almeida E, Cesario de Mello A, Ferreira de Santana C, et al: *Rev Port Farm* 38:21-23, 1988.
24. Sareen V, Jain S, Narula A: *Phytother Res* 9:139-141, 1995.

25. Almeida ME, Brandao MA, Guerra MO, et al: 1999, cited in Felicio AC, Chang CV, Brandao MA, et al: *Contraception* 66:289-293, 2002.

26. Guerra M: Personal communication, Feb 2003.

27. Souza ER, Guerra MO, Peters VM: cited in Felicio AC, Chang CV, Brandao MA, et al: *Contraception* 66:289-293, 2002.

28. Hullar TE, Sapers BL, Ridker PM, et al: *Am J Med* 106:267-268, 1999.

29. Block JB, Serpeck AA, Miller W, et al: *Cancer Chemother Rep* (Part 2) 4:27-28, 1974.

30. Estlander T, Jolanki R, Alanko K, et al: *Contact Dermatitis* 44:213-217, 2001.

31. Schulz KH, Garbe I, Hausen BM, et al: *Arch Dermatol Res* 258:41-52, 1977.

32. Morrison RK, Brown DE, Oleson JJ, et al: *Toxicol Appl Pharmacol* 17:1-11, 1970.

33. Schuerch AR, Wehrli W: *Eur J Biochem* 84:197-205, 1978.

34. Ferreira de Santana C, Gonclaves de Lima O, Leoncio d'Albuquerque I, et al: *Rev Inst Antibiot Recife* 8:89-94, 1968.

35. Oga S, Sekina T: *Rev Fac Farm Bioquim Univ Sao Paulo* 7:47-53, 1969.

36. Miranda FG, Vilar JC, Alves IA, et al: *BMC Pharmacol* 1:6, 2001.

37. Hakura A, Mochida H, Tsutsui Y, et al: *Chem Res Toxicol* 7:559-567, 1994.

PENNYROYAL

Botanical name: *Mentha pulegium* L.
Family: Labiatae
Plant part used: Aerial parts and essential oil

Safety Summary

Pregnancy category X: High risk of damage to the foetus (due to the toxicity of pulegone).
Lactation category X: Contraindicated in breast-feeding (due to the toxicity of pulegone).
Contraindications: Pregnancy and lactation. The oil should not be taken internally.
Warnings & precautions: Do not use excessive doses.
Adverse reactions: Rare allergic reactions.
Interactions: None required on current evidence.

Typical Therapeutic Use

Traditional indications of pennyroyal in Western herbal medicine include flatulent dyspepsia and common cold.[1] There is a traditional folk use in bringing on delayed menstruation (as an emmenagogue): this often implies a role as an abortifacient.

Actions

Carminative, spasmolytic, emmenagogue; topically astringent.

Key Constituents

An essential oil containing 60% to 90% pulegone, 10% to 20% menthol.[2] Pulegone is potentially epileptogenic.[3]

Adulteration

No adulterants known.

Typical Dosage Forms & Dosage

Typical adult dosage ranges:
- 3 to 12 g/day of dried herb or as an infusion
- 3 to 12 mL/day of 1:1 liquid extract

These are the recommended doses in the *British Herbal Pharmacopoeia* 1983. However, modern practice by herbalists is to use much lower doses:

typically 3 to 6 mL/day of a 1:5 tincture. The higher doses listed above are not recommended for high quality preparations.

Contraindications

Pennyroyal is contraindicated in pregnancy and lactation. The oil should not be taken internally.

Use in Pregnancy

Category X: High risk of damage to the foetus (due to the toxicity of pulegone).

Although traditionally used as an abortifacient, there are no studies elaborating on the nature of the effect on the womb, nor any teratogenic or other related toxicity data. Nevertheless, the risk of harm to mother or foetus if pennyroyal or its oil is used is at least as high as any systemic abortifacient, with the additional risks of damage to organ development and central nervous system in the foetus.

Use in Lactation

Lactation category X: Contraindicated in breast-feeding (due to the toxicity of pulegone).

Warnings & Precautions

Do not use excessive doses.

Effect on Ability to Drive or Operate Machinery

No adverse effects expected.

Adverse Reactions

An allergic reaction is possible, but rare. Central nervous system reactions that have been reported include lethargy, agitation and dizziness, seizures, and hallucinations. Adverse gastrointestinal reactions are common, including nausea, vomiting, abdominal pain, and diarrhoea. Toxic liver damage in the case of pennyroyal oil ingestion has included massive centrolobular hepatic necrosis and hepatomegaly.[4]

Interactions

None known.

Safety in Children

No information available, but its use is not advised.

Overdosage

Twenty-two cases of pennyroyal ingestion in humans suggested moderate to severe toxicity in patients who had been exposed to at least 10 mL of pennyroyal oil. In one fatal case, postmortem examination of a serum sample, which had been obtained 72 hours after the acute ingestion, identified 18 ng/mL of pulegone in serum and 1 ng/mL of menthofuran. N-acetylcysteine is a potentially useful antidote to pennyroyal poisoning.[5] (Pulegone, but not menthofuran, depletes hepatic glutathione. The toxicity of menthofuran is only slightly affected by glutathione depletion, suggesting that N-acetylcysteine may be most effective in the early phases of pennyroyal poisoning.[6]) In one case of ingestion of 30 mL of pennyroyal oil by a pregnant woman, symptoms included abdominal spasm, nausea, vomiting, alternating lethargy and agitated behaviour. Later, a kidney failure and a solid liver necrosis developed; death occurred 7 days later. For two similar cases, where doses were 10 and 15 mL of oil, there was vomiting, agitation, fainting, flank pain, and dermatitis, but no lasting toxic symptoms.[4]

Toxicology

Table 1 lists LD$_{50}$ data recorded for pennyroyal oil and its major constituent.[7,8]

The toxicology of pulegone and related substances has been extensively reviewed, and so only a selection of this information is provided below.[9]

The no observed adverse effect level (NOAEL) for pulegone by gavage in rats was measured at 20 mg/kg/day,[10] although another study, in which the pulegone was added to the rat's food, found the NOAEL to be 250 mg/kg.[11]

Oxidation of the allylic methyl groups of pulegone by cytochrome P450 enzymes forms the hepatotoxin menthofuran, which is oxidised further by cytochrome P450 to a gamma-ketoenal that reacts with nucleophilic groups on proteins to form covalent adducts, as well as mintlactones (mintlactone and isomintlactone).[12,13] Pulegone is hepatotoxic after intraperitoneal injection in mice[14] and oral ingestion in rats (at 400 mg/kg, including decreases in microsomal cytochrome P450 levels).[15]

High pressure liquid chromatography (HPLC) analysis of the collected urine from rats administered moderate levels of pulegone showed its metabolism to be extensive and complex. Contrary to previous studies where near lethal doses were used, all but one of the major metabolites are phase II rather than phase I metabolites.[16] This suggests that some toxicity studies, implicating the cytochrome P450 pathways[17] in producing toxic metabolites (such as the hepatotoxin menthofuran,[13,18,19] or p-cresol, a glutathione depletor[20]), may give misleading information about the fate of pulegone administered in lower doses.

Pulegone was negative for genotoxicity in concentrations up to 1 g/plate in *Salmonella typhimurium* test systems. Pulegone (2 μL) was weakly positive in the wing spot test of *Drosophila melanogaster*.[21]

Regulatory Status

See Table 2 for regulatory status in selected countries.

Table 1   **LD$_{50}$ Data Recorded for Pennyroyal Oil and Its Major Constituent**

Substance	Route, Model	LD$_{50}$ Value (mg/kg)	Reference
Pennyroyal oil	Oral, rats	220 to 580	7
Pulegone	Oral, rats	470	8

Table **2**   **Regulatory Status for Pennyroyal in Selected Countries**

Australia	Pennyroyal is included in Part 4 of Schedule 4 of the Therapeutic Goods Regulations. A listable good containing pennyroyal for oral use must not contain more than 150 mg of volatile oil components for its recommended daily dose.
UK & Europe	Pennyroyal is not included on the General Sale List. It was not included in the Commission E assessment.
US	Pennyroyal does not have generally recognised as safe (GRAS) status. However, it is freely available as a "dietary supplement" in the US under DSHEA legislation (Dietary Supplement Health and Education Act of 1994).

REFERENCES

1. British Herbal Medicine Association's Scientific Committee: *British herbal pharmacopoeia*, Bournemouth, 1983, BHMA, p 143.
2. Hefendehl FW: *Phytochemistry* 9:1985-1995, 1970.
3. Burkhard PR, Burkhardt K, Haenggeli CA, et al: *J Neurol* 246:667-670, 1999.
4. Boyd EL. In: De Smet PAGM, Keller K, Hansel R, et al, eds: *Adverse effects of herbal drugs*, vol 1, Berlin, 1992, Springer-Verlag, p. 152.
5. Anderson IB, Mullen WH, Meeker JE, et al: *Ann Intern Med* 124:726-734, 1996.
6. Chitturi S, Farrell GC: *J Gastroenterol Hepatol* 15:1093-1099, 2000.
7. Opdyke DLJ: *Food Cosmet Toxicol* 12:949-950, 1972.
8. Opdyke DLJ: *Food Cosmet Toxicol* 16:867-868, 1978.
9. Speijers GJA: *Pulegone and related substances*. WHO Food Additives Series 46, Geneva, 2001, World Health Organization, pp 221-243.
10. Thorup I, Wurtzen G, Carstensen J, et al: *Toxicol Lett* 19:207-210, 1983.
11. Imaizumi K, Hanada K, Mawartari K, et al: *J Agric Biol Chem* 49:2795-2796, 1985.
12. Nelson SD: *Drug Metab Rev* 27:147-177, 1995.
13. Khojasteh-Bakht SC, Chen W, Koenigs LL, et al: *Drug Metab Dispos* 27:574-580, 1999.
14. Mizutani T, Nomura H, Nakanishi K, et al: *Res Commun Chem Pathol Pharmacol* 58: 75-83, 1987.
15. Moorthy B, Madyastha P, Madyastha KM: *Toxicology* 55:327-337, 1989.
16. Chen LJ, Lebetkin EH, Burka LT: *Drug Metab Dispos* 29:1567-1577, 2001.
17. Madyastha P, Moorthy B, Vaidyanathan CS, et al: *Biochem Biophys Res Commun* 128: 921-927, 1985.
18. Madyastha KM, Gaikwad NW: *Xenobiotica* 28:723-734, 1998.
19. Nelson SD, McClanahan RH, Thomassen D, et al: *Xenobiotica* 22:1157-1164, 1992.
20. Madyastha KM, Raj CP: *Biochem Biophys Res Commun* 297:202-205, 2002.
21. Franzios G, Mirotsou M, Hatziapostolou E, et al: *J Agric Food Chem* 45:2690-2694, 1997.

PEPPERMINT

Botanical name: *Mentha* × *piperita* L.
Family: Labiatae
Plant part used: Leaf, distilled oil

Safety Summary

Pregnancy category B2: No increase in frequency of malformation or other harmful effects on the foetus from limited use in women. Animal studies are largely lacking.

Lactation category CC: Compatible with breast-feeding but use caution.

Contraindications: Gastro-oesophageal reflux. In principle, the use of herbs containing high levels of tannins is contraindicated or at least inappropriate in constipation, iron deficiency anaemia and malnutrition. Do not use during lactation without professional advice.

Warnings & precautions: The leaf is generally safe, but use of the oil can cause sensitivity reactions, especially in the mouth and airways, and especially in young children. Because of the tannin content of this herb, long-term use should be avoided and it should be used cautiously in highly inflamed or ulcerated conditions of the gastrointestinal tract.

Adverse reactions: For the oil: sensitivity reactions in mouth and airways, heartburn; anal burning from the enteric-coated oil. Possible irritation of the gastrointestinal tract in sensitive individuals due to the tannin content.

Interactions: Use the oil with care when taken together with powerful drugs whose impact might be affected by changes in absorption rate. Due to the tannin content, take peppermint leaf separately from oral thiamine, metal ion supplements or alkaloid-containing medications.

Typical Therapeutic Use

Controlled clinical trials with peppermint oil have generally shown gastrointestinal spasmolytic effects with few or no adverse side effects.[1-4] Inhaled peppermint oil has been shown to have a cooling effect on peripheral circulation in human volunteers compared with inhaled basil oil.[5] A menthol receptor on sensory nerves has been identified, which may modulate the cool sensation.[6]

Traditional uses of peppermint in Western herbal medicine include flatulent dyspepsia and colic, and dysmenorrhoea. It is also used as inhalation for respiratory conditions[7] and as a diaphoretic tea for colds and influenza.

Actions

Spasmolytic, carminative, cholagogue, antiemetic, antitussive, antimicrobial, sedative, diaphoretic. Locally: antiseptic, analgesic, antipruritic.

Key Constituents

Essential oil (0.5% to 4%), consisting of predominantly of menthol (35% to 45%) and (−)-menthone (10% to 30%),[8] but also including minor amounts of pulegone.

Flavonoids, tannins (6% to 12%), triterpenes, and bitter substances.

The *European Pharmacopoeia* 4.2 recommends that whole peppermint leaf contain not less than 12 mL/kg of essential oil, and the cut leaf contain not less than 9 mL/kg of essential oil. Because of the toxicity of pulegone, its safe concentration should be limited to less than 1% of the oil.[9]

Adulteration

Although many *Mentha* species are also used, notably *Mentha arvensis* and *M. spicata*, the cultivation of most peppermint makes confusion rare. Peppermint oil is liable to augmentation with extra menthol, synthetic or natural menthofuran and menthyl acetate.

Adulteration with *Mentha pulegium* may occur from wildcrafting.[10]

Typical Dosage Forms & Dosage

Typical adult dosage ranges are:
- 6 to 12 g/day of dried leaf or by infusion
- 1.5 to 4.5 mL/day of a 1:2 liquid extract or equivalent in tablet or capsule form
- 6 to 9 mL/day of a 1:5 tincture

Contraindications

Patients with oesophageal reflux symptoms should avoid peppermint, as it may decrease lower oesophageal sphincter pressure.[11] The Commission E suggests that peppermint oil is contraindicated for internal use in occlusion of the gallbladder passages, cholecystitis, and severe liver disease.[12] Peppermint oil should not be applied to the facial areas of babies and small children, and especially not around the nose. Do not use during lactation without professional advice.

In principle, the use of tannins is contraindicated or at least inappropriate in constipation, iron deficiency anaemia, and malnutrition.

Use in Pregnancy

Category B2: No increase in frequency of malformation or other harmful effects on the foetus from limited use in women. Animal studies are largely lacking.

A tea consisting of peppermint, *Urtica dioica*, *Glycyrrhiza glabra*, *Helichrysum arenarium* and a species of *Rosa* did not affect postnatal development or demonstrate embryotoxicity or teratogenicity when administered to rats.[13]

Teratogenic effects were not observed in mice, rats, hamsters and rabbits for menthol tested at maximum oral doses of 190, 220, 400 and 430 mg/kg/day, respectively.[14]

Use in Lactation

Category CC: Compatible with breastfeeding but use caution. The leaf is compatible with breastfeeding, but use of the oil should be discouraged. Caution should be exercised, because there is a view that use of peppermint may dry up milk secretions.

Warnings & Precautions

The Commission E advises that in the case of gallstones, peppermint can only be used under professional supervision.[15] Because of the tannin content of this herb, long-term use should be avoided (for both internal and topical use). Use cautiously in highly inflamed or ulcerated conditions of the gastrointestinal tract.

Effect on Ability to Drive or Operate Machinery

No adverse effects expected.

Adverse Reactions

Being a concentrated form, peppermint oil has been associated with mucosal ulcerations.[16,17] These are

consistent with the development of buccal contact sensitivity reactions to peppermint or menthol.[18,19] Three constituents of peppermint oil, α-pinene, limonene and phellandrene, also found in turpentine oil, are thought to be the primary sensitising agents.[20] Menthol inhalations can also cause breathlessness and laryngeal spasm in susceptible individuals.[21] This may be a particular risk in young children.

The use of non–enteric-coated oil preparations occasionally causes heartburn, especially in persons suffering from reflux oesophagitis.[22,23] Enteric-coated capsules may produce anal burning in patients with diarrhoea due to excreted peppermint oil.

Skin rashes, headache, bradycardia, muscle tremor, heartburn, and ataxia are rarely reported side effects associated with enteric-coated capsules of peppermint oil.

Menthol can cause jaundice in newborn babies. This has been linked to glucose-6-phosphate dehydrogenase deficiency in some cases.[24]

A case of exacerbation of urticaria and asthma after ingestion of menthol-containing lozenges has been reported.[25]

High doses of tannins lead to excessive astringency on mucous membranes, which has an irritating effect.

Interactions

There is evidence that topical use of menthol could enhance penetration of other agents, which could affect the use of other topical ingredients whose safety assessment is based on their lack of absorption.[9] Peppermint oil also slows intestinal transit in healthy volunteers[26]; this may slow the absorption rate, or increase the total absorption, of other drugs.

Peppermint tea reduced the absorption of iron by 84% from a bread meal (compared to a water control) in adult volunteers. The inhibition was dose dependent and related to its tannin content. Inhibition by black tea was 79% to 94%.[27] This indicates a potential interaction for concomitant administration of peppermint during iron intake. In anaemia and cases where iron supplementation is required, peppermint should not be taken simultaneously with meals or iron supplements.

Refer to the cranesbill root (*Geranium maculatum*) monograph for information regarding interactions of tannins.

Safety in Children

Direct application of peppermint oil preparations to the nasal area or chest of babies and small children must be avoided because of the risk of laryngeal and bronchial spasms. No adverse effects are expected from use of peppermint leaf.

Overdosage

Bradycardia has been reported in a patient addicted to menthol cigarettes[28] and fibrillation has been associated with the excessive consumption of peppermint-flavoured confectionery (up to 225 g/day).[29]

Excessive inhalation of mentholated products has caused reversible, undesirable effects, such as nausea, anorexia, cardiac problems, ataxia and other CNS problems, probably due to the presence of volatile menthol. See also the Adverse reactions section above.

No cases of overdosage are documented for peppermint leaf.

Toxicology

Table 1 lists LD$_{50}$ data recorded for the constituents of peppermint.[9,30]

Mice treated orally for 7 days with 4 g/kg of peppermint concentrate (4.2:1) did not show any macroscopic signs of toxicity.[31] Peppermint infusion (20 g/L) provided as drinking water did not produce nephrotoxicity in rats. However, *Mentha spicata* produced markedly nephrotoxic changes.[32]

Peppermint oil was given by mouth to four groups of 28 rats at dosage levels of 0, 10, 40 and 100 mg/kg per day for 90 days. At the highest dose,

histopathological changes consisting of cyst-like spaces scattered in the white matter of the cerebellum were seen. No other signs of encephalopathy were observed. Nephropathy was also seen in the male rats in the highest dose group. A no observed adverse effect level of 40 mg/kg/day body weight was determined.[33] Peppermint oil containing 1% to 2% pulegone was administered to rats (20 to 500 mg/kg/day) for 5 weeks. The rats showed no effects on general health, behaviour, or body weight, and the haematological and urinary parameters were normal. Histological examination revealed no specific pathological lesions.[34]

Repeated intradermal dosing with peppermint oil produced moderate and severe reactions in rabbits, although peppermint oil did not appear to be phototoxic.[9]

The estimated lethal dose for menthol in humans may be as low as 2 g; however there are reports of individuals surviving doses as high as 9 g.[35]

Menthone at dose levels in rats of 0, 200, 400 and 800 mg/kg body weight per day for 28 days led to a dose-dependent decrease in creatinine, and increases in alkaline phosphatase and bilirubin. The no-effect level for menthone in this study was lower than 200 mg/kg body weight per day.[36]

Refer to the pennyroyal (*Mentha pulegium*) monograph for toxicology and LD$_{50}$ values for pulegone. Refer to the cranesbill root (*Geranium maculatum*) monograph for information regarding interactions of tannins (see Interactions section).

Regulatory Status

See Table 2 for regulatory status in selected countries.

Peppermint is widely consumed as a herbal tea.

Table 1   **LD$_{50}$ Data Recorded for the Constituents of Peppermint**

Substance	Route, Model	LD$_{50}$ Value (g/kg)	Reference
Peppermint oil	Oral, mice	2.4	31
Peppermint oil	Oral, rat	4.4	31
Menthol	Oral, rat	3.3	32
Menthol	Oral, cat	0.8 to 1	32

Table **2**   **Regulatory Status for Peppermint in Selected Countries**

Australia	Peppermint is not included in Part 4 of Schedule 4 of the Therapeutic Goods Regulations.
UK & Germany	Peppermint is included on the General Sale List. Peppermint leaf is covered by a positive Commission E monograph.
	Peppermint is official in the *European Pharmacopoeia* 4.3.
US	Peppermint does have generally recognised as safe (GRAS) status. It is freely available as a "dietary supplement" in the US under DSHEA legislation (Dietary Supplement Health and Education Act of 1994).

REFERENCES

1. Madisch A, Heydenreich CJ, Wieland V, et al: *Arzneim Forsch* 49:925-932, 1999.
2. May B, Kohler S, Schneider B: *Aliment Pharmacol Ther* 14:1671-1677, 2000.
3. Micklefield G, Jung O, Greving I et al: *Phytother Res* 17:135-140, 2003.
4. Hiki N, Kurosaka H, Tatsutomi Y et al: *Gastrointest Endosc* 57:475-482, 2003.
5. Satoh T, Sugawara Y: *Anal Sci* 19:139-146, 2003.
6. Eccles R: *Curr Allergy Asthma Rep* 3:210-214, 2003.
7. British Herbal Medicine Association's Scientific Committee: *British herbal pharmacopoeia*, Bournemouth, 1983, BHMA, pp 141-142.
8. Wagner H, Bladt S: *Plant drug analysis: a thin layer chromatography atlas*, ed 2, Berlin, 1996, Springer-Verlag, p 156.
9. Nair B: *Int J Toxicol* 20(Suppl 3):61-73, 2001.
10. Blaschek W, Ebel S, Hackenthal E, et al: *HagerROM 2002: Hagers Handbuch der Drogen und Arzneistoffe*, Heidelberg, 2002, Springer.
11. Friedman G: *Gastroenterol Clin North Am* 20:313-324, 1991.
12. Blumenthal M, et al, eds: *The complete German Commission E monographs: therapeutic guide to herbal medicines*, Austin, 1998, American Botanical Council, pp 181-182.
13. Ubasheev IO, Lonshakova KS, Matkhanov EI, et al: *Khim Farm Zh* 22:445-450, 1988.
14. Fifty-first meeting of the Joint FAO/WHO Expert Committee on Food Additives (JECFA): *Safety evaluation of certain food additives*. WHO Food Additives Series no 42, Geneva, 1999, World Health Organization.
15. Blumenthal M, et al, eds: *The complete German Commission E monographs: therapeutic guide to herbal medicines*, Austin, 1998, American Botanical Council, pp 180-181.
16. Moghadam BK, Gier R, Thurlow T: *Cutis* 64:131-134, 1999.
17. Rogers SN, Pahor AL: *Dent Update* 22:36-37, 1995.
18. Morton CA, Garioch J, Todd P, et al: *Contact Dermatitis* 32:281-284 1995.
19. Sainio EL, Kanerva L: *Contact Dermatitis* 33:100-105, 1995.
20. Dooms-Goossens A, Degreef H, Holvoet C, et al: *Contact Dermatitis* 3:304-308, 1977.
21. Lässig W, Graupner I, Leonhardt H, et al: *Z Klin Med* 45:969-971, 1990.
22. Somerville KW, Richmond CR, Bell GD: *Br J Clin Pharmac* 18:638-640, 1984.
23. Nash P, Gould SR, Barnardo DE: *Br J Clin Pract* 40:292-293, 1986.
24. Owa JA: *Acta Paediatr Scand* 78:848-852, 1989.
25. Marlowe KF: *Am J Health Syst Pharm* 60:1657-1659, 2003.
26. Goerg, KJ, Spilker T: *Aliment Pharmacol Ther* 17:445-451, 2003.
27. Hurrell RF, Reddy M, Cook JD: *Br J Nutr* 81:289-295, 1999.
28. Luke E: *Lancet* 1:110-111, 1962.
29. Thomas JG: *Lancet* 1:222, 1962.
30. Opdyke DL: *Food Cosmet Toxicol* 14:471, 1976.
31. Della Loggia R, Tubaro A: *Fitoterapia* 61:215-221, 1990.
32. Akdogan M, Kilinc I, Oncu M, et al: *Hum Exp Toxicol* 22:213-219, 2003.
33. Spindler P, Madsen C: *Toxicol Lett* 62:215-220, 1992.
34. Mengs U, Stotzem CD: *Med Sci Res* 17:499-500, 1989.
35. De Smet PAGM, Keller K, Hansel R, et al, eds: *Adverse effects of herbal drugs*, vol 2. Berlin, 1992, Springer-Verlag, pp 171-178.
36. Madsen C, Wurtzen G, Carstensen J: *Toxicol Lett* 32:147-152, 1986.

POKE ROOT

Other common names: Pokeweed, pokeberry
Botanical names: *Phytolacca decandra* L. (*P. americana* L.)
Family: Phytolaccaceae
Plant part used: Root

Safety Summary

Pregnancy category D: Has caused or is associated with a substantial risk of causing foetal malformation or irreversible damage.
Lactation category X: Contraindicated in breast-feeding (on the basis of its potential toxicity).
Contraindications: Pregnancy, lactation, lymphocytic leukaemia and gastrointestinal irritation. Do not apply to broken or ulcerated skin.
Warnings & precautions: Do not exceed the recommended dose. Do not use for longer than 6 months. Avoid contact with the eyes. Liquid extracts and fresh plant tinctures are not recommended and should be used with extreme caution. The use of herbs rich in saponins is possibly inappropriate in coeliac disease, fat malabsorption and vitamins A, D, E, and K deficiency, and some upper digestive irritations. Caution in patients with preexisting cholestasis.
Adverse reactions: Nausea, abdominal pain, haematemesis, diarrhoea, hypotension, and tachycardia. Herbs rich in saponins may cause irritation of the gastric mucous membranes and reflux.
Interactions: Avoid concurrent use with immunosuppressive drugs.

Typical Therapeutic Use

Traditional uses of poke root in Western herbal medicine include lymphadenitis, mastitis, mumps, and inflammatory conditions of the upper respiratory tract, such as laryngitis and tonsillitis. Topically, it has been used for the treatment of mastitis and mammary abscess.[1] *Phytolacca americana* root is used in traditional Chinese medicine for generalised oedema with oliguria and constipation.[2]

Actions

Antiinflammatory, lymphatic, depurative, immune enhancing.

Key Constituents

Major constituents of the root of *Phytolacca americana* are triterpenoid saponins (phytolaccosides). Other constituents include sterols and traces of lectins (also known as poke weed mitogen). Antiviral proteins occur mainly in the seeds and leaves.[3]

Adulteration

No adulterants known.

Typical Dosage Forms & Dosage

Typical dosage ranges are:
- 0.18 to 0.9 g/day of the dried root or by decoction
- 0.3 to 1.5 mL/day of a 1:1 liquid extract[*]
- 0.15 to 0.7 mL of a 1:5 tincture per day or equivalent in tablet or capsule form
- 0.2 to 0.6 mL of a 1:10 tincture three times per day

Contraindications

Poke root is contraindicated in pregnancy, lactation, gastrointestinal irritation, and lymphocytic leukaemia (due to its mitogenic properties). Because of the irritant effect of the saponins, poke root should not be applied to broken or ulcerated skin.

Use in Pregnancy

Category D: Has caused or is associated with a substantial risk of causing foetal malformation or irreversible damage.

Poke root is contraindicated in pregnancy due to its potential toxicity. Mid-term abortifacient activity has been reported for the seeds (10 mg/kg), roots (20 mg/kg) and leaves (40 mg/kg) of *P. acinosa* (a species used in traditional Chinese medicine) after intraperitoneal administration to pregnant mice.[4] Abortion in cows has been described as a result of toxicity from the berries.[5] Use of the root as an abortifacient has been reported.[6]

---

[*] This dosage regime is excessive and dangerous, and was presumably developed from observing the use of denatured preparations.

Use in Lactation

Category X: Contraindicated in breastfeeding (on the basis of its potential toxicity).

Poke root is used topically in traditional Western medicine to treat mastitis.[1] Breast feeding infants should not be exposed to poke root applied topically to the breasts, so application to the nipple should be avoided.

Warnings & Precautions

Poke root tinctures may be safely prescribed if the recommended dosage is not exceeded. The maximum recommended dosage has been exceeded in some cases, with resultant toxic effects. Liquid extracts and fresh plant tinctures have the potential to cause poisoning because they are more active and may contain higher levels of poke weed mitogen. They should be used with extreme caution, if at all. Accurate measurement of dried plant tincture volumes is vital to ensure that the safe dosage is not exceeded. Topical application of poke root should be restricted to dried plant tinctures, and contact with the eyes should be avoided. In light of the potential risks, medium-term use of poke root up to 6 months is advised.

The use of herbs rich in saponins is possibly inappropriate in coeliac disease, fat malabsorption and vitamins A, D, E, and K deficiency, and some upper digestive irritations. Saponin-containing herbs are best kept to a minimum in patients with preexisting cholestasis.

Effect on Ability to Drive or Operate Machinery

No adverse effects expected.

Adverse Reactions

Individual responses to the ingestion of poke root plant parts appear to vary greatly and can be independent of the quantity of the plant part consumed.[7] Adverse reactions (possibly from mild overdose) include nausea, abdominal pain, haematemesis, diarrhoea, hypotension, and tachycardia.

Topical application of preparations derived from the green plant and root have produced inflammation of the skin.[8,9] Severe respiratory irritation and gastroenteritis have been described after occupational exposure to poke root dust by accidental inhalation.[10]

As with all herbs rich in saponins, oral use may cause irritation of the gastric mucous membranes, and reflux.

Interactions

Avoid concurrent use with immunosuppressive drugs.

Safety in Children

No information is available for poke root, but the recommended dosage should be adhered to and adjusted accordingly.

Preschool children are more likely to be poisoned by ingestion of the berries rather than by leaf or root.[11] Up to 10 raw berries can be considered harmless for adults and older children, but may lead to serious poisoning in infants.[12] A few fatal cases of poisoning in children from eating the fruit have been recorded, but it is not clear whether death was caused by the seed or the pulp.[6] Another source indicates that the reports of poisoning of children by the berries are not conclusive.[13]

Overdosage

Intoxication with poke root usually involves an initial burning sensation in the mouth and throat, followed a few hours later by nausea, repeated vomiting, salivation, profuse sweating, severe abdominal cramps, and watery or bloody diarrhoea. Other symptoms commonly include generalised weakness, headaches, dizziness, hypotension, and tachycardia. Urinary incontinence, confusion, unconsciousness, and tremors may also occur. The onset of symptoms usually occurs 2 to 4 hours after ingestion. Nonfatal cases usually recover within 24 to 48 hours with medical treatment.[5,11,14,15]

Poisonings occurred in North America during the 19th century following overdose of dried plant tinctures and ingestion of berries or roots mistaken for other vegetables. Fatalities were reported.[6,16] More recently, poisoning has mainly occurred from inappropriate use. An 18-year-old male died after eating a 4 to 5 inch piece of the root, mistaken for parsnip.[17] Nonfatal poisonings have occurred from drinking tea prepared by extracting the leaves and stems with boiling water,[18] eating fresh and/or cooked leaves,[19,20] mistakenly eating grated root,[21] or chewing on the fresh root.[14] In the last case, the patient's lymphocyte count increased nearly four-fold within one week of intoxication.[14]

A 43-year-old woman drank one cup of pow-dered poke root tea, which was prepared as per the label directions (approx. 1 g per cup of boiling water); she experienced overdosage symptoms such as nausea, abdominal pain, haematemesis, watery and bloody diarrhoea, hypotension, and tachycardia.[16]

Peripheral blood plasmacytosis (increase in the number of plasma cells) occurred in children exposed through oral ingestion to large amounts of berries, or by exposure of fresh cuts and abrasions to berry juice.[22] Large immature basophilic lympho-cytes appeared in the peripheral blood of two adults shortly after accidental exposure to a root extract (one through the conjunctiva and the other through a subcutaneous puncture wound).[23] *P. americana* extracts have demonstrated mitogenic effects in human peripheral blood cells in vitro.[24]

Parts of the plant are commonly assumed to be safe to eat when they are prepared properly; that is, when the berries have been cooked or when the young green shoots or leaves have been boiled in two changes of water.[5,11,14] However, poisonings have still occurred when these measures have been taken.[7,14,25]

A number of sources state that the root is con-sidered the most toxic part of the plant, although all parts are noted as toxic. Toxicity is said to increase as the plant matures, with the only exception being that the green berries are more toxic than the mature berries. Primary references are not pro-vided.[5,11,14] However, early animal studies with the berry extract report that it has milder toxic effects than the root.[6] Poisonings after consumption of the leaves, berries, or root have been reported in livestock.[6]

The main toxic components are the saponins,[26,27] which act as gastrointestinal irritants and probably account for the severe nausea, vomit-ing, and diarrhoea which accompany an overdose. Immunological changes are probably due to the lectins.[14,26] Poke root saponins are not considered to be cardiotoxic.[14] Cardiac effects may be second-ary to the increased vagal tone seen with severe gastrointestinal irritation.[19] To date, there have been no studies which correlate toxic effects with levels of particular saponins.

Toxicology

Table 1 lists LD_{50} data recorded for poke root extract and one of its key constituents.[26,28]

Saline suspensions of poke root extract pro-duced high rates of intraperitoneal lethality in mice, rats and guinea pigs. Intravenous injection to anaes-thetised cats markedly depressed respiratory and circulatory functions. Intragastric administration of dilute poke root extract produced violent vomiting in cats. Large oral doses of liquid extracts markedly impaired liver function, but not kidney function, in rabbits.[29] Reddening and irritation of the conjuncti-vae occurred after instillation of a saline suspension of poke root extract into rabbit eyes.[29]

Regulatory Status

See Table 2 for regulatory status in selected countries.

Table 1 　**LD_{50} Data Recorded for Poke Root Extract and a Key Constituent**

Substance	Route, Model	LD_{50} Value (mg/kg)	Reference
Saponin extract of *P. americana* root	i.p., mice	181	28
Saponin extract of *P. americana* root	i.p., rats	208	28
Acidic steroidal saponin from the root	i.p., mice	0.065	26

Table **2   Regulatory Status for Poke Root in Selected Countries**

Australia	Poke root is included in Part 4 of Schedule 4 of the Therapeutic Goods Regulations. The recommended daily dose must not exceed 1 mg of the dry herbal material.
China	Poke root is official in the *Pharmacopoeia of the People's Republic of China* 1997. The usual adult dosage, usually administered in the form of a decoction, is listed as 3 to 9 g.
UK & Germany	Poke root is listed on the General Sale List, with a maximum single oral dose of 120 mg. It was not included in the Commission E assessment.
US	Poke root does not have generally recognised as safe (GRAS) status. However, it is freely available as a "dietary supplement" in the US under DSHEA legislation (Dietary Supplement Health and Education Act of 1994).

REFERENCES

1. British Herbal Medicine Association's Scientific Committee: *British herbal pharmacopoeia*, Bournemouth, 1983, BHMA, p 157.

2. Pharmacopoeia Commission of the People's Republic of China: *Pharmacopoeia of the People's Republic of China*, English ed, vol I, Beijing, 1997, Chemical Industry Press, p 162.

3. Tang W, Eisenbrand G: *Chinese drugs of plant origin*, Berlin, 1992, Springer Verlag, pp 765-775.

4. Yeung HW, Feng Z, Li WW, et al: *J Ethnopharmacol* 21:31-35, 1987.

5. De Smet PAGM. In De Smet PAGM, Keller K, Hänsel R, et al, eds: *Adverse effects of herbal drugs*, vol 2, Berlin, 1993, Springer-Verlag, pp 253-261.

6. Watt JM, Breyer-Brandwijk MG: *The medicinal and poisonous plants of southern and eastern Africa: being an account of their medicinal and other uses, chemical composition, pharmacological effects and toxicology in man and animal*, ed 2, Edinburgh, 1962, Livingstone, pp 834-836.

7. Edwards N, Rodgers GC: *Vet Hum Toxicol* 24(Suppl):135-137, 1982.

8. Felter HW, Lloyd JU: *King's American dispensatory*, ed 18, rev 3, vol 2, first published 1905; reprinted Portland, 1983, Eclectic Medical Publications, pp 1471-1475.

9. Mitchell J, Rook A: *Botanical dermatology: plants and plant products injurious to the skin*, Vancouver, 1979, Greengrass, p 513.

10. Goldstein SW, Jenkins GL, Thompson MR: *J Am Pharm Assoc* 26:306-312, 1973.

11. Mack RB: *North Carolina Med J* 43:365, 1982.

12. Frohne D, Pfander HJ: *A colour atlas of poisonous plants: a handbook for pharmacists, doctors, toxicologists, and biologists*, translated from the 2nd German ed by Bisset NG. London, 1984, Wolfe Publishing, pp 166-167.

13. Kingsbury JM: *Poisonous plants for the United States and Canada*, Englewood Cliffs, 1964, Prentice Hall, pp 225-227.

14. Roberge R, Brader E, Martin ML, et al: *Ann Emerg Med* 15:470-473, 1986.

15. Kell SO: *Vet Hum Toxicol* 24(Suppl):138, 1982.

16. Lewis WH, Smith PR: *JAMA* 242:2759-2760, 1979.

17. Brooker J, Obar C, Courtemanche L: *J Toxicol Clin Toxicol* 39:549-550, 2001.

18. Jaeckle KA, Freemon FR: *South Med J* 74:639-640, 1981.

19. Hamilton RJ, Shih RD, Hoffman RS: *Vet Human Toxicol* 37:66-67, 1995.

20. Stein ZLG: *Am J Hosp Pharm* 36:1303, 1979.

21. Lawrence RA: *Vet Hum Toxicol* 32:369, 1990.

22. Barker BE, Rarnes P, LaMarche PH: *Pediatrics* 38:490-493, 1966.

23. Barker BE, Farnes P, Fanger H: *Lancet* 1:170, 1965.

24. Farnes P, Barker BE, Brownhill LE, et al: *Lancet* 2:1100-1101, 1964.

25. No authors listed: *MMWR Morb Mortal Wkly Rep* 30:65-67, 1981.

26. Ahmed ZF, Zufall CJ, Jenkins GL: *J Am Pharm Assoc* 38:443-448, 1949.

27. Woo WS, et al: *Planta Med* 34:87, 1978.

28. Woo WS, Shin KH, Kang SS: *Soul Taehakkyo Saengyak Yonguso Opjukjip* 15:103-106, 1976.

29. Macht DI: *J Am Pharm Assoc Sci Ed* 26:594-599, 1937.

PRICKLY ASH

Botanical names: *Zanthoxylum clava-herculis* L. (*Zanthoxylum macrophyllum* Nutt.), *Zanthoxylum americanum* Mill. Note: *Xanthoxylum* is a previous genus name for *Zanthoxylum*.
Family: Rutaceae
Plant part used: Stem bark

Safety Summary

Pregnancy category B2: No increase in frequency of malformation or other harmful effects on the foetus from limited use in women. Animal studies are lacking.
Lactation category C: Compatible with breastfeeding.
Contraindications: None required on current evidence.
Warnings & precautions: None required on current evidence.
Adverse reactions: None found in published literature.
Interactions: No precautions required on current evidence.

Typical Therapeutic Use

Two double-blind, placebo-controlled clinical trials have demonstrated that standardised prickly ash extract improved venous circulation in patients with varicose veins.[1] Traditional indications for prickly ash in Western herbal medicine include chronic rheumatic symptoms and peripheral circulatory insufficiency.[2]

Actions

Circulatory stimulant, diaphoretic, antirheumatic, sialogogue.

Key Constituents

Constituents of *Zanthoxylum clava-herculis* stem bark include alkaloids (such as chelerythrine, nitidine, and tembetarine),[3] lignans (asarinin), and an isobutylamide (neoherculin, also known as echinacein).[4] Berberine is not present.[3] *Z. americanum* stem bark contains the same alkaloids.[5]

Adulteration

King's American Dispensatory carries the warning not to confuse *Z. clava-herculis* bark with the bark of *Aralia spinosa*.[6] Prickly ash preparations lacking in alkylamides (as evidenced by a lack of tingling sensation on oral contact) are possibly prepared from *Aralia spinosa*.

Typical Dosage Forms & Dosage

Typical adult dosage ranges are:
- 3 to 9 g/day of dried stem bark or by decoction
- 3 to 9 mL/day of a 1:1 liquid extract
- 1.5 to 4.5 mL/day of a 1:2 liquid extract or equivalent in tablet or capsule form
- 6 to 15 mL/day of a 1:5 tincture

Contraindications

None known.

Use in Pregnancy

Category B2: No increase in frequency of malformation or other harmful effects on the foetus from limited use in women. Animal studies are lacking.

The *British Herbal Compendium* carries a contraindication for pregnancy.[4] This may be due to the presence of alkaloids. However, the Eclectic physicians who introduced this herb into western use do not caution against use in pregnancy.[6-8]

Use in Lactation

Category C: Compatible with breastfeeding.

Warnings & Precautions

None required.

Effect on Ability to Drive or Operate Machinery

No adverse effects expected.

Adverse Reactions

None known.

Interactions

None known.

Safety in Children

No information available, but adverse effects are not expected.

Overdosage

Poisoning has been observed in cattle believed to have grazed on the bark of Z. clava-herculis. Ingestion of parts of Z. americanum has been suspected as the cause of death in cattle and sheep. A neuromuscular blocking action could have contributed to the toxic effects.[9]

Toxicology

An extract of Zanthoxylum clava-herculis standardised for total alkaloids and magnoflorine content produced a good safety profile determined in subchronic, chronic, and acute toxicity assays. No more information is available.[1]

No toxic symptoms other than excessive salivation were observed in rats orally administered 500 mg/kg Z. clava-herculis bark extract. The bark was extracted successively with petroleum ether, ethyl ether, chloroform, and ethanol.[10]

Regulatory Status

See Table 1 for regulatory status in selected countries.

Table 1   **Regulatory Status for Prickly Ash in Selected Countries**

Australia	Prickly ash is not included in Part 4 of Schedule 4 of the Therapeutic Goods Regulations.
UK & Germany	Prickly ash is included on the General Sale List. It was not included in the Commission E assessment.
US	Prickly ash does have generally recognised as safe (GRAS) status. It is freely available as a "dietary supplement" in the US under DSHEA legislation (Dietary Supplement Health and Education Act of 1994).

REFERENCES

1. Jia Q, Qui Z, Nissanka A, et al: Phytomedicine 7(Suppl 2):46, 2000.
2. British Herbal Medicine Association's Scientific Committee: British herbal pharmacopoeia, Bournemouth, 1983, BHMA, p 237.
3. Fish F, Waterman PG: J Pharm Pharmacol 25(Suppl):115P-116P, 1973.
4. British Herbal Medicine Association: British herbal compendium, vol 1, Bournemouth, 1992, BHMA, pp 177-178.
5. Fish F, Gray AI, Waterman PG, et al: Lloydia 38:268-270, 1975.
6. Felter HW, Lloyd JU: King's American dispensatory, ed 18, rev 3, vol 2. First published 1905; reprinted Portland, 1983, Eclectic Medical Publications, pp 2087-2091.
7. Ellingwood F, Lloyd JU: American materia medica, therapeutics and pharmacognosy, ed 11, Naturopathic Medical Series: Botanical vol 2, Portland, 1983, Eclectic Medical Publications, pp 165-166.
8. Cook WH: The physio-medical dispensatory. First published 1869; reprinted Portland, 1985, Eclectic Medical Publications, pp 751-754.
9. Bowen JM, Cole RJ, Bedell D, et al: Am J Vet Res 57:1239-1244, 1996.
10. Jacobsen M: J Am Chem Soc 70:4234-4237, 1948.

PYGEUM

Botanical names: *Prunus africana* (Hook. f.) Kalkm. (formerly *Pygeum africanum* Hook. f.)
Family: Rosaceae
Plant part used: Bark

Safety Summary

Pregnancy category B2: No increase in frequency of malformation or other harmful effects on the foetus from limited use in women. Animal studies are lacking.
Lactation category ND: No data available.
Contraindications: None required on current evidence.
Warnings & precautions: None required on current evidence.
Adverse reactions: Occasional mild gastrointestinal upset.
Interactions: No precautions required on current evidence.

Typical Therapeutic Use

Pygeum bark extract has been used for the symptomatic treatment of mild and moderate benign prostatic hyperplasia in Europe since 1969.[1] A Cochrane review of 18 randomised controlled trials concluded that, compared to those receiving placebo, pygeum provided a moderately large improvement in urological symptoms and flow measures.[2]

Actions

Antiprostatic, antiinflammatory, antioedematous.

Key Constituents

Lipophilic extracts of pygeum bark contain phytosterols (such as β-sitosterol), pentacyclic terpenes (such as oleanolic and ursolic acids), and ferulic acid esters of fatty alcohols (such as n-docosanol and n-tetracosanol).[3-5] Extracts are usually standardised to contain 14% phytosterols and 0.5% n-docosanol.

Adulteration

This plant is listed as an endangered species[6,7] (it is listed in Appendix II of the Convention on International Trade in Endangered Species [CITES] as of May 2003), which increases the possibility of substitution. Research to 1993 indicates that bark harvested in Kivu, Zaire was probably a mixture of *Prunus africana* and *Prunus crassifolia* bark.[8]

Typical Dosage Forms & Dosage

The dose of standardised liposterolic extract of pygeum prescribed in clinical trials ranged from 75 to 200 mg/day. The extracts are standardised to contain 12% to 13% total sterols.[9] This daily dosage of extract corresponds to 15 to 40 g of original, dried bark.

Contraindications

None required on current evidence.

Use in Pregnancy

Category B2: No increase in frequency of malformation or other harmful effects on the foetus from limited use in women. Animal studies are lacking. Pygeum has been used predominately by men and is unlikely to be indicated for a pregnant woman.

Use in Lactation

Category ND: No data available.
As pygeum has been used predominately by men, there is a lack of information about its use by lactating woman.

Warnings & Precautions

None required.

Effect on Ability to Drive or Operate Machinery

No adverse effects expected.

Adverse Reactions

The Cochrane review described above concluded that adverse effects from pygeum treatment were mild and comparable to placebo. The dropout rate was similar to placebo or other controls. The most frequently reported adverse events were gastrointestinal.[2,9]

A case of protracted cholestatic hepatitis after the use of a herbal preparation was reported. The herbal preparation contained hydrangea, saw palmetto (*Serenoa serrulata*), *Pygeum africanum*, *Panax ginseng*, zinc picolinate, pyridoxine, alanine, glutamic acid, *Apis mellifica* pollen, and silica.[10] The ingredient causing the adverse reaction was not identified.

Interactions

None known.

Safety in Children

Given the current applications for pygeum in Western herbal medicine, use in children is not relevant.

Overdosage

No incidents found in published literature.

Toxicology

Acute and chronic toxicity tests in mice and rats found pygeum extract to be devoid of severe toxic effects (acute oral dosages: 1 to 6 g/kg in mice, 1 to 8 g/kg in rats; chronic oral dosages: 60 and 600 mg/kg for 11 months, in mice and rats respectively).[11,12] Pygeum extract was also well tolerated and with no adverse effects in dogs (375 mg/kg/day for 6 months). Pygeum extract (80 mg/kg/day) had no effect on the fertility of male rats and rabbits.[13]

An aqueous extract of pygeum was administered repeatedly at doses of 10, 100, and 1000 mg/kg/day to rats. The extract caused moderate rises in plasma alanine aminotransferase and creatine kinase, mainly at the 1000 mg/kg dosage.[14] Chloroform extract of pygeum did not cause toxicity in rats at oral doses of up to 1 g/kg/day for 8 weeks. However, the extract caused marked clinical signs, organ damage, and a 50% mortality rate at 3.3 g/kg/day for 6 days.[15]

In vitro and in vivo mutagenicity studies showed an absence of mutagenic and clastogenic potential.[13]

Regulatory Status

See Table 1 for regulatory status in selected countries.

Table 1 **Regulatory Status for Pygeum in Selected Countries**

Australia	Pygeum is not included in Part 4 of Schedule 4 of the Therapeutic Goods Regulations.
UK & Germany	Pygeum is not included on the General Sale List. It was not included in the Commission E assessment.
	Pygeum is official in the *British Pharmacopoeia* 2002 and the *European Pharmacopoeia* 4.3.
US	Pygeum does not have generally recognised as safe (GRAS) status. However, it is freely available as a "dietary supplement" in the US under DSHEA legislation (Dietary Supplement Health and Education Act of 1994).

REFERENCES

1. Marandola P, Jallous H, Bombardelli E, et al: *Fitoterapia* 68:195-204, 1997.
2. Wilt T, Ishani A, Mac Donald R, et al: *Cochrane Database Syst Rev* (1):CD001044, 2002.
3. Bombardelli E, Morazzoni P: *Fitoterapia* 68:205-218, 1997.
4. Catalano S, Ferretti M, Marsili A, et al: *J Nat Prod* 47:910, 1984.
5. Longo R: *Planta Med* 42:195-196, 1981.
6. Acworth J, Ewusi BN: *Med Plant Conserv* 5:15-18, 1999.
7. Dawson I: *Agroforest Today* 9:15-17, 1997.
8. Cunningham AB, Mbenkum FT: *Sustainability of harvesting Prunus africana bark in Cameroon. People and plants working paper*, Paris, May 1993, UNESCO.
9. Ishani A, MacDonald R, Nelson D, et al: *Am J Med* 109:654-664, 2000.
10. Hamid S, Bojter S, Vierling J: *Ann Intern Med* 127:169-170, 1997.
11. Rocchietta S: *Min Med* 68:4261-4264, 1977.
12. Latalski M, Spruch T, Obuchowska E: *Folia Morphol* 38:193-201, 1979.
13. Andro MC, Riffaud: *Curr Ther Res* 56:796-817, 1995.
14. Gathumbi PK, Mwangi JW, Njiro SM, et al: *Onderstepoort J Vet Res* 67:123-128, 2000.
15. Gathumbi PK, Mwangi JW, Mugera GM, et al: *Phytother Res* 16:244-247, 2002.

RASPBERRY LEAF

Other common name: Red raspberry leaf
Botanical name: *Rubus idaeus* L.
Family: Rosaceae
Plant part used: Leaf

Safety Summary

Pregnancy category A: No proven increase in the frequency of malformation or other harmful effects on the foetus despite consumption by a large number of women.
Lactation category C: Compatible with breastfeeding.
Contraindications: In principle, the use of herbs containing high levels of tannins is contraindicated, or at least inappropriate, in constipation, iron deficiency anaemia, and malnutrition.
Warnings & precautions: Because of the tannin content of this herb, long-term use should be avoided. Use cautiously in highly inflamed or ulcerated conditions of the gastrointestinal tract.
Adverse reactions: None found in published literature for raspberry leaf. A potential adverse reaction due to the high tannin content is irritation of the mouth and gastrointestinal tract.
Interactions: Take separately from oral thiamine, metal ion supplements, or alkaloid-containing medications.

Typical Therapeutic Use

Results from a retrospective, controlled study and a randomised, double-blind, placebo-controlled trial have suggested that raspberry leaf may shorten labour in pregnant women and reduce the need for medical intervention.[1,2] Traditional indications for raspberry leaf in Western herbal medicine include pregnancy (especially to facilitate parturition), diarrhoea, stomatitis, and tonsillitis.[3]

Actions

Astringent, partus praeparator, parturifacient, antidiarrhoeal.

Key Constituents

Constituents of raspberry leaf include flavonoids, gallotannins, and ellagitannins.[4]

Adulteration

Occasionally raspberry leaf is confused with bramble/blackberry leaf (*Rubus fruticosus*).[5]

Typical Dosage Forms & Dosage

Typical adult dosage ranges are:
- 12 to 24 g/day of dried leaf or by infusion
- 12 to 24 mL/day of a 1:1 liquid extract
- 4.5 to 14 mL/day of a 1:2 liquid extract or equivalent in tablet or capsule form

Contraindications

In principle, the use of tannins is contraindicated, or at least inappropriate, in constipation, iron deficiency anaemia, and malnutrition.

Use in Pregnancy

Category A: No proven increase in the frequency of malformation or other harmful effects on the foetus despite consumption by a large number of women.

No adverse effects are expected in pregnancy, but it is most appropriate to confine use to the second and third trimesters. This is because raspberry leaf has a reputation as a uterine stimulant, which is probably doubtful, except perhaps near term.

Results from a controlled, retrospective, observational study involving 108 women suggested that the consumption of raspberry leaf during pregnancy might shorten labour, reduce the likelihood of preterm and postterm labour and reduce the need for medical intervention. One woman ceased use of raspberry leaf during pregnancy after experiencing an increased frequency of Braxton Hicks contractions, and another woman ceased use after an episode of diarrhoea. Raspberry leaf could not be established as the cause in either case. The authors stated that the use of raspberry leaf appeared to be safe for pregnant women and their babies during pregnancy, labour and birth, and in the early postpartum period. Consumption of raspberry leaf commenced as early as 8 weeks' gestation, with the majority of women commencing at 30 to 34 weeks. The daily dosage ranged from 1 to 6 cups of tea or 1 to 8 tablets, with 3 cups of tea per day or 6 tablets per day being the most popular dosages. The weight of the tablets was not defined.[1]

The effect of raspberry leaf ingestion during pregnancy on birth outcome was assessed in a randomised, double-blind, placebo-controlled trial involving 192 women. Women in the treatment group received 1.2 g of raspberry leaf twice per day from 32 weeks of pregnancy to labour. Raspberry leaf did not shorten the first stage of labour. Clinically significant findings were a shortening of the second stage of labour (mean difference = 9.6 minutes) and a lower rate of forceps deliveries between the treatment group and control group (19.3% vs. 30.4%). Raspberry leaf was not found to cause adverse effects for mothers or babies. Side effects were reported by 32% of women in the raspberry leaf group and 25% of women in the placebo group. Most discomforts were pregnancy-related and included diarrhoea, constipation, nausea, vomiting, headaches, heartburn, strong uterine tightening, dizziness, and bloating.[2]

In a 1999 survey of certified nurse-midwives in the United States, raspberry leaf was reported to be used by 63% of the 90 respondents who used herbal medicine to stimulate labour. There were no reported complications from the use of raspberry leaf tea.[6]

Uterine contractions decreased in frequency and strength in three pregnant women given a crude raspberry leaf extract (about 1.3 to 2.6 g) in an early pharmacological study. Secondary contractions were also eliminated. A very slight fall in the systolic blood pressure was observed.[7]

Raspberry leaf has demonstrated a variable effect on uterine muscle tone in pharmacological experiments. Results imply a regulatory action on contractions. An aqueous extract contracted strips of pregnant (10 to 16 weeks) human uteri, but inhibited contractions in isolated pregnant rat uteri. However, the intrinsic rhythm of contraction of these tissues appeared to become more regular in most cases, and contractions were less frequent when they were observed over a 20-minute period in contact with the extract. Little or no effect was demonstrated in nonpregnant human uterine strips and isolated rat uteri.[8] A concentrate of raspberry leaf infusion induced uterine contraction in situ by intravenous administration to nonpregnant rabbits, but elicited uterine relaxation in situ in nonpregnant cats and one cat in late pregnancy. In isolated uteri (presumably nonpregnant), raspberry leaf caused contraction where there was little tone present, but induced relaxation when the uterus was toned.[9]

Use in Lactation

Category C: Compatible with breastfeeding.

Warnings & Precautions

Because of the tannin content of this herb, long-term use should be avoided (for both internal and topical use). Use cautiously in highly inflamed or ulcerated conditions of the gastrointestinal tract.

Effect on Ability to Drive or Operate Machinery

No adverse effects expected.

Adverse Reactions

None significantly attributed to raspberry leaf (see Use in pregnancy section). High doses of tannins lead to excessive astringency on mucous membranes, which has an irritating effect.

Interactions

Refer to the cranesbill root (*Geranium maculatum*) monograph for information regarding the interactions of tannins.

Safety in Children

No information available, but adverse effects are not expected if taken within the recommended dosage.

Overdosage

No incidents found in published literature. However, long-term use with high doses of tannins is to be avoided.

Toxicology

Raspberry leaf has very low toxicity. The intraperitoneal LD_{50} of raspberry leaf extract in mice was equivalent to 20 g/kg of dried leaf. No harmful effects were observed when raspberry leaf extract (about 2 g of dried leaf) was administered orally.[9]

Serum from a pregnant mare was incubated with aqueous raspberry leaf extract. Ovarian weight decreased when this mixture (containing 10 to 18 mg of dried raspberry leaf) was injected subcutaneously into female rats, whereas it increased with serum alone.[10] The relevance of this result to the in vivo action of raspberry leaf is unclear, and effects observed are probably due to the tannin content of raspberry leaf extract (which would bind and inactivate proteins in the serum).

Refer to the cranesbill root (*Geranium maculatum*) monograph for the toxicology of tannins.

Regulatory Status

See Table 1 for regulatory status in selected countries.

Table **1**   **Regulatory Status for Raspberry Leaf in Selected Countries**

Australia	Raspberry leaf is not included in Part 4 of Schedule 4 of the Therapeutic Goods Regulations.
UK & Germany	Raspberry is included on the General Sale List; however, the plant part is undefined. Raspberry leaf is covered by a negative Commission E monograph.
US	Raspberry leaf does not have generally recognised as safe (GRAS) status. However, it is freely available as a "dietary supplement" in the US under DSHEA legislation (Dietary Supplement Health and Education Act of 1994).

REFERENCES

1. Parsons M, Simpson M, Ponton T: *J Aust Coll Midwives* 12:20-25, 1999.
2. Simpson M, Parsons M, Greenwood J, et al: *J Midwifery Womens Health* 46:51-59, 2001.
3. British Herbal Medicine Association's Scientific Committee: *British herbal pharmacopoeia,* Bournemouth, 1983, BHMA, p 182.
4. Wagner H, Bladt S: *Plant drug analysis: a thin layer chromatography atlas,* ed 2, Berlin, 1996, Springer-Verlag, p 201.
5. Bisset NG (ed): *Herbal drugs and phytopharmaceuticals: a handbook for practice on a scientific basis,* Stuttgart, 1994, Medpharm Scientific Publishers, pp 434-436.
6. McFarlin BL, Gibson MH, O'Rear J, et al: *J Nurse Midwifery* 44:205-216, 1999.
7. Whitehouse B: *BMJ* 2:370-371, 1941.
8. Bamford DS, Percival RC, Tothill AU: *Br J Pharmacol* 40:161P-162P, 1970.
9. Burn JH, Withell ER: *Lancet* 2:1-3, 1941.
10. Graham RCB, Noble RL: *Endocrinology* 56:239-247, 1955.

REHMANNIA

Other common names: Di Huang, Chinese foxglove
Botanical name: *Rehmannia glutinosa* (Gaertn.) Libosch.
Family: Gesneriaceae
Plant part used: Root

Safety Summary

Pregnancy category B3: No increase in frequency of malformation or other harmful effects on the foetus from limited use in women. Evidence of increased foetal damage in animal studies exists, although the relevance to humans is unknown. In traditional Chinese medicine (TCM), uncured rehmannia is contraindicated in pregnant women with *deficient blood*, *deficient spleen,* or *deficient stomach.*
Lactation category C: Compatible with breastfeeding.
Contraindications: See the text below for TCM contraindications. Do not use during pregnancy without professional advice.
Warnings & precautions: None required on current evidence.
Adverse reactions: Mild oedema, diarrhoea, abdominal pain, dizziness, fatigue, and palpitations.
Interactions: No precautions required on current evidence.

Typical Therapeutic Use

Uncured* rehmannia is used in TCM to treat febrile diseases with reddened tongue and thirst, diabetes, spitting of blood, epistaxis, and skin eruptions.[1] Western uses of uncured rehmannia include inflammatory disorders involving the immune system (such as allergies and autoimmune disease) and to prevent the suppressive effect of corticosteroid drugs on endogenous levels of corticosteroids.[2] Cured* rehmannia is used in TCM in conditions such as fever, night sweats, anaemia, dizziness, palpitations, irregular menstruation, and uterine and postpartum bleeding.[1,3]

Actions

Antipyretic, adrenal tonic, antihaemorrhagic, antiinflammatory.

*In TCM, the uncured form of rehmannia consists of the dried root of *Rehmannia glutinosa.* The cured form consists of the clean, fresh root stewed in wine and subsequently dried.

Key Constituents

Constituents of rehmannia root include iridoid glycosides such as aucubin and catalpol (0.3% to 0.5%), rehmanniosides A-D,[4] and phenethylalcohol glycosides (acteoside),[5] jioglutosides, and rehmaglutins A-D.[6]

Adulteration

No information available.

Typical Dosage Forms & Dosage

Typical adult dosage ranges are:
- 9 to 15 g of dried (uncured) root per day by decoction
- 4.5 to 8.5 mL/day of a 1:2 liquid extract or equivalent in tablet or capsule form

Contraindications

TCM contraindications for uncured rehmannia are *damp phlegm* patterns, *deficient spleen* with dampness, and *deficient yang.*[7] Do not use during pregnancy without professional advice.

Use in Pregnancy

Category B3: No increase in frequency of malformation or other harmful effects on the foetus from limited use in women. Evidence of increased foetal damage in animal studies exists, although the relevance to humans is unknown.

Subcutaneous administration of rehmannia aqueous extract (0.1 to 0.4 mL/day) for 5 days decreased litter numbers in mice. This antifertility effect was not associated with systemic toxicity or interruption of the oestrus cycle.[8]

In TCM, uncured rehmannia is contraindicated in pregnant women with *deficient blood*, *deficient spleen*, or *deficient stomach.*[7]

Use in Lactation

Category C: Compatible with breastfeeding.

Warnings & Precautions

None required on current evidence.

Effect on Ability to Drive or Operate Machinery

No adverse effects expected.

Adverse Reactions

A small number of rheumatoid arthritis patients developed mild oedema during an uncontrolled trial.[9] Based on clinical trials in China, a minority of patients may develop diarrhoea, abdominal pain, dizziness, fatigue, and palpitations, which disappear spontaneously within a few days.[9] Overuse of cured rehmannia can lead to abdominal distension and loose stools.[3]

Two cases of liver toxicity[10,11] (one fatal) and two cases of elevated serum levels of a liver enzyme[12] were reported after the ingestion of preparations containing rehmannia used for the treatment of skin conditions. However, these formulations contained eight or more different Chinese herbs, and the herb or herbs responsible have not been identified. The adverse reactions were not ascribed conclusively to the treatment with Chinese herbs in all cases.[13]

Interactions

None known.

Safety in Children

No adverse effects expected at usual doses.

Overdosage

No incidents found in published literature.

Toxicology

Intragastric administration of either rehmannia decoction or an alcohol extract at a dose of 60 g/kg/day for 3 days did not cause adverse reactions in mice observed for 1 week. Rats were administered the same preparations by the same route at a dose of 18 g/kg and observed for 1.5 months. There were no significant changes in behaviour, body weight, serum nonprotein nitrogen, or hepatic or renal tissues.[14]

Uncured rehmannia did not demonstrate mutagenic potential in the Ames test or chromosomal aberration in in vivo assays. Similarly, cured rehmannia did not demonstrate mutagenic potential in the Ames test. However, it did demonstrate mutagenic potential in two in vivo assays when administered to mice by intraperitoneal injection at a dosage of 2 to 4 g/kg.[15]

Oral administration of rehmannia tended to increase levels of urea nitrogen, creatinine, methylguanidine, and guanidinosuccinic acid in rats with renal failure.[16]

A Chinese herbal formula (Man-Shen-Ling) which contains rehmannia did not exhibit toxic, mutagenic, teratogenic, or carcinogenic effects in acute and chronic toxicity tests in animal models.[17]

Regulatory Status

See Table 1 for regulatory status in selected countries.

Table 1   **Regulatory Status for Rehmannia in Selected Countries**

Australia	Rehmannia is not included in Part 4 of Schedule 4 of the Therapeutic Goods Regulations.
China	Rehmannia is official in the *Pharmacopoeia of the People's Republic of China* 1997. The usual adult dosage of fresh uncured rehmannia, usually administered in the form of a decoction, is listed as 12 to 30 g. The dosage of dried, uncured Rehmannia is 9 to 15 g, and 9 to 15 g for cured rehmannia.
UK & Germany	Rehmannia is not included on the General Sale List. It was not included in the Commission E assessment.
US	Rehmannia does not have generally recognised as safe (GRAS) status. However, it is freely available as a "dietary supplement" in the US under DSHEA legislation (Dietary Supplement Health and Education Act of 1994).

REFERENCES

1. Pharmacopoeia Commission of the People's Republic of China: *Pharmacopoeia of the People's Republic of China,* English ed, Beijing, 1997, Chemical Industry Press, pp 166-167.
2. Bone K: *Clinical applications of Ayurvedic and Chinese herbs,* Warwick, 1996, Phytotherapy Press, pp 52-54.
3. Bensky D, Gamble A: *Chinese herbal medicine materia medica,* Seattle, 1986, Eastland Press, pp 470-471.
4. Wagner H, Bladt S: *Plant drug analysis: a thin layer chromatography atlas,* ed 2, Berlin, 1996, Springer-Verlag, p 76.
5. Wagner H, Bauer R, Peigen X, et al: *Chinese drug monographs and analysis: Radix Rehmanniae – Dihuang,* vol 1, no. 3, Wald, 1996, Verlag fur Ganzheitliche Medizin Dr. Erich Wuhr GmbH.
6. Tang W, Eisenbrand G: *Chinese drugs of plant origin,* Berlin, 1992, Springer Verlag, pp 849-852.
7. Bensky D, Gamble A: *Chinese herbal medicine materia medica,* Seattle, 1986, Eastland Press, pp 95-97.
8. Matsui AS, Rogers J, Woo YK, et al: *Med Pharmacol Exp* 16:414-424, 1967.
9. Hu CS: *Chin Med J* 51:290, 1965.
10. Perharic-Walton L, Murray V: *Lancet* 340:674, 1992.
11. Kane JA, Kane SP, Jain S: *Gut* 36:146-147, 1995.
12. Sheehan MP, Atherton DJ: *Br J Dermatol* 130:488-493, 1994.
13. Rustin M, Atherton D: *Lancet* 340:673-674, 1992.
14. Chang HM, But PP: *Pharmacology and applications of Chinese materia medica,* vol 1, Singapore, 1987, World Scientific, p 465.
15. Yin XJ, Liu DX, Wang HC, et al: *Mutat Res* 260:73-82, 1991.
16. Yokozawa T, Fujioka K, Oura H, et al: *Phytother Res* 9:1-5, 1995.
17. Su ZZ, He YY, Chen G: *Chung Kuo Chung Hsi I Chieh Ho Tsa Chih* 13:259-260, 269-272, 1993.

ROSEMARY

Botanical name: *Rosmarinus officinalis* L.
Family: Labiatae
Plant part used: Leaf

Safety Summary

Pregnancy category B1: No increase in frequency of malformation or other harmful effects on the foetus from limited use in women. No evidence of increased foetal damage in animal studies.
Lactation category C: Compatible with breastfeeding.
Contraindications: None required on current evidence.
Warnings & precautions: None required on current evidence.
Adverse reactions: None found in published literature.
Interactions: Avoid concomitant intake with iron supplementation.

Typical Therapeutic Use

Traditional indications for rosemary in Western herbal medicine include dyspepsia, headache, depression associated with stress, debility, and cardiovascular weakness.[1]

Actions

Carminative, spasmolytic, antioxidant, antimicrobial, circulatory stimulant, hepatoprotective.

Key Constituents

Rosemary contains an essential oil (1% to 2%), the composition of which varies (three main chemotypes are found growing in Europe). The major constituents of rosemary essential oil are 1,8-cineole, alpha-pinene, and camphor. Other constituents include phenolic diterpenes (such as carnosol and carnosic acid), rosmarinic acid, flavonoids, and triterpenoids.[2-4] (Carnosic acid is also known as carnosolic acid or salvin, carnosol is also known as picrosalvin.)

Adulteration

Adulteration is not as common now as in former times. Adulterants included *Ledum palustre* (commonly named wild or marsh rosemary) and *Teucrium montanum*.[5]

Typical Dosage Forms & Dosage

Typical adult dosage ranges:
- 6 to 12 g/day of dried leaf or by infusion
- 6 to 12 mL/day of a 1:1 liquid extract
- 2 to 4.5 mL/day of a 1:2 liquid extract or equivalent in tablet or capsule form

Contraindications

None known.

Use in Pregnancy

Category B1: No increase in frequency of malformation or other harmful effects on the foetus from limited use in women. No evidence of increased foetal damage in animal studies.

Rosemary aqueous extract (corresponding to 13 mg solids/mL), made from leaf, flowers, and stem, was administered orally to rats in the preimplantation period (days 1 to 6) and organogenic period (days 6 to 15) of pregnancy. There was no change in the postimplantation loss, or number of malformations of term foetuses in either group compared to controls. For the preimplantation group, there was an increase in preimplantation loss, although the difference was not significant compared to the control group.[6]

However, rosemary has gained a reputation as being contraindicated during pregnancy, probably because of the content of the essential oil (the above study used an aqueous extract which would have contained low levels of essential oil).

Also, rosemary has been used as an abortifacient, with early reports of poisoning.[7] A 1925 reference indicated that rosemary was used to procure abortion, although in some cases rosemary was present in a complex mixture and a causal link was not established.[5]

The potential embryotoxic effect of rosemary oil has been attributed largely to its camphor content.[8] However, a study found that D-camphor elicited no evidence of teratogenicity when administered orally during the foetal period of organogenesis to pregnant rats, at doses up to 1000 mg/kg/day, and to pregnant rabbits at doses up to 681 mg/kg/day.[9]

Use in Lactation

Category C: Compatible with breastfeeding.

Rosemary contains an essential oil which may pass into breast milk and could thereby confer carminative activity.

Warnings & Precautions

None required on current evidence.

Effect on Ability to Drive or Operate Machinery

No adverse effects expected.

Adverse Reactions

Allergic contact dermatitis has been reported from contact with a rosemary extract and was attributed to the carnosol. However, allergy to carnosol is rare.[10] Cases of inflammation of the lips[11] and acute itchy vesicular exudative dermatitis[12] caused by contact allergy to rosemary oil and rosemary leaf, respectively, have been reported.

Interactions

Nonhaem iron absorption was significantly decreased in female volunteers who consumed a phenolic-rich extract of rosemary (8.2% by weight of polyphenols, including carnosic acid, carnosol, and rosmarinic acid) via a test meal.[13] This indicates a potential interaction for concomitant administration of rosemary during iron intake. In anaemia and cases where iron supplementation is required, rosemary should not be taken simultaneously with meals or iron supplements.

Safety in Children

No information available.

Overdosage

Large quantities of rosemary have been reported to cause poisoning in humans, although the exact dose is not documented.[5]

Toxicology

The LD_{50} value of 5 mL/kg was measured for oral dosage of rosemary essential oil in rats.[14] Toxic effects were not observed in rats and mice administered a single dose of an alcohol extract of rosemary (2 g/kg) by intraperitoneal injection.[15]

Rosemary methanolic extract produced glutathione (GSH adducts) in an in vitro assay developed to screen for the formation of electrophilic quinoid species upon bioactivation by the cytochrome P450 enzyme system. Several GSH adducts were detected, including the expected derivatives of rosmarinic acid.[16] In another study, rosemary extract blocked induced DNA adduct formation by strongly inhibiting cytochrome P450 activities and inducing the expression of glutathione S-transferase.[17] This suggests an antitoxic activity for rosemary via enhanced hepatic metabolism of xenobiotics. Rosemary extract decreased experimentally induced tumorigenesis in mice,[18] and rosemary extract, with carnosic acid and carnosol as the two major active ingredients, exhibited strong antimutagenic effects in the Ames tester strain TA102.[19]

Regulatory Status

See Table 1 for regulatory status in selected countries.

Rosemary is widely consumed as a condiment throughout the world.

Table 1   Regulatory Status for Rosemary in Selected Countries

Australia	Rosemary is not included in Part 4 of Schedule 4 of the Therapeutic Goods Regulations.
UK & Germany	Rosemary is included on the General Sale List. It is covered by a positive Commission E monograph. Rosemary is official in the *British Pharmacopoeia* 2002 and in the *European Pharmacopoeia* 4.3.
US	Rosemary does have generally recognised as safe (GRAS) status. It is freely available as a "dietary supplement" in the US under DSHEA legislation (Dietary Supplement Health and Education Act of 1994).

REFERENCES

1. British Herbal Medicine Association's Scientific Committee: *British herbal pharmacopoeia,* Bournemouth, 1983, BHMA, p 181.
2. Battaglia S: *The complete guide to aromatherapy,* Virginia, Queensland, 1995, The Perfect Potion, p 51.
3. Wagner H, Bladt S: *Plant drug analysis: a thin layer chromatography atlas,* ed 2, Berlin, 1996, Springer-Verlag, p 156.
4. Bisset NG, ed: *Herbal drugs and phytopharmaceuticals,* Stuttgart, 1994, Medpharm Scientific Publishers, pp 428-430.
5. Blaschek W, Ebel S, Hackenthal E, et al: *HagerROM 2002: Hagers Handbuch der Drogen und Arzneistoffe,* Heidelberg, 2002, Springer.
6. Lemonica IP, Damasceno DC, di-Stasi LC: *Braz J Med Biol Res* 29:223-227, 1996.
7. Gessner O: *Gift-und Arzneipflanzen von Mitteleuropa,* ed 3, Heidelberg, 1974, Carl Winter Universitatsverlag, p 304.
8. Tisserand R, Balacs T: *Essential oil safety: a guide for health care professionals,* Edinburgh, 1995, Churchill Livingstone, pp 106-107.
9. Leuschner J: *Arzneim Forsch* 47:124-128, 1997.
10. Hjorther AB, Christophersen C, Hausen BM, et al: *Contact Dermatitis* 37:99-100, 1997.
11. Guin JD: *Contact Dermatitis* 45:63, 2001.
12. Fernandez L, Duque S, Sanchez I, et al: *Contact Dermatitis* 37:248-249, 1997.
13. Samman S, Sandstrom B, Toft MB, et al: *Am J Clin Nutr* 73:607-612, 2001.
14. Opdyke DLJ: *Food Cosmet Toxicol* 12:977-978, 1974.
15. Mongold JJ, Camillieri S, Susplugas S, et al: *Plantes Med Phytother* 25:6-11, 1991.
16. Johnson BM, Bolton JL, van Breemen RB: *Chem Res Toxicol* 14:1546-1551, 2001.
17. Mace K, Offord EA, Harris CC, et al: *Arch Toxicol Suppl* 20:227-236, 1998.
18. Singletary KW, Nelshoppen JM: *Cancer Lett* 60:169-175, 1991.
19. Minnunni M, Wolleb U, Mueller O, et al: *Mutat Res* 269:193-200, 1992.

SAGE

Botanical name: *Salvia officinalis* L.
Family: Labiatae
Plant part used: Leaf

Safety Summary

Pregnancy category C: Has caused or is associated with a substantial risk of causing harmful effects on the foetus or neonate without causing malformations.
Lactation category X: Contraindicated in breastfeeding except to stop milk flow.
Contraindications: Pregnancy and lactation.
Warnings & precautions: Do not exceed recommended doses and avoid long-term use (except for low-thujone varieties).
Adverse reactions: Allergic reactions are possible.
Interactions: No precautions required on current evidence.

Typical Therapeutic Use

Traditional indications for sage in Western herbal medicine include inflammation of the mouth and throat, excessive perspiration, menopausal hot flushes, and flatulent dyspepsia.[1]

Actions

Spasmolytic, antiseptic, antihydrotic, astringent, antioxidant.

Key Constituents

Essential oil, up to 2.5%,[2] containing monoterpenoids such as α- and β-thujone (up to 60% and 10% respectively), camphor, and cineole, all having potentially epileptogenic properties.[3] Abietane diterpenoids such as carnosic acid, and its derivatives such as carnosol, are present, all with remarkably strong antioxidant properties.[4] Triterpenoids; flavonoids such as 5-methoxysalvigenin; and phenolic compounds such as rosmarinic acid have also been reported.[4]

Adulteration

Occasional substitution by other species of sage.

Typical Dosage Forms & Dosage

Typical adult dosage ranges are:
- 3 to 12 g/day of dried leaf or by infusion
- 3 to 12 mL/day of a 1:1 liquid extract
- 2 to 4.5 mL/day of a 1:2 liquid extract or equivalent in tablet or capsule form

Contraindications

Pregnancy and lactation.

Use in Pregnancy

Category C: Has caused or is associated with a substantial risk of causing harmful effects on the foetus or neonate without causing malformations.

Given the potential toxicity of thujone[5] and other constituents of the essential oil, there has been a general view that the use of the herb in any quantity should not be recommended during pregnancy or lactation. This is largely a theoretical concern, however.

Several types of sage leaf extract, including aqueous and ethanolic, were inactive when administered orally to rats (250 mg/kg, days 1 to 10 postcoitum) in an antiimplantation study.[6]

Use in Lactation

Category X: Contraindicated in breastfeeding except to stop milk flow. Sage has also been used topically for this effect.

Warnings & Precautions

Do not exceed recommended doses of alcoholic preparations of sage because of the presence of thujone. Caution with long-term use except in low-thujone varieties.[7]

Effect on Ability to Drive or Operate Machinery

No adverse effects expected.

Adverse Reactions

Occasional allergic reactions have been recorded after topical contact with sage products. Otherwise adverse effects are almost unknown at moderate doses.

Interactions

None known.

Safety in Children

No information available, but adverse effects are not expected if used within recommended doses.

Overdosage

After taking sage essential oil, a potent concentrate from the plant, symptoms are typically delayed for some minutes to hours. This is followed by recurrent bouts of vomiting, excessive salivation, and, notably, by epileptic spasms with cyanosis and the risk of tongue swallowing, each bout being separated by periods of atonicity. After two or three bouts, recovery takes place with amnesia for the events.[8]

Toxicology

Sage oil has been shown to have convulsive properties directly on the central nervous system in rats at doses above 0.5 g/kg, accounting for occasional reports of tonico-clonic convulsions associated with human intoxication. Terpene ketones, camphor, and thujone were identified as the most toxic constituents. The lethal dose of the oil was 3.2 g/kg. The substances were administered by intraperitoneal injection.[8] The acute oral LD_{50} of sage oil in rats is 2.6 g/kg.[9]

Refer also to the wormwood (*Artemisia absinthium*) monograph for toxicology information and LD_{50} values for thujone.

Regulatory Status

See Table 1 for regulatory status in selected countries.

Table 1   **Regulatory Status for Sage in Selected Countries**

Australia	Sage is not included in Part 4 of Schedule 4 of the Therapeutic Goods Regulations.
UK & Germany	Sage is included on the General Sale List. It is covered by a positive Commission E monograph. Sage is official in the *European Pharmacopoeia* 4.3.
US	Sage does have generally recognised as safe (GRAS) status. It is freely available as a "dietary supplement" in the US under DSHEA legislation (Dietary Supplement Health and Education Act of 1994).

REFERENCES

1. British Herbal Medicine Association's Scientific Committee: *British herbal pharmacopoeia*, Bournemouth, 1983, BHMA, pp 185-186.
2. Steinegger E, Hänsel R: *Pharmakognosie*, ed 5, Berlin-Heidelberg, 1992, Springer, pp 343-345.
3. Burkhard PR, Burkhardt K, Haenggeli CA, et al: *J Neurol* 246:667-670, 1999.
4. Miura K, Kikuzaki H, Nakatani N: *J Agric Food Chem* 50:1845-1851, 2002.
5. Pinto-Scognamiglio W: *Boll Chim Farm* 106:292-300, 1967.
6. Kamboj VP, Dhawan BN: *J Ethnopharmacol* 6:191-226, 1982.
7. Scientific Committee of ESCOP (European Scientific Cooperative on Phytotherapy): *ESCOP Monographs: Salviae folium*, UK, March 1996, ESCOP Secretariat.
8. Millet Y, Jouglard J, Steinmetz MD, et al: *Clin Toxicol* 18:1485-1498, 1981.
9. Opdyke DLJ: *Food Cosmet Toxicol* 12:987-988, 1974.

SAW PALMETTO

Botanical names: *Serenoa repens* (Bartr.) Small (*S. serrulata* (Michx.) Nichols., *Sabal serrulata* (Michx.) Nutt. ex Schult. & Schult. f., *Brahea serrulata* (Michx.) H. Wendl., *Corypha repens* Bartr.)
Family: Palmae
Plant part used: Fruit

Safety Summary

Pregnancy category B2: No increase in frequency of malformation or other harmful effects on the foetus from limited use in women. Animal studies are lacking.
Lactation category C: Compatible with breastfeeding.
Contraindications: None required on current evidence.
Warnings & precautions: Prostate cancer should be excluded before patients receive saw palmetto treatment as the herb treatment may mask the symptoms of this disease (but will not alter prostate-specific antigen [PSA] readings). Exercise caution for concurrent use with warfarin.
Adverse reactions: Minor side effects such as gastrointestinal problems have been recorded from clinical trials. Two case reports suggest possible anticoagulant activity, but more information is required.
Interactions: Caution with concurrent use of warfarin.

Typical Therapeutic Use

According to a recent Cochrane Review, current clinical evidence suggests that saw palmetto liposterolic extract provides mild to moderate improvement in urinary symptoms and flow measures in patients with benign prostatic hyperplasia.[1]

Traditional indications for saw palmetto in Western herbal medicine include prostatic hypertrophy and chronic or subacute cystitis.[2]

Actions

Antiinflammatory, male tonic, antiprostatic, spasmolytic, possibly antiandrogenic.

Key Constituents

Constituents of saw palmetto berries include free fatty acids, triglycerides, phytosterols (mainly β-sitosterol), flavonoids, and polysaccharides.[3]

Adulteration

No adulterants known.

Typical Dosage Forms & Dosage

Typical adult dosage ranges are:
- 1.5 to 3 g/day of dried fruit or by decoction
- 1.8 to 4.5 mL/day of a 1:1 liquid extract
- 2 to 4.5 mL/day of a 1:2 liquid extract or equivalent in tablet or capsule form
- 320 to 480 mg/day of the 10:1 liposterolic extract

Contraindications

None known.

Use in Pregnancy

Category B2: No increase in frequency of malformation or other harmful effects on the foetus from limited use in women. Animal studies are lacking. However, saw palmetto treatment is unlikely to be indicated in pregnant women.

Use in Lactation

Category C: Compatible with breastfeeding.

Addition of liposterolic extract at concentrations ranging from 1 to 10 μg/mL to Chinese hamster ovary cells completely inhibited the effects of prolactin, suggesting that saw palmetto may inhibit prolactin-induced hormonal effects.[4] However, the relevance of this research to normal human use is unclear.

Warnings & Precautions

Prostate cancer should be excluded before patients receive saw palmetto treatment, as the herb treatment may mask the symptoms of this disease (but will not alter PSA readings). Exercise caution for concurrent use with warfarin.

Effect on Ability to Drive or Operate Machinery

No adverse effects expected.

Adverse Reactions

Saw palmetto is well tolerated by most patients and causes relatively few side effects. Most side effects are minor gastrointestinal problems such as nausea, which are usually resolved when the herb is taken with meals.

In the double-blind study of Descotes and co-workers[5] there was no significant difference between the tolerability of active and placebo treatments. Only one patient discontinued active treatment with complaints of fatigue, depression, and stomach upset.

The large comparative study of Carraro and co-workers[6] found that gastrointestinal complaints were the most frequently reported adverse events with both saw palmetto and finasteride, but tended to occur more frequently with finasteride. As might be expected, decreased libido and impotence were also more common with finasteride treatment. Two deaths occurred during the trial (one in each group) and three serious adverse events occurred (two with saw palmetto, one with finasteride). None of these were deemed to be related to treatment. PSA was not changed by saw palmetto treatment, indicating that the herb is unlikely to interfere with the diagnostic value of this test.

The German Commission E lists stomach upsets as the only side effect from treatment with saw palmetto liposterolic extract.[7]

One case of haemorrhage during surgery, which was associated with intake of saw palmetto extract, has been reported.[8] A case of an elevated international normalised ratio (INR) of 2.1 was reported after a patient consumed tablets containing saw palmetto and pumpkin seed extracts and a small amount of vitamin E for 1 year (see below).[9]

A case of protracted cholestatic hepatitis after the use of a herbal and nutritional preparation has been reported. The herbal preparation contained saw palmetto, hydrangea, *Pygeum africanum*, *Panax ginseng*, zinc picolinate, pyridoxine, alanine, glutamic acid, *Apis mellifica* pollen, and silica.[10] The ingredient causing the adverse reaction was not identified.

Interactions

Caution with concurrent use of warfarin.

A 61-year-old man had long been treated with warfarin and simvastatin. His INR values had been stable around 2.4. Due to micturition difficulties he started to take a saw palmetto and pumpkin seed preparation, five tablets daily. After 6 days' treatment his INR increased to 3.4. The herbal product was discontinued and 1 week later the INR returned to its previous level.[9]

Safety in Children

No information available, but adverse effects are not expected.

Overdosage

No incidents found in published literature.

Toxicology

Published toxicological data on saw palmetto are limited. Brine shrimp lethality-directed fractionation of an ethanolic extract led to the isolation of two monoacylglycerides.[11] These compounds showed moderate biological activities in the brine shrimp lethality test and against renal and pancreatic human tumour cells in vitro; borderline cytotoxicity was exhibited against human prostatic cells.

The company Madaus has released toxicological data on their ethanolic extract.[12] The LD_{50} in the rat, mouse, and guinea pig is greater than 10 g/kg. High doses given to rats over 6 weeks (360 times the human therapeutic dose of about 5 mg/kg) did not cause adverse haematological, histological, or biochemical changes. A long-term study over 6 months in rats at 80 times the human dose again found no negative influences. The same dose administered to rats had no influence on fertility.

An ethanolic extract of saw palmetto tested negative in the Ames test (with and without microsomal activation).[13]

Regulatory Status

See Table 1 for regulatory status in selected countries.

Table **I**   **Regulatory Status for Saw Palmetto in Selected Countries**

Australia	Saw palmetto is not included in Part 4 of Schedule 4 of the Therapeutic Goods Regulations.
UK & Germany	Saw palmetto is included on the General Sale List. It is covered by a positive Commission E monograph.
US	Saw palmetto is official in the *United States Pharmacopeia-National Formulary* (USP 26-NF 21, 2003). Saw palmetto does not have generally recognised as safe (GRAS) status. However, it is freely available as a "dietary supplement" in the US under DSHEA legislation (Dietary Supplement Health and Education Act of 1994).

REFERENCES

1. Wilt T, Ishani A, MacDonald R: *Cochrane Database Syst Rev* (3):CD001423, 2002.
2. British Herbal Medicine Association's Scientific Committee: *British herbal pharmacopoeia,* Bournemouth, 1983, BHMA, pp 196-197.
3. Bombardelli E, Morazzoni P: *Fitoterapia* 68:99-113, 1997.
4. Vacher P, Prevarskaya N, Skryma R, et al: *J Biomed* Sci 2:357-365, 1995.
5. Descotes JL, Rambeaud JJ, Deschaseaux P, et al: *Clin Drug Invest* 9:291-297, 1995.
6. Carraro J-C, Raynaud J-P, Koch G, et al: *Prostate* 29:231-240, 1996.
7. Blumenthal M, et al, eds: *The complete German Commission E monographs: therapeutic guide to herbal medicines,* Austin, 1998, American Botanical Council, p 201.
8. Cheema P, El-Mefty O, Jazieh AR: *J Intern Med* 250:167-169, 2001.
9. Yue Q-Y, Jansson K: *J Am Geriatr Soc* 310:838, 2001.
10. Hamid S, Bojter S, Vierling J: *Ann Intern Med* 127:169-170, 1997.
11. Kondás J, Philipp V, Diószeghy G: *Orv Hetil* 138:419-421, 1997.
12. Prosta Urgenin Uno, *Zur Behandlung der BPH,* Koln, 1996, Madaus AG, p 33.
13. Degenring FH, Sokolowski A, Suter A, et al: *ESCOP EPJ* Issue 2 draft, available online: http://www.escop.com/epj2pdfs/weber4p.pdf (accessed May 2003).

SCHISANDRA

Other common names: Schizandra, wuweizi
Botanical names: *Schisandra chinensis* (Turcz.) Baill. (*Kadsura chinensis* Turcz.)
Family: Schisandraceae
Plant part used: Fruit

Safety Summary

Pregnancy category B1: No increase in frequency of malformation or other harmful effects on the foetus from limited use in women. No evidence of increased foetal damage in animal studies. (However, the herb is traditionally contraindicated in pregnancy, except to assist childbirth.)
Lactation category ND: No data available.
Contraindications: Early stages of cough or rash (traditional contraindication).
Warnings & precautions: Pregnancy (except at birth).
Adverse reactions: Mild gastrointestinal symptoms (nausea, heartburn, indigestion, stomach ache, anorexia) and headache.
Interactions: No precautions required on current evidence, although schisandra may accelerate the clearance of several drugs from the body due to its effects on phase I/II hepatic metabolism.

Typical Therapeutic Use

Schisandra has demonstrated therapeutic benefit in the treatment of chronic viral hepatitis[1] and improved physical performance, endurance, and resistance to the effects of stress[2] in controlled clinical trials. Schisandra extract and its constituents have been shown to enhance phase I/II hepatic metabolism in animal models.[3,4] Traditional indications for schisandra in traditional Chinese medicine (TCM) include spontaneous sweating, palpitations, and insomnia.[5]

Actions

Hepatoprotective, antioxidant, adaptogenic, nervine tonic, antitussive.

Key Constituents

Constituents of schisandra fruit include dibenzocyclooctene lignans (about 2% by weight), such as schisandrin, schisandrins A to C, and gomisin A,[6] and an essential oil (about 3%).[7]

Adulteration

Schisandra sphenanthera is the most commonly traded substitute for *S. chinensis*.[8] This is most likely due to it being recognised as medicinally interchangeable for *Schisandra chinensis* in TCM.[5,9] The fruits of other *Schisandra* spp. as well as the fruits of *Kadsura*, *Eunonymus*, and *Vitis* spp. have also been reported as substitutes.[8]

Typical Dosage Forms & Dosage

Typical adult dosage ranges are:
- 1.5 to 6 g/day of dried fruit by decoction
- 3.5 to 8.5 mL/day of a 1:2 liquid extract or equivalent in tablet or capsule form

Contraindications

According to TCM, schisandra is contraindicated in the early stages of cough or rash, in excess heat patterns,[10] peptic ulcer, excessive exercise, epileptic seizure, increased intracranial pressure, mental excitement, and hypertension.[9] (The latter contraindications were noted in a 1965 Chinese medical journal.) However, schisandra is likely to be of benefit in excessive exercise as it has adaptogenic and tonic activity, demonstrated in clinical studies.[8]

Use in Pregnancy

Category B1: No increase in frequency of malformation or other harmful effects on the foetus from limited use in women. No evidence of increased foetal damage in animal studies.

Schisandra tincture was used successfully to induce labour in 72 of 80 women with prolonged labour. The dose administered was 20 to 25 drops per hour for 3 hours of a 1:3 tincture for three consecutive days. No negative effects in terms of the postnatal health of the mother or child were observed.[11] Schisandra tincture (1:10, 30 to 40 drops, three times per day) improved cardiovascular symptoms in hypotensive pregnant women. The schisandra-treated group experienced fewer birth complications than the untreated women. No effects were observed on contraction or on labour.[12]

Oral administration of 105 to 500 mg/kg/day of schisandra extract (standardised to 2% schisandrins) to rats and mice did not result in foetotoxicity, changes in implantation efficiency, nor other measures of reproductive function.[13]

Schisandra preparations strengthened the rhythmic contractions of nonpregnant, pregnant, and postpartum uteri in isolated tissue and in vivo.[9] Subcutaneous injection of schisandra liquid extract (30 mg/kg) increased uterine contractility and tension in rabbits. This effect was enhanced when the dose was increased to 100 mg/kg.[11]

Use in Lactation

Category ND: No data available.

Warnings & Precautions

Schisandra is used to induce labour in TCM and has also strengthened uterine contractions (see above), hence it should only be used during pregnancy (other than to assist birth) if absolutely necessary.

Effect on Ability to Drive or Operate Machinery

No adverse effects expected.

Adverse Reactions

Mild gastrointestinal symptoms have been reported, such as heartburn, indigestion, stomach ache, and anorexia.[9] In one trial, 4 out of the 107 patients treated with the equivalent of 1.5 g/day of dried fruit developed mild and transient nausea, headache, and stomach ache.[1]

Interactions

No precautions required on current evidence, although schisandra may accelerate the clearance of several drugs from the body due to its effects on phase I/II hepatic metabolism.

Safety in Children

Schisandra (0.25 to 2 g), the 90% ethanol tincture (strength undefined, 30 to 40 drops) and the extract (0.5 g) have been used to treat infantile dysentery in clinical trials, with beneficial therapeutic effects.[9]

Overdosage

No incidents found in published literature.

Toxicology

Table 1 lists LD_{50} data recorded for schisandra extract and its constituents.[13-15]

It can be concluded that schisandra fruit has low toxicity. Only mild toxic effects, such as decreased activity, piloerection, and apathy, were observed in mice orally administered a schisandra ethanol extract (0.6 and 1.2 g/kg) for 10 days. Major organs and blood parameters were not significantly altered.[9] Similarly, schisandra fruit extract (standardised to 2% schisandrins) had no toxic effect on body weight, food intake, blood parameters, liver enzymes, or major organs after oral administration to piglets at daily doses of 0.07, 0.36, and 0.72 g/kg for 90 days.[13]

No fatalities resulted from single oral doses (2 g/kg) of schisandrins A, B, and C to mice. Fatalities occurred after intraperitoneal doses of 1 g/kg of schizandrins A and C and 2 g/kg of schisandrin B.[16] No toxic effects were observed after daily oral administration of schisandrin B to mice at a dose of 200 mg/kg for 30 days, nor to dogs at a dose of 10 mg/kg for 4 weeks.[9]

Increased benzo(α)pyrene (BaP) and aflatoxin mutagenicity were observed using the Ames assay with liver microsomes derived from mice fed a schisandra ethanol extract (5% of diet) for 14 days.[17] However, schisandra lignans have also been shown to decrease BaP mutagenicity in the Ames test.[18,19]

Feeding experiments in mice with the oil of schisandra fruit (10 to 15 g/kg) resulted in dyspnoea in 15 to 60 minutes, decreased activity, and then death 1 to 2 days later. However, these are very high doses. Oral administration of the essential oil (0.28 g/kg) to mice resulted in depression, dyspnoea, ataxia, and death within 1 to 3 hours.[9]

Regulatory Status

See Table 2 for regulatory status in selected countries.

Table 1 **LD$_{50}$ Data Recorded for Schisandra Extract and Its Constituents**

Substance	Route, Model	LD$_{50}$ Value	Reference
Schisandra petroleum ether extract (10% schisandrins)	Oral, mice	10.5 g/kg	14
Schisandra petroleum ether extract (40% schisandrins)	Oral, mice	2.8 g/kg	14
Schisandra (4:1) extract (standardised to 2% schisandrins)	Oral, rats	>21 g/kg	13
Schisandra petroleum ether extract (10% schisandrins)	i.p., mice	4.4 g/kg	14
Schisandrin	Oral, mice	777 mg/kg	15
Schisandrin	i.p., mice	390 mg/kg	15
Schisandrin	s.c., mice	500 mg/kg	15
Gomisin A	Oral, mice	1448 mg/kg	15
Gomisin A	i.p., mice	518 mg/kg	15
Gomisin A	s.c., mice	1861 mg/kg	15

Table 2 **Regulatory Status for Schisandra in Selected Countries**

Australia	Schisandra is not included in Part 4 of Schedule 4 of the Therapeutic Goods Regulations.
China	Schisandra is official in the *Pharmacopoeia of the People's Republic of China* 1997. The usual adult dosage, usually administered in the form of a decoction, is listed as 1.5 to 6 g.
UK & Germany	Schisandra is not included on the General Sale List. It was not included in the Commission E assessment.
US	Schisandra does not have generally recognised as safe (GRAS) status. However, it is freely available as a "dietary supplement" in the US under DSHEA legislation (Dietary Supplement Health and Education Act of 1994).

REFERENCES

1. Liu KT: Plenary lecture, *World Health Organization Seminar on the use of Medicinal Plants in Health Care,* Tokyo, Sept 1977. In: WHO Regional Office for the Western Pacific Final Report, Manila, 1977, pp 101-112.
2. Lupandin AV: *Fiziol Cheloveka* 16:114-119, 1990.
3. Ko KM, Ip SP, Poon MKT, et al: *Planta Medica* 61:134-137, 1995.
4. Lu H, Liu GT: *Chung Kuo Yao Li Hsueh Pao* 11:331-335, 1990.
5. Pharmacopoeia Commission of the People's Republic of China: *Pharmacopoeia of the People's Republic of China,* English ed, vol I, Beijing, 1997, Chemical Industry Press, p 77.
6. Hikino H, Kiso Y, Taguchi H, et al: *Planta Med* 50:213-218, 1984.
7. Hancke JL, Burgos RA, Ahumada F: *Fitoterapia* 70:451-471, 1999.
8. American Herbal Pharmacopoeia: *Schisandra berry—Schisandra chinensis: analytical, quality control, and therapeutic monograph,* Santa Cruz, October 1999, American Herbal Pharmacopoeia.
9. Chang HM, But PP: *Pharmacology and applications of Chinese materia medica,* vol I, Singapore, 1987, World Scientific, pp 199-209.
10. Bensky D, Gamble A: *Chinese herbal medicine materia medica,* Seattle, 1986, Eastland Press, p 542.
11. Trifonova AT: *Akush Ginekol* 4:19-22, 1954.
12. Gaistruk AN, Taranovskij KL: *Urg Probl Obstet Gynecol L'vov* 1:183-186, 1968.
13. Burgos RA, Hancke JL: Toxicological studies on *S. chinensis,* Instituto de Farmacologia, Facultad de Medinia Veterinaria, Universidad Austral de Chile, Valdivia, Chile, 1992, cited in Hancke JL, Burgos RA, Ahumada F: *Fitoterapia* 70:451-471, 1999.
14. Volicer L, Sramka M, Janku J, et al: *Arch Int Pharmacodyn* 163:249-262, 1966.
15. Maeda S, Sudo K, Aburada M, et al: *Yakugaku Zasshi* 101:1030-1041, 1981.
16. Bao TT, Liu GT, Song ZY, et al: *Chinese Med J* 93:41-47, 1980.
17. Hendrich S, Bjeldanes LF: *Food Chem Toxicol* 24:903-912, 1986.
18. Liu KT, Cresteil T, Columelli S, et al: *Chem Biol Interact* 39:315-330, 1982.
19. Liu KT, Lesca P: *Chem Biol Interact* 39:301-314, 1982.

SENNA

Other common names: Senna Alexandrian senna pods, Tinnevelly senna pods
Botanical names: *Cassia senna* L. (*C. acutifolia* Delile), *C. angustifolia* Vahl.
Family: Leguminosae (Caesalpinioideae)
Plant part used: Dried fruits (pods) and leaves

Safety Summary

Pregnancy category A: No proven increase in the frequency of malformation or other harmful effects on the foetus despite consumption by a large number of women.
Lactation category CC: Compatible with breast-feeding but use caution.
Contraindications: Inflammation or irritation of the bowel and digoxin prescription. Do not use during lactation without professional advice.
Warnings & precautions: For short-term use only; causes of chronic constipation and any other abdominal symptoms need to be investigated.
Adverse reactions: Griping colic, diarrhoea, potassium and fluid loss, possible hepatic reactions.
Interactions: Digoxin, thiazide diuretics, theoretically other remedies exacerbated by or causing potassium loss.

Typical Therapeutic Use

Efficacy of senna preparations as a laxative is comparable to lactulose in terminal cancer patients on opioids,[1] and appears more effective in other geriatric patients.[2,3] Traditional indications for senna leaf and pods in Western herbal medicine include constipation.[4]

Actions

Laxative. The leaves are reputed to be stronger than the pods.

Key Constituents

The prominent constituents are β-linked dianthrones, sennosides A and B, which are metabolised by gut bacteria to rhein anthrone and to rhein by oxidation; other anthracenes are also present in smaller quantities.

The *European Pharmacopoeia* 4.3 recommends that *C. acutifolia* or *C. angustifolia* leaf contains not less than 2.5% of hydroxyanthracene glycosides calculated as sennoside B. *Cassia acutifolia* pods should contain not less than 3.4% of hydroxyanthracene glycosides and *C. angustifolia* pods not less than 2.2% of hydroxyanthracene glycosides, in both cases calculated as sennoside B.

Adulteration

Adulteration of *C. acutifolia* and *C. angustifolia* leaves may occur with other medicinal *Cassia* species (e.g., *C. auriculata*, *C. italica*, and *C. holosericea*) and from other genera (e.g., *Solenosemma arghel*, *Coriaria myrtifolia*, and *Tephrosia purpurea*).[5]

Typical Dosage Forms & Dosage

Typical adult dosage ranges are:
- 1.5 to 6 g/day of dried leaf
- 0.5 to 2 g/day of dried pods
- 1.5 to 6 mL/day of a 1:2 liquid extract or equivalent in tablet or capsule form
- other preparations: equivalent to 15 to 30 mg daily of hydroxyanthracene derivatives, calculated as sennoside B

Contraindications

Senna should not be used in the case of diarrhoea, or inflammatory or other disease of the colon, lower small intestine, or appendix. It should be avoided with the prescription of digoxin or antiarrhythmic drugs, or in any case where heart disturbances are combined with the prescription of diuretics. It is not advisable to use senna or other stimulating laxatives where constipation is associated with an irritable or spastic bowel, or in any child under the age of 10 years. Do not use during lactation without professional advice.

Use in Pregnancy

Category A: No proven increase in the frequency of malformation or other harmful effects on the foetus despite consumption by a large number of women.

A 1992 review noted that the evidence from clinical studies indicates that treatment with senna does not involve any increased risk for the pregnancy or for the foetus. In 10 studies, women were treated with standardised senna preparations, a combination of senna and *Plantago ovata* seeds, and various anthranoids plus methylcellulose, over periods ranging from 2 weeks up to 9 months. Good laxative efficacy and few side effects (exclusively gastrointestinal) were observed. The senna and *P. ovata* combination was without any stimulating effect on uterine contractions, even in women with high-risk pregnancies. Experimental toxicological reproduction studies with sennosides have not revealed any abortifacient, teratogenic, or foetotoxic effects in rats and rabbits, even in large doses. Perinatal and postnatal development also proceeded normally. Sennosides did not show any stimulation of uterine contractions in pregnant sheep, and a slight inhibition of contraction frequency was observed in some ewes.[6]

Use in Lactation

Category CC: Compatible with breastfeeding but use caution.

A 1992 review noted, from the results of clinical observations of infants and analytical studies of breast milk, that treatment of lactating mothers with senna does not carry a risk of producing a laxative effect in the infant. Highly sensitive techniques (HPLC) can detect traces of rhein (metabolite of senna) in breast milk, but at amounts far smaller than the amounts required to produce a laxative effect.[7] The American Academy of Pediatrics has judged senna as compatible with breastfeeding.[8,9]

Warnings & Precautions

Senna is a stimulating laxative and should not be used for long periods and not beyond 2 weeks without expert supervision. Persistent constipation should be investigated and other appropriate treatment schedules initiated, in which occasional use of senna may be justified, but which should emphasise dietary changes, bulk laxatives, and exercises.

Senna should not be given when there are any undiagnosed abdominal symptoms.

Effect on Ability to Drive or Operate Machinery

No adverse effects expected.

Adverse Reactions

Diarrhoea: 4% of new cases of diarrhoea at gastroenterology clinics in the west and central belt of Scotland were found to be laxative induced.[10] Stimulating laxatives may induce griping pains and may best be given with carminative treatments.

Extended use is likely to lead to tolerance, with diminishing efficacy and the need for increased doses. Traditional views were that long-term use of stimulating laxatives led to intractable constipation, or "cathartic colon". No case of cathartic colon has been observed in prospective studies[11] or otherwise during the past few decades, and it can be assumed that it was probably caused by laxatives that are no longer in use (such as podophyllin).[12]

There are suggestions that anthraquinone laxatives are a risk factor in the development of urothelial cancer, but rationales have not been provided for these observations.[13]

Occupational exposure to senna is associated with widespread (over 15% of the workforce) contact allergic reactions, as elicited by skin prick tests and associated with symptoms of allergic rhinitis.[14]

Pseudomelanosis Coli and Colorectal Cancer

Long-term use of senna laxatives leads to chronic mucosal inflammation,[15] with the accumulation of melanic (pigmented) residues in leucocytes, and the apoptosis (death) of colon cells.[16] Research has supported the orthodox view, now challenged (see below) that pseudomelanosis coli is a reliable parameter of chronic laxative abuse over 9 to 12 months, and is specific for anthranoid drugs.[17] Rhein has been identified from in vitro studies as a possible factor via the secretion of nitric oxide.[18] The pigmented lesions in pseudomelanosis coli associated with anthranoid use are stable and disappear quickly after discontinuation of the treatment, without residual carcinogenicity and genotoxicity.[19]

A 1992 review notes that there is no profound evidence in experimental studies to suggest that senna has any specific harmful effects on neuronal structures in the colon, and that clinical studies in patients with long-term laxative abuse do not rule out the possibility that degenerative changes in the nerve plexus, if present, are the cause of chronic constipation and not the consequence of a toxic effect of a laxative. However, the possibility that laxatives might cause secondary lesions in the nerve plexus as a result of electrolyte shifts associated with long-term laxative abuse and diarrhoea cannot be excluded.[20]

Pseudomelanosis coli requires at least 4 months' consumption of anthranoid-containing laxatives before it develops, and it does not appear in every patient.[21] Pigmentation of the caecum in guinea pigs can be induced in a relatively short time by bisacodyl (stimulant laxative) and phenolphthalein (cathartic). Cases of non–anthranoid-induced pseudomelanosis coli have also been reported (assuming reliability of case history re. laxative use), and pigmentation of the intestinal wall can also be due to causes other than laxative intake (e.g., metabolic disorders).[21] Withdrawal tests with cascara (*Rhamnus purshiana*) have shown that the pigmentation is reversible within 5 to 15 months in a large proportion of patients,[21] and there is no evidence of its link to carcinogenicity or genotoxicity.[19]

Differentiation between melanosis coli, as a broad phenomenon of colonic pigmentation, and pseudomelanosis coli seems to be important. Following investigations of patients with melanosis coli, it is clear that laxative use is not the only causative factor.[22]

The ongoing toxicological debate is whether the pseudomelanosis coli associated with laxative use is a risk factor for colorectal cancer. Biopsies have shown that a single dose of sennosides can induce significant apoptosis, a change marked also by shorter crypts, and increased cell proliferation. This observation is seen to support the potential carcinogenic effect of sennosides.[23] There is even a suggestion that this short-term effect is compounded in severe melanosis coli, and thus presumably over longer-term use, by a breakdown in defences against carcinogenesis.[24]

Regulatory attitudes to the risks of senna laxatives, and some review articles,[25] appear to have been influenced by substantial studies in the early 1990s. In a retrospective study of 3049 patients who underwent diagnostic colorectal endoscopy, the incidence of pseudomelanosis coli was 3.13% in patients without pathological changes and 3.29% in those with colorectal cancer; much higher levels, 8.64%, were seen in those with polyps (colorectal adenomas). The authors were puzzled by this disparity and suspected poor records of colorectal cases. To pursue this they set up a prospective study of 1095 patients. Here the incidence of pseudomelanosis coli was 6.9% for patients with no abnormality seen on endoscopy, 9.8% for patients with adenomas, and 18.6% for patients with colorectal carcinomas. Colorectal can-

cer was thus judged as being three times more likely in the case of anthranoid laxative abuse.[26] However, the association between melanosis and anthranoid laxative abuse was assumed rather than specifically tested (see above for the discussion that this association is not tight). In addition, these findings have been contested in other research. A meta-analysis suggested a number of confounding factors, such as diet, and the different effects of various laxatives may have been overlooked.[27] In a large study on successive colonoscopies in over 2000 patients with colorectal cancer, no association was found with melanosis coli or laxative use.[28,29] A later study proposed that even an apparent increase in the number of adenomas in the case of melanosis coli was most likely due to the relative ease of identification of the polyps against a dark background.[30] A smaller, but rigorous, investigation of 55 surgical patients with sigmoid cancer, compared to other bowel inflammatory disease, and matched controls without intestinal disease found no evidence of an association between colon cancer (or precancerous lesions [aberrant crypt foci]) and constipation, laxative use, or the presence of melanosis coli.[31]

Interactions

Stimulating laxatives may decrease the gastrointestinal transit time and absorption of coadministered agents. Potassium deficiency (resulting from long-term laxative abuse) can potentiate the action of cardiac glycosides and may affect the action of antiarrhythmic agents. Potassium deficiency can be increased by concomitant use of thiazide diuretics, corticosteroids, and licorice root.[32,33] There is potential (but not established) interaction for the same reason with quinidine and licorice.

Safety in Children

For children under 10 years constipation is most often due to excessive activity of the bowel musculation and rarely to the relative atony that marks some later-onset constipation. It is therefore usually inappropriate to provide stimulating laxatives in this age group.

Using senna preparations in infants and young children is associated with rash, especially those in nappies (diapers), skin blisters in the perianal region, and even skin sloughing.[34]

Overdosage

Griping and diarrhoea are most likely symptoms of overdosage with anthraquinone laxatives. Consequent fluid and electrolyte losses (especially of potassium), metabolic alkalosis, and renal tubular damage may occur, and possible cardiac and neuromuscular dysfunction.[12] Treatment should include rehydration and electrolyte replacement.

Senna abuse was associated with severe finger clubbing and urinary secretion of aspartyl-glucosamine in one patient with anorexia nervosa.[35] Finger clubbing has been reported elsewhere as a consequence of senna abuse.[36]

Two cases of intermittent obstruction of the oesophagus, which subsided spontaneously, has been demonstrated for a senna preparation taken in excessive doses.[37]

Toxicology

The LD_{50} from a single oral dose of sennosides was approximately 5 g/kg in both mice and rats. Death was probably due to an extensive loss of water and electrolytes following massive diarrhoea. In subacute studies with rats (up to 20 mg/kg) and dogs (up to 500 mg/kg) sennosides caused no specific local or systemic toxicity. In a 6-month study with rats, sennosides were tolerated without specific toxic effects in doses up to 100 mg/kg. Effects secondary to chronic diarrhoea were observed.[38] The acute toxicity of a partially purified senna extract (20% sennosides) was 2.5 g/kg for oral administration in mice (higher than for administration of pure sennoside). The difference may be due to the presence of free aglycones in the extract.[39] However, toxicity data on anthranoid laxatives obtained in experimental animals cannot be extrapolated to humans. There is said to be a large difference in sensitivity between humans and rodents, the latter being about 100-fold less sensitive.[40]

The ESCOP monograph on senna refers to unpublished papers from the manufacturer of a leading senna preparation, Agiolax, demonstrating low toxicity of this product in animals, even lower for the whole extract than for purified glycosides. In a conference paper, it was reported that oral consumption of a senna preparation over 2 years had no carcinogenic effect on male and female rats.[41]

No influence on ileal and colonic mucosal cell proliferation has been observed in rats after long-term ingestion of anthraquinones.[42] Compared with danthron (1,8-dihydroxyanthraquinone, a synthetic anthraquinone), which affected neuropeptide levels, there appeared to be no significant effects of senna consumption over the long term on the gut wall in the rat.[43] No signs of intestinal mucosa injury were found in mice after long-term sennoside ingestion either, contrasting with the myenteric plexus abnormalities associated with the ingestion of danthron.[44] Danthron preparations are increasingly restricted because of the risk of hepatotoxicity. Although chronic senna use has been associated with hepatitis in one case,[45] there is also some evidence that anthraquinones may have some hepatoprotective activity.[46]

Regulatory Status

See Table 1 for regulatory status in selected countries.

Table 1 **Regulatory Status for Senna in Selected Countries**

Australia	Senna is not included in Part 4 of Schedule 4 of the Therapeutic Goods Regulations.
UK & Germany	Senna pods and leaf are included on the General Sale List. Senna leaf and the two varieties of senna pods are all covered by positive Commission E monographs. Senna leaf and the two varieties of senna pods are all official in the *British Pharmacopoeia* 2002 and the *European Pharmacopoeia* 4.3.
US	Senna leaf is official in the *United States Pharmacopeia-National Formulary* (USP 26-NF 21, 2003). Senna does not have generally recognised as safe (GRAS) status. It is freely available as a "dietary supplement" in the US under DSHEA legislation (Dietary Supplement Health and Education Act of 1994) but must carry the following warning label: "This product contains *Cassia* spp. (senna). Read and follow directions carefully.

Continued

Table **1**   **Regulatory Status for Senna in Selected Countries—Cont'd**

Do not use if you have or develop diarrhea, loose stools, or abdominal pain. Consult your physician if you have frequent diarrhea. If you are pregnant, nursing, taking medication, or have a medical condition, consult your physician before using this product."*

The California Department of Health Services Food and Drug Branch issued an emergency regulation 1 November 1996, requiring that all herb teas and dietary supplements containing herbs with stimulant laxative activity carry a warning label. The herbs included in this regulation include aloe (Aloe ferox and other related species), buckthorn bark and berry (Rhamnus catharticus), cascara sagrada bark (Rhamnus purshiana), rhubarb root (Rheum palmatum), and senna leaf and pod (Cassia acutifolia, C. angustifolia, C. senna). The ruling exempts herb products made from aloe leaf gel, which normally does not contain significant natural levels of anthraquinones. The new ruling went into effect 1 January 1997.[47]

REFERENCES

1. Agra Y, Sacristan A, Gonzalez M, et al: *J Pain Symptom Manage* 15:1-7, 1998.
2. Kinnunen O, Winblad I, Koistinen P, et al: *Pharmacology* 47(Suppl. 1):253-255, 1993.
3. Passmore AP, Wilson-Davies K, Stoker C, et al: *BMJ* 307:769-771, 1993.
4. British Herbal Medicine Association's Scientific Committee: *British herbal pharmacopoeia,* Bournemouth, 1983, BHMA, pp 49, 51.
5. Blaschek W, Ebel S, Hackenthal E, et al: *HagerROM 2002: Hagers Handbuch der Drogen und Arzneistoffe,* Heidelberg, 2002, Springer.
6. Leng-Peschlow E, ed: *Pharmacology* 44(Suppl. 1):20-22, 1992.
7. Leng-Peschlow E, ed: *Pharmacology* 44(Suppl. 1):23-25, 1992.
8. Hagemann TM: *J Hum Lact* 14:259-262, 1998.
9. American Academy of Pediatrics: *Pediatrics* 108:776-789, 2001.
10. Duncan A, Morris AJ, Cameron A, et al: *J R Soc Med* 85:203-205, 1992.
11. Gattuso JM, Kamm MA: *Drug Safety* 10:47-65, 1994.
12. Muller-Lissner SA: *Pharmacology* 47(Suppl. 1):138-145, 1993.
13. Bronder E, Klimpel A, Helmert U, et al: *Soz Praventivmed* 44:117-125, 1999.
14. Marks GB, Salome CM, Woolcock AJ: *Am Rev Respir Dis* 144:1065-1069, 1991.
15. Mitty RD, Wolfe GR, Cosman M: *Am J Gastroenterol* 92:707-708, 1997.
16. Benavides SH, Morgante PE, Monserrat AJ, et al: *Gastrointest Endosc* 46:131-138, 1997.
17. Willems M, van Buuren HR, de Krijger R: *Neth J Med* 61:22-24, 2003.
18. Raimondi F, Santoro P, Maiuri L, et al: *J Pediatr Gastroenterol Nutr* 34:529-534, 2002.
19. Krbavcic A, Pecar S, Schara M, et al: *Pharmazie* 53:336-338, 1998.
20. Leng-Peschlow E, ed: *Pharmacology* 44(Suppl. 1):26-29, 1992.
21. Leng-Peschlow E, ed: *Pharmacology* 44(Suppl. 1):33-35, 1992.
22. Byers RJ, Marsh P, Parkinson D, et al: *Histopathology* 30:160-164, 1997.
23. van Gorkom BA, Karrenbeld A, van Der Sluis T, et al: *Digestion* 61:113-120, 2000.
24. van Gorkom BA, Karrenbeld A, van Der Sluis T, et al: *J Pathol* 194:493-499, 2001.
25. van Gorkom BA, de Vries EG, Karrenbeld A, et al: *Aliment Pharmacol Ther* 13:443-452, 1999.
26. Siegers CP, von Hertzberg-Lottin E, Otte M, et al: *Gut* 34:1099-1101, 1993.
27. Sonnenberg A, Müller AD: *Pharmacology* 47(Suppl. 1):224-233, 1993.
28. Nusko G, Schneider B, Ernst H, et al: *Z Gastroenterol* 35:313-318, 1997.
29. Nusko G, Schneider B, Muller G, et al: *Pharmacology* 47(Suppl. 1):234-241, 1993.
30. Nusko G, Schneider B, Schneider I, et al: *Gut* 46:651-655, 2000.
31. Nascimbeni R, Donato F, Ghirardi M, et al: *Cancer Epidemiol Biomarkers Prev* 11:753-757, 2002.
32. Blumenthal M, et al, eds: *The complete German Commission E monographs: therapeutic guide to herbal medicines,* Austin, 1998, American Botanical Council, pp 80-81.
33. Scientific Committee of ESCOP (European Scientific Cooperative on Phytotherapy): *ESCOP monographs: Aloe capensis – Cape Aloes,* UK, June 1997, ESCOP Secretariat.
34. Spiller HA, Winter ML, Weber JA, et al: *Ann Pharmacother* 37:636-639, 2003.
35. Malmquist J, Ericsson B, Hulten-Nosslin MB, et al: *Postgrad Med J* 56:862-864, 1980.
36. Prior J, White I: *Lancet* 2:947, 1978.
37. Sauerbruch T, Kuntzen O, Unger W: *Endoscopy* 12:83-85, 1980.
38. Mengs U: *Pharmacology* 36(Suppl. 1):180-187, 1988.
39. Marvola M, Koponen A, Hiltunen R, et al: *J Pharm Pharmacol* 33:108-109, 1981.
40. van Os FH: *Pharmacology* 14(Suppl. 1):18-29, 1976.
41. Scientific Committee of ESCOP (European Scientific Cooperative on Phytotherapy): *ESCOP monographs: Sennae fructus acutifoliae.* UK, June 1997, ESCOP Secretariat.

42. Geboes K: *Verh K Acad Geneeskd Belg* 57:51-74, 1995.
43. Milner P, Belai A, Tomlinson A, et al: *J Pharm Pharmacol* 44:777-779, 1992.
44. Dufour P, Gendre P: *Pharmacology* 36(Suppl. 1):194-202, 1988.
45. Beuers U, Spengler U, Pape GR: *Lancet* 337:372-373, 1991.
46. Arosio B, Gagliano N, Fusaro LM, et al: *Pharmacol Toxicol* 87:229-233, 2000.
47. Blumenthal M: *HerbalGram* 39:26-27, 1997.

SHATAVARI

Botanical names: *Asparagus racemosus* Willd. (*Protasparagus racemosus* [Willd.] Oberm.)
Family: Asparagaceae (broadly Liliaceae)
Plant part used: Root

Safety Summary

Pregnancy category B2: No increase in frequency of malformation or other harmful effects on the foetus from limited use in women. Animal studies are lacking.
Lactation category C: Compatible with breastfeeding.
Contraindications: None required on current evidence.
Warnings & precautions: The use of herbs rich in saponins is possibly inappropriate in coeliac disease, fat malabsorption, and vitamins A, D, E and K deficiency, some upper digestive irritations, and topically to open wounds. Caution in patients with preexisting cholestasis.
Adverse reactions: Herbs rich in saponins may cause irritation of the gastric mucous membranes and reflux.
Interactions: No precautions required on current evidence.

Typical Therapeutic Use

Traditional indications for shatavari in Ayurvedic medicine include menopause, threatened miscarriage, to promote lactation, for sexual debility, and to promote conception in both sexes.[1-4]

Actions

Tonic, galactagogue, sexual tonic, adaptogenic, spasmolytic, antidiarrhoeal, diuretic.

Key Constituents

Constituents of shatavari root include steroidal saponins, including shatavarin-I[5]; alkaloids, including the pyrrolizidine alkaloid asparagamine A[6]; and mucilage.[7] (On the basis of its chemical structure, asparagamine A would not be expected to be toxic.)

Adulteration

No adulterants known.

Typical Dosage Forms & Dosage

Typical adult dosage ranges are:
- 20 to 30 g/day of dried root (lower doses are used by infusion or decoction)
- 4.5 to 8.5 mL/day of a 1:2 liquid extract or equivalent in tablet or capsule form

Contraindications

None known.

Use in Pregnancy

Category B2: No increase in frequency of malformation or other harmful effects on the foetus from limited use in women. Animal studies are lacking.

Shatavari is used in traditional Ayurvedic medicine to promote conception[1] and preparations based on shatavari are often recommended for threatened miscarriage.[2] However, folk use of shatavari root to promote abortion has been reported in an ethnobotanical study of the tribal peoples of the Bihar district of India.[8] This would presumably involve doses far in excess of those normally used.

Use in Lactation

Category C: Compatible with breastfeeding.

Shatavari is used in Ayurveda and the traditional medicine of South-East Asia to promote lactation.[3,9] One teaspoon (0.5 g) of shatavari powder is given with milk twice daily for insufficient lactation.[10]

In a multicentre, randomised, double-blind, placebo-controlled trial, a formulation containing 68% shatavari was administered to mothers with lactational inadequacy. The formulation was not found to be superior to placebo.[11]

In animal studies, oral administration of shatavari increased the weight of mammary lobulo-alveolar tissue[12] and corrected irregular, low milk yields.[13]

Warnings & Precautions

The use of herbs rich in saponins is possibly inappropriate in coeliac disease, fat malabsorption, and vitamins A, D, E and K deficiency, some upper digestive irritations, and topically to open wounds. Saponin-containing herbs are best kept to a minimum in patients with preexisting cholestasis.

Effect on Ability to Drive or Operate Machinery

No adverse effects expected.

Adverse Reactions

As with all saponin-containing herbs, oral use may cause irritation of the gastric mucous membranes and reflux.

Interactions

None known.

Safety in Children

Shatavari is used in South-East Asia for providing nourishment to children.[9]

Overdosage

No incidents found in published literature.

Toxicology

No acute toxic effects were observed after oral administration of shatavari extract (1 g/kg) to mice.[14] The oral LD_{50} of shatavari suspension (prepared by boiling the dried, powdered root in water without separating the insoluble part) was greater than 1 g/kg in rats and mice. No animals died and no toxic effects were observed. Similarly, no toxic effects were observed in rats and mice administered shatavari suspension for 15 to 30 days in subacute toxicity studies. No deleterious changes were detected in liver or renal function tests. The suspension was administered orally in doses ranging from 50 to 1000 mg/kg.[15]

After oral administration of shatavari, the livers of nonpregnant mice were larger and heavier than those of pregnant mice. The nonpregnant group also showed liver congestion, bile plugs, mild cellular degeneration, fibrosis, and leucocytic infiltration. Kupffer cell hyperplasia and nuclear enlargement were observed in both experimental groups.[16]

Regulatory Status

See Table 1 for regulatory status in selected countries.

Table **1**   **Regulatory Status for Shatavari in Selected Countries**

Australia	Shatavari is not included in Part 4 of Schedule 4 of the Therapeutic Goods Regulations.
UK & Germany	Shatavari is not included on the General Sale List. It was not included in the Commission E assessment.
US	Shatavari does not have generally recognised as safe (GRAS) status. However, it is freely available as a "dietary supplement" in the US under DSHEA legislation (Dietary Supplement Health and Education Act of 1994).

REFERENCES

1. Thakur RS, Puri HS, Husain A: *Major medicinal plants of India,* Lucknow, 1989, Central Institute of Medicinal and Aromatic Plants, pp 78-81.
2. Dev S: *Environ Health Perspect* 107:783-789, 1999.
3. Nadkarni AK: *Dr. K.M. Nadkarni's Indian materia medica,* ed 3, vol 1, first published 1954, reprinted Bombay, 1976, Popular Prakashan, pp 153-155.
4. Frawley D, Lad V: *The yoga of herbs: an Ayurvedic guide to herbal medicine,* ed 2, Santa Fe, 1988, Lotus Press, pp 183-184.
5. Hostettmann K, Marston A: *Chemistry and pharmacology of natural products: saponins,* Cambridge, 1995, Cambridge University Press, p 298.
6. Sekine T, Ikegami F, Fukasawa N, et al: *Perkin Transactions* 1:391-393, 1995.
7. Bharatiya Vidya Bhavan's Swami Prakashananda Ayurveda Research Centre: *Selected medicinal plants of India.* Bombay, 1992, Chemexcil, pp 43-46.
8. Tarafder CR: *J Econ Taxon Bot* 4:507-516, 1983.
9. World Health Organization: *The use of traditional medicine in primary health care: a manual for health workers in South-East Asia,* New Delhi, 1990, WHO Regional Office for South-East Asia, pp 9-10.
10. World Health Organization: *The use of traditional medicine in primary health care: a manual for health workers in South-East Asia,* New Delhi, 1990, WHO Regional Office for South-East Asia, p 132.

11. Sharma S, Ramji S, Kumari S, et al: *Indian Pediatr* 33:675-677, 1996.
12. Sabnis PB, Gaitonde BB, Jetmalani M: *Indian J Exp Biol* 6: 55-57, 1968.
13. Patel AB, Kanitkar UK: *Indian Vet J* 46:718-721, 1969.
14. Debelmas AM, Hache J: *Plant Med Phytother* 10:128-138, 1976.
15. Rege NN, Thatte UM, Dahanukar SA: *Phytother Res* 13:275-291, 1999.
16. Pandey SK, Sahay A: *Indian Drugs* 38:132-136, 2001.

SHEPHERD'S PURSE

Botanical name: *Capsella bursa-pastoris* (L.) Medik.
Family: Cruciferae
Plant part used: Aerial parts

Safety Summary

Pregnancy category B3: No increase in frequency of malformation or other harmful effects on the foetus from limited use in women. Evidence of increased foetal damage in animal studies exists, although the relevance to humans is unknown.
Lactation category CC: Compatible with breast-feeding but use caution.
Contraindications: None required on current evidence. Do not use during pregnancy or lactation without professional advice.
Warnings & precautions: Should not be taken in doses exceeding the maximum therapeutic range in the long term.
Adverse reactions: None found in published literature.
Interactions: No precautions required on current evidence.

Typical Therapeutic Use

Traditional indications for shepherd's purse in Western herbal medicine include uterine haemorrhage, menorrhagia, haematemesis, diarrhoea, and acute cystitis.[1]

Actions

Antihaemorrhagic, urinary antiseptic.

Key Constituents

The constituents of shepherd's purse have not been investigated extensively, and those isolated in early research require verification. Shepherd's purse contains flavonoids. An early study recorded the presence of sinigrin (a glucosinolate) in the whole plant,[2] although its presence has been disputed.[3] However, being a member of the Cruciferae family, shepherd's purse is likely to contain glucosinolates. The presence of saponins is doubted,[4] but the presence of amino acids (mainly proline, valine, and α-aminobutyric acid) in an aqueous ethanol extract has been verified.[5] However, the presence of the amino acids choline, acetylcholine, and tyramine recorded in 1888 to 1922 have not been confirmed.[6] The oxalic acid content of shepherd's purse leaves was considered moderate for a potential food item.[7]

Adulteration

No adulterants known.

Typical Dosage Forms & Dosage

Typical adult dosage ranges are:
- 3 to 12 g/day of dried aerial parts or by infusion
- 3 to 12 mL/day of a 1:1 liquid extract
- 3 to 6 mL/day of a 1:2 liquid extract or equivalent in tablet or capsule form

Contraindications

None known. Do not use during pregnancy or lactation without professional advice.

Use in Pregnancy

Category B3: No increase in frequency of malformation or other harmful effects on the foetus from limited use in women. Evidence of increased foetal damage in animal studies exists, although the relevance to humans is unknown.

Shepherd's purse (part unknown) is used by indigenous Bolivians to stimulate uterine contractions at birth.[8] A review of traditional Ayurvedic literature notes that shepherd's purse is listed as an abortifacient in three of the five sources checked. However, the definition of abortifacient was very broad and included emmenagogue, ecbolic (uterine contractor), and "antimetabolite".[9] One of these references indicates that a hot infusion of herb was used as an emmenagogue. Powdered herb mixed with a normal diet (25% to 50% concentration) was used to inhibit the oestrus cycle (probably of the rat).[10]

Several glucosinolates, including sinigrin, and some of their derivatives, were not teratogenic to rat foetuses when administered subcutaneously to the dams on day 8 and/or day 9 of gestation.[11] Placental transfer of glucosinolates and their metabolites may occur. Adverse effects in the newborn occurred for animals fed dietary levels of glucosinolates.[12] This level of glucosinolates is not likely to occur from normal therapeutic doses of shepherd's purse.

Shepherd's purse infusion (1 to 2 mg/mL) demonstrated some uterotonic activity with isolated uterine tissue.[13] Shepherd's purse had less activity than chamomile, which indicates that the activity was relatively mild. This contrasts with an early study in which strong contractile activity was demonstrated for extracts of dried and fresh plant material.[14] A fraction isolated from an ethanol extract of shepherd's purse exerted contractile activity on isolated rat uterus[15] and increased experimentally induced contractions in vivo (after intravenous injection).[16]

See also Toxicology section below.

Use in Lactation

Category CC: Compatible with breastfeeding but use caution.

Animal studies indicate that glucosinolates are excreted in breast milk[12] and may taint the milk.[17] Adverse effects were observed in newborns fed milk from goats that were given dietary levels of glucosinolates.[12] Shepherd's purse should be avoided if possible by lactating women, or used with caution.

Warnings & Precautions

Due to potential mutagenicity and goitrogenicity, herbs containing glucosinolates should not be taken in doses exceeding the maximum therapeutic range in the long term.

Effect on Ability to Drive or Operate Machinery

No adverse effects expected.

Adverse Reactions

None known for shepherd's purse.

Interactions

None known.

Safety in Children

No information available, but adverse effects are not expected.

Overdosage

No incidents found in published literature.

Toxicology

The LD_{50} value of 1 g/kg was obtained for a 90% ethanol extract of the whole plant which was administered i.p. to rats.[18] Fractions isolated from an ethanol extract of shepherd's purse showed low toxicity in mice.[16]

At a dietary level of 20%, shepherd's purse did not affect female fertility in guinea pigs. At 40% it impeded ovulation and produced temporary infertility in both females and males. It did not demonstrate oestrogenic activity.[19]

Shepherd's purse is occasionally recorded as causing stock poisoning.[2] Suspected nitrite poisoning occurred in pigs after ingestion of *Capsella bursa-pastoris* leaf.[20]

Sinigrin induced chromosome aberrations in vitro at concentrations above 2 mg/mL.[21]

Regulatory Status

See Table 1 for regulatory status in selected countries.

Table 1 **Regulatory Status for Shepherd's Purse in Selected Countries**

Australia	Shepherd's purse is not included in Part 4 of Schedule 4 of the Therapeutic Goods Regulations.
UK & Germany	Shepherd's purse is included on the General Sale List. It is covered by a positive Commission E monograph.
US	Shepherd's purse does not have generally recognised as safe (GRAS) status. However, it is freely available as a "dietary supplement" in the US under DSHEA legislation (Dietary Supplement Health and Education Act of 1994).

REFERENCES

1. British Herbal Medicine Association's Scientific Committee: *British herbal pharmacopoeia,* Bournemouth, 1983, BHMA, p 47.
2. Sabri NN, Sarg T, Seif El-Din AA: *Egypt J Pharm Sci* 16:521-522, 1975.
3. Blaschek W, Ebel S, Hackenthal E, et al: *HagerROM 2002: Hagers Handbuch der Drogen und Arzneistoffe,* Heidelberg, 2002, Springer.
4. Bisset NG, ed: *Herbal drugs and phytopharmaceuticals: a handbook for practice on a scientific basis,* Stuttgart, 1994, Medpharm Scientific Publishers, pp 112-114.
5. Maillard C, Barlatier A, Debrauwer L, et al: *Ann Pharm Fr* 46:211-216, 1988.
6. Kuroda K, Kaku T: *Lide Sci* 8:151-155, 1969.
7. Guil-Guerrero JL: *J Food Biochem* 23:283-294, 1999.
8. Bastien JW: *J Ethnopharmacol* 8:97-111, 1983.
9. Casey RCD: *Indian J Med Sci* 14:590-600, 1960.
10. de Laszlo H, Henshaw PS: *Science* 119:626-631, 1954.
11. Nishie K, Daxenbichler ME: *Food Cosmet Toxicol* 18:159-172, 1980.
12. Panter KE, James LF: *J Anim Sci* 68:892-904, 1990.
13. Shipochliev T: Vet *Med Nauki* 18:94-98, 1981.
14. Harste W: *Arch Pharm* 266:133-151, 1928.
15. Kuroda K, Takagi K: *Nature* 220:707-708, 1968.
16. Kuroda K, Takagi K: *Arch Int Pharmacodyn* 178:382-391, 1969.
17. Molfino RH: *Rev Farm* 89:7-17, 1947.
18. Sharma ML, Chandokhe N, Ghatak BJ, et al: *Indian J Exp Biol* 16:228-240, 1978.
19. East J: *J Endocrinol* 12:267-272, 1955.
20. Wiese WJ, Joubert JP: *J S Vet Assoc* 72:170-171, 2001.
21. Musk SR, Smith TK, Johnson IT: *Mutat Res* 348:19-23, 1995.

SIBERIAN GINSENG

Other common names: Eleuthero, Eleutherococcus
Botanical names: *Eleutherococcus senticosus* (Rupr. & Maxim.) Maxim. (*Acanthopanax senticosus* [Rupr. & Maxim.] Harms)
Family: Araliaceae
Plant part used: Root and rhizome

Safety Summary

Pregnancy category B1: No increase in frequency of malformation or other harmful effects on the foetus from limited use in women. No evidence of increased foetal damage in animal studies.
Lactation category C: Compatible with breastfeeding.
Contraindications: Acute phase of infections.
Warnings & precautions: The typically recommended regime for healthy people is a course of 6 weeks followed by a 2-week break.
Adverse reactions: Insomnia, palpitations, headache, tachycardia, pericardial pain, and hypertension have been reported in a few cases in patients with cardiovascular disorders.
Interactions: No precautions required on current evidence.

Typical Therapeutic Use

Siberian ginseng minimised the effects of environmental and occupational stress in a controlled trial,[1] improved physical strength in athletes in a randomised, placebo-controlled trial[2] and enhanced immune function in healthy individuals in a randomised, comparative trial.[3] Traditional indications for Siberian ginseng in Western herbal medicine and traditional Chinese medicine include temporary fatigue and general debility.[4,5]

Actions

Adaptogenic, immune modulating, tonic.

Key Constituents

Key constituents of Siberian ginseng root include the eleutherosides (a chemically diverse group of compounds), especially eleutheroside E. Minor constituents are triterpenoid saponins and glycans.[6-8] Total eleutheroside yields in the roots have been determined as being in the range 0.6% to 0.9%.[6]

Adulteration

Periploca sepium is recorded as a substitute for Siberian ginseng.[9,10]

Typical Dosage Forms & Dosage

Typical adult dosage ranges are:
- 2 to 3 g/day of dried root and rhizome or by decoction
- 2 to 8 mL/day of a 1:2 liquid extract or equivalent in tablet or capsule form

Contraindications

In accordance with Russian experiences, Siberian ginseng is best not used during the acute phase of infections. Some medical scientists and expert bodies[11,12] consider it to be contraindicated in hypertension, but it has also been used to treat hypertension.[13]

Use in Pregnancy

Category B1: No increase in frequency of malformation or other harmful effects on the foetus from limited use in women. No evidence of increased foetal damage in animal studies.

A case of neonatal androgenisation which was attributed to maternal use of "pure Siberian ginseng" has been reported.[14] Further follow-up research revealed that the product in question did not contain Siberian ginseng but instead contained *Periploca sepium*.[9,10] A pharmacological study of Siberian ginseng in rats observed no androgenic effects.[15]

Feeding experiments in several animal species have demonstrated an absence of teratogenicity and lack of adverse effects in both mothers and offspring.[16]

Use in Lactation

Category C: Compatible with breastfeeding.

No adverse effects on mothers and offspring were observed when Siberian ginseng 10% extract (10 mL/kg) was fed to minks from days 1 to 45 of the lactation period.[16]

Warnings & Precautions

The recommended regime for healthy people as an adaptogen is a course of 6 weeks followed by a

2-week break. This regime can be repeated for as long as is necessary. For the treatment of specific illnesses, continuous use is preferable.

Effect on Ability to Drive or Operate Machinery

No adverse effects expected.

Adverse Reactions

Russian studies on Siberian ginseng in over 2100 healthy volunteers and 2200 patients have noted a general absence of side effects. However, care should be exercised in patients with cardiovascular disorders since insomnia, palpitations, headache, tachycardia, pericardial pain, and hypertension have been reported in a few cases. Side-effects are more likely if normal doses are exceeded.[17]

"Ginseng abuse syndrome" with insomnia, diarrhoea, and hypertension has been described, but this study had many flaws.[18] Most notably it did not differentiate between Korean ginseng (*Panax ginseng*) and Siberian ginseng, and side effects appeared to be linked to excessive doses.

Interactions

A case of apparently elevated serum digoxin levels attributed to consumption of "Siberian ginseng" has been reported.[19] It was not conclusive as to whether the product caused a real increase in serum digoxin levels, as opposed to interference with the test method used. The researchers failed to test for eleutherosides to authenticate the product.

Siberian ginseng may interfere with drug-metabolising enzymes in the liver, but on current evidence this is unlikely. Aqueous and alcohol extracts of Siberian ginseng inhibited cytochrome P450 isozymes in vitro. Eleutherosides B and E showed no activity.[20]

Safety in Children

No information available, but adverse effects are not expected.

Overdosage

No incidents found in published literature, but see "ginseng abuse syndrome" above.

Toxicology

Table 1 lists LD_{50} data recorded for Siberian ginseng, indicating low toxicity.[16,21]

No toxic effects or deaths occurred when Siberian ginseng was fed to rats over their whole lifetime at many times the normal human dose,[16] or after oral administration of the ethanol extract (eleutherosides 10 mg/kg/day) for 2 months.[22] No pathological, histological, or cytotoxic changes were observed in the livers, brains, or kidneys of mice consuming Siberian ginseng infusion for up to 96 days. Aggressive behaviour was observed in mice drinking a concentrated extract containing sugar.[23] In vitro and in vivo tests with Siberian ginseng extract failed to reveal mutagenic or carcinogenic potential.[24]

Regulatory Status

See Table 2 for regulatory status in selected countries.

Table 1   **LD_{50} Data Recorded for Siberian Ginseng**

Substance	Route, Model	LD_{50} Value	Reference
Siberian ginseng root	Oral, mice	31 g/kg	16
Siberian ginseng root 33% ethanol extract	Oral, mice	14.5 g/kg	16
Siberian ginseng root extract	Oral, rats	10 mL/kg	21

Table **2** **Regulatory Status for Siberian Ginseng in Selected Countries**

Australia	Siberian ginseng is not included in Part 4 of Schedule 4 of the Therapeutic Goods Regulations.
China	Siberian ginseng is official in the *Pharmacopoeia of the People's Republic of China* 1997. The usual adult dosage, usually administered in the form of a decoction, is listed as 9 to 27 g.
UK & Germany	Siberian ginseng is not included on the General Sale List. It is covered by a positive Commission E monograph. Siberian ginseng is official in the *British Pharmacopoeia* 2002 and the *European Pharmacopoeia* 4.3.
US	Siberian ginseng is official in the *United States Pharmacopeia-National Formulary* (USP 26-NF 21, 2003). Siberian ginseng does not have generally recognised as safe (GRAS) status. However, it is freely available as a "dietary supplement" in the US under DSHEA legislation (Dietary Supplement Health and Education Act of 1994).

REFERENCES

1. Farnsworth NR, Kinghorn AD, Soefarto DD, et al: Siberian ginseng (*Eleutherococcus senticosus*): current status as an adaptogen. In Farnsworth NR, et al, eds: *Economic and medicinal plant research*, vol 1, London, 1985, Academic Press, p 178.
2. McNaughton L, Egan G, Caelli G: *Int Clin Nutr* Rev 9:32-35, 1989.
3. Szolomicki J, Samochowiec L, Wojcicki J, et al: *Phytother Res* 14:30-35, 2000.
4. British Herbal Medicine Association: *British herbal compendium*, Bournemouth, 1992, BHMA, pp 89-91.
5. Pharmacopoeia Commission of the People's Republic of China: *Pharmacopoeia of the People's Republic of China*, English ed, Beijing, 1997, Chemical Industry Press, pp 132-133.
6. Farnsworth NR, et al, eds: *Economic and medicinal plant research*, vol 1, London, 1985, Academic Press, p 157.
7. Segiet-Kujawa E, Kaloga M: *J Nat Prod* 54:1044-1048, 1991.
8. Hikino H, Takahashi M, Otake K, et al: *J Nat Prod* 49:293-297, 1986.
9. Awang DVC: *JAMA* 266:363, 1991.
10. Awang DVC: *JAMA* 265:1828, 1991.
11. Blumenthal M, et al, eds: *The complete German Commission E monographs: therapeutic guide to herbal medicines*, Austin, 1998, American Botanical Council, pp 124-125.
12. Dalinger OI: Central nervous stimulants - Tomsk 1986, pp 112-114, cited in De Smet PAGM, Keller K, Hansel R, et al, eds: *Adverse effects of herbal drugs*, vol 2, Berlin, 1993, Springer-Verlag, pp 163-164.
13. Farnsworth NR, et al, eds: *Economic and medicinal plant research*, vol 1, Academic Press, 1985, London, pp 179-191.
14. Koren G, Randor S, Martin S, et al: *JAMA* 264:2866, 1990.
15. Waller DP, Martin AM, Farnsworth NR, et al: *JAMA* 267:2329, 1992.
16. Farnsworth NR, et al, eds: *Economic and medicinal plant research*, vol 1, London, 1985, Academic Press, pp 164-166.
17. Farnsworth NR, et al, eds: *Economic and medicinal plant research*, vol 1, London, 1985, Academic Press, pp 179, 180-182, 187, 193, 195.
18. Siegel RK: *JAMA* 241:1614-1615, 1979.
19. MacRae S: *Can Med Assoc J* 155:293-295, 1996.
20. Harkey MR, Henderson GL, Zhou L, et al: *Altern Ther Health Med* 7:S14, 2001.
21. Kaemmerer K, Fink J: *Prakt Tierarzt* 61:748, 750-752, 754, 759-760, 1980.
22. Dardymov IV, Suprunov NI, Sokolenko LA: *Lek Sredstva Dal'nego Vostoka* 11:66-69, 1972.
23. Lewis WH, Zenger VE, Lynch RG: *J Ethnopharmacol* 8:209-214, 1983.
24. Hirosue T, Matsuzawa M, Kawai H, et al: *J Food Hyg Soc Jpn* 27:380-386, 1986.

SKULLCAP

Other common name: Scullcap
Botanical name: *Scutellaria lateriflora* L.
Family: Labiatae
Plant part used: Aerial parts

Safety Summary

Pregnancy category B2: No increase in frequency of malformation or other harmful effects on the foetus from limited use in women. Animal studies are lacking.
Lactation category C: Compatible with breastfeeding.
Contraindications: None required on current evidence.
Warnings & precautions: None required on current evidence.
Adverse reactions: Not likely from the authentic herb.
Interactions: No precautions required on current evidence.

Typical Therapeutic Use

Traditional indications for skullcap in Western herbal medicine include nervous tension, anxiety, insomnia, neuralgia, and epilepsy.[1,2]

Actions

Nervine tonic, spasmolytic, mild sedative.

Key Constituents

Key constituents of *Scutellaria lateriflora* aerial parts are flavonoids, including polyoxygenated flavones and their glycosides (including baicalein and baicalin).[3] Other constituents include cinnamic acid derivatives such as caffeic acid[3] and neoclerodane diterpenes (such as scutelaterins).[4] An essential oil containing sesquiterpenes is also present.[5]

Adulteration

Skullcap is frequently adulterated. Eclectic texts indicate adulteration with other *Scutellaria* species including *S. versicolor* and *S. canescens*. Other species considered of similar medicinal value include *S. galericulata*, *S. pilosa*, *S. integrifolia*, *S. hyssopifolia* and *S. minor*.[2,6] *Scutellaria serrata*, although medicinal, was considered inferior to *S. lateriflora*.[7] The British Pharmaceutical Codex of 1934 lists *S. galericulata* and *S. lateriflora* as medicinal, with *S. integrifolia* as a substitute.[8] Dried aerial parts of *S. galericulata* and *S. lateriflora* are difficult to distinguish morphologically.[9] The Dispensatory of the United States 1947 notes that skullcap "has been one of the most substituted and adulterated drugs in the materia medica".[10]

Of more concern is adulteration with potentially toxic plant species. Skullcap (*Scutellaria lateriflora*) is often adulterated on the European market. Commonly used substitutes for skullcap are species of *Teucrium*. In fact, so widespread was the adulteration that the macroscopic and microscopic description of skullcap cut herb in the *British herbal pharmacopoeia 1983* was "probably" for a species of *Teucrium*. Adulteration of commercial skullcap continued to be an issue in Europe, the United Kingdom, and the United States into the late 20th century.[11,12]

Typical Dosage Forms & Dosage

Typical adult dosage ranges are:
- 3 to 6 g/day of dried aerial parts or by infusion
- 6 to 12 mL/day of a 1:1 liquid extract
- 2 to 4.5 mL/day of a 1:2 liquid extract or equivalent in tablet or capsule form
- 3 to 6 mL/day of a 1:5 tincture

Contraindications

None known.

Use in Pregnancy

Category B2: No increase in frequency of malformation or other harmful effects on the foetus from limited use in women. Animal studies are lacking.

Eclectic texts indicate that a concentrated preparation of skullcap (referred to as scutellarin*) has been combined with other nervines and spasmolytics (resin/oleoresin of *Cimicifuga racemosa*, *Caulophyllum thalictroides*, and *Cypripedium pubescens*) for various female disorders in both pregnant and nonpregnant women.[2]

---

*Not to be confused with the flavonoid scutellarin, which is a minor flavonoid component of S. lateriflora aerial parts.[13]

Use in Lactation

Category C: Compatible with breastfeeding.

Warnings & Precautions

None required.

Effect on Ability to Drive or Operate Machinery

No adverse effects expected.

Adverse Reactions

A 26-year-old woman presented at hospital with chest pain. Her heart rate and blood pressure dropped temporarily during the course of monitoring and her urine digoxin level was 0.9 ng/mL (within the normal therapeutic range). Her only medication was a herbal preparation containing skullcap, black cohosh (Cimicifuga racemosa), lousewort (Pedicularis canadensis), hops (Humulus lupulus), valerian (Valeriana officinalis), and cayenne pepper (Capsicum annuum). The product was not available for analysis.[14]

Other adverse reactions have been reported for patients reportedly ingesting skullcap. However, there is doubt as to the botanical identity of the herb consumed.

Hepatotoxicity has been reported for tablets containing skullcap and valerian[15] and tablets that contained skullcap, mistletoe, kelp, wild lettuce, and motherwort[16] (although the presence of mistletoe was later questioned).[17] There is a possible link between the development of chronic active hepatitis and ingestion of herbal tablets in one reported case. The person was taking three herbal products: mistletoe; celery seed + guaiacum + burdock root + sarsaparilla; valerian + skullcap + passionflower and the following conventional medications: verapamil, chlordiazepoxide, thyroxine.[18]

The Welsh Drug Information Centre reported that it was informed of jaundice associated with ingestion of tablets containing skullcap only, skullcap in combination with valerian, and skullcap in combination with mistletoe. In four cases of hepatotoxicity resulting from these products, the authors were uncertain whether the patients had taken the tablets containing skullcap and valerian or the refor-

mulated product containing valerian, hops, asafoetida, and gentian.[15] A case was reported of hepatic failure in a man who was self-treating mild multiple sclerosis with zinc, skullcap tablets, and pau d'arco tablets. The authors postulated that the skullcap tablets were contaminated.[19]

A case of liver failure in a 45-year-old woman was reported. She had consumed more than 30 different herbal remedies, including chaparral, Jin Bu Huan, ephedra, valerian, skullcap, and barberry over the course of several months.[20] The content of the tablets and preparations was not verified, but chaparral and ephedra (see the monographs in this text) and Jin Bu Huan[21] are all known to cause hepatotoxicity.

The observed hepatotoxicity of the herbal tablets above is probably attributable to germander (Teucrium chamaedrys) or a closely related species, rather than most of the herbs mentioned, including skullcap. Germander has caused numerous cases of cytolytic hepatitis in France (more than 30 cases reported to 1997, including cases with positive rechallenge).[22,23] Case reports of hepatotoxicity caused by germander are not limited to T. chamaedrys,[24] other Teucrium spp. have caused hepatic failure.[25] One of the reported U.K. cases of skullcap-related hepatotoxicity was definitely due to T. canadense rather than skullcap.[24]

Interactions

None reported.

Safety in Children

Adverse effects are not expected if taken within the recommended dosage. Eclectic physicians recommended skullcap infusion to calm the teething child.[2]

Overdosage

Overdose of skullcap tincture is said to cause giddiness, stupor, confusion of mind, twitchings of the limbs, intermission of the pulse, and other symptoms indicative of epilepsy.[6] It is unclear whether two cases of skullcap poisoning, including one death, reported from the Riks Hospital in Norway in 1991 were due to skullcap, germander, or another herb.[26]

Toxicology

Neoclerodane diterpenes are present in many plant families.[27,28] They are bicyclic diterpenoids, the basic skeleton of which contains two substructures: C11-C16, and a decalin portion.[27] In the Labiatae there are three genera (*Teucrium*, *Scutellaria*, and *Ajuga*), whose aerial parts contain neoclerodane diterpenes. These diterpenes are typical taxonomic markers. Only three of the 200 diterpenes found in *Teucrium* occur in other genera (and not in *Scutellaria*). The *Scutellaria* diterpenes are present only in this genus (with the exception of one which is found in another family). The structures of the neoclerodanes in *Scutellaria* differ considerably from those isolated from *Teucrium*; particularly, those found in *Teucrium* frequently carry a furan group, and those from *Scutellaria* do not.[28]

The neoclerodane diterpene teucrin A was found to be responsible for the hepatotoxicity of germander after metabolic activation by cytochrome P450 3A (CYP3A). This has been shown both in vitro,[29] using hepatocytes, and in vivo (0.125 mg/kg, oral; furanoneoclerodane diterpenoid fraction).[30] The fraction produced hepatotoxicity similar to that observed in individuals who had consumed germander (midzonal hepatocyte necrosis). (Liver histology indicated that the hepatotoxicity [midzonal hepatocyte necrosis] of a given dose of freeze-dried extract of germander tea could be reproduced by administering the diterpenoid fraction [which contained almost 100% of the furanoneoclerodane diterpenoids of the germander tea dosage] at 10% of the tea dose. In both cases, the necrosis was observed in all animals.)

The authors suggested the following mechanism for the hepatotoxicity. The furanoneoclerodane diterpenoids may be activated by cytochrome P450 (especially CYP3A) into reactive metabolites (probably epoxides), which can be inactivated by glutathione conjugate formation, or may react with hepatic proteins leading to toxic hepatitis. Formation of reactive metabolites may also lead to immune reactions.[30]

In a further in vivo study, oral administration of teucrin A (150 mg/kg) was found to cause the same midzonal hepatic necrosis as that observed from germander extracts (2 to 4 g/kg ethanol extract, 0.5 g/kg acetone extract). It was further demonstrated that oxidation of the furan ring of teucrin A is involved in the initiation of hepatocellular injury. The authors point out that there may be other germander neoclerodane diterpenes and other structural groups contributing to the hepatotoxicity.[31] (A review published in 1987 noted that all the diterpenes from the *Teucrium* genus belonged to the neoclerodane group, and all contained the furan ring except for one in which the ring was oxidised.[32]) These two in vivo studies also demonstrated that slight differences in the source of plant material and extract preparation affected the dosage required to produce the hepatotoxicity.

Neoclerodane diterpenes have been isolated from skullcap and demonstrate similar hepatotoxic activity in vitro[33] as that obtained using the same model for germander diterpenes and teucrin A. These skullcap constituents caused apoptosis (programmed cell death).[29,34] The findings of the in vitro study were further investigated in an in vivo study. Intraperitoneal injection of the neoclerodane diterpenes from skullcap (20 mg) in mice caused activation of hepatic caspase 3 (an enzyme involved in potential DNA fragmentation). Liver histology revealed that, in one mouse, apoptosis without necrosis (pathological cell death) affected a few hepatocytes, in one mouse necrosis without apoptosis affected a few hepatocytes, and neither apoptosis nor necrosis was observed in the other 13 mice. In 16 mice treated with both skullcap diterpenes and a caspase inhibitor, apoptosis and necrosis were absent. All other fractions of the skullcap extract had no toxic activity. (*Scutellaria lateriflora* was obtained from a commercial herb supplier. The diterpenoids were verified as the neoclerodane diterpenes of skullcap [scutelaterins A, B, C] by thin-layer chromatography.)[33]

In terms of the hepatotoxicity demonstrated for neoclerodane diterpenes, the relevance of this to skullcap diterpenes is not clear. The skullcap neoclerodane diterpenes do not contain a furan ring (which is a structural requirement for the hepatotoxicity of teucrin A from germander) and hepatotoxicity has not been clearly demonstrated in vivo. Hepatotoxicity demonstrated in vivo for germander and its neoclerodane constituents is extensive and severe.

Regulatory Status

See Table 1 for regulatory status in selected countries.

Table **I**   **Regulatory Status for Skullcap in Selected Countries**

Australia	Skullcap is not included in Part 4 of Schedule 4 of the Therapeutic Goods Regulations.
UK & Germany	Skullcap is included on the General Sale List. It was not included in the Commission E assessment.
US	Skullcap does not have generally recognised as safe (GRAS) status. However, it is freely available as a "dietary supplement" in the US under DSHEA legislation (Dietary Supplement Health and Education Act of 1994).

REFERENCES

1. British Herbal Medicine Association's Scientific Committee: *British herbal pharmacopoeia,* Bournemouth, 1983, BHMA, pp 193-194.
2. Felter HW, Lloyd JU: *King's American dispensatory,* ed 18, rev. 3, vol 2, first published 1905, reprinted Portland, 1983, Eclectic Medical Publications, pp 1739-1741.
3. Gafner S, Batcha LL, Bergeron C, et al: *International Congress and 48th Annual Meeting of the Society for Medicinal Plant Research and the 6th International Congress on Ethnopharmacology of the International Society for Ethnopharmacology, Zurich, 3-7 September 2000,* Abstract P1E/08.
4. Bruno M: *Phytochem* 48:687-691, 1998.
5. Yaghmai MS: *Flavour Fragrance J* 3:27-31, 1988.
6. Grieve M: *A modern herbal,* New York, 1971, Dover Publications, pp 724-725.
7. Cook WH: *The physio-medical dispensatory,* first published 1869, reprinted Portland, 1985, Eclectic Medical Publications, pp 687-689.
8. Pharmaceutical Society of Great Britain: *British pharmaceutical codex 1934,* London, 1941, The Pharmaceutical Press, pp 941-942.
9. Hosokawa K, Minami M, Kawahara K, et al: *Planta Med* 66:270-272, 2000.
10. Osol A, Farrar GE, et al: *The dispensatory of the United States of America,* ed 24, Philadelphia, 1947, Lippincott, p 1580.
11. Mills SY: *The A-Z of modern herbalism,* London, 1989, Thorsons, pp 190-191.
12. Landes P, Adelson J: *HerbalGram* 2:3, 1985.
13. Lehmann R, Penman K, Leach D, et al: *International Congress and 48th Annual Meeting of the Society for Medicinal Plant Research and the 6th International Congress on Ethnopharmacology of the International Society for Ethnopharmacology, Zurich, 3-7 September 2000.* Abstract P1E/11.
14. Scheinost ME: *J Am Osteopathic Assoc* 101:444-446, 2001.
15. MacGregor FB, Abernethy VE, Dahabra S, et al: *BMJ* 299:1156-1157, 1989.
16. Harvey J, Colin-Jones DG: *BMJ (Clin Res Ed)* 282:186-187, 1981.
17. De Smet PAGM, Keller K, Hansel R, et al, eds: *Adverse effects of herbal drugs,* vol 2, Berlin, 1993, Springer-Verlag, pp 289-296.
18. Weeks GR, Proper JS: *Aust J Hosp Pharm* 19:155-157, 1989.
19. Hullar TE, Sapers BL, Ridker PM, et al: *Am J Med* 106:267-268, 1999.
20. American College of Gastroenterology 66th Annual Scientific Meeting: *Clinician Rev* 12:126, 131, 134, 2002.
21. McRae CA, Agarwal K, Mutimer D, et al: *Eur J Gastroenterol Hepatol* 14:559-562, 2002.
22. De Berardinis V, Moulin C, Maurice M, et al: *Mol Pharmacol* 58:542-551, 2000.
23. Castot A, Djezzar S, Deleau N, et al: *Therapie* 52:97-103, 1997.
24. De Smet PAGM, Keller K, Hansel R, et al, eds: *Adverse effects of herbal drugs,* vol 3, Berlin, 1997, Springer-Verlag, pp 137-144.
25. Mattei A, Rucay P, Samuel D, et al: *J Hepatol* 22:597, 1995.
26. Huxtable RJ: *Ann Intern Med* 117:165-166, 1992.
27. Bruno M, Piozzi F, Rosselli S: *Nat Prod Rep* 19:357-378, 2002.
28. Piozzi F: *Gazz Chim Ital* 127:537-544, 1997.
29. Lekehal M, Pessayre D, Lereau JM, et al: *Hepatology* 24:212-218, 1996.
30. Loeper J, Descatoire V, Letteron P, et al: *Gastroenterology* 106:464-472, 1994.
31. Kouzi SA, McMurtry RJ, Nelson SD: *Chem Res Toxicol* 7:850-856, 1994.
32. Piozzi F, Rodriguez B, Savona G: *Heterocycles* 25:807-841, 1987.
33. Haouzi D, Lekehal M, Moreau A, et al: *Hepatology* 32:303-311, 2000.
34. Fau D, Lekehal M, Farrell G, et al: *Gastroenterology* 113:1334-1346, 1997.

ST. JOHN'S WORT

Other common name: Hypericum
Botanical name: *Hypericum perforatum* L.
Family: Guttiferae
Plant part used: Aerial parts

Safety Summary

Pregnancy category B1: No increase in frequency of malformation or other harmful effects on the foetus from limited use in women. Evidence of increased foetal damage in animal studies exists, although the relevance to humans is unknown.

Lactation category CC: Compatible with breast-feeding but use caution.

Contraindications: Severe depression and see Interactions below. Do not use during lactation without professional advice.

Warnings & precautions: Known photosensitivity. Recommend against excessive exposure to full sun or artificial ultraviolet A (UVA) irradiation by patients taking high doses. Seek alternative treatment if a significant clinical response in depression is not apparent after 6 weeks. Discontinue use of St. John's wort at least 3 days prior to general anaesthesia. Also see Interactions below.

Adverse reactions: Most commonly: gastrointestinal symptoms; rarely: erythroderma, photosensitivity, delayed emergence from anaesthesia.

Interactions: Contraindicated with cyclosporin, digoxin, HIV nonnucleoside reverse transcriptase inhibitors and other protease inhibitors, irinotecan, and anticoagulant drugs. Caution is advised with photosensitising agents and selective serotonin reuptake inhibitors and other serotonergic agents, low-dose oral contraceptive pill, fexofenadine, mida-zolam, theophylline, simvastatin, and phenytoin.

Typical Therapeutic Use

A systematic review of clinical trials published in 2002 noted that St. John's wort extracts were superior over placebo (despite the negative results of two recently published American trials) for the treatment of mild to moderately depressed patients. St. John's wort demonstrated a therapeutic efficacy comparable to that of synthetic antidepressants.[1] Traditional indications for St. John's wort in Western herbal medicine include hysteria, nervous conditions with depression, neuralgia, and menopausal neurosis.[2,3]

Actions

Antidepressant, nervine tonic, antiviral, vulnerary, antimicrobial (topically).

Key Constituents

Key constituents of St. John's wort include the naph-thodianthrones (0.05% to 0.3%), especially hypericin and pseudohypericin (collectively referred to as total hypericin or hypericins), flavonoids, and phenolic compounds such as hyperforin.[4]

Adulteration

St. John's wort may be adulterated with other *Hypericum* spp.[5]

Typical Dosage Forms & Dosage

Typical adult dosage ranges are:
- 6 to 12 g/day of dried aerial parts or by infusion
- 6 to 12 mL/day of a 1:1 liquid extract
- 2 to 6 mL/day of a 1:2 liquid extract or equivalent in tablet or capsule form
- 900 mg/day of a concentrated extract (6:1) standardised to 0% to 3% of total hypericin

Contraindications

St. John's wort is not suitable for the treatment of serious depression with psychotic symptoms, suicidal risk, or signs and symptoms that are so severe that they do not allow the patient's family or work involvements to continue. However, in these cases, St. John's wort may be a valuable adjunct to other therapy, such as drug therapy and psychotherapy. Also see the Interactions section below. Do not use during lactation without professional advice.

Use in Pregnancy

Category B1: No increase in frequency of malformation or other harmful effects on the foetus from limited use in women. No evidence of increased foetal damage in animal studies, other than minor adverse effects observed at high doses in one study in mice. The relevance of this study to humans is unknown.

The dried herb administered orally to rats (1 g/kg/day) and rabbits (1.5 g/kg/day) did not adversely affect the health of the foetus or of the mother. The fertility of adult animals was not affected.[6] Maternal administration of St. John's wort (180 mg/kg/day) for 2 weeks before conception and throughout gestation did not affect the long-term growth and physical maturation of exposed mouse offspring.[7] A significant reduction in litter size and smaller offspring were observed in mice fed St. John's wort (136 mg/kg/day) prior to mating and throughout gestation.[8] Prenatal exposure to St. John's wort (180 mg/kg/day) in mice reduced male birth weight but did not affect long-term growth and physical development of exposed offspring.[9] Fertility, development of the embryo, prenatal and postnatal development were not influenced by oral administration of a standardised, aqueous methanol extract of St. John's wort (4:1 to 7:1) in rats and dogs (0.9 and 2.7 g/kg, for 26 weeks in both species).[10] A lack of toxicity was observed in mothers and offspring in a study in which rats were orally exposed to St. John's wort (up to 4.5 g/kg) from gestational day 3 until offspring weaning.[11]

At 24 weeks of her pregnancy a woman commenced St. John's wort (900 mg/day of a concentrated extract [6:1]) for treatment of depression, and took the preparation until 24 hours prior to delivery. She gave birth to a healthy baby whose physical examination and laboratory results were normal. The woman discontinued taking St. John's wort postpartum and initiated breastfeeding. The neonate developed jaundice on day 5. On day 20 the mother resumed St. John's wort (300 mg/day of the concentrated extract) and continued breastfeeding. Behavioural assessment of the baby at 4 and 33 days was normal.[12]

Use in Lactation

Category CC: Compatible with breastfeeding but use caution.

The constituents of St. John's wort penetrate the blood-brain barrier poorly and thus are likely to penetrate the breast milk compartment poorly as well.[13] A case study confirmed that hypericin did not pass into breast milk. Hyperforin is excreted at a low level. Hyperforin and hypericin were below the lower limit of quantification in the infant's plasma and no side effects were observed in the mother or infant.[14] A clinical study investigating St. John's wort intake during lactation found a statistically significant higher frequency of infant side effects (16.6%: colic, drowsiness, lethargy) for the mothers taking St. John's wort, compared to the frequency in those not exposed to the herb (two control groups, 0% and 3.3%: colic).[15]

Warnings & Precautions

Avoid in patients with known photosensitivity. Patients taking high doses of St. John's wort should not spend excessive amounts of time in the full sun and should avoid artificial UVA irradiation. Also see the Interactions section below.

Despite some concerns expressed in the literature, avoidance of foods that interact with monoamine oxidase–inhibiting drugs, such as tyramine-containing foods (cheeses, beer, wine) and drugs such as L-dopa, is not necessary.

If a significant response in depressive disorders is not apparent after 4 to 6 weeks, the treatment should be discontinued and other forms of treatment implemented. Practitioners should avoid dispensing the sediment from St. John's wort liquid extracts as it may be linked to adverse events.[16]

Effect on Ability to Drive or Operate Machinery

No adverse effects expected.

Adverse Reactions

Reviews assessing clinical trials to 1998 indicate that the tolerability of St. John's wort was good in randomised, controlled trials. Few adverse effects were noted. Postmarketing surveillance studies reported only rare and mild side effects. The proportion of patients reporting side effects for St. John's wort single preparation was 26.3%, compared to 44.7% for standard antidepressant drugs. Gastrointestinal symptoms were the most common adverse reactions recorded.[17,18] The most common adverse events (1 per 300,000 treated cases) among the spontaneous reports in the official German register to 2000 relate to reactions of the skin exposed to light.[19]

Reports of adverse reactions should be considered in the context of usage. St. John's wort extracts, used either as self-medication or as a prescribed antidepressant, accounted for 111 million daily doses sold in Germany in 1997, and the total European sales figure in 1998 amounted to US$6 billion.[20,21]

Table 1 documents adverse reactions information from clinical studies and case reports.[16,19,22-58]

Pharmacokinetic studies suggest that the phototoxic threshold level of hypericin is not reached with the normal doses of St. John's wort used for the oral treatment of depression.[63]

Interactions

Avoid prescribing St. John's wort if patients are taking the following drugs:

Table **1**   **Clinical Study Information and Case Reports of Adverse Reactions Possibly Associated with St. John's Wort or Hypericin Intake**

Case Reports/Clinical Studies	Adverse Reaction	Ref.
GENERAL		
Clinical study, 1990; 26 HIV patients; St. John's wort extract (containing 1 mg/day hypericin, 4 months)	Mild reversible liver enzyme elevations* in 5 patients, which returned to baseline after 1 month without hypericin	22
1 case, 1997; St. John's wort (dosage undefined) for 2 weeks prior to symptoms	Adynamic ileus, resolved gradually after discontinuation	23
1 case, 1998; St. John's wort (dosage not specified)	Multiple side effects, including rhinitis, mydriasis, flushing, headache, hyperventilation, palpitations, tremor	24
1 case, 2000; St. John's wort (dosage undefined) for 4 days prior to reaction, also taking a tricyclic antidepressant	Erythroderma on light-exposed and nonexposed areas	25
1 case, 2001; St. John's wort extract (0.9 g/day, 5 months), also taking olanzapine (atypical antipsychotic)	Hair loss	26
1 case, 2002; St. John's wort (dosage unspecified, for 1 week), had consumed aged cheeses and red wine prior to reaction	Hypertension, delirium	27
1 case, 2002; St. John's wort tablets (increased dose to 3 g/day, 3 months)	Delayed emergence from anaesthesia	28
1 case, 2000; St. John's wort (dosage unspecified, for 6 months)	Cardiovascular collapse during anaesthesia	29
1 case, 2003; St. John's wort tablets (5.4 g/day [of herb] corresponding to extract containing 0.3% hypericin, taken for 32 days)	Withdrawal syndrome	30
Retrospective case-control study (4 of 37 patients had taken St. John's wort), 2001; probable association with St. John's wort intake but further investigation required[†]	Elevated thyroid stimulating hormone	31
SEROTONIN SYNDROME?		
1 case, 2001; St. John's wort product (equivalent to 6 g/day dried herb, hypericin 3 mg/day; 2 months), also taking clonazepam (benzodiazepine); history of major depression, manic symptoms following treatment with selective serotonin reuptake inhibitor, heavy alcohol use	Flushing, diaphoresis, agitation, weakness of the legs, dry mouth, tightness in the chest, inability to focus	26

Continued

Table **I**   **Clinical Study Information and Case Reports of Adverse Reactions Possibly Associated with St. John's Wort or Hypericin Intake—cont'd**

Case Reports/Clinical Studies	Adverse Reaction	Ref.
I case, 2002; St. John's wort extract (0.45 g/day, 10 days), also taking buspirone (anxiolytic; serotonin receptor agonist); history of anxiety disorder	Nervousness, aggressiveness, hyperactivity, insomnia, blurred vision, confusion, disorientation	32

MANIA AND PSYCHOSIS

14 cases, 1998 to 2002; in those with and without a history of psychiatric illness including previous mania; St. John's wort taken in unspecified, normal and high doses, and in two cases with other supplements (ginkgo, valerian, melatonin), in four cases with, or just after, orthodox drugs	Mania	33-41
3 cases, 2000 to 2001; St. John's wort, no other medication; Alzheimer disease (1), schizophrenia (2)	Psychotic episode	42, 43

PHOTOSENSITIVITY

3 clinical studies; HIV and hepatitis C patients; oral hypericin in doses from 0.05 to 0.5 mg/kg/day‡	Mild to moderate, reversible photosensitivity	44-47
Clinical study, volunteers; threshold dose: St. John's wort extract containing 5 to 10 mg of hypericin	Mild increase in photosensitisation§	19
I case, 2001; St. John's wort at the time of laser treatment	Developed severe phototoxic reaction to laser light	48
I case, 1997; St. John's wort extract for a period of 3 years	Recurring elevated itching erythematous lesions in light-exposed areas; reversible and confirmed by provocation test	49
3 cases, 2000; one patient had lupus, one had psoriasis; St. John's wort oil used topically and orally; St. John's wort cream; St. John's wort pills (dosage unspecified).	Phototoxic reaction upon exposure to sunlight or, in one case, after phototherapy commenced	50

NEURAL HYPERSENSITIVITY

I case, 1998; St. John's wort (ground, whole plant, 500 mg/day for 4 weeks)	Subacute polyneuropathy	51
I case, 1998; St. John's wort (dosage not specified)	Hyperaesthesia	24
4 cases, 1997; St. John's wort high hypericin liquid extract‖	Sensory nerve hypersensitivity	16

SEXUAL DYSFUNCTION

I case, 2000; St. John's wort tablets (4 × 0.9 mg/day, for I week)	Erectile dysfunction and orgasmic delay¶	52
I case, 2001; St. John's wort taken for 9 months; history of psychiatric illness	Diminution of libido	53

Table 1   **Clinical Study Information and Case Reports of Adverse Reactions Possibly Associated with St. John's Wort or Hypericin Intake—cont'd**

Case Reports/Clinical Studies	Adverse Reaction	Ref.
ORGAN REJECTION		
6 cases, 1999 to 2001; St. John's wort taken concomitantly with cyclosporin	Tissue rejection as a result of a herb–drug interaction	54-58

*In another clinical study hypericin had no effect on liver enzymes.[45]

†This study has been criticised for design limitations, not adding meaningful scientific information to assess a potential association, and that no association was demonstrated.[59]

‡In two trials the phototoxic reaction involved areas exposed to light, in another trial the participants were advised to cover and protect their skin and to avoid excessive exposure to the sun. This higher dose would not likely be achieved by normal therapeutic doses of St. John's wort.

§Two clinical trials with volunteers have shown no significant changes of erythema threshold levels following exposure to UV radiation, visible light, and solar-stimulated radiation,[60] no significant change in UVB photosensitivity, but a moderate increase in UVA photosensitivity[61,62] for oral intake of St. John's wort extract (4.5 to 5.4 mg/day hypericin for 7 to 15 days). There was also an increased UVA photosensitivity in the subgroup of light-sensitive skin types.[62]

‖Based on the clinical experience of some Australian practitioners, there is evidence to suggest that these patients ingested St. John's wort preparations from late-harvested herb, which contained high levels of resinous constituents which would not normally be ingested (e.g., the sediment in a liquid extract). This can be avoided by not dispensing the sediment and by using St. John's wort harvested before or at the onset of full flowering.[16]

¶This reaction had also been induced in the patient by administration of sertraline (100 mg/day) several days earlier.

- immune suppressants (cyclosporin),[56,64-71]
- cardiac glycosides (digoxin) – for doses of St. John's wort greater than 1 g/day (dried herb equivalent),[72-74]
- HIV nonnucleoside reverse transcriptase inhibitors (nevirapine),[75]
- other HIV protease inhibitors (indinavir),[76]
- chemotherapeutic drugs (irinotecan),[77,78]
- anticoagulants (warfarin, phenprocoumon).[79,80]

Caution is advised in prescribing St. John's wort if patients are taking the following drugs:

- selective serotonin reuptake inhibitors (paroxetine, trazodone, sertraline)[81-85] and other serotonergic agents (nefazodone, venlafaxine)[84,86]
- very low dose oral contraceptive pill,[87,88]
- amitriptyline (tricyclic antidepressant),[89]
- fexofenadine (antihistamine),[90]
- midazolam (benzodiazepine),[91]
- theophylline (bronchodilator),[92]
- the 3-hydroxy-3-methylglutaryl coenzyme A (HMG-CoA) reductase inhibitor simvastatin (but pravastatin was unaffected),[93]
- phenytoin (theoretical concern),[94-96]
- photosensitising agents (delta-aminolaevulinic acid).[97]

No interactions have been observed between St. John's wort and the following:

- alcohol (in terms of cognitive capabilities, observed in a clinical trial),[98]
- tolbutamide (pharmacokinetic studies, healthy volunteers),[91]
- carbamazepine (pharmacokinetic studies, healthy volunteers),[99,100]
- cimetidine (pharmacokinetic study, healthy volunteers),[100]
- alprazolam (pharmacokinetic study, but only taken for 3 days),[101]
- dextromethorphan (pharmacokinetic study, but only taken for 3 days).[101]

A brief episode of acute delirium occurred in a woman taking loperamide (an opioid-based antidiarrhoeal agent), St. John's wort, and valerian.[102]

Two cases have been reported of a favourable interaction of St. John's wort with orthodox medication (phenothiazine antipsychotics, amitriptyline, and a tetracyclic antidepressant) in severe depressive states.[103] (In Chapter 6, see also Table 6-1 on herb-drug interaction.)

Safety in Children

St. John's wort was trialled successfully for the treatment of depression and psychovegetative disturbances in 101 children under 12 years old. Tolerability was good and no adverse events were reported.[104]

Overdosage

Overdose with St. John's wort in humans has not been reported. Phototoxicity could be expected to occur. Livestock poisoning due to St. John's wort has been reported in Australia, North Africa, Europe, the United States, New Zealand, and Iraq.[105]

Hypericism is a state of sensitivity to sunlight caused by the ingestion of certain *Hypericum* species rich in hypericin-type pigments that are transferred by the bloodstream to the skin. As a disease of livestock, it affects unpigmented portions of the skin of sheep, cattle, horses, goats, and pigs, depressing the central nervous system and rendering them hypersensitive to temperature change and handling. Goats are the most resistant.[106,107] *Hypericum perforatum* is more phototoxic to grazing animals if ingested at flowering than when young or dry. The minimum phototoxic dose of foliage for cattle and sheep is approximately 1% and 4% of live weight, respectively (i.e., 10 and 40 g/kg). Variation in susceptibility was observed within a herd.[106] Intragastric doses of 3 g/kg or more of dried *H. perforatum* aerial parts produced photosensitisation in 4- to 6-month-old calves. The first symptoms appeared 3 to 4 hours after exposure to the sun. Two calves which had been give the same dose but not exposed to sunlight passed soft faeces but showed no other clinical signs. A single dose of

1 g/kg produced no detectable effect when the calves were exposed to sunlight.[108]

Toxicology

Table 2 lists LD_{50} data recorded for extracts of St. John's wort flowers and indicates low acute toxicity.[109]

No signs of toxicity were observed following oral administration of the dried herb to rats (up to 2 g/kg/day for 1 year; up to 3 g/kg/day for 28 days) and to dogs (up to 2 g/kg/day for 1 year).[6] No toxicity was observed in rats fed ground, dried, fully flowering St. John's wort at 10% of their diet for 12 days, followed by 5% for another 107 days.[110]

Tolerance levels of <10 g/kg (wet weight of *H. perforatum*, eaten at the flowering stage) and <2.65 mg/kg for hypericin were demonstrated in sheep.[111]

Feeding freshly cut *H. perforatum* (4 to 16 g/kg/day, for 14 days) to sheep resulted in dermal and ocular effects (including blindness), hyperthermia, diarrhoea, with possible haemolytic anaemia and damage to the kidneys and liver. The severity of the effects increased with duration of exposure but not with dose.[105]

The no observed adverse effect level following single oral administration of a standardised, aqueous methanol extract of St. John's wort (4:1 to 7:1) was measured at >5 g/kg. Unspecific toxic symptoms, including slight load damage to the liver and kidneys, were observed after administration of 0.9 and 2.7 g/kg of extract (4:1 to 7:1), for 26 weeks in both toxicological models (probably rats and dogs).[10]

Toxic effects on testicular function were observed in groups of mice fed either St. John's wort (4 g/kg) or hypericin (200 mg/kg).[112]

Genotoxicity tests (in vitro and in vivo) showed no mutagenic effects following administration of

Table **2 LD_{50} Data Recorded for Extracts of St. John's Wort Flowers**

Substance	Route, Model	LD_{50} Value	Reference
Polyphenol fraction of St. John's wort flowers	i.p., mice	780 mg/kg	109
Lipophilic fraction of St. John's wort flowers	i.p., mice	4.3 g/kg	109
Water fraction of St. John's wort flowers	i.p., mice	2.8 g/kg	109

St. John's wort aqueous ethanol extract.[113] An antimutagenic effect was observed for St. John's wort in an in vitro assay using *Escherichia coli*.[114]

Regulatory Status

See Table 3 for regulatory status in selected countries.

Table **3** **Regulatory Status for St. John's Wort in Selected Countries**

Australia	St. John's wort is included in Part 4 of Schedule 4 of the Therapeutic Goods Regulations. The requirement for listing (automatic registration) is that, if the preparation is not a homoeopathic preparation and the proposed route of administration is oral, the label must include the following warning: "St. John's Wort affects the way some prescription medicines work. Consult your doctor".
UK & Germany	St. John's wort for external use is included on the General Sale List. It is covered by a positive Commission E monograph. St. John's wort is official in the *British Pharmacopoeia* 2002 and the *European Pharmacopoeia* 4.3.
US	St. John's wort is official in the *United States Pharmacopeia-National Formulary* (USP 26-NF 21, 2003). St. John's wort does not have generally recognised as safe (GRAS) status. However, it is freely available as a "dietary supplement" in the US under DSHEA legislation (Dietary Supplement Health and Education Act of 1994).

REFERENCES

1. Laakmann G, Jahn G, Schule C: *Nervenarzt* 73:600-612, 2002.
2. British Herbal Medicine Association's Scientific Committee: *British herbal pharmacopoeia*, Bournemouth, 1983, BHMA, pp 115-116.
3. Felter HW, Lloyd JU: *King's American dispensatory*, ed 18, rev 3, vol 2, first published 1905, reprinted, Portland, 1983, Eclectic Medical Publications, pp 1038-1039.
4. Bisset NG, ed: *Herbal drugs and phytopharmaceuticals: a handbook for practice on a scientific basis*, Stuttgart, 1994, Medpharm Scientific Publishers, pp 273-275.
5. American Herbal Pharmacopoeia: *St. John's wort – Hypericum perforatum: quality control, analytical and therapeutic monograph*, Santa Cruz, July 1997, American Herbal Pharmacopoeia.
6. *Psychotonin M: product information*, Darmstadt, 1992, Steigerwald Arzneimittelwerk GmbH.
7. Rayburn WF, Gonzalez CL, Christensen HD, et al: *Am J Obstet Gynecol* 184:191-195, 2001.
8. Gonzalez CL, Stewart JD, Rayburn WF, et al: *Neurotoxicol Teratol* 20:369, 1998.
9. Christensen HD, Rayburn WF, Coleman FH, et al: *Teratology* 59:411, 1999.
10. Leuschner J: *2nd International Congress on Phytomedicine, Munich, 11-14 September, 1996*, Abstract SL-80.
11. Cada AM, Hansen DK, LaBorde JB, et al: *Nutr Neurosci* 4:135-141, 2001.
12. Grush LR, Nierenberg A, Keefe B, et al: *JAMA* 280:1566, 1998.
13. McKenna DJ, Jones K, Hughes K, et al: *Botanical medicines: the desk reference for major herbal supplements*, ed 2, New York, 2002, Haworth Herbal Press, p 966.
14. Klier CM, Schafer MR, Schmid-Siegel B, et al: *Pharmacopsychiatry* 35:29-30, 2002.
15. Lee A, Minhas R, Shinya I: *Clin Pharmacol Therapeut* 67:130, Abstract No. PII-64, 2000.
16. Mills S, Bone K: *Principles and practice of phytotherapy: modern herbal medicine*, Edinburgh, 2000, Churchill Livingstone, p 550.
17. Linde K, Mulrow CD: *Cochrane Database Syst Rev* (2):CD000448, 2000.
18. Ernst E, Rand JI, Barnes J, et al: *Eur J Clin Pharmacol* 54:589-594, 1998.
19. Schulz V: *Schweiz Rundsch Med Prax* 89:2131-2140, 2000.
20. Ernst E: *Lancet* 354:2014-2016, 1999.
21. Wentworth JM, Agostini M, Love J, et al: *J Endocrinol* 166:R11-R16, 2000.
22. Cooper WC, James J: *Int Conf AIDS* 6:369 (abstract no. 2063), 1990.
23. Tran TL: *Curr Clin Strategies* 125:1022-1087, 1997.
24. Rey JM, Walter G: *Med J Aust* 169:583-586, 1998.
25. Holme SA, Roberts DL: *Br J Dermatol* 143:1127-1128, 2000.
26. Parker V, Wong AH, Boon HS, et al: *Can J Psychiatry* 46:77-79, 2001.
27. Patel S, Robinson R, Burk M: *Am J Med* 112:507-508, 2002.
28. Crowe S, McKeating K: *Anesthesiology* 96:1025-1027, 2002.
29. Irefin S, Sprung J: *J Clin Anesth* 12:498-499, 2000.
30. Dean AJ, Moses GM, Vernon JM: *Ann Pharmacother* 37:150, 2003.

31. Ferko N, Levine MA: *Pharmacotherapy* 21:1574-1578, 2001.
32. Dannawi M: *J Psychopharmacol* 16:401, 2002.
33. Nierenberg AA, Burt T, Matthews J, et al: *Biol Psychiatry* 46:1707-1708, 1999.
34. Moses EL, Mallinger AG: *J Clin Psychopharmacol* 20:115-117, 2000.
35. Guzelcan Y, Scholte WF, Assies J, et al: *Ned Tijdschr Geneeskd* 145:1943-1945, 2001.
36. Fahmi M, Huang C, Schweitzer L: *World J Biol Psychiatry* 3:58-59, 2002.
37. Spinella M, Eaton LA: *Brain Inj* 16:359-367, 2002.
38. Schneck C: *J Clin Psychiatry* 59:689, 1998.
39. O'Breasail AM, Argouarch S: *Can J Psychiatry* 43:746-747, 1998.
40. Nierenberg AA, Burt T, Matthews J, et al: *Biol Psychiatry* 46:1707-1708, 1999.
41. Barbenel DM, Yusufi B, O'Shea D, et al: *J Psychopharmacol* 14:84-86, 2000.
42. Laird RD, Webb M: *J Herb Pharmacother* 1:81-87, 2001.
43. Lal S, Iskandar H: *CMAJ* 163:262-263, 2000.
44. Pitisuttithum P, Migasena S, Suntharasamai P, et al: *Int Conf AIDS* 11:285 (abstract no. Tu-B-2121), 1996.
45. [No authors listed] *TreatmentUpdate* 12:4-5, 2001.
46. Gulick RM, McAuliffe V, Holden-Wiltse J, et al: *Ann Intern Med* 130:510-514, 1999.
47. Jacobson JM, Feinman L, Liebes L, et al: *Antimicrob Agents Chemother* 45:517-524, 2001.
48. Cotterill JA: *J Cosmet Laser Ther* 3:159-160, 2001.
49. Golsch S, Vocks E, Rakoski J, et al: *Hautarzt* 48:249-252, 1997.
50. Lane-Brown MM: *Med J Aust* 172:302, 2000.
51. Bove GM: *Lancet* 352:1121-1122, 1998.
52. Assalian P: *J Sex Marital Ther* 26:357-358, 2000.
53. Bhopal JS: *Can J Psychiatry* 46:456-457, 2001.
54. Bon S, Hartmann K, Kuhn M: *Schweiz Apoth* 16:535-536, 1999.
55. Ruschitzka F, Meier PJ, Turina M, et al: *Lancet* 355:548-549, 2000.
56. Karliova M, Treichel U, Malago M, et al: *J Hepatol* 33:853-855, 2000.
57. Barone GW, Gurley BJ, Ketel BL, et al: *Ann Pharmacother* 34:1013-1016, 2000.
58. Turton-Weeks SM, Barone GW, Gurley BJ, et al: *Prog Transplant* 11:116-120, 2001.
59. Hauben M: *Pharmacotherapy* 22:673-675, 2002.
60. Schempp CM, Muller K, Winghofer B, et al: *Arch Dermatol* 137:512-513, 2001.
61. Brockmoller J, Reum T, Bauer S, et al: *Pharmacopsychiatry* 30:94-101, 1997.
62. Roots I, Reum T, Brockmoller J, et al: *2nd International Congress on Phytomedicine, Munich, 11-14 September,* 1996.
63. Schempp CM, Muller KA, Winghofer B, et al: *Hautarzt* 53:316-321, 2002.
64. Ahmed SM, Banner NR, Dubrey SW: *J Heart Lung Transplant* 20:795, 2001.
65. Mai I, Kruger H, Budde K, et al: *Int J Clin Pharmacol Ther* 38:500-502, 2000.
66. Rey JM, Walter G: *Med J Aust* 169:583-586, 1998.
67. Barone GW, Gurley BJ, Ketel BL, et al: *Transplantation* 71:239-241, 2001.
68. Beer AM, Ostermann T: *Med Klin* 96:480-483, 2001.
69. Breidenbach T, Kliem V, Burg M, et al: *Transplantation* 69:2229-2230, 2000.
70. Breidenbach T, Hoffmann MW, Becker T, et al: *Lancet* 355:1912, 2000.
71. Moschella C, Jaber BL: *Am J Kidney Dis* 38:1105-1107, 2001.
72. Johne A, Brockmoller J, Bauer S, et al: *Clin Pharmacol Ther* 66:338-345, 1999.
73. Uehleke B, Mueller SC, Uehleke B, et al: *Phytomedicine* 7(Suppl. 2):20, 2000.
74. Durr D, Stieger B, Kullak-Ublick GA, et al: *Clin Pharmacol Ther* 68:598-604, 2000.
75. de Maat MMR, Hoetelmans RMW, Mathot RAA, et al: *AIDS* 15:420-421, 2001.
76. Piscitelli SC, Burstein AH, Chaitt D, et al: *Lancet* 355:547-548, 2000.
77. Mathijssen RH, Verweij J, de Bruijn P, et al: *J Natl Cancer Inst* 94:1247-1249, 2002.
78. Mansky PJ, Straus SE: *J Natl Cancer Inst* 94:1187-1188, 2002.
79. Yue QY, Bergquist C, Gerden B: *Lancet* 355:576-577, 2000.
80. Maurer A, Johne A, Bauer S, et al: *Eur J Clin Pharmacol* 55:A22, 1999.
81. Gordon JB: *Am Fam Phys* 57:950, 953, 1998.
82. Demott K: *Clinical Psychiatry News* 26:28, 1998.
83. Barbenel DM, Yusufi B, O'Shea D, et al: *J Psychopharmacol* 14:84-86, 2000.
84. Lantz MS, Buchalter E, Giambanco V: *J Geriatr Psychiatry Neurol* 12:7-10, 1999.
85. Waksman JC, Heard K, Jolliff H, et al: *Clin Toxicol* 38:521, 2000.
86. Prost N, Tichadou L, Rodor F, et al: *Presse Med* 29:1285-1286, 2000.
87. Bon S, Hartmann K, Kuhn M: *Schweiz Apoth* 16:535-536, 1999.
88. Yue QY, Bergquist C, Gerden B: *Lancet* 355:576-577, 2000.
89. Johne A, Schmider J, Brockmoller J, et al: *J Clin Psychopharmacol* 22:46-54, 2002.
90. Wang Z, Hamman MA, Huang SM, et al: *Clin Pharmacol Ther* 71:414-420, 2002.
91. Wang Z, Gorski JC, Hamman MA, et al: *Clin Pharmacol Ther* 70:317-326, 2001.
92. Nebel A, Schneider BJ, Baker RK, et al: *Ann Pharmacother* 33:502, 1999.
93. Sugimoto K, Ohmori M, Tsuruoka S, et al: *Clin Pharmacol Ther* 70:518-524, 2001.
94. Australian Therapeutic Goods Administration, Media Release, March 2000.
95. Breckenridge A: *Message from Committee on Safety of Medicines,* London, 29 February 2000, Medicines Control Agency.

96. Henney JE: *JAMA* 283:1679, 2000.

97. Ladner DP, Klein SD, Steiner RA, et al: *Br J Dermatol* 144:916-918, 2001.

98. Schmidt U, Harrer G, Kuhn U, et al: *Nervenheilkunde* 12:314-319, 1993.

99. Burstein AH, Horton RL, Dunn T, et al: *Clin Pharmacol Ther* 68:605-612, 2000.

100. Donath F, Johne A, Maurer A, et al: Cited in Uehleke B: *Report on the 6th International Scientific ESCOP Symposium, Bonn, Beethovenhalle, 10-11 May*, 2001.

101. Markowitz JS, DeVane CL, Boulton DW, et al: *Life Sci* 66:PL133-PL139, 2000.

102. Khawaja IS, Marotta RF, Lippmann S: *Psychiatr Serv* 50:969-970, 1999.

103. Schlich DF, Braukmann F, Schenk N: *Psycho* 13:440-447, 1987.

104. Hubner WD, Kirste T: *Phytother Res* 15:367-370, 2001.

105. Kako MD, al-Sultan II, Saleem AN: *Vet Hum Toxicol* 35:298-300, 1993.

106. Campbell MH, Delfosse ES: *J Aust Institute Agric Sci* 50:63-73, 1984.

107. Southwell IA, Campbell MH: *Phytochem* 30:475-478, 1991.

108. Araya OS, Ford EJH: *J Comp Pathol* 91:135-142, 1981.

109. Evstifeeva TA, Sibiriak SV: *Eksp Klin Farmakol* 59:51-54, 1996.

110. Garrett BJ, Cheeke PR, Miranda CL, et al: *Toxicol Lett* 10:183-188, 1982.

111. Bourke CA: *Aust Vet J* 78:483-488, 2000.

112. MohiAldeen KA, Khalil ABA: *Iraqi J Vet Sci* 14:A1-A8, 2001.

113. Okpanyi SN, Lidzba H, Scholl BG, et al: *Arzneim Forsch* 40:851-855, 1990.

114. Vukovic-Gacic B, Simic D: *Basic Life Sci* 61:269-277, 1993.

ST. MARY'S THISTLE

Other common name: Milk thistle
Botanical names: *Silybum marianum* (L.) Gaertn.
(*Carduus marianus* L.)
Family: Compositae
Plant part used: Fruit (sometimes referred to as seed)

Safety Summary

Pregnancy category B1: No increase in frequency of malformation or other harmful effects on the foetus from limited use in women. No evidence of increased foetal damage in animal studies.
Lactation category C: Compatible with breastfeeding.
Contraindications: Known allergy.
Warnings & precautions: Caution in patients with known hypersensitivity to plants in the Compositae family.
Adverse reactions: Rare cases of anaphylaxis have been reported.
Interactions: No precautions required on current evidence.

Typical Therapeutic Use

Controlled, double-blind clinical trials have demonstrated benefit for the concentrated extract of St. Mary's thistle in the treatment of toxic liver damage, chronic inflammatory liver disease, and hepatic cirrhosis.[1]

Traditional indications for St. Mary's thistle in Western herbal medicine include liver and gallbladder problems, including jaundice, hepatitis, and gallstones.[2,3]

Actions

Hepatoprotective, hepatic trophorestorative, antioxidant, choleretic.

Key Constituents

Constituents of St. Mary's thistle seed include flavanolignans (1.5% to 3%): silybin, silychristin, silydianin, and 2,3-dehydro derivatives. These flavanolignans are collectively known as silymarin.[4] The concentrated extract containing 70% to 80% silymarin is also referred to as "silymarin" in the literature.

Adulteration

No adulterants known.

Typical Dosage Forms & Dosage

Typical adult dosage ranges are:
- 4.5 to 8.5 mL/day of a 1:1 liquid extract
- 200 to 600 mg/day of a concentrated extract in tablet or capsule form standardised to 70% to 80% silymarin

Contraindications

Contraindicated in those with known sensitivity.

Use in Pregnancy

Category B1: No increase in frequency of malformation or other harmful effects on the foetus from limited use in women. No evidence of increased foetal damage in animal studies.

Oral administration of silymarin extract (100 mg/kg/day from days 8 to 17 of gestation in rabbits; 1 g/kg/day from days 8 to 12 in rats) failed to demonstrate teratogenic effects compared to controls.[5] A silymarin phospholipid compound demonstrated a foetoprotective effect against ethanol-induced behavioural deficits in rats.[6]

Use in Lactation

Category C: Compatible with breastfeeding.

Warnings & Precautions

Caution in patients with known hypersensitivity to plants in the Compositae family.

Effect on Ability to Drive or Operate Machinery

No adverse effects expected.

Adverse Reactions

Drug monitoring studies in 1995, investigating the concentrated extract (70% to 80% silymarin), indicated that adverse effects were recorded in 1% of patients, mainly as mild gastrointestinal complaints.[7,8]

A mild laxative effect was occasionally observed with St. Mary's thistle preparations.[9]

A systematic review identified adverse effects from St. Mary's thistle documented in 18 reports (which included seven randomised clinical trials, six cohort studies, and five case reports) and involving more than 7000 participants. (Research obtained to July 1999.) Three adverse effects were noted[10]:

- gastroenteritis associated with "collapse" from a combination containing St. Mary's thistle, with recurrent symptoms after rechallenge[11]
- anaphylactic reactions (two cases after ingestion of tea or standardised extract, respectively).[12,13]

Gastrointestinal symptoms were the most common adverse effect reported. Overall, their frequency was low, ranging from 2% to 10% in controlled trials, which was similar to that of placebo. Other adverse effects included dermatological symptoms and headaches, which were similar in frequency between placebo and treatment groups.[10]

Interactions

Oral administration of silymarin (100 mg/kg/day) to rats resulted in a significant increase in the activity of the mixed-function oxidation system (cytochrome P450; aminopyrine demethylation, *p*-nitroanisole demethylation). However, an experimentally induced reduction in activities of the mixed-function oxidation system and glucose-6-phosphatase could not be prevented by pretreatment with silymarin. In human volunteers, treatment with silymarin (210 mg/day for 28 days) had no influence on the metabolism of aminopyrine and phenylbutazone.[14]

Concentrated St. Mary's thistle extract at commonly administered doses did not interfere with indinavir therapy in patients with HIV.[15] Silymarin had no effect on reducing the drug-induced eleva-tion of serum alanine aminotransferase but reduced gastrointestinal and cholinergic adverse effects of tacrine in patients with Alzheimer's disease.[16]

Silybin has demonstrated pronounced iron-chelating activity in vitro.[17] However, whether this would result in enhanced or impaired iron absorption is unclear at this stage.

Safety in Children

No information available, but adverse effects are not expected. Children administered silymarin (200 mg/day for 30 days) showed no adverse clinical or biochemical effects.[18]

Overdosage

No incidents found in published literature.

Toxicology

The acute toxicology of silymarin is very low. Oral doses up to 20 g/kg/day for 7 days in mice and a single dose of 1 g/kg in dogs resulted in no mortality or signs of adverse effects. In chronic toxicity studies, rats treated orally with silymarin (1 g/kg/day for 15 days and 100 mg/kg/day for 22 weeks) did not demonstrate significant differences compared to control animals.[5]

Silymarin is capable of inducing DNA damage (measured as strand breaks in human cells) and inhibiting human cell growth. Toxicity was only seen at high micromolar concentrations (levels that are unlikely to be achieved in humans).[19]

Regulatory Status

See Table 1 for regulatory status in selected countries.

Table 1　**Regulatory Status for St. Mary's Thistle in Selected Countries**

Australia	St. Mary's thistle is not included in Part 4 of Schedule 4 of the Therapeutic Goods Regulations.
UK & Germany	St. Mary's thistle is included on the General Sale List. It is covered by a positive Commission E monograph.
US	St. Mary's thistle is official in the *United States Pharmacopeia-National Formulary* (USP 26-NF 21, 2003). St. Mary's thistle does not have generally recognised as safe (GRAS) status. However, it is freely available as a "dietary supplement" in the US under DSHEA legislation (Dietary Supplement Health and Education Act of 1994).

REFERENCES

1. Mills S, Bone K: *Principles and practice of phytotherapy: modern herbal medicine*, Edinburgh, 2000, Churchill Livingstone, pp 557-560.
2. Madaus G: *Lehrbuch der Biologischen Heilmettel*, vol I, Hildesheim, 1976, Georg Olms Verlag, pp 830-836.
3. Grieve M: *A modern herbal*, New York, 1971, Dover Publications, p 797.
4. Wagner H, Bladt S: *Plant drug analysis: a thin layer chromatography atlas*, ed 2, Berlin, 1996, Springer-Verlag, p 204.
5. Hahn G, Lehmann HD, Kurten M, et al: *Arzneim-Forsch* 18:698-704, 1968.
6. Busby A, Grange L la, Edwards J, et al: *J Herbal Pharmacother* 2:39-47, 2002.
7. Albrecht M, Frerick H, Kuhn H, et al: *Z Klin Med* 47:87-92, 1992.
8. Grungreiff K, Albrecht M, Strenge-Hesse A: *Med Welt* 46:222-227, 1995.
9. Blumenthal M, et al, eds: *The complete German Commission E monographs: therapeutic guide to herbal medicines*, Austin, 1998, American Botanical Council, pp 169-170.
10. Jacobs BP, Dennehy C, Ramirez G, et al: *Am J Med* 113:506-515, 2002.
11. ADRAC: *Med J Aust* 170:218-219, 1999.
12. Geier J, Fuchs T, Wahl R: *Allergolog* 13:387-388, 1990.
13. Mironets VI, Krasovskaia EA, Polishchuk II: *Vrach Delo* 7:86-87, 1990.
14. Leber HW, Knauff S: *Arzneim-Forsch* 26:1603-1605, 1976.
15. Piscitelli SC, Formentini E, Burstein AH, et al: *Pharmacotherapy* 22:551-556, 2002.
16. Allain H, Schuck S, Lebreton S, et al: *Dement Geriatr Cogn Disorder* 10:181-185, 1999.
17. Borsari M, Gabbi C, Ghelfi F, et al: *J Inorg Biochem* 85:123-129, 2001.
18. Mingrino F, Tosti U, Anania S, et al: *Minerva Pediatr* 31:451-456, 1979.
19. Duthie SJ, Johnson W, Dobson VL: *Mutat Res* 390:141-151, 1997.

TANSY

Botanical names: *Tanacetum vulgare* L. (*Chrysanthemum vulgare* [L.] Bernh)
Family: Compositae
Plant part used: Aerial parts

Safety Summary

Pregnancy category D: Has caused or is associated with a substantial risk of causing foetal malformation or irreversible damage.
Lactation category X: Contraindicated in breastfeeding (on the basis of the potential toxicity of the essential oil of tansy).
Contraindications: Pregnancy and lactation.
Warnings & precautions: Avoid in patients with known hypersensitivity to plants in the Compositae family. Do not exceed the recommended dosage range.
Adverse reactions: None found in published literature for doses taken within the recommended therapeutic range.
Interactions: No precautions required on current evidence.

Typical Therapeutic Use

Traditional indications for tansy in Western herbal medicine include nematode infestation, dyspepsia, amenorrhoea, and topically for scabies and swellings.[1,2]

Actions

Anthelmintic, carminative, spasmolytic, emmenagogue.

Key Constituents

The composition of the essential oil (and other constituents) varies with geographical location, chemotype, seasonal changes, and extraction method. More than 100 volatile monoterpenes and sesquiterpenes have been identified.[3,4] There are many chemotypes of tansy, a few are rich in β-thujone, many contain camphor.[3]

A survey in 1969 found the following levels of thujone in various tansy preparations of different origins: 1.8 to 167 mg/L (infusion), 9 mg/g (powder), and 0.4 mg/g (tincture).[5]

Other constituents include sesquiterpene lactones (including parthenolide), flavones, and sesquiterpene alcohols.[4,6]

Adulteration

Tanacetum vulgare should be distinguished from the highly poisonous plant tansy ragwort (*Senecio jacobaea*) which has a similar appearance.[7]

Typical Dosage Forms & Dosage

Typical adult dosage ranges are:
- 3 to 6 g/day of dried aerial parts or by infusion (use not recommended at these dosage levels)
- 3 to 6 mL/day of a 1:1 liquid extract (use not recommended at these dosage levels)
- 2 to 4.5 mL/day of a 1:5 tincture (safe dosage) or equivalent in tablet or capsule form

Contraindications

Contraindicated in pregnancy due to the presence of thujone.[1] Tansy is also contraindicated in lactation.

Use in Pregnancy

Category D: Has caused or is associated with a substantial risk of causing foetal malformation or irreversible damage.

Circumstantial evidence has linked tansy to cattle abortions, although animals rarely eat it.[8] Tansy oil has been used as an abortifacient by women, almost always with fatal results.[2,9,10] It is most likely that any abortifacient activity of tansy oil is due to a toxic effect, not a direct effect on the uterus.

Use of tansy herb as an abortifacient has also been reported.[10,11] Warm infusion of tansy was indicated in Eclectic texts for "tardy labour pains".[2]

Tansy oil did not stimulate contractions of uterine strips.[12] A herbal tea consisting of flowers of *Helichrysum arenarium* and tansy, peppermint and nettle leaf, licorice root, and *Rosa* spp. fruit had no adverse effect on rat embryos and foetuses or on postnatal development.[13]

Use in Lactation

Category X: Contraindicated in breastfeeding (on the basis of the potential toxicity of the essential oil of tansy).

Tansy imparts a bitter taste to the milk of cows that eat it.[14] Thujone produces a bitter taste in human milk.[15]

Warnings & Precautions

Avoid in patients with known hypersensitivity to plants in the Compositae family. Tansy has elicited positive reactions in the patch testing of Compositae-allergic patients.[16] A positive response was given by 3.1% to 4.5% of individuals tested with a Compositae plant mixture. Further testing with the single species indicated a high percentage of positive response for tansy.[17,18] Sesquiterpene lactones are considered to be responsible for the sensitisation and for cross-reactions with other Compositae plants.[19]

Tansy should not be taken in high doses over a prolonged period of time. Caution is advised in epilepsy due to the convulsant activity of thujone in the essential oil.

Effect on Ability to Drive or Operate Machinery

No adverse effects expected.

Adverse Reactions

Allergic contact dermatitis has been reported. There is an early report of severe dermatitis caused by ingestion of a tansy extract intended for desensitisation.[20]

Interactions

None known.

Safety in Children

No information available, but caution is advised. Tansy has been used traditionally for worm infestation in children.[1,2]

Overdosage

There are early reports of cases of human poisoning with tansy.[14] Fatal cases of poisoning from infusions of tansy have been reported.[5] Death from ingestion of tansy oil is recorded.[2] A case of poisoning from ingestion of tansy leaf tea in Switzerland has been reported recently.[21]

Toxicology

The toxicity of tansy will depend upon the chemotype and amount of constituents such as thujone. Although undefined, the studies shown in Table 1 probably used material containing thujone.[20,22]

A 1912 reference reports that cattle appear to have been poisoned by ingestion of tansy.[14]

Refer to the wormwood (*Artemisia absinthium*) monograph for toxicology and LD_{50} values for thujone.

Regulatory Status

See Table 2 for regulatory status in selected countries.

Table 1   **LD_{50} Data Recorded for Tansy**

Substance	Route, Model	LD_{50} Value	Reference
Tansy essential oil	Oral, dogs	3 mg/kg	20
Tansy essential oil	Oral, rats	1.15 g/kg	20
Tansy chloroform extract (1.7:1)	i.p., rats	285 mg/kg	22

Table **2**   **Regulatory Status for Tansy in Selected Countries**

Australia	Tansy is included in Schedule 4 of the SUSDP (Standard for the Uniform Scheduling of Drugs and Poisons), except in preparations containing <0.8% of oil of tansy. It is not included in Part 4 of Schedule 4 of the Therapeutic Goods Regulations.
UK & Germany	Tansy is not included on the General Sale List. It is covered by a negative Commission E monograph.
US	Tansy does not have generally recognised as safe (GRAS) status. However, it is freely available as a "dietary supplement" in the US under DSHEA legislation (Dietary Supplement Health and Education Act of 1994).

REFERENCES

1. British Herbal Medicine Association's Scientific Committee: *British herbal pharmacopoeia*, Bournemouth, 1983, BHMA, pp 205-206.
2. Felter HW, Lloyd JU: *King's American dispensatory*, ed 18, rev 3, vol 2, first published 1905, reprinted Portland, 1983, Eclectic Medical Publications, pp 1912-1913.
3. Keskitalo M, Pehu E, Simon JE, *Biochem Syst Ecol* 29:267-285, 2001.
4. Appendino G, Gariboldi P, Nano GM, *Phytochemistry* 22:509-512, 1983.
5. Jaspersen-Schib R: *Schweiz Apoth Ztg* 107:271-276, 1969.
6. Schinella GR, Giner RM, Recio MC, et al: *J Pharm Pharmacol* 50:1069-1074, 1998.
7. Burrill LC, Callihan RH, Parker R, et al: *Pacific Northwest Cooperative Extension Publication*, No. pnw175, 1994.
8. Mitich LW: *Weed Technol* 6:242-244, 1992.
9. Felter HW, Lloyd JU: *King's American dispensatory*, ed 18, rev 3, vol 2, first published 1905, reprinted Portland, 1983, Eclectic Medical Publications, p 1394.
10. Blaschek W, Ebel S, Hackenthal E, et al: *HagerROM 2002: Hagers Handbuch der Drogen und Arzneistoffe*, Heidelberg, 2002, Springer.
11. Gessner O: *Gift- und Arzneipflanzen von Mitteleuropa*, ed 3, Heidelberg, 1974, Carl Winter Universitatsverlag, pp 253-255.
12. Macht DI: *J Pharmacol Exp Therapeut* 4:547-552, 1912.
13. Ubasheev IO, Lonshakova KS, Matkhanov EI, et al: *Khim Farm Zh* 22:445-450, 1988.
14. Long HC: *Plants poisonous to live stock*, ed 2, revised, Cambridge, 1924, Cambridge University Press, pp 43-44.
15. Kobal G: *Electroencephalogr Clin Neurophysiol* 62:449-454, 1985.
16. Paulsen E, Andersen KE, Hausen BM: *Contact Dermatitis* 45:197-204, 2001.
17. Hausen BM: *Am J Contact Dermatitis* 7:94-99, 1996.
18. Paulsen E, Andersen KE, Hausen BM: *Contact Dermatitis* 29:6-10, 1993.
19. Hausen BM: *Dermatol* 159:1-11, 1979.
20. Opdyke DLJ: *Food Cosmet Toxicol* 14:869-871, 1976.
21. Jaspersen-Schib R, Theus L, Guirguis-Oeschger M, et al: *Schweiz Med Wochenschr* 126: 1085-1098, 1996.
22. Mordujovich-Buschiazzo P, Balsa EM, Buschiazzo HO: *Fitoterapia* 67:319-322, 1996.

THUJA

THUJA

Other common names: Arbor-vitae, tree of life, American white cedar
Botanical name: Thuja occidentalis L.
Family: Cuppressaceae
Plant part used: Leaf

Safety Summary

Pregnancy category D: Has caused or is associated with a substantial risk of causing foetal malformation or irreversible damage.
Lactation category X: Contraindicated in breast-feeding (on the basis of the potential toxicity of the essential oil of thuja).
Contraindications: Pregnancy and lactation.
Warnings & precautions: Do not exceed the recommended dosage range. Caution is advised for patients with underlying defects in hepatic haem synthesis and for those with epilepsy.
Adverse reactions: May cause headache when taken in high doses.
Interactions: No precautions required on current evidence.

Typical Therapeutic Use

Traditional indications for thuja in Western herbal medicine include bronchitis, warts, amenorrhoea, psoriasis, rheumatism, and uterine carcinoma. It is also applied to genital and anal warts.[1]

Actions

Antimicrobial, depurative, antiviral, antifungal.

Key Constituents

Thuja contains an essential oil consisting mainly of α-thujone (31% to 65%), β-thujone (8% to 15%), and fenchone (7% to 15%).[2] The chemical composition of the essential oil varies from tree to tree.[3] The essential oil content varies depending upon the season, but typically the herb contains 1.4% to 4%.[4] Percolation with 30% ethanol (v/v) produced a thujone yield of 37% (extract to dried herb). (The dried herb contained 3.8% essential oil of which 20% was thujone.) Increasing the ethanol content during percolation or using distillation increased the thujone yield substantially.[5] Thuja plicata contains a greater proportion of thujone in its essential oil than T. occidentalis.[6]

Adulteration

Morphological distinction between Thuja spp. is very difficult. Other species of Thuja (e.g., T. plicata) and species of Chamaecyparis may be mistaken for Thuja occidentalis.[4]

Typical Dosage Forms & Dosage

Typical adult dosage ranges are:
- 3 to 6 g/day of dried leaf or by infusion (use not recommended at these dosage levels)
- 6 mL/day of a 1:1 liquid extract (use not recommended at these dosage levels)
- 1 to 3 mL/day of a 1:5 tincture (safe dosage) or equivalent in tablet or capsule form
- 3 to 6 mL/day of a 1:10 tincture (safe dosage)

Contraindications

Pregnancy and lactation.

Use in Pregnancy

Category D: Has caused or is associated with a substantial risk of causing foetal malformation or irreversible damage.

Thuja infusion, tincture, and essential oil have been used as abortifacients in humans[7,8] (see also Overdosage section). Thuja may cause abortion by stimulating uterine contractions.[1] Thuja stimulated contractions in isolated uteri.[9] Anovulatory activity was not demonstrated in rabbits receiving an aqueous ethanol extract of thuja (whole plant, 100 mg/kg, oral). In this model ovulation was induced by copper acetate,[10] therefore anovulatory activity is likely to mean that ovulation was inhibited under these circumstances.

Anovulatory activity was also demonstrated in vivo in an early study for T. occidentalis leaf.[11]

Use in Lactation

Category X: Contraindicated in breastfeeding (on the basis of the potential toxicity of the essential oil of thuja).

Warnings & Precautions

Thuja should not be taken in high doses over a prolonged period of time. Caution is advised in epilepsy due to the convulsant activity of thujone in the essential oil.

α-Thujone demonstrated porphyrogenic properties in vitro and is theoretically hazardous to patients with underlying defects in hepatic haem synthesis, such as in acute hepatic porphyrias.[12]

Effect on Ability to Drive or Operate Machinery

No adverse effects expected.

Adverse Reactions

High doses of thuja may cause headache, which is attributed to the thujone content.[13]

Contact allergy to thuja has occurred in men working with it (such as dermatitis, pharyngitis, and bronchitis)[14] and from therapeutic use of the extract.[15] Erythema multiforme–like reactions have been reported in two patients who used thuja essential oil topically.[16]

Interactions

None known.

Safety in Children

No information available, but use should be restricted to the recommended dosage.

Overdosage

Intoxications have resulted from the ingestion of aqueous decoctions of thujone-containing plants for their supposed abortifacient action.[17] A review found that only 8 of the 18 reported poisonings with thuja from 1980 to 1992 could be evaluated, and concerned mostly babies that had chewed the leaves/branches.[4]

Several cases of poisoning from thuja oil have been recorded in which epileptiform convulsions occurred,[7,17] and death has followed its use as an abortifacient.[7] In one case of poisoning, the dosage of thuja oil ingested was a single dose of 10 mL, and in another case, 20 drops twice a day for 5 days.[17] Sixteen drops of thuja oil taken by a girl aged 15 caused unconsciousness followed by spasms and convulsions, with subsequent gastrointestinal irritation.[18]

Toxicology

Table 1 lists LD_{50} data recorded for thuja.[19,20]

Refer to the wormwood (*Artemisia absinthium*) monograph for toxicology and LD_{50} values for thujone.

Poisoning has occurred in horses eating the branches.[21]

Three tinctures of thuja did not induce mutagenesis in the *Salmonella*/mammalian microsome assay or the SOS-chromotest, even with metabolisation.[8]

Regulatory Status

See Table 2 for regulatory status in selected countries.

Table 1   **LD_{50} Data Recorded for Thuja**

Substance	Route, Model	LD_{50} Value (mg/kg)	Reference
Thuja essential oil	Oral, rats	83	19
Thuja tincture (1:10)	Oral, mice	440	20

Table **2**   **Regulatory Status for Thuja in Selected Countries**

Australia	Thuja is not included in Part 4 of Schedule 4 of the Therapeutic Goods Regulations.
UK & Germany	Thuja is not included on the General Sale List. It was not included in the Commission E assessment.
US	Thuja does not have generally recognised as safe (GRAS) status. However, it is freely available as a "dietary supplement" in the US under DSHEA legislation (Dietary Supplement Health and Education Act of 1994).

REFERENCES

1. British Herbal Medicine Association's Scientific Committee: *British herbal pharmacopoeia*, Bournemouth, 1983, BHMA, pp 210-211.
2. Tisserand R, Balacs T: *Essential oil safety: a guide for health care professionals*, Edinburgh, 1995, Churchill Livingstone, p 175.
3. Kamdem PD: *J Essent Oil Res* 5:279-282, 1993.
4. Blaschek W, Ebel S, Hackenthal E, et al: *HagerROM 2002: Hagers Handbuch der Drogen und Arzneistoffe*, Heidelberg, 2002, Springer.
5. Tegtmeier M, Harnischfeger G: *Eur J Pharm Biopharm* 40:337-340, 1994.
6. Banthorpe DV, Davies HS, Gatford C, et al: *Planta Med* 23:64-69, 1973.
7. Jungmichel G: *Dtsch Z Gesamte Gerichtl Med* 17:449, 1932.
8. Valsa JO, Felzenszwalb I: *Braz J Biol* 61:329-332, 2001.
9. Prochnow L: *Arch Int Pharmacodyn* 21:313-319, 1906.
10. Kamboj VP, Dhawan BN: *J Ethnopharmacol* 6:191-226, 1982.
11. Chaudhury RR: *Spec Rep Ser Indian Counc Med Res* 55:3-19, 1966.
12. Bonkovsky HL, Cable EE, Cable JW, et al: *Biochem Pharmacol* 43:2359-2368, 1992.
13. Zeylstra H: *Course material*, Tunbridge Wells, UK, 1983, College of Phytotherapy.
14. Mitchell J, Rook A: *Botanical dermatology: plants and plant products injurious to the skin*, Greengrass, 1979, Vancouver, p 244.
15. Grimm I: *Allergol* 14:272-274, 1991.
16. Puig L, Fernandez-Figueras MT, Montero MA, et al: *Contact Dermatitis* 33:329-332, 1995.
17. Millet Y, Jouglard J, Steinmetz MD, et al: *Clin Toxicol* 18:1485-1498, 1981.
18. Grieve M: *A modern herbal*, New York, 1971, Dover Publications, pp 176-178.
19. Opdyke DL: *Food Cosmet Toxicol* 12:843-844, 1974.
20. Lagarto Parra A, Silva Yhebra R, Guerra Sardinas I, et al: *Phytomed* 8:395-400, 2001.
21. Gessner O: *Gift- und Arzneipflanzen von Mitteleuropa*, ed 3, Heidelberg, 1974, Carl Winter Universitatsverlag, pp 251-253.

THYME

Botanical name: *Thymus vulgaris* L., *Thymus zygis* L.
Family: Labiatae
Plant part used: Leaf and flower

Safety Summary

Pregnancy category B2: No increase in frequency of malformation or other harmful effects on the foetus from limited use in women. Animal studies are lacking.
Lactation category C: Compatible with breastfeeding.
Contraindications: None required on current evidence.
Warnings & precautions: None required on current evidence.
Adverse reactions: Occasional allergic reactions.
Interactions: No precautions required on current evidence.

Typical Therapeutic Use

Traditional indications for thyme in Western herbal medicine include bronchitis, asthma, dyspepsia, and inflammation of the mouth and throat.[1]

The essential oil was effective against head lice in clinical trials.[2]

Actions

Expectorant, spasmolytic, antimicrobial, antioxidant.

Key Constituents

Essential oil containing antimicrobial and antioxidant[3,4] phenols, predominantly thymol and/or carvacrol[5] (up to 51% and 4% respectively of the essential oil,[6] but varying considerably with the many chemotypes of thyme), and their corresponding monoterpene hydrocarbon precursors (p-cymene and gamma-terpinene); the strongly antioxidant carnosol, rosmanols, galdosol, and carnosic acid[7]; flavonoids; acetophenone glycosides[8]; salicylates[9]; and a polysaccharide[10] with anticomplementary properties.[11]

Adulteration

Adulteration occurs rarely, with Moroccan thyme such as *Thymus satureioides* and wild thyme (*T. ser-*

pyllium).[12,13] There are several subspecies of *T. vulgaris* that do not have high levels of phenols and could be regarded as inferior substitutes.

There is innate protection against aflatoxin contamination,[14] and potentially preservative properties against other fungi[15] and some bacterial strains,[16] especially anaerobes such as *E. coli*,[17] *Campylobacter jejuni*, *Salmonella enteritidis*, *Staphylococcus aureus,* and *Listeria*.[18]

Typical Dosage Forms & Dosage

Typical adult dosage ranges are:
- 3 to 12 g/day of dried aerial parts or by infusion
- 2 to 6 mL/day of a 1:2 liquid extract or equivalent in tablet or capsule form
- 6 to 18 mL/day of a 1:5 tincture

Topical use: 5% infusion as a gargle or mouthwash.

Contraindications

None known.

Use in Pregnancy

Category B2: No increase in frequency of malformation or other harmful effects on the foetus from limited use in women. Animal studies are lacking.

A 1913 German reference indicates that thyme leaf has been used as an abortifacient.[19] A paste consisting of soap, potassium iodide, thymol, and astringents was used topically by doctors into the 1970s to procure abortion by an irritant action. However, it was regarded as carrying a high risk, with a number of maternal deaths attributed to its use.[20] Ingestion of large doses of thymol (>1 g) may produce abortion.[21]

Phyto-oestrogenic activity has been reported with in vitro competitive binding to oestradiol and progesterone receptors.[22]

Use in Lactation

Category C: Compatible with breastfeeding.

Warnings & Precautions

None required.

Effect on Ability to Drive or Operate Machinery

No adverse effects expected.

Adverse Reactions

Occasional cases of airborne contact dermatitis have been reported in farmers and other workers exposed to thyme dust.[23] One case of systemic allergy to thyme and other Labiates has been reported.[24] Five per cent of patients with crural ulceration were found to be positive on patch testing to thyme oil, perhaps present in dressings and topical treatments.[25]

Interactions

None known.

Safety in Children

Thyme oil should not be applied near the mouth and nose of infants and young children, as it can provoke a dangerous reflex breathing spasm.[26]

Otherwise, no adverse effects from thyme are expected.

Overdosage

No incidents found in published literature.

Toxicology

The LD_{50} of the essential oil by oral route in rats was reported variously as 2.84 g/kg and 4.7 g/kg.[27,28]

Oral doses (0.5 to 3.0 g/kg) of concentrated thyme extract (equivalent to 4.3 to 26.0 g/kg thyme) produced decreased locomotor activity and slight slowing down of respiration in mice. An increase in liver and testes weight was observed after chronic administration for 3 months (100 mg/kg, equivalent to 0.9 g/kg dried plant per day). Spermatotoxic activity was not demonstrated.[29] Thyme oil had no mutagenic or DNA-damaging activity in the Ames or *Bacillus subtilis* rec-assay.[30] Thymol was not mutagenic in the Ames assay.[31]

Regulatory Status

See Table 1 for regulatory status in selected countries.

Table 1   **Regulatory Status for Thyme in Selected Countries**

Australia	Thyme is not included in Part 4 of Schedule 4 of the Therapeutic Goods Regulations.
UK & Germany	Thyme is included on the General Sale List. It is covered by a positive Commission E monograph. Thyme is official in the *European Pharmacopoeia* 4.3.
US	Thyme does have generally recognised as safe (GRAS) status. It is freely available as a "dietary supplement" in the US under DSHEA legislation (Dietary Supplement Health and Education Act of 1994).

REFERENCES

1. British Herbal Medicine Association's Scientific Committee: *British herbal pharmacopoeia*, Bournemouth, 1983, BHMA, pp 212-213.
2. Veal L: *Complement Ther Nurs Midwifery* 2:97-101, 1996.
3. Lee KG, Shibamoto T: *J Agric Food Chem* 50:4947-4952, 2002.
4. Takacsova M, Pribela A, Faktorova M: *Nahrung* 39:241-243, 1995.
5. Cosentino S, Tuberoso CI, Pisano B, et al: *Lett Appl Microbiol* 29:130-135, 1999.
6. Hudaib M, Speroni E, Di Pietra AM, et al: *J Pharm Biomed Anal* 29:691-700, 2002.
7. Miura K, Kikuzaki H, Nakatani N: *J Agric Food Chem* 50:1845-1851, 2002.
8. Wang M, Kikuzaki H, Lin CC, et al: *J Agric Food Chem* 47:1911-1914, 1999.
9. Swain AR, Dutton SP, Trusswell AS: *J Am Diet Assoc* 85:950-960, 1985.
10. Chun H, Shin DH, Hong BS, et al: *Biol Pharm Bull* 24:941-946, 2001.
11. Chun H, Jun WJ, Shin DH, et al: *Chem Pharm Bull (Tokyo)* 49:762-764, 2001.
12. Blaschek W, Ebel S, Hackenthal E, et al: *HagerROM 2002: Hagers Handbuch der Drogen und Arzneistoffe*, Heidelberg, 2002, Springer.
13. Bisset NG, ed: *Herbal drugs and phytopharmaceuticals: a handbook for practice on a scientific basis*, Stuttgart,

1994, Medpharm Scientific Publishers, pp 470-472, 493-495.

14. Llewellyn GC, Burkett ML, Eadie T: *J Assoc Off Anal Chem* 64:955-960, 1981.

15. Soliman KM, Badeaa RI: *Food Chem Toxicol* 40:1669-1675, 2002.

16. Manou I, Bouillard L, Devleeschouwer MJ, et al: *J Appl Microbiol* 84:368-376, 1998.

17. Marino M, Bersani C, Comi G: *J Food Prot* 62:1017-1023, 1999.

18. Smith-Palmer A, Stewart J, Fyfe L: *Lett Appl Microbiol* 26:118-122, 1998.

19. Watt JM, Breyer-Brandwijk MG: *The medicinal and poisonous plants of southern and eastern Africa: being an account of their medicinal and other uses, chemical composition, pharmacological effects and toxicology in man and animal*, ed 2, Edinburgh, 1962, Livingstone, pp 528-529.

20. No authors listed: *Br Med J* 2:70, 1976.

21. Sollmann T: *A manual of pharmacology and its applications to therapeutics and toxicology*, ed 7, Philadelphia, 1948, WB Saunders, p 190.

22. Zava DT, Dollbaum CM, Blen M: *Proc Soc Exp Biol Med* 217:369-378, 1998.

23. Spiewak R, Skorska C, Dutkiewicz J: *Contact Dermatitis* 44:235-239, 2001.

24. Benito M, Jorro G, Morales C, et al: *Ann Allergy Asthma Immunol* 76:416-418, 1996.

25. Le Roy R, Grosshans E, Foussereau J: *Derm Beruf Umwelt* 29:168-170, 1981.

26. Naumann HH. In Dost FH, Leiber B: *Menthol and menthol-containing external remedies*, Stuttgart, 1967, Thieme, pp 99-107.

27. Skramlik E: *Pharmazie* 14:435-445, 1959.

28. Opdyke DLJ: *Food Cosmet Toxicol* 12:1003-1004, 1974.

29. Qureshi S, Shah AH, Al-Yahya MA, et al: *Fitotherapia* 62:319-323, 1991.

30. Zani F, Massimo G, Benvenuti S, et al: *Planta Med* 57:237-241, 1991.

31. Azizan A, Blevins RD: *Arch Environ Contam Toxicol* 28:248-258, 1995.

TRIBULUS LEAF

Other common name: Puncture vine
Botanical name: *Tribulus terrestris* L.
Family: Zygophyllaceae
Plant part used: Aerial parts

Safety Summary

Pregnancy category B3: No increase in frequency of malformation or other harmful effects on the foetus from limited use in women. Evidence of increased foetal damage in animal studies exists, although the relevance to humans is unknown.
Lactation category CC: Compatible with breast-feeding but use caution.
Contraindications: None required on current evidence. Do not use during pregnancy or lactation without professional advice.
Warnings & precautions: The use of herbs rich in saponins is possibly inappropriate in coeliac disease, fat malabsorption, and vitamins A, D, E, and K deficiency, some upper digestive irritations, and topically to open wounds. Caution in patients with preexisting cholestasis.
Adverse reactions: Herbs rich in saponins may cause irritation of the gastric mucous membranes and reflux.
Interactions: No precautions required on current evidence.

Typical Therapeutic Use

In open label clinical trials, tribulus leaf has demonstrated benefit for the treatment of male infertility and impotence, female infertility, and menopausal symptoms.[1-9]

There is little information available on the traditional use of tribulus leaf. In Ayurveda, the plant and fruit have been used to treat spermatorrhoea, gonorrhoea, impotence, uterine disorders after parturition, cystitis, painful urination, kidney stones, and gout.[10] The fruit is also used in traditional Chinese medicine (TCM).[11]

Actions

Tonic, aphrodisiac, oestrogenic in females (indirectly), androgenic in males (indirectly), fertility agent.

Key Constituents

The key constituents of tribulus leaf include the steroidal saponins, mainly furostanol glycosides (including protodioscin and protogracillin) and small quantities of spirostanol glycosides.[12-14] An analytical study published in 1956 reported the isolation of crude saponins in yields of 0.5% to 2% of dry mass of *Tribulus terrestris* plant.[15] Other constituents include phytosterols (β-sitosterol),[16] and possibly small quantities of harmala alkaloids[17] (although their presence is in doubt).

Adulteration

The root or fruit are often substituted for the leaf in modern products, but are unlikely to have the same therapeutic profile. A tribulus leaf product designated for performance enhancement was found to contain anabolic steroids.[18]

Typical Dosage Forms & Dosage

Typical adult dosage ranges are:
- 750 to 1500 mg/day of a concentrated extract standardised to contain 45% furostanol saponins calculated as protodioscin

Contraindications

None required on current evidence. Do not use during pregnancy or lactation without professional advice.

Use in Pregnancy

Category B3: No increase in frequency of malformation or other harmful effects on the foetus from limited use in women. Evidence of increased foetal damage in animal studies exists, although the relevance to humans is unknown.

According to TCM, tribulus fruit should be used with caution in pregnancy.[11]

Preliminary experiments with penned ewes fed *Tribulus terrestris* from days 85 to 130 of gestation indicated that lamb survival was decreased. Intravenous infusion of the ewe with an ethanolic extract of *T. terrestris* was noted to sometimes cause a decrease of foetal heart rate. In another experiment, five ewes began consuming 300 to 400 g of dried powdered *Tribulus terrestris* leaf (which was equivalent to at least 900 to 1200 g of the fresh plant) at days 103 to 112 of gestation and were then exposed to it for the next 18 to 44 days. No consistent change in foetal blood pressure or heart rate was observed following the ingestion of tribulus. The incidence of foetal breathing movements was significantly lower compared with the lucerne-fed group. This may indicate there was an effect on the functional maturation of some pathways in the central nervous system. Despite this, foetal growth and postnatal survival were not impaired.[19]

Use in Lactation

Category CC: Compatible with breastfeeding but use caution.

Warnings & Precautions

While it is unlikely that normal human doses of tribulus would cause the cholestasis observed in some animals after grazing on this plant, this possibility should be considered in unexplained cases of cholestasis in patients taking tribulus. Saponin-containing herbs are best kept to a minimum in patients with preexisting cholestasis.

The use of herbs rich in saponins is possibly inappropriate in coeliac disease, fat malabsorption, and vitamins A, D, E, and K deficiency, some upper digestive irritations and topically to open wounds.

Effect on Ability to Drive or Operate Machinery

No adverse effects expected.

Adverse Reactions

As with all herbs rich in saponins, oral use may cause irritation of the gastric mucous membranes and reflux.

Interactions

None known.

Safety in Children

No information available.

Overdosage

No incidents found in published literature for tribulus leaf.

Toxicology

LD_{50} values for oral administration of tribulus leaf extract in both mice and rats were greater than 10 g/kg, indicating very low toxicity. No lethality, change in behaviour or changes in biochemical indices were observed in rats given oral doses ranging from 75 to 300 mg/kg for 30 and 90 days, or dogs receiving 75 mg/kg for 180 days.[20] There was no evidence of induced carcinogenicity after oral administration of tribulus leaf extract at 50 or 150 mg/kg/day for 93 weeks in rats.[21]

Tribulus staggers is a unique neuromuscular disorder in sheep. Although its cause was suggested to be due to the accumulation of harmala alkaloids over a period of time, their presence in the plant was not confirmed using more sophisticated analytical techniques.[17,22] A photosensitisation reaction known as geeldikkop has been reported in livestock after consumption of tribulus.[23-25] Cholestasis is believed to play a role in the development of this disorder. These reactions have not been observed in humans, and are highly unlikely at the recommended dosage.

Regulatory Status

See Table 1 for regulatory status in selected countries.

Table 1   **Regulatory Status for Tribulus Leaf in Selected Countries**

Australia	Tribulus leaf is not included in Part 4 of Schedule 4 of the Therapeutic Goods Regulations.
UK & Germany	Tribulus leaf is not included on the General Sale List. It was not included in the Commission E assessment.
US	Tribulus leaf does not have generally recognised as safe (GRAS) status. However, it is freely available as a "dietary supplement" in the US under DSHEA legislation (Dietary Supplement Health and Education Act of 1994).

REFERENCES

1. Protich M, Tsvetkov D, Nalbanski B, et al: *Akush Ginekol* 22:326-329, 1983.
2. Kumanov F, Bozadzhieva E, Andreeva M, et al: *Savr Med* 4:211-215, 1982.
3. Viktorov IV, Kaloyanov AL, Lilov L, et al: MBI: Medicobiologic Information 1982. Cited in Zarkova S: *Tribestan: experimental and clinical investigations*, Sofia, Bulgaria, Chemical Pharmaceutical Research Institute.
4. Nikolova V, Stanislavov R: *Dokl Bolg Akad Nauk* 53:113-116, 2000.
5. Stanislavov R, Nikolova V: *Dokl Bolg Akad Nauk* 53:107-110, 2000.
6. Nikolaeva LF, Dedov II, Kurbanov VA: *Kardiologiia* 26:82-85, 1986.
7. Sankaran JR: *J Natl Integ Med Ass* 26:315-317, 1984.
8. Misra DN, Shukla GD: *Indian Med Gaz* 118:322-324, 1984.
9. Zarkova S: *Tribestan: experimental and clinical investigations*, Sofia, Bulgaria, Chemical Pharmaceutical Research Institute.
10. Kapoor LD: *CRC handbook of Ayurvedic medicinal plants*, Boca Raton, 1990, CRC Press, pp 325-326.
11. Bensky D, Gamble A: *Chinese herbal medicine materia medica*, Seattle, 1986, Eastland Press, pp 607-608.
12. Gjulemetowa R, Tomowa M, Simowa M, et al: *Pharmazie* 37:296, 1982.
13. Tomova M, Gyulemetova R, Zarkova S, et al: *Int Conf Chem Biotechnol Biol Act Nat Prod* (proc) 1st, 3:298-302, 1981.
14. Yan W, Ohtani K, Kasai R et al: *Phytochem* 42:1417-1422, 1996.
15. Enslin PR, Wells RJ: *S Afr Indust Chem* 10:96-97, 101, 1956.
16. Mahato SB, Sahu NP, Ganguly AN, et al: *J Chem Soc Perk Trans* 1:2405-2410, 1981.
17. Bourke CA, Stevens GR, Carrigan MJ: *Aust Vet J* 69:163-165, 1992.
18. Geyer H, Mareck-Engelke U, Reinhart U, et al: *Dtsch Z Sportmed* 51:378-382, 2000.
19. Walker D, Bird A, Flora T, et al: *Reprod Fertil Dev* 4:135-144, 1992.
20. Tanev G, Zarkova S: Toxicological studies on tribestan. Cited in Zarkova S: *Tribestan: experimental and clinical investigations*, Sofia, Bulgaria, Chemical Pharmaceutical Research Institute.
21. Gendzhev Z: *Tr Nauchnoizsled Khim Farm Inst* 15:241-250, 1985.
22. Lehmann R, Penman K: Private communication, 2002, MediHerb Research Laboratory, University of Queensland, St. Lucia, Queensland 4072, Australia.
23. Tapia MO, Giordano MA, Gueper HG: *Vet Hum Toxicol* 36:311-313, 1994.
24. Glastonbury JR, Doughty FR, Whitaker SJ, et al: *Aust Vet J* 61:314-316, 1984.
25. Waller GR, Yamasaki K, eds: *Saponins used in food and agriculture*. Part of series: *Advances in experimental medicine and biology*, vol 405, New York, 1996, Plenum Press, pp 381-382.

TURMERIC

Botanical names: *Curcuma longa* L. (*C. domestica* Val.)
Family: Zingiberaceae
Plant part used: Rhizome

Safety Summary

Pregnancy category A: No proven increase in the frequency of malformation or other harmful effects on the foetus despite consumption by a large number of women.
Lactation category C: Compatible with breastfeeding.
Contraindications: Obstruction of the biliary tract. Professional advice should be sought before using in patients with gallstones.
Warnings & precautions: Do not prescribe high doses long term. Patients applying topical doses should not be exposed to excessive sunlight.
Adverse reactions: Contact dermatitis, frequent bowel movements and mild gastric discomfort.
Interactions: It is preferable not to prescribe high doses (greater than 15 g/day) of turmeric concomitantly with antiplatelet or anticoagulant medication.

Typical Therapeutic Use

Turmeric demonstrated therapeutic benefit as an adjuvant therapy for precancerous conditions[1] and for gastric ulcers[2] in controlled trials. Benefits for dyspepsia[3] were observed in a randomised, double-blind, placebo-controlled trial. Traditional uses of turmeric in Western herbal medicine include jaundice and use as an aromatic stimulant.[4] Other traditional uses of turmeric include liver disorders, the common cold and fever in Ayurvedic medicine[5,6] and jaundice and amenorrhoea in traditional Chinese medicine (TCM).[7]

Actions

Antiinflammatory, antiplatelet, antioxidant, hypolipidaemic, choleretic, antimicrobial, carminative, depurative.

Key Constituents

Key constituents of turmeric rhizome include an essential oil (0.3% to 5%) containing sesquiterpene ketones and curcuminoids (3% to 5%), including curcumin and methoxylated curcumins.[8,9]

Adulteration

Confusion with *Curcuma xanthorrhiza* (Javanese turmeric) or *C. zedoaria* (zedoary) occurs rarely.[10,11] *C. aromatica* is often used as a medicinally interchangeable species in TCM.[7,12] Powdered turmeric is sometimes adulterated with synthetic dyes.[13]

Typical Dosage Forms & Dosage

Typical adult dosage ranges are:
- 1 to 4 g/day of dried rhizome powder
- 3 to 9 g/day of dried rhizome as an infusion
- 5 to 14 mL/day of a 1:1 liquid extract or equivalent in tablet or capsule form

Contraindications

According to the Commission E, turmeric is contraindicated where there is obstruction of the biliary tract and should be used only after seeking professional advice if gallstones are present.[14]

Use in Pregnancy

Category A: No proven increase in the frequency of malformation or other harmful effects on the foetus despite consumption by a large number of women as an item of diet. Turmeric decoction is traditionally used in Ayurvedic medicine to treat vomiting of pregnancy.[5] In the traditional medicine of Indonesia[15] and Fiji,[16] turmeric is given at parturition.

Oral administration of high doses of turmeric extract (100 mg/kg/day and 200 mg/kg/day) did not exhibit significant anovulatory activity in rabbits, but oral administration of the same doses to mice during the first week of pregnancy reduced the number of implantations and the number of pups delivered at term. No teratogenic effects were observed.[17] However, when turmeric (0.5% of diet) or curcumin (0.015% of diet) were fed to mice for 12 weeks there were no significant effects on the pregnancy rate, number of live and dead embryos, and number of implantations.[18,19] Similarly, no reproductive toxicity or teratogenic effects were observed in rats fed turmeric (50 mg/kg/day) for 52 weeks[20] or rats and rabbits fed curcumin (600 mg/kg/day and 1600 mg/kg/day) from days 6 to 15 postcoitus.[19]

Oral administration of very high doses of ethanol extract (15 g/kg) of *Curcuma* spp. used in TCM (*C. aromatica, C. zedoaria,* or *C. wenyujin*) prevented implantation or led to abortion in mice.[21] Similar antifertility effects were demonstrated with the essential oil administered by intraperitoneal, subcutaneous or intravaginal routes in mice and rabbits.[22] It is uncertain whether this research has any relevance to women wishing to conceive.

Turmeric rhizome decoction and extract had a stimulant effect on isolated uteri of mice and guinea pigs and on uterine fistulae of rabbits.[23]

Use in Lactation

Category C: Compatible with breastfeeding.

In the Fijian traditional medicine, turmeric is taken by new mothers to promote lactation.[16]

Warnings & Precautions

Do not prescribe high doses long term, or concomitantly with antiplatelet or anticoagulant medication.[24,25] Care should be exercised with women wishing to conceive and patients complaining of hair loss. Turmeric has traditional use as a topical depilatory[26,27] and hair loss has been reported in feeding experiments with rats.[28] However, the relevance of this research to human use is uncertain.

Patients applying topical doses of turmeric should not be exposed to excessive sunlight. Curcumin has demonstrated phototoxic effects in vitro.[25]

Effect on Ability to Drive or Operate Machinery

No adverse effects expected.

Adverse Reactions

Two cases of allergic contact dermatitis (due to curcumin in one case[29] and occupational use of turmeric in the other[26]) have been reported. A 2001 review of the literature concluded that allergic reactions to turmeric are rare.[30]

Generally, turmeric and curcumin have been well tolerated in clinical trials after oral and topical administration. One incident of localised itchiness was reported in a trial following topical application.[31] Frequent bowel movements and mild gastric discomfort may occur in individual patients.[7]

Interactions

Do not prescribe high doses (greater than 15 g/day) of turmeric concomitantly with antiplatelet or anticoagulant medication. Antiplatelet activity has been demonstrated in in vitro and in vivo studies, mainly with curcumin, suggesting turmeric may potentiate the effects of these medications.[25]

Safety in Children

No information available, but adverse effects are not expected.

Overdosage

No incidents found in published literature.

Toxicology

Table 1 lists LD_{50} data recorded for various fractions of turmeric, indicating low toxicity.[20,32,33]

In acute toxicity studies, no toxic effects were observed when either turmeric powder (2.5 g/kg and 30% of diet), an ethanol extract (0.3 to 3 g/kg) and curcumin (1 to 5 g/kg) were orally administered to mice, rats, guinea pigs, and monkeys.[19,34-37]

No toxic effects were observed in chronic oral toxicity studies of turmeric powder (0.1% to 10% of diet and 500 mg/kg/day) for up to 52 weeks, a hydroalcoholic extract (4 mg/kg/day) for 4 weeks, a petroleum ether extract (1 and 2 g/kg) for 4 weeks and curcumin (0.1% to 2% of diet; 400 to 800 mg/kg) for 8 to 13 weeks in mice, rats, and monkeys.[18-20,32,38,39]

Reduced weight gain due to decreased food intake was observed in rats fed turmeric powder (10% of diet) for 8 weeks. This effect was not found in the groups fed lower concentrations and was attributed to a change in the taste of the food.[38] However, reduced weight gain without an apparent reduction in food intake together with hair loss were observed in another study involving rats fed the same dietary concentration of turmeric for 4 to 7 weeks.[28]

Turmeric extract (0.05% to 0.25% of diet) and turmeric powder (0.2% to 5% of diet) caused some cases of hepatotoxicity when fed to mice for 14 days or longer.[40,41] The mouse is probably a susceptible species for turmeric-induced toxicity. Guinea pigs fed turmeric (500 mg/kg/day) or the alcohol extract (70 mg/kg/day) for 90 days showed no significant changes from controls, apart from reduced liver weight.[19]

Oral administration of a concentrated ethanolic extract of turmeric (100 mg/kg/day) for 90 days to mice significantly increased sperm motility, heart, lung, and caudae epididymis weights and significantly decreased red and white blood cell levels. No spermatotoxic effects were observed.[35] Subcutaneous injection of an alcohol extract (0.1 mL/day) to immature male rats for 10 days resulted in a significant decrease in testis weight and testosterone concentration.[26]

Administration of turmeric (4 g/kg) and curcumin (0.4 g/kg) for 14 to 21 days to lactating mice significantly elevated cytochrome b5 and cytochrome P450 levels in mothers and pups.[42]

Curcumin increased the formation of stomach ulcers in rats at a dose of 100 mg/kg, but not at 50 mg/kg, after oral administration for 6 days.[43] Lower doses of curcumin and turmeric have been shown to protect against ulceration.[44,45] The ulcerogenic effect was attributed to the reduced mucin secretion which also occurred at the higher dosage.[43]

Thyroid enlargement, pericholangitis, and epithelial changes in the kidney and bladder were observed in pigs fed turmeric oleoresin (296 and 1551 mg/kg/day) for 102 to 109 days. Reduced weight gain due to decreased food intake was observed only in the higher dose group.[46] Turmeric oleoresin consists mainly of curcuminoids and essential oil.

Undiluted turmeric oil was slightly irritating to rabbit skin in vivo after topical application, but was not irritating or photosensitising to hairless mice. Turmeric essential oil (4% in petroleum) was not irritating to the skin or sensitising in human volunteers.[33]

A turmeric ethanol extract and curcumin demonstrated cytotoxic effects after direct contact with mammalian cells in vitro, including chromosomal separation and breakage, mitotic arrest, and growth inhibition,[47-50] and a turmeric methanol extract demonstrated chromosomal damage in vivo in mice after intraperitoneal administration at a dose of approximately 6 g/kg of turmeric.[51] However, turmeric powder, the alcohol extract, oleoresin, and curcumin were not mutagenic in vitro in the Ames test,[52,53] and turmeric powder (0.5% of the diet and 1.25 to 5 g/kg) and curcumin (0.015% of the diet) were not mutagenic in vivo after oral administration.[18,19,54] Absence of mutagenicity in vitro was also reported for a turmeric ethanol extract following activation with caecal microorganisms.[55] Turmeric ethanol extract exhibited mutagenic activity in the Ames test in one study,[i] but not in another.[52]

Turmeric ethanol extract did not demonstrate toxicity in the brine shrimp assay.[56]

Regulatory Status

See Table 2 for regulatory status in selected countries.

Turmeric is widely consumed as a condiment throughout the world.

Table 1   **LD$_{50}$ Data Recorded for Various Fractions of Turmeric**

Substance	Route, Model	LD$_{50}$ Value (g/kg)	Reference
Turmeric petroleum ether extract	Oral, rats	12.2	32
Turmeric oleoresin	Oral, mice & rats	>10	20
Turmeric oil	Oral, rats	>5	33
Turmeric essential oil	Dermal, rabbits	>5	33

Table **2   Regulatory Status for Turmeric in Selected Countries**

Australia	Turmeric is not included in Part 4 of Schedule 4 of the Therapeutic Goods Regulations.
China	Turmeric is official in the *Pharmacopoeia of the People's Republic of China*, 1997. The usual adult dosage, usually administered in the form of a decoction, is listed as 3 to 9 g.
UK & Germany	Turmeric is not included on the General Sale List. It is covered by a positive Commission E monograph.
US	Turmeric does have generally recognised as safe (GRAS) status. It is freely available as a "dietary supplement" in the US under DSHEA legislation (Dietary Supplement Health and Education Act of 1994).

REFERENCES

1. Hastak K, Lubri N, Jakhi SD, et al: *Cancer Lett* 116:265-269, 1997.
2. Intanonta A, Meteeveeravongsa S, Viboonvipa P, et al: Report submitted to Primary Health Care Office. Thailand, 1986, The Ministry of Public Health.
3. Thamlikitkul MD, Bunyapraphatsara N, Dechatiwongse T, et al: *J Med Assoc Thai* 72:613-620, 1989.
4. Grieve M: *A modern herbal*, vol II, New York, 1971, Dover Publications, p 823.
5. Chopra RN, Chopra IC, Handa KL, et al: *Chopra's indigenous drugs of India*, ed 2, 1958; reprinted Calcutta, 1982, Academic Publishers, pp 325-327.
6. Kapoor LD: *CRC handbook of Ayurvedic medicinal plants*, Boca Raton, 1990, CRC Press, pp 149-150.
7. Chang HM, But PP: *Pharmacology and applications of Chinese materia medica*, vol 2, Singapore, 1987, World Scientific, pp 936-939.
8. Wagner H, Bladt S: *Plant drug analysis: a thin layer chromatography atlas*, ed 2, Berlin, 1996, Springer-Verlag, p 159.
9. Blaschek W, Ebel S, Hackenthal E, et al: *HagerROM 2002: Hagers Handbuch der Drogen und Arzneistoffe*, Heidelberg, 2002, Springer.
10. Bisset NG, ed: *Herbal drugs and phytopharmaceuticals: a handbook for practice on a scientific basis*, Stuttgart, 1994, Medpharm Scientific Publishers, pp 173-175.
11. Sen AR, Gupta PS, Dastidar NG: *Analyst* 99:153-155, 1974.
12. Raghuveer KG, Govindarajan VS: *J Assoc Off Anal Chem* 62:1333-1337, 1979.
13. Salmen R, Pedersen BF, Malterud KE: *Z Lebensm Unters Forsch* 184:33-34, 1987.
14. Blumenthal M, et al, eds: *The complete German Commission E monographs: therapeutic guide to herbal medicines*, Austin, 1998, American Botanical Council, p 222.
15. Dharma AP: *Indonesian medicinal plants*, Jakarta, 1987, Balai Pustaka, pp 148-149.
16. Cambie RC, Ash J: *Fijian medicinal plants*, 1994, CSIRO Australia, pp 64-65.
17. Garg SK: *Planta Med* 26:225-227, 1974.
18. Vijayalaxmi: *Mutat Res* 79:125-132, 1980.
19. Govindarajan VS: *Crit Rev Food Sci Nutr* 12:199-301, 1980.
20. Francis FJ: *Food Chem Safety* 173-206, 2002.
21. Chen ZZ, et al: Cited in *Abst Chin Med* 2:247-269, 1988.
22. An YX, et al: Cited in *Abst Chin Med* 2:247-269, 1988.
23. Zhang YZ: *Chin Med J* 5:400, 1955.
24. Blaschek W, Ebel S, Hackenthal E, et al: *HagerROM 2002: Hagers Handbuch der Drogen und Arzneistoffe*, Heidelberg, 2002, Springer.
25. Mills S, Bone K: *Principles and practice of phytotherapy: modern herbal medicine*, Edinburgh, 2000, Churchill Livingstone, pp 569-580.
26. Rao AJ, Kotagi SG: *IRCS Med Sci* 12:500-501, 1984.
27. Goh CL, Ng SK: *Contact Dermatitis* 17:186, 1987.
28. Patil TN, Srinivasan M: *Indian J Exp Biol* 9:167-169, 1971.
29. Hata M, Sasaki E, Ota M, et al: *Contact Dermatitis* 36:107-108, 1997.
30. Lucas CD, Hallagan JB, Taylor SL: *Adv Food Nutr Res* 43:195-216, 2001.
31. Kuttan R, Sudheeran PC, Josph CD: *Tumori* 73:29-31, 1987.
32. Arora RB, Basu N, Kapoor V, et al: *Indian J Med Res* 59:1289-1295, 1971.
33. Opdyke DLJ, Letizia C: *Food Chem Toxicol* 21:839-840, 1983.
34. Shankar TNB, Shantha NV, Ramesh HP, et al: *Indian J Exp Biol* 18:73-75, 1980.
35. Qureshi S, Shah AH, Ageel AM: *Planta Med* 58:124-127, 1992.
36. Srimal RC, Dhawan BN: *J Pharm Pharmacol* 25:447-452, 1973.
37. Wahlström B, Blennow G: *Acta Pharmacol Toxicol (Copenh)* 43:86-92, 1978.
38. Sambaiah K, Ratankumar S, Kamanna VS, et al: *J Food Sci Technol* 19:187-190, 1982.
39. Miquel J, Martinez M, Diez A, et al: *Age* 18:171-174, 1995.
40. Deshpande SS, Lalitha VS, Ingle AD, et al: *Toxicology Lett* 95:183-193, 1998.
41. Kandarkar SV, Sawant SS, Ingle AD, et al: *Indian J Exp Biol* 36:675-679, 1998.
42. Singh A, Singh SP, Bamezai R: *Cancer Lett* 96:87-93, 1995.
43. Gupta B, Kulshrestha VK, Srivastava RK, et al: *Indian J Med Res* 71:806-814, 1980.

44. Sinha M, Mukherjee BP, Mukherjee B, et al: *Indian J Pharmacol* 6:87-90, 1974.

45. Rafatullah S, Tariq M, Al-Yahya MA, et al: *J Ethnopharmacol* 29:25-34, 1990.

46. Billie N, Larsen JC, Hansen EV, et al: *Food Chem Toxicol* 23:967-973, 1985.

47. Goodpasture CE, Arrighi FE: *Food Cosmet Toxicol* 14:9-14, 1976.

48. Kuttan R, Bhanumathy P, Nirmala K, et al: *Cancer Lett* 29:197-202, 1985.

49. Blasiak J, Trzeciak A, Malecka-Panas E, et al: *Teratog Carcinog Mutagen* 19:19-31, 1999.

50. Donatus IA, Vermeulen S, Vermeulen NPE: *Biochem Pharmacol* 39:1869-1875, 1990.

51. Jain AK, Tezuka H, Kada T, et al: *Curr Sci* 56:1005–1006, 1987.

52. Nagabhushan M, Bhide SV: *Nutr Cancer* 8: 201-210, 1986.

53. Jensen NJ: *Mutat Res* 105:393-396, 1982.

54. Abraham SK, Kesavan PC: *Mutat Res* 136:85-88, 1984.

55. Shah RG, Netrawali MS: *Bull Environ Contam Toxicol* 40:350-357, 1988.

56. Mahmoud I, Alkofahi A, Abdelaziz A: *Int J Pharmacognosy* 30:81-85, 1992.

TYLOPHORA

Other common names: Indian ipecac, Indian lobelia
Botanical names: *Tylophora indica* (Burm. f.) Merr.
(*T. asthmatica* [L. f.] Wight & Arn.)
Family: Asclepiadaceae
Plant part used: Leaf

Safety Summary

Pregnancy category C: Has caused or is associated with a substantial risk of causing harmful effects on the foetus or neonate without causing malformations (due to its strong pharmacological activity).
Lactation category X: Contraindicated in breast-feeding.
Contraindications: Contraindicated in pregnancy and lactation.
Warnings & precautions: Short-term, intermittent use is recommended.
Adverse reactions: Sore mouth, loss of taste for salt, nausea and vomiting.
Interactions: No precautions required on current evidence.

Typical Therapeutic Use

Tylophora has demonstrated therapeutic benefit in the treatment of asthma in randomised, double-blind, placebo-controlled trials.[1-3] Traditional indications for tylophora in Ayurveda include bronchial asthma,[4] chronic bronchitis, catarrh, dysentery, and as an emetic.[5]

Actions

Antiasthmatic, antiinflammatory, immune depressant, antiallergic, emetic.

Key Constituents

The leaves of tylophora contain several alkaloids including tylophorine and tylophorinine. Tylophorine and tylophorinine levels are highest in the leaves during the flowering period of a rainy season (up to 0.5%).[6]

Adulteration

No adulterants known.

Typical Dosage Forms & Dosage

Typical adult dosage ranges are:
- 0.6 to 2 g/day of dried leaf or by infusion
- 1 to 2 mL/day of a 1:5 tincture for the first 10 to 14 days of each calendar month

Contraindications

Due to the strong pharmacological activity of tylophora, it is best avoided in pregnancy and lactation.

Use in Pregnancy

Category C: Has caused or is associated with a substantial risk of causing harmful effects on the foetus or neonate without causing malformations.

A review of the traditional Ayurvedic literature notes that tylophora (part and dose undefined) is listed as an abortifacient in one of the five sources checked. However, the definition of abortifacient was very broad and included emmenagogue, ecbolic (uterine contractor) and "antimetabolite".[7]

Use in Lactation

Category X: Contraindicated in breastfeeding.

Warnings & Precautions

It is generally recommended that tylophora be taken as a short-term, intermittent treatment because of potential immunosuppressive effects.

Effect on Ability to Drive or Operate Machinery

No adverse effects expected.

Adverse Reactions

Side effects of sore mouth, loss of taste for salt, and/or nausea and vomiting have been reported in randomised, double-blind, placebo-controlled trials.[1,2] These occurred in 52.6% of asthma patients receiving one chopped fresh leaf of tylophora per day, compared to 8.7% of those receiving placebo. They were only present for the 6 days when the leaf was being taken.[1] The frequency and severity of side effects were less when the alcohol extract was prescribed. Only 16.3% of asthma patients receiving the extract (40 mg/day) for 6 days reported side effects compared to 6.6% in the placebo group.[2] Nausea and vomiting may occur even at a low dose and especially in sensitive individuals.

A case of occupational dermatitis caused by working with extracts of tylophora alkaloids has been reported.[5]

Interactions

None known.

Safety in Children

No information available.

Overdosage

Three cases of fatal poisoning have been recorded in India after consumption of the plant or plant juice to treat gonorrhoea. Death occurred within 24 hours and symptoms of poisoning included acrid feeling in the mouth and throat, nausea, vomiting, purging, convulsions, and unconsciousness.[8]

Toxicology

The oral LD_{50} for ethanol extract of tylophora leaf was measured at 350 mg/kg in mice.[9]

Oral administration of single doses of a pure alkaloid fraction of tylophora (12.5 to 100 mg/kg) to rats caused inactivity, respiratory distress, salivation, nasal discharge, and diarrhoea. The oral LD_{50} was 35.32 mg/kg. In subacute oral toxicity studies over 15 days, doses of 1.25 mg/kg/day and 2.5 mg/kg/day did not produce signs of poisoning or death in rats. Doses above this level did produce fatalities (100% mortality within 7 days at 10 mg/kg/day). Liver enzyme activity significantly increased and was associated with morphological changes in the liver. Marked changes in the morphology of seminiferous tubules and spermatogenic activity were also observed.[10] The minimum lethal dose of tylophorine in frogs was 0.4 g/mg body weight. Tylophorine was nonirritant when applied topically to skin and conjunctiva, and had little or no local irritant reaction when injected subcutaneously and intramuscularly in mice and guinea pigs. Cardiac depressant activity has also been observed in animal experiments.[5]

Regulatory Status

See Table 1 for regulatory status in selected countries.

Table 1   **Regulatory Status for Tylophora in Selected Countries**

Australia	Tylophora is not included in Part 4 of Schedule 4 of the Therapeutic Goods Regulations.
UK & Germany	Tylophora is not included on the General Sale List. It was not included in the Commission E assessment.
US	Tylophora does not have generally recognised as safe (GRAS) status. However, it is freely available as a "dietary supplement" in the US under DSHEA legislation (Dietary Supplement Health and Education Act of 1994).

REFERENCES

1. Shivpuri DN, Menon MPS, Prakash D: *J Allergy* 43:145-150, 1969.
2. Shivpuri DN, Singhal SC, Parkash D: *Ann Allergy* 30:407-412, 1972.
3. Thiruvengadam KV, Haranath K, Sudarsan S et al: *J Indian Med Assoc* 71:172-176, 1978.
4. Nadkarni AK: *Dr KM Nadkarni's Indian materia medica*, ed 3, vol 2, Bombay, 1976, Popular Prakashan, p 332.
5. Chopra RN, Chopra IC, Handa KL, et al: *Chopra's indigenous drugs of India*, ed 2, 1958; reprinted Calcutta, 1982, Academic Publishers, pp 431-433, 689.
6. Karnick CR: *Planta Med* 27:333-336, 1975.
7. Casey RCD: *Indian J Med Sci* 14:590-600, 1960.
8. Chopra RN, Badhwar RL, Ghosh S: *Poisonous plants of India*, vol I, New Delhi, 1965, Indian Council of Agricultural Research, pp 585-587.
9. Atal CK, Sharma ML, Kaul A, et al: *J Ethnopharmacol* 18:133-141, 1986.
10. Dikshith TSS, Raizada RB, Mulchandani NB: *Indian J Exp Biol* 28:208-212, 1990.

VALERIAN

Botanical name: *Valeriana officinalis* L.
Family: Valerianaceae
Plant part used: Root and rhizome

Safety Summary

Pregnancy category B1: No increase in frequency of malformation or other harmful effects on the foetus from limited use in women. No evidence of increased foetal damage in animal studies.
Lactation category CC: Compatible with breast-feeding, but use caution.
Contraindications: None required on current evidence. Do not use during lactation without professional advice.
Warnings & precautions: In principle, herbal sedatives are best avoided in depression and insomnia marked by increasing restlessness during the early hours of the morning. Prescription of herbal sedatives should ideally be limited in duration. May slightly reduce vigilance.
Adverse reactions: Only minor adverse effects credibly reported.
Interactions: No clear evidence of interactions in current literature.

Typical Therapeutic Use

Clinical trials have supported use of valerian in improving sleep[1,2] (although there is some contention about the conclusiveness of these data[3]). Traditional indications for valerian in Western herbal medicine include insomnia, nervous tension, excitability, cramping, and migraine.[4]

Actions

Mild sedative, anxiolytic, spasmolytic, hypnotic.

Key Constituents

An essential oil containing monoterpenes (e.g., camphene and the pinenes) and sesquiterpenes. Sesquiterpene carboxylic acids (including valerenic acid and derivatives)[5]; gamma-aminobutyric acid (GABA).[6] Valepotriates are also present. Their decomposition products, baldrinals, can also be present, especially in aqueous–ethanolic extracts.[7,8] A lignan, hydroxypinoresinol, has been detected and

shown to competitively bind receptors sensitive to benzodiazepine.[9]

Adulteration

Adulteration can occur with other species of *Valeriana* such as *Valeriana wallichii* DC. (*Valeriana jatamansi* Jones, Indian valerian).[10,11] It was noted that valerian root can be adulterated with the poison *Veratrum album*.[12] *Valeriana officinalis* is a protected plant in France and wildcrafting is prohibited in Bulgaria.[13]

Typical Dosage Forms & Dosage

Typical adult dosage ranges are:
- 3 to 9 g/day of dried root and rhizome or by infusion
- 2 to 6 mL/day of a 1:2 liquid extract or equivalent in tablet or capsule form
- 9 to 15 mL/day of a 1:5 tincture

Contraindications

None known. Do not use during lactation without professional advice.

Use in Pregnancy

Category B1: No increase in frequency of malformation or other harmful effects on the foetus from limited use in women. No evidence of increased foetal damage in animal studies.

No problems were noted in three cases of intentional overdose with 2 to 5 g of valerian during weeks 3 to 10 of pregnancy.[14]

Very high oral doses of valerian (2.79 g/kg/day) reduced placental weights at days 1 to 8 and days 8 to 15 of gestation in rats. The foetal weights showed no significant changes compared to controls. The percentage of implantation loss and litter size were not significantly different from controls and major malformations were relatively rare. The herb was administered as an ethanol extract and the dose administered was the highest possible in which ethanol remained below the teratogenic threshold.[15]

There was no alteration in the fertility of female rats after oral administration of a mixture of valepotriates (6 to 24 mg/day, for 30 days). In another study, the valepotriate mixture was given from the first to the 19th day of pregnancy (6 to 24 mg/day), and did not effect foetotoxicity or external forma- tion. However, internal examination revealed an increase in the number of retarded ossifications after the higher doses (12 and 24 mg/kg).[16]

Use in Lactation

Category CC: Compatible with breastfeeding, but use caution.

Warnings & Precautions

In principle, herbal sedatives are best avoided in depression and insomnia marked by increasing rest- lessness during the early hours of the morning. Prescription of herbal sedatives should ideally be limited in duration. A very slight impairment of vigi- lance was noted in one study (see below).

Effect on Ability to Drive or Operate Machinery

Residual sedative effects were examined in a con- trolled study of 20 healthy volunteers, assigned to four groups receiving the following medication in single dose: tablets of valerian and hops (*Humulus lupulus*), valerian syrup, flunitrazepam, or placebo. Objectively measurable impairment of perform- ance on the morning after medication occurred only in the flunitrazepam group. Fifty percent of volunteers in the flunitrazepam group reported mild side effects compared with 10% from the other groups. Subjective perception of sleep quality was improved in all three medication groups compared to placebo. A very slight impairment of vigilance after taking valerian syrup was statistically significant, as was a retardation in the processing of complex information for the valerian tablets. It was suggested that herbal remedies offer a viable alternative to benzodiazepines with regard to impairment of vigilance on the morning after ingestion.[17]

Evidence from clinical trials to 1996 indicates that valerian does not cause excessive sedation.[18]

Adverse Reactions

A literature search of clinical trial data confirmed that there were few adverse effects reported in the short term.[19] Remarkably, in a randomised placebo- controlled, crossover study demonstrating the effi- cacy of valerian after long-term use in reducing insomnia, an extremely low number of adverse events occurred during valerian treatment—sub- stantially less than placebo.[20]

Only one minor stomach reaction was observed in a randomised, double-blind, controlled clinical trial with a product containing valerian and hops (*Humulus lupulus*).[21] In another study, 600 mg/day of concentrated valerian extract (LI 156) was at least as efficacious as 10 mg/day oxazepam in a double- blind, randomised comparison involving 202 patients. Over 6 weeks, adverse events occurred in 28.4% of patients receiving valerian extract and 36.0% of those receiving oxazepam. All adverse events were rated as mild to moderate.[22]

Three cases of "vivid dreams" were the only side effect reported in 19 patients observed taking valer- ian over 6 weeks in a controlled study.[23]

Unusual reports of toxic reactions to valerian root in Israel include nephrotoxicity, headaches, chest tightness, mydriasis, abdominal pain, and tremor.[24] In the absence of additional information, the link of these adverse reactions to valerian intake is highly suspect.

Reports of a link with valerian intake and liver damage in four cases[25] were not sustained, but the impression has been left in the literature.[26] (The product may have contained germander [*Teucrium chamaedrys*] masquerading as skullcap [*Scutellaria lateriflora*].[25] Refer to the skullcap monograph.) Acute hepatitis was reported in 1999 in a woman taking homoeopathic medications and valerian tea. Viral markers were negative and there was no evi- dence of autoimmune liver disease. A link to valer- ian intake was not established.[27]

A patient taking multiple medications experi- enced serious cardiac complications and delirium following a surgical procedure.[28] He had self-med- icated for "many years" with valerian root extract (0.53 to 2 g per dose, 5 times daily). However, due to his multiple medications, valerian could not be linked causally to his symptoms. It is possible that these other factors increased the risk of a with- drawal reaction.

Minor short-term hepatotoxic reactions to valerian have been impugned from observations of reactions to a proprietary mixture combining valerian with hyoscine and cyproheptadine; how- ever, direct evidence was not found and other ele- ments in the formula make any such assessment unsafe.[29]

Interactions

There are no data clearly identifying interactions between valerian and other drugs.

Speculative suggestions that valerian may potentiate antiepileptic prescriptions[30] have not been supported. Potentiation of anaesthetics has been postulated as a theoretical concern[31]; and many other published interactions, such as with sedatives, seem wholly speculative and even alarmist.[32]

A brief episode of acute delirium occurred in a woman taking loperamide (an opioid-based antidiarrhoeal agent), St. John's wort (Hypericum perforatum), and valerian.[33]

Compounding effects on mental symptoms in alcohol abusers have been adduced from a 51-year-old woman consuming alcohol (about 0.3 gallon/day of wine for more than 2 years), valerian tablets (approx. 2 to 4 g/day, 2 years) and Ginkgo biloba (unknown amount, unknown duration), who presented with fainting and psychosis. Alcohol intake was increased prior to the incident.[34]

Safety in Children

No information available. However, it is recommended that valerian be avoided in children under 3 years of age.[35]

Overdosage

A 1998 letter assessed 24 patients who were treated in a medical unit after taking an overdose of over-the-counter "valerian products". In 13 patients, other agents were involved. The amounts of valerian ingested were estimated in 23 patients and ranged from 0.15 to 4.5 g. Six patients developed vomiting. The clinical problems were mainly CNS depression and anticholinergic poisoning. One patient required ventilatory support and developed aspiration pneumonia. In 17 patients, liver function tests were performed and all were normal. All patients made a complete recovery.[36] A close reading of this letter shows that the culprit was not valerian at all. As well as containing valerian, the product contained the drugs hyoscine, hydrobromide, and cyproheptadine hydrochloride, which would readily explain the symptoms observed on overdose.

Valerian root at a dose of approximately 20 times the recommended dose caused benign symptoms (fatigue, abdominal cramp, chest tightness, lightheadedness, hand tremor, and mydriasis) which disappeared within 24 hours.[37]

Injection of an alcoholic valerian extract in one case of abuse led to transient fevers, pains and stiffness, headache, and mild liver function abnormalities. These may have been due to the presence of endotoxin in the injected material. The person recovered over the following 3 days.[38]

Toxicology

Table 1 lists LD_{50} data recorded for valerian extract and essential oil.[39,40]

Studies involving large doses of valerian extract (600 mg/kg/day; undefined extract strength, 1.5% valtrates) over 30 days in rats showed unremarkable adverse effects.[41]

No acute toxicity was found for the valepotriates valtrate, didrovaltrate and acevaltrate in mice after oral administration up to 4.6 g/kg.[42]

Valepotriates developed mutagenic activity only in the presence of S9 mix in the Salmonella/microsome test and the SOS-chromotest. Baldrinal and homobaldrinal showed mutagenic effects in both tests with and without metabolic activation.[43]

Regulatory Status

See Table 2 for regulatory status in selected countries.

Table 1   **LD_{50} Data Recorded for Valerian Extract and Essential Oil**

Substance	Route, Model	LD_{50} Value (g/kg)	Reference
Valerian extract*	i.p., mice	3.3	39
Valerian essential oil	Oral, rats	15	40

* Extracted with ether, then 90% ethanol to produce a 9.5:1 extract.

Table **2**   **Regulatory Status of Valerian in Selected Countries**

Australia	Valerian is not included in Part 4 of Schedule 4 of the Therapeutic Goods Regulations.
UK & Germany	Valerian is included on the UK General Sale List. It is covered by a positive Commission E monograph. Valerian is official in the *European Pharmacopoeia* 4.3.
US	Valerian is official in the *United States Pharmacopeia-National Formulary* (USP 26-NF 21, 2003). Valerian does not have generally recognised as safe (GRAS) status. However, it is freely available as a "dietary supplement" in the US under DSHEA legislation (Dietary Supplement Health and Education Act of 1994).

REFERENCES

1. Dominguez RA, Bravo-Valverde RL, Kaplowitz BR, et al: *Cultur Divers Ethnic Minor Psychol* 6:84-92, 2000.
2. Vorbach EU, Gortelmeyer R, Bruning J: *Psychopharmakotherapie* 3:109-115, 1996.
3. Stevinson C, Ernst E: *Sleep Med* 1: 91-99, 2000.
4. British Herbal Medicine Association's Scientific Committee: *British herbal pharmacopoeia*, Bournemouth, 1983, BHMA, pp 225-226.
5. Wagner H, Bladt S: *Plant drug analysis: a thin layer chromatography atlas*, ed 2, Berlin, 1996, Springer-Verlag, p 342.
6. Lapke C, Nündel M, Wendel G, et al: *Planta Med* 59(Suppl):627, 1993.
7. De Smet PAGM, Keller K, Hansel R, et al, eds: *Adverse effects of herbal drugs*, vol 3, Berlin, 1997, Springer-Verlag, p 166.
8. Bos R, Hendriks H, Scheffer JJC, et al: *Phytomedicine* 5:219-225, 1998.
9. Houghton PJ: *J Pharm Pharmacol* 51:505-512, 1999.
10. Bisset NG, ed: *Herbal drugs and phytopharmaceuticals: a handbook for practice on a scientific basis*, Stuttgart, 1994, Medpharm Scientific Publishers, pp 513-516.
11. American Herbal Pharmacopoeia: *Valerian root – Valeriana officinalis: analytical, quality control, and therapeutic monograph*, Santa Cruz, April 1999, American Herbal Pharmacopoeia.
12. Blaschek W, Ebel S, Hackenthal E, et al: *HagerROM 2002: Hagers Handbuch der Drogen und Arzneistoffe*, Heidelberg, 2002, Springer.
13. Lange D: *Europe's medicinal and aromatic plants: their use, trade and conservation*, Cambridge, 1998, TRAFFIC International, p XXVI.
14. Czeizel AE, Tomcsik M, Timar L: *Obstet Gynecol* 90:195-201, 1997.
15. Yao M, Brown-Woodman PDC, Ritchie H: *Birth Defects Res* (Part A) 67:141-147, Abstract 9, 2003.
16. Tufik S, Fujita K, Seabra Mde L, et al: *J Ethnopharmacol* 41:39-44, 1994.
17. Gerhard U, Linnenbrink N, Georghiadou C, et al: *Schweiz Rundsch Med Prax* 85: 473-481, 1996.
18. Mills S, Bone K: *Principles and practice of phytotherapy: modern herbal medicine*, Edinburgh, 2000, Churchill Livingstone, pp 581-589.
19. Pallesen S, Bjorvatn B, Nordhus IH, et al: *Tidsskr Nor Laegeforen* 122:2857-2859, 2002.
20. Donath F, Quispe S, Diefenbach K, et al: *Pharmacopsychiatry* 33:47-53, 2000.
21. Schmitz M, Jackel M: *Wien Med Wochenschr* 148:291-298, 1998.
22. Ziegler G, Ploch M, Miettinen-Baumann A, et al: *Eur J Med Res* 7:480-486, 2002.
23. Wheatley D: *Hum Psychopharmacol* 16:353-356, 2001.
24. Boniel T, Dannon P: *Harefuah* 140:780-783, 805, 2001.
25. MacGregor FB, Abernethy VE, Dahabra S, et al: *BMJ* 299:1156-1157, 1989.
26. Shepherd C: *BMJ* 306:1477, 1993.
27. Mennecier D, Saloum T, Dourthe PM, et al: *Presse Med* 28:966, 1999.
28. Garges HP, Varia I, Doraiswamy PM: *JAMA* 280:1566-1567, 1998.
29. Chan TY, Tang CH, Critchley JA: *Postgrad Med J* 71: 227-228, 1995.
30. Spinella M: *Epilepsy Behav* 2:524-532, 2001.
31. Ang-Lee MK, Moss J, Yuan CS: *JAMA* 286:208-216, 2001.
32. Abebe W: *Clin Pharm Ther* 27:391-401, 2002.
33. Khawaja IS, Marotta RF, Lippmann S: *Psychiatr Serv* 50:969-970, 1999.
34. Chen D, Klesmer J, Giovanniello A, et al: *Am J Addict* 11:75-77, 2002.
35. Schilcher H: *Phytotherapie in der Kinderheilkunde*, ed 2, Stuttgart, 1992, Wissenschaftliche Verlagsgesellschaft, pp 60–61.
36. Chan TY: *Int J Clin Pharmcol Ther* 36:569, 1998.
37. Willey LB, Mady SP, Cobaugh DJ, et al: *Vet Hum Toxicol* 37:364-365, 1995.
38. Mullins ME, Horowitz BZ: *Vet Hum Toxicol* 40:290-291, 1998.
39. Rosecrans JA, Defeo JJ, Youngken HW Jr: *J Pharm Sci* 50:240-244, 1961.
40. Skramlik E: *Pharmazie* 14:435-445, 1959.
41. Fehri B, Aiache JM, Boukef K, et al: *J Pharm Belg* 46:165-176, 1991.
42. Eickstedt KW, Rahman S: *Arzneim Forsch* 19:316-319, 1969.
43. von der Hude W, Scheutwinkel-Reich M, Braun R: *Mutat Res* 169:23-27, 1986.

WHITE HOREHOUND

Botanical name: *Marrubium vulgare* L.
Family: Labiatae
Plant part used: Aerial parts

Safety Summary

Pregnancy category B3: No increase in frequency of malformation or other harmful effects on the foetus from limited use in women. Evidence of increased foetal damage in animal studies exists, although the relevance to humans is unknown.

Lactation category C: Compatible with breastfeeding.

Contraindications: None required on current evidence. Do not use during pregnancy without professional advice.

Warnings & precautions: None required on current evidence.

Adverse reactions: None expected.

Interactions: No precautions required on current evidence.

Typical Therapeutic Use

Traditional uses of white horehound in Western herbal medicine include bronchitis, whooping cough, nonproductive cough, dyspepsia, and poor appetite.[1,2]

Actions

Expectorant, spasmolytic, bitter tonic.

Key Constituents

The aerial parts of white horehound contain bitter principles, including the diterpene marrubiin (0.1% to 1%) and flavonoids.[3]

Adulteration

White horehound has been adulterated with other *Marrubium* spp. such as *M. incanum*, *M. peregrinum*, *M. remotum* (*M. vulgare* × *M. peregrinum*), *M. anisodon*, and *M. candidissimum*.[4-6] Black horehound (*Ballota nigra*) as well as *Ballota hirsuta* have been adulterants.[4]

Typical Dosage Forms & Dosage

Typical adult dosage ranges are:
- 3 to 6 g/day of dried aerial parts or by infusion
- 3 to 6 mL/day of a 1:1 liquid extract
- 2 to 6 mL/day of a 1:2 liquid extract or equivalent in tablet or capsule form
- 9 to 36 mL/day of a 1:5 tincture

Contraindications

None known. Do not use during pregnancy without professional advice.

Use in Pregnancy

Category B3: No increase in frequency of malformation or other harmful effects on the foetus from limited use in women. Evidence of increased foetal damage in animal studies exists, although the relevance to humans is unknown.

Oral administration of white horehound decoction (2 mL/kg) to two pregnant guinea pigs resulted in four stillborn animals. This activity was not demonstrated in rats and mice.[7] The fresh plant juice is said to assist in discharging the placenta.[8]

Use in Lactation

Category C: Compatible with breastfeeding.

Warnings & Precautions

None required.

Effect on Ability to Drive or Operate Machinery

No adverse effects expected.

Adverse Reactions

Taken in large doses, white horehound is purgative.[9] The juice of the plant can cause contact dermatitis.[10]

Interactions

None reported.

Safety in Children

No information available, but adverse effects are not expected.

Overdosage

No incidents found in published literature, although overdosage may produce purgation.

Toxicology

In large doses, marrubiin disturbed heart rhythm.[8] Early studies note a decrease in the amplitude of heart contraction and lowering of blood pressure in isolated frog's heart for aqueous and alcoholic extracts.[11] However, in a more recent study, water extract of white horehound orally administered to normotensive rats had no effect on systolic blood pressure. Blood pressure was lowered in hypertensive rats.[12]

An extract of white horehound tested negative for in vitro mutagenic activity in the Ames test.[13]

Regulatory Status

See Table 1 for regulatory status in selected countries.

Table 1 **Regulatory Status for White Horehound in Selected Countries**

Australia	White horehound is not included in Part 4 of Schedule 4 of the Therapeutic Goods Regulations.
UK & Germany	White horehound is included on the General Sale List. It is covered by a positive Commission E monograph.
US	White horehound does have generally recognised as safe (GRAS) status and it is freely available as a "dietary supplement" in the US under DSHEA legislation (Dietary Supplement Health and Education Act of 1994).

REFERENCES

1. British Herbal Medicine Association's Scientific Committee: *British herbal pharmacopoeia*, Bournemouth, 1983, BHMA, pp 137-138.
2. British Herbal Medicine Association: *British herbal compendium*, vol 1, Bournemouth, 1992, BHMA, pp 218-220.
3. Wagner H, Bladt S: *Plant drug analysis: a thin layer chromatography atlas*, ed 2, Berlin, 1996, Springer-Verlag, p 77.
4. Bisset NG, ed: *Herbal drugs and phytopharmaceuticals*, Stuttgart, 1994, Medpharm Scientific Publishers, pp 317-318.
5. Osol A, Farrar GE, et al: *The dispensatory of the United States of America*, ed 24, Lippincott, Philadelphia, 1947, p 1515.
6. Blaschek W, Ebel S, Hackenthal E, et al: *HagerROM 2002: Hagers Handbuch der Drogen und Arzneistoffe*, Heidelberg, 2002, Springer.
7. Kchouk M, Chadli A: *Arch Inst Pasteur Tunis* 40:129-132, 1963.
8. Gessner O: *Gift-und Arzneipflanzen von Mitteleuropa*, ed 3, Heidelberg, 1974, Carl Winter Universitatsverlag, pp 337-338.
9. Grieve M: *A modern herbal*, New York, 1971, Dover Publications, p 416.
10. Mitchell J, Rook A: *Botanical dermatology: plants and plant products injurious to the skin*, Vancouver, 1979, Greengrass, p 362.
11. Aliev RK, Aliev AM: *Uch Zap Azerb Gos* 9:69-75, 1956.
12. El Bardai S, Lyoussi B, Wibo M, et al: *Clin Exp Hypertens* 23:329-343, 2001.
13. Schimmer O, Kruger A, Paulini H, et al: *Pharmazie* 49:448-451, 1994.

WILD CHERRY

Other common name: Black cherry
Botanical name: *Prunus serotina* Ehrh.
Family: Rosaceae
Plant part used: Bark

Safety Summary

Pregnancy category B3: No increase in frequency of malformation or other harmful effects on the foetus from limited use in women. Evidence of increased foetal damage in animal studies exists, although the relevance to humans is unknown.
Lactation category C: Compatible with breastfeeding.
Contraindications: None required on current evidence. Do not use during pregnancy without professional advice.
Warnings & precautions: Use only as needed and limit use as soon as practical. Long-term therapy is not advisable.
Adverse reactions: None found in published literature.
Interactions: No precautions required on current evidence.

Typical Therapeutic Use

Traditional indications for wild cherry bark in Western herbal medicine include the irritable and persistent cough of bronchitis, whooping cough, and nervous dyspepsia.[1]

Actions

Antitussive, mild sedative, astringent.

Key Constituents

Wild cherry bark contains a cyanogenic glycoside (prunasin), the amount of which varies with the time of collection, thickness, and type of bark,[2] and is typically 0.02% to 0.03%.[3] Prunasin is hydrolysed by a β-glucosidase into hydrocyanic acid, glucose, and benzaldehyde.[2,4] Spontaneous release of hydrogen cyanide from the plant depends on the presence of a specific glucosidase and water. The enzymes are extracellular and gain access to the glucosidase after physical disruption of the cell. The reaction is enhanced if the plant is soaked in water after crushing.[5]

Adulteration

Barks from other species of *Prunus* are occasionally substituted for the official species and an inferior form of the official bark has been observed in commerce.[6] Substitutes in the United States for *P. serotina* have included *P. virginiana* and *P. demissa*.[7] (Note: *P. virginiana* L. is likely to be an adulterant, but *P. virginiana* Mill. is an old botanical synonym for *P. serotina*.)

Typical Dosage Forms & Dosage

Typical adult dosage ranges are:
- 1.5 to 6 g/day of dried bark or by infusion
- 3 to 6 mL/day of a 1:1 liquid extract
- 2 to 4.5 mL/day of a 1:2 liquid extract or equivalent in tablet or capsule form

Contraindications

None known. Do not use during pregnancy without professional advice.

Use in Pregnancy

Category B3: No increase in frequency of malformation or other harmful effects on the foetus from limited use in women. Evidence of increased foetal damage in animal studies exists, although the relevance to humans is unknown (see below).

Malformation occurred after ingestion of *Prunus serotina* leaves, bark and fruit by pregnant sows.[8]

Use in Lactation

Category C: Compatible with breastfeeding.

Warnings & Precautions

Antitussives should be used only as needed and limited as soon as practical. Long-term therapy with antitussives is not advisable, particularly those that contain (albeit low) levels of cyanide.

Effect on Ability to Drive or Operate Machinery

No adverse effects expected.

Table I   **LD$_{50}$ Data Recorded for Withania**

Substance	Route, Model	LD$_{50}$ Value (g/kg)	Reference
Withania root aqueous extract	Oral, mice and rats	>1	21
Withania root alcohol extract	i.p., rats	1.26	22

reproductive organs, liver, kidneys, or adrenal glands. It was concluded that the effects were not due to changes in testosterone levels or toxicity.[26] In contrast, healthy males (aged 50 to 59 years) prescribed therapeutic doses of withania (3 g/day) for 1 year in a randomised, double-blind, placebo-controlled clinical trial reported an increase in their sexual performance.[1]

Regulatory Status

See Table 2 for regulatory status in selected countries.

Table **2**   **Regulatory Status for Withania in Selected Countries**

Australia	Withania is not included in Part 4 of Schedule 4 of the Therapeutic Goods Regulations.
UK & Germany	Withania is not included on the General Sale List. It was not included in the Commission E assessment.
US	Withania does not have generally recognised as safe (GRAS) status. However, it is freely available as a "dietary supplement" in the US under DSHEA legislation (Dietary Supplement Health and Education Act of 1994).

REFERENCES

1. Kuppurajan K, Rajagopalan SS, Sitaraman R, et al: *J Res Ayu Sid* 1:247-258, 1980.
2. Venkataraghavan S, Seshadri C, Sundaresan TP, et al: *J Res Ayu Sid* 1:370-385, 1980.
3. Kapoor LD: *CRC handbook of Ayurvedic medicinal plants*, Boca Raton, 1990, CRC Press, pp 337-338.
4. Wagner H, Norr H, Winterhoff H: *Phytomedicine* 1:63-76, 1994.
5. Atal CK, Gupta OP, Raghunathan K, et al: *Pharmacognosy and phytochemistry of Withania somnifera (Linn) Dunal (Ashwagandha)*, New Delhi, 1975, Central Council for Research in Indian Medicine and Homoeopathy, pp 47-53.
6. American Herbal Pharmacopoeia: *Ashwagandha root— Withania somnifera: analytical, quality control, and therapeutic monograph*, Santa Cruz, April 2000, American Herbal Pharmacopoeia.
7. Casey RCD: *Indian J Med Sci* 14:590-600, 1960.
8. Merzouki A, Ed-derfoufi F, Molero Mesa J: *J Ethnopharmacol* 73:501-503, 2000.
9. Garg LC, Parasar GC: *Planta Med* 13:46-47, 1965.
10. Singh S, Kumar S: *Withania somnifera: the Indian ginseng Ashwagandha*, Lucknow, 1998, Central Institute of Medicinal and Aromatic Plants (CIMAP), pp 131-177.
11. Lehmann R, Penman K: Information on file. St. Lucia, Queensland 4072, Australia, 2003 MediHerb Research Laboratory, University of Queensland.
12. Sharma S, Dahanukar S, Karandikar SM: *Indian Drugs* 23:133-139, 1985.
13. World Health Organization: *The use of traditional medicine in primary health care: a manual for health workers in south-east Asia*, New Delhi, 1990, WHO Regional Office for South-East Asia, pp 96-97.
14. World Health Organization: *The use of traditional medicine in primary health care: a manual for health workers in south-east Asia*, New Delhi, 1990, WHO Regional Office for South-East Asia, p 132.
15. Shelukar PS, Dakshinkar NP, Sarode DB, et al: *Indian Vet J* 77:605-607, 2000.
16. Selukar PS, Dakshinkar NP, Sarode DB: *Indian Vet J* 78:249-250, 2001.
17. Mishra LC, Singh BB, Dagenais S. *Altern Med Rev* 5:334-346, 2000.
18. Chandha E, ed: *The wealth of India: a dictionary of Indian raw materials and industrial products*, vol 10, New Delhi, 1976, Council of Scientific and Industrial Research. Cited in American Herbal Pharmacopoeia: *Ashwagandha root – Withania somnifera: analytical, quality control, and therapeutic monograph*, Santa Cruz, April 2000, American Herbal Pharmacopoeia.
19. Kulkarni SK, George B, Mathur R: *Phytother Res* 12:451-453, 1998.
20. Mehta AK, Binkley P, Gandhi SS, et al: *Indian J Med Res* 94:312-315, 1991.
21. Rege NN, Thatte UM, Dahanukar SA: *Phytother Res* 13:275-291, 1999.

22. Sharada AC, Soloman FE, Devi PU: *Int J Pharmacog* 31:205-212, 1993.

23. Dhuley JN: *J Ethnopharmacol* 70:57-63, 2000.

24. Singh N, Singh SP, Nath R, et al: *Int J Crude Drug Res* 24:90-100, 1986.

25. Arseculeratne SN, Gunatilaka AA, Panabokke RG: *J Ethnopharmacol* 13:323-335, 1985.

26. Ilayperuma I, Ratnasooriya WD, Weerasooriya TR: *Asian J Androl* 4:295-298, 2002.

WORMWOOD

Botanical name: *Artemisia absinthium* L.
Family: Compositae
Plant part used: Aerial parts

Safety Summary

Pregnancy category D: Has caused or is associated with a substantial risk of causing foetal malformation or irreversible damage.
Lactation category X: Contraindicated in breast-feeding (on the basis of the potential toxicity of the essential oil of wormwood).
Contraindications: Pregnancy and lactation, hyperacidity, known sensitivity to wormwood or the Compositae family.
Warnings & precautions: Do not exceed the recommended dosage range. Caution is advised for patients with underlying defects in hepatic haem synthesis, and for patients with known hypersensitivity to plants in the Compositae family.
Adverse reactions: Hypersensitivity reactions have occurred.
Interactions: No precautions required on current evidence.

Typical Therapeutic Use

Traditional indications for wormwood in Western herbal medicine include anorexia, atonic dyspepsia, and worm infestation.[1]

Actions

Bitter tonic, anthelmintic, antiparasitic.

Key Constituents

Constituents of the aerial parts of wormwood include bitter substances (sesquiterpene lactones, mainly absinthin) and an essential oil (0.2% to 1.5%) containing mainly terpenes. The composition of the essential oil varies depending upon geographical location,[2] but typically contains mainly β-thujone (46%) and linalyl acetate (28%) and a small amount of α-thujone.[3] α-Thujone and β-thujone are isomers and, although not always defined as such in the quoted literature, "thujone" is a mixture of both isomers.

Adulteration

Occasionally, wormwood is adulterated with *Artemisia vulgaris* (mugwort).[2]

Typical Dosage Forms & Dosage

Typical adult dosage ranges are:
- 3 to 6 g/day of dried aerial parts or by infusion (use not recommended at these dosage levels)
- 3 to 6 mL/day of a 1:1 liquid extract (use not recommended at these dosage levels)
- 0.7 to 3 mL/day of a 1:5 tincture* (safe dosages), or equivalent in tablet or capsule form

A review of toxicological information regarding thujone and thujone-containing liquors published in 1964 estimated that an oral daily dose of 1.25 mg/kg thujone can be consumed without health risk.[4] The estimated amount of thujone exposure from good quality commercial tinctures taken at the recommended dosage is 0.005 to 0.021 mg/day,[5] which is around four orders of magnitude below this estimated safe level (1.25 mg/kg = 87.5 mg for an adult weighing 70 kg). Moreover, this safe exposure level is based on consistent intake via food and beverages, whereas the wormwood tincture is only recommended for short-term use.

Contraindications

Pregnancy and lactation, hyperacidity.[6]

Persons with known sensitivity to wormwood or other members of the Compositae family (such as ragweed, daisies, and chrysanthemums) should avoid use of wormwood.

Use in Pregnancy

Category D: Has caused or is associated with a substantial risk of causing foetal malformation or irreversible damage.

Significant antiimplantation activity was demonstrated after administration of wormwood ethanol extract to rats.[7] Abuse with high doses of wormwood (presumably oil) resulting in toxic effects or death has been reported in the context of its use to procure abortion.[8]

---

*Doses at the high end of the dosage range are for short-term use only.

Use in Lactation

Category X: Contraindicated in breastfeeding (on the basis of the potential toxicity of the essential oil of wormwood).

Warnings & Precautions

Do not exceed the recommended dosage range.

α-Thujone demonstrated porphyrogenic properties in vitro and is theoretically hazardous to patients with underlying defects in hepatic haem synthesis, such as in acute hepatic porphyrias.[9]

The likelihood of wormwood preparations causing an allergic reaction is low, but caution is advised in patients with known hypersensitivity to plants in the Compositae family.

Effect on Ability to Drive or Operate Machinery

No adverse effects expected.

Adverse Reactions

Wormwood pollen is an allergen and has caused hypersensitivity symptoms in the upper airways of humans.[10] Contact allergy from the flowers has been reported. The flowers may have greater sensitising capacity than the leaves.[11]

Interactions

None known.

Safety in Children

No information available.

Overdosage

Ingestion of wormwood oil (10 and 60 mL) has been reported in two cases. It caused altered mental status, seizures, and secondary complications including rhabdomyolysis, hyperthermia, and aspiration in one case,[12] and seizures, rhabdomyolysis, and acute renal failure in the other.[13]

Wormwood (or rather thujone) was blamed for the adverse effects arising from (excessive) ingestion of absinthe, a liqueur popular in late 19th century Europe. Absinthe was usually manufactured from a number of herbs including wormwood and *Acorus calamus* and typically contained 0.26 g/L thujone, not to mention other terpenes. Regular consumption of absinthe caused stomach irritation and eventually general upset of the nervous system. Convulsions resembling epilepsy were observed in humans and induced in animals from toxic doses of absinthe. Animal studies indicated that the alcohol content alone was not responsible for the toxicity observed from chronic doses. By 1915, absinthe was banned or restricted in many countries.[14,15] Colouring agents such as copper sulphate and antimony chloride, which were added to absinthe (as adulterants) may have also contributed to the toxicity.[16] Too frequent or excessive use of absinthe could produce headache,[15] which may have been due to the presence of thujone.

Intoxications have resulted from the ingestion of an aqueous decoction of thujone-containing plants, for their supposed abortifacient action.[17] Death by overdose has been reported for wormwood.[8]

Toxicology

Table 1 lists LD$_{50}$ data recorded for wormwood extract and its constituents.[4,18-22]

Oral administration of a total dose of 15.3 g of powdered wormwood over a period of 18 months diminished the life expectancy and the growth of rats, but did not cause liver damage or tumour formation.[23] Hexane-, chloroform- and water-soluble extracts were well tolerated orally in rabbits up to the highest administered dose of 1.6 g/kg. No mortality occurred.[24] Large does of "essence of absinthe" produced seizures in dogs.[25]

Oral thujone is convulsive, psychotropic and lethal to mice at 0.25 g/kg.[26] α-Thujone is more toxic than β-thujone in mice[22] and the fruit fly.[21] Both α-thujone and β-thujone are convulsants,[27] and their toxicity is primarily attributable to their action as noncompetitive blockers of the γ-aminobutyric acid–gated chloride channel.[21] Chronic oral administration of thujone leads to fatty degeneration of the liver.[4]

An extract of wormwood tested negative for in vitro mutagenic activity in the Ames test.[28]

Regulatory Status

See Table 2 for regulatory status in selected countries.

Table **1**　**LD$_{50}$ Data Recorded for Wormwood Extract and Its Constituents**

Substance	Route, Model	LD$_{50}$ Value	Reference
Wormwood liquid extract (1:3)	Oral, mice	2.5 g/kg	18
Wormwood whole plant, ethanol extract	i.p., rats	1 g/kg	19
Wormwood essential oil	Oral, rats	96 mg/kg	20
α-Thujone	i.p., mice	45 mg/kg	21
α-Thujone	s.c., mice	87.5 mg/kg	22
β-Thujone	s.c., mice	442.2 mg/kg	22
α- and β-Thujone mixture	s.c., mice	134.2 mg/kg	22
α- and β-Thujone mixture	Oral, rats	192 mg/kg	4
α- and β-Thujone mixture	Oral, mice	230 mg/kg	4

Table **2**　**Regulatory Status for Wormwood in Selected Countries**

Australia	Wormwood is not included in Part 4 of Schedule 4 of the Therapeutic Goods Regulations. However, it is subject to control under the Customs Import/Export Legislation, and permission is required when importing the herb.
UK & Germany	Wormwood is not included on the General Sale List. It is covered by a positive Commission E monograph. Wormwood is official in the *European Pharmacopoeia* 4.3.
US	Wormwood does not have generally recognised as safe (GRAS) status. However, it is freely available as a "dietary supplement" in the US under DSHEA legislation (Dietary Supplement Health and Education Act of 1994).

REFERENCES

1. British Herbal Medicine Association's Scientific Committee: *British herbal pharmacopoeia*, Bournemouth, 1983, BHMA, p 32.
2. Bisset NG, ed: *Herbal drugs and phytopharmaceuticals*, Stuttgart, 1994, Medpharm Scientific Publishers, pp 45-48.
3. Lawrence B: *Perfum Flav* 17:32, 1992.
4. Pinto-Scognamiglio W: *Boll Chim Farm* 106:292-300, 1967.
5. Lehmann R, Penman K: Information on file, University of Queensland, St Lucia, Queensland, Australia, 2003, MediHerb Research Laboratory.
6. Scientific Committee of ESCOP (European Scientific Cooperative on Phytotherapy): *ESCOP monographs: Absinthii herba*, UK, July 1997, European Scientific Cooperative on Phytotherapy Secretariat.
7. Rao VSN, Menezes AMS, Gadelha MGT: *Fitoterapia* 59:17-20, 1988.
8. Gessner O: *Gift-und Arzneipflanzen von Mitteleuropa*, ed 3, Heidelberg, 1974, Carl Winter Universitatsverlag, pp 258-260.
9. Bonkovsky HL, Cable EE, Cable JW, et al: *Biochem Pharmacol* 43:2359-2368, 1992.
10. Gniazdowska B, Doroszewska G, Doroszewski W: *Pneumonol Alergol Pol* 61:367-372, 1993.
11. Mitchell J, Rook A: *Botanical dermatology: plants and plant products injurious to the skin*, Vancouver, 1979, Greengrass, p 190.
12. Berlin R, Smilkstein M: *J Toxicol Clin Toxicol* 34:583, 1996.
13. Weisbord SD, Soule JB, Kimmel PL: *N Engl J Med* 337:825-827, 1997.
14. Strang J, Arnold WN, Peters T: *BMJ* 319:1590-1592, 1999.
15. Albert-Puleo M: *Econ Bot* 32:65-74, 1978.
16. Blaschek W, Ebel S, Hackenthal E, et al: *HagerROM 2002: Hagers Handbuch der Drogen und Arzneistoffe*, Heidelberg, 2002, Springer.
17. Millet Y, Jouglard J, Steinmetz MD, et al: *Clin Toxicol* 18:1485-1498, 1981.
18. Lagarto Parra A, Silva Yhebra R, Guerra Sardinas I, et al. *Phytomedicine* 8: 395-400, 2001.
19. Sharma ML, Chandokhe N, Ghatak BJ, et al: *Indian J Exp Biol* 16: 228-240, 1978.
20. Opdyke DL: *Food Cosmet Toxicol* 13:721-722, 1975.
21. Hold KM, Sirisoma NS, Ikeda T, et al: *Proc Natl Acad Sci U S A* 97:3826-3831, 2000.
22. Rice KC, Wilson RS: *J Med Chem* 19:1054-1057, 1976.

23. Schmahl D: *Z Krebsforsch* 61:227-229, 1956.
24. Khattak SG, Gilani SN, Ikram M: *J Ethnopharmacol* 14:45-51, 1985.
25. Magnan V: *Lancet* 2:410-412, 1874.
26. Le Boursi B, Soenen AM: *Food Cosmet Toxicol* 11:1-9, 1973.
27. Sirisoma NS, Hold KM, Casida JE: *J Agric Food Chem* 49:1915-1921, 2001.
28. Schimmer O, Kruger A, Paulini H et al: *Pharmazie* 49:448-451, 1994

YARROW

Other common name: Milfoil
Botanical name: *Achillea millefolium* L.
Family: Compositae
Plant part used: Aerial parts collected during the flowering period

Safety Summary

Pregnancy category B3: No increase in frequency of malformation or other harmful effects on the foetus from limited use in women. Evidence of increased foetal damage in animal studies exists, although the relevance to humans is unknown.

Lactation category CC: Compatible with breast-feeding but use caution.

Contraindications: Known allergy. Do not use during pregnancy or lactation without professional advice.

Warnings & precautions: Avoid in known sensitivity to plants of the Compositae family.

Adverse reactions: Allergic reactions are possible.

Interactions: No precautions required on current evidence.

Typical Therapeutic Use

Traditional indications for yarrow in Western herbal medicine include fever management, the common cold, control of excessive bleeding, diarrhoea, and menstrual problems.[1]

It has been used in Europe in the treatment and rehabilitation of chronic hepatitis.[2]

Actions

Diaphoretic, antipyretic, antiinflammatory, spasmolytic, aromatic bitter, haemostatic, hypotensive, emmenagogue.

Key Constituents

The *European Pharmacopoeia* recommends that dried flowering tops of yarrow contain at least 2 mL/kg of essential oil and not less than 0.02% of proazulenes, expressed as chamazulene. The chemical profile of the essential oil varies, depending upon its origin, subspecies, and chromosome number.[3,4]

Other constituents may include achimillic acids A, B, and C,[5] α-peroxyachifolid,[6] 3-β-hydroxy-11-α, 13-dihydro-costunolide, desacetylmatricarin, leucodin, achillin, 8-α-angeloxy-leucodin, and 8-α-angeloxy-achillin[7]; sterols; a triterpene: α-amyrin[8]; flavones: apigenin, luteolin, 5-hydroxy-3,6,7,4'-tetramethoxyflavone, artemetin, and casticin[9]; and alkamides.[10]

Adulteration

Various other *Achillea* species and chemical races (chemotypes) of *Achillea millefolium* may be found in any sample of yarrow.

Typical Dosage Forms & Dosage

Typical adult dosage ranges are:
- 6 to 12 g/day of dried aerial parts or by infusion
- 3 to 6 mL/day of a 1:1 liquid extract
- 2 to 6 mL/day of a 1:2 liquid extract or equivalent in tablet or capsule form
- 6 to 12 mL/day of a 1:5 tincture

Contraindications

Known hypersensitivity (rare) to yarrow or other Compositae. Do not use during pregnancy or lactation without professional advice.

Use in Pregnancy

Category B3: No increase in frequency of malformation or other harmful effects on the foetus from limited use in women. Evidence of increased foetal damage in animal studies exists, although the relevance to humans is unknown. Reported to have abortifacient properties in animals[11]—this may relate to varieties relatively high in thujone. There is no evidence of harm in humans.

Very high oral doses of yarrow (2.8 g/kg/day) reduced foetal weights when administered to rats from days 1 to 8 and days 8 to 15 of gestation. Placental weight was increased in the days 1 to 8 gestation period. No increase in preimplantation or postimplantation loss occurred and there was no significant difference in the number of external or internal malformations between the treatment and control groups. Yarrow had no effect on the ossification of the skeleton. The herb was administered as an ethanolic extract and the dose administered was the highest possible in which ethanol remained below the teratogenic threshold.[12]

Use in Lactation

Category CC: Compatible with breastfeeding but use caution. Avoid high doses during breastfeeding.

Warnings & Precautions

Avoid in patients with known hypersensitivity to plants in the Compositae family (such as feverfew).

Effect on Ability to Drive or Operate Machinery

No adverse effects expected.

Adverse Reactions

Contact reactions to Compositae, including yarrow, are well known.[13] Fifty percent of Compositae-sensitive subjects (3.1% of a sample of 3851 individuals) have been shown to be yarrow sensitive.[14] In further investigations, a sesquiterperpene lactone α-peroxyachifolid has been identified as a likely sensitiser; however, the experimental patches produced were not exacerbated by UV irradiation.[15] There are few data on adverse reactions from oral consumption of yarrow.

Interactions

None known.

Safety in Children

No information available, but adverse effects are not expected.

Overdosage

No incidents found in published literature.

Toxicology

Table 1 lists LD_{50} data recorded for yarrow.[16]

Guinea pigs were sensitised to crude extracts of the whole plant and the flowers of A. millefolium. A. millefolium tea was weakly genotoxic in a somatic mutation and recombination test using Drosophila melanogaster. In clinical tests, topical product formulations containing 2% yarrow extract were generally not irritating or phototoxic.[17]

Regulatory Status

See Table 2 for regulatory status in selected countries.

Table 1   **LD_{50} Data Recorded for Yarrow**

Substance	Route, Model	LD_{50} Value (g/kg)	Reference
Yarrow	Oral, mice	3.65	16
Yarrow	s.c., rats	16.86	16

Table 2   **Regulatory Status for Yarrow in Selected Countries**

Australia	Yarrow is not included in Part 4 of Schedule 4 of the Therapeutic Goods Regulations.
UK & Germany	Yarrow is included on the General Sale List. It is covered by a positive Commission E monograph. Yarrow is official in the European Pharmacopoeia 4.3.
US	Yarrow does not have generally recognised as safe (GRAS) status. However, it is freely available as a "dietary supplement" in the US under DSHEA legislation (Dietary Supplement Health and Education Act of 1994).

REFERENCES

1. British Herbal Medicine Association's Scientific Committee: *British herbal pharmacopoeia*, Bournemouth, 1983, BHMA, p 145.
2. Harnyk TP: *Lik Sprava* 7-8:168-170, 1999.
3. Bisset NG, ed: *Herbal drugs and phytopharmaceuticals: a handbook for practice on a scientific basis*, Stuttgart, 1994, Medpharm Scientific Publishers, pp 342-343.
4. British Herbal Medicine Association: *British herbal compendium*, vol 1, Bournemouth, 1992, BHMA, pp 227-229.
5. Tozyo T, Yoshimura Y, Sakurai K, et al: *Chem Pharm Bull (Tokyo)* 42:1096-1100, 1994.
6. Rucker G, Manns D, Breuer J: *Arch Pharm (Weinheim)* 324:979-981, 1991.
7. Glasl S, Mucaji P, Werner I, et al: *Z Naturforsch [C]* 57:976-982, 2002.
8. Chandler RF, Hooper SN, Hooper DL, et al: *J Pharm Sci* 71:690-693, 1982.
9. Falk AJ, Smolenski SJ, Bauer L et al: *J Pharm Sci* 64:1838-1842, 1975.
10. Muller-Jakic B, Breu W, Probstle A et al: *Planta Med* 60:37-40, 1994.
11. Farnsworth NR: *J Pharm Sci* 64:5355-5398, 1975.
12. Boswell-Ruys CL, Ritchie HE, Brown-Woodman PDC: *Birth Defects Res* (Part A) 67:141-147, abstract 8, 2003.
13. Davies MG, Kersey PJ: *Contact Dermatitis* 14:256-257, 1986.
14. Hausen BM: *Am J Contact Dermatitis* 7:94-99, 1996.
15. Hausen BM, Breuer J, Weglewski J, et al: *Contact Dermatitis* 24:274-280, 1991.
16. Newall CA, Anderson LA, Phillipson JD: *Herbal medicines*, London, 1996, Pharmaceutical Press, p 272.
17. [No authors listed]: *Int J Toxicol* 20(Suppl 2):79-84, 2001.

YELLOW DOCK

Other common name: Curled dock
Botanical name: *Rumex crispus* L.
Family: Polygonaceae
Plant part used: Root

Safety Summary

Pregnancy category B2: No increase in frequency of malformation or other harmful effects on the foetus from limited use in women. Animal studies are lacking.

Lactation category CC: Compatible with breastfeeding but use caution (due to the presence of anthraquinone glycosides).

Contraindications: Anthraquinone-containing laxatives are contraindicated in ileus (intestinal obstruction). Do not use during lactation without professional advice.

Warnings & precautions: Depuratives can in some cases be provocative to skin disease.

Adverse reactions: None found in published literature.

Interactions: Excessive use may add to the potassium depletion caused by agents such as thiazide diuretics and licorice.

Typical Therapeutic Use

Traditional indications for yellow dock in Western herbal medicine include chronic skin disease (especially psoriasis), obstructive jaundice, and constipation.[1]

Actions

Mild laxative, cholagogue, depurative.

Key Constituents

The root of *Rumex crispus* contains moderate levels of anthraquinone glycosides (such as chrysophanol, emodin, frangulin, and chrysophanein).[2,3] Total anthraquinone glycosides were measured at 1.2% in one study,[4] and in another study the concentration of anthraquinones increased from 0.35% to 0.91% during the vegetation period.[5]

Adulteration

No adulterants known.

Typical Dosage Forms & Dosage

Typical adult dosage ranges are:
- 6 to 12 g/day of dried root or by decoction
- 6 to 12 mL/day of a 1:1 liquid extract
- 2 to 4.5 mL/day of a 1:2 liquid extract or equivalent in tablet or capsule form
- 3 to 6 mL/day of a 1:5 tincture

Contraindications

Anthraquinone-containing laxatives are contraindicated in ileus (intestinal obstruction). Do not use during lactation without professional advice.

Use in Pregnancy

Category B2: No increase in frequency of malformation or other harmful effects on the foetus from limited use in women. Animal studies are lacking.

In traditional Chinese medicine, anthraquinone-containing herbs such as rhubarb are contraindicated in pregnancy because they promote a downward movement of energy.

Use in Lactation

Category CC: Compatible with breastfeeding but use caution.

Small amounts of anthraquinone metabolites may be excreted in the breast milk. In the case of senna, significant quantities of anthraquinone metabolites were not detected.[6] The American Academy of Pediatrics has judged senna as compatible with breastfeeding,[7,8] so it is likely that yellow dock, which contains a lower level of anthraquinones, would also be compatible.

Warnings & Precautions

Prolonged use of stimulating laxative is undesirable. However, the laxative action of yellow dock is very mild. Depuratives can be provocative to skin disease. Care needs to be taken to reduce the prospect of major exacerbations.

Effect on Ability to Drive or Operate Machinery

No adverse effects expected.

Adverse Reactions

None expected for yellow dock taken at the recommended dosage. For a discussion of the adverse reactions associated with anthraquinone use, refer to the senna (*Cassia* spp.) monograph.

Interactions

None expected if taken within the recommended dosage. Theoretically, anthraquinone-containing herbs can interact with the following drugs, due to the loss of potassium: thiazide diuretics, corticosteroids, licorice (*Glycyrrhiza glabra*), digoxin, and antiarrhythmic drugs. These interactions are unlikely to occur with normal therapeutic doses of yellow dock, due to the moderate level of anthraquinone glycosides present.

Safety in Children

No information available, but adverse effects are not expected.

Overdosage

No incidents were found in published literature concerning poisoning from the root of *Rumex crispus*. However, the leaf has caused fatal poisoning in sheep[9] and in a 53-year-old man who ingested a large quantity as a salad vegetable.[10] These fatal effects were due to the presence of oxalate,[9] which is only present in significant quantities in the leaf.

Toxicology

The toxicity of *Rumex crispus* root extracts in the brine shrimp assay increased significantly with increasing concentrations of anthraquinone glycosides.[5]

Refer to the senna (*Cassia* spp.) monograph for general information about the toxicology of anthraquinones.

Regulatory Status

See Table 1 for regulatory status in selected countries.

Table 1   Regulatory Status for Yellow Dock in Selected Countries

Australia	Yellow dock is not included in Part 4 of Schedule 4 of the Therapeutic Goods Regulations.
UK & Germany	Yellow dock is included on the General Sale List. It was not included in the Commission E assessment.
US	Yellow dock does not have generally recognised as safe (GRAS) status. However, it is freely available as a "dietary supplement" in the US under DSHEA legislation (Dietary Supplement Health and Education Act of 1994).

REFERENCES

1. British Herbal Medicine Association's Scientific Committee: *British herbal pharmacopoeia*, Bournemouth, 1983, BHMA, p 183.
2. Gunaydin K, Topcu G, Ion RM: *Nat Prod Lett* 16:65-70, 2002.
3. Sayed MD, Balbaa SI, Afifi MSA: *Egypt J Pharm Sci* 15:1-10, 1974.
4. Demirezer LO: *Pharmazie* 49:378-379, 1994.
5. Demirezer LO, Kuruuzum A: *Z Naturforsch C Biosci* 50:461-462, 1995.
6. Leng-Peschlow E, ed: *Pharmacology* 44(Suppl 1): 23-25, 1992.
7. Hagemann TM: *J Hum Lact* 1998; 14: 259-262.
8. American Academy of Pediatrics: *Pediatrics* 108:776-789, 2001.
9. Panciera R, Martin T, Burrows GE: *J Am Vet Med Assoc* 196:1981-1984, 1990.
10. Reig R, Sanz P, Blanche C, et al: *Vet Hum Toxicol* 32:468-470, 1991.

ZIZYPHUS SEED

Other common names: Ziziphus, spiny jujube, sour Chinese date seed
Botanical names: *Ziziphus jujuba* Mill. var. *spinosa* (Bunge) Hu ex H.F. Chou (*Ziziphus zizyphus* [L.] Karst.)
Note: Ziziphus is also spelt Zizyphus
Family: Rhamnaceae
Plant part used: Seed

Safety Summary

Pregnancy category B2: No increase in frequency of malformation or other harmful effects on the foetus from limited use in women. Animal studies are lacking.
Lactation category C: Compatible with breastfeeding.
Contraindications: None known.
Warnings & precautions: Caution in patients with severe diarrhoea.
Adverse reactions: Chills, fever, and joint pain.
Interactions: No precautions required on current evidence.

Typical Therapeutic Use

A traditional Chinese medicine (TCM) formula containing zizyphus seed (45.5% by dried weight) demonstrated therapeutic benefit in patients suffering anxiety symptoms[1] and sleep disorders[2] in controlled trials. Indications for zizyphus seed in TCM include insomnia, palpitations with anxiety, excessive sweating due to debility, and night sweats.[3,4]

Actions

Hypnotic, mild sedative, hypotensive, anxiolytic.

Key Constituents

Constituents of zizyphus seed include dammarane-type saponins (0.2%), known as jujubosides A and B, and a flavone C-glycoside called spinosin.[5]

Adulteration

No adulterants known.

Typical Dosage Forms & Dosage

Typical adult dosage ranges are:

- 9 to 15 g/day of dried seed by decoction
- 6 to 11.5 mL/day of a 1:2 liquid extract or equivalent in tablet or capsule form

Contraindications

None known.

Use in Pregnancy

Category B2: No increase in frequency of malformation or other harmful effects on the foetus from limited use in women. Animal studies are lacking.

Use in Lactation

Category C: Compatible with breastfeeding.

Warnings & Precautions

In TCM, the use of zizyphus seed is cautioned in patients with severe diarrhoea or *excess heat*.[4]

Effect on Ability to Drive or Operate Machinery

No adverse effects expected.

Adverse Reactions

A 30-year-old woman experienced chills, fever, and joint pain, which was attributed to taking *Ziziphus spinosa* seeds (dose not defined).[6]

Interactions

None known.

Safety in Children

No information available, but adverse effects are not expected.

Overdosage

No incidents found in published literature.

Toxicology

Zizyphus seed has exhibited low toxicity when administered orally. Mice receiving zizyphus seed decoction (50 g/kg) showed no signs of toxicity, and intragastric administration of 15 g/mL of the soluble extract at 1 mL/20 g did not cause any fatalities. Chronic administration of zizyphus seed to rats produced marginal toxicity.[7]

Toxicity increases when zizyphus seed is administered by injection, but the relative toxicity is still quite low. The intraperitoneal LD_{50} of zizyphus seed decoction was 14.3 g/kg in rats. Subcutaneous injec-

tion of a 50% ethanol extract (20 g/kg) was lethal to mice within 30 to 60 min, and intravenous injection of a 50% decoction (0.1 to 0.2 mL per mouse) resulted in immediate death.[7]

Regulatory Status

See Table 1 for regulatory status in selected countries.

Table 1　**Regulatory Status for Zizyphus Seed in Selected Countries**

Australia	Zizyphus seed is not included in Part 4 of Schedule 4 of the Therapeutic Goods Regulations.
China	Zizyphus seed is official in the *Pharmacopoeia of the People's Republic of China* 1997. The usual adult dosage, usually administered in the form of a decoction, is listed as 9 to 15 g.
UK & Germany	Zizyphus seed is not included on the General Sale List. It was not included in the Commission E assessment.
US	Zizyphus seed does not have generally recognised as safe (GRAS) status. However, it is freely available as a "dietary supplement" in the US under DSHEA legislation (Dietary Supplement Health and Education Act of 1994).

REFERENCES

1. Chen HC, Hsieh MT, Shibuya TK: *Int J Clin Pharmacol Ther Toxicol* 24:646-650, 1986.
2. Chen HC, Hsieh MT: *Clin Ther* 7:334-337, 1985.
3. Pharmacopoeia Commission of the People's Republic of China: *Pharmacopoeia of the People's Republic of China*, English ed, vol I, Beijing, 1997, Chemical Industry Press, pp 226-227.
4. Bensky D, Gamble A: *Chinese herbal medicine materia medica*, Seattle, 1986, Eastland Press, pp 580-581.
5. Tang W, Eisenbrand G: *Chinese drugs of plant origin*, Berlin, 1992, Springer-Verlag, pp 1017-1024.
6. Zhang L, Wang H: *China J Chin Materia Med* 14:116, 1989.
7. Chang HM, But PP: *Pharmacology and applications of Chinese materia medica*, vol 2, Singapore, 1987, World Scientific, pp 1221-1223.

Appendix A

Herb Listing by Pregnancy and Lactation Categories

Pregnancy Categories*

A Bilberry fruit, chamomile—German, cranberry, echinacea, garlic, ginger, ginseng, licorice, raspberry leaf, senna, turmeric

B1 Astragalus, blue flag, boswellia, bupleurum, burdock, butcher's broom, chaste tree, codonopsis, evening primrose oil, ginkgo, goat's rue, gotu kola, hawthorn leaf & flower, kava, myrrh, passionflower, rosemary, schisandra, Siberian ginseng, St. John's wort, St. Mary's thistle, valerian, willow bark, withania

B2 Bacopa, black cohosh, black haw, black walnut, bladderwrack, buchu, calendula, California poppy, cascara, celery seed, chickweed, cleavers, corn silk, couch grass, cramp bark, cranesbill root, damiana, dandelion, devil's claw, elder flower, elecampane, euphorbia, eyebright, false unicorn, fringe tree, gentian, globe artichoke, golden rod, grindelia, gymnema, hops, horsetail, hydrangea, lavender, lemon balm, lime flowers, marshmallow, mullein, nettle, peppermint, prickly ash, pygeum, saw palmetto, shatavari, skullcap, thyme, wild lettuce, willow herb, yellow dock, zizyphus seed

B3 Aloe, andrographis, bittersweet, crataeva, ephedra, fennel, fenugreek, feverfew, horsechestnut, meadowsweet, motherwort, rehmannia, shepherd's purse, tribulus leaf, white horehound, wild cherry, yarrow

C Barberry & Indian barberry, bearberry, bugleweed & gypsywort, chaparral, dong quai, golden seal, greater celandine, guggul, Oregon grape, pasque flower, sage, tylophora

D Blue cohosh, cat's claw, Jamaica dogwood, pau d'arco, poke root, tansy, thuja, wormwood

X Arnica, boldo, pennyroyal

Lactation Categories†

ND Andrographis, astragalus, black walnut, damiana, feverfew, ginkgo, gymnema, pygeum, schisandra, willow herb

C Bacopa, bilberry fruit, black haw, blue flag, boswellia, bupleurum, burdock, butcher's broom, calendula, chamomile—German, chaste tree, chickweed, cleavers, codonopsis, corn silk, couch grass, cramp bark, cranberry, cranesbill root, dandelion, devil's claw, dong quai, echinacea, elder flower, euphorbia, evening primrose oil, eyebright, false unicorn, fennel, fenugreek, fringe tree, garlic, gentian, ginger, ginseng, globe artichoke, goat's rue, golden rod, gotu kola, grindelia, hawthorn leaf & flower, horsetail, hydrangea, lavender, lemon balm, licorice, lime flowers, marshmallow, motherwort, mullein, nettle, passionflower, prickly ash, raspberry leaf, rehmannia, rosemary, saw palmetto, shatavari, Siberian ginseng, skullcap, St. Mary's thistle, thyme, turmeric, white horehound, wild cherry, withania, zizyphus seed

CC Aloe, bladderwrack, buchu, California poppy, cascara, cat's claw, celery seed, crataeva, hops, horsechestnut, kava, meadowsweet, myrrh, pau d'arco, peppermint, senna, shepherd's purse, St. John's wort, tribulus leaf, valerian, wild lettuce, yarrow, yellow dock

Herb Listing by Pregnancy and Lactation Categories—cont'd

SD Barberry & Indian barberry, bearberry, bittersweet, black cohosh, elecampane, ephedra, golden seal, greater celandine, guggul, Jamaica dogwood, Oregon grape, pasque flower, willow bark

X Arnica, blue cohosh, boldo, bugleweed & gypsywort, chaparral, pennyroyal, poke root, sage, tansy, thuja, tylophora, wormwood

Pregnancy category

A: No proven increase in the frequency of malformation or other harmful effects on the foetus despite consumption by a large number of women.

B1: No increase in frequency of malformation or other harmful effects on the foetus from limited use in women. No evidence of increased foetal damage in animal studies.

B2: No increase in frequency of malformation or other harmful effects on the foetus from limited use in women. Animal studies are lacking.

B3: No increase in frequency of malformation or other harmful effects on the foetus from limited use in women. Evidence of increased foetal damage in animal studies exists, although the relevance to humans is unknown.

C: Has caused or is associated with a substantial risk of causing harmful effects on the foetus or neonate without causing malformations.

D: Has caused or is associated with a substantial risk of causing foetal malformation or irreversible damage.

X: High risk of damage to the foetus.

†Lactation category

ND: No data available.

C: Compatible with breastfeeding.

CC: Compatible with breastfeeding but use caution.

SD: Strongly discouraged in breastfeeding.

X: Contraindicated in breastfeeding.

APPENDIX B

Pregnancy and Lactation Categories Listing by Herb

Herb	Pregnancy category*	Lactation category[†]
Aloe	B3	CC
Andrographis	B3	ND
Arnica	X	X
Astragalus	B1	ND
Bacopa	B2	C
Barberry & Indian barberry	C	SD
Bearberry	C	SD
Bilberry fruit	A	C
Bittersweet	B3	SD
Black cohosh	B2	SD
Black haw	B2	C
Black walnut	B2	ND
Bladderwrack	B2	CC
Blue cohosh	D	X
Blue flag	B1	C
Boldo	X	X
Boswellia	B1	C
Buchu	B2	CC
Bugleweed & gypsywort	C	X
Bupleurum	B1	C
Burdock	B1	C
Butcher's broom	B1	C
Calendula	B2	C
California poppy	B2	CC
Cascara	B2	CC
Cat's claw	D	CC

Pregnancy and Lactation Categories Listing by Herb—cont'd

Herb	Pregnancy category*	Lactation category†
Celery seed	B2	CC
Chamomile, German	A	C
Chaparral	C	X
Chaste tree	B1	C
Chickweed	B2	C
Cleavers	B2	C
Codonopsis	B1	C
Corn silk	B2	C
Couch grass	B2	C
Cramp bark	B2	C
Cranberry	A	C
Cranesbill root	B2	C
Crataeva	B3	CC
Damiana	B2	ND
Dandelion	B2	C
Devil's claw	B2	C
Dong quai	C	C
Echinacea	A	C
Elder flower	B2	C
Elecampane	B2	SD
Ephedra	B3	SD
Euphorbia	B2	C
Evening primrose oil	B1	C
Eyebright	B2	C
False unicorn	B2	C
Fennel	B3	C
Fenugreek	B3	C
Feverfew	B3	ND
Fringe tree	B2	C
Garlic	A	C
Gentian	B2	C
Ginger	A	C
Ginkgo	B1	ND
Ginseng	A	C
Globe artichoke	B2	C

Continued

Pregnancy and Lactation Categories Listing by Herb—cont'd

Herb	Pregnancy category*	Lactation category†
Goat's rue	B1	C
Golden rod	B2	C
Golden seal	C	SD
Gotu kola	B1	C
Greater celandine	C	SD
Grindelia	B2	C
Guggul	C	SD
Gymnema	B2	ND
Hawthorn leaf & flower	B1	C
Hops	B2	CC
Horsechestnut	B3	CC
Horsetail	B2	C
Hydrangea	B2	C
Jamaica dogwood	D	SD
Kava	B1	CC
Lavender	B2	C
Lemon balm	B2	C
Licorice	A	C
Lime flowers	B2	C
Marshmallow	B2	C
Meadowsweet	B3	CC
Motherwort	B3	C
Mullein	B2	C
Myrrh	B1	CC
Nettle	B2	C
Oregon grape	C	SD
Pasque flower	C	SD
Passionflower	B1	C
Pau d'arco	D	CC
Pennyroyal	X	X
Peppermint	B2	CC
Poke root	D	X
Prickly ash	B2	C
Pygeum	B2	ND
Raspberry leaf	A	C

Pregnancy and Lactation Categories Listing by Herb—cont'd

Herb	Pregnancy category*	Lactation category†
Rehmannia	B3	C
Rosemary	B1	C
Sage	C	X
Saw palmetto	B2	C
Schisandra	B1	ND
Senna	A	CC
Shatavari	B2	C
Shepherd's purse	B3	CC
Siberian ginseng	B1	C
Skullcap	B2	C
St. John's wort	B1	CC
St. Mary's thistle	B1	C
Tansy	D	X
Thuja	D	X
Thyme	B2	C
Tribulus leaf	B3	CC
Turmeric	A	C
Tylophora	C	X
Valerian	B1	CC
White horehound	B3	C
Wild cherry	B3	C
Wild lettuce	B2	CC
Willow bark	B1	SD
Willow herb	B2	ND
Withania	B1	C
Wormwood	D	X
Yarrow	B3	CC
Yellow dock	B2	CC
Zizyphus seed	B2	C

Pregnancy category

A: No proven increase in the frequency of malformation or other harmful effects on the foetus despite consumption by a large number of women.

B1: No increase in frequency of malformation or other harmful effects on the foetus from limited use in women. No evidence of increased foetal damage in animal studies.

B2: No increase in frequency of malformation or other harmful effects on the foetus from limited use in women. Animal studies are lacking.

Continued

Pregnancy and Lactation Categories Listing by Herb—cont'd

B3: No increase in frequency of malformation or other harmful effects on the foetus from limited use in women. Evidence of increased foetal damage in animal studies exists, although the relevance to humans is unknown.

C: Has caused or is associated with a substantial risk of causing harmful effects on the foetus or neonate without causing malformations.

D: Has caused or is associated with a substantial risk of causing foetal malformation or irreversible damage.

X: High risk of damage to the foetus.

†*Lactation category*

ND: No data available.

C: Compatible with breastfeeding.

CC: Compatible with breastfeeding but use caution.

SD: Strongly discouraged in breastfeeding.

X: Contraindicated in breastfeeding.

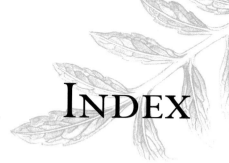

INDEX

Note: Page numbers followed by a indicate appendices; b, boxes; f, figures; t, tables.

WILLOW HERB

Other common name: Epilobium
Botanical names: *Epilobium parviflorum* Schreb., *E. montanum* L., *E. collinum* S. G. Gmel., *E. roseum* Schreb.
Family: Onagraceae
Plant part used: Aerial parts

Safety Summary

Pregnancy category B2: No increase in frequency of malformation or other harmful effects on the foetus from limited use in women.
Lactation category ND: No data available.
Contraindications: In principle, the use of herbs containing high levels of tannins is contraindicated or at least inappropriate in constipation, iron deficiency anaemia, and malnutrition.
Warnings & precautions: Because of the tannin content of this herb, long-term use should be avoided. Use cautiously in highly inflamed or ulcerated conditions of the gastrointestinal tract.
Adverse reactions: None found in published literature for willow herb. A potential adverse reaction due to the high tannin content is irritation of the mouth and gastrointestinal tract.
Interactions: Take separately from oral thiamine, metal ion supplements, or alkaloid-containing medications.

Typical Therapeutic Use

Traditional uses of willow herb in Western herbal medicine include chronic disorders of the prostate, especially obstruction to urination caused by prostatic enlargement.[1]

Actions

Antiprostatic.

Key Constituents

Epilobium parviflorum herb contains phenolic compounds (including the ellagitannin oenothein B), flavonoids (especially myricitrin), triterpenes, and sterols.[2,3] Large amounts of gallic acid derivatives are present.[4] Oenothein B is a large hydrolysable tannin.

Adulteration

Epilobium hirsutum and *E. angustifolium* are considered to be adulterants.[4] Hybridisation within *Epilobium* makes recognition of medicinal species difficult.[5] Poisoning by *E. hirsutum* in a 3-year-old boy was reported in 1897.[6] Authentication of correct botanical species is very difficult.[4] (Myricitrin is the main flavonoid constituent of a number of *Epilobium* species including *E. parviflorum*, *E. roseum,* and *E. hirsutum,* but is found in lower concentrations in *E. angustifolium*.[3]) There is a historical record of *Salix nigra* leaf presented for sale as willow herb.[7]

Typical Dosage Forms & Dosage

Typical adult dosage ranges are:
- 1 teaspoon of dried aerial parts per 0.25 litre (as an infusion), twice per day
- 3 to 6 mL/day of a 1:2 liquid extract or equivalent in tablet or capsule form

Contraindications

In principle, the use of tannins is contraindicated or at least inappropriate in constipation, iron deficiency anaemia, and malnutrition.

Use in Pregnancy

Category B2: No increase in frequency of malformation or other harmful effects on the foetus from limited use in women. Animal studies are lacking. Willow herb has been used mainly by men.

Use in Lactation

Category ND: No data available.
As willow herb has been used predominately by men, there is a lack of information about its use by lactating women.

Warnings & Precautions

Because of the tannin content of this herb, long-term use should be avoided (for both internal and topical use). Use cautiously in highly inflamed or ulcerated conditions of the gastrointestinal tract.

Effect on Ability to Drive or Operate Machinery

No adverse effects expected.

Adverse Reactions

The likelihood of willow herb causing an allergy is low. High doses of tannins lead to excessive astringency on mucous membranes, which has an irritating effect.

Interactions

None known for willow herb. Refer to the cranesbill root (*Geranium maculatum*) monograph for information regarding the interactions of tannins.

Safety in Children

No information available, but adverse effects are not expected if taken within the recommended dosage. Given the current applications for willow herb in Western herbal medicine, use in children is not relevant.

Overdosage

No incidents known for medicinal willow herb. However, long-term use with high doses of tannins is to be avoided.

Toxicology

The LD_{50} value of 200 mg/kg was obtained from i.p. administration of ethanol extract of aerial parts of willow herb in rats.[8]

Oral administration of water extract of *Epilobium angustifolium* decreased the weight of seminal vesicles of male rats. In testosterone-stimulated castrated rats, an increased weight of all accessory sexual organs was observed.[9] (*E. angustifolium* is not, however, medicinal willow herb and is considered an adulterant.)

Refer to the cranesbill root (*Geranium maculatum*) monograph for the toxicology of tannins.

Regulatory Status

See Table 1 for regulatory status in selected countries.

Table 1   **Regulatory Status for Willow Herb in Selected Countries**

Australia	Willow herb is not included in Part 4 of Schedule 4 of the Therapeutic Goods Regulations.
UK & Germany	Willow herb is not included on the General Sale List. It was not included in the Commission E assessment.
US	Willow herb does not have generally recognised as safe (GRAS) status. However, it is freely available as a "dietary supplement" in the US under DSHEA legislation (Dietary Supplement Health and Education Act of 1994).

REFERENCES

1. Weiss RF: *Herbal medicine*, English ed. Beaconsfield, 1988, Beaconsfield Publishers, p 256.
2. Nowak R, Krzaczek T: *Herba Pol* 44:5-10, 1998.
3. Ducrey B, Wolfender JL, Marston A, et al: *Phytochem* 38:129-137, 1995.
4. Bisset NG, ed: *Herbal drugs and phytopharmaceuticals: a handbook for practice on a scientific basis*, Stuttgart, 1994, Medpharm Scientific Publishers, pp 185-187.
5. Blaschek W, Ebel S, Hackenthal E, et al: *HagerROM 2002: Hagers Handbuch der Drogen und Arzneistoffe*, Heidelberg, 2002, Springer.
6. Felter HW, Lloyd JU: *King's American dispensatory*, ed 18, rev 3, vol 1; first published 1905: reprinted Portland, 1983, Eclectic Medical Publications, p 712.
7. Lloyd JU: *Druggist Circ* 59:87-90, 1915.
8. Sharma ML, Chandokhe N, Ghatak BJ, et al: *Indian J Exp Biol* 16:228-240, 1978.
9. Hiermann A, Bucar F: *J Ethnopharmacol* 55:179-183, 1997.

WITHANIA

Other common names: Ashwagandha, Ashwaganda
Botanical names: *Withania somnifera* (L.) Dunal
(*W. sicula* Lojac., *Physalis somnifera* L.)
Family: Solanaceae
Plant part used: Root

Safety Summary

Pregnancy category B1: No increase in frequency
of malformation or other harmful effects on the
foetus from limited use in women. No evidence of
increased foetal damage in animal studies.
Lactation category C: Compatible with breastfeeding.
Contraindications: None required on current evidence.
Warnings & precautions: None required on current evidence.
Adverse reactions: High doses may cause gastrointestinal upset, diarrhoea and vomiting.
Interactions: No precautions required on current evidence.

Typical Therapeutic Use

Withania has demonstrated therapeutic benefit in
conditions associated with ageing (including male
sexual inadequacy)[1] and in promoting growth in
children[2] in randomised, double-blind, placebo-
controlled trials. Traditional uses of withania in
Ayurvedic medicine include general debility, senile
debility, as an aphrodisiac, and for wasting in
children.[3]

Actions

Tonic, adaptogenic, mild sedative, antiinflammatory,
immune modulating, antianaemic.

Key Constituents

Major constituents of withania root include steroidal
compounds (lactones and glycosides),[4] including the
withanolides, and alkaloids.[5]

Adulteration

Withania coagulans has been reported to be both a
substitute and an adulterant of *W. somnifera*.[6]

Typical Dosage Forms & Dosage

Typical adult dosage ranges are:
- 3 to 6 g/day of dried root or by decoction
- 5 to 13 mL/day of a 1:2 liquid extract or equivalent in tablet or capsule form

Contraindications

None known.

Use in Pregnancy

Category B1: No increase in frequency of malformation or other harmful effects on the foetus from
limited use in women. No evidence of increased
foetal damage in animal studies.

A review of traditional Ayurvedic literature notes
that withania (part and dose undefined) is listed as
an abortifacient in three of the five sources checked.
However, the definition of abortifacient was very
broad and included emmenagogue, ecbolic (uterine
contractor) and "antimetabolite".[7] A 1952 publication notes that withania root powder is used in
Casablanca for abortion.[8] In West Pakistan, withania
root is used to cause abortion. It has also been used
to tone the uterus in women who habitually miscarry and to remove retained placenta.[9] In contrast,
another traditional source notes its use as a nutrient
and tonic for pregnant women,[3] and the animal
study below would suggest that it is safe during pregnancy. The confusion over safety in pregnancy from
traditional use may arise from the use of different
plant parts. Withania leaf has a very different phytochemical content compared to the root.[10,11]

Rats orally administered withania whole plant
decoction (100 mg/kg/day for 8 months) had comparable litter sizes and frequency of pregnancy to
controls, but produced progeny with higher average
body weight (indicating perhaps tonic activity).[12]
Withania root powder (25 mg/day for 10 days)
administered orally to male and female mice that
were later paired for mating resulted in decreased
litter size and produced some infertility (this indicates a potential antifertility effect but does not
imply harm during pregnancy).[9]

Use in Lactation

Category C: Compatible with breastfeeding.

Withania is used to promote lactation in Ayurvedic medicine and the traditional medicine of south-east Asia.[3,13] One teaspoon (0.5 g) of withania powder may be given twice daily with milk for insufficient lactation.[14]

Withania improved milk yield and quality in lactating cows.[15,16] Rats orally administered withania whole plant decoction (100 mg/kg/day) throughout their lactation period produced offspring with higher average body weight.[12]

Warnings & Precautions

None required.

Effect on Ability to Drive or Operate Machinery

No adverse effects expected.

Adverse Reactions

A review of the literature to 2000 concluded that constituents of withania exhibit a variety of therapeutic effects with little or no associated toxicity.[17]

High doses have been reported to cause gastrointestinal upset, diarrhoea, and vomiting,[18] which may be due to its steroidal saponin content.

Interactions

Withania extract may enhance the effect of benzodiazepines. Oral administration of withania extract (100 mg/kg) to rats reduced the effective dose of benzodiazepines, whilst providing a protective effect in experimentally induced epilepsy.[19] Withania enhanced the binding of a benzodiazepine to the $GABA_A$ receptor in vitro.[20] However, this interaction is speculative at this stage and has not been included in the safety summary above.

Safety in Children

Adverse events were not reported in a randomised, double-blind, placebo-controlled trial in which healthy children were orally administered 2 g per day of withania for 60 days.[2] Withania is traditionally used in Ayurvedic medicine to treat failure to thrive in children.[3]

Overdosage

No incidents found in published literature.

Toxicology

Table 1 lists LD_{50} data recorded for withania, which indicates low to moderate toxicity.[21,22]

Single intraperitoneal injections of a withania root alcohol extract were lethal to mice within 24 hours at doses above 1.1 g/kg (100% mortality at 1.5 g/kg), demonstrating low toxicity. In subacute toxicity studies, intraperitoneal administration of the extract (100 mg/kg/day) for 30 days significantly reduced spleen, thymus, and adrenal gland weights in male rats and significantly increased blood acid phosphatase activity in both sexes.[22] In contrast, no toxic effects were observed in rats and mice orally administered withania root aqueous extract (50 to 1000 mg/kg/day) for up to 4 weeks,[21] or in rats orally administered undefined withania root extract at 100 mg/kg/day for 180 days.[23] Catecholamine levels increased in cardiac and aortic tissues and decreased in the adrenal glands when withania root (100 and 200 mg/kg/day) was administered orally for 30 days.[23]

Oral administration of withania whole plant extract (200 mg/kg/day) for 7 months had no significant effect on mortality in mice.[24] Histopathological lesions were observed in the liver, lungs, and kidneys of mice fed very high doses of withania whole plant (20% w/w of diet; approximately 5 g/rat/day) for 10 to 14 days.[25] However, organ histopathology was not observed when rats were orally administered withania whole plant decoction at 250 mg/kg/day for 4 weeks. Adrenal weight decreased and liver and lung weights increased. Also, no toxic effects were observed when the decoction was orally administered at a dose of 100 mg/kg/day for 8 months.[12]

Male rats orally administered methanol extract of withania root at dose of 3 g/kg (much greater than 10 times the human therapeutic dose) for 7 days failed to ejaculate during the treatment period and for at least 7 days after and demonstrated reduced sexual performance, with sexual vigour and behaviour indicative of penile erectile dysfunction and reduced libido. There was no significant effect on serum liver enzymes, urea nitrogen, seminal fluid pH, or the gross appearance and weight of the

Adverse Reactions

None known.

Interactions

None known.

Safety in Children

No information available, but adverse effects are not expected.

Overdosage

No incidents found in published literature for poisoning with wild cherry bark. Livestock have been poisoned by ingestion of the leaves and sometimes seeds.[9-11] Children have died after ingestion of the kernel, by chewing twigs or drinking a tea made from the leaves.[10]

Toxicology

Although hydrocyanic acid (cyanide) is a poison, oral intake of prunasin is not necessarily toxic, as hydrolysis in the digestive tract or by the liver leads to a slow release of very low levels of hydrocyanic acid, which can be detoxified readily by the body.[12] The lethal dose of hydrocyanic acid derived from wild cherry leaves is approximately 2 mg/kg for livestock.[9]

Regulatory Status

See Table 1 for regulatory status in selected countries.

Table **1** **Regulatory Status for Wild Cherry in Selected Countries**

Australia	Wild cherry is not included in Part 4 of Schedule 4 of the Therapeutic Goods Regulations.
UK & Germany	Wild cherry is included on the General Sale List. It was not included in the Commission E assessment.
US	Wild cherry does have generally recognised as safe (GRAS) status. It is freely available as a "dietary supplement" in the US under DSHEA legislation (Dietary Supplement Health and Education Act of 1994).

REFERENCES

1. British Herbal Medicine Association's Scientific Committee: *British herbal pharmacopoeia*, Bournemouth, 1983, BHMA, pp 171-172.
2. Leung AY, Foster S: *Encyclopedia of common natural ingredients used in food, drugs and cosmetics*, ed 2, New York–Chichester, 1996, John Wiley, pp 155-156.
3. Bruneton J: *Pharmacognosy, phytochemistry, medicinal plants*, Paris, 1995, Lavoisier Publishing, p 170.
4. Mills S, Bone K: *Principles and practice of phytotherapy: modern herbal medicine*, Edinburgh, 2000, Churchill Livingstone, pp 25-26.
5. Liener IE, ed: *Toxic constituents of plant foodstuffs*, New York, 1980, Academic Press, p 147.
6. Pharmaceutical Society of Great Britain: *British pharmaceutical codex 1934*, London, 1941, The Pharmaceutical Press, pp 855-857.
7. Osol A, Farrar GE, et al: *The dispensatory of the United States of America*, ed 24, Philadelphia, 1947, Lippincott, pp 254-256.
8. Selby LA, Menges RW, Houser EC, et al: *Arch Environ Health* 22:496-501, 1971.
9. Kingsbury JM: *Poisonous plants for the United States and Canada*, Englewood Cliffs, 1964, Prentice Hall, pp 365-366.
10. Mulligan GA, Munro DB: *Can J Plant Sci* 61:977-992, 1981.
11. Enge EH: *J Am Vet Med Assoc* 47:123-124, 1939.
12. Mills S, Bone K: *Principles and practice of phytotherapy: modern herbal medicine*, Edinburgh, 2000, Churchill Livingstone, p 25.

WILD LETTUCE

Botanical name: *Lactuca virosa* L.
Family: Compositae
Plant part used: Dried leaf

Safety Summary

Pregnancy category B2: No increase in frequency of malformation or other harmful effects on the foetus from limited use in women. Animal studies are lacking.

Lactation category CC: Compatible with breast-feeding, but use caution.

Contraindications: Patients with known sensitivity to the Compositae family. Do not use during lactation without professional advice.

Warnings & precautions: In principle, herbal sedatives are best avoided in depression and insomnia marked by increasing restlessness during the early hours of the morning. Prescription of herbal sedatives should ideally be limited in duration. Avoid in patients with known hypersensitivity to plants in the Compositae family.

Adverse reactions: Allergic reactions

Interactions: No precautions required on current evidence.

Typical Therapeutic Use

Traditional indications for wild lettuce in Western herbal medicine include restlessness, insomnia, muscular pains, and irritable cough.[1]

There are some reports of hypotensive and CNS effects in experimental models.[2]

Actions

Mild sedative, antitussive.

Key Constituents

Wild lettuce leaf contains a latex that consists of sesquiterpene lactones (including lactucopicrin) and lactucerin (also known as lactucone, which is a mixture of acetates of α- and β-lactucerol and related triterpenes). Other constituents include flavonoids and coumarins. Traces of hyoscyamine were reported around 1900 in the fresh herb but were not detected in the dried latex or the dried herb.[3]

Although the constituents of the dried latex (known as lactucarium) have a reputation for opiate activity, this is likely to be only slight. The presence of the psychoactive constituent, N-methyl-β-phenethylamine has been suggested but not confirmed.[4]

Adulteration

Adulteration with *Sonchus oleraceus* L., *Dipsacus silvester* Huds. and other *Lactuca* species, in particular *Lactuca serriola* L., has occurred.[5]

Typical Dosage Forms & Dosage

Typical adult dosage ranges are:
- 1.5 to 12 g/day of dried leaf or by infusion
- 1.5 to 12 mL/day of a 1:1 liquid extract

Contraindications

Patients with known sensitivity to the Compositae family. Do not use during lactation without professional advice.

Use in Pregnancy

Category B2: No increase in frequency of malformation or other harmful effects on the foetus from limited use in women. Animal studies are lacking.

Use in Lactation

Category CC: Compatible with breastfeeding, but use caution.

Warnings & Precautions

In principle, herbal sedatives are best avoided in depression and insomnia marked by increasing restlessness during the early hours of the morning. Prescription of herbal sedatives should ideally be limited in duration. Avoid in patients with known hypersensitivity to plants in the Compositae family.

Effect on Ability to Drive or Operate Machinery

No adverse effects expected.

624

Adverse Reactions

Cases of allergy after contact with and oral consumption of lettuce and chicory have been reported.[6] In one epidemiological study, 19% of gardeners are known to react to a number of Compositae family, including feverfew (*Tanacetum parthenium*) and *Senecio* species, a liability closely associated with a history of atopic conditions in childhood, hayfever, and long-term exposure.[7] No cross-reactivity was found with ryegrass and birch pollen,[8] although mugwort (*Artemisia vulgaris*) has been identified as a cross-sensitiser.[9] Lettuce has been shown to share common allergens with carrot, although these are less potent. These findings may have some importance in patients with food-related symptoms, such as atopic dermatitis, because leaving lettuce in their diets may aggravate the condition.[10]

Interactions

None known.

Safety in Children

No information available.

Overdosage

Injection by two drug users of an aqueous wild lettuce extract led to fevers, chills, generalised stiffness and pains, headache, leucocytosis, and mild liver function abnormalities that resolved over 3 days.[11]

Toxicology

No information available.

Regulatory Status

See Table 1 for regulatory status in selected countries.

Table 1 **Regulatory Status for Wild Lettuce in Selected Countries**

Australia	Wild lettuce is not included in Part 4 of Schedule 4 of the Therapeutic Goods Regulations.
UK & Germany	Wild lettuce is included on the General Sale List. It was not included in the Commission E assessment.
US	Wild lettuce does not have generally recognised as safe (GRAS) status. However, it is freely available as a "dietary supplement" in the US under DSHEA legislation (Dietary Supplement Health and Education Act of 1994).

REFERENCES

1. British Herbal Medicine Association's Scientific Committee: *British herbal pharmacopoeia*, Bournemouth, 1983, BHMA, p 126.
2. Fong HH, Farnsworth NR, Henry LK, et al: *Lloydia* 35:35-48, 1972.
3. British Herbal Medicine Association: *British herbal compendium*, Bournemouth, 1992, BHMA, pp 222-223.
4. Huang ZJ, Kinghorn AD, Farnsworth NR: *J Pharm Sci* 71:270-271, 1982.
5. Blaschek W, Ebel S, Hackenthal E, et al: *HagerROM 2002: Hagers Handbuch der Drogen und Arzneistoffe*, Heidelberg, 2002, Springer.
6. Krook G: *Contact Dermatitis* 3:27-36, 1977.
7. Paulsen E, Sogaard J, Andersen KE: *Contact Dermatitis* 38:140-146, 1998.
8. Cadot P, Kochuyt AM, Deman R, et al: *Clin Exp Allergy* 26:940-944, 1996.
9. Vila L, Sanchez G, Sanz ML, et al: *Clin Exp Allergy* 28:1031-1035, 1998.
10. Helbling A, Schwartz HJ, Lopez M, et al: *Allergy Proc* 15:33-38, 1994.
11. Mullins ME, Horowitz BZ: *Vet Hum Toxicol* 40:290-291, 1998.

WILLOW BARK

Other common names: White willow, European willow

Botanical names: *Salix* spp. including *S. alba* L., *S. daphnoides* Vill., *S. purpurea* L. and *S. fragilis* L.

Family: Salicaceae

Plant part used: Bark

Safety Summary

Pregnancy category B1: No increase in frequency of malformation or other harmful effects on the foetus from limited use in women. No evidence of increased foetal damage in animal studies.

Lactation category SD: Strongly discouraged in breastfeeding.

Contraindications: Contraindicated in those with known allergy or hypersensitivity to salicylates and in glucose-6-phosphate dehydrogenase deficient patients. In principle, the use of herbs containing high levels of tannins is contraindicated or at least inappropriate in constipation, iron deficiency anaemia, and malnutrition. Do not use during lactation without professional advice.

Warnings & precautions: Use with caution in lactating women and in patients taking anticoagulants or synthetic salicylates. Because of the tannin content of this herb, long-term use should be avoided. Use cautiously in highly inflamed or ulcerated conditions of the gastrointestinal tract. Prescribe with caution for pain in children. Other precautions are neurological disease, depression and psychosis, liver and kidney disease, history of allergic or anaphylactic reactions. Long-term therapy with analgesics is not advisable.

Adverse reactions: Stomach ache, nausea, headache, dizziness, tiredness, sweating, skin rash, and allergic reactions. A potential adverse reaction due to the high tannin content is irritation of the mouth and gastrointestinal tract.

Interactions: May mildly potentiate the effects of anticoagulants. Take separately from oral thiamine, metal ion supplements, or alkaloid-containing medications. Do not prescribe concomitantly with powerful analgesics (theoretical concern).

Typical Therapeutic Use

Willow bark has demonstrated analgesic activity in patients with chronic low back pain and patients with osteoarthritis in randomised, double-blind, placebo-controlled trials.[1-3] Traditional indications for willow bark in Western herbal medicine include muscular and arthritic pain, gouty arthritis and ankylosing spondylitis.[4]

Actions

Antiinflammatory, analgesic, antirheumatic, antipyretic.

Key Constituents

Constituents of willow bark include phenolic glycosides (2.5% to 11%, such as salicin and salicin esters), flavonoids and condensed tannins (8% to 20%).[5,6] The total salicin content (after hydrolysis) varies according to the species.[6,7]

Adulteration

No adulterants known.

Typical Dosage Forms & Dosage

Typical adult dosage ranges are:
- 3 to 9 g/day of dried bark or by decoction
- 3.5 to 7 mL/day of a 1:2 liquid extract or equivalent in tablet or capsule form
- 15 to 24 mL/day of a 1:5 tincture
- standardised extract containing 120 to 240 mg/day of salicin and corresponding to about 10 to 20 g original dried bark

Contraindications

Contraindicated in those with known allergy or hypersensitivity to salicylates and in glucose-6-phosphate dehydrogenase (G6PD) deficient patients (in this condition, salicylic acid causes haemolytic anaemia). In principle, the use of tannins is contraindicated or at least inappropriate in constipation, iron deficiency anaemia, and malnutrition. Do not use during lactation without professional advice.

Use in Pregnancy

Category B1: No increase in frequency of malformation or other harmful effects on the foetus from limited use in women. No evidence of increased foetal damage in animal studies.

A combination of willow bark and primula root extracts did not have teratogenic effects in rabbits and no negative effects were observed on reproductive function in female rats.[8] Salicylates can cross the placenta and acetylsalicylic acid (aspirin) has been shown to be teratogenic in animals, although there is no conclusive evidence that aspirin causes malformations in humans.[9] Moreover, the salicylates in willow bark do not have the same pharmacology as aspirin.[10]

Willow bark demonstrated anovulatory activity in vivo in an early study.[11] The relevance of this research to human use is unclear.

Use in Lactation

Category SD: Strongly discouraged in breastfeeding.

Not advisable during lactation, since salicylates are excreted in the breast milk[9] and hypersensitivity reactions may occur.

Warnings & Precautions

Use with caution in lactating women and in patients combining willow bark with anticoagulants or synthetic salicylates (refer to Use in pregnancy, Use in lactation, and Interactions sections). Willow bark cannot be substituted for aspirin for the prevention of stroke or myocardial infarction. Clinicians should be aware of the possibility of Reye's syndrome (refer to Safety in children section below).

Because of the tannin content of this herb, long-term use should be avoided (for both internal and topical use). Use cautiously in highly inflamed or ulcerated conditions of the gastrointestinal tract.

The following conditions should be approached with caution when using herbal analgesics: concurrent prescription of powerful analgesics; pain in children; neurological disease; depression and psychosis; liver and kidney disease; history of allergic or anaphylactic reactions. Long-term therapy with analgesics is not advisable.

Effect on Ability to Drive or Operate Machinery

No adverse effects expected.

Adverse Reactions

A 2002 review of clinical trials found that 3.8% to 35.8% of 420 patients treated with willow bark extracts (containing 120 mg/day or 240 mg/day salicin) reported mild adverse events compared to 2.8% to 35.2% of patients who received placebo.[12] In an earlier review, mild adverse events were reported in 3.7% of 733 patients and volunteers treated with three different preparations containing willow bark.[13] The adverse events reported included stomach ache, nausea, headache, dizziness, tiredness, sweating, skin rash, and allergic reactions.[12,13]

Salicin was used similarly to aspirin with a recommended dosage of 0.3 to 1 g. At this dosage it often produces skin rashes.[14]

High doses of tannins lead to excessive astringency on mucous membranes, which has an irritating effect. Gastrointestinal side effects due to willow bark have been attributed to the high tannin content rather than the salicylate glycosides.[15] Oral administration of salicin (1.4 g/kg) to rats did not cause gastric injury.[16]

Acute salicylate poisoning is not expected from the use of willow bark as the salicylate dose, administered in the form of salicylate glycosides, is relatively low. Hypersensitivity reactions, which include symptoms such as rhinitis, urticaria, bronchoconstriction, asthma, and collapse, can occur from a few milligrams of aspirin and therefore are possible from the administration of willow bark, but the danger is not classed as high.[15]

A patient with G6PD deficiency presented with acute massive intravascular haemolysis. The patient had been taking a diuretic medication and a herbal combination that contained *Salix caprea*. As salicin is metabolised to salicylic acid and salicylic acid is a known inducer of haemolysis in G6PD deficient patients, it was speculated that the herbal preparation might be responsible for the reaction. However the herbal preparation was not analysed for its salicin content.[17]

Interactions

Willow bark may potentiate mildly the effects of anticoagulants, including warfarin. A clinical study observed very mild but significant antiplatelet activity in patients after the consumption of willow bark extract (standardised to 240 mg/day salicin) for 4 weeks.[18]

As a precaution, do not prescribe concomitantly with powerful analgesics. Refer to the cranesbill root (*Geranium maculatum*) monograph for information regarding the interactions of tannins.

Safety in Children

Clinicians should be aware of the possibility of Reye's syndrome, an acute sepsis-like illness encountered exclusively in children below 15 years of age. The cause is unknown, although viral agents and drugs, especially salicylate derivatives, have been implicated.[19] However, it is unknown if the salicylates in willow bark are capable of causing this reaction.

Overdosage

No incidents were found in the published literature regarding willow bark. Overdose resulting from acute ingestion of aspirin (6.5 to 9.8 g) usually produces a serum salicylate level of 300 mg/L or greater.[20] More than 50 g per day of salicin would need to be ingested in order to achieve this blood level of salicylate.[2] Long-term use with high doses of tannins is to be avoided.

Toxicology

In acute toxicity studies, the LD_{50} of a liquid willow bark ethanol extract was 28 mL/kg in mice.[21] No toxic effects were observed in rats orally administered a combination of willow bark and primula root extracts for 13 weeks.[8]

Refer to the cranesbill root (*Geranium maculatum*) monograph for the toxicology of tannins.

Regulatory Status

See Table 1 for regulatory status in selected countries.

Table 1   **Regulatory Status for Willow Bark in Selected Countries**

Australia	Willow bark is not included in Part 4 of Schedule 4 of the Therapeutic Goods Regulations.
UK & Germany	Willow bark is included on the General Sale List. It is covered by a positive Commission E monograph. Willow bark is official in the *European Pharmacopoeia* 4.3.
US	Willow bark does not have generally recognised as safe (GRAS) status. However, it is freely available as a "dietary supplement" in the US under DSHEA legislation (Dietary Supplement Health and Education Act of 1994).

REFERENCES

1. Schaffner W. In Chrubasik S, Wink M, eds: *Rheumatherapie mit Phytopharmaka*, Stuttgart, 1997, Hippokrates Verlag, pp 125-127.
2. Schmid B, Ludtke R, Selbmann HK, et al: *Phytother Res* 15:344-350, 2001.
3. Chrubasik S, Eisenberg E, Balan E, et al: *Am J Med* 109:9-14, 2000.
4. British Herbal Medicine Association's Scientific Committee: *British herbal pharmacopoeia*, Bournemouth, 1983, BHMA, pp 184-185.
5. British Herbal Medicine Association: *British herbal compendium*, Bournemouth, 1992, BHMA, pp 224-226.
6. American Herbal Pharmacopoeia: *Willow bark — Salix spp.: analytical, quality control, and therapeutic monograph*, Santa Cruz, December 1999, American Herbal Pharmacopoeia.
7. Wagner H, Bladt S: *Plant drug analysis: a thin layer chromatography atlas*, ed 2, Berlin, 1996, Springer-Verlag, p 250.
8. Leslie G, Salmon G: *Swiss Med* 1:43-45, 1979.
9. *E-MIMS* version 4.00.0457, Havas MediMedia International, St. Leonards, 2000.
10. Bone K, Morgan M: *Townsend Letter for Doctors and Patients* 226:65-68, 2002.
11. Chaudhury RR: *Spec Rep Ser Indian Counc Med Res* 55:3-19, 1966.
12. Marz RW, Kemper F: *Wien Med Wochenschr* 152:354-359, 2002.
13. Scientific Committee of ESCOP (European Scientific Cooperative on Phytotherapy): *ESCOP monographs: Salicis cortex*, UK, July 1997, European Scientific Cooperative on Phytotherapy Secretariat.
14. Reynolds JEF, ed: *Martindale: the extra pharmacopoeia*, ed 26, London, 1973, The Pharmaceutical Press, p 256.
15. Hansel R, Haas H: *Therapie mit Phytopharmaka*, Berlin, 1984, Springer-Verlag, pp 234-235.
16. Akao T, Yoshino T, Kobashi K, et al: *Planta Med* 68:714-718, 2002.
17. Baker S, Thomas PS: *Lancet* 1:1039-1040, 1987.
18. Krivoy N, Pavlotzky E, Chrubasik S, et al: *Planta Med* 67:209-212, 2001.
19. Isselbacher KJ, Podolsky DK. In Harrison TR, Fauci AS, eds: *Harrison's principles of internal medicine*, ed 14 CD-ROM, New York, 1998, McGraw-Hill.
20. Munson PL, Mueller RA, Breese GR, eds: *Principles of pharmacology: basic concepts and clinical applications*, New York, 1995, Chapman & Hall, p 1167.
21. Leslie G: *Medita* 10:31-37, 1978.